Nanomedicine, Volume I: Basic Capabilities

Nanomedicine, Volume I: Basic Capabilities

Robert A. Freitas Jr.
Research Fellow
Institute for Molecular Manufacturing
Palo Alto, California, U.S.A.

CRC Press
Taylor & Francis Group
Boca Raton London New York

CRC Press is an imprint of the
Taylor & Francis Group, an **informa** business

Nanomedicine, Volume I: Basic Capabilities

First published 1999 by Landes Bioscience

Published 2018 by CRC Press
Taylor & Francis Group
6000 Broken Sound Parkway NW, Suite 300
Boca Raton, FL 33487-2742

ISBN 13: 978-1-57059-680-3 (pbk)

Visit the Taylor & Francis Web site at
http://www.taylorandfrancis.com

and the CRC Press Web site at
http://www.crcpress.com

Library of Congress Cataloging-in-Publication Data

Nanomedicine, volume I: Basic capabilities by Robert A. Freitas Jr.
ISBN 1-57059-645-X (alk. paper)
CIP information applied for but not received at time of publishing.

for Library of Congress CIP

To Nancy, Barbara, and Bob

sine qua non

CONTENTS

FIGURES

1. The Prospect of Nanomedicine

2. Pathways to Molecular Manufacturing

3. Molecular Transport and Sortation

4. Nanosensors and Nanoscale Scanning

5. Shapes and Metaphoric Surfaces

6. Power

7. Communication

8. Navigation

9. Manipulation and Locomotion

TABLES

9. Manipulation and Locomotion

10. Other Basic Capabilities

FOREWORD

K. Eric Drexler, Ph.D.
Institute for Molecular Manufacturing

The coming ability to carry out targeted medical procedures at the molecular level will bring unprecedented power to the practice of medicine. Within a few short decades we can expect a major revolution in how the human body is healed. *Nanomedicine* lays the foundations for understanding this revolution and points to where it is taking us.

Throughout science and technology, the race to obtain complete control of the structure of matter is gaining speed and focus. From chemistry to biotechnology, from applied physics to software, increasing resources are being brought to bear on the goal of nanotechnology. The term nanotechnology is used to describe a variety of nanoscale technologies. More precise for present purposes is molecular nanotechnology: the ability to construct objects with atomic-scale control. In lay terms, this is often called "building atom-by-atom"; more accurately, it means being able to bond every atom into a specific, designed location within a larger structure.

It is easy to see that such an ability could lead to, for example, the construction of stronger, more reliable materials, and smaller, faster computer chips. One can also anticipate improved versions of the molecular machines found in nature, similar to today's work in redesigning enzymes. More advanced work should eventually enable the building of molecular machine systems -- micron-scale and even macro-scale systems of novel molecular machines, performing complex operations as do the natural molecular machine systems in living things. Such systems could in principle manufacture large numbers of atomically-precise products—a process known as molecular manufacturing.

For those with a medical or biological background, a description of such powerful technological abilities at the molecular scale raises questions regarding the potential for applications in living systems, including the human body. The responsible use of technology demands that these interactions be considered in advance of widespread deployment.

For millennia, physicians and their predecessors have worked to aid the human body in its efforts to heal and repair itself. Slowly at first, and with accelerating speed, new methods and instruments have been added to the physician's toolkit -- microsurgical techniques for physically removing problematic tissue and reconfiguring healthy tissue, antibiotics for jamming the molecular machinery of unwanted bacteria, gene chips for rapid identification of genetic sequences.

In most cases, however, physicians must chiefly rely on the body's self-repair capabilities. If these fail, external efforts are hopeless. We cannot today put the component parts of human cells exactly where they should be, and configure them as they should be to form a healthy physiological state. There are no tools for working, precisely and with three-dimensional control, at the molecular level.

Nanomedicine points the way to these advances, which will arm physicians with the most important new tools in medicine since the discovery of antibiotics. The comprehensive development of nanomedicine will dominate medical technology research during the first half of the 21st century, and perhaps beyond.

These are not high-risk predictions, but merely the extension of currently-observable progress in biological and medical research. Advances in understanding living systems in general, and the human body in particular, have arrived at astounding speed over the past three decades and show no signs of slowing down. The completion of the Human Genome Project, once thought almost impossibly ambitious, is now widely regarded as both routine and destined to revolutionize medicine. What was visionary a short time ago is now a minimum baseline expectation.

We can expect this now-familiar pattern to be repeated in the field of nanomedicine. So often a goal, achievable in theory but considered at first to be far too difficult, within a few decades becomes first an active goal, and then an achievement.

Given its revolutionary potential, it is not too soon to examine the goals and potential consequences of nanomedicine. Provided that this work is firmly grounded in today's science—assuming no new scientific principles, but only the gradual accumulation and application of new data—we can be confident that our calculations will give reasonable, even conservative, results.

Of course, not all physicians will choose to join in examining the future of medicine. This is not only understandable, but quite reasonable for those who must treat patients today, with the methods available today. Nor is the medical researcher, working to improve today's pharmaceuticals, spurred on by the knowledge that his or her success—no matter how dramatic—will eventually be superseded. In both cases, what can be done today, or next year, is the most appropriate focus.

But only a fraction of today's physicians and researchers need look ahead for the entire field of medicine to benefit. Those practitioners who plan to continue their careers into the timeframe when nanomedical developments are expected to arrive—e.g., younger physicians and researchers, certainly those now in medical and graduate programs—can incrementally speed the development process, while simultaneously positioning their own work for best effect, if they have a sound idea of where the field of medicine is heading. Those farther along in their careers will be better able to direct research resources today, if the goals of nanomedicine are better understood. *Nanomedicine* helps us to frame the research issues that must be addressed, and to take better-directed steps on the path toward medical nanotechnology.

Finding the right theoretician to describe the foundations of such a field is difficult. The research requires a high degree of multidisciplinary ability—not the typical result of academic programs which reward specialization. A multidisciplinary group might serve, but would likely fail to provide the necessary conceptual integration.

Rather, the ideal author would be a careful researcher with a broad scientific background—in particular, one willing and able to tackle a daunting task requiring a decade of concentrated full-time research, constructing a technical exposition that may ultimately span thousands of pages and citations. Robert Freitas brings all these qualities and more to this challenging project.

Some aspects of the book will initially seem controversial. For example, the advent of nanomedicine will redefine the very concept of "disease" (Section 1.2.2). Today's medicine is limited to removing tissue, replacing it with transplants and artificial materials, or helping it repair itself. Current repair techniques require that the tissue be metabolizing and functioning, so inactive or structurally intact but non-functioning tissue is declared "dead." Nanotechnology will let us repair non-functioning tissue, leading us to reexamine the concept of clinical death used in medicine today.

This process of redefinition itself is not new in the field of medicine. It has happened many times before and is central to the goal of extending the frontiers of health into new territory. The advance of the physician's reach down to control at the nanoscale is just one more step on the long evolutionary pathway of medical history.

Also controversial will be the question of how nanomedical techniques should be used. Science discovers natural laws and facts, and technology extends the limits of what was possible with unaltered natural systems. But science and technology do not speak to the issues of what is morally or ethically correct—they can only help to frame the context of those discussions. Seemingly simple questions such as who is sick and who is well, how much we can do for them, and how much it will cost, require a fundamental understanding of the underlying scientific and technical limits of what is possible. Beyond that, the dialogue must include value judgments, and increasingly—if the economic and environmental costs can be handled responsibly—the answers have been provided by the customer, here, the patient.

There is a growing body of humanitarian, religious, and political work in the field of bioethics. A purpose of the present volume is to help frame the issues with a better understanding of what will be possible technically and economically. Thus, it can provide an essential ingredient for responsible ethical discussions while itself staying within the bounds of scientific and engineering analysis.

Leaving aside the substantive ethical debates to come, the technical case presented in *Nanomedicine* is sure to spark controversy on its own. Those who disagree with the thrust of this book may find segments which, taken out of context, appear unsupported or overstated. This is almost unavoidable in the writing of any book, much less one as ambitious as *Nanomedicine*. Yet the ideas in this book are supported, as presented in their intended context, and criticisms of them will be most valuable if they keep this context linked to the discussion.

Both the author and publisher of *Nanomedicine* have graciously agreed to publish the entire book online, accessible at no charge, to better enable debate on, and evolution of, this work. Published critiques, to serve the advance of knowledge, should include a reference to the online location of this material, enabling readers to probe questions in more depth. Online tools now allow third-party annotation of online texts, enabling all concerned parties to contribute to a reasoned discussion of the technical issues raised here. Robert Freitas and I invite readers of this volume to participate in this discussion, with the goal of furthering the evolution of knowledge in the new and vital field of nanomedicine.

PREFACE & ACKNOWLEDGMENTS

Molecular nanotechnology has been defined as the three-dimensional positional control of molecular structure to create materials and devices to molecular precision. The human body is comprised of molecules, hence the availability of molecular nanotechnology will permit dramatic progress in human medical services. More than just an extension of "molecular medicine," nanomedicine will employ molecular machine systems to address medical problems, and will use molecular knowledge to maintain and improve human health at the molecular scale. Nanomedicine will have extraordinary and far-reaching implications for the medical profession, for the definition of disease, for the diagnosis and treatment of medical conditions including aging, for our very personal relationships with our own bodies, and ultimately for the improvement and extension of natural human biological structure and function.

Nanomedicine, the book, will be published in three Volumes over the course of several years. The present Volume is the first in this series. Readers wishing to keep abreast of the latest developments may visit the nanomedicine website maintained by the Foresight Institute (http://www.foresight.org/Nanomedicine/index.html) and may visit http://www.nanomedicine.com, the first commercial Internet domain exclusively devoted to nanomedicine and the online home of this document. To date, the author has expended ~19,000 man-hours, plus ~1000 man-hours by reviewers, a total of ~10 man-years of effort.

To hold the book to a manageable length, most technical discussions have been greatly abbreviated, usually omitting lengthy historical surveys and extensive derivations or proofs of formulas, but providing useful pointers to the relevant specialist literature. Equations are presented, whenever possible, with sufficient qualifications to enable the reader to determine the extent of applicability in a given circumstance; however, complete derivations are rarely provided. Care should be taken in applying these mathematical relationships, since in some cases their applicability to submicron systems, while anticipated, has not yet been definitively established by experiment. With more than 270 mathematical equations in this Volume, it was impossible to maintain strict usage consistency of variables across Chapters, although some effort was made to achieve such consistency within individual Chapters. Clarity is enhanced by defining all variables and constants near or immediately after each usage in an equation. In this book, the symbol "~" signifies "approximately," and scientific exponential notation appears throughout. Cubic volumes are sometimes specified as, for example, $(1\ \mathrm{nm})^3$ to signify a $1\ \mathrm{nm}^3$ block. Conversions among various units (which were chosen to maximize interdisciplinary understanding) are summarized in Appendix A; common abbreviations, measurement units, and prefixes employed in the text may also be found in Appendix A.

References [####] are used in this book to denote the source of:

1. a direct quotation (enclosed in quotes),
2. a lightly or heavily paraphrased passage (footnoted but not enclosed in quotes), or
3. a specific datum.

Citations are also employed to indicate sources of additional information on a given topic, especially literature review papers. The author apologizes in advance for any inadvertent instances of unattributed usage of previously published material; such events should be few but should be brought to the author's immediate attention for correction in a future edition of this work. An attempt was made to cite primary sources whenever possible, but some references are made to secondary sources believed by the author to be reliable. Unreferenced in-text attributions to specific named people generally refer to comments made by a technical reviewer of the manuscript, as a personal communication.

Acknowledgments

Naturally I am replete with gratitude to many people and organizations, but my first thanks must go to K. Eric Drexler. I honor Eric for his original vision of the revolution in future medicine that molecular nanotechnology will inevitably bring; for patiently yet doggedly pursuing that vision during the long hard years when this position was not yet scientifically popular; and for describing the inspirational concept of cellular repair machines in his popular writings[8,9] and then offering detailed technical engineering analysis of molecular machine components, devices, and systems in *Nanosystems*,[10] a textbook which has established high standards of scholarship and has paved the way for all future research in this area.

Next, I would like to thank the following 77 people for providing useful references, preprints, publications or information, helpful discussions or newsgroup postings, personal communications, or other assistance related to the project: Rehal Bhojani, Forrest Bishop, Frank Boehm, Jonathan Boswell, Robert J. Bradbury, Claud A. Bramblett, Donald W. Brenner, Fred and Linda Chamberlain, Thomas M.S. Chang, M.D., Scott R. Chubb, Sharon Churchill, Philip G. Collins, Andrew Czarn, Jerry A. Darsey, Thomas Donaldson, K. Eric Drexler, William L. Dye, Mark Dyer, Robert I. Eachus, James von Ehr, James C. Ellenbogen, Gregory M. Fahy, David R. Forrest, Berry Fowler, M.D., John Gilmore, James L. Halperin, Jie Han, Barbara and Danny Haukedalen, Dan Heidel, Tad Hogg, Neil Jacobstein, Ted Kaehler, Jeffrey D. Kooistra, Tobias A. Knoch, Markus Krummenacker, Ronald G. Landes, M.D., Kevin Leung, Eric W. Lewis, M.D.,

James B. Lewis, David Mathes, Ralph C. Merkle, Richard Nakka, Philippe Van Nedervelde, Vik Olliver, Michael Park, Christine L. Peterson, Christopher J. Phoenix, Frederik Pohl, Virginia Postrel, Patrick Salsbury, Tilman E. Schaffer, J. David Schall, Nadrian C. Seeman, Paul E. Sheehan, Brian Shock, John A. Sidles, Richard Smith, Jeffrey Soreff, Edmund Storms, Carey Sublette, Richard P. Terra, Tihamer Toth-Fejel, James M. Tour, Werner Trabesinger, Robert E. Tuzun, Ty S. Twibell, Francisco Valdes, William Ware, James Brent Wood, Christian P. Worth; four anonymous referees of early versions of my now-published "respirocytes"[1400] paper; and, finally, the one person whose name I have inadvertently but inexcusably omitted.

I also thank Conrad Schneiker[153] for his highly useful summary of the early history of nanotechnology, which I leaned on rather heavily in Section 1.3.2; Roy Porter, from whose excellent history of medicine[2204] I borrowed extensively in Section 1.2.1; W.J. Bishop, whose fine book on the history of surgery[2158] provided most of the material for the first six paragraphs of Chapter 1, and substantial material for Section 1.2.1 as well; and the Foresight Institute for establishing and maintaining the first nanomedicine website, under the technically-savvy webmastering of James B. Lewis.

I extend my heartfelt thanks to the 48 individuals listed below who reviewed or commented on all or part of various Chapters in Volume I (total number in parentheses): Douglas Berger, M.D. (1), Forrest Bishop (2), Robert J. Bradbury (8), David Brin (1), Fred Chamberlain (2), Linda Chamberlain (1), Gino J. Coviello (2), Andrew Czarn (1), Thomas Donaldson (1), K. Eric Drexler (6), William L. Dye (2), Martin Edelstein (1), Gregory M. Fahy (2), Steven S. Flitman, M.D. (1), Tim Freeman (1), Thomas W. Gage (2), Al Globus (2), J. Storrs Hall (2), Jan H. Hoh (1), Christopher Jones (3), Tanya Jones (2), Ted Kaehler (1), Tobias A. Knoch (1), Markus Krummenacker (7), Sarma Lakkaraju (1), Ronald G. Landes, M.D. (10), Eugene Leitl (1), James B. Lewis (8), James Logajan (5), David Mathes (4), Thomas McKendree (3), Ralph C. Merkle (10), Hans Moravec (1), Max More (1), Kenneth Philipson, M.D. (1), Christopher J. Phoenix (10), Virginia Postrel (1), Edward M. Reifman, D.D.S. (1), Edward A. Rietman (6), Markus Roberts (1), Patrick Salsbury (3), Salvatore Santoli (3), Bruce Smith (4), Steven S. Smith (1), Jeffrey Soreff (8), Tihamer Toth-Fejel (3), James M. Tour (1), and Steven C. Vetter (1). These reviewers are to be lauded for undertaking a difficult task and should be held blameless for any errors that remain in the manuscript; the author is solely responsible for all errors of fact or judgement within these pages. Reports of errata may be transmitted by mail to the author at the following physical address: Robert A. Freitas Jr., Institute for Molecular Manufacturing, 555 Bryant Street, Suite 253, Palo Alto, CA 94301 USA; or electronically to the author at the following Internet address: rfreitas@imm.org.

My special thanks go to Robert J. Bradbury and Markus Krummenacker for particularly lengthy and detailed Chapter reviews, and for illuminating the often shadowy boundaries between biotechnology and nanotechnology; to Jeffrey Soreff for his stunningly insightful commentary and analysis of the most difficult technical concepts (on occasions almost too numerous to count), for his advice on equations and technical phraseology, and for several capsule descriptions of recent research results that are reported in Chapter 2; to Chris Phoenix for reading the entire manuscript with alacrity; to Ralph C. Merkle for his many years of sage technical advice and his unwavering encouragement when it was needed most; and to K. Eric Drexler and Ralph C. Merkle for generously contributing the Foreword and Afterword, respectively, to this Volume.

My very special thanks go to James L. Halperin, Ralph C. Merkle, many anonymous Senior Associates of the Foresight Institute, and other friends, family, and colleagues who generously provided financial support which enabled the author to complete this Volume; and to the Foresight Institute for establishing the Nanomedicine Book Fund.

I thank my publisher, Ronald G. Landes, M.D., for having the perspicacity to recognize the potential significance of nanomedicine, the trust in the author to impose no major constraints on substance, length or time, the fortitude to publish an unusual book of uncertain marketability in a difficult business environment, and the audacity to dare to present the material contained herein to medical and publishing colleagues for their serious consideration. I also applaud Cynthia Dworaczyk, Michelle Wamsley, Penny King, and the rest of the staff of Landes Bioscience for their excellent and professional work on this project, and Andreas Passens for the cover art.

Finally, and most importantly, I wish to thank my wife, Nancy Ann Freitas, and my parents, Robert A. Freitas Sr. and Barbara Lee Freitas, without whose help, understanding, and encouragement this book could not have been written.

Robert A. Freitas Jr.
Research Fellow
Institute for Molecular Manufacturing
15 April 1999

No new findings will ever be made if we rest content with the findings of the past. Besides, a man who follows someone else not only doesn't find anything, he is not even looking. "But surely you are going to walk in your predecessors' footsteps?" Yes indeed, I shall use the old road, but if I find a shorter and easier one I shall open it up. The men who pioneered the old routes are leaders, not our masters. Truth lies open to everyone. There has yet to be a monopoly of truth. And there is plenty of it left for future generations too.

— Seneca, the Younger (4 BC - 65 AD)

We are like children standing on the shoulders of a giant, for we can see all that the giant can see, and a little more.

— Guy de Chauliac, Chirurgia Magna, 1362

The human mind is often so awkward and ill-regulated in the career of invention that it is at first diffident, and then despises itself. For it appears at first incredible that any such discovery should be made, and when it has been made, it appears incredible that it should so long have escaped men's research. All which affords good reason for the hope that a vast mass of inventions yet remains, which may be deduced not only from the investigation of new modes of operation, but also from transferring, comparing, and applying these already known, by the method of what we have termed literate experience.

— Francis Bacon, Novum Organum: Aphorisms on the Interpretation of Nature and the Empire of Man, 1620

CHAPTER 1

The Prospect of Nanomedicine

1.1 A Noble Enterprise

The history of disease is vastly older than that of humankind itself. Indeed, disease and parasitism have been inseparable companions to life since the dawn of life on Earth. Fossilized bacteria similar to those responsible for many infections that afflict people today have been found in geological formations that are 500 million years old. Fossil shells dating from an era almost equally remote show clear evidence of disturbance by injury and parasites. Examination of the skeletons of long-extinct dinosaurs and other great reptiles show that these creatures suffered from fractures, bone tumors, arthritis, osteomyelitis, dental caries and other diseases that still plague us in the 20th century. While available fossil evidence is largely limited to changes observable in bones and teeth, it is probably safe to assume that disease processes were equally prevalent in the soft organs and tissues that have not been geologically preserved, and that the general pattern of disease has not changed in its essentials during the hundreds of millions of years that animal life has existed on this planet.[2158]

Since its first appearance on the prehistoric stage millions of years ago, the human body has also been constantly subject to assault and injury, invasion by parasites, extremes of heat and cold, and infections. Early man probably suffered from a number of diseases due to nutritional factors and body chemistry disorders. For example, the poor condition of the teeth of an 18-year old Australopithecus who lived 1.75 million years ago, found at Olduvai Gorge by Louis Leakey[2187,2188] in 1959, suggests that the hominid had a disease that lasted for many months — most likely gastro-enteritis due to malnutrition — with three major attacks of the disease at the ages of two, four, and four and a half.[2186] Diseases that may date back more than 25 million years to the ape ancestors of modern apes and man[2190,2191] are amoebic dysentery, malaria,[2189] pinworm infections, syphilis, yaws,[2199] and yellow fever. Diseases which may have appeared and evolved with man[2198] include leprosy and typhoid; certain modern diseases such as cholera, measles,[2196,2197] mumps, smallpox, whooping cough, and the common cold require large concentrated populations to support them, thus probably could not have existed in the prehistoric era.[2186,2191-2195]

As for cancer, Java man, first discovered by Dutch anatomist Eugene Dubois in 1891 and considered to be half a million years old, had a morbid growth on his femur. It is likely that bone cancer and other forms of cancer have existed from the earliest times. The remains of Neanderthal, a competing species to *Homo sapiens* that roamed through Europe, Africa, and the Near East during the last glacial period ~75,000 years ago, show clear evidence of arthritis, tooth loss, and suppurative bone disease. (The high rate of broken bones and early death suggests that Neanderthals engaged in more close-quarter combat with large animals than did modern humans, who had figured out safer strategies.[2329]) Human bones unearthed from the New Stone Age period reveal that Neolithic man suffered from arthritis, congenital dislocations and fractures, sinusitis, tuberculosis of the spine, and tumors.[2158]

In considering the question of how our earliest ancestors dealt with these conditions, we are on somewhat uncertain ground, since little direct evidence has been preserved. Anthropologists point out that in pre-Neanderthal hunter-gatherer tribes, a sick or lame person is a serious handicap to a group on the move. In the event of major illness or mortal wounds, sufferers may either leave the group, be abandoned, or, as with lepers in medieval Europe, may be ritually expelled, becoming "culturally dead" before they are biologically dead. Early hunter-gatherer hominid bands were more likely to abandon their seriously sick than to succor them,[2204] although Cro-Magnons and Neanderthals evidently were the first to care for their wounded and disabled, and to bury their dead.[2341-2343]

But moderate wounds, bruises, fractures, or foreign bodies such as arrowheads or thorns are tangible things that demand attention. Thus the art of surgery must first have originated as a response to immediate crises. The first and most obvious course of action of a wounded man would be to protect the site of injury from the influence of external forces or agents. For this there was, and remains to this day, only one means — the application of a dressing. Many observations were made and many substances tried, and in time a body of experience was accumulated and passed on orally to others for use in similar emergencies, eventually creating a considerable sum of inherited empirical knowledge. It is believed that the art of dressing wounds long constituted the whole of medicine — the use of internal remedies or herbs, and use of the knife or fire, came much later.[2158]

Present-day primitive and folk medicines provide additional clues to early medical practice. For example, many early peoples developed effective methods to control bleeding — the use of cobwebs is an ancient folk remedy, as is the application of tourniquets, packing with absorbent materials, the laying on of snow or, at the other temperature extreme, the application of cautery by hot knife or spear.[2158,2204] The Masai and Akamba tribes treated sword wounds by slapping on a poultice of cow dung and dust. The suturing of wounds is practiced by some primitive peoples and may have been known to prehistoric man. Bone needles furnished with an eye have been found in paleolithic deposits in France and England, and some Indian tribes suture with threads of sinew or bone needles (the needles are left in and the thread is twisted around them). One of the strangest suturing techniques, observed among primitive tribal cultures in such widely separated places as India, East Africa and Brazil, is the sealing of wounds, especially abdominal wounds, using termites or ants. The edges of the wound are drawn closely together and the insect is allowed to bite through them both, firmly securing the flesh on two sides. Once attached, the insect's body is severed, allowing only the jaws to remain in place, holding the wound shut.[2158]

While able to deal with wounds, early man did not admit the existence of disease from "natural causes". Internal diseases were generally ascribed to malevolent influences exercised by a supernatural entity or a human enemy. As centuries passed, many internal diseases were eventually recognized and simple treatments empirically established — for example, Celsus (ca. 30 AD), a Roman medical writer, described ligature (tying off blood vessels), suturing the large intestine, eye operations such as couching for cataract, tonsillectomy, and bladder surgery to remove stones.[2200] But the rational basis for internal medicine awaited basic physiological knowledge such as the circulation of the blood, finally proven by William Harvey (1578-1657) in 1628, and the discovery and acceptance of the theory of infection by microorganisms in the 1800s. Throughout most of human history, life has been short indeed — Table 1.1 shows the average age of death for a sampling of persons buried in Roman times. (Some variation may represent regional differences in burial practices.) Even by the 17th century, more than half of all children never lived past the age of ten, often succumbing to diseases such as cholera, diphtheria, scarlet fever, or whooping cough, or being scarred for life by smallpox. It was a common and widely accepted fact of life that people would die at all ages, although wealthy families could leave town every year during the cholera season.[1724]

One of the constant missions of human civilization has been the avoidance and elimination of animals that prey on humans. Cave-dwelling carnivorous saber-toothed tigers, having occupied the upper echelons of the food chain for 30-35 million years, finally became extinct not more than about ten thousand years ago, most likely at the hands of newly-arrived human hunters crossing the Siberian land bridge into post-Pleistocene North America.[2186] As late as medieval times, wolves ranged freely over Europe, remaining abundant in France through 1500 AD — in winter, audacious wolf packs would enter Paris and eat children, dogs, and even adults who were alone on the streets.[1724] With technological advances, extant tiger and wolf species are now largely confined to artificial habitats or isolated nature preserves and no longer pose any serious threat to human health. People in most places are not eaten by wolves; indeed today, a few venturesome individuals actually keep and breed wolves with dogs, as pets.

Bacteria are among the last remaining "wild animals" on Earth that threaten man. As our instrumentalities continue to progress from the macroscale to the microscale, and finally to the molecular or nanoscale, all of the remaining natural "wild things" that endanger human life and health — whether viruses, bacteria, protozoa, metazoan parasites,[3253,3254] or even our own pathological native cells — will be confined and tamed, reconstructed or eliminated. Using smaller tools, we hunt smaller prey. As with sabertooths in the post-Neolithic era, and with wolves in post-medieval times, people of the 21st century will no longer fear or need suffer predation by wild microbes or tumor cells run amok.

Humanity is poised at the brink of completion of one of its greatest and most noble enterprises. Early in the 21st century, our growing abilities to swiftly repair most traumatic physical injuries, eliminate pathogens, and alleviate suffering using molecular tools will begin to coalesce in a new medical paradigm called nanomedicine. Nanomedicine may be broadly defined as the comprehensive monitoring, control, construction, repair, defense, and improvement of all human biological systems, working from the molecular level, using engineered nanodevices and nanostructures.

Table 1.1. Average Age of Death of Persons Buried in Roman Times[2201]

Burial Location	Average Age of Death
City of Rome	29.9 years
Iberia	31.4 years
Britain	32.5 years
Germany	35.0 years
North Africa	46.7 years

In this book we shall explore in preliminary fashion a few of the technical details, specific requirements, and physical limitations of these engineered nanodevices, and the meaning of nanomedicine within the context of the traditional healing arts. Since at this writing these nanodevices cannot yet be built, our subject matter is of necessity somewhat speculative, albeit thoroughly grounded in the best scientific and engineering knowledge currently available. Medical philosopher Edmond A. Murphy notes that "to the physician, the more remote the area of speculation from the welfare of the patient, the more clearly [this speculation] must be shown to give promise of ultimate benefit".[2228] The author believes that nanomedicine clearly meets, indeed vastly exceeds, this stringent requirement for relevance and utility.

After the manner of many contemporary medical school programs, the present trilogy progresses from a general emphasis on basic science and engineering capabilities in Volume I, to nanomedical tools and systems in Volume II, leading finally to a sharp focus on clinical nanomedicine in Volume III.

1.2 Current Medical Practice

In order to fully appreciate the changes that nanomedicine will inevitably bring, it is useful first to review the history and development of current medical practice. As Winston Churchill once remarked: "The further backward you look, the further forward you can see." The author unapologetically favors what medical anthropologists would regard as the "Western" healing tradition. The great medical theorist Otto E. Guttentag[2234] agreed: "Contemporary Western medicine involves a type of healing that potentially and actually exceeds all other approaches in maintaining that optimal status of selfhood we call being healthy and in eliminating that reduced status of selfhood we call being sick."

After summarizing the history of scientific medicine and placing nanomedicine in its proper historical context (Section 1.2.1), we define exactly what is meant by "medicine" and present a new model for "disease" (Section 1.2.2). The modern medical treatment methodology is examined in light of the changes that will be wrought by nanomedicine (Section 1.2.3), and this is followed by a discussion of several important issues in the evolution of medical bedside practice (Section 1.2.4) and the changing view of the human body (Section 1.2.5).

Many fascinating and important practical issues such as medical privacy rights, patient compliance, medical ethics and bioethics per se, nursing, the role of medical bureaucracies in the doctor-patient interaction, and the question of medical causality[2230] are not addressed here or are deferred to Chapter 31.

1.2.1 The Evolution of Scientific Medicine

A study of the history of "scientific" or Western medical practice suggests a continuity in certain aspects of the medical paradigm[292] even since ancient times — as for instance the basic precepts of observation and diagnosis, followed by treatment — but reveals changes in attitudes, techniques, and instrumentalities, and a gradual evolution in the epistemology and ontology of medical logic. Figure 1.1 presents a simple model of this historical progression, the details of which will soon become clear. Note that 2010 is marked as a possible date for the first applications of nanomedicine. These will most likely be ex vivo applications only — in vivo nanomedical treatments may come much later.

Another important reason to study the history of medicine[3192] is to gain a deeper appreciation of the long, hard struggle to improve human health, a struggle that is expected finally to culminate in victory in the 21st century. If the ~10 billion people that have ever lived survived an average of 40 years and spent 5% of their lives in sickness or physical misery from disease, then ~200 trillion man-hours of suffering have been paid to achieve this remarkable result, a not inconsiderable price.

There is no pretense to completeness here. For example, Chinese, Indian and Islamic contributions are omitted, not because they are unimportant, but because they did not significantly alter the evolutionary pathway of the Western medical paradigm. A great deal of physiology, pathology, neurology, systematics, and many other important medical-related disciplines are also neglected in the interest of brevity. Much of the following discussion, including most of the anecdotal quotations, is liberally and appreciatively drawn from comprehensive works by W.J. Bishop,[2158] Roy Porter,[2204,2205] William H. McNeill,[2206] and the *Cecil Textbook of Medicine.*[2207]

1.2.1.1 Prehistoric Medicine

The elementary nature of prehistorical medical practice has already been mentioned. There is direct evidence that Stone Age man used a natural fungus as a treatment for intestinal parasites.[3244] Besides basic wound-tending, the practice of circumcision is an age-old form of simple surgery with a rational, if sometimes controversial, hygienic basis.

An even more dramatic surgical operation, for which there is considerable prehistoric fossil evidence, is trephining the skull to remove a round piece of bone from it. This can be done using flint instruments, either by gradually scratching through the skin and bones of the skull, getting gradually deeper and deeper, or by drilling a series of small holes in a circle in the skull, then cutting the small bridges between to remove a disk of bone. Skulls have been found with multiple holes. The additional fact that some hole edges show callus formation (evidence of healing) indicates survival of the patient. Trephined skulls have been found in Western Europe, including England, North Africa, Asia, the East Indies, New Zealand, and the Americas from Alaska in the north down through the continent to Peru in the south. The practice was probably regarded as therapeutic, either to remove a depressed fracture, to try to cure mental illness, or to relieve severe headache or epilepsy, presumably by letting out the demon possessing the patient.

1.2.1.2 Ancient Mesopotamian Medicine

The first written records, which came from ancient Babylon and Egypt, contain the earliest references to medical care, obviously codifying earlier practices no record of which has survived. The medicine of the Sumerians of Mesopotamia from ca. 3000 BC was primarily religious. The Mesopotamian peoples saw the hands of the gods in everything. Disease was caused by spirit invasion, sorcery, malice, or the breaking of taboos, and sickness was both judgement and punishment. An Assyrian text circa 650 BC describes epileptic symptoms within a demonological framework: "If at the time of the possession, his mind is awake, the demon can be driven out; if at the time of his possession his mind is not so aware, the demon cannot be driven out." Headaches, neck pain, intestinal ailments and impotence were read as omens. The appropriate remedy was to identify the demons responsible and expel them by spells or incantations.

But medicine also had an empirical component, with some sicknesses being ascribed to cold, dust and dryness, putrefaction, malnutrition, venereal infection and other natural causes. The Babylonians drew on an extensive pragmatic materia medica — some 120 mineral drugs and twice that number of vegetable items are listed in surviving tablets. Alongside various fats, oils, honey,* wax, and milk, were many active ingredients that included mustard, oleander and hellebore (a plant in the buttercup family that is a violent gastrointestinal poison, hence acts as a powerful purgative, though it is lethal in high doses). Colocynth, senna and castor oil were used as laxatives, while wound dressings were compounded with dried wine dregs, salt, oil, beer, juniper, mud or fat, blended with alkali and herbs. With the discovery of distillation, the

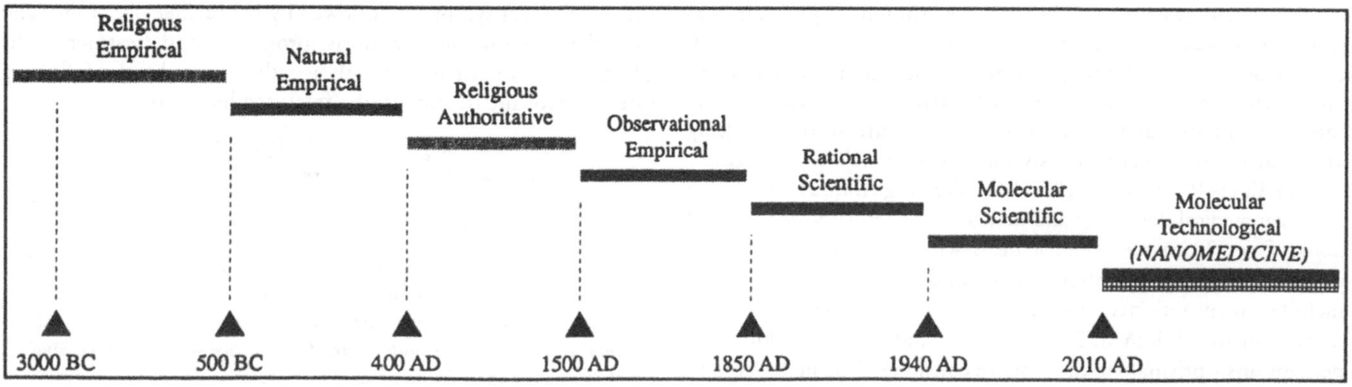

Fig. 1.1. Evolution of the paradigm of scientific medicine.

**Honey also was known to the ancients as a preservative agent. The corpses of military leaders who had died far from home and needed to be transported long distances were often immersed in honey to prevent decomposition. Famous historical examples from later Greek and Roman times include the Spartan commander Agesilaus (d. 362 BC) and Alexander the Great (d. 323 BC).*[2333,3259]

Mesopotamians made essence of cedar and other volatile oils. Turpentine, asafetida, henbane, myrrh, mint, poppy, fig, and mandrake are also mentioned. Dog dung and other fecal ingredients were used to drive off demons.

Surgical conditions such as wounds, fractures and abscesses were also treated by Mesopotamian surgeons. Practitioners were priests, and after 2000 BC, they were ruled by the strict laws included in the Code of Hammurabi. The Code laid down rewards for success and severe punishment for failure, and contained laws relating to medical practice which show that medicine and surgery were highly organized professions. Fees were regulated on a sliding scale of rewards based on the patient's rank, and severe penalties were laid down for failure:

"Concerning the wounds resulting from operations it is written: if a physician shall produce on anyone a severe wound with a bronze operating knife and cure him, or if he shall open an abscess with the operating knife and preserve the eye of the patient, he usually shall receive 10 shekels of silver [more than a craftsman's annual pay]; if it is a slave, his master shall usually pay 2 shekels of silver to the physician."

"If a physician shall make a severe wound with an operating knife and kill him, or shall open an abscess with an operating knife and destroy the eye, his hands shall be cut off."

"If a physician shall make a severe wound with a bronze operating knife on the slave of a free man and kill him, he shall replace the slave with another slave. If he shall open an abscess with a bronze operating knife and destroy the eye, he shall pay the half of the value of the slave."

The Hammurabic Code also mentions the Gallabu, or barber-surgeons, whose province was minor surgery, including dentistry and the branding of slaves. If Herodotus (ca. 485-425 BC) may be believed, Babylonian medicine must have declined in the 5th century BC. Herodotus states that there were no physicians, but that the people brought their sick into the marketplace in order that passers-by might make suggestions or offer cures.

1.2.1.3 Ancient Egyptian Medicine

The civilization of ancient Egypt dates from around 3000 BC. As in Mesopotamia, ancient Egyptian medicine was religious-empirical. An examination of the preserved bodies of members of the Royal family has provided much information on the diseases of ancient Egypt, including congenital deformities such as clubfoot, dental caries, gallstones, bladder and kidney stones, rheumatoid arthritis, mastoiditis, numerous eye diseases, and bone fractures, some of which show treatment by quite sophisticated splinting. Other evidence suggests that the average ancient Egyptian was extremely diseased. For example, a weaver who died in the 11th century BC, aged 14-18 years, evidently suffered from schistosomiasis, tapeworm likely associated with malnutrition, anthracosis of the lungs presumably due to environmental pollution from cooking and heating, pulmonary silicosis, and possibly malaria and fleas.

The Ebers Papyrus (ca. 1550 BC), deriving from Thebes, is the principal medical document and may be the oldest surviving medical book. Over 20 meters long, it deals with scores of diseases and proposes remedies involving spells and incantations, but also includes many rational treatments. The Ebers Papyrus covers 15 diseases of the abdomen, 29 of the eyes, and 18 of the skin, and, perhaps unsurprisingly to the modern consumer, lists no fewer than 21 cough treatments. About 700 drugs and 800 formulations are mentioned, mainly involving herbs but also including mineral and animal remedies. For example, to cure night blindness the patient should eat fried ox liver — possibly a tried-and-tested procedure, since liver is rich in Vitamin A,[749] lack of which causes the illness. Eye disorders were also common, for example:

"To drive away inflammation of the eyes, grind the stems of the juniper of Byblos, steep them in water, apply to the eyes of the sick person and he will be quickly cured. To cure granulations of the eye, prepare a remedy of cyllyrium, verdigris, onions, blue vitriol, powdered wood, and mix and apply to the eyes."

For stomach ailments, a decoction of cumin, goose-fat and milk was recommended, but other remedies sound more exotic, including a drink prepared from black ass testicles. A mixture of vulva and penis extracts and black lizard was supposed to cure baldness. Also good for hair growth was a compound of hippopotamus, lion, crocodile, goose, snake and ibex fat — merely assembling these ingredients might promise a hair-raising experience! Egyptian medicine credited many vegetables and fruits with healing properties, and also tree products such as sycamore bark and resins such as myrrh, frankincense and manna. As in Mesopotamia, plant extracts — notably senna, colocynth and castor oil — were employed as purgatives, and oil of camomile to improve digestion. Recipes included ox spleen, pig's brain, stag's horn, honey-sweetened tortoise gall, and the blood and fats of various animals. Antimony, copper salts, alum, and other minerals were recommended as astringents or disinfectants. Containing ingredients from leeks to lapis lazuli — including garlic, onion, tamarisk, cereals, spices, condiments, resins, gums, dates, hellebore, opium and cannabis — compound drugs were administered in the form of pills, ointments, poultices, fumigations, inhalations, gargles and suppositories; they might even be blown into the urethra through a tube. Among the most interesting of the healers whose names have been recorded for posterity are Peseshet, head female physician or overseer, proof of the existence, as in Mesopotamia, of female healers; and Iri, Keeper of the Royal Rectum, presumably the pharaoh's enema expert.

The Edwin Smith Papyrus (ca. 1600 BC), discovered by its American namesake at Luxor in 1862, may be the world's earliest surviving surgical text, and contains material probably derived from even more ancient times. The "book of wounds" comprises 48 case reports, which commence with the top of the head and proceed systematically downward — nose, face, ears, neck and chest, mysteriously stopping in mid-sentence at the spine, presumably when the scribe was interrupted at his work. The only surgical conditions treated were wounds, fractures, abscesses, and circumcisions. In the Papyrus, the method of presentation is first to set out the title or the chief symptom, followed by the further symptoms, and then the examination, diagnosis, prognosis, and treatment. The advice given is entirely rational, as will be seen by the following directions for the treatment of a fractured humerus:

"Instructions concerning a Break in his Upper Arm. If thou examinest a man having a break in his upper arm, and thou findest his upper arm hanging down, separated from its fellow, thou shouldst say concerning him: One having a break in his upper arm. An ailment which I will treat."

"Thou shouldst place him prostrate on his back, with something folded between his two shoulder blades; thou shouldst spread out with his two shoulders in order to stretch apart his upper arm until that break falls into its place. Thou shouldst make for him two splints of linen, and thou shouldst apply for him one of them both on the inside of his arm, and the other of them both on the underside of his arm. Thou shouldst bind it with ymrw [an unidentified mineral substance], and treat it afterward with honey every day until he recovers."

An interesting point in the case histories is that after the diagnosis the writer gives a decision about his further course of action. The verdict may take one of three forms: (1) an ailment which I will treat; (2) an ailment with which I will contend; and (3) an ailment not to be treated. Like modern military triage, the "hopeless" patient is left to his inevitable fate. This guarded attitude on the part of the medical man was widespread in antiquity. While present-day doctors generally do everything possible to alleviate symptoms to the very end, even when the patient has no chance of recovery, the view in ancient times was that hopeless cases were not to be touched. This attitude was entirely practical. A doctor in attendance at the courts of ancient Egypt might expect rich rewards if his patient recovered, but if a patient died under his care, the unfortunate physician ran a grave risk of impalement.

1.2.1.4 Ancient Greek Medicine

By 1000 BC the communities later collectively known as the Greeks were emerging around the Aegean Sea. How much medical knowledge they took from Egypt remains controversial, but the contrasts between the two are striking. Little is known of Greek medicine before the appearance of written texts in the 5th century BC. Archaic Greece had its folk healers, including priest healers employing divination and herbs. From early times (the first Olympic games were recorded in 776 BC), the love of athletics produced instructors in exercise, bathing, massage, gymnastics and diet. The Homeric epics (ca. 600 BC) offer glimpses of early Greek medicine. Scholars count 147 cases of battle wounds in the *Iliad*, including 106 spear thrusts, 17 sword slashes, 12 arrow shots, and 12 sling shots. Among the arrow wound survivors was King Menelaus of Sparta, whose physician extracted the arrow, sucked out the blood and applied a salve. As with other medical interventions in Homer, this shows no Egyptian influence, supporting the idea that, even if Greek practice owed much to Egypt, it rapidly went its own way.

Various Greek gods and heroes were identified with health and disease, the chief being Asclepius, who even had the power to raise the dead. A heroic warrior and blameless physician, Asclepius was the son of Apollo, sired upon a mortal mother, who was taught herbal remedies by Chiron and then generously used them to heal humans. Incensed at being cheated of death, Hades, the ruler of the underworld, appealed to the supreme god, Zeus, who obligingly dispatched Asclepius with a thunderbolt, though he was later elevated to godhood. A different version appears in Homer, who portrays Asclepius as a tribal chief and a skilled wound healer whose sons became physicians and were called Asclepiads, and from whom all Asclepian practitioners descended. As the tutelary god of medicine, Asclepius is usually portrayed with a beard, staff and snake — the origin of the caduceus symbol of the modern physician, with its two snakes intertwined, double-helix like, on a winged staff. The god was often shown accompanied by his daughters, Hygeia (health or hygiene) and Panacea (cure-all).

For all that, Hippocratic medicine, the foundation of Greek written medicine, explicitly grounds the art upon a quite different basis — a healing system independent of the supernatural and built upon natural philosophy. The beginnings of true medical science in the West were established when the reliance on superstition that underpinned tribal medicine was replaced by civilized and rational curiosity about the cause of illness. The growth of civilized thought allowed for argument on medical cause and cure, with great doctrinal multiplicity. The separation of medicine from religion reveals another distinctive feature of Greek healing: its openness, a quality characteristic of Greek intellectual activity in general, owing to political diversity. There was no imperial Hammurabic Code and, unlike Egypt, no state medical bureaucracy, nor were there examinations or professional qualifications. Those calling themselves doctors (iatroi) had to compete with bone-setters, exorcists, root-cutters, incantatory priests, gymnasts, and showmen, exposed to the quips of playwrights and the criticism of philosophers. Medicine was open to all.

Empedocles (fl. 450 BC) may have been the first to advance some of the key physiological doctrines in Greek medicine, including innate heat as the source of living processes such as digestion, the cooling function of breathing, and the notion that the liver makes the blood that nourishes the tissues. His contemporary, Alcmaeon of Croton (fl. 470 BC), believed that the brain, not the heart, was the chief organ of sensation. Alcmaeon's examination of the eyeball led him to discern the optic nerve leading into the skull, a genuine observational basis. He gave similar explanations for the sensations of hearing and smelling, because the ear and nostrils suggested passages leading to the brain. Most of such knowledge depended heavily on wound observation and animal dissection, for in the classical period the dignity of the human body forbade dissection.

All we know for sure of Hippocrates (ca. 460-377 BC), who "taught all that were prepared to pay," is that he was born on the island of Cos and lived a long and virtuous life. The sixty or so works comprising the Hippocratic Corpus (ca. 440-340 BC) derive from a variety of hands, and, as with the books of the Bible, they became jumbled up, fragmented, then pasted together again in antiquity. What is now called the Corpus was gathered around 250 BC in the Library at Alexandria, with further texts added later still. Some volumes are philosophical, others are teaching texts or case notes. What unites them all is the conviction that health and disease are capable of explanation by reasoning about nature, independently of supernatural interference. Man is governed by the same physical laws as the cosmos, hence medicine must be an understanding, empirical and rational, of the workings of the body in its natural environment. Anticipating modern medicine, appeal to reason, rather than to rules or to supernatural forces, gives Hippocratic medicine its distinctiveness. It was also patient- rather than disease-centered; the Hippocratics specialized in medicine by the bedside, prizing trust-based clinical relations:

> *"Make frequent visits; be especially careful in your examinations, counteracting the things wherein you have been deceived at the changes. Thus you will know the case more easily, and at the same time you will also be more at your ease. For instability is characteristic of the humours, and so they may also be easily altered by nature and by chance."*
>
> *"...Keep a watch also on the faults of the patients, which often make them lie about the taking of things prescribed. For through not taking disagreeable drinks, purgative or other, they sometimes die. What they have done never results in a confession, but the blame is thrown upon the physician."*

The Hippocratics promulgated the idea of "vis medicatrix naturae," or the power of nature to cure itself, and thus the belief that there was a natural tendency for things to get better on their own. This tendency could be aided by providing a beneficial environment for the patient and by improving physical function with a regimen of suitable diet, lifestyle, and exercise — the diatetica. In extreme cases, further aids to recovery could be sought. Stubbornly offending "humors" could be removed with the help of venesection (phlebotomy or bloodletting) and purgatives, sudorifics applied to induce sweating, and diuretics to increase urination. But the Hippocratic physician was extremely reluctant to administer drugs of any kind, because the physician's goal was to aid nature in healing the body.

Hippocratics scorned heroic interventions and left risky procedures to others. Their Oath (Chapter 31) explicitly forbade cutting, even for stones, and other texts reserved surgery for those used to handling war wounds. Surgery was regarded as an inferior trade, the work of the hand rather than the head, a fact reflected in its name: "surgery" derives from the Latin "chirurgia," which comes from the Greek "cheiros" (hand) and "ergon" (work); surgery was handiwork. Hippocratic surgical texts were thus conservative in outlook, encouraging a tradition in which doctors sought to treat complaints first through management, occasionally through drugs, and finally, if need be, by surgical intervention.

The art of diagnosis involved creating a profile of the patient's lifestyle, work and dietary habits, partly by asking questions and partly by the use of trained senses:

"When you examine the patient, inquire into all particulars; first how the head is...then examine if the hypochondrium [abdomen beneath lower ribs] and sides be free of pain, for...if there be pain in the side, and along with the pain either cough, tormina [painful intestinal colic] or bellyache, the bowels should be opened with clysters [enema].... The Physician should ascertain whether the patient be apt to faint when he is raised up, and whether his breathing is free..."

Hippocratics prided themselves on their clinical acuity, being quick to pick up telltale symptoms, as with the facies hippocratica, the facial look of those dying from long-continued illness or cholera: "a protrusive nose, hollow eyes, sunken temples, cold ears that are drawn in with the lobes turned outward, the forehead's skin rough and tense like parchment, and the whole face greenish or black or blue-grey or leaden." Experience was condensed into aphorisms, as for instance: "When sleep puts an end to delirium, it is a good sign."

The technique most prized among Hippocratics was the art of prognosis — a secular version of the priestly and oracular prognostications of earlier medicine, and bearing some analogy to the 20th century weatherman, who can give a bright or gloomy forecast but is powerless to change it. Noted one Hippocratic text:[2240]

"It appears to me a most excellent thing for the physician to cultivate Prognosis; for by foreseeing and foretelling, in the presence of the sick, the present, the past, and the future, and explaining the omissions which patients have been guilty of, he will be the more readily believed to be acquainted with the circumstances of the sick; so that men will have confidence to entrust themselves to such a physician.... Thus a man will be the more esteemed to be a good physician...from having long anticipated everything; and by seeing and announcing beforehand those who will live and those who will die."

The ultimate significance of Hippocratic medicine was twofold. First, it carved out a lofty role for the selfless physician which would serve as a lasting model for professional identity and conduct. Second, it taught that an understanding of sickness required an understanding of nature.

1.2.1.5 Ancient Alexandrian Medicine

Soon after the death of Aristotle (d. 322 BC) and his most famous pupil, Alexander the Great (d. 323 BC), a great medical school was founded in Egypt at the court of King Ptolemy, at his capital, Alexandria, at the mouth of the Nile. The King's main cultural creations were the Alexandrian Library* and the Museum (Sanctuary of the Muses), which installed Greek learning in a new Egyptian environment — Archimedes, Euclid, and the astronomer Ptolemy were soon to teach there. The Library became a wonder of the scholarly world, eventually containing, it was said, 700,000 manuscripts, and other facilities including an observatory, zoological gardens, lecture halls and rooms for research.

The two earliest teachers at the Alexandrian medical school were also its greatest — Herophilus of Chalcedon (ca. 330-260 BC) and his contemporary, Erasistratus of Chios (ca. 330-255 BC). Their writings having been lost, we know about them only through later physicians. Herophilus was the first to dissect cadavers in public. He was a student of Praxagoras of Cos (fl. 340 BC), who had improved Aristotelian anatomy by distinguishing arteries from veins, but who saw the arteries as air tubes, similar to the trachea and bronchi, a common error because arteries are devoid of blood in corpses. Herophilus observed that the coats of arteries were much thicker than those of the veins, thus he speculated that the arteries were filled not with air but with blood. Herophilus wrote at least eleven treatises, discovering and naming the prostate and the duodenum (from the Greek for twelve fingers, the length of gut he found). He also wrote on the pulse as a diagnostic guide and on therapeutics, ophthalmology, dietetics, and midwifery. He recognized the brain as the central organ of the nervous system and the seat of intelligence, extending the knowledge of the parts of the brain, certain of which still bear titles translated from those given by him. He was the first to grasp the nature of the nerves, which he distinguished as motor and sensory, though he did not separate them clearly from tendons. Erasistratus surmised that every organ is formed of a three-fold system of "vessels" — veins, arteries, and nerves, dividing indefinitely. These, plaited together, were postulated to make up the tissues. In the brain, Erasistratus observed convolutions, noting that they were more elaborate in man than in animals and associating this with higher intelligence. He distinguished between cerebrum and cerebellum, and is often regarded as an early mechanist because of his model of bodily processes — for instance, digestion involved the stomach grinding food. He was opposed to intrusive remedies such as venesection, and his favorite therapeutic measures were regulated exercise, diet, and the vapor bath — very much in the Hippocratic tradition.

1.2.1.6 Ancient Roman Medicine

Roman tradition held that one was better off without doctors. According to Cato (234-149 BC), citizens had no need of professional physicians because Romans were hale and hearty, unlike the effete Greeks. Apparently Romans enjoyed bad-mouthing Greek physicians. Thus the Romans despised medicine as a profession but this did not prevent them from making use of Greek physicians or even of the services of their own slaves. Galen of Pergamum (130-200 AD) tells us that in his time, large cities such as Rome and Alexandria swarmed with specialists who also travelled about from place to place. Martial (40-104 AD) mentions some of them in an epigram: "Cascellius extracts and repairs bad teeth; you, Hyginus, cauterize ingrowing eyelashes; Fannius cures a relaxed uvula without cutting; Eros removes brand marks from slaves; Hermes is a very Podalirius for ruptures." Under the Empire, military medicine was highly organized — every cohort had its surgeon, and surgeons of a higher grade were attached to the legions as consultants. Army surgeons ranked as noncombatants and enjoyed many privileges.

In the Roman empire, the earliest scientific teacher was a Greek, Asclepiades of Bithynia (124-40 BC). Asclepiades ridiculed the Hippocratic expectant attitude as a mere "meditation on death," and urged active measures that the cure might be "seemly, swift and

**Part of the Library was wrecked by fire in 48 BC during riots sparked by the arrival of Julius Caesar. Much later, Christian leaders encouraged the destruction of the Temple of Muses. As legend has it, in 415 AD the last resident scholar, the female mathematician Hypatia, was hauled out of the Museum by Christian fanatics and beaten to death (or her flesh was ripped off using clamshells, by another account). The 7th century Muslim conquest of the city resulted in the final destruction of the Library.*

sure." Though outside the mainstream, his medical practice is interesting as a modification of the atomic or corpuscular theory, according to which disease results from an irregular or inharmonious motion of the corpuscles of the body. His pupils were numerous, constituting the Methodical school, but his available therapeutic tools were few — he trusted mainly to changes of diet, friction, bathing, exercise, and occasionally emetics, bleeding, and wine. He was also the first to use music in the treatment of the insane.

Back in the mainstream, Galen of Pergamum (130-200 AD) provided the final medical synthesis of antiquity and the effective medical standard for the next 13 centuries. His first medical appointment was as surgeon to the Roman gladiators. He later traveled to Rome and wrote extensively on anatomy, physiology and practical medicine. His fame is due in part to his prolific pen — some 350 authentic titles ranging in topic from the soul to bloodletting polemics survive, about as much as all Greek medical writings together. Galen was a flamboyant character. One of his party tricks, revealing his genius for self-advertisement as well as experiment, was to sever the nerves in the neck of a pig. As these were severed, one by one, the pig continued to squeal; but when Galen cut one of the laryngeal nerves the squealing stopped, impressing the crowd.

Galen justified venesection in terms of his elaborate pulse lore. Written in the early 170s, his sixteen books on the pulse were divided into four treatises, each four books long. In one of these treatises, he explains how to take the pulse and to interpret it, raising key questions, for example: How was it possible to tell whether a pulse was full, rapid, or rhythmical? Such questions he resolved partly from experience and partly by reference to earlier authorities. Galen developed a characteristic physiological scheme that remained in vogue until the 17th century. It supposes three types of so-called spirits associated with three types of the activity of living things. These were the natural spirits formed in the liver and distributed by the veins, the vital spirits formed in the heart and distributed by the arteries, and the animal spirits formed in the brain and distributed by the nerves. Galen's system was an admirable if factually flawed working hypothesis, based on much experimental evidence, and he presented his work as "perfecting" the legacy of Hippocrates.

As in Greece, medicine remained personal in Rome. No medical degrees were conferred or qualifications required. In the absence of colleges and universities, the private face-to-face nature of medical instruction encouraged fluidity and diversity, Students attached themselves to an individual teacher, sitting at his feet and accompanying him on his rounds. Many different sorts of medical care were available, and self-help was universal. Celsus' *On Medicine* was written for a non-professional readership as willing to wield the scalpel as the plough. Disease explanations changed little. Public authorities still ascribed famines and pestilences to the gods, and Galen was silent on contagion. The essential trilogy of classical medicine remained dietetics, exercise, and drugs, accompanied by light surgery.

1.2.1.7 Medicine in the Middle Ages

The passage from the glorious days of Rome to the Middle Ages was often violent, especially in the West, with wave after wave of barbarian onslaughts from the East. These culminated in the sack of the Eternal City by Alaric's Goths in 410 AD, which effectively ended the western empire and frayed the thread of learned medicine. Thus Galen had no effective successor. Indeed, medieval medicine may be summed up as a corrupted version of Galenism. The true scientific tradition did not reappear in the West until the 16th century, after a lengthy incubation in the Islamic world. For example, in England the Venerable Bede (ca. 672-735) and his monks possessed many medical writings, and knowledge of plant remedies was extensive, but the English healer used chants and charms, predicated on the belief that certain diseases and bad luck were caused by darts shot by elves, while other ailments involved a "great worm," a term applied to snakes, insects, and dragons.

By contrast with the naturalist focus of Hippocratic and Galenic medicine, healing became more authoritarian and intertwined with religion, for the rising Church taught that there was a supernatural plan and purpose to everything, including sickness and death. Christian and Jewish healing traditions became more prominent. Disease could be cured by prayers or by invoking the names of saints, by exorcism, by amulets or number magic, or by transferring the sickness to animals, plants, or to the soil. Certain maladies such as leprosy were associated with the Almighty's punishments for sin, according to the Book of Leviticus:

> *"When a man shall have in the skin of his flesh a rising [a swelling], a scab, or bright spot, and it be in the skin of his flesh like the plague [the spots] of leprosy...and the plague in sight be deeper than the skin of his flesh it is a plague of leprosy: and the priest shall look on him, and pronounce him unclean."*

Such polluting diseases were curable by the Lord alone, encouraging some Jewish people to reject human medicine in favor of the divine, citing the fate of King Asa (ca. 914-874 BC), who "sought not the Lord, but his physicians," and whose foot sores consequently worsened, and he died. On the other hand, while Jewish dietary rituals (e.g. kosher food) are principally expressions of religious precepts about pollution and purification, a useful practical effect is to limit exposure to foodborne diseases such as trichinosis.[2215]

Many of the distinguished surgeons of the Middle Ages were clerics, but the practice of medicine and surgery by members of the Church was not favored by the hierarchy. Many laws were passed against the practice of medicine for worldly profit. In 1215 the Fourth Lateran Council forbade all sub-deacons, deacons, or priests to practice that part of surgery that had to do with burning and cutting. Finally, Pope Honorius III (d. 1216) prohibited all persons in holy orders from practicing medicine in any form, which meant that the educated classes were prohibited from performing any type of surgery.

In Europe in the Middle Ages, practitioners unsuccessfully sought to cure wounds by treating only the weapons that caused them, using an ointment on the offending knife or sword known as a weapon salve. Physicians practiced urine-gazing (uroscopy), but proper chemical analysis of urine did not develop until the 18th century. Medieval medicine is the source of many humorous "remedies" in contemporary diatribes against modern medicine — such as being strapped into a halter and walked around a pigsty three times for mumps, drinking water from the skull of a bishop to treat rheumatism, or nuzzling a mouse to cure the common cold.[2216] But we must recognize that such treatments were not put forth as reasonable science. Rather, they serve as a reminder of the results of injecting mystical or religious elements into medicine as a substitute for good science.

The Middle Ages are also remarkable for their plagues, which became more numerous as people crowded closer and closer together in urban centers of increasing population density. Plague records from China during this period often show 50%-70% mortality rates, and China probably served as the original source of the greatest of the bubonic plagues that swept through Europe in the 14th century, known as the Black Death. The disease broke out in 1346 among the armies of a Mongol prince who laid siege to the trading city of Caffa in the Crimea. This compelled his withdrawal, but not before the disease had entered Caffa, whence it rapidly spread by ship throughout the Mediterranean.

The initial shock in 1346-1350 was severe. Die-offs varied widely, with some small communities experiencing total extinction and others, such as Milan, being spared entirely. The lethal effect of the plague may have been enhanced by the fact that it was propagated not solely by the bites of fleas carried on infected rodents, but also was transmitted person to person as a result of inhaling bacillus-filled droplets that had been coughed or sneezed into the air by an infected individual. Lung infections of this kind were observed to be 100% lethal in Manchuria in 1921, the only time modern medicine has directly observed airborne plague communication, so it is tempting to assume a similar mortality for pneumonic plague in 14th century Europe. Mortality rates for sufferers from bubonic infection transmitted by flea bite varies from 30% to 90%. All told, the best estimate of European plague-induced mortality is that about one-third of the population died during the initial five-year period.

The plague returned in the 1360s, the 1370s, and thereafter, and European population declined irregularly as a result, reaching a low point in England sometime between 1440-1480.[2210] People learned to minimize infection risk via quarantine, a practice which stemmed from Biblical passages prescribing the ostracism of lepers. Plague sufferers were treated as though they were temporary lepers, with a standard 40-day quarantine for people and incoming ships at all major ports. However, since the role of fleas and rats in disease propagation remained unknown until the end of the 19th century, quarantine measures were often ineffectual. Through the 17th century, occasional plague outbreaks that carried off up to a third or a half of a city's population in a single year were considered normal.[2211] For example, Venetian statistics show that in 1575-77 and again in 1630-31, a third or more of the city's population died of plague.[2212]

Pre-modern medicine was powerless against bubonic plague. Before antibiotics reduced the disease to triviality in 1943, the average mortality rate was 60%-70% of those affected, despite all that the best hospital care could accomplish.[2213] The last recorded outbreak of plague that ran its course without benefit of penicillin and related antibiotics (which destroy the infection rapidly) occurred in Burma in 1947, with 78% lethality.[2214]

1.2.1.8 Renaissance and Pre-Modern Medicine

While internal medicine languished through the Middle Ages, the surgeons of the Renaissance gained wide experience during the many religious wars of the period. They had many new problems to face, including the treatment of wounds caused by firearms. The French had employed gunpowder at the siege of Puiguillaume in 1338, and cannon were used by the English at the Battle of Crecy in 1346. Gunshot wounds at that time were caused by large missiles of low velocity that caused ragged wounds and carried pieces of clothing into the tissues. These wounds were severe and very liable to become septic. The universal belief among contemporary surgeons was that gunpowder itself was venomous. To neutralize the effect of this venom, the general practice was to cauterize the wound by injecting boiling oil.

The first man to break away from this old doctrine was Ambroise Pare (1510-90). Pare came to Paris in 1532 as an apprentice to a barber-surgeon and then moved to the great Hotel Dieu as resident surgeon. In that immense medieval hospital, the only one in Paris at the time, he gained great experience, and in 1536 he began his career as a military surgeon. As described in his book *The Apologie and Treatise*, he recounts how, during his first campaign as a greenhorn military surgeon in Turin in 1537, he had run out of boiling oil, the established treatment for gunpowder wounds, just after French troops had captured the castle of Villaine. So in place of boiling oil, he applied:

> *"...a digestive of yolk of eggs, oil of roses, and turpentine. In the night I could not sleep in quiet, fearing some default in not cauterizing, that I should find those to whom I had not used the burning oil dead impoisoned; which made me rise very early to visit them, where beyond my expectation I found those to whom I had applied my digestive medicine, to feel little pain, and their wounds without inflammation or tumour, having rested reasonable well in the night; the other to whom was used the said burning oil, I found them feverish with great pain and tumour about the edges of their wounds. And then I resolved with myself never so cruelly to burn poor men wounded with gunshot."*

Pare also went on to show that bleeding after amputations should be arrested, not by the terrible method of the indiscriminate use of the red-hot cautery, but by simple tying of the blood vessels. His most famous phrase, so reminiscent of the old Hippocratic school of thought, was: "I dressed the wound, and God healed him."

In 1633 appeared the earliest book on first-aid for the injured, by one Stephen Bradwell, although the proffered advice sounds impractical and a bit odd to modern ears. For example, the treatment for the "Biting of a Madde Dogge" is to throw the patient into water. "In doing this, if he cannot swim, after he hath swallowed a good quantity of water, take him out again. But if he be skilful in swimming, hold him under the water a little while till he have taken in some pretty quantity." This procedure may not be wholly irrational — standard 20th century first aid for dog bites includes a thorough cleansing of the wound with water.

Venesection remained a popular 17th century universal remedy. As described by the surgeon Richard Wiseman (1622-1676), "a gentleman of about thirty years of age coming out of Hertfordshire through Tottenham and riding upon the causeway near an inn, one emptying a chamber pot out of the window as he was passing by, his horse started and rushed violently between a signpost and a tree which supported part of the sign. The poor gentleman was beaten off his horse and lay stunned upon the ground." A barber-surgeon was hastily summoned but nothing much was done for the injured man until Wiseman arrived, whereupon:

> *"I found the gentleman lying upon the ground, the people and chirurgeon gazing upon him. I felt his pulse much oppressed, the right brow bruised and inquired whether they had bled him blood. The chirurgeon replied that he had opened a vein in his arm but it would not bleed. I replied, we must make him bleed through it by splitting his veins. Turning his head on one side, I saw the jugular vein on the bruised side turgid and opened it. He bled freely. After I had taken about twelve ounces, the blood ran down from his arm which had been opened before and would not bleed. We bled him till he came to life, and then he raved and struggled with us."*

The patient's injuries were dressed and he was subjected to further bleedings, but evidently made a good recovery.

Even by the 18th century, the traditional surgeon's day-to-day business eschewed high-risk operations like amputations; rather, it was a round of minor procedures such as venesection, lancing boils, dressing skin abrasions, pulling teeth, managing whitlows, trussing ruptures, and treating skin ulcers. The fatality rates of these procedures were low, for surgeons understood their limits, and the repertoire of operations they attempted was small, because of the well-known risks of trauma, blood loss, and sepsis. Internal disorders were treated not by the knife but by medicines and management, since major internal surgery was unthinkable before anesthetics and antiseptic procedures. Improvements did occur in certain operations such as lithotomy. William Cheselden (1688-1752), a great British surgeon of the 18th century, perfected a technique which enabled him to remove a stone in the bladder in one minute (his record time was 54 seconds), thus reducing mortality from about 50% to under 10%. Cheselden's results were not bettered until almost the end of the 19th century.

In the 17th century, internal medical treatment was frequently overdone on those affluent enough to afford it. Critics often denounced physicians as meddlesome, capriciously practicing an often dangerous polypharmacy — a blunderbuss approach. The deathbed of Charles II (1630-1685) of England was a conspicuous case of such medical overkill; after the king had suffered a stroke, his doctors moved in, and Sir Raymond Crawfurd (1865-1938) recreated the scene:

> *"Sixteen ounces of blood were removed from a vein in his right arm with immediate good effect. As was the approved practice at this time, the King was allowed to remain in the chair in which the convulsions seized him. His teeth were held forcibly open to prevent him biting his tongue. The regimen was, as Roger North pithily describes it, first to get him to wake, and then to keep him from sleeping. Urgent messages had been dispatched to the King's numerous personal physicians, who quickly came flocking to his assistance; they were summoned regardless of distinctions of creed and politics, and they came. They ordered cupping-glasses to be applied to his shoulders forthwith, and deep scarification to be carried out, by which they succeeded in removing another eight ounces of blood. A strong antimonial emetic was administered, but as the King could be got to swallow only a small portion of it, they determined to render assistance doubly sure by a full dose of Sulphate of Zinc. Strong purgatives were given, and supplemented by a succession of clysters. The hair was shorn close, and pungent blistering agents were applied all over his head. And as though this were not enough, the red-hot cautery was requisitioned as well."*

One of the dozen attending physicians noted with pride that "nothing was left untried"; the King graciously apologized for being "an unconscionable time a-dying."

Meanwhile, the common citizen experienced poor health exacerbated by the many new dangers attending the Industrial Revolution. In 1775, Percivall Pott (1714-1788) pointed out that boy chimneysweeps developed scrotal cancer, due to soot irritation. In his *Condition of the Working Classes in England* (1844), Friedrich Engels (1820-1895), a Manchester factory owner as well as Karl Marx's collaborator, described workers who were "pale, lank, narrow-chested, hollow-eyed ghosts," cooped up in houses that were mere "kennels to sleep and die in." In 1832, the Leeds physician Charles Turner Thackrah (1795-1833) published *The Effects of Arts, Trades, and Professions on Health and Longevity*, documenting the diseases and disabilities of various occupations. Apart from factory workers, among those most exposed to harmful substances were cornmillers, maltsters, coffee-roasters, snuff-makers, rag-pickers, papermakers and feather-dressers. Tailors were so subject to anal fistulas that they set up their own "fistula clubs." Thackrah's overall verdict was bleak: "Not 10% of the inhabitants of large towns enjoy full health."

The single worst malady cultivated in populous cities was tuberculosis (TB), a disease characterized by fever, night sweats, and hemoptysis (coughing up blood), called "consumption" because victims were almost literally consumed. By 1800 TB was proclaimed the most common disease, and in 1815 Thomas Young (1773-1829) surmised that tuberculosis brought a premature death to one in four in the general population. Autopsies conducted in the chief Paris hospitals recorded TB as the cause of death in some 40% of cases. In the continental U.S. as late as 1890, the corresponding percentage was about 13%, and tuberculosis was still the leading cause of death (Table 1.2), though the data are partially suspect because cases of lung cancer were sometimes reported as "consumption".[2226]

Table 1.2. Leading Causes of Death in the United States, 1890 vs. 1990

(crude annual death rate per 100,000 of population)[2208,2209]

Cause of Death	1890 Death Rate per 100,000	1990 Death Rate per 100,000
Consumption (TB)	245.4	0.7
Pneumonia	186.9	31.1
Heart disease	121.8	310.4
Diarrheal diseases	104.1	~ 0
Debility and atrophy	88.6	N/A
Infantile cholera	79.7	~ 0
Bronchitis	74.4	1.7
Diphtheria	70.1	~ 0
Kidney diseases	59.7	8.8
Meningitis	49.1	0.4
Apoplexy (stroke)	49.0	57.9
Cancer	47.9	203.2
Typhoid Fever	46.3	~ 0
Old age	44.9	N/A
Brain diseases	30.9	N/A
Croup	27.6	~ 0
Malaria	19.2	0.002
Influenza	6.2	0.8
Other	~ 488.2	248.8
All Causes	**~ 1840.0**	**863.8**

One important 18th century improvement in internal medicine which decisively saved many lives was the introduction of inoculation and vaccination against smallpox. Smallpox, "the speckled monster," had become virulent throughout Europe and in bad years accounted for about 10% of all deaths; Queen Mary of England (1662-1694), Louis XV of France (1710-1774), and Queen Anne's son and sole surviving direct heir (d. 1700) died of it. Doctors had long been aware of the immunizing properties of an attack, and smallpox inoculation seems to have been known and practiced for centuries at a folk level throughout Arabia, North Africa, Persia, and India. Reports of a more elaborate Chinese method, involving the insertion of a suitable infected swab of cotton inside the patient's nostril, reached London in 1700. But it was a report from Mary Wortley Montagu (1689-1762), wife of the British consul in Constantinople, that Turkish women held smallpox parties at which they routinely performed inoculations with the aim to induce a mild dose so as to confer lifelong protection without pockmarking, that hastened acceptance in the rural medical community. The usual method was to transfer the infection by introducing matter from a smallpox pustule into a slight wound made in the patient's skin. Occasionally the patient developed a severe case of smallpox from such treatment, and some died. But usually the symptoms were slight — a few score of pox only — and immunity proved equivalent to that resulting from contracting the disease naturally.

Edward Jenner (1749-1823), an English country doctor who performed such inoculations, noticed that cowpox, a cattle disease occasionally contracted by humans, particularly dairy maids, also conferred immunity against smallpox. Suspecting that it might be possible to produce this immunity by arm-to-arm inoculation from the cowpox pustule, and surmising it would be safer than inoculation from smallpox pustules directly, since in humans cowpox was benign, Jenner tried the experiment, and it worked. In 1798 he published his discovery in *An Inquiry into the Causes and Effects of the Variolae Vaccinae*. By 1799 over 5000 individuals had been vaccinated in England and abroad the practice was taken up remarkably swiftly, being made compulsory in Sweden and supported by Napoleon, who had his army vaccinated. For the first time in history, organized medicine began to contribute to human population growth in a statistically significant fashion.

The Napoleonic Wars spurred new attempts to treat battle-wounded soldiers in a more timely manner. Traditionally, the wounded were left on the field unattended until the end of battle, but Napoleon's chief surgeon Dominique Jean Larrey (1766-1842) introduced the use of rudimentary carts called ambulances volantes (little more than horsedrawn rickshaws) as the first "ambulances" to evacuate and transport wounded soldiers from the field to nearby aid stations, even while the battle raged on. In 1792, Larrey organized the first air evacuation, by hot air balloon.

The use of ambulances didn't catch on until the late 1800s; until then, anyone injured in the streets of Paris, London, New York or Boston depended on the kindness of strangers or a nearby business shop for a place to rest until a doctor could be summoned.[2287] The first "modern" ambulance appeared in the city of Cincinnati in 1865, but the first true city ambulance system was developed in association with Bellevue Hospital in New York City in 1866, receiving 1500 requests for transport in its first three years of service.[2294] These horse-drawn ambulances, usually provided by local mortuaries, carried a driver and a surgeon, who was on board mainly to pronounce a patient's death at the scene or upon arrival at the hospital, since little could be done for the seriously injured.[2287] The surgeon kept meticulous notes on the ride, recording the time of the call, transport and arrival times, and any other details that "a coroner's jury might possibly require".[2294]

The period also saw the development of many simple diagnostic tools that are taken for granted today. For example, a French physician, Rene Theophile Hyacinthe Laennec (1781-1826), in his *Treatise On Mediate Auscultation* (1819), described pathological lesions found in the chest at autopsy and showed how they correlated with disease detected in living patients, establishing for the first time the modern concept of clinicopathological correlation, the cornerstone of modern diagnosis. Laennec also developed an instrument that he named a "stethoscope" to assist him in his examination of patients, especially female patients, against whose chests the direct placing of a male ear was socially taboo. The original device was a straight wooden tube; by mid-century rubber tubing was introduced to create a flexible monaural stethoscope, and in 1852 an American physician, George P. Cammann (1804-1863), devised our familiar two-ear instrument.

The clinical thermometer is of like vintage. Galileo (1564-1642) invented the first thermometer in the late 16th century, but it was not applied to medicine. Early medical thermometers in the 18th century were a foot long and difficult to use at the bedside, and were reportedly carried under the arm "as one might carry a gun." The short clinical thermometer was devised by Sir Clifford Allbutt (1836-1925) in the 1860s, and was widely used during the American Civil War (1861-1865). The classical work in temperature diagnostics was Carl Wunderlich's (1815-1877) *The Temperature in Diseases*, published in 1868, which presented data on nearly 25,000 patients and analyzed temperature variations in 32 diseases, showing that temperature readings could differentiate fevers. Other devices emerged later to measure pulse and blood pressure. In 1854, Karl Vierordt (1818-1884) created the sphygmograph, a pulse recorder usable for routine monitoring on humans. Blood pressure was measured using the familiar inflatable band wrapped around the upper arm, called the sphygmomanometer, whose basic design was established in 1896 by Scipione Riva-Rocci (1863-1937). The hypodermic syringe was invented in 1853.

Biochemistry also began to play an increasing diagnostic function. In the 18th century, Matthew Dobson (d. 1784) developed tests for diabetes. In 1827, Richard Bright (1789-1858) showed show the kidney complaint subsequently called Bright's disease could be diagnosed by a single, simple chemical test. Chemical analysis was crucial to Alfred Becquerel's (1814-1862) urinalysis studies in 1841, establishing the average amounts of water, urea, uric acid, lactic acid, albumin, and inorganic salts secreted over 24 hours, and correlating these with various disease conditions. In 1859, Alfred Garrod (1819-1907) devised a simple chemical test pathognomonic for gout.

1.2.1.9 Fully Invasive Surgery

The fully invasive surgery of the 19th and 20th centuries rests upon the triple foundation of anatomy, anesthesia, and asepsis. Each has an interesting story, described below, presaging the emergence of the rational-scientific approach to medical treatment.

1.2.1.9.1 Anatomy

In surgical practice, lack of accurate anatomical knowledge had long been a great obstacle. Dissection of the human body was first practiced systematically at the great medical school of Alexandria, which flourished from about 300 BC until the death of the last ruler of Ptolemaic Egypt, Cleopatra, in 30 BC. After the decline of Alexandria, dissection was carried on at a few other centers in the Middle East, but in the first two centuries of the Christian era human bodies were replaced on the dissection table by those of apes and other animals. The anatomical knowledge gained by Galen and others from the dissection of animals was an adequate guide for the simple operative procedures carried out at this time because the abdomen, the chest, and the head were rarely opened by the surgeon's knife.

Anatomical demonstrations of a kind were introduced into some Italian medical schools early in the 14th century but their main purpose was to serve as an aid in memorizing what Galen had written a thousand years before. During the late Middle Ages, and for a long time after, the procedure was for the professor to read from some second- or third-hand manuscript version of Galen while a demonstrator pointed to the part under discussion with a wand. As the text of Galen was often based on the dissection of an ape or pig, there were naturally many occasions when the anatomical structure under examination did not correspond with Galen's description.

Some of the great artists took up the scientific study of anatomy, but the true founder of modern anatomy was Andreas Vesalius (1514-1564), a native of Brussels who studied medicine in Paris and later taught surgery and anatomy at Padua and Bologna. Vesalius was filled with a passionate desire for anatomical study, and many stories are told of the great risks which he took in obtaining material, including, it is reported, graverobbing. On one occasion he stole the skeleton of a criminal which was hanging on a gallows outside the city wall of Louvain and the trophy proved of great value in his studies. His public dissections during his seven years in Padua drew enormous crowds of students. In 1543 he published his 355-page great work, *De Humani Corporis Fabrica Libri Septem* (*On the Fabric of the Human Body*), the outstanding and precise illustrations in which were copied and plagiarized by scholars for more than 100 years, and could be used for teaching even today. For the first time in the history of medicine, doctors had at their disposal a detailed and accurate anatomical text with illustrations from the hand of a great artist. This book is the foundation stone of anatomy — indeed of all modern medicine — because without a sound knowledge of the structure of the body there can be no real understanding of the body's functions in health and disease.

A tremendous shortage of dead human bodies for dissection, to teach anatomy, remained a problem for centuries. In Edinburgh in 1827, an old man died in William Hare's (1792-1870) boarding-house; assisted by his lodger William Burke (1792-1829), the two men bypassed the grave and sold the body directly to anatomists. Spurred by success, they turned to murder, luring victims and suffocating them to avoid signs of violence. Sixteen were done to death and their bodies sold, fetching 7 pounds apiece, before Burke and Hare were brought to justice in 1829. Hare turned King's evidence and Burke was hanged. The last cadaver was found in the dissecting room of a respected anatomist, Robert Knox (1791-1862). Despite his cries of innocence, an incensed crowd burned down his house and he fled to London, his career in ruins, and eventually Knox died in obscurity.

To help pass the English Anatomy Act of 1832 (which awarded to doctors the "unclaimed bodies" of paupers) and to dispel public concern about dissection, the body of the great English philosopher and jurist, Jeremy Bentham (1748-1832), in accordance with his directions, was dissected in the presence of his friends. The skeleton was then reconstructed, supplied with a wax head to replace the original (which had been mummified), dressed in Bentham's own clothes and set upright in a glass-fronted case. Both this effigy and the head are preserved at University College, London, to this day.

1.2.1.9.2 Anesthesia

Pain did not prevent surgery but made it almost unbearable, and the accompanying trauma often proved dangerous. Before the anesthetic era, which commenced in the late 1840s, surgical operations were agonizing. Of course, if the patient had a broken leg or a major wound, there was no choice but submit to a surgeon's knife. But non-emergency elective operations would only be undergone if the condition itself was so painful or life-threatening that the victim could even consider allowing surgery. In this event, patients would choose a surgeon with the best reputation for quickness — a limb might be removed or a bladder stone evacuated in a couple of minutes. Progress in technique was often rapid. For example, in 1824, Astley Cooper (1768-1841) took 20 minutes to amputate a leg through the hip joint; ten years later, James Syme (1799-1870) was doing it in just 90 seconds.

In pre-anesthetic days, operations were rushed through at lightning speed and under conditions of appalling difficulty. The most hardened surgeons had to steel themselves to perform operations which they knew would cause agony to their patients and nerve-wracking distress to themselves. It is hard for any 20th century inhabitant of an industrialized nation to imagine what a major surgical operation must have meant to the patient in the days before anesthesia. The following is a personal account by a male patient who suffered the removal of a stone from the bladder by Henry Cline (1750-1827), surgeon to St. Thomas's Hospital and one of the leading operators of the day, on 30 December 1811, just three decades before the widespread adoption of anesthesia:

> *"My habit and constitution being good it required little preparation of body, and my mind was made up. When all parties had arrived I retired to my room for a minute, bent my knee in silent adoration and submission, and returning to the surgeons conducted them to the apartment in which the preparations had been made. The bandages &c. having been adjusted I was prepared to receive a shock of pain of extreme violence and so much had I overrated it, that the first incision did not even make me wince although I had declared that it was not my intention to restrain such impulse, convinced that such effort of restraint could only lead to additional exhaustion. At subsequent moments, therefore I did cry out under the pain, but was allowed to have gone through the operation with great firmness."*
>
> *"The forcing up of the staff prior to the introduction of the gorget gave me the first real pain, but this instantly subsided after the incision of the bladder was made, the rush of urine appeared to relieve it and soothe the wound."*
>
> *"When the forceps was introduced the pain was again very considerable and every movement of the instrument in endeavoring to find the stone increased. Still, however, my mind was firm and confident, and, although anxious, I was yet alive to what was going on. After several ineffectual attempts to grasp the stone I heard the operator say in the lowest whisper, "It is a little awkward, it lies under my hand. Give me the curved forceps," upon which he withdrew the others. Here, I think, I asked if there was anything wrong — or something to that purport — and was reanimated by the reply conveyed in the kindest manner, "Be patient, Sir, it will soon be over." When the other forceps was introduced I had again to undergo the searching for the stone and heard Mr. Cline say, "I have got it." I had probably by this time conceived that the worst was over; but when the necessary force was applied to withdraw the stone the sensation was such as I cannot find words to describe. In addition to the positive pain there was something peculiar in the feel. The bladder embraced the stone as firmly as the stone was itself grasped by the forceps; it seemed as if the whole organ was about to be torn out. The duration, however, of this really trying part of the operation was short and when the words "Now, Sir, it is all over" struck my ear, the ejaculation of "Thank God! Thank God!" was uttered with a fervency and fulness of heart which can only be conceived....I never heard what was the precise duration of the operation but conceive it to have been between twelve and fifteen minutes."*

And now, a woman's point of view. In 1810, Napoleon's famed military doctor Dominique Jean Larrey performed a radical mastectomy without anesthetic on the popular female novelist Fanny Burney (1752-1840). Burney later wrote a long account of the operation which, despite the excruciating agony, she believed had nevertheless saved her life:

> *"M. Dubois placed me upon the Mattress, & spread a cambric handkerchief upon my face. It was transparent, however, & I saw through it that the Bed stead was instantly surrounded by the 7 men and my nurse. I refused to be held; but when, bright through the cambric, I saw the glitter of polished steel — I closed my eyes...*
>
> *"Yet — when the dreadful steel was plunged into the breast — cutting through veins — arteries — flesh — nerves — I needed no injunctions not to restrain my cries. I began a scream that lasted unintermittingly during the whole time of the incision — & I almost marvel that it rings not in my Ears still! so excruciating was the agony.*
>
> *"When the wound was made, & the instrument was withdrawn, the pain seemed undiminished, for the air that suddenly rushed into those delicate parts felt like a mass of minute but sharp & forked poniards [small pointed daggers], that were tearing at the edges of the wound. But when again I felt the instrument, describing a curve, cutting against the grain, if I may so say, while the flesh resisted in a manner so forcible as to oppose & tire the hand of the operator, who was forced to change from the right to the left — then, indeed, I thought I must have expired, I attempted no more to open my eyes.... The instrument the second time withdrawn, I concluded the operation over — Oh no! presently the terrible cutting was renewed — & worse than ever, to separate the bottom, the foundation of the dreadful gland from the parts to which it adhered...yet again all was not over...."*

This chilling account continued for several more pages.

When did the practice of anesthesia begin? *The Herbal of Dioscorides* (ca. 40-90 AD) contains specific directions for giving a decoction (boiled extraction) of mandragora "to such as shall be cut or cauterized," one of the earliest references to surgical anesthesia. Bernard de Gordon (ca. 1260-1308) tells us that the Salernitans rubbed up poppy seed and henbane and used them as a plaster to deaden the sensibility of a part to be cauterized. Arnold of Villanova (1235-1311) gives the following recipe:

> *"To produce sleep so profound that the patient may be cut and will feel nothing, as though he were dead, take of opium, mandragora bark, and henbane root equal parts, pound them together and mix with water. When you want to sew or cut a man, dip a rag in this and put it to his forehead and nostrils. He will soon sleep so deeply that you may do what you will. To wake him up, dip the rag in strong vinegar."*

Some of the surgical textbooks of the Middle Ages contain references to anesthetic sponges which were prepared by soaking them in various herbs reputed to have soporific properties. The favorite herb for this purpose was the mandrake. Another simple method of producing analgesia used intermittently from early times was compression. Writing in 1564 about the various uses of the tourniquet, the French surgeon Ambrose Pare noted that "it much dulls the sense of the part by stupefying it." Amusingly, reliable witnesses claim that as late as the 19th century, a method of anesthesia practiced at the Imperial Court of China was to "knock the patient out by a sudden blow on the jaw."

The almost complete absence of any mention of pain-relieving drugs in medical literature of the post-medieval period is not easy to explain. It is, however, probable that the action of crude concoctions employed in early times was very uncertain, and that drugged sleep often ended in death. The active ingredients of the many herbs used in medicine had not been isolated and it would have been very difficult to regulate dosages reliably.

The story of inhalation anesthesia begins in 1799 when Sir Humphry Davy (1778-1829) recorded the effects produced by the inhalation of nitrous oxide. He breathed various concentrations of the gas and noted that a headache and the pain associated with the cutting of a wisdom tooth were relieved. Demonstrations of the effects of nitrous oxide were frequently given, bladders filled with "laughing gas" being passed around at lectures. Gas inhalation became a popular party game. A little book of 1839 contains a description of the "irresistibly ridiculous" sight of a large room filled with persons each of whom was sucking from a bladder. As the gas began to take effect, "some jumped over the tables and chairs; some were bent on making speeches; some were very much inclined to fight; and one young gentleman persisted in attempting to kiss the ladies." At about the same time, "ether frolics" became equally popular.

In January 1842, William E. Clarke (b. 1818), a young American physician of Rochester, New York, who had acquired some knowledge of ether by attendance at ether frolics, administered the chemical on a towel to a Miss Hobbie who then had one of her teeth extracted painlessly. So far as is known this was the first use of ether for a dental or surgical operation. In March 1842, Crawford W. Long (1815-1878) of Danielville, Georgia, who had also witnessed ether frolics "enjoying sweet kisses from the girls," successfully removed a small tumor from the neck of a patient under the influence of ether. Horace Wells (1815-1848), a dentist of Hartford, Connecticut, attended a public demonstration of the effects of nitrous oxide in December 1844, and the day after he administered the gas to himself and had one of his own teeth pulled out by a colleague. Afterwards, Wells wrote: "I didn't feel it so much as the prick of a pin." His former partner, William Thomas Green Morton (1819-1868), also introduced ether into his dental practice in 1846. By February 1847, the Lancet and other medical journals were reporting anesthetic operations from all parts of Great Britain, and ether had been used in most European countries. In June 1847 the news reached South Africa and a leg was amputated painlessly by W.G. Atherstone of Grahamstown.

Sir James Young Simpson (1811-1870), professor of surgery at Edinburgh, introduced chloroform in 1847. Tradition has it that Simpson had been testing chemicals with his assistants when somebody upset a bottle of chloroform; upon bringing in dinner, Simpson's wife found them all asleep. Unlike ether, chloroform did not irritate the lungs or cause vomiting, and was powerful and easy to administer. In April 1853, Queen Victoria (1819-1901) took chloroform for the birth of Prince Leopold; John Snow (1813-1858) administered the anesthetic. Protests followed — some objections were religious (e.g., the Bible taught that women were supposed to bring forth in "travail and pain"*) but most were medical, putatively on grounds of safety but ringing with naturophilia (Section 1.3.4): "In no case could it be justifiable to administer chloroform in perfectly ordinary labor," complained the Lancet. Incredibly, some early 19th century surgeons believed that using anesthesia for an operation would weaken a patient's character.

Of course, general anesthesia could indeed prove dangerous, and deep unconsciousness was unnecessary for less invasive procedures, so the search was on for substances that would numb a particular area for local surgery. Cocaine was isolated in 1859 and was first used in ophthalmologic procedures by Carl Koller (1857-1944). Cocaine became the first widely-used local anesthetic, synthesized in 1885 by the Merck drug company.

1.2.1.9.3 Germ Theory and Antisepsis

By the middle of the 19th century, pain had been banished from surgical operations, but one grave danger still faced every patient submitting himself to the surgeon's knife. This was the ever-present risk of sepsis (infection). Hospital diseases such as erysipelas, pyemia, septicemia and gangrene, were rife. In the 1850s the death rate after amputations varied from 25%-60% in different countries and in military practice it reached the appalling figure of 75%-90%. The first ovariotomies, which were the first abdominal operations performed on a fairly large scale, had a mortality rate of more than 30% even in the most expert hands. That all these diseases were due to some form of "contagion" had long been suspected, but the general view was that whatever agent was responsible was generated spontaneously in wounds. Alternatively, it was theorized that air itself was responsible for suppuration and many attempts were made to exclude the air from wounds by means of elaborate dressings.

Some medical men had postulated the existence of minute particles in the air which carried contagion, the so-called "germ theory." In 1546, Girolamo Fracastoro of Verona (1478-1553) proposed "seminaria, the seeds of disease which multiply rapidly and propagate their life," minute bodies passing unseen from the infector to the infected by contact, by clothing or utensils, and by infection at a distance through the air.

What made the germ theory of contagion so difficult to accept was that no one could see the supposed microbes. Magnifying lenses were used in ancient times, and by the beginning of the 17th century

Others pointed to Genesis 2:21, where Adam is put to sleep as the rib is taken for Eve.

they had been combined in a tube to make the compound microscope. The first man to employ the microscope in investigating the causes of diseases was probably Athanasius Kircher (1601-1680), a learned Jesuit priest. In 1658 Kircher described experiments upon the nature of putrefaction, showing how maggots and other living creatures developed in decaying matter. He also claimed to have found in the blood of plague-stricken patients "countless masses of small worms, invisible to the naked eye." It is impossible that he could have seen the plague bacillus with the very low power microscopes at his disposal, but he may have seen some of the larger microorganisms and his statements about the doctrine of contagion are even more explicit than those of Fracastoro.

The great pioneer of modern microscopy was Anthoni van Leeuwenhoek (1632-1723), a Dutch linen draper, who ground his own lenses and made hundreds of microscopes. Few of his instruments provided a magnification of more than 160X but he is generally credited as making the first observations of germs, reported in his communications to the Royal Society in London. Leeuwenhoek was the first to describe spermatozoa and he gave the first complete account of the red blood corpuscles in 1674; he also found that the film from his own teeth contained "little animals, more numerous than all the people in the Netherlands."

In 1847, Ignaz Philipp Semmelweis (1818-1865), an assistant at the Vienna General Hospital in the maternity clinic (the world's largest at the time), was investigating the 29% postpartum mortality rate among women in Ward One, where births were handled by medical students, vs. a 3% rate in Ward Two where births were handled by midwifery pupils. Semmelweis noticed that the appearances of these deaths from puerperal fever looked the same as those observed in the body of an older colleague, forensic medicine Professor Jakob Kolletschka (1803-1847), who had died from a dissection wound suffered in the clinic. He correctly surmised that the postpartum deaths were caused by infection from "putrid particles" carried on the hands of medical students who often shuttled back and forth between the labor wards, the obstetrical clinic, and the autopsy room where dissections were performed. Semmelweis instituted a simple routine of hand-washing with water solutions of chloride of lime, which promptly reduced mortality to 1.27%. Unfortunately, his ideas were met with fierce opposition by the conservative medical community in Vienna, who subjected him to laughter and ridicule. In disgust, Semmelweis left Austria for Budapest. There he became head of the obstetrical division of St. Rochus Hospital, where puerperal fever mortality rates were reduced to below 1% after Semmelweis introduced chlorinated water disinfection.

The man who elucidated the true nature of infection, founded the science of bacteriology, and paved the way for Lister and the antiseptic system in surgery was Louis Pasteur (1822-1895). Pasteur was led to his great discoveries regarding bacteria and other microorganisms by his investigations into the process of fermentation. He showed conclusively that fermentation was brought about by some external agent entering the wine. He proved by painstaking experiments under rigorously controlled conditions that meat and fluids like blood did not putrefy if they were kept in such a way that all air was excluded from them. By taking samples of air at different levels Pasteur showed that contamination became less with increasing altitude. Then he proved that the contaminating agents were living organisms (bacteria) which were everywhere — in every room, in the air, on every article of clothing, on furniture, on the ground, and on the skin. He showed that putrefaction was caused by the presence of bacteria and that this applied to putrefaction in foods (milk, wine, and meat), urine, and in wounds.

The application of Pasteur's discoveries to surgical practice was the work of Joseph Lister (1827-1912), a young English surgeon who had concluded that it must also be bacteria that caused the suppuration, pus and gangrene which plagued the surgical wards of those days. He determined to prevent the access of organisms by killing them in or on the surface of the wound. Pasteur had shown that heat could kill microbes, but it was impossible to apply heat to a wound without burning the patient, so some chemical substance had to be found. After trying various chemical agents he finally selected carbolic acid, and he insisted that everything which touched the wound, the dressings, the instruments and the fingers, should be treated with this antiseptic. He even produced an antiseptic atmosphere by means of a carbolic spray. The clinical results of Lister's first antiseptic system in 1865 included 11 compound fracture cases with only one death, a 9% mortality rate, marking a watershed between the primitive and modern eras of surgery.

Throughout the 19th century, the arguments continued as to whether microorganisms seen in a sick patient were merely coincidental with the illness, or resulted from the changes brought about by the illness itself. In 1882 the German microbiologist Robert Koch (1843-1910) formulated three famous postulates to guide scientists searching for disease-causing microbes. Koch argued that to prove an organism causes a disease, microbiologists must show that the organism occurs in every case of the disease; that it is never found as a harmless parasite associated with another disease; and that once the organism is isolated from the body and grown in laboratory culture, it can be introduced into a new host and produce the disease again. (An oft-stated fourth postulate, that the microbe must be isolated again from the second host, was not part of Koch's original formulation.[2202])* Koch and his pupils discovered specific bacillary causes for various diseases, including anthrax, cholera, tuberculosis, gonorrhea, diphtheria, leprosy, typhoid, trypanosomiasis, and malaria.

The theory that specific germs could cause specific disease remained contentious until the beginning of the 20th century. Many scientists of great repute rejected Koch's conclusions, with one scientist confidently asserting that "no microbe found in the living blood of any animal was pathogenic." In one celebrated case, Max von Pettenkofer of Bavaria (1818-1901), a distinguished 19th century experimental hygienist, induced Koch to send him a sample of his cholera vibrios culture and then wrote a letter back to Koch in 1892, as follows:

> *"Herr Doctor Pettenkofer presents his compliments to Herr Doctor Professor Koch and thanks him for the flask containing the so-called cholera vibrios, which he was kind enough to send. Herr Doctor Pettenkofer has now drunk the entire contents and is happy to be able to inform Herr Doctor Professor Koch that he remains in his usual good health."*

Apparently Pettenkofer, aged 74 at the time he wrote the letter, survived this cholera exposure quite well, perhaps possessing the high stomach acidity which sometimes neutralizes the bacillus, though he shot himself to death in Munich 9 years later.

Skeptics notwithstanding, microbes were key. Enormous new vistas now lay open, as surgeons could confidently make an incision through intact skin without incurring an extreme risk of wound infection. The next step was to progress beyond killing wound

Koch's postulates are still valuable, especially as ideals, but many diseases do not conform to them so they are no longer considered the essential basis of diagnosis that they once were.[2202]

bacteria with chemical antiseptics, to the prevention of bacterial contamination by eliminating bacteria in the operating theater — aseptic surgery. The use of steam sterilization of instruments, dressings and gowns, the wearing of masks, caps and gloves, air filtration and the other rituals of the operating theater of today were introduced over the decades following Lister's efforts.

Anesthesia and antisepsis enabled surgeons to carry out procedures that had formerly been quite beyond them, including long operations inside the head, the abdomen and the pelvis. Theodor Billroth of Vienna (1829-1894) resected the esophagus in 1872, parts of the intestines in 1878, and the pyloric end of the stomach in 1881. Billroth also made the first complete excision of the larynx. The first successful repair of a gunshot wound on a major artery was performed in Chicago by John B. Murphy (1857-1916) in 1897; Ludwig Rehn (1849-1930) of Frankfurt am Main performed the first successful repair of a cardiac injury in Germany in the same year.

Writing in 1874, Sir John Eric Erichsen (1818-1896), Professor of Surgery at University College, London, had predicted that "the abdomen, the chest, and the brain would be forever shut from the intrusions of the wise and humane surgeon." By the time of Erichsen's death 22 years later, surgeons had successfully removed from patients the stomach and large parts of the intestines, a whole lung had been excised, and a brain tumor had been extirpated. These operations were not mere feats of surgical showmanship; they saved the lives and restored the health of thousands of human beings.

1.2.1.10 Cells and Tissues

The doctrine of the essential cellular nature of living things was established by 1840. Modern cell theory[3223] began in botany. The Jena botanist Matthias Schleiden (1804-1881) observed that plants were aggregates of cells, existing as self-reproducing living units. Exploring analogies between animals and plants in structure and growth, Theodor Schwann (1810-1882) took up the idea, maintaining that all these phenomena could also be demonstrated in animal structures. Thus living cells were basic to living things, and cells incorporated a nucleus and an outer membrane.

Jacob Henle (1809-85) applied cell biology to man. His three-volume *Handbuch der systematischem Anatomie des Menschen (Handbook of Systematic Human Anatomy)* (1866-1871) addressed the body from an architectural standpoint, describing its macro- and microscopic structure. Henle discovered kidney tubules and was the first to describe the muscular coat of the arteries, the minute anatomy of the eye and various skin structures, earning him a reputation as the Vesalius of histology (the study of tissues). Physiologists stressed organ and tissue function — Claude Bernard (1813-1878) emphasized the experimental method in establishing biological knowledge and urged that medical practice should be grounded in such knowledge.

Histology was raised to the status of an independent science by the Swiss microanatomist Albert von Kolliker (1817-1905), who wrote the first textbook on the subject, *Handbuch der Gewebelehre des Menschen (Handbook of the Tissues of Man)* (1852). The medical implications of cell theory were taken up by Rudolph Virchow (1821-1902), who dominated German biomedical research for half a century. Virchow extended the cell concept to diseased tissues; his *Die Cellularpathologie (Cellular Pathology)* (1858) analyzed such tissues from the point of view of cell formation and cell structure. Virchow initiated the idea that the body may be regarded as a "cell state in which every cell is a citizen." Disease is often but civil war, and white cells are likened to scavengers or police. Virchow maintained that cells always arose from pre-existing cells through cellular division. Since Kolliker and Virchow, the study of the intimate structure and workings of the cells themselves, as distinct from the tissues, has become a separate science, cytology, further extended to the study of cells in disease, or cytopathology (Chapter 21).

1.2.1.11 Blood Transfusions

Vague references to blood transfusion are found in medieval writings, though physicians historically were far more concerned with taking blood out of the body than with putting it back in. For example, one story tells of an attempt to prolong the life of Pope Innocent VIII (d. 1492) by means of a blood transfusion. By one account, a Jewish physician transfused the aged Pontiff with blood from three small boys, who each received one ducat as their reward; but another account says the blood was drunk, not infused. One of the earliest proposals to transfuse blood was by Andreas Libavius (1540-1616), a physician of Halle in Saxony, in 1615.

The first serious attempts at blood transfusion were made in England and France. In 1657 Sir Christopher Wren (1632-1723) carried out numerous experiments on the injection of liquids into the veins of animals. Richard Lower (1631-1691) of Oxford carried out the first successful transfusion from artery to vein between two dogs in 1665, a feat repeated by the French physician Jean-Baptiste Denys (1625-1704), who went on to attempt transfusion of blood from one kind of animal into another. Finally, before the Royal Society in 1667, Lower transfused a human youth, 15 years of age, from a sheep. The patient was greatly improved and the only ill effect was a feeling of great heat along his arm; subsequent patients were not so lucky. Blood transfusions from lambs and calves to humans continued to be tried in the mid 17th century, but were not very successful, and in 1670 were finally forbidden by law in England.

The first known transfusion of human blood into an already moribund person was attempted by James Blundell in 1818, and on several other occasions during the 1820s, with poor results. Transfusion was carried out on a small scale during the American Civil War, but technical difficulties connected with premature clotting and the occurrence of accidents arising from the use of incompatible blood prevented the rapid acceptance of the process. The cause of many of the untoward effects of blood transfusion was finally explained in 1901 when the presence of agglutinins and iso-agglutinins in the blood was demonstrated by Karl Landsteiner (1868-1943) in Vienna, winning him the Nobel Prize in 1930; in 1907, the four main blood groups were determined by Jan Jansky (1873-1921) of Prague. Rhesus factor was later identified by two American scientists, Philip Levine (1900-1987) and Rufus Stetson (1886-1967). These advances were of fundamental importance and it became possible in the 20th century to eliminate most of the fatalities due to incompatibility, allowing blood transfusions to be practiced reliably and with uniformly good results.

1.2.1.12 20th Century Medicine

The 20th century saw more discoveries and advances in medical science than all previous centuries combined. In this period, medicine became more powerful than ever before as scientists gained knowledge of matters and processes of illness that, at the beginning of the century, were still unknown or mysterious. Unlike the mere palliatives of earlier eras, 20th century physicians could actually cure some diseases, reverse some physical traumas, and save many lives that could not be saved before.

In the first half of the 20th century, the rational scientific paradigm that arose in the 19th century was pursued and extended. Acceptance of the germ theory of infection and the discovery of leukocytes led to the rapid emergence of immunology. This allowed

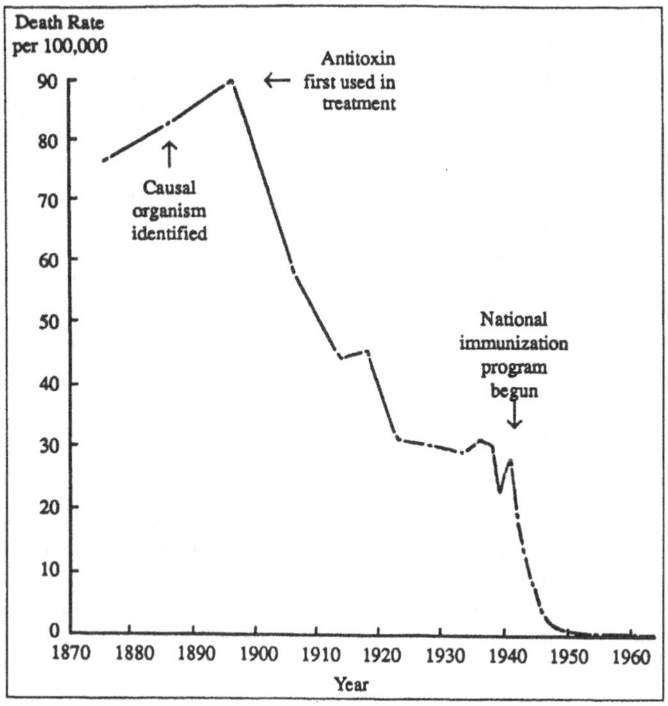

Fig. 1.2. Deaths due to Diptheria in England and Wales (children under 15).[2231]

medical scientists to produce protective vaccines and antisera which largely eliminated many diseases that were previously prevalent and dangerous, including whooping cough, measles, and diphtheria — the first truly effective medical treatments (Figure 1.2). Acceptance of the germ theory also led to the discovery of filterable viruses (organisms that could pass through the pores of all known filters) in the 1890s, and subsequently to the identification of viruses as specific causes of yellow fever, smallpox, typhus (a Rickettsia organism), measles, poliomyelitis, rabies, and viral meningitis. Biochemists synthesized vitamins which were recognized as essential constituents of a healthy diet, thus allowing the elimination of vitamin deficiency diseases such as scurvy, rickets, osteomalacia, beriberi, pellagra, xerophthalmia, nyctalopia, and pernicious anemia, via dietary supplements. Many metabolic diseases became treatable due to biochemical investigations; for example, the discovery of insulin in 1921 by the Canadian physiologists Sir Frederick Banting (1891-1941) and Charles Best (1899-1978) rapidly transformed diabetes from an invariably and often rapidly fatal disease into one that could be at least partially controlled, allowing sufferers many years of good life.

Blood group specification made transfusions convenient, facilitating dramatic advances in many branches of medicine, especially surgery. The first report of a successful autotransplant of a kidney into the neck of a dog was performed by Emerich Ullmann (1861-1937) in 1902. The first successful kidney graft between identical twins was performed in 1954 by Joseph E. Murray (b. 1919), who received a Nobel Prize for his work. The first heart transplantation in man was achieved by Christiaan Barnard (b. 1922) in 1967. Results were poor at first, but the use of new anti-rejection techniques such as the drug cyclosporin in the late 1970s, aided by advances in immunology, greatly improved the success of this and other organ transplants. By 1987, a total of ~7000 human hearts had been transplanted. At the close of the 20th century, heart, lung, heart-lung, and liver transplants were standard procedures, while grafts of small intestine and pancreas (the latter for refractory diabetes) were under active clinical investigation.

Two pivotal events transformed scientific medicine from a merely rational basis to a molecular basis, thus laying the groundwork for 21st century nanomedicine. The first pivotal event was the drug revolution, among which the most useful and spectacular were the antibiotics introduced between 1935-1945 and widely used ever since. Antibiotics are significant because they actively interfere with microbial metabolism and growth at the molecular level. The first antibiotic drugs were the sulphonamides, in 1935. Then penicillin became available in the 1940s, initially in very small quantities, then mass-produced by Pfizer during and after World War II, as a result of the research work of Alexander Fleming (1888-1955), Howard Florey (1898-1968) and Ernst Chain (1906-1979). In 1943, Selman A. Waksman (1888-1973) discovered streptomycin, the first effective anti-tuberculosis drug, for which he received the 1952 Nobel Prize. For the first time, physicians had true cures for many diseases, especially the most common bacterial diseases. Antifungal, anti-parasitic, and antiviral drugs of more limited effectiveness soon followed.

The 20th century also produced drugs that altered mood and levels of consciousness. Barbiturates were first introduced in 1903 (e.g. barbitone or Veronal), followed by phenobarbitone (Luminal) in 1912 and Evipan, the barbiturate anesthetic, in 1932. By mid-century these highly addictive drugs began to be replaced by the somewhat less-addictive benzodiazepines, including Valium and Librium. Tranquilizers, largely the phenothiazines such as chlorpromazine (Thorazine) and antimanics such as lithium carbonate, came to be widely used in psychiatry as effective medications for major mental illnesses including schizophrenia and manic depression.

The second pivotal event was the genetics revolution, starting with the discovery in 1953 of the information-carrying double-helix structure of DNA by Francis Crick (b. 1916) and John B. Watson (b. 1928) [2974-2975], followed in the 1980s by the ability to chemically read the genetic code, isolate specific genes and clone them for further study. In the mid-1980s, the Human Genome Project (Chapter 20) was launched, with the objective of fully sequencing every gene in the human genome. The first phase of this project neared completion as the 20th century drew to a close.[2322]

Molecular biology became the premier scientific discipline of the latter 20th century.[2217] By 1998, the compositions of organs, tissues, cells, organelles, and membranes had been defined, and the biosynthesis and catabolism of hundreds of compounds had been elucidated. The regulation of body processes was described at progressively finer levels in biochemical language. Many pharmacologic agents were finally understood in terms of specific molecular loci and mechanisms of action. Advances were particularly rapid in immunology, virology, cellular biology, peptide research, and structural biology. A beginning was made in explaining human behavior in mechanistic terms, as more and more chemical mediators and pharmacologic modifiers were discovered. In biology, these disciplines developed porous boundaries with related disciplines such as physiology, pharmacology, neurosciences, biochemistry and biophysics. All entered a phase of confluence, employing the common language of chemistry.

Thus the late 20th century is best regarded as the molecular age of basic biological science.[2207] The molecular influence pervades all the traditional disciplines underlying clinical medicine. As of February 1999, one source[2998] listed exactly 1446 genetic disorders, most of which could be linked to a specific human chromosome;

another source[2999] stated that ~4000 genetic disorders were known in 1998. There were more than 575 known abnormal human hemoglobins, and for each of these the precise structural defect in the DNA of the mutant gene could be defined. Knowledge of membrane, cytoplasmic, and nuclear receptors for hormones and drugs was exploding, with old as well as new diseases being defined in terms of receptor abnormalities — for example, type II hypercholesterolemia and nephrogenic diabetes insipidus. Recognition of opiate receptors led to the discovery of endogenous peptides (endorphins) with analgesic activity. Their localization promised further understanding of the limbic system, affective states, and addictions. Defects in a subcellular organelle, the peroxisome, were known to be responsible for a growing list of important genetic afflictions such as Refsum disease, Zellweger syndrome, and X-linked adrenoleukodystrophy. The genetic defect responsible for Huntington's disease was discovered, and in the 1990s the genetic defects responsible for many other important neurological disorders were becoming known, including forms of Alzheimer's disease, Charcot-Marie-Tooth disease, and common blinding retinal degenerative disorders such as retinitis pigmentosa, Leber's hereditary optic neuropathy, Norrie's disease, and choroideremia.[2218]

DNA sequencing techniques and restriction endonucleases permitted precise identification of the exact structural alteration of the gene in an increasing number of hereditary diseases. For example, Burkitt's lymphoma is characterized by a translocation of the distal end of the long arm of chromosome 8 to loci on chromosomes 14, 22, or 2.[2219] Gene therapy — both pharmacologic modification of specific gene action and physical replacement of damaged genetic segments — became possible in experimental systems. Complete maps of the entire genomes of 18 microbial species had been compiled and published by the end of 1998, with more than 60 others in progress.[2345] In 1992, wrote the conservative *Cecil Textbook of Medicine*:[2207] "The expansion of the knowledge bank of the past quarter century justifies great optimism for the eventual control and cure of major diseases and the possible elimination of premature death from illness."

Global changes in progressive aging dysfunction were shown to be strongly related to declining secretion of growth hormone by Rudman[2976] in 1990. Shortly thereafter, anti-aging medicine was recognized as a distinct discipline and was promoted by the American Academy of Anti-Aging Medicine (A^4M), a group[2981] that claimed >6000 physician and scientist members worldwide by 1998 and had held numerous conferences.[2977] In a book on the subject,[2979] Ronald Klatz,[2978-2980] A^4M's president, first comprehensively documented the implications of Rudman's work.

While biological science was vaulting forward into the molecular realm at a blistering pace, biomedical engineering lagged considerably behind, though many remarkable successes had been achieved since mid-century. Radiology expanded with sophisticated radiotherapy, ultrasound, scanning and imaging techniques (e.g., CAT, PET, NMR), with submillimeter resolution in living tissues. Surgical instruments became less damaging and less invasive; minimally invasive techniques used OK (orifice and keyhole) surgery and surgery performed under the "eye" of a scan. Fetuses could be screened for abnormality and surgery then performed upon them inside the womb, or they could be removed temporarily from the womb and then returned to continue gestating, after surgery. Prospective parents with fertility difficulties could make use of a wide range of therapies including in vitro fertilization. Implantable pacemakers, defibrillators, and ventricular assist devices were commonplace, and in 1998 artificial wearable/implantable and full/partial replacements for lungs, heart, kidney, liver, and pancreas were either available, in clinical trials, or under development (Volume III). Electron microscopes with 200,000X magnifications allowed many details of internal cellular and viral structures to be resolved as early as 1946; by 1998, atomic-force (AFM) and scanning-tunneling microscopy (STM) permitted direct tactile examination of individual biomolecules in fixed cells.

As the 20th century drew to a close, a few preliminary efforts had been made to apply the molecular approach to medical diagnostic and clinical tools. Biotechnology was one avenue being pursued, with the rational design of artificial enzymes and specified-ligand binding sites having already been achieved in certain limited cases, and the beginnings of gene therapy as noted earlier. Carbon fullerenes (Section 2.3.2) had been used to create a water-soluble inhibitor of HIV protease,[2633,2634] and had other biological applications.[2642] AFM-based force-amplified biological sensors[2313] could detect defined biological species such as cells, proteins, toxins, and DNA at concentrations as low as 10^{-18} M (~1/mm^3), and automated laboratory systems for sorting and handling individual cells[2314] and viruses[3219] were commonplace. Biotech companies such as Physiome Sciences of Princeton NJ had developed three-dimensional computer models of the heart and other organs. Physiome's heart model was based on detailed molecular, biochemical, cellular and anatomical information, including submodels of all the different cell types found in the heart embodying knowledge of the function of each cell type in healthy and diseased hearts, and information on gene function and the causes and effects of congestive heart failure, arrhythmias and heart attacks. Other cell biochemistry simulators included E-CELL (http://www.e-cell.org) and the Virtual Cell (http://www.nrcam.uchc.edu).[3199] There was also much progress and interest in nanostructure analysis and nanomaterials fabrication for medical and biological purposes, with research groups emerging at major universities such as the Cornell Nanofabrication Facility, the University of Michigan Center for Biologic Nanotechnology, the Rice University Center for Nanoscale Science and Technology, the CalTech Materials and Process Simulation Center, the Washington University Nanotechnology Center (St. Louis, MO), the USC Laboratory for Molecular Robotics, the UCLA Exotic Materials Center, the Institute for Molecular Medicine of the University of Oxford, and at many biotechnology-oriented corporations such as Nanogen and Affymetrix.

However, the greatest medical revolution of all awaits the ability to engineer and fabricate whole devices and systems at the molecular scale. Along this course lies nanotechnology and molecular manufacturing, a deep well from which nanomedicine will inevitably spring.

1.2.1.13 21st Century Medicine

It is always somewhat presumptuous to attempt to predict the future, but in this case we are on solid ground because most of the prerequisite historical processes are already in motion and all of them appear to be clearly pointing in the same direction.

Medical historian Roy Porter notes that the 19th century saw the establishment of what we think of as scientific medicine. From about the middle of that century the textbooks and the attitudes they reveal are recognizable as not being very different from modern ones. Before that, medical books were clearly written to address a different mind-set.

But human health is fundamentally biological, and biology is fundamentally molecular. As a result, throughout the 20th century scientific medicine began its transformation from a merely rational basis to a fully molecular basis. First, antibiotics that interfered with pathogens at the molecular level were introduced. Next, the ongoing

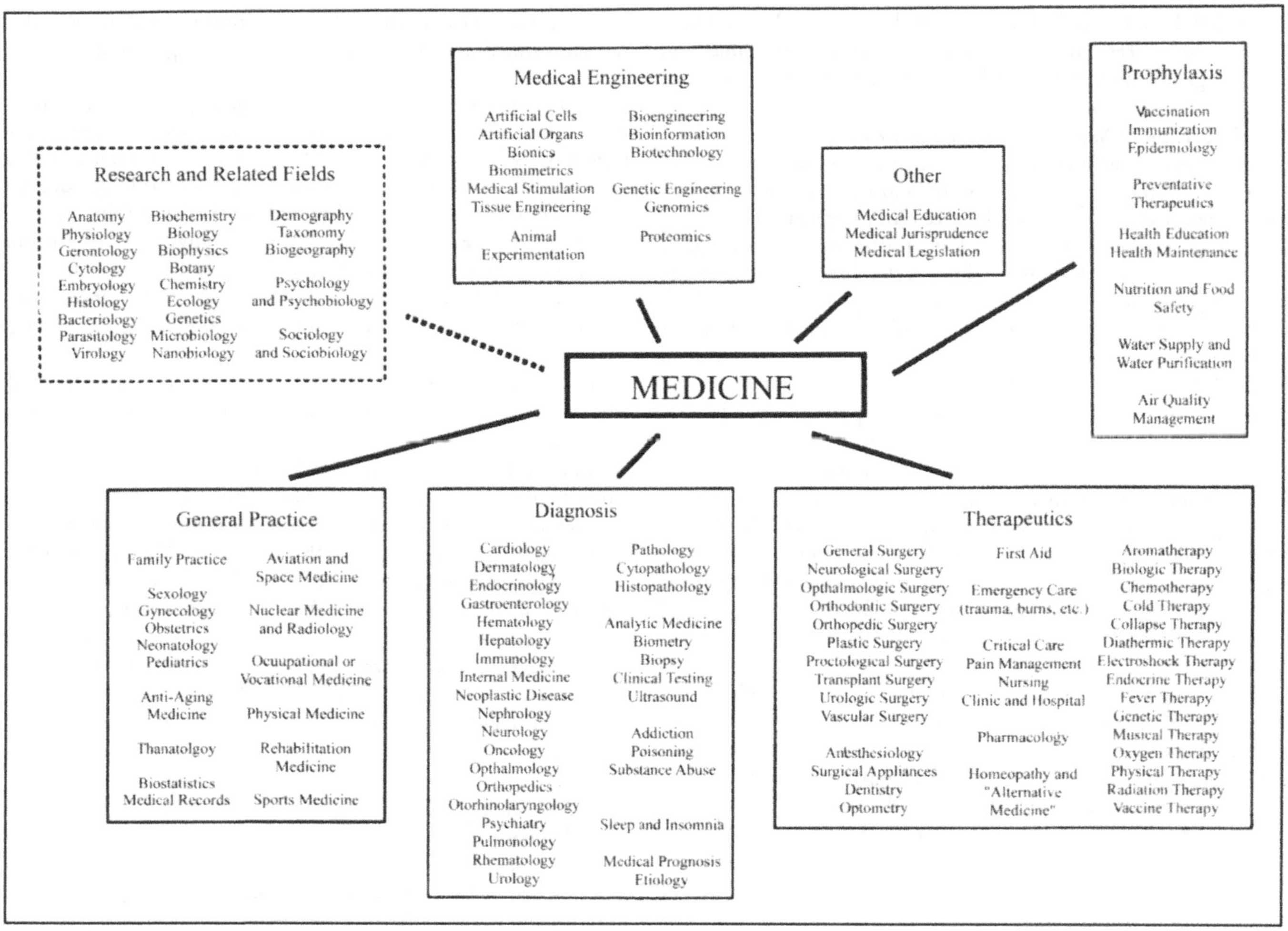

Fig. 1.3. Branches of medicine and associated disciplines.

revolutions in genomics, proteomics and bioinformatics[2321] provided detailed and precise knowledge of the workings of the human body at the molecular level. Our understanding of life advanced from organs, to tissues, to cells, and finally to molecules, in the 20th century. By the early 21st century, the entire human genome will be mapped. This map will inferentially incorporate a complete catalog of all human proteins, lipids, carbohydrates, nucleoproteins and other molecules, including full sequence, structure, and much functional information. Only some systemic functional knowledge, particularly neurological, may still be lacking by that time.

This deep molecular familiarity with the human body, along with simultaneous nanotechnological engineering advances (Chapter 2), will set the stage for a shift from today's molecular scientific medicine in which fundamental new discoveries are constantly being made, to a molecular technologic medicine in which the molecular basis of life, by then well-known, is manipulated to produce specific desired results. The comprehensive knowledge of human molecular structure so painstakingly acquired during the 20th and early 21st centuries will be used in the 21st century to design medically-active microscopic machines. These machines, rather than being tasked primarily with voyages of pure discovery, will instead most often be sent on missions of cellular inspection, repair, and reconstruction. In the coming century, the principal focus will shift from medical science to medical engineering. Nanomedicine will involve designing and building a vast proliferation of incredibly efficacious molecular devices, and then deploying these devices in patients to establish and maintain a continuous state of human healthiness.

The very earliest nanotechnology-based biomedical systems may be used to help resolve many difficult scientific questions that remain. They may also be employed to assist in the brute-force analysis of the most difficult three-dimensional structures among the 100,000-odd proteins of which the human body is comprised, or to help ascertain the precise function of each such protein. But much of this effort should be complete within the next 20-30 years because the reference human body has a finite parts list, and these parts are already being sequenced, geometered and archived at an ever-increasing pace. Once these parts are known, then the reference human being as a biological system is at least physically specified to completeness at the molecular level. Thereafter, nanotechnology-based discovery will consist principally of examining a particular sick or injured patient to determine how he or she deviates from molecular reference structures, with the physician then interpreting these deviations in light of their possible contribution to, or detraction from, the general health and the explicit preferences of the patient.

In brief, nanomedicine will employ molecular machine systems to address medical problems, and will use molecular knowledge to maintain human health at the molecular scale.

1.2.2 Volitional Normative Model of Disease

What, exactly, is "medicine"? Dictionaries give several definitions, ranging from the very restrictive to the most general, as follows: "a drug or remedy";[2223,2224] "any substance used for treating disease";[2220] "any drug or other substance used in treating disease, healing, or relieving pain";[2221] "in a restricted sense, that branch of the healing art dealing with internal diseases";[2220] "treatment of disease by medical, as distinguished from surgical, treatment";[2223] "the branch of this science and art that makes use of drugs, diet, etc., as distinguished especially from surgery and obstetrics";[2221] "the study and treatment of general diseases or those affecting the internal parts of the body";[2224] "the science of treating disease, the healing art";[2220] "the art and science of preventing or curing disease";[2224] "the act of maintenance of health, and prevention and treatment of disease and illness";[2223] "the department of knowledge and practice dealing with disease and its treatment";[2222] or, most generally, "the science and art of diagnosing, treating, curing, and preventing disease, relieving pain, and improving and preserving health".[2221] In this book, we shall adopt the latter, maximally-inclusive, definition of "medicine" (Figure 1.3).

Reviewing Figure 1.3, the contemporary physician might at first be inclined to relegate molecular approaches to some minor subfield, perhaps "nanoanalytics," "nanogenomics," or "nanotherapeutics." This would be a serious mistake, because the application of molecular approaches to health care will significantly impact virtually every category of laboratory and clinical practice across the board. Thus we are led to the broadest possible conception of nanomedicine as "the science and technology of diagnosing, treating, and preventing disease and traumatic injury, of relieving pain, and of preserving and improving human health, using molecular tools and molecular knowledge of the human body."

This brings us to the question of "disease," a complex term whose meaning is still hotly debated among medical academics.[2225-2230] Figure 1.4 shows the results of a survey of four different groups of people who were read a list of common diagnostic terms and then asked if they would rate the condition as a disease. Illnesses due to microorganisms, or conditions in which the doctor's contribution to the diagnosis was important, were most likely to be called a disease, but if the cause was a known physical or chemical agent the condition was less likely to be regarded as disease; general practitioners also had the broadest definition of disease.

No less than eight different types of disease concepts are held by at least some people currently engaging in clinical reasoning and practice, including:[2226,2227]

1. *Disease Nominalism* — A disease is whatever physicians say is a disease. This approach avoids understanding and forestalls inquiry, rather than furthering it.

2. *Disease Relativism* — A disease is identified or labeled in accordance with explicit or implicit social norms and values at a particular time. In 19th century Japan, for example, armpit odor was considered a disease and its treatment constituted a medical specialty. Similarly, 19th-century Western culture regarded masturbation as a disease, and in the 18th century, some conveniently identified a disease called drapetomania, the "abnormally strong and irrational desire of a slave to be free."[2205] Various non-Western cultures having widespread parasitic infection may consider the lack of infection to be abnormal, thus not regarding those who are infected as suffering from disease.

3. *Sociocultural Disease* — Societies may possess a concept of disease that differs from the concepts of other societies, but the concept may also differ from that held by medical practitioners within the society itself. For instance, hypercholesterolemia is regarded as a disease condition by doctors but not by the lay public; medical treatment may be justified, but persons with hypercholesterolemia may not seek treatment, even when told of the condition. Conversely, there may be sociocultural pressure to recognize a particular condition as a disease requiring treatment, such as alcoholism and gambling.

4. *Statistical Disease* — A condition is a disease when it is abnormal, where abnormal is defined as a specific deviation from a statistically-defined norm. This approach has many flaws. For example, a statistical concept makes it impossible to regard an entire population as having a disease. Thus tooth decay, which is virtually universal in humans, is not abnormal; those lacking it are abnormal, thus are "diseased" by this definition. More reasonably, a future highly-aseptic society might regard bacterium-infested 20th century humans (who contain in their bodies more foreign microbes than native cells; Section 8.5.1) as massively infected. Another flaw is that many statistical measurables such as body temperature and blood pressure are continuous variables with bell-shaped distributions, so cutoff thresholds between "normal" and "abnormal" seem highly arbitrary.

5. *Infectious Agency* — Disease is caused by a microbial infectious agent. Besides excluding systemic failures of bodily systems, this view is unsatisfactory because the same agent can produce very different illnesses. For instance, infection with hemolytic *Streptococcus* can produce diseases as different as erysipelas and puerperal fever, and Epstein-Barr virus is implicated in diseases as varied as Burkitt's lymphoma, glandular fever, and naso-pharyngeal carcinoma.[2227]

6. *Disease Realism* — Diseases have a real, substantial existence regardless of social norms and values, and exist independent of whether they are discovered, named, recognized, classified, or diagnosed. Diseases are not inventions and may be identified with the operations of biological systems, providing a reductionistic account of diseases in terms of system components and subprocesses, even down to the molecular level. One major problem with this view is that theories may change over time — almost every 19th century scientific theory was either rejected or highly modified in the 20th century. If the identification of disease is connected with theories, then a change in theories may alter what is viewed as a disease. For example, the 19th century obsession with constipation was reflected in the disease labelled "autointoxication," in which the contents of the large bowel were believed to poison the body. Consequently much unnecessary attention was paid to laxatives and purgatives and, when surgery of the abdomen became possible toward the end of the century, operations to remove the colon became fashionable in both England and America.[2205]

7. *Disease Idealism* — Disease is the lack of health, where health is characterized as the optimum functioning of biological systems. Every real system inevitably falls short of the optimum in its actual functioning. But by comparing large numbers of systems, we can formulate standards that a particular system ought to satisfy, in order to be the best of its kind. Thus "health" becomes a kind of

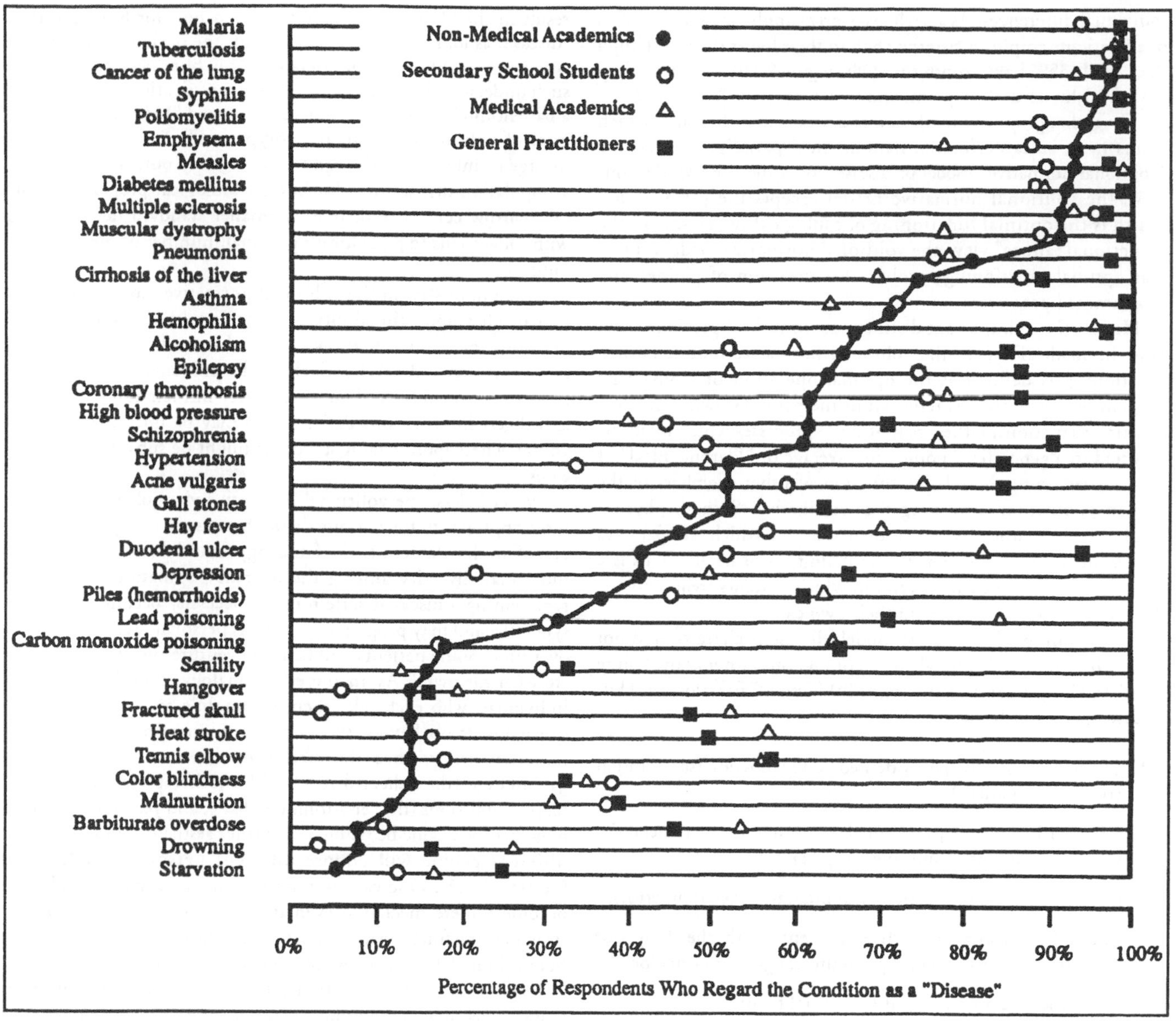

Fig. 1.4. Opinion survey: what is disease? (modified from Campbell,Scadding, and Roberts[2232])

Platonic ideal that real organisms approximate, and everyone is a less than perfect physical specimen. Since we are all flawed to some extent, disease is a matter of degree, a more or less extreme variation from the normative ideal of perfect functioning. This could be combined with the statistical approach, thus characterizing disease as a statistical variation from the ideal. But this view, like the statistical, suffers from arbitrary thresholds that must be drawn to qualify a measurable function as representing a diseased condition.

8. *Functional Failure* — Organisms and the cells that constitute them are complex organized systems that display phenomena (e.g. homeostasis) resulting from acting upon a program of information. Programs acquired and developed during evolution, encoded in DNA, control the processes of the system. Through biomedical research, we write out the program of a process as an explicit set (or network) of instructions. There are completely self-contained "closed" genetic programs, and there are "open" genetic programs that require an interaction between the programmed system and the environment, e.g. learning or conditioning. Normal functioning is thus the operation of biologically programmed processes, e.g. natural functioning, and disease may be characterized as the failure of normal functioning. One difficulty with this view is that it enshrines the natural (Section 1.3.4) as the benchmark of health, but it is difficult to regard as diseased a natural brunette who has dyed her hair blonde in contravention of the natural program, and it is quite reasonable to regard the mere possession of an appendix as a disease condition, even though the natural program operates so as to perpetuate this troublesome organ.* A second weakness of this view is that disease is still defined against population norms of functionality, ignoring

** The vermiform appendix may have some minor immune function, but it is clearly nonessential and can kill when infected. Yet natural selection has not eliminated it. Indeed, there is evidence for positive selection due to the following accident of physiological evolution. Appendicitis results when inflammation causes swelling, compressing the artery supplying blood to the appendix. High bloodflow protects against bacterial growth, so any reduction aids infection, creating more swelling; if flow is completely cut off, bacteria multiply rapidly until the organ bursts. A slender appendix is especially susceptible, so untreated appendicitis applies positive selective pressure to maintain a larger appendix.[2185]*

individual differences. As a perhaps overly simplistic example, 65% of all patients employ a cisterna chyli in their lower thoracic lymph duct, while 35% have no cisterna chyli (Figure 8.10) — which group has a healthy natural program, and which group is "diseased"?

The author proposes a ninth view of disease, a new alternative which seems most suitable for the nanomedical paradigm, called the "volitional normative" model of disease. As in the "disease idealism" view, the volitional normative model accepts the premise that health is the optimal functioning of biological systems. Like the "functional failure" view, the volitional normative model assumes that optimal functioning involves the operation of biologically programmed processes.

However, two important distinctions from these previous views must be made. First, in the volitional normative model, normal functioning is defined as the optimal operation of biologically programmed processes as reflected in the patient's own individual genetic instructions, rather than of those processes which might be reflected in a generalized population average or "Platonic ideal" of such instructions; the relative function of other members of the human population is no longer determinative. Second, physical condition is regarded as a volitional state, in which the patient's desires are a crucial element in the definition of health. This is a continuation of the current trend in which patients frequently see themselves as active partners in their own care.

In the volitional normative model, disease is characterized not just as the failure of "optimal" functioning, but rather as the failure of either (a) "optimal" functioning or (b) "desired" functioning. Thus disease may result from:

1. a failure to correctly specify desired bodily function (specification error by the patient),
2. a flawed biological program design that doesn't meet the specifications (programming design error),
3. flawed execution of the biological program (execution error),
4. external interference by disease agents with the design or execution of the biological program (exogenous error), or
5. traumatic injury or accident (structural failure).

In the early years of nanomedicine, volitional physical states will customarily reflect "default" values which may differ only insignificantly from the patient's original or natural biological programming. With a more mature nanomedicine, the patient may gain the ability to substitute alternative natural programs for many of his original natural programs. For example, the genes responsible for appendix morphology or for sickle cell expression might be replaced with genes that encode other phenotypes, such as the phenotype of an appendix-free cecum or a phenotype for statistically typical human erythrocytes.* Many persons will go further, electing an artificial genetic structure which, say, eliminates age-related diminution of the secretion of human growth hormone and other essential endocrines. (The graduated secretion of powerful proteolytic enzymes, perhaps targeted for gene-expression in appropriate organs, may reverse and control the accumulation of highly crosslinked collagenaceous debris; by 1998, many members of the mainstream medical community were already starting to regard aging as a treatable condition.)[2310,2976-2981] On the other hand, a congenitally blind patient might desire, for whatever personal reasons, to retain his blindness. Hence his genetic programs that result in the blindness phenotype would not, for him, constitute "disease" as long as he fully understands the options and outcomes that are available to him. (Retaining his blindness while lacking such understanding might constitute a specification error, and such a patient might then be considered "diseased.") Whether the broad pool of volitional human phenotypes will tend to converge or diverge is unknown, although the most likely outcome is probably a population distribution (of human biological programs) with a tall, narrow central peak (e.g., a smaller standard deviation) but with longer tails (e.g., exhibiting a small number of more extreme outliers).

One minor flaw in the volitional normative model of disease is that it relies upon the ability of patients to make fully informed decisions concerning their own physical state. The model crucially involves desires and beliefs, which can be irrational, especially during mental illness, and people normally vary in their ability to acquire and digest information. Patients also may be unconscious or too young, whereupon default standards might be substituted in some cases.

Nevertheless, the volitional normative view of disease appears most appropriate for nanomedicine because it recognizes that the era of molecular control of biology could bring considerable molecular diversity among the human population. Conditions representing a diseased state must of necessity become more idiosyncratic, and may progressively vary as personal preferences evolve over time. Some patients will be more venturesome than others — "to each his own." As an imperfect analogy, consider a group of individuals who each take their automobile to a mechanic. One driver insists on having the carburetion and timing adjusted for maximum performance (the "racer"); another driver prefers optimum gas mileage (the "cheapskate"); still another prefers minimizing tailpipe emissions (the "environmentalist"); and yet another requires only that the engine be painted blue (the "aesthete"). In like manner, different people will choose different personal specifications (Section 1.2.5). One can only hope that the physician will never become a mere mechanic even in an era of near-perfect human structural and functional information; an automobile conveys a body, but the human body conveys the soul. Agrees theorist Guttentag:[2234] "The physician-patient relationship is ontologically different from that of a maintenance engineer to a machine or a veterinarian to an animal."

1.2.3 Treatment Methodology

The availability of advanced nanomedical instrumentalities should not significantly alter the classical medical treatment methodology, although the patient experiences and outcomes will be greatly improved. Treatment in the nanomedical era will become faster and more accurate, efficient, and effective. In clinical practice, patient treatment customarily includes up to six distinguishable phases: examination, diagnosis, prognosis, treatment, validation, and prophylaxis. Let us consider each of these, in turn.

1.2.3.1 Examination

The first step in any treatment process is the examination of the patient, including the individual's medical history, personal functional and structural baseline, and current complaints. In classical medicine, interview and observation have long been the cornerstone of examination. In ancient times this was limited to obvious

It is often pointed out that sickle cell is advantageous in malaria-infested countries because the trait confers resistance to malaria. This flaw-tolerant view makes a virtue of necessity—a direct cure for malaria will undoubtedly be more efficient. Sickle cell is disadvantageous in hypoxic conditions, which is why no one with this trait can hold a civil airline pilot's license.[2227]

manifestations and simple constellations of observables, such as the Hippocratic facies, the four signs of inflammation noted by Celsus, or pulse rate and fever. Clinicians recognize that the traditional taking and interpreting of oral medical histories from new patients is a subtle and complex art,[2235] although some aspects of this process might be automated using voice recognition and text preinterpretation software, somewhat easing the physician's burden.

Advancing technology has also brought a plethora of tests that contribute to accurate diagnosis, including auscultation, microscopy and clinical bacteriology in the 19th century, and radiological scanning, clinical biochemistry, genetic testing, and minimally invasive exploratory surgery in the 20th century.[2694]

In the 21st century, new tools for nanomedical testing and observation (Chapter 18) will include clinical in vivo cytography; real-time whole-body microbiotic surveys; immediate access to laboratory-quality data on the patient (e.g. blood tests such as blood counts, dissolved gases and solutes, vitamin and ion assays); physiological function and challenge tests; tissue composition including direct organelle counts in specified tissue populations; quantitative flowcharts of in cyto secondary messenger molecules, extracellular hormones and neuropeptides; per-compartment cytoglucose inventories; and so forth. Before a proper diagnosis can be made, the physician must also establish the patient's personal functional and structural baseline against which any deviations can be noted and corrected, in keeping with the volitional normative model of disease (Section 1.2.2).

The capabilities of nanomedical testing are explored at length in Chapter 18. By way of introduction, it is instructive to think about a trivial class of test procedures that might be used to diagnose a simple infectious disease at several different levels of technological competence. Let us consider a patient who presents with signs and symptoms that are nonspecific in nature but which suggest an infectious process — e.g. nasal congestion, mild fever, discomfort and cough. The initial signs are due in part to the body's inflammatory response and in part to the infectious agent itself. The diagnostic goal is to identify the infectious agent.

In the late 20th century, the usual procedure would be to culture a sample taken from the patient, in the microbiology laboratory, using various broths, petri plates, and biochemical tests. Some infectious agents are easy to demonstrate. Beta hemolytic streptococci from a throat swab will grow overnight on a blood agar plate, and colony counts for *E. coli* in a urine sample are available in 24 hours. A throat culture that the lab reports as a mixed culture causes no excitement, and a single isolate of *Staphylococcus epidermidis* in a blood culture is usually regarded as a skin contaminant.

Moving up to a higher level of technological competence, biotechnologists describe an ideal diagnostic scenario which takes a molecular approach to the diagnosis of infectious disease using recombinant DNA technology. This approach was not yet possible in 1996 when first suggested,[2233] but was regarded as a reasonable and likely future application* of biotechnology in the early 21st century given rapid progress in single-molecule DNA assay techniques:[2682]

"A patient presents in the clinic with mild fever, nasal congestion, discomfort, and cough. A swab of his throat is taken. Instead of culture to identify abnormal microorganisms by their pattern of growth, the sample is analyzed by recombinant DNA techniques. The cotton throat swab is mixed with a cocktail of DNA probes. Enzymes that digest and release the DNA from both host cells and invading bacteria make the DNA in the sample immediately available for hybridization to the probes. The swab is swirled in the liquid mix of the prepackaged test kit for 1 minute. The liquid is then poured through a column that separates hybridized DNA molecules (bacterial target DNA sequences bound to probe DNA) from all other debris [taking several minutes]. A chemiluminescence detection system for the probes shows two of several possible colors indicating mixed infection. The diagnostic result, available in 10 minutes, indicates a Rhinovirus of a strain known to be epidemic in the geographic area. A significant superinfection with a penicillin-resistant streptococcus is also identified. With a definitive diagnosis, the patient is started on the appropriate antibiotic."

How might nanomedicine handle this test? In the nanomedical era, taking and analyzing microbial samples will be much simpler for the practitioner. Such analysis will be as quick and convenient as the electronic measurement of body temperature using a tympanic thermometer in a late 20th-century clinical office or hospital. As described in Chapter 18, the physician faces the patient and pulls from his pocket a lightweight handheld device resembling a pocket calculator. He unsnaps a self-sterilizing cordless pencil-sized probe from the side of the device and inserts the business end of the probe into the patient's opened mouth in the manner of a tongue depressor. The ramifying probe tip contains billions of nanoscale molecular assay receptors mounted on hundreds of self-guiding retractile stalks. Each receptor is sensitive to one of thousands of specific bacterial membrane or viral capsid ligands (Section 4.2).** An acoustic echolocation transceiver provides gross spatial mapping. The patient says "Ahh," and a few seconds later a three-dimensional color-coded map of the throat area appears on the display panel that is held in the doctor's hand. A bright spot marks the exact location where the first samples are being taken. Underneath the color map scrolls a continuously updated microflora count, listing in the leftmost column the names of the ten most numerous microbial and viral species that have been detected, key biochemical marker codes in the middle column, and measured population counts in the right column. The number counts flip up and down a bit as the physician directs probe stalks to various locations in the pharynx to obtain a representative sampling, with special attention to sores or any signs of exudate. After a few more seconds, the data for two of the bacterial species suddenly highlight in red, indicating the distinctive molecular signatures of specific toxins or pathological variants. One of these two species is a known, and unwelcome, hostile pathogen. The diagnosis is completed, the infectious agent is promptly exterminated (Chapter 19),[3233] and a resurvey with the probe several minutes afterwards reveals no evidence of the pathogen.

1.2.3.2 Diagnosis

Diagnosis is the determination of the cause and nature of a disease in order to provide a logical basis for treatment and prognosis. Traditionally the diagnostic process begins with a thorough history taken from the patient and a relevant physical examination. Often this sufficed to make a confident diagnosis, but the cause of some illnesses remained uncertain without recourse to additional information such as blood tests or radiological examinations. Nanotechnology-based diagnosis (Chapter 18) will consist principally of examining the patient to determine how he or she deviates from autogenous reference structures and functions, and then interpreting those deviations as healthy or unhealthy for that patient.

**In 1997, kits were being manufactured in Moscow, Russia, that allowed routine PCR diagnosis of multiple microorganisms in both clinical and agricultural settings [R. Bradbury, personal communication, 1999], and by 1998 PCR detection of bacteria in <10 minutes was well-known.[3226]*

***Inexpensive biosensor devices capable of detecting* Salmonella *contamination in meat and poultry were already commercially available in 1998.*

In the 20th century, diagnoses frequently involved a high degree of uncertainty, largely due to the general lack of comprehensive molecular diagnostic tools. Thus diagnosis would be guided by statistical analyses; one branch of decision analysis, called utility analysis, even allowed the patient to participate in the decisionmaking process.[2227] When the correct decision is unclear, urges one textbook, it is well to remember time-honored Hippocratic aphorisms such as "first, do no harm" and "common things occur commonly." The eminent Canadian physician Sir William Osler (1849-1919) lamented that "errors of judgement must occur in the practice of an art which consists largely in balancing probabilities." Most doctors would prefer to understand the root cause of medical problems rather than adopt mere statistical approaches.

Nanomedical tools will vastly reduce diagnostic uncertainty. Using nanomedical instrumentalities, doctors will gain access to unprecedented amounts of information about their patients including in-office comprehensive genotyping and real-time whole-body scans for particular bacterial coat markers, tumor cell antigens, mineral deposits, suspected toxins, hormone imbalances of genetic or lifestyle origin, and other specified molecules, producing three-dimensional maps of desired targets with submillimeter spatial resolution. Embedded in vivo nanomedical data archives (Section 10.2.5, Chapter 19) can provide onboard storage of regularly updated self-diagnostic scans, reducing to a minimum the need for symptomatic interview data from patients who may be unconscious, inarticulate, or verbose, who may have limited powers of self-analysis or self-observation and who may have forgotten, suppressed, or amplified descriptions of symptoms.

Of course, physicians do not require an exhaustive survey of the entire body of each patient to molecular detail to make a valid diagnosis. In any particular case, it is the function of the trained medical mind to quickly ascertain where and where not to look in molecular detail. But in the nanomedical era, powerful tools will be available to allow the practitioner to examine almost any portion of a patient in as much detail as desired, right down to the molecular level, with results available in seconds or minutes, and at reasonable cost (e.g. Section 2.4.2).

1.2.3.3 Prognosis and Treatment

Prognosis is a judgement or forecast, based upon a correct diagnosis, of the future course of a disease or injury, and of the patient's prospects for partial or full recovery. Guttentag[2234] identifies prognosis as "the predicted course of the reduced state of the patient's psychosomatic freedom of action," and treatment as "the physician's ability to intervene."

But prognosis is a function of treatment as well as disease. From the post-Hippocratic era through the 18th century, treatments were almost purely empirical and often did more harm than good. During the 19th and early 20th centuries, treatments were scientific but largely homeostatic — the medical intervention was rational but served mainly to assist the body in healing itself. Throughout the remainder of the 20th century, truly curative treatments began to rescue some patients from conditions from which their unaided bodies would not have been able to recover. Although conventional biotechnology will enable some important tissue and cellular replacement treatments by the early 21st century, nanomedicine will enable major reconstructive and restorative procedures at the tissue, cellular and molecular levels and will employ active antibiotic devices. The prognosis will almost always be good, except in cases of severe neural damage and a few other specialized circumstances. Therapeutic treatments will be selected to reverse all pathological effects of disease or injury, with a minimum of pain, discomfort, side-effects, intrusiveness and time, and with a maximum of effectiveness, efficiency, and likelihood of success, though of course some tradeoffs will always exist. Nanomedicine also will excel in the correction of molecular defects of a kind which Nature has no predesigned tools — such as the breakdown and removal of intracellular lipofuscin (for which there appear to be no natural enzymes) and the removal of indigestible waste products which interfere with neuronal axon transport.

As in Section 1.2.3.1, we may compare the therapeutic response to a simple infection at several different levels of technological competence. Consider a patient who has been diagnosed with eastern equine encephalitis, a mosquito- or tick-borne arbovirus. In the 20th century, there was no specific treatment for this disease. Care was generally supportive, with the doctor attempting to maintain the patient's heart and lung function while the infection ran its course. The prognosis was poor. There was a 50%-75% mortality rate with frequent sequelae including seizures and paralysis, especially in children.[2180]

Biotechnologists proposed a molecular approach to therapeutics using recombinant DNA technology that was not yet possible in 1996 but was regarded as likely by the early 21st century:[2233]

> *"A patient enters the hospital with high fever and intense headaches. A spinal fluid tap is submitted to the molecular microbiology lab. After screening for several viruses, a species of equine encephalitis virus is identified that is endemic to a location recently visited by the patient. A call to the Centers for Disease Control results in the emergency delivery of a new antiviral agent. Antisense oligonucleotides are injected into the cerebral spinal fluid. These small DNA pieces bind directly to the virus and block its further proliferation. A temporary reservoir giving access to the cerebrospinal fluid is placed and infusion of this therapeutic molecular inhibitor of the virus continues for 5 days until signs of encephalitis have passed."*

The nanomedical therapy? As before, a nanomedical cure for eastern equine encephalitis may be far simpler, less painful and a great deal quicker. A single therapeutic dose consisting of ~0.1 cm^3 of isotonic saline fluid containing ~10 billion active micron-size virucidal nanodevices, a 10% volumetric nanodevice suspension, is injected into the cerebrospinal fluid. Each therapeutic nanorobot has chemical sensors that can unambiguously recognize fluidborne or in cyto arbovirus particles and, once recognition has occurred, destroy them and also reverse the cellular damage. A nanorobot population of this size should be able to destroy all viral particles and effect needed repairs in at most an hour (Chapter 19),[3233] after which the devices are programmed and equipped either to eliminate themselves from the body (Chapter 16) or to be manually exfused (e.g., nanapheresis; Section 10.3.6).

1.2.3.4 Validation and Prophylaxis

A proper therapeutic protocol will include a procedure for follow-up to ensure that the prescribed treatment was correctly executed with good results. This step is often neglected in order to save costs and may be considered unimportant by some practitioners because approximately 80%-90% of all illnesses which take patients to the doctor are self-curing or self-limiting.[2205] For example, the common cold, most infectious diseases and many minor injuries are problems that usually will resolve on their own even with no treatment. In these cases the purpose of treatment is not to provide a cure, but rather to speed the healing process, improve comfort, and avoid complications. Many nanomedical treatments will require supervision and will run quickly to completion, thus follow-up may come back into vogue. Validation may also be viewed as a post-treatment re-diagnosis to ensure that no disease remains present in the patient.

Prophylaxis is the prevention of disease, typically including patient education, immunization programs, amelioration of occupational hazards, and other preventive and public health measures. In a treatment environment that is rich in effective antibacterial instrumentalities, those microbes which survive will evolve to produce only modest or negligible symptoms that are insufficiently annoying to motivate a patient to seek professional therapeutic relief. It is well-known that bacteria can modify their behavior over time. For example, syphilis had a much more fulminating course in the Middle Ages than it has in the 20th century. Some future strain of the syphilitic microbe might produce negligible symptoms, but we should still insist on its eradication because of its potential to revert to its earlier virulence if allowed to spread unchecked in a more benign form. Preventative procedures may also be needed to discover, diagnose, and treat apparently symptomless diseases, and a variety of molecular-based physiological malfunctions and structural micropathologies may require nanoscale tools in order to detect them.

With medical conditions that require ongoing supervision and adjustment, such as maintaining optimum hormone balance and minimal accumulation of molecular debris (e.g. anti-aging medicine), nanoscale monitoring stations may act as onboard cellular guidance systems, stimulating or suppressing endocrine secretion as necessary to preserve an ideal state of equilibrium. In some cases, direct manufacture of compounds not easily produced by ribosomes or other biological organelles may be required.

1.2.4 Evolution of Bedside Practice

The relationship between physician and patient has been evolving in response to the rapidly changing medical environment. Two of the most important trends are the decline of traditional holism (with a concomitant increase in specialization) and the rise of therapeutic customization in medical practice.

1.2.4.1 Specialization and Holistic Medicine

Holism is a philosophy which holds that individuals function as complete units that cannot be reduced merely to the sum of their parts.[2223] It is unarguable that a simplistic reductionist view of the patient which ignores the complex interactions among the many cells, tissues, organs, and systems constituting the human body is deeply flawed. For example, an understanding of the molecular basis of the contractile proteins of heart muscle will not alone tell us how heart muscle cells will look or act; knowing only about the parts of something is not sufficient to predict the behavior of the whole.[2239] However, traditional concepts of holistic medicine go well beyond such basic systems philosophy — incorporating requirements for a consideration of all physical, emotional, social, spiritual, environmental and economic needs of the patient.

N. Jewson[2203] and others[2205] have decried the modern shift away from holistic medicine, which is asserted to have taken place in three historical phases in the West. The initial phase is identified as the practice of "bedside medicine," where wealthy fee-paying clients in the 17th and 18th centuries helped shape their own diagnosis and treatment by medical practitioners in an holistic manner. Aspects of the patient's emotional and spiritual life were seen as central by the practitioner in making a diagnosis, since most physical treatments were only palliative and so the doctor had to focus on nonphysical supportive measures. This frame of reference was progressively replaced during the 19th century with the trend toward "hospital medicine," wherein physicians concentrated on generic classifications of diseases that were manifested in the patient, moving doctors away from the earlier focus on the individual as a whole person. The 20th century saw the development of "laboratory medicine," which moved diagnosis and therapy even further away from the whole patient, "who came to be medically conceived as little more than a depersonalized object, comprised of a complex of cells."

A more charitable view is that physicians have increasingly specialized in treating those physical diseases for which effective treatments may be readily specified, leaving nonphysical and nontreatable issues for psychiatrists, social workers, fitness coaches, priests, lawyers, or other professionals to deal with. In the 21st century this operational specialization may become complete, since nanomedicine phenomenologically regards the human body as an intricately structured machine with trillions of complex interacting parts, with each part (and each subsystem of parts) subject to individual scrutiny, repair, and possibly replacement by artificial technological means. In this new medical cosmology, the concept of the whole patient almost completely dissolves into a data-intensive whirlwind of molecular detail at the cellular, tissue, organ, and systemic levels.

And yet, as in a bygone era, patients once again will help to shape their own diagnosis and treatment at the hands of medical practitioners who begin to apply the volitional normative model of disease (Section 1.2.2) in their practices. This may breathe new life into the age-old medical school dictum to "treat the patient as a person" and to "focus on the sick person" rather than exclusively on the body.[2230]

The availability of extremely powerful and transforming molecular technologies also argues for a return to the romantic and perhaps quaint concept of a single doctor taking care of a single patient. The potential for interactions among highly potent nanorobotic instrumentalities argues for diagnostic and therapeutic "gatekeeping" by a single trusted practitioner in whom strategic treatment responsibility is vested — in partnership, of course, with the patient.

1.2.4.2 Customized Diagnosis and Therapeutics

In science the objective is to understand the individual occurrence by means of a general law; in medical practice, knowledge of what is generally the case does not tell the physician how to treat a particular patient. Thus the problem of how to proceed from the prototypic case to the individual instance remains to be solved in a systematic manner by the practitioner.[2230]

The practitioner of "bedside medicine" in the 17th and 18th centuries had few curative and almost no customized tools at his disposal — perhaps a few dozen basic surgical techniques, performed septically, hazardously, and without anesthesia, and a drug/herbal formulary consisting of a few hundred substances. For instance, the *Edinburgh Pharmacopoeia* of 1803 listed only 222 simples while the *London Pharmacopoeia* of 1809 listed fewer than 200 items, most of which had variable, uncertain, minimal, or nonspecific potency. A few more options became available to the 19th century medical practitioner, including complex surgical techniques for specific conditions that could be performed aseptically with anesthesia and a good chance for success, a somewhat broader and more efficacious pharmacopeia, vaccines targeted to several diseases, and an improving diagnostic ability. By the 20th century, the physician could prescribe from among tens of thousands of specific drugs to target specific bacterial, viral, fungal, or parasitic infections; select from among a very precise array of anesthetic agents, chosen to avoid allergic responses in particular patients; perform a wide variety of noninvasive tests and scans for diagnostic purposes to identify very specific conditions; and perform minimally invasive surgeries directed at many arbitrary tissue masses as small as 1 mm^3 in volume. The first glimmerings of personalized genetic therapies also began to appear.

With the arrival of nanomedicine in the 21st century, the treatment paradigm will complete its transition from coarse-grained, one-size-fits-all, slow-acting methods to molecularly-precise, completely customized, speedy and highly-efficacious procedures and instrumentalities. The irregular shotgun pattern of 18th century palliatives will evolve during the early 21st century into a penetrating and perfectly tailored hail of "magic bullets" each targeting an individual cell or group of cells unique to the individual patient. The 19th century herbalist John Ayrton Paris could have been describing the nanomedical future in his popular textbook *Pharmacologia*, 1840 edition, when he wrote:

> *"If [a physician] prescribes upon truly scientific principles, he will rarely in the course of his practice compose two formulae that shall, in every respect, be perfectly similar, for the plain reason that he will never meet with two cases exactly alike. Now let me ask what constitutes the essential difference between the true physician and his counterfeit — between the philosopher and the empiric? Simply this — that the latter exhibits the same medicine in every disease, however widely each may differ from the other in its symptoms and character; while the former examines, in the spirit of philosophic analysis, all the existing peculiarities of his patient, and of his discord...and then adapts with a sound discretion and with a correct judgement of his medicinal agents, such means as may best be calculated to control and correct the patient's morbid condition."*

1.2.4.3 The Physician-Patient Relationship

Many other aspects of the physician-patient relationship, especially as this relationship may evolve in the coming era of nanomedicine, are important and worthy of extensive discussion. One such issue is the obligation of both parties in the partnership to tell the truth. The patient as a fellow human being has every right to know the truth about his or her biological condition, but other considerations may enter into the fulfillment of this obligation.[2234] Patients have a quite natural anxiety about their own possible death, and it has been claimed that this anxiety implies that no one can be truly objective toward his or her own body.[2236] Guttentag[2234] observes that "telling an unwelcome truth to the unprepared is as ill-conceived as trying to hide the truth from the prepared."

In the nanomedical era, the sheer number of "truths" that may become available for disclosure will increase enormously even as the terminal prognosis becomes rare. For example, each human being is believed to possess at least 4-10 potentially serious genetic defects; up to 1% of human DNA is of exogenous viral origin, and as much as 10% of the genome consists of transposons, discrete sequences that are positionally mobile among the chromosomes (Chapter 20). Should something be done about this, or not? What should the average patient make of the news that his physician has discovered exactly 57 submicron-scale lamellar defects scattered throughout the compact bone of the caudal epiphysis of the patient's right humerus? In the nanomedical era, people will gain the ability to specify their own physical structure to minute detail, but many patients will not be ready, willing, or able to assume responsibility for this knowledge. Thus there is no ideal substitute for the doctor's interpretative abilities and judgements on the patient's behalf as to the personal significance of specific diagnostic information. As the great clinician Thomas Addis observed in another context:[2237] "Honesty with patients requires thought and discipline and effort."

Perhaps the single most important aspect of the physician-patient relationship, in any century, is the humanistic quality of the good doctor. The patient seeks a physician who cares about him as a person and will diagnose and prescribe in a sensitive and compassionate manner, accepting some degree of obligation to the patient. Speaking to medical students, J.C. Bennett[2238] describes the implicit social contract between doctor and patient that will still apply in the nanomedical era, as it does today:

> *"To receive medical care, patients must trust their bodies and their very lives to physicians, and so to be in an honest position to give medical care, physicians must earn such radical trust. Mere technical treatment of disease does not suffice. Patients must be able reasonably to believe that their physicians care about them in an extraordinarily personal way. This exchange of care for trust, while not identical to friendship or love, is equally binding. From it develops an interdependence that is far from unwholesome; rather, it potentiates care and promotes healing. Our late twentieth century sophistication and technologic orientation have too often cost us warmth, humor, and humanity, leaving us in social isolation. We do far better as professionals to err on the side of being human with our patients, than to try to play deus ex machina, the god from the machine."*

1.2.5 Changing View of the Human Body

How does a patient regard his or her own body, and how might this most intimate of all relationships change in the nanomedical era? The so-called dualist theory of the human compound, as originally developed by Descartes and widely accepted today by the ordinary person, holds that the human being consists of two separate kinds of thing: the body and the mind or soul. The body acts as a host or receptacle for the mind. The mind, often called "the ghost in the machine," is manifested by the brain, which it uses (via the bodily senses) to acquire and store information about the world and to integrate this with its genetically-driven imperative to live, thus resolving internal conflicts among action-choices and expressing these in what we (in our consciousness) experience as decisive action.

Scientific medicine has concentrated primarily on the body. The ancient Roman physician Galen first dissected and vivisected a variety of animals to increase his knowledge of anatomy and physiology, and dissection became increasingly important in the training of physicians and surgeons, and in painting and sculpture, during the Renaissance. By the late 20th century, dissection had reached the molecular level, with the insides of the human cell and nucleus being taken apart and examined by molecular biologists, literally receptor by receptor. Dissection and the mechanistic understanding it provides have led some to decry what they regard as the modern "soulless" view of the human body as a mere machine.

In the nanomedical era, even the most diehard reductionist must come to see the human body not merely as a heap of parts but rather as a finely tuned vehicle that is owned and piloted by a single human mind. As with automobiles, some body-owners will be more diligent about maintenance, regular tuneups, and paint jobs than other body-owners. Some will crave the latest upgrades, while others may prefer a more conservative model that reliably gets them around town. At either extreme, all human vices and virtues will be on full display, though one may perhaps anticipate an increasing pride of corporeal ownership if for no other reason than because maintenance and repair will become quick, convenient, and inexpensive.

From this simple analogy of body-and-mind to car-and-driver, it might at first appear that the advent of nanomedical technology will confirm and strengthen the traditional dualist conception of the body. But closer inspection reveals that the analogy is at best incomplete, and at worst deeply flawed. This is because mind, first being necessarily embedded in physical structure and relying upon that structure for its faithful execution, and second, this physical structure now being manipulable at the molecular level, enters also into the purview of our mechanic. Both car and driver may be modified in the shop. Speaking allegorically, it is as if the driver, after getting his car a tuneup, emerges from the shop no longer favoring chocolate but enjoying vanilla instead, or now preferring jazz over classical, the opposite of before. Such psychological changes may be either volitional or emergent.

Until the late 20th century, human progress was measured almost exclusively in terms of externalities. Food was gathered, then sown, then manufactured. Shelters had no running water, then gained outhouses, then indoor plumbing. Natural lighting and campfires gave way to candles, then oil lamps, then electric illumination. Finger-counting yielded first to the abacus, then the mechanical adding machine, and finally to the digital computer. But throughout all of history, the human body itself has remained largely untouched by progress. We have always regarded our bodies, evolved by natural selection, as fundamentally inviolate and immutable — subject perhaps to various natural or traumatic degradations, but rarely to any significant intrinsic improvement on the timescale of human civilization.

Now we are set to embark upon an era in which our natural physiological equipment may for the first time in history become capable of being altered, improved, augmented, or rendered more comfortable or convenient, due to advances in medical technology. The physical human body may be one of the last bastions of "naturalness" (Section 1.3.4). It will also be one of the last elements in our common worldview to be modernized.

Our subjective experience of reality will shift by subtle degrees. For instance, all objective information about our physical surroundings has traditionally arrived in the conscious mind via the various natural senses such as hearing, sight, and smell. In the nanomedical era, machine-mediated sensory modalities may permit direct perception of physical phenomena well removed from our bodies in both time and space, or which are qualitatively or quantitatively inaccessible to our original natural senses. Perception will gradually expand to incorporate nonphysical phenomena including abstract models of mental software, purely artificial constructs of simulated or enhanced realities,[2991] and even the mental states of others. Such new perceptions will inevitably alter the way our minds process information.

But the winds of change will sweep deeper still, into our very souls. Like ants oblivious to the collective purpose of their colony, the billions of neurons in the human brain are all busily buzzing, wholly ignorant of the emergent plan. This is the physical, mechanical world of our electrochemical hardware. People also have thoughts, feelings, emotions, and volitions, a higher level in the data processing hierarchy which in turn is equally oblivious of the brain cells. We can happily think while being totally unaware of any help from our neurons. But nanomedicine will give us unprecedented systemic multilevel access to our internal physical and mental states, including real-time operating parameters of our own organs, tissues, and cells, and, if desired, the activities of small groups of (or even individual) neurons. Diverse parts of our selves previously closed to our attention may slowly conjoin and enter our conscious awareness.

Will this access promote an integrated identity or lead to hopeless confusion, or worse? Marvin Minsky, in his collection of essays *The Society of Mind*,[2982] persuasively argues that our selves or identities are in fact networks of semi-autonomous neurological "agencies" which sometimes cooperate and sometimes compete with one another. We think of ourselves as singular "persons," but we also experience "conflicting desires" and "differing viewpoints" within our minds that are, in Minsky's view, a direct experience of the multiplicity of our brain's neurostructures. Other models of the human mind[2988-2990,3728] suggest that our internal mental states, prospectively transparent via nanomedical augmentation,[2992,2993] are diverse and intricate; Julian Jaynes[2983] is one of many writers who have drawn attention to profound dichotomies between the two cerebral hemispheres. The component-oriented personality models of Freud (e.g. ego/id/superego),[2984] Jung (e.g. archetypes),[2985] and Rank (e.g. will/counterwill),[2986] and the identification of 4541 distinct personality traits by Allport and Odbert[2987] warn us that full access to our brain's architecture could be perilous.

More seriously, most of us suppose that we are endowed with free will. But if choices by free will are simply the resolution of conflicts of neurological subsystems, and we become consciously aware of those subsystems and are able to intervene in their processes, do we run the risk of runaway instabilities at the deepest levels of what we presently call our "minds"? Will we find that these instabilities are profound counterparts to the maladies we currently designate as epilepsy, or psychosomatic illnesses? In any redesigns of our brains which would involve opening doors to, quite literally, the ultrastructure of our thoughts, we could become "naked to ourselves" in ways that we can only vaguely speculate about at present. Along with any other dangers we might encounter, this will raise entirely new issues of the proper role of psychotherapy and the sanctity of personal privacy.[2996]

Repairs to the brain may be carefully monitored to ensure quality control and to verify intended results, as already proposed in another context.[3000] Major modifications might be strictly regulated, both to prevent abuse by unscrupulous third parties and also to forestall accidental or volitional alterations that could render the patient a significant threat to society. Nanomedical alterations to the brain and other physical systems may give us vastly expanded freedom to be who we choose to be (Section 1.3.4), along with increased responsibility to make wise and informed choices. The ethical and legal aspects of these questions, as well as the scientific and psychological ones, are extremely important and should be thoroughly debated in the years and decades that lie ahead.

1.3 The Nanomedical Perspective

1.3.1 Nanomedicine and Molecular Nanotechnology

A mature nanomedicine will require the ability to build structures and devices to atomic precision, hence molecular nanotechnology and molecular manufacturing are key enabling technologies for nanomedicine. The prefix "nano-" (from the Greek root nanos, or dwarf) means one-billionth (10^{-9}) of something. The term "nanotechnology" refers most generally to technology on the scale of a billionth of a meter, or a nanometer (a nanometer is ~6 carbon atoms wide). Similarly, the words "nanomachine," "nanorobot," "nanomotor" and "nanocomputer" may refer to complex engineered objects fabricated by positioning matter with molecular control.

Molecular engineering was discussed as an extension of bulk technologies in the 1960s and 1970s by von Hippel,[2245] von Foester,[2246] and Zingsheim.[2247] The phrase "Nano-Technology" was first used in print in 1974 by N. Taniguchi[2241] to refer to the increasingly precise machining and finishing of materials, progressing from larger to smaller scales and ultimately to nanoscale tolerances, following in the path of Feynman's proposed "top-down" approach,[156] a schemata which persisted in Taniguchi's thinking throughout the 1980s[282] and 1990s.[2242] In 1981, K.E. Drexler[182] described a new "bottom-up" approach involving molecular manipulation and molecular engineering in the context of building molecular machines and molecular devices with atomic precision, a fundamentally different mind-set. Drexler again described molecular technology[311] in 1982 and molecular mechanical devices[2243] in 1983, first using the word "nanotechnology" in 1985[259] and 1986[8] as synonymous with molecular technology, finally settling upon "molecular nanotechnology" in 1991[9] and "molecular machine systems" in 1992[279] to clarify that his concept involved working devices constructed with atomic precision, as distinguished from nanostructured bulk materials, micromachinery, polymeric self-assembly, pure biotechnology, nanolithography, Langmuir-Blodgett thin films, and the like.[154,3262] Drexler's definition — molecular nanotechnology as the three-dimensional positional control of atomic and molecular structure to create materials and devices with molecular precision — is the usage adopted in this book. The first known use of the term "nanomedicine" was in 1991 by Drexler, Peterson, and Pergamit in their popular book *Unbounding the Future.*[9]

Is molecular nanotechnology possible? This question is explicitly addressed in Chapter 2, but the bottom line is that molecular nanotechnology violates no physical laws and there exist many possible technical paths leading to useful results.[10] Even by 1985, for example, G. Yamamoto[164] had reported on molecular gears, describing "compounds that exist in conformations which are regarded as static meshed gears with two-toothed and three-toothed wheels and some of them behave as dynamic gears." H. Iwamura[163] prepared a system that formed a chain of beveled molecular gears with ~GHz rotation rates. In 1998, it was generally accepted that molecular nanotechnology would be developed, although there was still some disagreement about how long it would take.

It is often noted that molecular biological systems are themselves nanomachines, constituting an existence proof for molecular nanotechnology.[8-10,3261] Indeed, biotechnology is one possible implementation pathway for molecular nanotechnology that is being pursued (Section 2.3.1). Table 1.3 reveals the close functional correspondence between the macroscale components of everyday machines and the molecular components of natural biological systems. Such comparisons have a long history. For example, Marcello Malpighi (1628-1694), a professor of medicine in Pisa who discovered the fine structure of the lungs and the capillaries using the microscope,[2204] once observed that "our bodies are composed of strings, thread, beams, levers, cloth, flowing fluids, cisterns, ducts, filters, sieves, and other similar mechanisms."

Parallels to living systems as molecular machines were drawn by Changeau,[162] McClaire,[2248] Laing,[2249-2251] Drexler,[182] and Mitchell,[2252] inspiring early thinking in molecular manufacturing. For example, in 1991 Drexler[9] observed:

"Technology-as-we-know-it is a product of industry, of manufacturing and chemical engineering. Industry-as-we-know-it takes things from nature — ore from mountains, trees from forests — and coerces them into forms that someone considers useful. Trees become lumber, then houses. Mountains become rubble, then molten iron, then steel, then cars. Sand becomes a purified gas, then silicon, then chips. And so it goes. Each process is crude, based on cutting, stirring, baking, spraying, etching, grinding, and the like."

"Trees, though, are not crude. To make wood and leaves, they neither cut, stir, bake, spray, etch, nor grind. Instead, they gather solar energy using molecular electronic devices, the photosynthetic reaction centers of chloroplasts. They use that energy to drive molecular machines — active devices with moving parts of precise, molecular structure — which process carbon dioxide and water into oxygen and molecular building blocks. They use other molecular machines to join these molecular building blocks to form roots, trunks, branches, twigs, solar collectors, and more molecular machinery. Every tree makes leaves, and each leaf is more sophisticated than a spacecraft, more finely patterned than the latest chip from Silicon Valley. They do all this without noise, heat, toxic fumes, or human labor, and they consume pollutants as they go. Viewed this way, trees are high technology. Chips and rockets are not."

Table 1.3. Comparison of Macroscale and Biomolecular Components and Functions[182]

Macroscale Device	Device Function	Biomolecular Examples
Struts, beams, casings	Transmit force, hold positions	Microtubules, cellulose
Cables	Transmit tension	Collagen
Fasteners, glue	Connect parts	Intermolecular forces
Solenoids, actuators	Move things	Conformation-changing proteins, actin/myosin
Motors	Turn shafts	Flagellar motor
Drive shafts	Transmit torque	Bacterial flagella
Bearings	Support moving parts	Sigma bonds
Containers	Hold fluids	Vesicles
Pumps	Move fluids	Flagella, membrane proteins
Conveyor belts	Move components	RNA moved by fixed ribosome (partial analog)
Clamps	Hold workpieces	Enzymatic binding sites
Tools	Modify workpieces	Metallic complexes, functional groups
Production lines	Construct devices	Enzyme systems, ribosomes
Numerical control systems	Store and read programs	Genetic system

Contemplating applications of nanotechnology to medicine, Brian Wowk[261] concluded that 20th century physicians were in a predicament similar to that which would be faced by 18th-century engineers trying to maintain a 20th-century automobile — repairs would be crude at best, and breakdowns inevitable:

"Like primitive engineers faced with advanced technology, medicine must 'catch up' with the technology level of the human body before it can become really effective. What is the technology level? Since the human body is basically an extremely complex system of interacting molecules (i.e., a molecular machine), the technology required to truly understand and repair the body is molecular machine technology — nanotechnology. A natural consequence of [our achieving] this level of technology will be the ability to analyze and repair the human body

as completely and effectively as we can repair any conventional machine today."

In *Engines of Creation*,[8] Drexler drew inspiration from the cell's eye view to recognize that nanotechnology could bring a fundamental breakthrough in medicine. Noting that 20th century physicians relied chiefly on surgery and drugs to treat illness, Drexler explained:

"Surgeons have advanced from stitching wounds and amputating limbs to repairing hearts and reattaching limbs. Using microscopes and fine tools, they join delicate blood vessels and nerves. Yet even the best microsurgeon cannot cut and stitch finer tissue structures. Modern scalpels and sutures are simply too coarse for repairing capillaries, cells, and molecules. Consider 'delicate' surgery from a cell's perspective. A huge blade sweeps down, chopping blindly past and through the molecular machinery of a crowd of cells, slaughtering thousands. Later, a great obelisk plunges through the divided crowd, dragging a cable as wide as a freight train behind it to rope the crowd together again. From a cell's perspective, even the most delicate surgery, performed with exquisite knives and great skill, is still a butcher job. Only the ability of cells to abandon their dead, regroup, and multiply makes healing possible."

"Drug therapy, unlike surgery, deals with the finest structures in cells. Drug molecules are simple molecular devices. Many affect specific molecules in cells. Morphine molecules, for example, bind to certain receptor molecules in brain cells, affecting the neural impulses that signal pain. Insulin, beta blockers, and other drugs fit other receptors. But drug molecules work without direction. Once dumped into the body, they tumble and bump around in solution haphazardly until they bump a target molecule, fit, and stick, affecting its function. Drug molecules affect tissues at the molecular level, but they are too simple to sense, plan, and act. Molecular machines directed by nanocomputers will offer physicians another choice. They will combine sensors, programs, and molecular tools to form systems able to examine and repair the ultimate components of individual cells. They will bring surgical control to the molecular domain."

By the end of the 20th century, mainstream military (DoD), NIH, NSF, and other U.S. government and international groups had begun to seriously consider the potential future applications of molecular nanotechnology in medicine. For example, in 1997 a panel of U.S. Department of Defense health science experts known as Military Health Service Systems (MHSS) 2020 concluded in its final report:[1095]

"If a breakthrough to a [molecular] assembler occurs within ten to fifteen years, an entirely new field of nanomedicine will emerge by 2020. Initial applications will be focused outside the body in areas such as diagnostics and pharmaceutical manufacturing. The most powerful uses would eventually be within the body. Possible applications include programmable immune machines that travel through the bloodstream, supplementing the natural immune system; cell herding machines to stimulate rapid healing and tissue reconstruction; and cell repair machines to perform genetic surgery."

The present book takes as its starting point the assumption that the mass production of nanomachines at modest cost is technically feasible (Chapter 2), and then explores the medical implications of this assumption. Proposed systems presented in this trilogy are intended not as final engineering blueprints but merely as points of departure for further analysis and refinement. All designs and projected capabilities are, for the most part, conservatively drawn with generous safety margins, leaving a considerable volume of design space yet to be explored by more intrepid future investigators.

1.3.2 Nanomedicine: History of the Idea

Conclusive proof of the existence of atoms was not obtained until the close of the 19th century. This may explain why the idea of nanomedicine is an exclusively 20th century phenomenon. The first hint of it may be found in a famous 1929 essay written by J.D. Bernal:[2972]

"The discoveries of the twentieth century, particularly the micro-mechanics of the Quantum Theory which touch on the nature of matter itself, are far more fundamental and must in time produce far more important results. The first step will be the development of new materials and new processes in which physics, chemistry and mechanics will be inextricably fused. The stage should soon be reached when materials can be produced which are not merely modifications of what nature has given us in the way of stones, metals, woods and fibers, but are made to specifications of a molecular architecture. Already we know all the varieties of atoms; we are beginning to know the forces that bind them together; soon we shall be doing this in a way to suit our own purposes. The result — not so very distant — will probably be the passing of the age of metals and all that it implies — mines, furnaces, and engines of massive construction. Instead we should have a world of fabric materials, light and elastic, strong only for the purposes for which they are being used, a world which will imitate the balanced perfection of a living body."

Development of the concept of nanomedicine has followed two principal paths[2244] which Richard Smalley has termed "wet nanotechnology" in the biological tradition, and "dry nanotechnology" in the mechanical tradition. Both approaches were presaged in speculative fiction. The following abbreviated history focuses on nanomedicine largely to the exclusion of broader issues in molecular engineering, manufacturing and nanoscopy, and includes a number of inspirational, speculative, or fictional early references from non-refereed sources.

We will first consider the biotechnology approach (Section 1.3.2.1), followed by the molecular nanotechnology approach (Sections 1.3.2.2-3), and then these two approaches will be contrasted and compared in Section 1.3.3.

1.3.2.1 The Biological Tradition

The general idea of biological engineering stretches back at least to the mid-19th century, but the first science fiction story involving actual genetic engineering was "Proteus Island" (1936), written by the chemical engineer Stanley Weinbaum. Artificial engineered organisms subsequently appeared in minor roles in several stories, a notable example being the familiars employed by the fake witches in Fritz Leiber's "Gather, Darkness!" (1943), and A.E. van Vogt used "gene transformation" to create the superman in "Slan" (1940). The first artificially evolved creatures appeared in Theodore Sturgeon's "Microcosmic God" (1941), wherein a biochemist established conditions allowing accelerated artificial evolution, creating the Neoterics, a submillimeter-sized race of intelligent hypermetabolic creatures which could accomplish tasks very rapidly. The first artificially designed microcreatures appeared in James Blish's "Surface Tension" (1952). In this story, crash-landed dying human astronauts create a completely new form of humanity — tiny men and women reduced to protozoan size — who are seeded in the pools and puddles at the surface of the new planet, and who go on to master the biotechnology necessary to travel from one water puddle to another.

The scientific tradition of biological nanomachines for medical purposes began in 1964 when Robert Ettinger, an early cryonics pioneer, suggested that cellular-level or even molecular-level repair might be developed for life extension. Ettinger[157] speculated that "...surgeon machines, working 24 hours a day for decades or even centuries, will tenderly restore the frozen brains, cell by cell, or even molecule by molecule in critical areas."

In 1965, the synthesis of artificial life was publicly proposed as a national goal by the president of the American Chemical Society, Professor Charles Price, who pointed out that many new types of life might be made, not "mere imitations" of biology as we know it.[153]

In 1967, Isaac Asimov[2257] suggested the future possibility of "factories...where the working machinery consists of submicroscopic nucleic acids" and that a "repertoire of hundreds or thousands of complex enzymes" could be used to "bring about chemical reactions more conveniently than any methods now used" and also for "helping to construct life."

In 1968, G.R. Taylor[2258] cited the possibilities for genetic engineering and genetic surgery: "The microsurgery of DNA may possibly be achieved by physical methods: fine beams of radiation (probably laser light or pulsed X-rays) may be used to slice through the DNA molecule at desired points." He also cited predictions that bacteria would soon be programmed.

In 1969, J. White[2259] suggested that a modified virus could be used as a cell repair machine: "It has been proposed that appropriate genetic information be introduced by means of artificially constructed virus particles into a congenitally defective cell for remedy; similar means may be used for the more general case of repair. The repair program must use means such as protein synthesis and metabolic pathways to diagnose and repair any damage... [Information] can be preserved by specifying that the repair program incorporate appropriate RNA tapes into itself..."

In 1970, Jeon et al[158] carried out "the reassembly of *Amoeba proteus* from its major components: namely nucleus, cytoplasm, and cell membrane," taken from three different cells.

In 1972, Ettinger[160] proposed using genetic engineering to make microscopic biorobots: "Genetic engineering's most sensational impact will concern the modification of humans, but it will have other uses as well. Some of the "robots" that will serve us will need to be nanominiaturized." Existing organisms could be modified to make biologically-based programmable biorobots for medical applications: "If we can design sufficiently complex behavior patterns into microscopically small organisms, there are obvious and endless possibilities, some of the most important in the medical area. Perhaps we can carry guardian and scavenger organisms in the blood, superior to the leukocytes and other agents of our human heritage, that will efficiently hunt down and clean out a wide variety of hostile or damaging invaders." Computerized cellular repair machines "must use means such as protein synthesis and metabolic pathways to diagnose and repair any damage...[Information] can be preserved by specifying that the repair program incorporate appropriate RNA tapes into itself...." Also in 1972, Danielli [2260] described various possibilities for generating new life forms via "life-synthesis" and genetic engineering, noting that "macromolecular engineering" might enable the development of very powerful and compact macromolecular computer systems.

In 1974, Halacy[2261] noted "some rather inglorious ways" to use "the miracle of artificial life," including potential capabilities for growing diverse items ranging from computers to airplanes. Morowitz[159] suggested cooling cells to cryogenic temperatures in order to analyze and determine their structure. Artificial cells could also be assembled at such temperatures and then be set in motion by thawing. Morowitz further reported that microsurgery experiments on amoebas "have been most dramatic. Cell fractions from four different animals can be injected into the eviscerated ghost of a fifth amoeba, and a living functioning organism results."

In 1975, Richard Laing[2250] described the theoretical possibility of molecular machine self-replicators using molecular (data) tapes based on the idea of universal Turing machines, examining several ways that such "artificial organisms" might replicate themselves as "a vehicle for the exploration of broad biological possibilities."

In 1976, Donaldson[2262] presented the first detailed (and quite ambitious) list of biotechnological techniques that appeared necessary to achieve cell repair and might prove feasible, writing at a time that predated many current capabilities such as automated protein/DNA sequencing and synthesis, and most knowledge of restrictions on cellular developmental pathways and genetic programs and networks. For repair at the level of the cell, Donaldson's techniques would have included:

1. The ability to design enzymes to produce specific repair functions such as renaturing denatured proteins, joining broken lipoprotein complexes, annealing broken strands of DNA or RNA, reading proteins of existing or special types onto RNA and replicating them, and giving a cell the ability to metabolize new substrates, use novel cofactors, or construct essential amino acids;

2. Specially constructed bacteria or macrophages able to replicate themselves, spread throughout a specific target tissue, and carry out specific repairs according to the programs designed into their DNA/RNA; these could be designed to operate at unnatural temperatures or to utilize metabolic pathways not presently found in nature;

3. The abilities to re-introduce lost DNA or lost organelles such as mitochondria into a cell, to introduce entirely new forms of organelles perhaps to perform specific repair functions, and to introduce new metabolic capacities into a cell;

4. The ability to modify at will the developmental program of a cell, as for instance to induce postmitotic cells such as neurons to divide,* according to a specific program, forming daughter cells with specific properties; and

5. Several different types of repair bacteria able to work together in an integrated fashion, and linked together by chemical means (e.g. hormones), so as to apply optimal repairs to every body cell in order to (A) diagnose the precise nature of the damage, call other repair bacteria to its location, and report to the attending doctor that new types of repair bacteria other than those already introduced are needed, and (B) identify structures which must be preserved (e.g. memory) and reconstruct them if necessary.

For repairs at the level of the whole organism, Donaldson offered the following rather aggressive biological nanotechnology techniques:

1. Understanding the physiology of aging combined with the ability to reverse it;

* *It is now known that genetic programs to allow postmitotic cell division do not exist for many cells, although in theory artificial programs could possibly be devised. Stem cells may differentiate, and in some cases cells may be induced to de-differentiate back to stem cells thus allowing subsequent division and re-differentiation — but losing, in the case of neurons, the existing neural connections.*

2. Control over growth and development, including the ability to program types of growth and development which do not naturally occur, such as growth of new eyes or other organs which have been lost or damaged, growth of an entire and well-formed body from a head alone, and regrowth of injured or lost brain tissue; and
3. Nonpermanent "substitute organs" which will take over from others which have been lost, including (A) the ability to keep a given tissue alive and healthy in vitro for an indefinite time and similar abilities for a body part, and (B) temporary replacements for any body organ which may have been lost. These would be used to support the body while new organs were growing, e.g. as "metabolic crutches." This capacity specifically includes the ability to make temporary replacements for diffuse systems such as the vascular or nervous systems. For instance, a specially created "plant" would grow an entire vascular system into the patient, down to replacement for the capillaries and venules from a single seed, always introducing its fibrils between cells and destroying none or very little of the original structure.

The last of these is a description of a (clearly speculative) "repair net," a concept which Donaldson may have been the first to propose in 1976. A whole-body repair net was later termed a "chrysalis",[161,1724] and twelve years later, in 1988, Donaldson provided an artist's conception and an additional description of these proposed biotechnological instrumentalities:[1724]

> *"Severe crushing or mangling injuries require us to provide a new vascular system. The repair device might resemble a fungus, growing mycelia into the injured tissue. A repair net would grow into a [crushed] limb, guided by recognition of the injured cells and a plan for how the limb should look after repair....[In the most severe injuries,] a chrysalis first envelops the patient, then enters in between all his cells. It disassembles the patient, surrounding each cell with its own repair machinery and vascular system. The geometry already preserves information about locations of the patient's cells. If necessary, morphogen chemical gradients could also retain this information. A patient would [locally] swell up to 10 times original diameter. After repair, the chrysalis withdraws the same way it entered."*

In 1977, Darwin[2263] further developed the theme of tissue repair and cellular repair biomachines, independently proposing a modified white blood cell to perform repair functions.

In 1981, Asimov[2264] suggested that we "consider the bacteria. These are tiny living things made up of single cells far smaller than the cells in plants and animals....[We] can, by properly designing these tiniest slaves of ours, use them to reshape the world itself and build it close to our hearts' desire." More importantly, Donaldson[161] elaborated on his earlier discussion[2262] of how cryonically suspended human beings might be repaired. He extended the earlier concepts of Ettinger[160] and White,[2259] concluding that "with such hybrid technology as micro-miniature biological-mechanical machines the size of viruses" and related technology, "it seems unlikely that (to repair a single cell) there would be any difficulty at all in principle to carrying out any imaginable repair." He estimated that about 10 programmable cell-repair biomachines could be introduced into a cell that was under repair without causing too much mechanical disruption. In 1988, Donaldson[1724] described artificial macrophages that "can carry control machinery to recognize target cells, responding only to them, or responding differently depending upon cell type or cell conditions. They can still work even if the target cell isn't functioning (unlike viruses), rebuild target cell machinery other than the genes, and transfer many more genes up to an entire copy of the patient's genome." They can also "communicate with one another [and] release diffusible chemicals to guide one another's behavior."

By the 1990s, bioengineered viruses of various types and certain other vectors were routinely being used in experimental genetic therapies[3001-3011] as a means to target and penetrate certain cell populations, with the objective of inserting therapeutic DNA sequences into the nucleus of human target cells in vivo. Retrovirally-altered lymphocytes (T cells) began to be injected into humans for therapeutic purposes. Another example of an engineered cell in therapeutics was the use of genetically modified cerebral endothelial cell vectors to attack glioblastoma, which was being pursued by Neurotech (in Paris) in 1998. Engineered bacteria were being pursued by Vion Pharmaceuticals in collaboration with Yale University.[3038] In their "Tumor Amplified Protein Expression Therapy" program, antibiotic-sensitive *Salmonella typhimurium* (food poisoning) bacteria were attenuated by removing the genes that produce purines vital to bacterial growth. The tamed strain (cell line VNP20009) could not long survive in healthy tissue, but quickly multiplied ~1000-fold inside tumors, which are rich in purines. The next step would be to add genes to the bacterium to produce anticancer proteins that can shrink tumors, or to modify the bacteria to deliver various enzymes, genes, or prodrugs for tumor cell growth regulation. The engineered bacteria were available in multiple serotypes (Section 8.5.2) to avoid potential immune response in the host. Phase I human clinical trials were expected to begin in 1999 using clinical dosages produced in 50-liter fermenters, and other possible bacterial vector species were being examined.

Micro-biorobotics was still regarded by many in the biotechnology community as a highly speculative topic in 1998. Glen A. Evans[3014] described the possible construction of synthetic genomes and artificial organisms. His proposed strategy involves determining or designing the DNA sequence for the genome, synthesizing and assembling the genome, introducing the synthetic DNA into an enucleated pluripotent host cell, then introducing the host cell into an organism. Evans foresees the high throughput "read-out" of gene products discovered through genomic sequencing, rapid construction of designer genes and genomes, automated designer vector synthesis for gene replacement/insertional mutagenesis, and finally the construction of synthetic genomes and artificial organisms. Robert Bradbury[3015] has considered requirements and costs for genome synthesis and replacement. For example, Bradbury estimates genome synthesis costs by assuming a projected ~\$0.03/base for DNA synthesis (compared to ~\$0.80-\$1.00/base-micromole in 1999), with ~20,000 expressed genes per biorobotic cell with an average gene size of ~3000 bases, giving a ~60 megabase expressed genome per biorobotic cell (1 chromosome) and a raw synthesis cost of ~\$3 million per designer cell line (excluding design costs). There has also been discussion of "chemical reaction automata" as precursors for synthetic organisms,[3016] synthetic lifeforms[3263] and "nanobiology",[3017] "biorobotics",[3079-3081] "cell rovers",[3241] microbial engineering,[1962,3248,3543,3544] lymphocyte engineering,[965] and artificial chromosomes (Chapter 20), and cell engineering (Chapter 21) is rapidly gaining popularity.

1.3.2.2 The Mechanical Tradition

The late science fiction author Robert A. Heinlein[155] nearly invented the concept of molecular nanotechnology in 1942 when he suggested a process for manipulating microscopic structures. Heinlein envisioned the extensive use of life-size teleoperator hands, called "waldoes," complete with sensory feedback for full, remote-controlled telepresence. His fictional hero, Waldo, used a collection of these mechanical teleoperated hands for building and operating a series of ever-smaller sets of such mechanical hands. The smallest mechanical hands, "hardly an eighth of an inch across," were equipped with micro-surgical instruments and stereo "scanners," and were used to "manipulate living nerve tissue, [to examine] its performance in situ," and to perform neurosurgery. Eric Frank Russell's 1947 story "Hobbyist" described a fabrication process with "atom fed to atom like brick after brick to build a house." In 1955, Russell's serial "Call Him Dead," also published in *Astounding Science Fiction*, had a virus-based alien intelligence that spread through contact with blood or saliva; the story features a "microforger," a man who makes "surgical and manipulatory instruments so tiny they can be used to operate on a bacillus." Also in the mechanical tradition, Isaac Asimov's "Fantastic Voyage"[339,340] in 1966 took its miniaturized human crew in a miniaturized submarine through the bloodstream of a human patient on a mission of repair.

Heinlein, Russell, and Asimov overlooked the full implications of their ideas, and most scientists were unsympathetic — for example, in 1952 Erwin Schrodinger wrote that we would never experiment with just one electron, atom, or molecule.[3197] But by the early 1960s, several scientists had reinvented similar approaches to micromanipulation and miniaturization, this time extending their reach into the nanotechnology domain. The first and most famous of these scientists was the Nobel physicist Richard P. Feynman. In his remarkably prescient 1959 talk "There's Plenty of Room at the Bottom," Feynman[156] proposed employing machine tools to make smaller machine tools, these to be used in turn to make still smaller machine tools, and so on all the way down to the atomic level. Feynman prophetically concluded that this is "a development which I think cannot be avoided." Such nanomachine tools, nanorobots and nanodevices could ultimately be used to develop a wide range of submicron instrumentation and manufacturing tools, i.e., nanotechnology. Feynman's suggested applications for these tools included producing vast quantities of ultrasmall computers and various micro- and nano-robots.

Feynman was clearly aware of the potential medical applications of the new technology he was proposing. After discussing his ideas with a colleague, Feynman offered the first known proposal for a nanomedical procedure to cure heart disease: "A friend of mine (Albert R. Hibbs) suggests a very interesting possibility for relatively small machines. He says that, although it is a very wild idea, it would be interesting in surgery if you could swallow the surgeon. You put the mechanical surgeon inside the blood vessel and it goes into the heart and looks around. (Of course the information has to be fed out.) It finds out which valve is the faulty one and takes a little knife and slices it out. Other small machines might be permanently incorporated in the body to assist some inadequately functioning organ."[156] Later in his historic lecture, Feynman urged us to consider the possibility, in connection with biological cells, "that we can manufacture an object that maneuvers at that level!"

In 1961, K.R. Shoulders[2265] rejected the use of biological building blocks, even though biological "processes do work, and they can do so in a garbage can without supervision." He saw them as too limited environmentally and too difficult to control with available technology. Instead, he sought to directly produce much simpler, more powerful and rugged nanostructure arrays, operating at video frequency rates, which in turn could ultimately aid in their own replication. In 1965, Shoulders[2266] reported the actual operation of micromanipulators able to position tiny items with 10 nm accuracy while under direct observation by field ion microscopy.

In 1970, Volkenstein[2267] noted that "the creation of a nonmacromolecular system which would act as a model for living organisms is definitely possible" but could not arise by itself, and that the macromolecularity of present organisms is not essential, but due to their evolutionary origins. Taking some poetic license, he added: "Consequently, the cybernetic nonmacromolecular machine, which simulates life, could have been and can be created on earth only by man. Then it could perfect itself without limits." T. Nemes[2268] discussed artificial self-replicating machines and described how to construct "an automatic lathe able to reproduce itself," a concept apparently developed before von Neumann's work on machine replication.[1985]

In 1981, Drexler[182] suggested the construction of mechanically deterministic nanodevices using biological parts; these devices could inspect cells at the molecular level and also repair cellular tissues that had been damaged during cryonic suspension. In 1982, Drexler[311] described cell repair machines even more clearly in the mechanical tradition, in a popular publication.

By 1983, Drexler[2253] began privately circulating a draft technical paper entitled "Cell Repair Machines" which investigated for the first time, in some detail, whether an advanced mechanical-based nanotechnology would "permit construction of systems of molecular-scale sensors, computers, and manipulators able to enter and repair cells; the nature of the computational algorithms and magnitude of the computational resources needed to guide repairs; and the physical capabilities and constraints important to the repair process [in order to] sketch the conceptual design of a cell repair system based on a mature molecular technology."

Peterson[2254] notes that "medical applications were explored by Drexler during the early 1980s but the medical community was not ready for the concept." A technical paper by Drexler, invited by an editor at the *Journal of the American Medical Association*, was dismissed by a referee as "science fiction."

In 1985, G. Feinberg[2269] proposed using short-wavelength coherent laser energy to power and communicate with "nanosensors that could be implanted into the human body. They could...[monitor] various physiological functions from subcellular molecules up through tissues and organs...essential in determining some of the mechanisms involved in growth and aging."

In a 1985 book entitled *Robotics*, edited by Marvin Minsky (a well-known computer scientist and artificial intelligence pioneer), Minsky briefly described how fully-automatic cellular repair machines might work, following Drexler's vision:

> *"Suppose that we could design a repair machine so small that it could repair an artery from the inside! The first such machines might be the size of fleas. (There is room for a great deal of machinery in something the size of a flea — as the body of the flea itself testifies.) These micromachines could crawl into all but the smallest blood vessels, clear out debris, and reline the walls with suitable materials yet to be invented. Later generations of micromachines could be even smaller, perhaps no larger than the body cells they repair. These minuscule machines would be mass-produced by the billions, either by larger machines or by techniques of making them reproduce themselves. Perhaps these biological janitors would even be implanted in our bodies to remain there as permanent maintenance workers, just like many biological cells that already serve such purposes."*

> *"Today the idea of such a technology may seem fantastic, yet many of the circuits in our computers are already smaller than many of our bodies' cells. Let's try, for a moment, to look ahead to: mass production of highly intelligent machines; gigantic advances in miniaturization; a technology so advanced that these machines reproduce themselves without our help. Fantastic? Not at all. Even the simplest algae and bacteria can do that. True, they're not intelligent, but each of them contains enough computerlike machinery and memory to do those things. So, to build bacteria-size*

computers should be perfectly feasible, once we have the necessary microtechnology. Some day we'll have the means to build artificial, cell-like machines with all those capabilities."[202]

R.A. Freitas Jr.[204] also contributed a chapter to Minsky's 1985 book, offering the following suggestion for remote-controlled incisionless nanosurgery: "One possibility is the concept of remote-controlled medical mites made feasible by modern micromachinery technology. Some medical mites would be like microminiature submarines, released inside the human body for internal sensing. Other mites could float, crawl, or swim through major arteries in the human body and perform on-site repairs from within, controlled by radio link under direction of a skilled telemicrosurgeon."

In 1986, Drexler published *Engines of Creation*,[8] a popular text with two chapters devoted to discussions of cellular repair machines. Drexler further expounded upon the topic of cellular repair machines in articles published in 1985,[259] 1986,[310] 1987,[165] and 1989,[72] and his concepts were described by Brian Wowk in 1988[261] and in a Time-Life book in 1989.[2256] Cellular repair machines are explored at length in Chapter 21.

In 1988, A.K. Dewdney[18] reported an early nanomedical concept of an artery-cleaning nanorobot that he attributed to Drexler, accompanied by an artist's conception with the caption "a nanomachine swimming through a capillary attacks a fat deposit." (A preferable nanorobotic design for this purpose, the endotheliocyte, is presented in Chapter 22.)

1.3.2.3 Nanomedicine in the 1990s

Despite the tremendous importance of molecular nanotechnology, a published 1993 literature review of robotics in health care included not a single reference to nanotechnology or to nanomedicine.[2255] At this writing in 1998, the list of original post-1989 technical and popular nonfiction works that deal with nanomedical topics in the mechanical tradition is short enough to permit virtually an exhaustive listing, including Beardsley,[122] Bova,[2973] Coombs and Robinson,[570] Crawford,[2270] Drexler,[9,10,2397] DuCharme,[358] Emanuelson,[3270] Fahy,[27,215,224,322,2271] Fiedler and Reynolds,[70] Freitas,[19,2300,1400] Kaehler,[2272] Klatz and Kahn,[2979] Kurzweil,[2309] Lampton,[168,330] Merkle,[258,262,306,888] Merrill,[3487] Minsky,[132] More,[2992,2993] Ostman,[2284] Reifman,[2273] and Wowk and Darwin.[20] The first nanomedical device design technical paper was published in 1998 by Freitas in the biotechnology journal *Artificial Cells*,[1400] and the present trilogy (*Nanomedicine*) is the first book-length technical treatment of the medical implications of molecular nanotechnology.

The author again must caution enthusiasts that the full capabilities of these machines will not be realized without a great deal of sweat and toil by legions of well-funded and dedicated researchers working for many decades to develop the technology. One purpose of this book is to help motivate this future work.

1.3.3 Biotechnology and Molecular Nanotechnology

Some pragmatic readers may be wondering what is so special about molecular nanotechnology, that existing or anticipated biotechnology could not accomplish just as well? After all, biotechnology is already an established medical capability. It has real applications and real products already on the market. Reflecting upon the future possibility of sophisticated mechanical medical nanorobots equipped with powerful nanocomputers, in 1989, one well-known cryobiologist[215] mused that "what is not clear is just what need we would have for such devices." The simplest answer, suggested by Figure 1.5, is that each of the three contemporary branches of

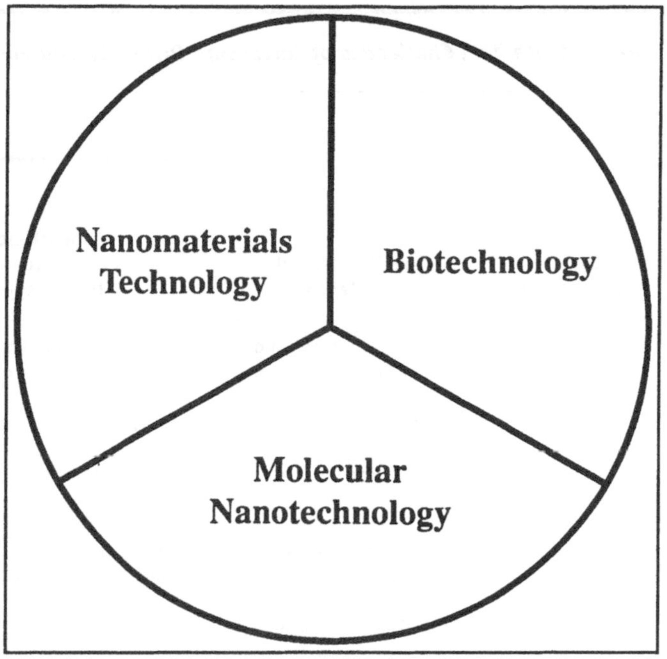

Fig. 1.5. Three contemporary branches of "nanotechnology."

"nanotechnology" offers something of unique value to the practice of medicine.

Nanoscale materials technology[3221,3222,3262] has already found widespread use in medicine, including biocompatible materials and analytical techniques,[341] surgical and dental practice, nerve cell research using intracellular electrodes, biostructures research and biomolecular research using near-field optical microscopy, scanning-probe microscopy and optical tweezers, and vaccine design,[570] and also many 20th century bulk chemical and biochemical manufacturing techniques along with much of classical pharmacology.

As for "biotechnology," the original meaning of this word contemplated "the application of biological systems and organisms to technical and industrial processes".[2223] In recent times, the field has expanded to include genetic engineering and now takes as its ultimate goal no less than the engineering of all biological systems, even completely artificial organic living systems, using biological instrumentalities.

The third branch, molecular nanotechnology, takes as its purview the engineering of all complex mechanical systems constructed from the molecular level — potentially offering new tools for medical practice, the principal subject of this book. Observes G.M. Fahy,[2271] "the difference between nanotechnologists and biotechnologists is that the former do not restrict themselves to the biological limitations of the latter, and they are much more ambitious about the kinds of accomplishments that they want to achieve."

Doctors can utilize solutions to medical problems from all three approaches. As noted earlier, 80-90% of medical complaints resolve themselves via natural homeostatic processes, or without the necessary involvement of active biotechnological or molecular-nanotechnological agents. But by employing biotechnology, the range and efficacy of treatment options greatly increases. With molecular nanotechnology, the range, efficacy, comfort and speed of possible medical treatments again expands enormously. Molecular nanotechnology is essential when the damage to the human body is extremely subtle, highly selective, or time-critical (as in head traumas, burns, or fast-spreading diseases), or when the damage is very

Table 1.4. Medical Challenges of Increasing Difficulty and Possible Approaches

Increasing Efficacy →

Level of Difficulty	Specific Medical Challenge	Homeostatic or Nanomaterials Technology	Biotechnology Approach	Molecular Nanotechnology Approach
I	**Minor Symptoms and Minor Physical Trauma**	Herbal preparation, minor surgery, passage of time	Symptomatic suppression pharmacology	Pharmacytes, zippocytes, respirocytes, etc.
II	**Infectious Agents**	Natural immune system	Antibiotics and vaccines	Nanobiotics
III	**Mutation and Cell Disease**	Natural immune system Major surgery	Molecular diagnostics and treatments; gene therapies	Nanobiotics Cell repair machines
IV	**Health Maintainance and Aging**	Vitamins, good diet, exercise, moderation and "clean living"	Gene therapy to enhance self-repair and immune function	Whole-body cyto-assay Cell repair machines
V	**Major Organ Replacement or Repair**	Organ transplantation Major surgery	Stem cell & tissue engineering; embryonic gene reactivation	Cell mills, tissue mills, organ mills, nanosurgery
VI	**Morpho-Engineering**	Cosmetic surgery	Control of natural morphogenetic systems	Nanosurgery Chromatin editors
VII	**Emergency Care; Restoration of Nonhomeostatic Tissue**	Emergency major surgery Prosthesis or bionics	Biological repair nets Bioengineered immune cells	Traumapods Warm biostasis
VIII	**Augmentation of Natural Structure or Function**	Prosthesis or bionics	Cross-species and artificial morphogenetic supplementation	Cell engineering devices Autogenous control

massive, overwhelming the body's natural defenses and repair mechanisms.

Table 1.4, inspired by an earlier discussion from G.M. Fahy,[215] makes these options more explicit. At every difficulty level, most classes of medical problems may be resolved with varying efficacy within the homeostatic/nanomaterials, biotechnological, or molecular-nanotechnological approaches. As the chosen technology becomes more precise, active, and controllable, the range of options broadens and the quality of the options improves. Thus the question is not whether molecular nanotechnology is required to accomplish a given medical objective. In many cases, it is not — though of course there are some things that only biotechnology and molecular nanotechnology can do, and some other things that only molecular nanotechnology can do. Rather, the important question is which approach offers a superior solution to a given medical problem, using any reasonable metric of treatment efficacy. For virtually every class of medical challenge, a mature molecular nanotechnology offers a wider and more effective range of treatment options than any other approach.

It is quite possible to imagine an advanced biotechnology that uses an engineered white cell, fibroblast, or macrophage chassis, energized by native oxygen and glucose (Section 6.3.4) and modified mitochondrial powerplants, driven by pseudopodia, cilia or flagella (Section 9.4), communicating and navigating via biochemical signals (Sections 7.2.1 and 8.4.3), and even incorporating onboard digital biocomputers (Section 10.2.3) to make microscopic biorobots. Principal arguments favoring the biotechnology approach for medical purposes are: (1) that we are already somewhat familiar with such systems, after half a century of intensive molecular biology research; (2) that we have already "built" precursor systems, such as a whole living amoeba constructed from five distinct parts,[159] bioengineered viruses[3003] and bacteria[2018,3038] as DNA insertion devices, and natural replication stimulated in genetically engineered starter microbes; (3) that biocompatibility will not be a major issue since fibroblasts (which express no HLA Class II antigens, hence stimulate no rejection response; Section 8.5.2.1) could be used as the starter material; (4) that both engineered viruses[2326,2327] and bacteria are already in wide commercial and research use; and (5) the greater complexity of self-repair in mechanical systems, should it be needed. Many believe that the development pathway to early biorobots may be considerably shorter than for the mechanical nanorobots of the molecular nanotechnology approach, for which in 1998 not a single working prototype yet existed, even in research laboratories.

It is also possible to imagine a molecular nanotechnology that uses mechanical nanorobotic systems. Such systems will have many constitutional differences from biological-based systems. For instance, mechanical systems will transport parts, materials, energy and instructions via fixed channels, whereas most (but not all) biological systems operate by diffusion.[2244] Mechanical systems will have structures constrained by specific geometries, whereas biological systems have structures defined by patterns of containment and interconnection — the shape of a membrane compartment in a cell matters less than its continuity and the contents of the volume it defines.[2244] Mechanical systems will be deterministically manufactured by operations analogous to manual construction, whereas engineered ribosomes will self-assemble via diffusion and stochastic matching of complementary parts;[2244] in other words, biology uses recipes, while mechanical systems use blueprints.[2022] Cells grow, with their parts adapting to one another; mechanical nanorobots may be constructed from parts of fixed structure.[2244] Biology uses self-repair; mechanical systems generally do not[2022] — largely because self-repair (by component exchange) will not be needed in molecular mechanical systems, whose designs may be made more simple by relying upon high component redundancy[10] (Chapter 13). These and other differences imply a number of important advantages that mechanical-based medical systems will enjoy over biological-based medical systems, which, taken together, strongly suggest that predominantly mechanical nanosystems may be the approach of choice for a mature medical nanotechnology. The advantages of molecular nanotechnology (e.g. the mechanical tradition) are many:

1. *Speed of Medical Treatment* — Doctors may be surprised by the incredible quickness of nanorobotic action when compared to the speeds available from fibroblasts or leukocytes. Normal homeostatic processes such as dermal wound repair via natural fibroblasts may require weeks to run to completion. Typical fibroblast movements occur at 0.1-1 microns/sec (Section 9.4), but mechanical nanomanipulators can operate at 1-10 cm/sec speeds (Section 9.3.1) or faster, a speed advantage of 4-5 orders of magnitude. Even the strongest biological fibers (e.g. intermediate filaments) have a failure strength 3 orders of magnitude below the strongest mechanical fibers (e.g. fullerene nanotubes; Table 9.3). Biological cilia beat at ~30 Hz while mechanical nanocilia may cycle up to ~20 MHz, though practical power restrictions and other considerations may limit them to the ~10 KHz range for most of the time (Section 9.3.1). Flexible mechanical surfaces can complete a morphing motion in ~0.1 millisec, compared to the ~100 millisec snapback time for pinched red cell membrane (Section 5.3.1.4), again a thousandfold advantage in speed. Thus we expect that mechanical therapeutic systems can reach their targets up to ~10,000 times faster, all else equal, and treatments which require ~10^5 sec for a biological system may need only ~10^2 sec for a mechanical system;[3233] tachyiatria improves both patient and physician comfort. In either biological or mechanical systems, large numbers of devices of comparable physical size (e.g. ~microns) may be employed to do the work, so numbers alone cannot offset the mechanical speed advantage.

2. *Power Density and Transduction* — Biological cells typically employ power densities of 10^3-10^4 W/m^3, with maximum densities of ~10^6 W/m^3 in honeybee flight muscle cells and bacterial flagellar motors (Table 6.8). By contrast, nanomechanical power systems can produce power densities of 10^9-10^{12} W/m^3 (Section 6.3), an advantage of 10^3-10^8 for mechanical over biological systems. By 1998, conducting polymer-based actuators generated 20-100 times the force for a given cross-sectional area as mammalian skeletal muscle.[2388] Additionally, amoebic locomotion in motile cells requires diffusion-limited cytoskeletal disassembly and reassembly to achieve movement; mechanical motility systems may employ simple cable-pulling, winches, or ratchets, which are faster and more direct. Some biological energy transducers are reversible, but muscle contraction is irreversible — not only cannot muscle actively re-expand, but stretching it doesn't make it produce much useful chemical energy. In contrast, electric motors can be run backwards to generate electricity, forcing pistons makes them pump, and loudspeakers can be used as microphones.[2022]

3. *Superior Building Materials* — Typical biological materials have tensile failure strengths in the 10^6-10^7 N/m^2 range, with the strongest biological materials such as wet compact bone having a failure strength of ~10^8 N/m^2, all of which compare poorly to ~10^9 N/m^2 for good steel, ~10^{10} N/m^2 for sapphire, and ~10^{11} N/m^2 for diamond and carbon fullerenes (Table 9.3), again showing a 10^3-10^5 advantage for mechanical systems that use nonbiological materials. Nonbiological materials can be much stiffer, permitting the application of higher forces with greater precision of movement, and they also tend to remain stable over a larger range of temperature, pressure, salinity and pH. Proteins are heat sensitive in part because much of the functionality of their structure is due to noncovalent bonds involved in folding, which are broken more easily at higher temperatures; in diamond, sapphire, and many other rigid materials, structural shape is covalently fixed, hence is far more temperature-stable. Most proteins tend to become dysfunctional at cryogenic temperatures, unlike diamond-based mechanical structures (Section 10.5). Biomaterials are not ruled out for all nanomechanical systems, but represent only a small subset of the materials that can be used in nanorobots. Mechanical systems can employ a wider variety of atoms and molecular structures in their design and construction, with novel functional forms that might be difficult to implement in a biological system such as steam engines (Section 6.3.1) or nuclear power (Section 6.3.7). As another example, an application requiring the most effective bulk thermal conduction possible should use diamond, the best conductor available, not some biomaterial with inferior thermal performance.

4. *Nondegradation of Treatment Agents* — Diagnostic and therapeutic agents constructed of biomaterials generally are biodegradable in vivo, although there is a major branch of pharmacology devoted to designing drugs that are moderately non-biodegradable — anti-sense DNA analogues with unusual backbone linkages and peptide nucleic acids (PNAs) are difficult to break down. However, suitably designed nanorobotic agents constructed of nonbiological materials are not biodegradable. An engineered fibroblast may not stimulate an immune response when transplanted into a foreign host, but its biomolecules are subject to chemical attack in vivo by free radicals, acids, and enzymes. Even "mirror" biomolecules or "Doppelganger proteins"[2285] comprised exclusively of unnatural D-amino acids have a lifetime of only ~5 days inside the human body.[2286] Nonbiological materials such as diamond and sapphire are highly resistant to chemical breakdown or leukocytic degradation in vivo, and pathogenic biological entities cannot easily evolve useful attack strategies against these materials (Section 9.3.5.3.6).

5. *Control of Nanomedical Treatment* — Present-day biotechnological entities are not programmable and cannot be switched on and off conditionally during task execution. A digital biocomputer, while possible in theory, represents a considerable conceptual departure from the usual biological paradigm. Even assuming that a digital biocomputer could be installed in a fibroblast, and that appropriate effector mechanisms could be attached, such a system would necessarily have slower clock cycles, less capacious memory per unit volume, and longer data access times, implying less diversity of action, poorer control, and less complex executable programs than would be available in nanoscale electromechanical computer systems (Section 10.2). The mechanical approach emphasizes precise control of action, including control of physical placement, timing, strength, structure, and interactions with other (especially biological) entities. The biological approach emphasizes the use of poorly controlled natural structures, needlessly sacrificing huge blocks of the available functionality and design space.

6. *Nanodevice Versatility* — Mechanical systems can readily incorporate biological elements if necessary, but artificial biological

systems can incorporate nonbiological materials such as carbon nanotubes or diamond/sapphire structural elements only with difficulty, in part because biology has a more limited repertoire of "effector" mechanisms. Artificial biological systems cannot easily incorporate nonbiological materials where desired because natural biological assembly methods make no provisions for these materials either in the coded instructions in DNA or in the attachment chemistries. Rebuilding or reconstructing the human body with nonbiological components (e.g. fullerene encabled bone for bone damaged in an accident; Chapters 24 and 30), or augmentation of human body function with unnatural abilities or features (e.g. autogenous paracrine control; Chapter 12), will be very difficult or impossible to achieve using purely biotechnological means.

7. *Avoiding Overspecialization* — M. Krummenacker notes that one of the most glaring shortcomings of bacteria and other naturally occurring molecular machinery — when viewed as systems subject to further engineering — is the rather limited range of molecular substrates they can utilize. For example, bacterial enzymes are highly specialized devices, with very narrow substrate specificities. Thousands of different enzymes are needed in each organism, and the substance classes capable of digestion are limited to some sugars, various amino acids including proteins that can be degraded by excreted proteases, lipids, and a few other smallish oxygen-functionalized carbon molecules such as glycerol and ethanol. Some bacteria can metabolize CO_2 and a handful of aromatic compounds, but there is a vast range of organic chemicals that most bacteria cannot degrade or manufacture. A much smaller set of substantially more general molecular tools can probably be designed using the mechanical approach; mechanosynthesis can fabricate and assemble, or disassemble, a far wider range of molecular structures than are available to the cellular machinery of life.

8. *Faster and More Precise Diagnosis* — The analytic function of medical diagnosis requires rapid communication between the injected devices and the attending physician. If limited to chemical messaging, biotechnology devices will require minutes or hours to complete each diagnostic loop. Nanomachines, with their more diverse set of input-output mechanisms (Chapter 7), can outmessage the results of in vivo reconnaissance or testing literally in seconds. Such nanomachines can also run more tests of greater variety in less time. Mechanical nanoinstruments, including molecule-by-molecule disassemblers (Chapter 19), will make comprehensive cell mapping and cell interaction analysis possible. Bacterial resistance can be assayed at the molecular level, allowing new treatment agents to more easily be composed, manufactured and immediately deployed (Chapter 19).

9. *More Sensitive Response Threshold for High-Speed Action* — Unlike natural systems, an entire population of nanobiotic devices can be triggered globally by just a single local detection of the target antigen or pathogen. The natural immune system takes $>10^5$ sec to become fully engaged after exposure to a systemic pathogen or other antigen-presenting intruder. A biotechnologically enhanced immune system that can employ the fastest natural unit replication time ($\sim 10^3$ sec for some bacteria) will require $\sim 10^4$ sec for full deployment post-exposure. By contrast, a nanobiotic immune system (Chapter 19) can probably be fully engaged (though not finished) in at most two blood circulation times, or $\sim 10^2$ sec.[3233]

10. *More Reliable Operation* — Engineered macrophages would probably individually operate less reliably than mechanical nanorobots. Many pathogens, such as *Listeria monocytogenes* and *Trypanosoma cruzi*, are known to be able to escape from phagocytic vacuoles into the cytoplasm;[2165] while biotech drugs or cell manufactured proteins could be developed to prevent this (e.g. cold therapy drugs are entry-point blockers), nanorobotic trapping mechanisms can be more secure (Section 10.4.2). Proteins assembled by natural ribosomes typically incorporate one error per $\sim 10^4$ amino acids placed; current gene and protein synthesizing machines utilizing biotechnological processes have similar error rates. A molecular nanotechnology approach will improve error rates by at least a millionfold[10] (Chapter 20). Mechanical systems can also incorporate sensors to determine if and when a particular task needs to be done, or when a task has been completed. Finally, it is unlikely that natural organisms will be able to infiltrate mechanical nanorobots or to co-opt their functions. By contrast, a biological-based robot could be diverted or defeated by microbes that can piggyback on its metabolism, interfere with its normal workings, or even incorporate the device wholesale into their own structures, causing the engineered biomachine to perform some new or different function than was originally intended. There are many examples of such co-option among natural biological systems, including the protozoan mixotrichs found in the termite gut that have assimilated bacteria into their bodies for use as motive engines,[2025-2027] and the nudibranch mollusks (marine snails without shells) that steal nematocysts (stinging cells) away from coelenterates such as jellyfish (i.e. a Portuguese man-of-war) and incorporate the stingers as defensive armaments in their own skins,[2295] a process which S. Vogel[2022] has called "stealing loaded guns from the army."

11. *Verification of Progress and Treatment* — Using a variety of communication modalities, nanorobots can report back to the attending physician, with digital precision, a summary of diagnostically- or therapeutically-relevant data describing exactly what was found, and what was done, and what problems were encountered, in every cell visited. A biological-based approach relying upon chemical messaging is necessarily slow with limited signaling capacity. Also unlike mechanical nanorobots, biotechnological systems generally cannot monitor their own functions while working, and, except for a few highly specialized DNA proofreading systems, cannot directly inspect their work while it is in progress or after it is finished.

12. *Minimum Side Effects* — Almost all drugs have side effects, such as conventional cancer chemotherapy which causes hair loss and vomiting, although computer-designed drugs (Chapter 18) have high specificity and relatively few side effects. Carefully tailored cancer vaccines under development in the late 1990s were expected unavoidably to affect some healthy cells. Even well-targeted drugs are distributed to unintended tissues and organs in low concentrations,[1492] although some bacteria can target certain organs fairly reliably without being able to distinguish individual cells. By contrast, mechanical nanorobots may be targeted with virtually 100% accuracy to specific organs, tissues, or even individual cellular addresses within the human body (Chapter 8). Such nanorobots should have few if any side effects, and will remain safe even in large dosages because their actions can be digitally self-regulated using rigorous control protocols (Chapter 12) that affirmatively prohibit device activation unless all necessary preconditions have been, and continuously remain, satisfied. G.M. Fahy[2271] has noted that these possibilities could transform "drugs" into "programmable machines with a range of sensory, decision-making, and effector capabilities [that] might avoid side effects and allergic reactions...attaining almost complete specificity of

action....Designed smart pharmaceuticals might activate themselves only when, where, and if needed." Additionally, nanorobots may be programmed to excuse themselves from the site of action, or even from the body, after a treatment is completed; by contrast, spent biorobotic elements containing ingested foreign materials may have more limited post-treatment mobility, thus lingering at the worksite causing inflammation when naturally degraded or removed.*

13. *Reduced Replicator Danger* — Drexler[2244] points out that living systems are evolved systems, while nanomechanical replicators would be designed: "The former are shaped to serve the goal of their own survival and replication in a natural environment, whereas the latter will be shaped (whether well or poorly) to serve human goals, perhaps in an artificial environment." Genetic engineering involves not design of replicators from scratch, but tinkering with the molecular machinery of existing bioreplicators. Since bioreplicators were not designed, they are not necessarily structured in ways that lend themselves to complete understanding, and processes based on diffusion and matching allow complex nonlocal interactions that can be hard to trace. Bioreplicators can be crippled, but having evolved in nature, they resemble systems that can survive in nature. Typically, they are able to exchange genetic information with wild organisms, raising the possibility of the introduction of new, unconstrained replicators in the natural environment. Having evolved to evolve, they have a capacity for further evolution — to serve their own survival, not human goals.[2244] For example, even when stripped of key pieces of DNA to interfere with its replication powers, a live attenuated AIDS vaccine can slowly recover its virulence and can attack immune cells.[2939] R. Bradbury suggests that artificial biorobots could incorporate multiple fail-safe mechanisms including required external essential nutrients or suicide suppressors, self-destruct triggers, countdown timers like telomeres, and engineering to reject foreign DNA (the basis for restriction enzymes), but it remains logically easier for a system with inchoate capacity to evolve to resume doing so, than for a system which has never had this capability to spontaneously develop it.

In contrast, nanomechanical replicators (e.g. assemblers; Section 2.4.2) will be designed from scratch and thus will differ fundamentally from biological systems. The parts and structures of designed mechanical systems will be known, and the relationships among their parts will also be designed and fixed. More important, nanoreplicators will be fundamentally alien to the biosphere, unrelated to anything that has evolved to survive in nature. Certainly the capacity to fail can appear by accident, and emergent capabilities cannot be completely ruled out, but engineering experience shows that the ability to perform complex organized activities (such as replication in a natural environment) does not normally appear spontaneously.[2244] Also, and purely as a geometrical consideration, adding a new part inside a densely organized geometric structure (as would be found in a nanomachine) typically requires changes in the relative positions of many other parts, and hence corresponding adjustments in design. Adding a part inside a densely organized topological structure (as found in living systems) typically leaves topologies unchanged — room can be made by stretching and shifting other parts, with no change in their essential design,[2244] hence permitting easier modification to biological structures by exogenous agencies.

Note that mechanical medical nanodevices need not be capable of replication. There is no requirement for replication in vivo; such replication would be needlessly dangerous, and adding this capability would reduce effectiveness in carrying out the primary medical task. Analogously, viral vectors employed in genetic therapies are modified to be "incapable" of replication.

14. *Assured Patentability* — Microscopic biorobots, unavoidably derived from natural biological material, may someday be deemed unpatentable under a general prohibition on "genetic colonialism" or other emerging legal doctrines.[2323] In contrast, mechanical nanorobots, being fully-artificial and designed machines, should always be patentable provided they satisfy the customary legal criteria.

1.3.4 Naturophilia

As already noted (Section 1.3.1), living things in general and the human body in particular are awesome examples of a powerful and intricately woven natural molecular technology to which human engineers, in 1998, still aspire. But embracing Nature is not the same as finding her perfect. Today, the word "natural" has acquired a strong connotation of rightness, even of sanctity. For most of human history, notes biologist Steven Vogel,[2022] "the natural and human worlds stood opposed. Nature was something to be tamed and utilized; we had the ordinary attitude of organisms toward other species. Nowadays the natural world intrudes far less but gets venerated far more. And why not? When one's meat is bought in a store, when locusts don't threaten one's corn crop, when central heating and plumbing are the norm, the aesthetics of nature hold greater appeal." And so we embrace the natural rectitude or moral superiority of nature's ways, a kind of pantheism which may be called ethical naturalism,[2299] biophilia,[2296] or naturophilia.

Many great minds have fallen prey to naturophilia. In the 4th century BC, Aristotle wrote[2297] that "if one way be better than another, that you may be sure is Nature's way." In the 15th century, we have from Leonardo da Vinci:[2298] "Human ingenuity may make various inventions, but it will never devise any inventions more beautiful, nor more simple, nor more to the purpose than Nature does; because in her inventions nothing is wanting and nothing is superfluous."

However, as Virginia Postrel notes in *The Future and Its Enemies*:[2299] "If nature is itself a dynamic process rather than a static end, then there is no single form of 'the natural.' An evolving, open-ended nature may impose practical constraints, but it cannot dictate eternal standards. It cannot determine what is good. The distinction between the artificial and the natural must lie not in their source — human or not — but in their characteristics, in the way they relate to the world around them."

According to the dictionary, "artificial" usually means "made by man, rather than occurring in nature." More usefully, Herbert Simon[2301] defines the artificial as that which is designed, expresses goals, and possesses external purposes. The artificial is controlled and serves its creators' purposes, subject to the universal laws of physics. Kevin Kelly[381] defines the natural as "out of control." Nature is evolved, not designed, and serves no goal or external purpose save its own survival. Nature, lacking intent, is amoral — it simply is.[2299] By building the artificial, observes Postrel, "we do not overthrow nature, but cooperate with it, using nature's own art to create new

---

**R. Bradbury notes that artificial eukaryotic biorobots may possess an apoptotic pathway (Section 10.4.1.1) which could be activated to permit clean and natural self-destruction that avoids inflammation in surrounding tissues. Artificial prokaryotic biorobots could also be designed for human biocompatibility; by replacing bacterial genes with generic human genes, such a device may be undetectable to the immune system.*

natural forms. Our artifice alters the path of nature, but it does not end it, for nature has no stopping point, no final shape. It is a process, not an end."

Some naturophilist writers have decried the increasing "medicalization of society" in which formerly natural functions have come to be regarded as medical conditions requiring intervention or treatment.[2204,2302-2308] However, history suggests that naturophilia is usually undermined by any new medical technology that offers clear, safe, and immediate benefits to patients. For example, prior to 1842, intense pain was viewed as the natural outcome of being cut with a scalpel during surgery. It had always been so — how could it ever be otherwise? The invention of anesthesia in 1842 (Section 1.2.1.9.2) suddenly altered this natural outcome and replaced it with a less painful artificial outcome, despite anguished cries from naturophiles within the medical community that eliminating pain might somehow diminish the human character.

Another example of a widely-accepted medicalization of normal function is childbirth, a quite natural activity that can nevertheless be very dangerous to the mother's health. Precise prehistoric death rates are unknown, although archeological evidence shows that Neandertal females tended to die before the age of 30 due to hazards of childbirth.[2339,2340] In the worst 19th century maternity hospitals the natural death rate from childbirth was 9-10%, falling to a very artificial 0.4% rate in England by 1930 and to less than 0.01% in the U.S. during the 1990s. As a result, it now seems "natural" for a woman always to survive childbirth, even though the reverse may have been true for most of human history. Warns historian Roy Porter:[2204] "We should certainly not hanker after some mythic golden age when women gave birth naturally, painlessly, and safely; the most appalling Western maternal death rate today is among the Faith Assembly religious sect in Indiana, who reject orthodox medicine and practice home births; their perinatal mortality is 92 times greater than in Indiana as a whole."

A disease seems "natural" to those who suffer from it when no treatment exists. But once a treatment is discovered and is widely employed, the disease becomes rare and its absence now becomes "natural." To those in the past, writes K.E. Drexler,[9] "the idea of cutting people open with knives painlessly would have seemed miraculous, but surgical anesthesia is now routine. Likewise with bacterial infections and antibiotics, with the eradication of smallpox, and the vaccine for polio: each tamed a deadly terror, and each is now half-forgotten history. What amazes one generation seems obvious and even boring to the next. The first baby born after each breakthrough grows up wondering what all the excitement was about." In the next century, says Charles Sheffield,[343] "our descendants will look on angiograms, upper and lower GIs, and biopsies the way we regard the prospect of surgery without anesthetics."

Future generations who take for granted an all-pervasive nanomedicine in their lives may look aghast upon the 20th century, wondering among other things how we managed to retain productive focus given the constant annoyance of our numerous undiagnosed minor disease states. Most of these diseases are not yet recognized as such, and many are still regarded as "natural" and not worthy of treatment. In a few decades, this may change. Some examples:

1. *Addictions* — In 1998, many people laugh off seemingly harmless addictions to chocolate (chocoholics), fats or sugar (sweet tooth), food (gluttony), nicotine (smokers), caffeine (coffee and cola drinkers), work (workaholics), exercise (runner's high), telling falsehoods (pathological liars), gambling (wagerphilia), stealing (kleptomania), medical treatments (hypochondria), marriage (polygamy), power-seeking (domination), skydiving or bungee-jumping (thrillseeking), superstition (astrology), shopping (spendoholics), driving cars that kill 40,000 Americans per year (mobilophilia), unusual sexual preferences (bestiality), sexual activity (nymphomania, satyriasis), or pregnancy (gravidophilia). Without making any value judgements, it is highly likely that most or all of these addictions have genetic or physiological components which, once properly modified, can greatly reduce or eliminate the addiction if so desired. Many on the list are already suspected to have genetic components, much like schizophrenia, drug abuse, bulimia, and alcoholism (dipsomania).

2. *Allergies and Intolerances* — A food allergy[2997] is an allergic reaction to a particular food, although true food allergies are much rarer than is generally believed.[1604] In the cases of milk, eggs, shellfish, nuts, wheat, soybeans, and chocolate, sufferers may lack an enzyme necessary for digesting the substance. In other cases, dust particles, plant pollens, pet danders, drugs, or foods may be allergens for natural IgE-mediated immunosensitivity. Intolerance, a much more common condition, is any undesirable effect of eating a particular food, including gastrointestinal distress, gas, nausea, diarrhea, or other problems. Urticaria (hives), angioedema and even mild anaphylaxis are common reactions to various drugs, insect stings or bites, allergy shots, or certain foods, particularly eggs, shellfish, nuts and fruits. Physical allergies to ordinary stimuli such as cold, sunlight, heat, pollen, pet dander, or minor injury can produce itching, skin blotches, pimples, and hives.

3. *Minor Physical Annoyances* — In a world where most major medical maladies are readily treated, numerous minor medical conditions which today escape our notice will rise up from obscurity and present themselves annoyingly to our conscious minds, demanding attention. These conditions may be of several kinds. First is cosmetics, including small moles, freckles and blemishes on the skin; broken fingernails or unevenly-growing cuticles; minor skin reddenings or pimples; old childhood scars, wrinkled skin, birthmarks or stretch marks; unwanted hair growth in unusual places, or differential hair color or texture growing in patches; fingerprint patterns that are aesthetically unappealing; and mismatched leg lengths, hands with different left/right ring sizes, an asymmetrical face, or lopsided breasts. Second is minor aches and pains, which may include headaches; eyebrow hairs trapped in the eyeball conjunctiva; bent-hair pain (folliculalgia); dyspepsia; creaking limb joints and stomach growling; ingrown nails and hairs; earwax plugs and temporary tinnitis; chapped lips, canker sores and heat rashes; stuffy nose or gritty eyes upon rising in the morning; dermal chafing marks from elastic bands in clothing; minor flatulence; PMS (premenstrual syndrome); a leg or arm "falling asleep" in certain postures; nervous tics, itches, and twitches; uncracked knuckles, stiff neck, or backache; blocked middle ear following descent from high altitude; restless leg syndrome (akathisia); rotationally-induced dizziness, as on an amusement park ride; or rock-and-roll neck, wherein active musical performers or listeners bob their heads violently, rupturing small blood vessels in the neck. Third is minor physical or functional flaws, such as poor stream during male urination, female papillary leakage, colorblindness, snoring, unpleasant body odors, nosebleeds, declining visual or aural acuity, handedness (currently ~90% dextromanual, ~10% sinistromanual,[3136,3137] mild strabismus (eyeball misalignment), bad moods (neurotransmitter imbalances), or post-intoxication hangover.

4. *Undiscovered Infectious Agents* — Peptic ulcers once were thought to result from a stressful life, a purely natural response to a lifestyle choice. Then it was found that the major cause of ulcers is the

presence of *Helicobacter pylori* bacteria in the stomach. Bacteria have been implicated in some cases of atherosclerosis[2970] and Alzheimer's disease,[2971] and nanobacteria have been proposed as possible nucleation sites for kidney stones.[2149] Other seemingly natural but undesirable conditions may also be due to undiscovered microbial agents,[3237] especially since bacteria outnumber tissue cells in our highly infested 20th century bodies by more than 10:1 (Section 8.5.1).

5. *Unwanted Syndromes* — Syndromes are groups of related symptoms and signs of disordered function that define a disease whose cause remains unknown, that is, idiopathic. A good example is irritable bowel syndrome (IBS), which affects up to 20% of the adult U.S. population and includes symptoms of abdominal distention and pain, with more frequent and looser stools. Many are unaware they are afflicted. In 1998 there was no known cause or simple complete treatment for this still "natural" disease.[3713-3717] Even more mysterious than IBS is our general activity level — some people seem to have high-energy personalities, while others have more phlegmatic low-energy personalities. Either may be regarded as "natural," but nanomedicine can probably bring this ill-defined neurophysiological variable under human control. The need to sleep is another imperfectly understood syndrome. It is experienced by everyone and thus was universally regarded as "natural" in the 20th century. Physiological short sleepers[2122] were unusual, insomnia or asomnia[3273] was thought of as an abnormal state, and there were a few anecdotal but medically undocumented instances of total nonsomnia, such as the celebrated case of Al Herpin.[2312]

6. *Psychological Traits* — Psychological traits which, if identified by a patient as undesirable, might be subject to genetic or physiological modification could include: sexual preference (6-10% of the adult population is homosexual);[1604] shyness or boldness;[2332] acquisitive or altruistic propensity; misanthropy or philanthropy; theistic or atheistic orientation; loquacity or dourness; childhood imprinting; criminal propensity (up to 1-5% of the population); various recognized personality disorders that affect ~10% of the population[2122] such as antisocial, paranoid, schizotypal, histrionic, narcissistic, avoidant, dependent, obsessive-compulsive, and passive-aggressive disorders; panic attacks (experienced at least once by ~33% of all adults each year);[1604] and phobic disorders such as social phobias (~13% of the population), specific phobias including fear of large animals (zoophobia), snakes (ophidiophobia), spiders (arachnophobia), needles (belonephobia,[3272] ~10%), the dark (noctiphobia or scotophobia), or strangers (xenophobia) (total ~5.7%), the fear of blood or hemophobia (~5%), agoraphobia (~2.8%),[1604] and other unusual phobias[2223] such as the fears of certain colors (chromophobia), daylight (phengophobia), girls (parthenophobia), men (androphobia), stars in the sky (siderophobia), the number thirteen (triskaidekaphobia), and even the fear of developing a phobia (phobophobia).

The above sampling of minor afflictions, almost all considered "natural" in 1998, may come to be regarded as commonplace correctable medical conditions in the nanomedical era. By the time such petty annoyances are deemed worthy of immediate treatment, biotechnology and nanomedicine already will have defeated the most fearsome illnesses of the late 20th century[2310] and will have moved on to other challenges.[2311,2864,2973] Naturophiles may dissent, but the emerging trend from medical biotechnology is to characterize health, not as a static standard, but rather as a condition defined by the lives that people want to lead. Affirming the volitional normative model of disease (Section 1.2.2), Virginia Postrel concludes:[2299]

"Different goals will produce different choices about trade-offs and standards. What makes a condition unhealthy is not that it is unnatural but that it interferes with human purposes. Revering nature [would mean] sacrificing the purposes of individuals to preserve the world as given. It [would require] that we force people to live with biological conditions that trouble them, whether diseases such as cystic fibrosis or schizophrenia, disabilities such as myopia or crooked teeth, or simply less beauty, intelligence, happiness, or grace than could be achieved through artifice. In a world where it's no big deal to take hormone therapy, Viagra, or Prozac, to have a face lift, or to know a child's sex before birth, a world in which even such radical interventions as sex-change operations and heart transplants have failed to turn society upside down, it is extremely difficult to argue that medical innovations are dangerous simply because they fool Mother Nature."

1.4 Background and Brief Overview of This Book

The publication of *Nanosystems*[10] in 1992 laid a strong technical foundation for the field of molecular manufacturing. Such technology was already known to have major implications for medicine.[8,9] Still lacking, however, was an overview and synthesis of the interactions between molecular machine systems and living systems, particularly human living systems.

With *Nanosystems* as the intellectual cornerstone, research on *Nanomedicine*, originally intended to be a single volume, began in 1994. It quickly became clear that the field of nanomedicine would be even more interdisciplinary than molecular manufacturing, in part because of the many essential interfaces between mechanical nanosystems and living systems. This realization prompted ramification of the book into multiple volumes, allowing the field to be defined from diverse technical orientations. Additionally, the need to consider all major aspects of nanomedical device design and operations demanded a substantial increase in the intended length of the work, a regrettable but necessary circumstance for which the author apologizes in advance.

As a result, *Nanomedicine* has become a three-volume technical work with 31 chapters. Its intended audience is technical and professional people who are seriously interested in the future of medical technology. The three Volumes build upon each other cumulatively. The first Volume, now complete, describes basic capabilities common to all medical nanodevices, and the physical, chemical, thermodynamic, mechanical, and biological limits of such devices. Its primary audience is physical scientists, chemists, biochemists, and biomedical engineers engaged in basic research. The second Volume, still in progress, deals with aspects of device control and configuration, biocompatibility and safety issues, and basic nanomedical components and simple systems. Its primary audience is systems and control engineers, research physiologists, clinical laboratory analysts, biotechnologists, and biomedical engineers doing applied research. The third Volume, also in progress, discusses specific treatments for specific conditions and injuries, using nanomedical technology in the context of clinical (e.g. doctor-patient) situations. Its primary audience is clinical specialists and research physicians, and interested general practitioners.

The first molecular assemblers (Chapter 2) may be able to build only very simple nanomechanical systems, possibly only from very highly ordered substrates with significant rate-limiting intermediate steps, and only in very small numbers, so the earliest functional nanomachines may be laboratory curiosities. As assembler technology slowly improves, progressively more complex and capable nanomachines will be manufactured in vastly larger numbers. This book primarily investigates the rational design and operation of these more complex and capable nanomachines, and assumes that cubic centimeter quantities (e.g. ~10^{12} micron-sized nanorobots) will not be unreasonably expensive to manufacture (Section 2.4.2) and thus can be therapeutically deployed routinely by future doctors.

Volume I of *Nanomedicine, Basic Capabilities,* describes the set of basic capabilities of molecular machine systems that may be required by many, if not most, medical nanorobotic devices. These include the abilities to recognize, sort and transport important molecules (Chapter 3); sense the environment (Chapter 4); alter shape or surface texture (Chapter 5); generate onboard energy to power effective robotic functions (Chapter 6); communicate with doctors, patients, and other nanorobots (Chapter 7); navigate throughout the human body, i.e. determining somatographic or cytographic location within vessels, organs, tissues, or cells (Chapter 8); manipulate microscopic objects and move about inside a human body (Chapter 9); and timekeep, perform computations, disable living cells and viruses, and operate at various pressures and temperatures (Chapter 10).

Volume II of *Nanomedicine, Systems and Operations,* considers system-level technical requirements in the design and operation of medical nanodevices. Part 1 describes aspects of nanomedical operations and configurations, including scaling factors and general design principles (Chapter 11); control issues including teleoperation and haptic controllers, swarm motions, autogenous control systems, and various operational protocols (Chapter 12); repair, replacement, and reliability issues (Chapter 13); and molecular machine systems design issues such as tradeoffs between special-purpose and general purpose architectures, and deployment configurations such as nano-organs, medical utility fogs, and replicators (Chapter 14). Part 2 deals with a multitude of issues involving clinical safety and performance, specifically medical nanorobot biocompatibility including immunoreactivity and thrombogenicity (Chapter 15); methods of nanorobotic ingress and egress from the human body (Chapter 16); and possible nanodevice failure modes, environmental interactions, side effects of nanomedical treatments, iatrogenic factors, nanodevice software bugs, and other safety issues (Chapter 17). Part 3 summarizes various classes of medical nanosystems, including instruments, tools, and diagnostic systems (Chapter 18); specific medical nanorobot devices (Chapter 19); rapid mechanical reading and editing of chromatin and protein macromolecules (Chapter 20); and various complex nanorobotic systems that will make possible advanced cytopathology and cell repair, tissue and organ manufacturing, and personal defensive systems (Chapter 21).

Volume III of *Nanomedicine, Applications,* describes the full range of nanomedical applications which employ molecular nanotechnology inside the human body, from the perspective of a future practitioner in an era of widely available nanomedicine. Proof-of-concept designs for whole nanodevices, artificial nano-organs, and nanomedical treatments include rapid cardiovascular repair (Chapter 22); treatments for pathogenic disease and cancer, with epidemiological considerations (Chapter 23); responses to various physical traumas, burns and radiation exposures, and new methods of first aid, surgery, and emergency or critical care (Chapter 24); neurography, spinal restoration and brain repair (Chapter 25); improved nutrition and digestion (Chapter 26); sex, reproduction, and population issues (Chapter 27); cosmetics, recreation, veterinary and space medicine (Chapter 28); the control of aging processes, eliminating most causes of death prevalent in the 20th century, and strategies for biostasis (Chapter 29); and human augmentation systems (Chapter 30). The Volume concludes with a discussion of the sociology of nanomedicine, regulatory issues, nanotechnology implementation timelines, and some speculations on the future of hospitals, pharmaceutical companies, and the medical profession (Chapter 31).

CHAPTER 2

Pathways to Molecular Manufacturing

2.1 Is Molecular Manufacturing Possible?

Most contemporary industrial fabrication processes are based on "top-down" technologies, wherein small objects are sawn or machined from larger objects, or small features are imposed on larger objects, in either case by removing unwanted matter. The results of such processes may be small, such as micron-featured integrated circuits, or very large, such as jet aircraft, but in most cases the material is being processed in chunks far larger than molecular scale.

Molecular manufacturing, on the other hand, represents a "bottom-up" technology. Desired products will be built directly by "assembler" machines, molecule by molecule, making larger and larger objects with atomic precision. The results of such processes may also be very small or very large, much as biology builds both micron-sized bacteria and 100-meter tall sequoia trees. However, since assemblers add matter only where it is intended, little need be removed and hence there may be minimal waste during the process. By guiding with precision the assembly of molecules and supramolecular structures, such a manufacturing system could construct an extraordinarily wide range of products of unprecedented quality and performance.

In 1959, the Nobel physicist Richard P. Feynman[156] observed that:

> *"The principles of physics, as far as I can see, do not speak against the possibility of maneuvering things atom by atom. It is not an attempt to violate any laws; it is something, in principle, that can be done; but, in practice, it has not been done because we are too big . . . Ultimately, we can do chemical synthesis."*
>
> *"A chemist comes to us and says, "Look, I want a molecule that has the atoms arranged thus and so; make me that molecule." The chemist does a mysterious thing when he wants to make a molecule. He sees that it has got that ring, so he mixes this and that, and he shakes it, and he fiddles around. And, at the end of a difficult process, he usually does succeed in synthesizing what he wants."*
>
> *"But it is interesting that it would be, in principle, possible (I think) for a physicist to synthesize any chemical substance that the chemist writes down. Give the orders and the physicist synthesizes it. How? Put the atoms down where the chemist says, and so you make the substance. The problems of chemistry and biology can be greatly helped if our ability to see what we are doing, and to do things on an atomic level, is ultimately developed—a development which I think cannot be avoided."*

Nearly 40 years after Feynman's famous "Plenty of Room at the Bottom" speech, and a decade after Drexler's original proposal[8-10] for a bottom-up approach to machine-building using molecular assemblers, Nobel chemist Richard Smalley also largely agreed that this objective should prove feasible. Noted Smalley:[2389] "On a length scale of more than one nanometer, the mechanical robot assembler metaphor envisioned by Drexler almost certainly will work..."

Many skeptical questions arise when one first encounters the ideas of molecular nanotechnology and molecular assemblers (Section 2.4.2). It is useful to keep in mind the proven feasibility of such systems in the biological tradition (Section 1.3.2.1) over billions of years of natural evolution. In one sense, molecular nanotechnology will be a refinement and expansion upon how nature works at the molecular scale. Nature's examples, such as human beings, certainly answer the most basic skeptical questions, such as: Can macroscopic objects be built from molecular scale processes? (Yes, thanks to cellular replication.) Are molecular objects stable? (Of course; the human population alone contains $>10^{29}$ reasonably stable and quite functional ribosomal "nanomachines"). Observes Nobel chemist Jean-Marie Lehn:[765] "The chemist finds illustration, inspiration and stimulation in natural processes, as well as confidence and reassurance since they are proof that such highly complex systems can indeed be achieved on the basis of molecular components."

What about quantum effects? The uncertainty principle makes electron positions somewhat fuzzy, but the atom as a whole has a comparatively definite position set by the relatively great mass of the atomic nucleus. The quantum probability function of electrons in atoms tends to drop off exponentially with distance outside the atom, giving atoms a moderately sharp "edge". Mathematically, the positional uncertainty of a single carbon atom of mass $m_C = 2 \times 10^{-26}$ kg bound in a single C-C bond of stiffness[10] $k_C = 440$ N/m may be crudely estimated from the classical vibrational frequency $\nu_C = (k_C / m_C)^{1/2} = 1.5 \times 10^{14}$ Hz. This sets the zero-point vibrational bond energy $E_C = h \, \nu_C / 2 = 4.9 \times 10^{-20}$ J $= k_C \, \Delta X_C^2 / 2$ where $h = 6.63 \times 10^{-34}$ J-sec (Planck's constant) and $\Delta X_C \sim 0.015$ nm is the maximum classical amplitude of the bound carbon atom (roughly the same as the 3 dB point for the gaussian wavefunction, notes J. Soreff). Thus ΔX_C is just ~5% of the typical atomic electron cloud diameter of ~0.3 nm, imposing only a modest additional constraint on the fabrication and stability of nanomechanical structures. (Even in most liquids at their boiling points, each molecule is free to move only ~0.07 nm from its average position.)[2036]

How about the effects of Brownian bombardment on nanomachines? Describing a nanomechanical component as a harmonic oscillator embedded in a gas, Drexler[10] notes: "At equilibrium, an impinging gas molecule is as likely to absorb energy as to deliver it, and so molecular bombardment has no net effect on the amplitude of vibration. How a system is coupled to a thermal bath can affect its detailed dynamics, but not the statistical distribution of dynamical quantities." Nanomachines must also obey the laws of thermodynamics. Nanorobots cannot be used as a "Maxwell's demon"[2349,2350]—energy must be expended to do useful work; there can be no free lunch.[2611]

Will high-energy radiation damage nanomachines? Radiation can break chemical bonds and disrupt molecular machines.[8] The annual failure rate for a properly designed ~1 micron^3 molecular machine (containing many billions of atoms) can be made as low as several percent.[10] This estimate is derived from a consideration of all known thermal, photochemical, radiation, and other damage mechanisms, but the dominant error mechanism that appears difficult to substantially reduce is damage caused by background radiation. Failure rates are not zero, but are nonetheless remarkable by today's standards (Chapter 13), especially given error detection and correction at the module level.

During nanodevice fabrication, the problems of crossbonding and reactive intermediates pose additional constraints that must be dealt with using appropriate assembler designs. Specifically, assemblers with rigid positioning components operating in vacuo can restrict reactive intermediates and molecular tool tips to desired locations with a precision of at least ~0.1 nm (Section 9.3.1.4), or slightly less than an atomic diameter. Within the confines of an evacuated or "eutactic" assembler workspace, the location of every structural atom may be known to within the uncertainty created by thermal noise. Internal structural components may possess relatively high stiffness, so positional uncertainty caused by thermal noise may be small. In the classical analysis, positional variance $\Delta X^2 = kT / k_s$, where k = 1.381 x 10^{-21} J/kelvin (Boltzmann's constant), T is temperature in kelvins, and k_s is component stiffness, typically ≥10 N/m for nanometer-scale diamondoid components,[10] hence the standard deviation of component position is ~0.02 nm at room temperature, or ~0.01 nm at cryogenic (e.g., LN_2) temperatures. By employing sufficiently stiff mechanisms the position of every structural atom in the system can be known to within a fraction of an atomic diameter with high reliability and without the need for explicit positional sensing.* Steric tool hindrance—in molecular manufacturing, the conical volume occupied by a tool tip or manipulator platform—is a technical design problem that may be overcome by using sufficiently stiff tools or multi-tip tools, working in vacuo. Additionally, while some synthetic methods might involve the manipulation of individual atoms by appropriate tools, such as the hydrogen abstraction tool which removes a single selected hydrogen atom from a diamondoid surface (Section 2.3.3), other reactions will involve small clusters of atoms or larger molecular components (Section 2.4.1).

What about friction[2896] and wear among nanomechanical components? Properly designed molecular machines lack wear mechanisms, although other damage mechanisms remain.[2243] Dry bearings with atomically precise surfaces can have negligible static friction[3243] and wear, and very low dynamic friction or drag.[10] Nanomechanical components are better viewed as moving smoothly in a force field than as sliding subject to friction. For example, total drag power dissipated by an isolated molecular sleeve bearing of radius 2 nm spinning at 1 MHz is dominated by band-stiffness scattering, amounting to ≤0.000004 picowatts (pW) (Eqn. 6.4), very small compared to the 1-1000 pW power draw that will be typical of micron-size medical nanorobots (Section 6.5.3). The strong precise surfaces of nanomachines experience no change during a typical operational cycle, hence zero wear. Within the single-point failure model (Chapter 13), the first step in a wear process (e.g., a dislocated atom) is regarded as fatal, hence cumulative wear plays no role in determining device lifetimes.[10] In eutactic nanomachines, contaminants of all kinds are rigorously excluded. The equivalent of wear particles cannot appear until the device has failed. On this scale, repulsive fields provide "lubrication" and an oil molecule would be a contaminant object, not a lubricant.

The general conclusion is that molecular nanotechnology violates no physical laws. In 1998, it was generally accepted that molecular nanotechnology will be developed, although there remains some disagreement about how long it will take. To progress from today's limited capabilities to the complex nanorobots described later in this trilogy will clearly require a great deal of research and development effort. Still, the proper question is no longer "if" but "when." This Chapter presents a few of the many possible technical paths leading to a working molecular assembler that were being discussed in 1998. The reader is strongly urged to consult the most current literature for the latest results. Section 2.2 briefly summarizes the conventional top-down approaches to nanotechnology. Section 2.3 describes several possible direct bottom-up pathways to molecular manufacturing including biotechnology, supramolecular chemistry, and scanning probes. Gimzewski and Joachim[3200] note that "bottom-up approaches to nanofabrication may one day compete with conventional top-down approaches in providing nanotechnologies for the next millenium. Top-down refers to increasing miniaturization through extension of existing microfabrication schemes, [whereas] the bottom-up scenario is one of ever-increasing complexity at the molecular level while maintaining control on an atom-by-atom basis". Section 2.4 surveys molecular mechanical components and design work on molecular assemblers and molecular manufacturing systems from the perspective of 1998.

2.2 Top-Down Approaches to Nanotechnology

Nanotechnology was first proposed by Nobel physicist Richard Feynman in December 1959, in a talk[156] in which he also issued a seemingly "impossible" challenge to build a working electric motor no larger than a 1/64th-inch (400-micron) cube, backed by a $1000 prize to spur interest in the new field. Just 11 months later, engineer William McLellan had constructed a 250-microgram 2000-rpm motor out of 13 separate parts and collected his reward.[300,355] (McLellan's entire motor is only as big as the period at the end of this sentence.)[355] In 1995, a $250,000 Feynman Grand Prize (Section 2.4.2) was made available, this time sponsored by the Foresight Institute, for any engineer who could build the first programmable nanometer-scale robotic arm. How long will it take for history to repeat?

In his famous 1959 talk, Feynman proposed the prototypical top-down strategy for building complex nanomachinery—essentially a completely teleoperated machine shop, including mills, lathes, drills, presses, cutters, and the like, plus master-slave grippers to allow the human operator to move parts and materials around the workshop.

To build a nanomachine using Feynman's scheme, the operator first directs a macroscale machine shop to fabricate an exact copy of itself, but four times smaller in size. After this work is done, and all machines are verified to be working properly and as expected, the reduced-scale machine shop would be used to build a copy of itself, another factor of four smaller but a factor of 16 tinier[156] than the original machine shop. This process of fabricating progressively smaller machine shops proceeds until a machine shop capable of manipulations at the nanoscale is produced. The final result is a nanomachine shop capable of reconstructing itself, or of producing

Medical nanorobots may be built to atomic precision, but once built and deployed such devices often will not perform molecularly precise movements during normal functions and may frequently rely upon sensor-based motion control; Section 9.3.3.

any other useful nanoscale output product stream that is physically possible to manufacture, using molecular feedstock.

As Feynman describes the process:[156]

> *"When I make my first set of slave hands at one-fourth scale, I am going to make ten sets. I make ten sets of hands, and I wire them to my original levers so they each do exactly the same thing at the same time in parallel. Now, when I am making my new devices one-quarter again as small, I let each one manufacture ten copies, so that I would have a hundred hands at the 1/16th size.... If I made a billion little lathes, each 1/4000th the scale of a regular lathe, there are plenty of materials and space available because in the billion little ones there is less than two percent of the materials in one big lathe. It doesn't cost anything for materials, you see. So I want to build a billion tiny factories, models of each other, which are manufacturing simultaneously, drilling holes, stamping parts, and so on."*

> *"As we go down in size, there are a number of interesting problems that arise. All things do not simply scale down in proportion. There is the problem that materials stick together by the molecular (van der Waals) attractions. There will be several problems of this nature that we will have to be ready to design for.... [But] if we go down far enough, all of our devices can be mass produced so that they are absolutely perfect copies of one another. We cannot build two large machines so that the dimensions are exactly the same. But if your machine is only 100 atoms high, you only have to get it correct to one-half of one percent to make sure the other machine is exactly the same size—namely, 100 atoms high!"*

Progress is being made on Feynman's top-down approach in a relatively new engineering field known as Micro Electro-Mechanical Systems or MEMS, originally an extension of chip-etch technology rather than micromanipulation. Conventional purely-electronic devices fabricated on silicon chips with ~0.2 micron features must be coupled to external systems to produce mechanical effects, but MEMS devices integrate mechanical components directly with electrical circuitry. Thus while microelectronic chips merely route electrons, microelectromechanical systems give the electronics immediate access to control applications, enabling single microdevices to interact directly with the physical world.

Generic microsystems research has proven to be a rewarding activity for two decades, with each successively smaller motor or machine widely publicized.[2865] The field gathered momentum after the first working micromotors were demonstrated in the late 1980s by groups at Berkeley and MIT. By 1990, tiny electrostatic motors with 100-micron rotors displayed operating speeds of ~250 Hz[556] and operating lifetimes of ~10^6 revolutions.[2363] A new *Journal of Micromechanics and Microengineering* appeared in 1991, followed by the *Journal of Microelectromechanical Systems* in 1992 and the first MEMS Application Symposium in Tokyo in June 1996. By the mid-1990s, Sandia's Microelectronics Development Laboratory,[2356] one of the most prominent vendors of micromachines, could mass-produce planar micromechanical devices smaller than ~1 mm^2, incorporating motors with gears and cogs each no thicker than a human hair and turning at speeds of >4000 Hz. Wobble micromotors such as those fabricated in silicon by the University of Utah's micromachine lab demonstrated very little friction or abrasion, with measured operating lifetimes in excess of 300 million revolutions.[2366] (Diamond coatings could further reduce friction by an order of magnitude over silicon,[2545] and the wear rate of polycrystalline diamond is known to be ~10^4 times lower than for silicon.)[2852]

MEMS research has produced multi-micron-scale accelerometers,[2382-2384] diverse microsensors (e.g., blood pressure microsensors attached to cardiac catheters), microscale cantilevers and jointed crank mechanisms,[2380] 5-micron barbs,[2371] flow microvalves and pressure microtransducers,[544,2373] micropistons and micropumps,[2373] microgear trains,[2379] microactuators[545] and piezo-driven micromotors,[2381] micromirrors and microshutters,[546,1062,1974] Fresnel lens microarrays,[2374] microgyroscopes,[1383] a 2-mm long combustion chamber suitable for turbine use[2377] (making possible a 1 cm^3 gas-turbine generator that would deliver 50 W of power or 0.2 N of thrust),[2378] and multidevice microsystems[2372] that were available customized or off-the-shelf in mass quantities by 1998. Laser beams[2375] and ion beams[2376] were used to carve ~300-micron diameter gears with 50-micron wide teeth in solid diamond. Microelectrodeposition and microcontact printing readily produced topologically complex 3-D microstructures with 1-10 micron feature sizes.[2364] Colloidal templating yielded 0.7-1 micron diameter hollow silica spheres with wall thicknesses from tens to hundreds of nanometers,[2368] 10-25 nm trenches,[2357] or 4-nm thick graphite sheet layers tiled on spherical surfaces ~0.2 microns in diameter.[2369] A CAD/CAM desktop micromanufacturing system invented at Lincoln Laboratory in Lexington, MA, machined three-dimensional structures, including spheres, in silicon, using computer-controlled laser/chemical etching of cubic-micron voxels at the rate of ~20,000 voxels/sec.[2367]

By 1998, smaller (~100 nm) accelerometers were being developed by such companies as Analog Devices in the U.S. and Daimler-Benz in Germany, and electronic control systems such as microswitches and microrelays were available commercially from several companies including Integrated Micromachines of California. Micromachining was a well-developed engineering discipline.[2696] Westinghouse Science and Technology Center used MEMS sensors to build a miniaturized mass spectrometer. Micro-opto-mechanical systems were under development. Chemists were proposing[121] and building[1222,1228] Integrated Chemical Synthesizers consisting of millimeter to micron-sized chemical reactors, designed for specific applications, along with associated devices for moving reactant and product streams (pumps), mixing reactants (reaction chambers), analyzing streams, and separating products (separation chambers), constructed conventionally using silicon substrates and photolithographic techniques to form the desired structures but also utilizing the high selectivity of biological molecules such as enzymes and antibodies to fabricate sensors. MEMS had also led to the development of microgrippers that could manipulate individual 2.7-micron polystyrene spheres, dried red blood cells of similar size, and various protozoa.[1267] Market Intelligence Research Corp. of Mountain View, CA, estimated a total worldwide budget for micromachine research and development of $995 million in 1992 and over $3 billion by 1998.[357] Systems Planning Corporation of Arlington, VA, projected that the microsystems industry could be worth more than $14 billion annually by 2001.[1259]

Some MEMS research followed surprising directions. For example, in the mid-1990s MEMS engineers at the University of Tokyo Department of Mechanical Engineering fabricated an 8-hinge, 8-plate wing microstructure capable of independent flight through the air.[1573-1576,2353] The structure was fabricated by traditional silicon micromachining techniques and was then released from the wafer surface, with the initially flat sections lifted into flight position using a micromanipulation system with glass probes several microns in diameter. Each wing was ~500 microns square; applying 300 VAC at 10 KHz caused resonant vibration and the flapping amplitude of the wings exceeded 30°.[2353] In another 4-wing configuration,[1574] the flapping resonance frequency was ~150 Hz and the device freely flew up and down a thin glass pole when placed in an alternating electromagnetic field. Another bi-wing design made of magnetized nickel coated silicon measuring 2000 x 10,000 microns successfully flew without power supply cables and guides in the manner of a butterfly or mosquito, when an alternating magnetic field strength of >400 oersted and 12 Hz was applied;[1576] a similar device with 320 x 800 micron wings also flew in a 300 Hz magnetic field.[1575] "If we release the silicon mosquito from the silicon chip, it flies off and we cannot find it again," complained researcher H. Miura. "It's very small, like dust." MEMS "gnat robots" have also been described.[1250]

Using electron-beam (e-beam) lithography, in 1997 researchers at the Cornell University Nanofabrication Facility built what they believed were the world's smallest mechanical devices, including a 4-micron-wide Fabry-Perot interferometer and, just for fun, the world's smallest guitar, carved out of crystalline silicon and no larger than a single human cell.[2354] The "nanoguitar" was 10 microns long and 2 microns wide, with six strings each ~50 nm (~200 atoms) wide that would probably resonate at >10-100 MHz if plucked. Presentation of the nanoguitar enthralled the public, surprising at least one Cornell researcher (in another lab) who remarked that "anyone with a sufficiently advanced e-beam lithography system could make it. I make 50 nanometer silicon objects routinely. Doesn't seem like a big deal to me, but evidently most people have no idea what we're capable of these days."

Direct-write e-beam lithography uses a tightly-focused beam of electrons, steered by electromagnetic deflectors, to trace out patterns on a wafer resist surface. The electrons chemically alter the resist, which is then etched away, leaving the desired pattern. By 1998, e-beam spot sizes had been focused to less than 1 nm, and 5-nm beam widths were routine, although forward scattering of the electrons imposed a limit of resist exposure resolution of ~10 nm for e-beams[2358] and ~5 nm for focused ion beams.[1259] E-beam writing times were very slow—for example, 80 hours were required to carve a single photolithography mask for a 1G DRAM, though much of this time was required for proximity calculations by the AI (artificial intelligence) software [E.A. Rietman, personal communication, 1999] (a better approach is to use a neural net).[3012] By 1998, an electron interferometer containing atomically smooth mirrors spaced a few atomic layers apart had been fabricated,[3183] and in 1999, careful electron-energy-loss spectroscopy experiments revealed that silicon dioxide must be at least 4 atoms (~0.7 nm) thick to act as a conventional electrical insulator.[3295]

Atom lithography, employing a low-energy neutral atomic beam (usually Na or Cr) cooled and collimated by optical molasses, then concentrated at the nodes of the standing wave formed by the superposition of a laser beam and its reflection, was predicted also eventually to allow surface deposition of 5-10 nm features.[2355,2370,2838-2841] The first directional atomic beam (of sodium) with a ~0.002 radian beamspread and ~femtogram pulses (~26 million atoms, or ~(100 nm)^3, per pulse) was demonstrated in early 1999, with one commentator noting that "the longer dream...is atomic holography...[that] could combine beams of atoms to build a 3D solid object".[3173] At the same time, another group achieved a continuous stream of rubidium atoms lasting up to ~0.1 sec in duration, with a beam radius potentially as small as ~1 nm.[3205] Current-carrying wires have been used to guide cold lithium atoms "just as optical fibers guide light";[3182] the first curved focusing atom mirror also was demonstrated in early 1999.[2925] By 1998, the speculative possibility of quantum-mechanical micromanipulation also had been described.[6]

Other approaches offered comparable results. For instance, engineers at the University of Minnesota NanoStructure Laboratory used nanoimprint lithography (NIL) in 1996 to etch out patterns of lines, grooves and circles as small as 25 nanometers in a polymer,[2357] and by 1998 NIL had been demonstrated in nanoscale quantum-wire, quantum-dot, and ring transistors with feature sizes below 10 nm.[2358] Nanochannel array glasses containing 33-nm capillaries arranged in a 2-D hexagonal close packing configuration at a number density of ~300/micron^2 had been available since 1992.[2365]

Thus by 1998, top-down MEMS techniques could in theory already make nanoscale (though not atomically precise) parts. Might these techniques also produce assemblies of such parts, creating complex machines? Very simple mobile robots of ~1 cm^3 volume were commonplace,[2361,2362] so for a more challenging demonstration of MEMS' ability to manufacture complete working microrobots, in 1994 Japanese researchers at Nippondenso Co., Ltd. fabricated a 1/1000th-scale working electric car.[2351,2352] As small as a grain of rice, the micro-car was a 1/1000-scale replica of the Toyota Motor Corp's first automobile, the 1936 Model AA sedan (Fig. 2.1). The tiny vehicle incorporated 24 parts, including tires, wheels, axles, headlights and taillights, bumpers, a spare tire, and hubcaps carrying the company name inscribed in microscopic letters, all manually assembled using a mechanical micromanipulator of the type generally used for cell handling in biological research (Chapter 21). In part because of this handcrafting, each microcar cost more to build than a full-size modern luxury automobile.

The Nippondenso microcar was 4800 microns long, 1800 microns wide, and 1800 microns high, consisting of a chassis, a shell body, and a 5-part electromagnetic step motor measuring 700 microns in diameter with a ~0.07-tesla magnet penetrated by an axle 150 microns thick and 1900 microns long. Power was supplied through thin (18 micron) copper wires, carrying 20 mA at 3 volts. The motor developed a peak torque of 1.3 x 10^{-6} N-m (mean 7 x 10^{-7} N-m) at a mean frequency of ~100 Hz (peak frequency ~700 Hz), propelling the car forward across a level surface at a top speed of 10 cm/sec. Some internal wear of the rotating parts was visible after ~2000 sec of continuous operation; the addition of ~0.1 microgram of lubricant to the wheel microbearings caused the mechanism to seize due to lubricant viscosity. The microcar body was a 30-micron thick 20-milligram shell, fabricated with features as small as ~2 microns using modeling and casting, N/C machine cutting, mold etching, submicron diamond-powder polishing, and nickel and gold plating processes. Measured average roughness of machined and final polished surfaces was 130 nm and 26 nm, respectively. The shell captured all features as small as 2 mm on the original full-size automobile body. Each tire was 690 microns in

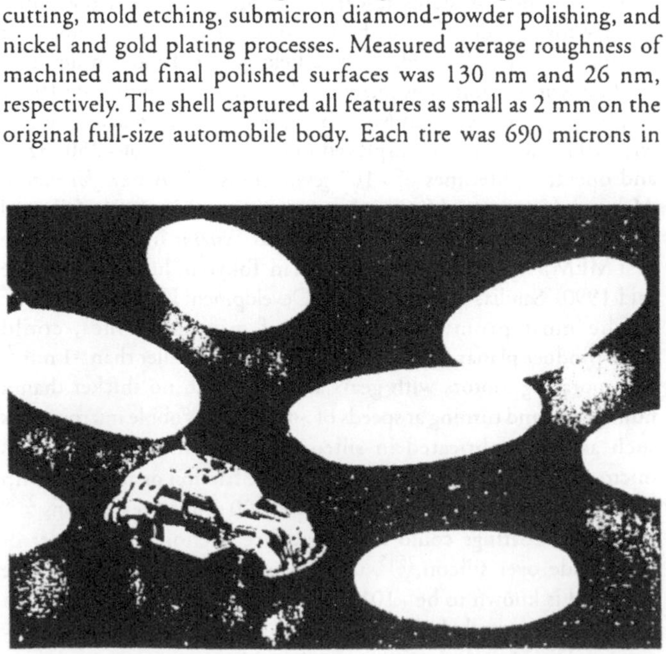

Fig. 2.1. The Nippondenso Microcar—smaller than a grain of rice. (Photo courtesy of Nippondenso Co., Ltd.)[2352]

diameter and 170 microns wide. The license plate was 10 microns thick, 380 microns wide and 190 microns high. Nippondenso subsequently used similar manufacturing techniques to build a prototype of a capsule intended to crawl through tiny pipes in a power plant or chemical plant like an inchworm, hunting for cracks. In 1999, three Japanese electronics companies announced the creation of a 0.42-gram, 5-mm long "ant size" robot reportedly able to lift 0.8-gram loads and to move at ~2 mm/sec, as part of the government's ongoing Micro Machine Project.[3258]

By 1998, micromanipulators with high placement precision had been demonstrated in various laboratories around the world. For example, the Spider-II micromanipulation robot employed bimorphic piezoactuators within a 260-micron cubic work volume and a three-axis gripper placement accuracy of 8 nm.[2359] A microassembly robot using stick-and-slip actuators had 5-nm resolution over a 200-nm scanning range with a maximum speed of 4 mm/sec and 0.4% repeatability at 10 KHz, delivering a maximum driving force of 155 mN and rigidity of 6.3 N/micron.[2360]

In terms of system size, micromachined MEMS devices (typically ~10^{-13} m^3 in volume) lie exactly intermediate between the macroscale world (~10^{-4} m^3) and the nanoscale world (~10^{-22} m^3). The medical nanorobots described in this book generally will have dimensions, precisions, and component part sizes ~1000-fold smaller than the Nippondenso microcar, which itself was, in turn, ~1000-fold smaller than a macroscale automobile. It is difficult to see how MEMS techniques involving statistical materials deposition and removal could fabricate parts to better than ~10 nm feature sizes or tolerances, or could position parts during assembly to much better than ~10 nm spatial resolution, nor does it appear likely that MEMS techniques, on their own, can manufacture or position any structure to atomic precision. However, this does not rule out the possible use of MEMS techniques to fabricate crude useful parts for subsequent "finishing" to atomic precision by other techniques, or to facilitate the assembly of nanoscale components (of atomic precision or otherwise) that have been fabricated or subassembled by other means (Section 2.3).

2.3 Bottom-Up Pathways to Molecular Manufacturing

To manufacture machines of any kind generally requires two primary capabilities—fabrication of parts, and assembly of parts. As will be shown below, by 1998 at least a primitive parts fabrication and parts assembly capability had been demonstrated at the molecular level using three different enabling technologies:[2889] biotechnology (Section 2.3.1), supramolecular chemistry (Section 2.3.2), and scanning probes (Section 2.3.3). This Section reviews the most preliminary steps and basic approaches to molecular manufacturing. Consideration of more complex nanoscale components and assemblies is deferred to Section 2.4. The primary focus here is on bridging technologies that may lie between what can already be done and what is desired to be done—specifically, the manufacture of mechanical nanorobots. The reader is again cautioned that in 1998 this field was experiencing an explosion of interest and pathbreaking research efforts, so the current literature should be consulted for the latest results.

2.3.1 Biotechnology

The first broad category of enabling technology for molecular manufacturing in the mechanical tradition is biotechnology.[10,322] Molecular biologists study and modify systems of molecular machines, and genetic engineers reprogram these systems, sometimes to build novel molecular objects having complex functions. By 1998, biotechnologists could make almost any DNA sequence or polypeptide chain desired (though not extremely long aperiodic ones), assemble "devices" such as artificial chromosomes and viruses, and were actively pursuing gene therapy, all of which are examples of molecular engineering. While earlier writers had suggested that biomolecules could be used as mechanical components,[2414] Drexler[182] evidently was the first to point out, in 1981, that complex devices resembling biomolecular motors, actuators, bearings, and structural components could be combined to build versatile molecular machine systems analogous to machine systems in the macroscopic world (Table 1.3). "Development of the ability to design protein molecules," Drexler wrote, "will open a path to the fabrication of devices to complex atomic specifications, thus sidestepping obstacles facing conventional microtechnology. This path will involve construction of molecular machinery able to position reactive groups to atomic precision."

Perhaps the best-known biological example of such molecular machinery is the ribosome (Fig. 2.2; see also Section 8.5.3.4), the only freely programmable nanoscale assembler already in existence.* In nature, ~8000 nm^3 ribosomes act as general-purpose factories building diverse varieties of proteins by bonding amino acids together in precise sequences under instructions provided by a strand of messenger RNA (mRNA) copied from the host DNA, powered by the decomposition of adenosine triphosphate (ATP) to adenosine diphosphate (ADP). Each ribosome is a compact ribonucleoprotein particle consisting of two subunits, with each subunit consisting of

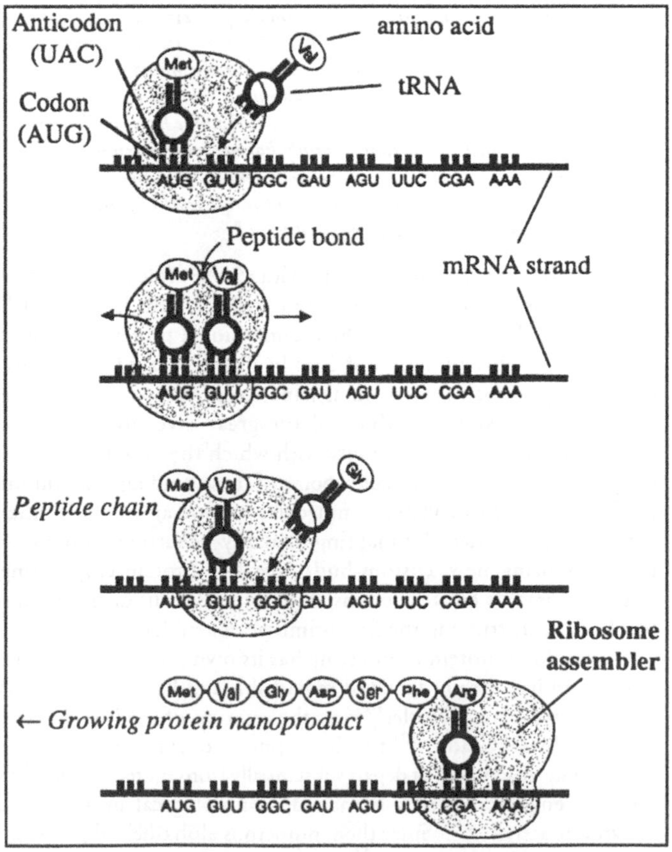

Fig. 2.2. The ribosome acts as a programmable nanoscale assembler of protein nanoproducts (redrawn from Ball[382]).

D. Heidel notes that there are three distinct types of ribosome—eubacterial, archaebacterial and eukaryotic—and multiple subvarieties among the ~10^8 different species on Earth; additionally, other bioassembler units such as poly-ketide synthetases[3224] also exist but these enzymes generally only make one type of product per assembly.

several proteins associated with a long RNA molecule (rRNA). Biotechnology can employ the ribosomal machinery of bacteria to produce novel proteins, which proteins then might serve as components of larger molecular structures.[182]

Of course, such biological mechanisms have been disparaged as "slip-shod devices working in spite of haphazard design." Dan Heidel, a University of Washington biomimetics engineer, agrees that biological systems are sloppy but observes that they are designed to tolerate it, and offers high praise for the lowly ribosome:

"The average ribosome sits in an aqueous environment surrounded by thousands of cosolutes at concentrations just a hair's breadth from precipitating out of solution. The ribosome itself consists of three RNA molecules that spontaneously fold into floppy spaghetti noodle piles of chemically active groups surrounded by >50 proteins of similarly dubious structure. The other solutes are bombarding this motley assemblage at tens to hundreds of miles an hour and the solvating water molecules are a constantly shifting and unpredictable network of hydrogen bonds and polar ionic charges constantly impinging upon the ribosome. The ribosome must recognize one particular cognate transfer RNA (tRNA) for the codon in its A-site out of ~60 other nearly identical tRNAs. This particular tRNA must be discriminated from all its tRNA brethren along with whatever other solutes can fit into the A-site pocket using only three base pairs for discrimination. In fact, most codons use only two of the three base pairs for recognition so some tRNAs are recognized by as few as 4 hydrogen bonds. All of this requires sub-Angstrom precision in the active sites but since the ribosome is a massive complex of sub-units held together by only ionic, hydrogen, hydrophobic and Van der Waals bonds, it's like getting sub-millimeter accuracy from points on a bunch of taped-together water balloons being rolled down a staircase."

"This ridiculous machine can assemble proteins at a 20 Hz subunit-incorporation frequency with a 10^{-3} error rate. Ribosomes are even more impressive when one considers that the number of amino acids in each ribosome's own protein subunits combined with the 10^{-3} protein assembly error rate ensures that each ribosome has several errors in it and that each cell almost certainly has no two ribosomes exactly alike. I dare any engineer on this planet to rationally design an assembler at any scale that is able to operate at a comparable level of performance under similarly adverse operating conditions."

Thus ribosomes can manufacture, with >99.9% fidelity to arbitrary specifications, linear strings of amino acids of great length which may then fold up to produce three-dimensional protein structures performing a broad range of highly differentiated functions, providing good analogs for working nanomachines capable of forming self-assembling systems. Much of the great diversity of protein activity flows from the selectivity with which they bind to specific receptor sites on other molecules. Some of these binding mechanisms might be copied to construct molecular robotic arms, while other devices could be made by adapting naturally-occurring proteins, or by synthesizing new, custom-built ones.[2393] Protein engineering might be used to create proteins with desired qualities as building blocks for constructing the first primitive assemblers.

The field of protein engineering has its own journal of the same name, and has already achieved remarkable results in the synthesis of novel structures. Drexler[10] cites the creation of the first de novo structure by DeGrado,[2394] the development of synthetic branched protein-like structures that depart substantially from protein models,[2395] and the engineering of a branched, nonbiological protein with enzymatic activity.[2396] Since then, numerous alpha-helical peptides* have been designed de novo,[2410-2413] a 20-residue artificial peptide exhibiting designed beta-sheet secondary structure has been created,[2398] and various peptide analogs have also been synthesized.[2399] By 1998, advances in computational techniques allowed the design of precise side-chain packing in proteins with naturally occurring backbone structures, and the study of de novo backbone structures had begun.[2400] The catalytic task space[766] was being laboriously investigated at the molecular level—for example, one study of comparative enzyme structures revealed that changing as few as four amino acids converted an oleate 12-desaturase to an oleate hydroxylase, and as few as six substitutions could convert an oleate hydroxylase into an oleate desaturase.[2401] To further expand the toolkit, Mills[2431] and Fahy[322] proposed exploiting the degeneracy of the genetic code (wherein amino acids are specified by up to 6 different codons; Chapter 20) by assigning some codons to unnatural amino acids, allowing the creation of artificial proteins with unprecedented structural or catalytic properties. With 61 usable codons available, there is room for up to 41 novel amino acids in addition to the natural 20 amino acids; unnatural amino acids have been introduced into beta-lactamase and T4 lysozyme enzymes in a site-directed fashion, using artificial tRNAs and mRNAs in an in vitro translation system,[2402,2403] and into an engineered peptide as a reporter group.[2412] Additionally, artificial novel base pairs can be incorporated enzymatically into DNA[2404,2607,2932] and other schemes are possible.[2676] By incorporating one additional base pair, the number of possible codons is expanded from $4^3 = 64$ codons to $6^3 = 216$ codons, potentially allowing up to 193 novel amino acids to be incorporated into artificial protein structures—or at least 48 new amino acids assuming that present levels of redundancy are retained and the existing 4-letter code is kept as a subset for "upward compatibility".[2431] If the genetic alphabet is increased to eight bases ($8^3 = 512$ codons), the number of available codons for novel amino acid-like molecules increases to as many as 489.[322]

One of the greatest challenges in protein engineering (where one objective is to create functional, atomically-precise 3-D aperiodic structures) has been the difficulty of protein fold design, because individual amino acids have no strong, natural complementarity.[2392] In 1998, Duan and Kollman[2324] successfully folded a solvated 36-residue (~12,000-atom) protein fragment (i.e., a peptide) by molecular dynamics simulation into a structure that resembles an intermediate native state. During a 1-microsec simulation, the chain folded during 150 nanosec into a compact structure resembling the intermediate native state, as known by NMR, then unfolded and refolded again for a shorter period. In 1998, whole-protein folding to the final stable native state had not yet been computed deterministically using molecular dynamics—the real protein will fold and refold hundreds of times before it stumbles into the stable conformation with the lowest free energy[2405]—but research pursuing this objective was active and ongoing.[2406,2407] Structural changes that occur during protein function (e.g., enzymatic action) were also being avidly studied.[2408]

A different protein-based approach to near-atomically-precise 3-D structures avoids the folding problem by making use of semi-rigid protein nanoshells of deterministic size and shape to guide the ordered assembly of inorganic particles. For example, the capsid of the cowpea chlorotic mottle virus, a protein container with a 28-nm external diameter and an 18-nm internal cavity diameter, is composed of 180 identical coat protein subunits arranged on an icosahedral lattice. Each subunit presents at least nine basic residues (arginine and lysine) to the interior of the cavity, creating a positively charged interior surface which provides an interface for inorganic crystal nucleation and growth, while the outer capsid surface is not highly charged. In one experiment,[2391] the empty capsid shell was found to act as a spatially selective nucleation catalyst in paratungstate mineralization, in addition to its role as a size- and shape-constrained

*Chains of amino acids shorter than ~100 residues are customarily called peptides; longer chains are proteins.

reaction vessel. Noted the authors: "The range of viral morphology and size allow great flexibility for adapting this methodology to control the size and shape of the entrapped material, which is limited only by access to the protein interior and could include inorganic and organic species. The electrostatic environment within the cavity could be altered by site-directed mutagenesis to induce additional specific interactions."

It may also be possible to borrow various existing protein devices (Table 1.3) and apply them to new uses. The bacteriophage DNA injection system (Section 9.2.4) is self-assembling and could be engineered for other applications. Vogel[2425,2426] has attached kinesin motors to flat surfaces in straight grooves; when ATP was added, the motors were activated, passing 25-nm wide microtubules hand over hand down the line in the manner of a ciliary array (Section 9.3.4). Montemagno[2278,2426] genetically engineered the 12-nm wide ATPase molecular rotary motor so that one end would adhere to a metal surface and the other end would provide an attachment site for 1-micron fluorescent streptavidin-coated bead payloads. When ATP was added, each bead individually attached to a biomotor in the motor array began twirling at ~10 Hz, generating a >100 pN force. Bead rotation was maintained continuously for more than 2 hours, indicating the high reliability of these ~100% efficient self-assembling biomotors. Montemagno explains that his laboratory's "long-term goal is the integration of the F_1-ATPase biological motor with nano-electromechanical systems (NEMS) to create a new class of hybrid nanomechanical devices." Other natural nanomotors such as the self-assembling bacterial flagellar motor[578-581] and the hexagonal "packaging RNA" or pRNA pumping mechanism that packs DNA into the capsid shell of the bacteriophage Phi 29[1723] are also being intensively studied.

Yet another material which allows moderately well-defined three-dimensional nanoassemblies is DNA. The ideas behind DNA nanotechnology have been around since 1980,[2414] but activity in this field accelerated in the 1990s after numerous experimental difficulties were surmounted. Horn and Urdea[2606] reported branched and forked DNA polymers. Niemeyer[1905] and Smith[2430] exploited DNA specificity to generate regular protein arrays, and both[2430,2444,2544] suggested using self-assembled DNA as an early material for molecular nanotechnology. Shi and Bergstrom[2416] attached DNA single strands to rigid organic linkers, showing that cyclical forms of various sizes could be formed with these molecules. Mirkin's group[1904] attached DNA molecules to 13-nm colloidal gold particles with ~6 nm particle spacings, with the goal of assembling nanoparticles into macroscopic materials; Alivisatos, Schultz and colleagues[2415] used DNA to organize 1.4-nm gold nanocrystals in arrays with 2-10 nm spacings. In either case, the specificity of DNA pairing should allow the construction of complex geometries since the use of colloidal particles can potentially add structural elements (which are more rigid than any polymer strand) to the set of building blocks for nanometer-scale structures—although to take full advantage of this capability would require particles which are atomically precise and which possess several chemically distinct anchoring points on each particle. Damha has synthesized V-shaped and Y-shaped branched RNA molecules,[2566,2567] branching RNA dendrimers with "forked" and "lariat" shaped RNA intermediates,[2568] and even trihelical DNA.[2569] Henderson and coworkers[2706,2707] have designed a simple DNA decamer that can form an extended linear staggered quadruplex array reaching lengths of >1000 nm, and have made branched oligonucleotides that template the synthesis of their branched "G-wires"; depending on the ratio of linear to branched building blocks, extensive DNA arrays with differing connectivities but irregular interstices can be created.[2704]

In 1998 the most intensive work on three-dimensional engineered DNA structures was taking place in Nadrian Seeman's laboratory in the New York University Department of Chemistry. Seeman originally conceived the idea of rigid 3-D DNA structures in the early 1980s,[2414,2419] while examining DNA strands that had arranged themselves into unusual four-armed Holliday junctions.[3154] Seeman recognized that DNA had many advantages as a construction material for nanomechanical structures.[1916] First, each double-strand DNA with a single-strand overhang has a "sticky end," so the intermolecular interaction between two strands with sticky ends is readily programmed (due to base-pair specificity) and reliably predicted, and the local structure at the interface is known (sticky ends associate to form B-DNA). Second, arbitrary sequences are readily manufactured using conventional biotechnological techniques. Third, DNA can be manipulated and modified by a large variety of enzymes, including DNA ligase, restriction endonucleases, kinases and exonucleases. Fourth, DNA is a stiff polymer in 1-3 turn lengths[2421] and has an external code that can be read by proteins and nucleic acids.[2422]

During the 1980s, Seeman worked to develop strands of DNA that would zip themselves up into more and more complex shapes. Seeman made junctions with five and six arms, then squares,[2417] stick-figure cubes comprised of 480 nucleotides,[1914] and a truncated octahedron containing 2550 nucleotides and a molecular weight of ~790,000 daltons.[1915] The cubes (Fig. 2.3) were synthesized in solution, but Seeman switched to a solid-support-based methodology[2418] in 1992, greatly improving control by allowing construction of one edge at a time and isolating the growing objects from one another, allowing massively parallel construction of objects with far greater control of the synthesis sequence. By the mid-1990s, most Platonic (tetrahedron, cube, octahedron, dodecahedron, and icosahedron), Archimedean (e.g., truncated Platonics, semiregular prisms and prismoids, cuboctahedron, etc.), Catalan (linked rings and complex knots), and irregular polyhedra could be constructed as nanoscale DNA stick figures.

Seeman's DNA strands that formed the frame figures were strong enough to serve as girders in a molecular framework, but the junctions were too floppy. In 1993 Seeman discovered the more rigid antiparallel DNA "double crossover" motif,[1920] which in 1996 he used to design and build a stiff double junction to keep his structures from sagging.[2420] The next goal was to bring together a large number of stick figures to form large arrays or cage-shaped DNA crystals that could then be used as frameworks for the assembly of other molecules into pre-established patterns. These DNA molecules would serve as the scaffolding upon which new materials having precise molecular structure could be assembled.

In 1998, Erik Winfree and colleagues in Seeman's laboratory reported the design and construction of two-dimensional DNA crystals using self-assembling double crossover molecules.[1970] Repeating array units were approximately 2 nm x 4 nm x 16 nm in size, and examination of the array with an Atomic Force Microscope (AFM) revealed domains of up to 500,000 interconnected units, showing that the self-assembly process (Section 2.3.2) could be very reliable under ideal conditions. While the work described the construction of two- and four-unit lattices, the number of component tiles that could be used in the repeat unit did not appear to be limited to such small numbers, suggesting that complex patterns could be assembled into periodic arrays, which might also serve as templates for nanomechanical assembly. Noted the authors: "Because oligonucleotide synthesis can readily incorporate modified bases at arbitrary positions, it should be possible to control the structure within the periodic group by decoration with chemical groups, catalysts, enzymes and other proteins, metallic nanoclusters,

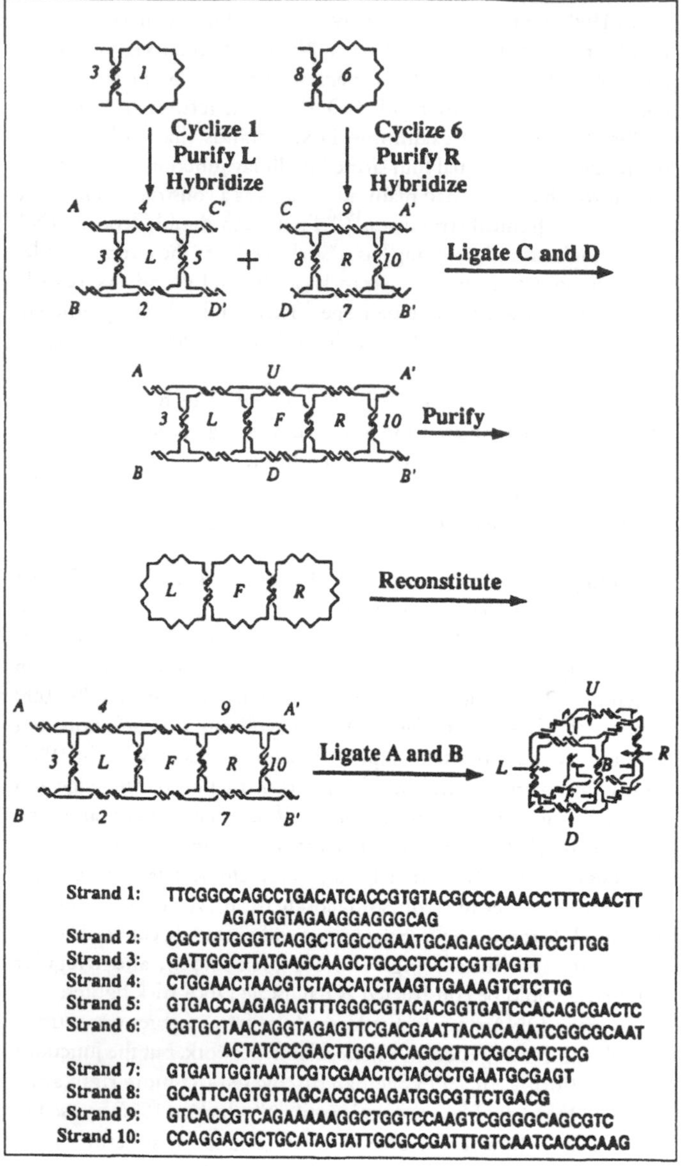

Strand 1:	TTCGGCCAGCCTGACATCACCGTGTACGCCCAAACCTTTCAACTT AGATGGTAGAAGGAGGGCAG
Strand 2:	CGCTGTGGGTCAGGCTGGCCGAATGCAGAGCCAATCCTTGG
Strand 3:	GATTGGCTTATGAGCAAGCTGCCCTCCTCGTTAGTT
Strand 4:	CTGGAACTAACGTCTACCATCTAAGTTGAAAGTCTCTTG
Strand 5:	GTGACCAAGAGAGTTTGGGCGTACACGGTGATCCACAGCGACTC
Strand 6:	CGTGCTAACAGGTAGAGTTCGACGAATTACACAAATCGGCGCAAT ACTATCCCGACTTGGACCAGCCTTTCGCCATCTCG
Strand 7:	GTGATTGGTAATTCGTCGAACTCTACCCTGAATGCGAGT
Strand 8:	GCATTCAGTGTTAGCACGCGAGATGGCGTTCTGACG
Strand 9:	GTCACCGTCAGAAAAAGGCTGGTCCAAGTCGGGGCAGCGTC
Strand 10:	CCAGGACGCTGCATAGTATTGCGCCGATTTGTCAATCACCCAAG

Fig. 2.3. Synthetic scheme used to build 3-dimensional DNA cubes in solution phase (redrawn from Chen and Seeman[1914]).

conducting silver clusters, DNA enzymes, or other DNA nanostructures such as polyhedra." In these experiments, DNA hairpin turns incorporated within selected units inside their structures were visible as topographic features under AFM imaging, proving the ability to build predictable, atomically precise 2-D crystals with design control over every lattice point. Since the density of lattice points was much sparser than atomic spacings, this DNA self-assembly technology could be paired with atomically precise synthesis of diverse nanoscale subassemblies so that each unique double crossover unit in a pattern could be decorated with a unique subassembly of comparable size, possibly allowing the construction of mechanical nanocomputers[1970] and other nanomachinery.

In early 1999, Seeman reported yet another breakthrough—the construction of a mechanical DNA-based device that is a possible prototype for a nanoscale robotic arm.[2409] The mechanism has two rigid arms a few nanometers long that can be rotated between fixed positions by introducing a positively charged cobalt compound into the solution surrounding the molecules, causing the bridge region to be converted from the normal B-DNA structure to the unusual Z-DNA structure. The free ends of the arms shift position by ~2.0 nm during the structural conversion. Explained Seeman: "Using synthetic DNA as a building material, we have constructed a controllable molecular mechanical system. In the long-term, the work will have implications for the development of nanoscale robots and for molecular manufacturing."

DNA can also serve as an assembly jig in solution phase. Bruce Smith and colleagues[2423] are devising a method for the assembly and covalent linkage of proteins into specific orientations and arrangements as determined by the hybridization of DNA attached to the proteins, called DNA-Guided Assembly of Proteins (DGAP). In this method, multiple DNA sequences would be attached to specific positions on the surface of each protein, and complementary sequences would bind, forcing protein building blocks (possibly including biomolecular motors, structural protein fibers, antibodies, enzymes, or other existing functional proteins) together in specific desired combinations and configurations, which would then be stabilized by covalent interprotein linkages. This technique could also be applied to non-protein components that can be functionalized at multiple sites with site-specific DNA sequences, although proteins, at least initially, may be more convenient building blocks due to their size, their surface chemistry, the wide variety of functions and mechanical properties they can confer on the resulting assemblies, and the many existing techniques for introducing designed or artificially evolved modifications into natural proteins of known structure. (In 1998, custom DNA and peptide sequences could be ordered online.)[2424] Methods for covalently attaching functional proteins to a DNA backbone in a specified manner at ~8.5 nm (25 base-pair) intervals,[2430] addressable protein targeting in macromolecular assembly,[2544] and "protein stitchery"[2848] were being explored by others. Drexler[3208] notes that evolution has not maximized the stability of natural proteins, and that substantially greater stability may be engineered by various means (e.g., increasing folding stability by >100 Kcal/mole).

2.3.2 Molecular and Supramolecular Chemistry

A second broad category of enabling technology for molecular manufacturing includes molecular chemistry—the conscious design of completely artificial, nonbiological chemical structures that could potentially serve as molecular "parts" or which have specific devicelike functionality.[10,322] For example, catalysts may very loosely "be thought of as rudimentary assemblers that are slightly programmable through changes in the reaction milieu (i.e., changes in pH, temperature, etc.)".[2603] The number of natural molecular "parts" is immense—perhaps a few hundred thousand bio-organic compounds have been separated, purified and identified—but by 15 February 1999 chemists had already registered 19,245,458 well-characterized artificial molecules or other "substances" in the CAS Registry.[2863] Synthesis of natural molecules containing ~100 atoms (e.g., a ~1 nm^3 molecular "part"), using methods of classical organic synthesis often requiring ~1 synthesis step per atom with ~90% yield per step,[2553] was state-of-the-art in 1998.

"What is exciting about modern nanotechnology," says Nobel chemist Roald Hoffmann,[3174] "is (a) the marriage of chemical synthetic talent with a direction provided by 'device-driven' ingenuity coming from engineering, and (b) a certain kind of courage provided by those incentives, to make arrays of atoms and molecules that ordinary, no, extraordinary chemists just wouldn't have thought of trying. Now they're pushed to do so. And of course they will. They can do anything."

Molecular chemists study how small numbers of atoms combine covalently with each other to produce molecules with a wide variety of different properties. Supramolecular chemists are primarily concerned with the much weaker noncovalent forces that can arise between molecules—such as hydrogen bonds and van der Waals interactions—that can be sufficient to bind collections of molecules tightly enough to form functional nanometer-sized structures. Supramolecular chemistry[765,2445,2446] studies "chemistry beyond the molecule"[765] or "the chemistry of the noncovalent bond".[2523] Its subject matter includes atomically precise supermolecules (well-defined discrete oligomolecular species resulting from the intermolecular association of a few components, such as a receptor and its substrate) and polymer-like supramolecular assemblies (polymolecular entities that result from the spontaneous association of a large undefined number of components).

Self-assembly is a key concept in supramolecular chemistry[2433,2455,2456,2491,2527] as it is in nature,[2968] allowing the manufacture of large numbers of compound objects simultaneously and in parallel, rather than sequentially. Molecular self-assembly is a strategy for nanofabrication that involves designing molecules and supramolecular entities so that complementarity causes them to aggregate into desired structures. Self-assembly of atomically precise supermolecules thus demands well-defined adhesion between selected molecules, which may require steric (shape and size) complementarity, interactional complementarity, large contact areas, multiple interaction sites, and strong overall binding.[765]

G.M. Whitesides[2433] explains that self-assembly has a number of advantages as a strategy. First, it carries out many of the most difficult steps in nanofabrication—those involving the smallest atomic-level modifications of structure—using the very highly developed techniques of synthetic chemistry. Second, it draws from the enormous wealth of examples in biology for inspiration; self-assembly is one of the most important strategies used in biology for the development of complex, functional structures, such as the well-studied examples of complex biomachine self-assembly of whole bacteriophage virions[1179,1180,2434,2435] and flagellar rotor motors[216,581,1397] from their smaller molecular "parts". Third, self-assembly can incorporate biological structures directly as components in the final systems. Fourth, self-assembly requires target structures to be among the most thermodynamically stable available to the system, thus tends to produce structures that are relatively defect-free and self-healing. As Lehn[765] points out: "By increasing the size of its entities, nanochemistry works its way upward towards microlithography and microphysical engineering, which, by further and further miniaturization, strive to produce ever smaller elements". Hierarchical self-assembly of many billions of micron-scale spherical components into a periodic honeycomb-structured photonic crystal optical device ~30 microns thick and ~1 cm^2 in area was demonstrated in 1998.[2461]

There is a wide range of different molecular systems that can self-assemble, including those which form ordered monomolecular structures by the coordination of molecules to surfaces,[2609] called self-assembled monolayers (SAMs),[2433,2455,2565] self-assembling thin films[2455,2564] and Langmuir-Blodgett films,[2608] and self-organizing nanostructures.[123,2563] In these systems, a single layer of molecules affixed to a surface allows both thickness and composition in the vertical axis to be adjusted to 0.1-nm by controlling the structure of the molecules comprising the monolayer, although control of in-plane dimensions to <100 nm is very difficult. Fluidic self-assembly of microscale parts[1150] and the dynamics of Brownian self-assembly[2889] have also been described, and the theory of designable self-assembling molecular machine structures is beginning to be addressed.[2956]

Another approach using solid-phase peptide synthesis and a massively convergent self assembly process was employed by M.R. Ghadiri and colleagues,[2436-2440] who designed and synthesized a number of self-assembling peptide-based nanotubes using cyclic peptides with an even number of alternating D- and L-amino acids for the building blocks of the nanotubes. The alternating stereochemistry of the cyclic peptides allowed all the side chains of the amino acids to be pointing outwards which would not be possible in an ordinary all L-cyclic peptide. In this conformation, the amide backbone can H-bond in a direction perpendicular to the plane of the cyclic peptide. The stacking of two cyclic peptides forms an H-bonding network resembling an anti-parallel beta-sheet[2441] as is commonly found in natural proteins. The H-bonding lattice quickly propagates perpendicular to the plane of the cyclic peptide, forming a tubular microcrystalline structure with 0.75-nm pores, or, in another experiment, 1.3-nm pores.[2442] Another group of nanotubes was designed with a highly hydrophobic outer surface and a hydrophilic inner pore. These nanotubes were easily inserted into a lipid bilayer and have been shown to be highly efficient ion channels;[1177,2440] nanotubes with slightly larger pores transport small molecules such as glucose as well.[2443] Stable flat nanodisks with diameters continuously (chemically) adjustable from 30-3000 nm have been self-assembled in surfactant solutions.[2934]

Self-assembled crystalline solids such as zeolites[2447,2468,2469] incompletely fill space, leaving substantial voids that may be occupied by solvent molecules or other guest molecules, producing solid-state host-guest complexes known as clathrates (from the Latin *clathratus*, meaning "enclosed by the bars of a grating"). MacNicol and co-workers[2453] reported the first rationally designed clathrate host in 1978, but the first true de novo design of an organic clathrate was in 1991[2454] and involved the formation of an extensive three-dimensional diamond-like porous lattice built from a single Tinkertoy-type subunit containing four tetrahedrally arrayed pyridone groups that acted as connectors to assemble the units together in a well-defined geometry. However, the crystal was held together only by weak hydrogen bonds and the links had a rotational degree of freedom, rendering the exact crystal molecular arrangement unpredictable.[2850] Engineered nanoporous molecular crystals can provide molecular-scale voids with controlled sizes, shapes, and embedded chemical environments at resolutions of 0.3-4.0 nm.[430,431,695,1522,2447-2449] Other self-assembling crystal structures have been described[2494,2561] including the crystal engineering of diamondoid networks,[2678] template-directed colloidal crystallization or colloidal epitaxy,[2837] organic templating to form crystalline zeolite-type structures with ordering lengths <3 nm,[2892] 3-D polymer channels with chemically functionalizable channel linings,[2921] and micromolding combined with templating and cooperative assembly of block copolymers (Section 3.5.7.1) to produce hierarchical ordering over discrete and tunable characteristic length scales of ~10 nm, ~100 nm, and ~1000 nm in a single body.[2893]

Dendrimers,[2470,2531,2580-2591] also known as arborols or fractal polymers, are a well-known set of self-assembling structures[2610] that possibly could be used as tools to assist in the assembly of early nanomachines. Dendrimers are large regularly-branching macromolecules resembling fractal patterns, made by an iterative process in which small linear molecules are allowed to bind to each other at a certain number of sites along their length, building up branches upon branches with each iteration working outward from a core molecule having at least two chemically reactive arms, somewhat mimicking tree growth (e.g., Fig. 2.20C). Different core molecules or building-block chains produce macromolecules with different shapes, and the outer surface can be terminated with chemical groups of specific functionality, producing hundreds of differently-surfaced branched molecules[2471] that have already found use in medical research.[2671] Growth is regulated, so size can be accurately controlled—dendrimers are typically a few nanometers wide but have been constructed with masses exceeding a million protons (~10^5 atoms) and with diameters larger than 30 nm. In 1999, convergent assembly of specified 6-mer dendrimers, via trimerization of precursor dimer "parts," was demonstrated.[3275]

Autocatalysis or self-replication (Section 2.4.2 and Chapter 14) is yet another approach to the chemical self-assembly of subunits. In 1989, J. Rebek[131,2450-2452] reported the synthesis of supermolecules that could generate copies of themselves when placed in a sea of simpler molecular parts, with each component part consisting of up to a few dozen atoms. Molecular self-replication has continued to be studied by others.[2524-2526,2602] Ghadiri[2457] reported a self-replicating peptide in 1996, and by 1998 his laboratory had moved on to studies of more complex autocatalytic cycle networks.[2458-2460] It is unknown how complex such assembly cycles may be made, but Ghadiri was investigating a self-replicating 256-component molecular ecosystem incorporating ~32,000 possible binary interactions,[2601] in 1998.

By 1998, chemists had already synthesized a vast variety of simple molecular parts of which only a tiny sampling can be mentioned here. For instance, carbon rings have been linked edge-on or by corners to create propeller-shaped molecules called propellanes[2497] (Fig. 2.4) or rotanes (Fig. 2.5), or stacked with short hydrocarbon links to make gear-looking molecules such as cyclophane[2493] and superphane (Fig. 2.6). Hydrocarbon molecular polyhedra in the shape of triangular (e.g., triangulane[2571]), cubic (e.g., cubane, first made by P. Eaton in 1964[2570]), pentagonal and hexagonal prisms, collectively known as prismanes, have been created (Fig. 2.7), along with more unusual geometrical forms such as paddlane, housane, basketane, churchane, pagodane, and bivalvane[382] (Fig. 2.8; one carbon atom at each vertex). Cryptands,[2479] spherands,[2492] cryptaspherands and carcerands,[410] corannulene baskets,[2639] and calixarenes[411] are bowl-shaped molecules whose benzene ring walls hold their cavities rigid. The bowl rim of a calixarene (Fig. 2.9) can be lined with chemical groups to determine which guests it will accept, or two bowls can be bonded together,[2547] making a hollow nanoscale reaction vessel, and various molecular cages and capsules with precise sizes and characteristics have been assembled.[1262,2549-2551] A variety of nonchiral and chiral square molecules have been synthesized,[2473,2543] as well as molecular "bottlebrushes";[2475] DNA-polymer constant-force springs;[2476,2477] the ferric wheel (Fig. 2.10);[2552] molecular barrels[2558] and molecular tennis balls;[2551] various helical,[2554-2556,2569,2605,2638] boxlike,[2559] and other hollow organic[2572] structures; molecular "turnstiles"[2573] and "molecular tweezers";[2677] simple and complex trefoil knot molecules;[2562] and stable carbyne* molecular rods with chains lengths up to ~300 carbon atoms having alternating single and triple covalent bonds.[317] Chemists are justifiably awed by the creation of structures like the ferric wheel; "for me," observed Nobel chemist Roald Hoffmann,[125] "this molecule provides a spiritual high....The molecule is beautiful because its symmetry reaches directly into the soul, [playing] a note on a Platonic ideal."

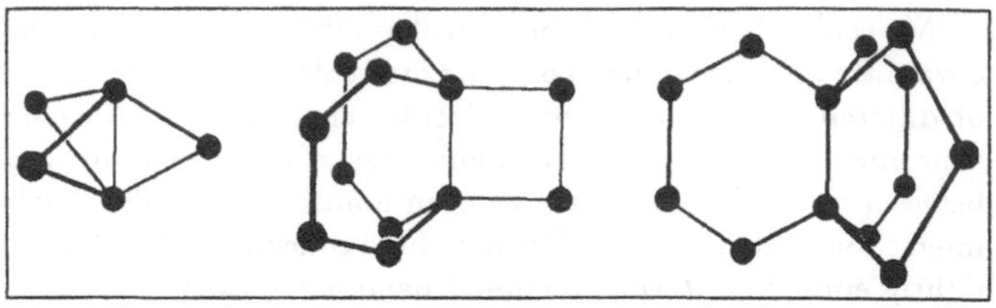

Fig. 2.4. Propellanes (H atoms not shown).[382]

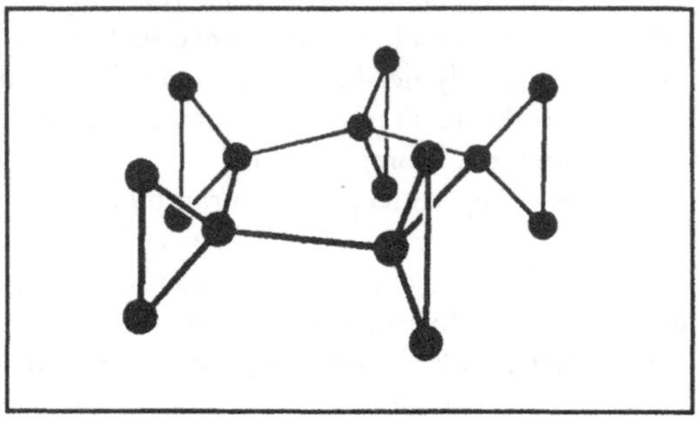

Fig. 2.5. Rotanes (H atoms not shown).[382]

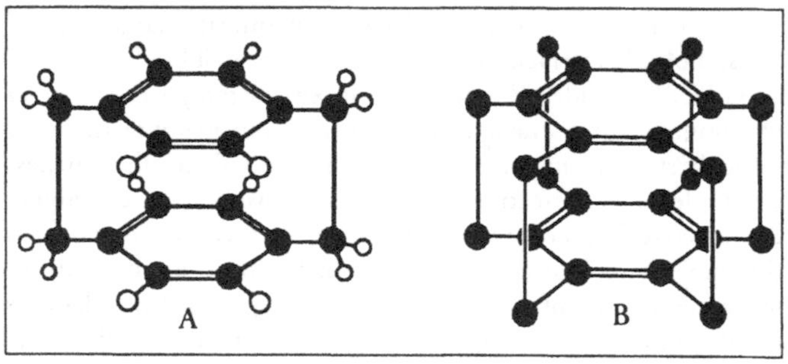

Fig. 2.6. (A) Cyclophane; (B) Superphane (H atoms not shown).[382]

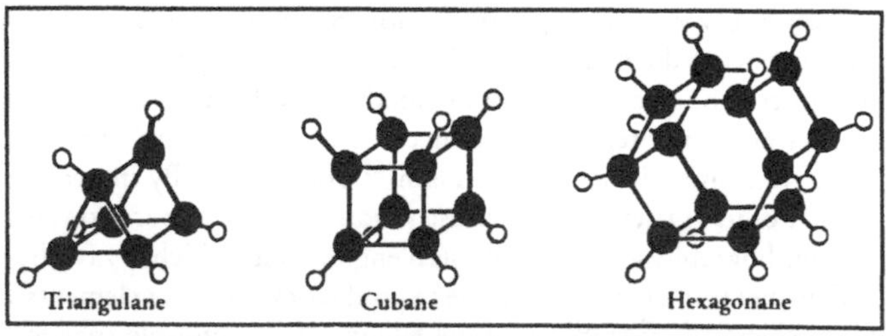

Fig. 2.7. The prismanes.[382]

Molecular gear systems first became a popular object of chemical study during the 1980s. For example, G. Yamamoto[164] described "compounds that exist in conformations which are regarded as static meshed gears with two-toothed and three-toothed wheels and some of them behave as dynamic gears." H. Iwamura[163] prepared one system that formed a chain of beveled molecular gears with ~GHz rotation rates, and another "doubly connected bevel gear system...[Transfer] of information from one end of the molecular system to the other end could take place in large molecules via cooperativity of the torsional motions of the chain." Kurt Mislow[2472]

*In chemical nomenclature, hydrocarbons with single carbon-carbon bonds are "-anes," double bonds make "-enes," and triple bonds make "-ynes."

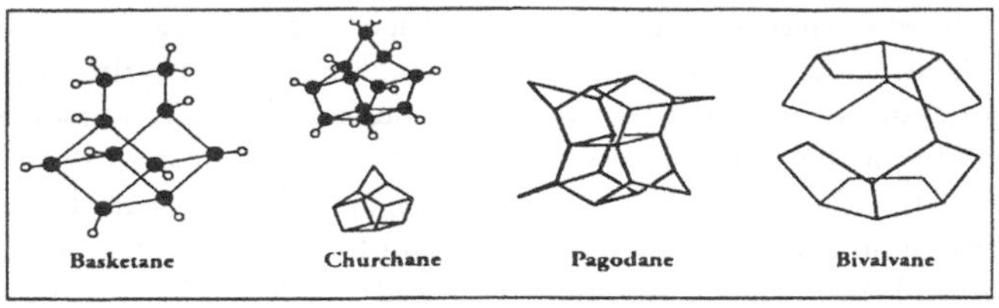

Fig. 2.8. Other unusual molecular "parts".[382]

gave numerous examples of molecular gear systems that he had synthesized using the methods of traditional solution chemistry, which "resemble to an astonishing degree the coupled rotations of macroscopic mechanical gears." He added: "It is possible to imagine a role for these and similar mechanical devices, molecules with tiny gears, motors, levers, etc., in the nanotechnology of the future."

In 1998, Gimzewski and coworkers[2474] synthesized and observed a 1.5-nm diameter gearlike single molecule (hexa-tert-butyl decacyclene) rotating within a supramolecular bearing (a void in a 2-D lattice) at room temperature on the surface of a Cu{100} lattice. The authors suggest that added non-thermal noise (e.g., temperature differences produced by tunnel current heating of the rotor) could be rectified by asymmetries in the rotor/neighbor potential energy curve, allowing the rotor to turn unidirectionally. Says Gimzewski: "Our wheel is frictionless in the conventional sense of the word, and it doesn't wear out." Gimzewski's experimental work confirms Drexler's calculations[10] that van der Waals bearings can operate in molecular systems, that multi-atomic bearing surfaces with higher load capacities than sigma bond bearings can be built, that these bearings can run with no lubricants, and that such bearings have sufficiently low energy barriers to allow turning by thermal vibrations alone.

By 1998, limited control of the mechanical action of molecular parts had been demonstrated. For example, in 1994 T. Ross Kelly's group created a "paddlewheel" molecule (a spinning propeller-shaped wheel) with a built-in chemically-controlled brake. In solution, the wheel spins freely, but when Hg^{++} ions are added, a blocking ligand physically rotates into a new position (tripping the brake) and stopping the rotation; removal of the mercury causes the wheel to resume spinning.[17] In 1997, Kelly's group used similar techniques to synthesize the first molecular ratchet,[2546] a propeller with three benzene-ring "blades" that serve as gear teeth. A row of four rings (the pawl) sits between two of the blades, such that the propeller cannot turn without pushing it aside; because of a twist in the pawl, it is easier to turn clockwise than counterclockwise under thermal agitation, providing mechanical rectification without net motion or energy extraction.[2611] Shinkai and colleagues[382,2478] fabricated a pair of molecular tongs for grasping metal ions that uses two crown ether rings as the jaws, linked by two benzene rings joined through two double-bonded nitrogen atoms (Fig. 2.11). Irradiation with ultraviolet light induces photoisomerization of the double bond between the nitrogen atoms, closing the jaws; heat reverses the process, opening the jaws. In related systems, collectively called "butterfly molecules," irradiation with visible light or pH changes can also induce opening. Seeman's chemically-operated mechanical DNA system[2409] provides similar control of molecular mechanical movement (Section 2.3.1). Numerous controllable molecular electronics devices and possible nanocomputer components are reviewed in Section 10.2.

Noncovalent self-assembly of molecular parts has also been demonstrated. For example, Fraser Stoddart and colleagues[1805,2482-2484] have extensively investigated the rotaxanes,[2481] molecules in which one part is threaded through a hole or loop in another, and kept from unthreading by end-groups, like a ring trapped on a barbell. In one system (Fig. 10.8), a ring-shaped molecule slides freely along a shaft-like chain molecule, moving back and forth between

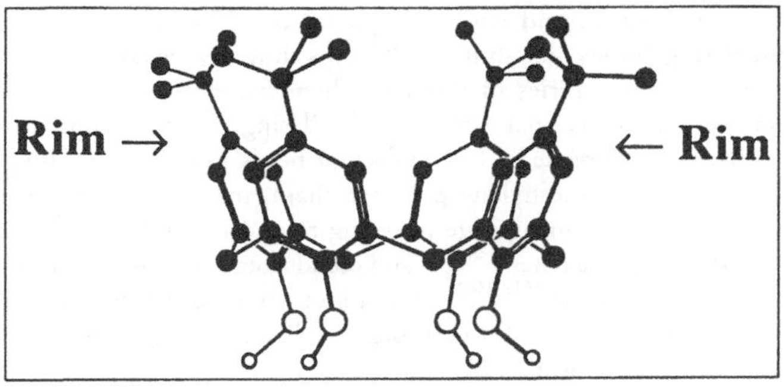

Fig. 2.9. Calixarene.[382]

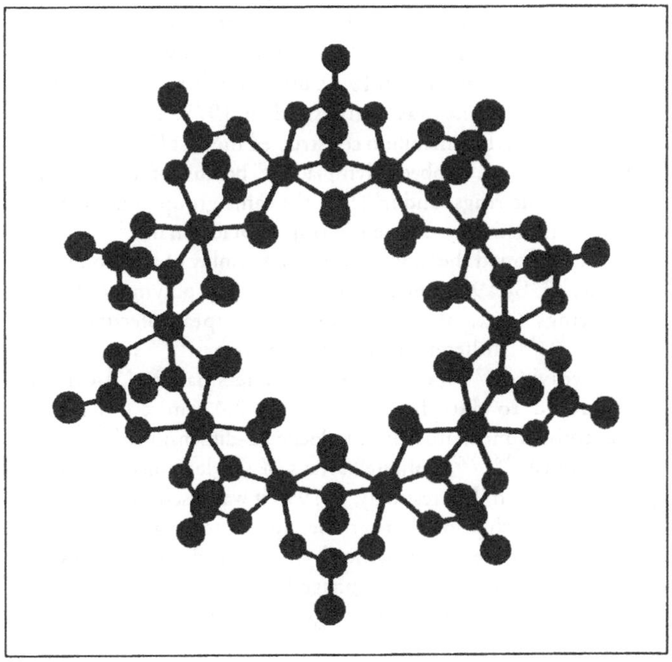

Fig. 2.10. Ferric wheel (Fe, O, C atoms shown; H, Cl atoms not shown).[2552]

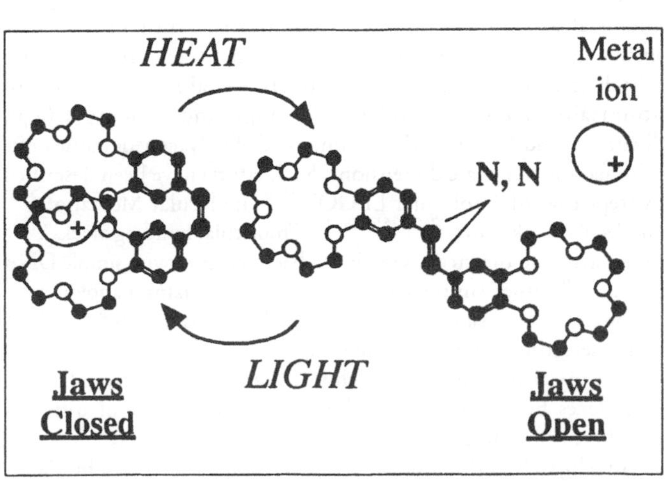

Fig. 2.11. "Butterfly Molecule" used as molecular tongs.[382]

stations at either end with a frequency of ~500 Hz, making an oscillating "molecular shuttle".[2483] This shuttling behavior can be controlled by a series of different chemical, electrochemical, or photochemical external stimuli.[2484,3541] Using a different approach, G. Wenz[2487] threaded ~120 molecular beads onto a single, long, poly-iminooligomethylene polymer chain, making a "molecular necklace." Other groups are pursuing related research[2522,2529,2530] regarding [n]-rotaxanes[2538,2539] and pseudorotaxanes (mechanically-threaded molecules),[2541,2542] while still others are using the necklace technique as a means, for example, of self-assembling ~2 nm wide cyclodextrin nanotubes.[2488]

Another interesting molecular system that can be made entirely by self-assembly is the catenanes,[2481] which have two or more closed rings joined like the links of a chain. The rings are mechanically linked—there are no covalent bonds between separate links. The first [2]-catenane (2 linked rings) was constructed by Edel Wasserman of AT&T Bell Laboratories in 1960, using simple hydrocarbon rings; the first [3]-catenane was synthesized in 1977. In 1994, Fraser Stoddart and David Amabilino constructed the first [5]-catenane,[2485] having ~372 atoms, dubbed "olympiadane" because of its resemblance to the Olympic rings, and in 1997 the same group announced the first deterministically-ordered 7-ring heptacatenane;[2535] another group later reported the spontaneous self-assembly of a 10-component catenane.[3285] By 1998, much research on larger polymeric chains of linked rings (e.g., oligocatenanes[2532]), supramolecular "daisy chains",[2533,2534] fullerene-containing catenanes,[2536] and supramolecular weaving[2537] was in progress. The smallest [2]-catenane constructed to date has dimensions 0.4 nm x 0.6 nm.[2528] Self-assembled mechanically-interlocked 2-dimensional[2595-2597] and 3-dimensional[2598,2599] "infinite" arrays of single molecular ringlike species are known. Interestingly, in 1998 it was discovered that many viral coats (which also self-assemble) appear to be a 2-dimensional "chain-mail" weave of mechanically-interlocked protein rings—for instance, the spherical bacteriophage HK97 capsid shell consists of exactly 72 interlinked protein rings, specifically 60 hexamers and 12 pentamers.[2486]

Complex molecular parts also can be built up from simpler molecular parts by covalent bonding as low-symmetry shape-invariant molecular object polymers,[2692] or via processes variously known as modular chemistry,[2498,2499] heterosupramolecular chemistry,[3220] chemical assembly,[3541] or structure-directed synthesis[2489,2490]—including the well-known Diels-Alder reactions[2557] (e.g., see Fig. 2.20F) which may be employed repetitively to fabricate a series of atomically-precise molecular rods, rings, and nanocages (e.g., "beltenes" and "collarenes"[2489]) composed of polyacenequinone units with nanometer-scale dimensions. Such efforts have been described as steps toward "molecular LEGO",[2489] "molecular Meccano",[2480] "molecular Tinkertoys",[2509-2516,2842] or "molecular building blocks".[2850] Some structure-directed assembly has been achieved with simple DNA forms.[1916] Other simple techniques for synthesizing nanowires,[643] nanorods,[2672,2710] nanotubes,[1411,2673,2674,2862] and nanocages,[2640,2675,2862] or for selecting polymers for length,[2686] are well-known.

For instance, Jean-Marie Lehn[2679] has created rectangular grid complexes by mixing rodlike ligands that make use of different numbers of binding sites—one example is a 4 x 5 array consisting of nine ligands and 20 metal ions, nanoscale grids which he claims might one day find use "as components within a futuristic information storage and processing nanotechnology". C.M. Drain[2680,2681] has described a 21-component (5 nm)^2 square array of nine porphyrins tethered together by 12 palladium ions shaped like a four-pane window. The structure is built from three different kinds of porphyrins—(1) an X-shaped unit that coordinates to four metal ions, forming the center of the array, (2) a T-shaped unit that coordinates to three metals and forms each side of the array, and (3) an L-shaped unit that coordinates to only two metals and forms each corner of the array. When these components are placed in solution in the correct ratio, they form the square array within a half hour at room temperature with about 90% yield. The same porphyrin units can be combined in different ratios and induced to form wires or tapes. The properties of such arrays can be fine-tuned by choosing the appropriate metal ion linker and functionalized porphyrin unit.[2679]

Jeffrey Moore has investigated a three-dimensional nanoscaffolding comprised of a molecular lattice that could serve as a framework for catalysts, photosynthetic molecules, or more complex molecular devices. Moore's original objective was to synthesize modular building blocks with physical and chemical properties that would dictate a "programmed assembly" protocol for "nanoarchitectures".[2574-2579] The characteristics of each modular unit shaped the weak intermolecular attractions—electrostatic, van der Waals, and hydrogen-bonding forces—between it and its neighbors so that units would array themselves in a larger structure with the desired spacing and geometry. Moore's group first linked phenylacetylene subunits into oligomers of various lengths which bend and twist like wire sculptures until their ends meet to form closed polyhedral molecules—the basic scaffold components (of which there were at least half a dozen shapes). These building blocks then self-assembled or folded[2555] into geometries at least partly controlled by designed hydrogen-bonding interactions. The molecular polyhedra each possessed several phenylene groups, "chemical handles" upon which other molecular groups could be hung. Moore then focused on ~10-nm dendrimeric forms[2580-2585] and later began attaching photosensitive antenna molecules to these structures.[2586-2591] By 1997, Moore had begun investigating norbornadiene on Si{100} in an effort to develop ways to covalently attach molecules onto surfaces with sub-nanometer spatial precision,[2592,2593] and had suggested a packing model for interpenetrated diamondoid structures.[2594] Robson's group[2846] has also investigated possible scaffolding molecules.

Josef Michl is attempting to build a molecular construction kit using molecular rods and connectors, pursuing an explicit vision of "molecular Tinkertoys"[2509-2516] by working with simple molecular structures that form stiff, flexible rods. Michl has assembled rods from a mixture of carbon-boron molecules (e.g., 10-vertex or 12-vertex carboranes[2495]) and carbon-hydrogen molecules, providing fine control over the total rod length. The rods are built up from more primitive molecular parts, such as propellane (a strained form of C_5H_6) and cubane (a strained form of C_8H_8), to make "staffanes"[2500-2510] which are a series of cage units in a linear series (Fig. 2.12). (Strained molecules are constructed with bonds that are forced out of their normal angles, as for example 90° in the case of cubane, compared with carbon's normal orientation of 109.5°.) Michl has fabricated rods whose lengths vary from 0.5 nm to 2.5 nm, in precise 0.1-nm steps. There are other ways of making rod-like molecules, but Michl's are highly inert, do not absorb visible or UV light, are stable up to at least 200°C, and do not react with the oxygen in air even at high temperatures.[2496]

Related work is underway in Michl's laboratory on connectors to join the rods together.[2496] Metal atoms would be the simplest

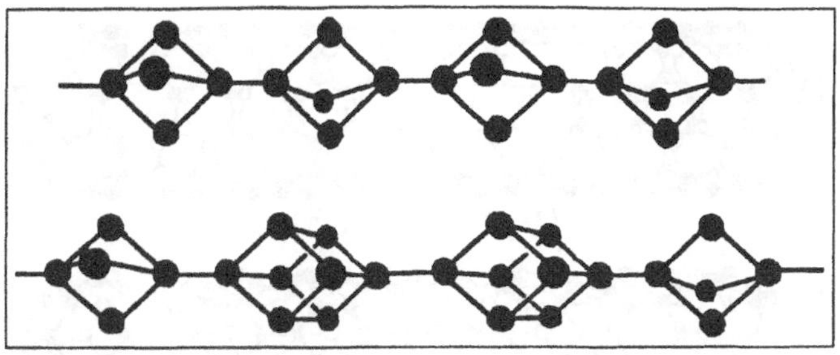

Fig. 2.12. "Staffane" rigid rods of different lengths for a molecular kit (H atoms not shown; redrawn from Pease[2496]).

solution, offering the useful quality of strong joints that can be easily disassembled. Different metals give different binding geometrics—square, octahedral, and so on. Many of the connectors are metal-containing species; some are symmetrically trisubstituted or hexasubstituted benzenes or tetrasubstituted cyclobutadiene complexes. Michl must build the right chemical groups onto the rod termini to make them adhere to the connectors as desired. In one example,[2496] tiny crosses were built by attaching carboxylate groups to one end of the staffanes, allowing them to bind to a connector made of two rhodium atoms. The groups at the other end of the rods were converted to an ester group, which doesn't bind to rhodium, and so the crosses self-assembled correctly. Michl has also fabricated "star connectors" in which the rods are built into the molecules as covalently bonded arms of a star. For instance, one 3-arm star connector uses three large carboranes coupled to a central benzene ring, allowing a pedestal to be attached vertically to the benzene ring via a ruthenium "sandwich" bond.[2496] Additional devices could be installed on this molecular scaffolding, such as optically active molecules or even molecular mechanical "windmills".[2516] Nanoscale square[2517-2519] and hexagonal[2520,2521] planar grids have been fabricated. Extensive ab initio quantum mechanical calculations accompany the experimental work and aid in the interpretation of the results. Michl's ultimate goal is "the production of thin layers of solids of completely controlled aperiodic structure consisting of an inert covalent scaffolding carrying selected active groups."

G. Leach and colleagues[2705] used computers to simulate various diamond and graphite nanostruts using molecular dynamics calculations, analyzing solid rectangular struts with varying aspect ratios, cross-sections, terminating atoms (for diamond), potential energy functions, and temperatures. The most dramatic differences were seen between struts with 100:1 aspect ratios and struts with lower (10:1 or 1:1) aspect ratios—the diamond strut with a 100:1 aspect ratio and a unit cell (~0.4 nm)^2) cross-section begins to curl (with end-to-end distance decreasing 1.2 nm after 20 picosec) due to thermal vibration (both at 150 K and 300 K), while a unit strut with an aspect ratio of 10:1 or a 100:1 strut with a (1 nm)^2 cross-section showed end-to-end length fluctuations of only ~0.1 nm. The authors concluded that support struts with a cross section of at least (1 nm)^2 would be sufficient to keep both end-to-end distance and transverse fluctuations below ~0.1 nm in struts with 10:1 aspect ratios. Other work by the same group[2664] claims that many nanomachine designs may actually perform better than molecular dynamics results might suggest, or may require fewer atoms for the same positional stability.[2705] The elastic and wear characteristics of diamond are being studied computationally by others.[2764,2900,2901]

No discussion of molecular "parts" could be complete without mention of the fullerenes,* first discovered in 1985[2612,2613] and vigorously investigated ever since.[522,523,1308,1821,2619,2636,2637,2702] Fullerenes are one of the three known allotropic forms of carbon. In graphite, the most common allotrope, carbon atoms are arranged in hexagonal rings and strongly bonded into parallel planar sheets, with much weaker bonding between the sheets, giving graphite its excellent lubricating properties. In diamond, the second allotropic form, carbon atoms are arranged in a symmetric, tetrahedral structure, giving immense strength. Exposed to air, both diamond surfaces and graphite edges are quickly coated or "passivated" with hydrogen or other atoms that tie up the dangling bonds. In fullerenes, the third allotropic form, carbon atoms form large and hollow cage-like structures, often roughly spherical or tubular, made up of closed curved one-atom-thick sheets of carbon atoms arranged in a number of five-, six-, and higher-membered rings. Interestingly, the fullerenes need no passivating hydrogens or other atoms to satisfy their chemical bonding requirements at the surface—in this sense, "fullerenes are the first and only stable forms of pure, finite carbon".[522]

A new journal, *Fullerene Science and Technology*, appeared in 1993, and by the mid-1990s ~3000 papers on fullerenes and their properties had been published and 149 fullerene-related patents had been issued in the U.S. alone (through 1996). By 1998, an incredible variety of fullerenes of many shapes and sizes had been synthesized.

The original fullerene, C_{60}, consists of exactly 60 carbon atoms arranged in a soccer-ball structure (Fig. 2.13; lone carbon atom at each vertex) with 20 hexagons and 12 pentagons (with each pentagon entirely surrounded by hexagons). In theory, small molecules such as H_2 or CO, and probably CH_4, would fit inside C_{60}.[2628] A slightly larger variant, C_{70}, is the same except that an extra belt of carbon atoms has been inserted around the equator. Smaller (Fig. 2.14) and

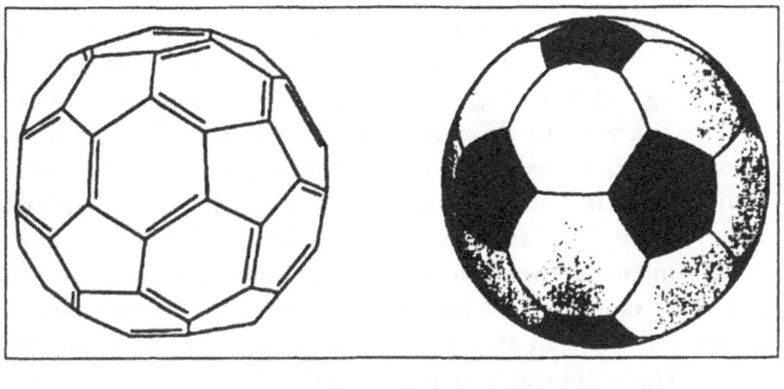

Fig. 2.13. C_{60} fullerene "buckyball" and a soccer ball.[382]

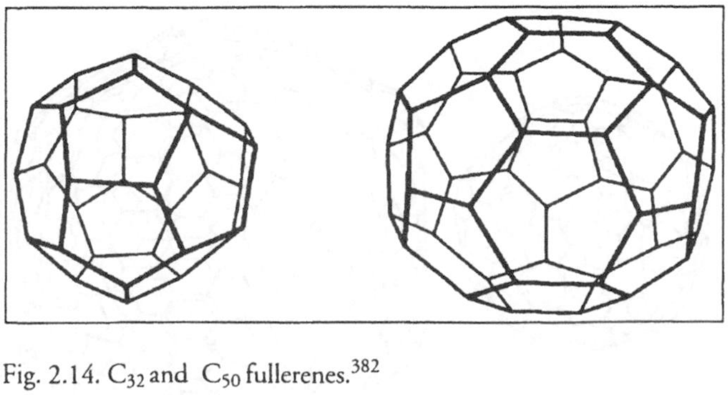

Fig. 2.14. C_{32} and C_{50} fullerenes.[382]

**The first fullerene to be discovered, the spherical C_{60} molecule, was originally named "buckminsterfullerene" by its discoverers, due to the molecule's similarity to the geodesic domes designed by the famous American architect and engineer, Buckminster Fuller (1895-1983). The name has since been shortened by common usage to "fullerenes," although spherical or tubular fullerenes are sometimes informally called "buckyballs" and "buckytubes," again reflecting the original provenance.*

larger (Fig. 2.15) variants have been observed; as cages get bigger, the corners (where the 12 pentagons needed for closure reside) get sharper. The topologically smallest possible fullerene is a dodecahedron consisting of 12 pentagons and 20 carbon atoms, but the ring isomer of C_{20} (a hoop of single carbons) is apparently energetically favored over the bowl or spherical (fullerene) isomers; in 1998, C_{28} was the smallest fullerene that had been observed experimentally,[2614] and C_{36} could be made in significant quantities by arc-discharge.[2910] The approximate diameter (measured to atomic centers) of a spheroidal fullerene of formula C_n is $D_{ball} \sim 1.1\ (n/60)^{1/2}$ nanometers.[2615] In 1998, purified C_{60} cost $27.50/gm (99.5% pure) or $60/gm (99.9%), C_{70} $250/gm (98%), and C_{84} $3,750/gm (90%) from Dynamic Enterprises Ltd. of London.

Insertion of many additional equatorial belts of carbon atoms (incorporated as hexagons) into a spheroidal fullerene results in a long cylinder with graphite-like ("graphene") walls and spherical endcaps, making a class of fullerenes known as the capsular fullerenes or single-walled carbon nanotubes (SWNT) that come in many sizes and chiral forms (Fig. 2.16).[2626,2651,2652,2857] The molecular form of carbon nanotubes has been likened to rolled chicken wire. SWNTs may be synthesized by vaporizing graphite spiked with 1% catalyst from the nickel, cobalt and iron group above 3000°C, then allowing the vapor to slowly condense. Tubes form because the metal atoms interact with dangling bonds at the end of a tube, favoring tube extension over hemispherical capping by newly arriving carbon vapor atoms. (For any given mass number, ball-shaped fullerenes are energetically favored over tube-shaped fullerenes during high-temperature synthesis in the absence of catalyst.[2615]) SWNTs typically self-assemble in 1.1 nm wide tubes, although smaller single-walled nanotubes and larger single-walled and multi-walled nested nanotubes[2626] exist. SWNT carbon atoms are bonded in virtually flawless hexagonal arrays. Simulations show that isolated flaws migrate to the ends of the tube and are eliminated, a phenomenon known as "self-healing".[1746] Single-molecule nanotubes of $C_{1,000,000}$ or larger, with lengths >100,000 times longer than their widths (e.g., ~1 mm long), had been synthesized by 1998. While graphite is a very brittle material, the graphene walls of a carbon nanotube are quite resilient. Computer simulations and experiments confirm that nanotubes kink when bent (Fig. 2.17), then snap back when released.[2661] Nanotube diameter is $D_{tube} = 0.078\ (n^2 + nm + m^2)^{1/2}$ nanometers, where (n, m) is the "rollup vector" defined by the number of steps required for a repeat pattern along two crystallographic cylinder wall axes. The cohesive energy per atom required to curve a flat graphene sheet into a cylinder[1308] is $E_{rollup} = (13\ \text{zJ-nm}^2 / D_{tube}^2)$. (1 zeptojoule (zJ) = 10^{-21} joules.) As an example, a (10,10)

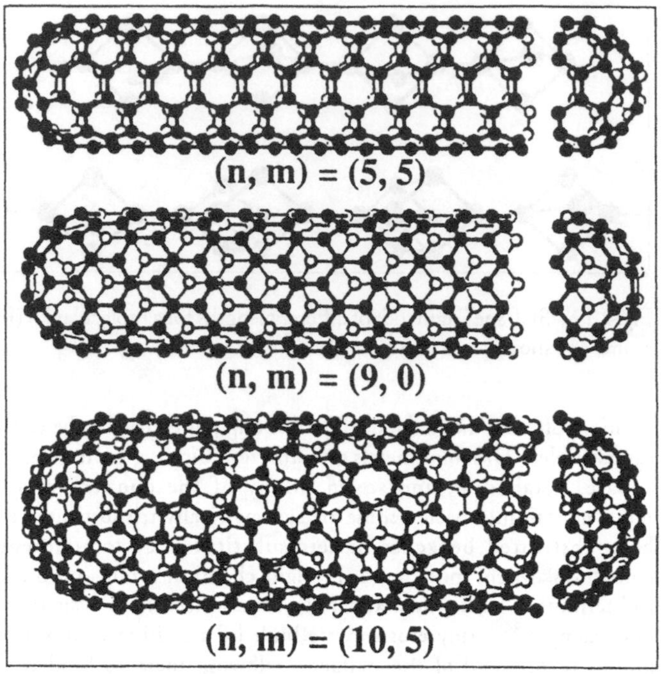

Fig. 2.16. Single-walled carbon nanotubes.[1308]

nanotube has D_{tube} = 1.36 nm and E_{rollup} = 7 zJ/atom. Young's modulus for individual SWNTs, assuming a hollow (open-ring) cross-section, has been estimated as high as ~5.5×10^{12} N/m^2;[2659] elastic bending modulus (measured as 1×10^{12} to 0.1×10^{12} N/m^2) decreases sharply with increasing diameter (from 8-40 nm).[3023] In 1998, purified carbon single-walled nanotubes were available via the Internet for $1400/gm from Tubes@Rice, or for $200/gm at lesser purity from CarboLex.

From spatial geometry, it is known that hexagonal tiling produces flat sections (like cylinder walls), and inserting pentagons into an hexagonal array produces positive curvature (like spheres), making endcaps. But 7-sided heptagons can also be inserted into hexagonal arrays to induce negative curvature,[1308,2651] thus permitting concave surface deformations such as saddle-shaped fullerenes[1308] (Fig. 2.18) or possibly helical tubular structures.[2635] Indeed, note Colbert and Smalley, "the use of hexagonal, pentagonal, and heptagonal substructures are sufficient to produce caged carbon structures of any topology".[2643] Nature makes use of this same geometrical principle in the radiolarians,[520] tiny protozoans with fullerene-like siliceous skeletons, and in the conical nucleoprotein core particle of the HIV-1

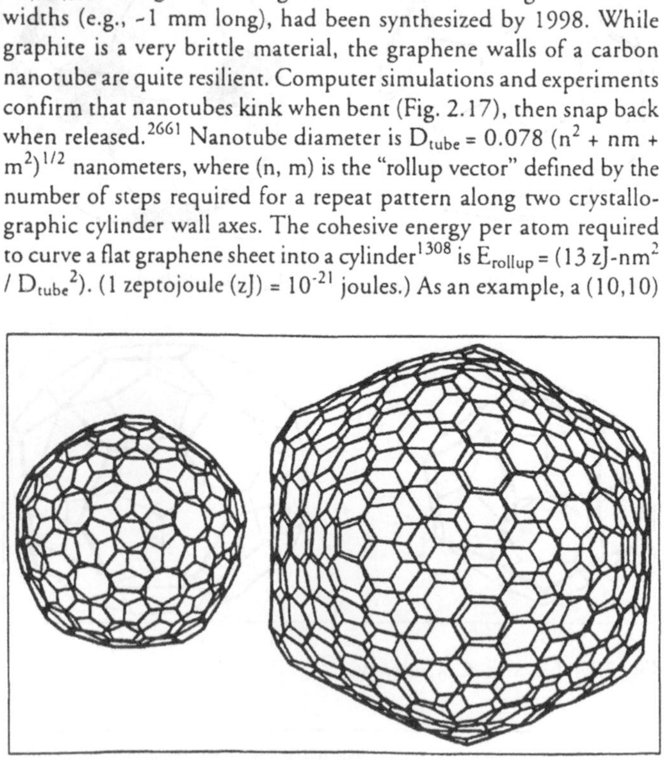

Fig. 2.15. C_{240} and C_{540} fullerenes.[382]

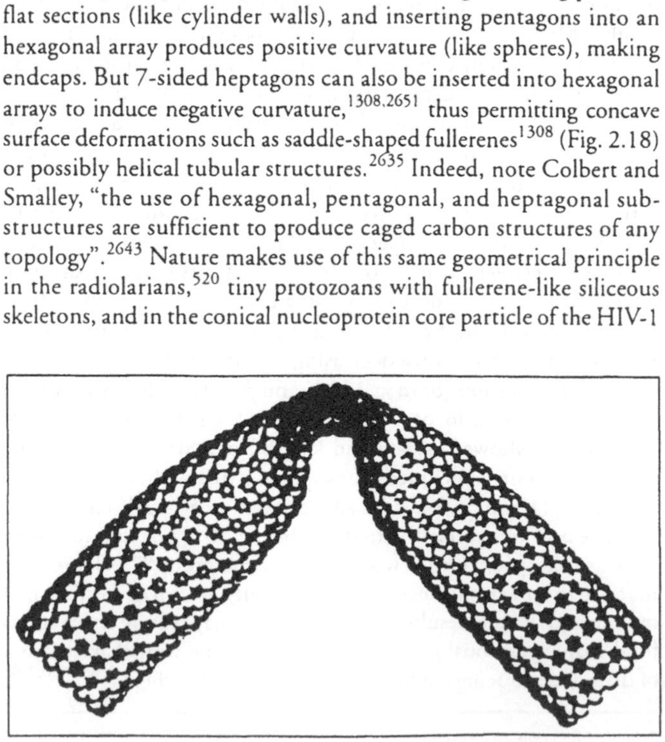

Fig. 2.17. Carbon nanotubes kink when bent.[2661]

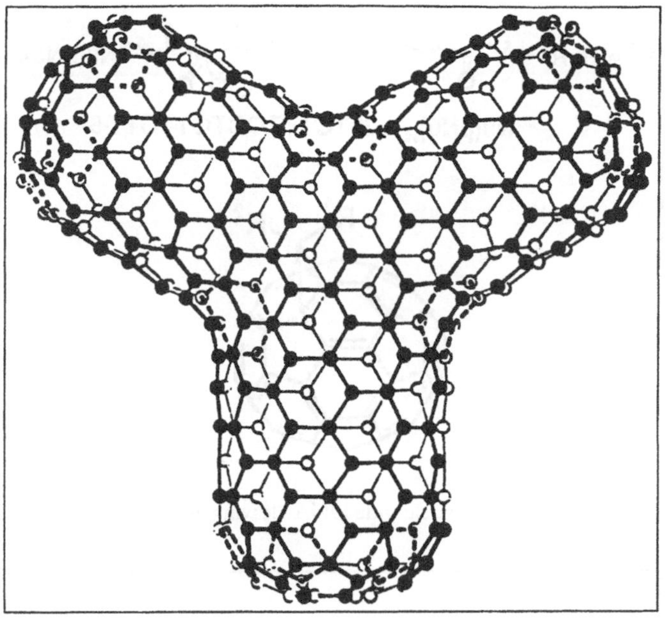

Fig. 2.18. One possible saddle-shaped fullerene.[1308]

virus[2684] (Fig. 2.19).* R. Smalley observes that a graphene sheet has the highest tensile strength of any known 2-dimensional network, and the packing density of atoms in the sheet (e.g., atoms/m^2) is higher than any other network made of any atoms in the periodic table and higher than the packing density in any 2-dimensional slice through any 3-dimensional object—even diamond which has the highest known 3-D packing density. Hence the graphene sheet is effectively impermeable under normal chemical conditions.

Carbon nanotubes have also been observed with a variety of end-cap shapes[2650] and with tubes that reduced[2651] or increased[2658] their diameter for some distance before terminating. Toroidal fullerenes can be produced experimentally;[2632,2657,3206] cone-like,[2652,2653,2684,2688] spindle-like,[2654] and helical[2655-2657] fullerene objects have also been examined. By 1998, the mechanical properties of fullerenes and carbon nanotubes were being extensively investigated[2277,2629,2659-2661,2715-2719,2903-2905] and there were experimental demonstrations of:

1. a limited ability to cut fullerene nanotubes to specific desired lengths;[1525,2685,2855]
2. dissolving derivatized SWNTs in common organic solvents;[2164]
3. the synthesis of self-oriented nanotube arrays;[2691] and
4. the trapping of individual C_{60} molecules in a perforated Langmuir-Blodgett film "workpiece holder"[2630] (though an even simpler means for producing 2-nm hole arrays with 7-8 nm hole spacings was later reported[2631]).

Nanotubes were also being investigated as nanoscale sensor components.[2908,2909,3023]

Given an ability to synthesize a wide variety of fullerene shapes and sizes, the next task is to find ways to join them together in specific desired molecular architectures. Two hydrogens were readily added to fullerene carbon atoms, making specific isomers of $C_{60}H_2$ and $C_{70}H_2$,[2616,2617] and in the 1990s fullerene chemistry began to be explored.[2618,2619,2649,2906] A little more than a decade after the discovery of C_{60}, gram quantities of buckyballs became widely available[2627] for chemical experimentation. Progress in covalent fullerene chemistry exploded.[2624] By the late 1990s, fullerene surfaces could be regioselectively functionalized in many interesting ways, including (Fig. 2.20):

A. a fullerene dimer,[2625]

B. a fullerene-polyester polymer,[2621]

C. a fullerene dendrimer,[2620]

D. a fullerene-rotaxane[2622] and catenane,[2536]

E. a fullerene-nucleotide DNA cleaving agent,[2623]

F. a Diels-Alder fullerene adduct that is very stable against cycloreversion,[2624] and

G. 3-dimensional extended polymeric multifullerene forms such as acetylenic macro-rings[2624] and DNA/fullerene hybrid materials.[3024]

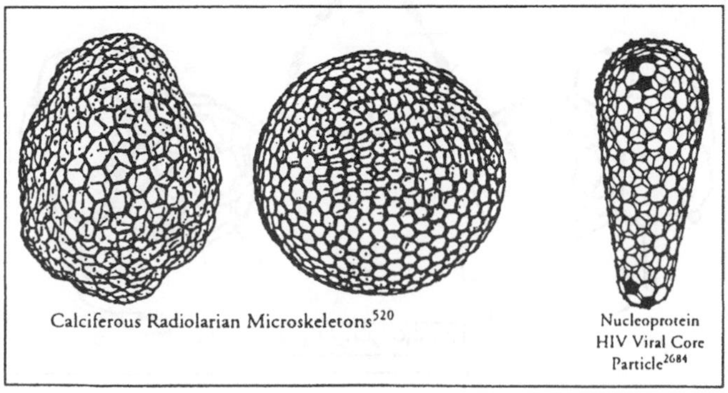

Fig. 2.19. Biological "fullerenes".

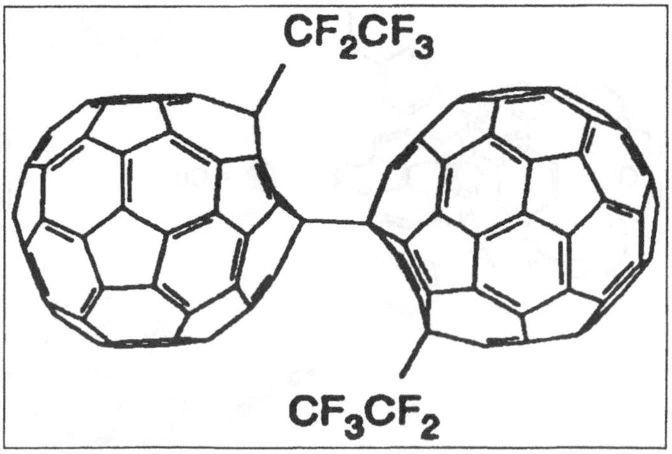

Fig. 2.20A. Fullerene dimer.[2625]

**Interestingly, conical hexagonal lattices with narrow endcaps that are closed using P pentagons are required by Euler's theorem to have a quantized cone angle θ defined by sin(θ/2) = 1 - (P/6) for P = 0, 1, ... , 6; minimum cone angle is 19.2° at P = 5.*[2684]

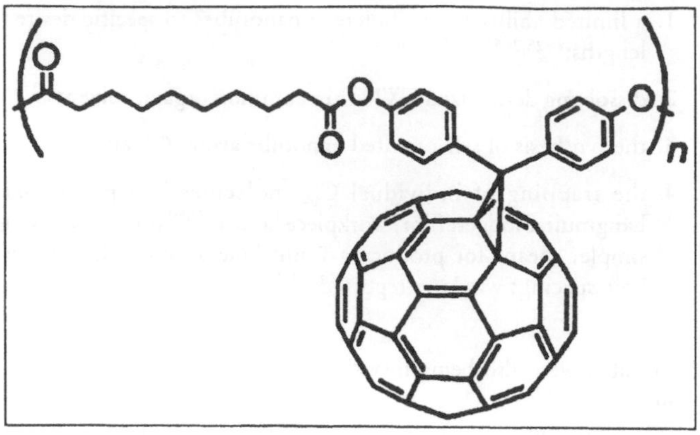

Fig. 2.20B. Fullerene polyester polymer.[2621]

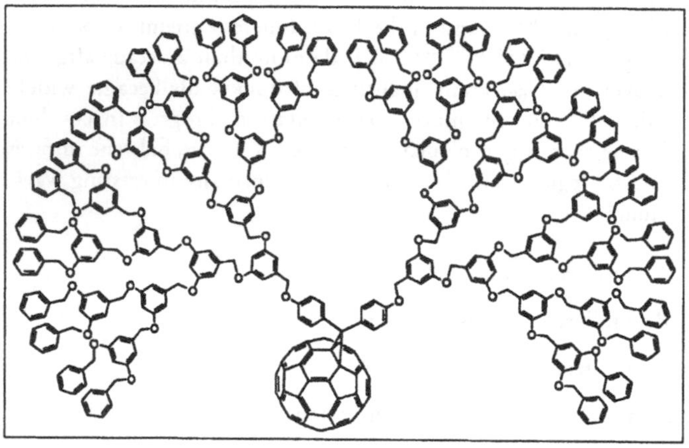

Fig. 2.20C. Fullerene dendrimer.[2620]

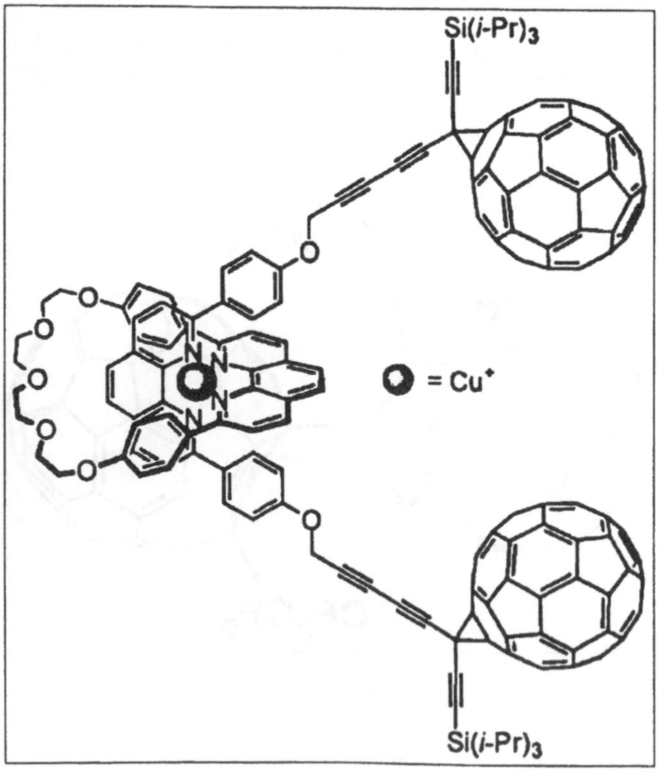

Fig. 2.20D. Fullerene rotaxane.[2622]

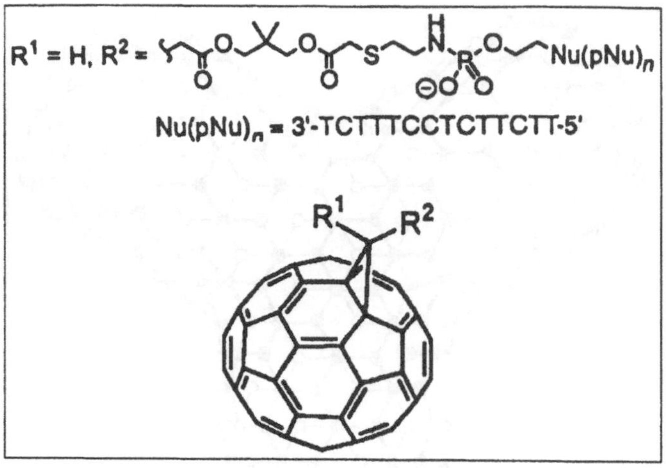

Fig. 2.20E. Fullerene-nucleotide DNA cleaving agent.[2623]

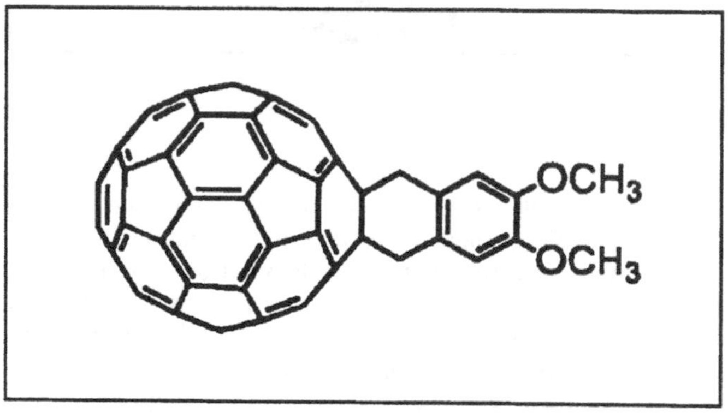

Fig. 2.20F. Stable Diels-Alder fullerene adduct.[2624]

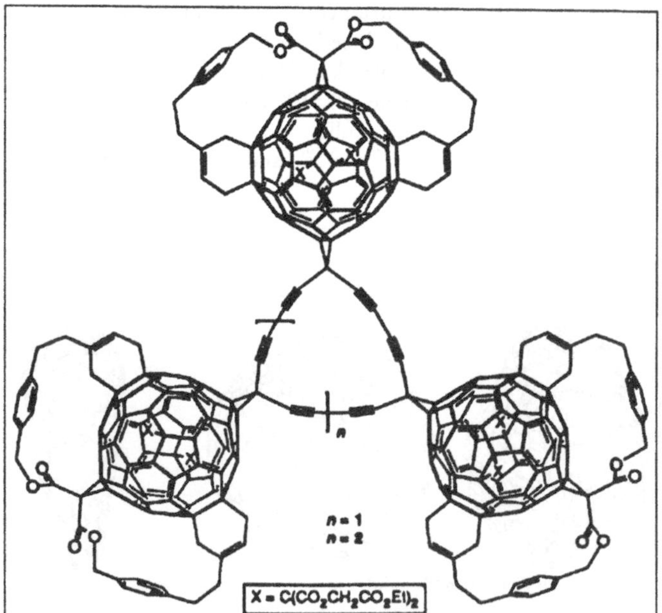

Fig. 2.20G. Extended fullerene polymers.[2624]

Theory[2665] and experiment[2666] suggest that SWNTs may be joined at 30° angles to create complex structures, including helices and three-way nanotube junctions[1308,2614] as suggested by Figure 2.18.

In 1998, the idea of using fullerenes as "Tinkertoys" for molecular construction was just starting to be considered.[2643] For example, given the synthesis of C_{60} exohedral monoadducts and multiple adducts described above, it may be possible to fabricate simple gears by bonding rigid ligands onto the external surfaces of carbon nanotubes in the manner of gear teeth,[2644-2646] although the chemical synthesis of nanotubes with precisely positioned teeth will not be easy.[2667] Given the success in 1996 of IBM scientists[2647] in positioning individual organic molecules (each having a total of 173 atoms and a 1.5-nm diameter) at room temperature by purely mechanical means, it might also be possible to align and maintain these molecular gear teeth in atomically precise meshed positions. If this could be done, would such devices actually work in the manner of macroscale gears?

J. Han and colleagues at NASA/Ames[2648] performed a detailed 2000-atom molecular dynamics simulation to investigate the properties of molecular gears fashioned from carbon nanotubes with teeth added via a benzyne reaction known to occur with C_{60}. Computationally, one gear is powered by forcing the atoms near the end of the nanotube to rotate (Fig. 2.21), and a second gear is allowed to rotate by keeping the atoms near the end of its nanotube constrained to a cylinder (i.e., the ends of the shaft were constrained to not elongate but were allowed to move within a plane transverse to the tube symmetry axis). The meshing aromatic gear teeth transfer angular momentum from the powered gear to the driven gear. Each gear is made of a 1.1-nm diameter (14, 0) nanotube with seven benzyne teeth. The spacing between two nanotubes is 1.8 nm and the smallest distance between a tooth atom and a tube atom is ~0.4 nm. The results show that the gears can operate up to 70 GHz in vacuo at room temperature without overheating or slipping. As rotational speed rises above 150 GHz, the gears overheat and begin to slip with tooth tilting up to 20°, but no bond or tooth breaking occurs up to at least 3000 K and slipping gears can always be returned to proper operation by lowering the temperature or the rotation rate. A related nanotube gear system (5-8 sprockets, 290-464 atoms) simulated by Robertson and colleagues[2670] at the Naval Research Laboratory (NRL) showed similar overheating at 500 GHz but was stable when accelerated to only 20 GHz.

The NASA group also simulated several other types of nanotube-based gear systems. For instance, a rack and pinion system (Fig. 2.22) was designed using a gear made from a (14, 0) nanotube with teeth separated by two hexagon rings and a shaft made from a (9, 9) tube with teeth separated by three rings. Gear and shaft are 1.94 nm apart, with tooth face normal to the radial direction of nanotube (14, 0) for the gear, but in the axis direction of nanotube (9, 9) for the shaft. The gear could receive power, driving the shaft, or vice versa, and worked well for shaft translational velocities up to ~100 m/sec. (Most devices described in Drexler[10] typically move at ≤1 m/sec.) Since shaft mass is almost twice gear mass, it takes more power for the gear to drive the shaft. In another simulation involving a large 1.4-nm gear coupled to a smaller 0.8-nm gear (Fig. 2.23), the large gear drives the smaller gear smoothly, but if power is instead applied to the smaller gear at a sufficiently large acceleration, then the smaller gear does not drive the larger one but instead "bounces back and forth several times, like elastic collisions of a small ball between two boards."

Another research group at Oak Ridge National Laboratory (ORNL) used classical molecular dynamics to investigate the properties of molecular bearings consisting of an inner and an outer carbon nanotube.[2662,2663] The graphite bearings ranged in size from inner shafts between 0.4-1.6 nm in diameter up to 12 nm long, and outer cylinders between 1.0-2.3 nm in diameter up to 4 nm long. The original simulations[2662] found excessive vibrational motion, but subsequent work using a more complete quantum approach[2663,2664] found that under certain conditions the nanobearing is "frictionless" and undergoes superrotation, a classical dynamical behavior reminiscent of superfluidity. The regime of superrotary motion is somewhat restricted when the nanobearing is under load, which suggests that a very careful design is required to ensure optimum performance.

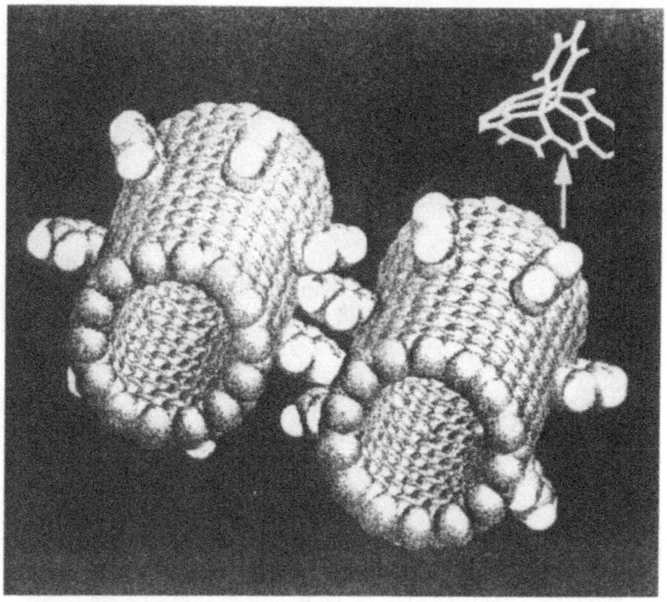

Fig. 2.21. Computer simulation of fullerene nanogears of the same size (courtesy of Al Globus, NASA/Ames).[2648,2667]

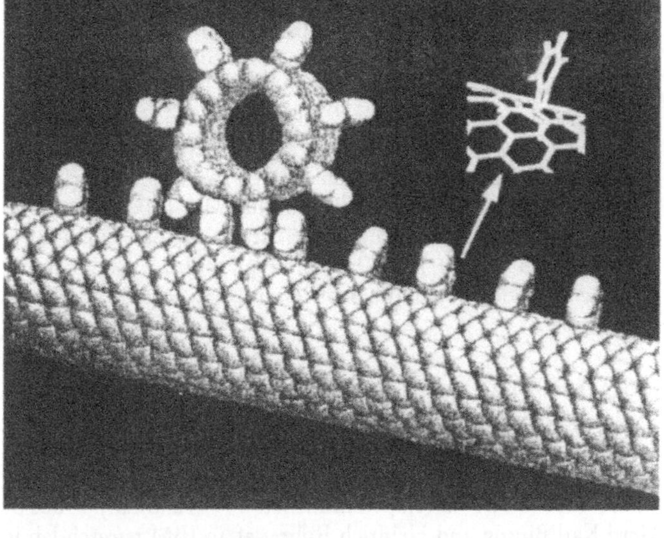

Fig. 2.22. Computer simulation of fullerene rack and pinion system (courtesy of Al Globus, NASA/Ames).[2648,2667]

The ORNL group simulated a fullerene motor[2668] consisting of two concentric graphite cylinders (shaft and sleeve) with one positive and one negative electric charge attached to the shaft. Rotational motion of the shaft was induced by applying one, or sometimes two, oscillating laser fields. The shaft cycled between periods of

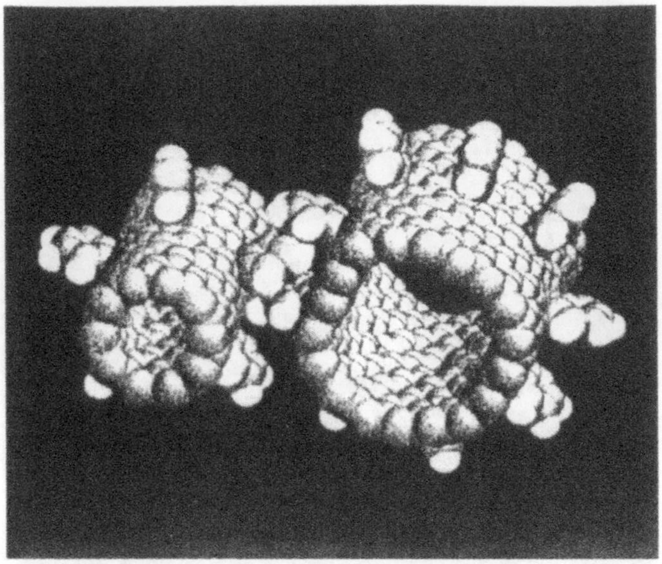

Fig. 2.23. Computer simulation of fullerene nanogears of different sizes (courtesy of Al Globus, NASA/Ames).[2648,2667]

undesirable rotational pendulum-like behavior and good unidirectional motor-like behavior. The NASA/Ames group simulated a pulsed-laser-powered carbon nanotube gear-motor system which rotated consistently in one direction, although that direction could be either clockwise or counterclockwise.[2667]

G. Leach and colleagues[2705] also simulated various carbon nanotubes treated as nanostruts using molecular dynamics calculations, as described earlier for diamondoid block struts. The conclusions were similar though less severe. Nanotubes with 100:1 aspect ratio and 0.8-nm diameter at 300 K experienced periodic oscillations in length of ~0.4 nm at ~122 GHz, although multiple modes clearly were being excited; nanotubes of lesser aspect varied by at most ~0.04 nm.

2.3.3 Scanning Probe Technology

The third general pathway leading to molecular manufacturing involves a technology known as scanning probe microscopes (SPMs).[1093,2728-2730] The first of the SPMs was the Scanning Tunneling Microscope (STM) developed in the late 1970s and early 1980s by Gerd Karl Binnig and Heinrich Rohrer at an IBM research lab in Zurich, Switzerland,[2731-2735] earning these scientists, along with Ernst Ruska, the 1986 Nobel in Physics. The STM was initially used as an imaging device, capable of resolving individual atoms by recording the quantum tunneling current that occurs when an extremely sharp conductive probe tip (usually tungsten, nickel, gold, or PtIr) is brought to within about one atomic diameter of an atom, and then adjusting the position of the tip to maintain a constant current as the tip is scanned over a bumpy atomic surface (Fig. 2.24). A height change as small as 0.1 nm can cause tunneling current to double. The tip is connected to an arm that is moved in three dimensions by stiff ceramic piezoelectric transducers that provide sub-nanometer positional control. If the tip is atomically sharp, then the tunneling current is effectively confined to a region within ~0.1 nm of the point on the surface directly beneath the tip, thus the record of tip adjustments generates an atomic-scale topographic map of the surface. STM tips can scan samples at ~KHz frequencies, although slower scans are used for very rough surfaces. In some

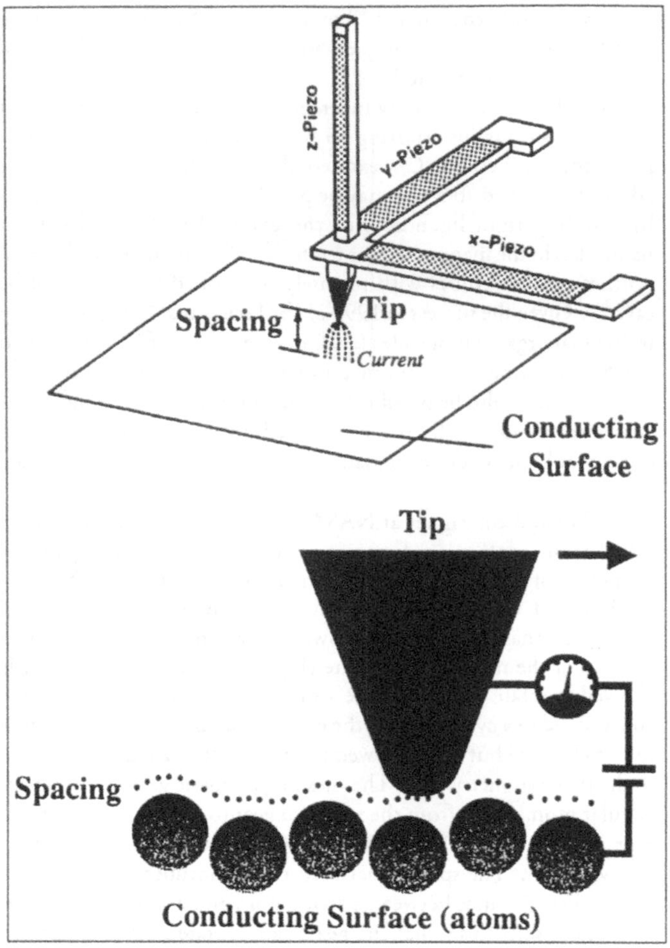

Fig. 2.24. Schematic of scanning tunneling microscope (STM) (redrawn from Drexler[72] and Foster[2788]).

modern STMs (e.g., the DI Nanoscope), the sample is moved while the tip is held stationary.

A major limitation of the STM was that it only worked with conducting materials such as metals or semiconductors, but not with insulators or biological structures such as DNA.[1066,2775] To remedy this situation, in 1986 Binnig, Quate and Gerber developed the Atomic Force Microscope (AFM)[445] which is sensitive directly to the forces between the tip and the sample, rather than a tunneling current. An AFM can operate in at least three modes. In "attractive" or non-contact mode (NC-AFM, 0.01-1 N/m force constant), the tip is held some tens of nanometers above the sample surface where it experiences the attractive combination of van der Waals, electrostatic, or magnetostatic forces. In "repulsive" or contact mode (C-AFM, 0.01-1 N/m force constant), the tip is pressed close enough to the surface for tip and sample electron clouds to overlap, generating a repulsive electrostatic force of ~10 nN, much like the stylus riding a groove in a record player. There is also intermittent-contact mode (IC-AFM, 0.01-1 N/m force constant), which is sometimes called "tapping" mode. In any of these modes, a topographic map of the surface is generated by recording the up-and-down motions of the cantilever arm as the tip is scanned. These motions may be measured either by the deflection of a light spot reflected from a mirrored surface on the cantilever or by tiny changes in voltage generated by piezoelectric transducers attached to the moving cantilever arm.

Typical AFM cantilevers have lengths of 100-400 microns, widths of 20-50 microns, and thicknesses between 0.4 to several microns. AFM tips may be positioned with ~0.01 nm precision, compressive loads as small as 1-10 pN are routinely measured,[433,450,2757,2758] and the tips may be operated even in liquids.[2898]

S. Vetter notes that STM technology has also improved, reaching resolutions of ~0.001 nm in the z direction (vertical) and ~0.01 nm in the xy plane, well beyond atomic resolution. The STM remains the instrument with the best resolution. The conducting-surface limitation has been overcome in some cases by coating the target with an extremely thin conducting layer, developing tips with multiple electrodes, and coating a conducting substrate with a sample so thin as to allow enough conduction even if the sample is characterized as an insulator in bulk.

By 1998, the growing family of SPMs included at least forty types of instruments and techniques that relied on interactions between a scanned surface and a nearby probe. Different instruments measured different forces and thus could be used to characterize different properties of the surface.[2758] For example, friction force microscopes (FFMs), magnetic force microscopes (MFMs), shear force microscopes (ShFMs), scanning capacitance microscopes (SCMs), scanning conducting ion microscopes, chemical force microscopes,[2755,2756] and electrostatic force microscopes (EFMs) measured frictional drag or other binding forces. Magnetic resonance force microscopes (MRFM)[2776,2929] used a field generated from a small magnet mounted on the tip of the cantilever arm to probe nuclear magnetic moments in a small region on the surface of the sample, imaging atom types and even detecting the spin of a single electron. By the mid-1990s, AFMs were already a $100 million/year industry[2777] and SPMs generally were an off-the-shelf technology costing up to $50,000-$500,000 for complete systems, with the whole industry worth up to ~$0.5 billion annually. (Low-performance "homebrew," student,[2712] and science-fair STMs have been built for as little as $50.[2778])

How might SPMs be used for molecular manufacturing? In the crudest approach, SPMs might be employed as nanoscale milling machines to carve out "nanoparts" from appropriate substrates. For example, Kim and Lieber[16] used an AFM to perform nanomachining operations on a molybdenum trioxide crystal—applying a 100 nN load at the tip, they milled a triangular-shaped 50-nm planar chunk from the crystal, then slid the part 200 nm across the work surface by pushing it with the AFM tip. Sheehan and Lieber[1737,2779] milled a 50-nm rectangular part and two other parts with concavities complementary to the rectangle by mechanically etching a MoO_3 layer deposited atop an MoS_2 surface by pressing down with an AFM tip at a 50 nN load. Like a numerical-controlled machine tool, the AFM motions could be programmed to perform a series of steps, like automatically carving the chemical formula "MoO_3" into the crystal.[2779] Nanoparts with features as narrow as 10 nm can be nanomilled in a limited set of materials [P.E. Sheehan, personal communication, 1995]. In theory, large arrays of independently-controlled SPM tips (see below) could be operated in parallel to carve out great numbers of similar objects simultaneously, though such objects would of course not be atomically identical without further "finishing." AFM tips have also been used to bulldoze nanoscale lines and rectangular <10-nm features into non-conducting photoresist,[2752-2754] perform "dip-pen" AFM nanolithography,[2780] form grooves,[2781] and fabricate a single-electron transistor via an STM nano-oxidation process.[2782] A carbon nanotube affixed to an AFM tip was used as a pencil to write 10-nm-wide features onto silicon substrates at ~0.5 mm/sec:[2711] An electric field issues from the nanotube, removing hydrogen atoms from a hydrogen monolayer atop a silicon base; the exposed silicon surface oxidized, producing narrow SiO_2 tracks.

Perhaps more significantly, SPMs have been employed in an increasingly sophisticated manner to manipulate individual atoms and small clusters of atoms. The possibility of modifying surfaces with scanning probe tips was evident from the earliest years of STM research, since inadvertent contact between tips and surfaces routinely caused such modifications,[10] and the possibility of transferring material between tip and sample had already been discussed.[2783] Suggestions for controlled surface modification soon appeared,[2784] and in 1985 Becker and Golovchencko[2785] used voltage pulses on an STM tip to pluck a single germanium atom from the {111} surface of a sample. In 1988, J. Foster and colleagues[2786] at IBM Almaden pinned small organic molecules to a graphite surface by applying a small electrical pulse through an STM. Additional pulses enlarged or erased this molecular feature, and often split the organic molecule into smaller pieces, though not in a controlled manner. Other workers used an STM to dump small clusters of gold atoms on a platinum surface,[2736-2739] clusters of copper atoms on a gold surface,[2787] and molecules of tungsten carbide from a supply flowing over a surface.[2788] Others reported positioning carbon monoxide molecules and platinum atoms on platinum surfaces,[278] moving clusters and single atoms of silicon across a silicon surface at room temperature,[2746-2751] and fabricating via STM a "molecular corral"[2789] or "quantum corral"[2790]—a ring of atoms so small that the enclosed electrons were forced to exhibit quantum behavior. In 1999, Tomanek and Kral[3266] proposed an atomic fountain pen in which a carbon nanotube filled with atoms is electrically induced to release these atoms, one by one every 15 microsec, onto the work surface.

More precise control was achieved by Eigler and Schweizer[278] at IBM Almaden in 1989, when they used an STM to position 35 individual xenon atoms on a nickel surface to spell out the corporate logo "IBM" (Fig. 2.25). To accomplish this, a bias voltage was applied to weaken the adsorption of each atom to its nickel substrate, then each atom was dragged, one by one, to the desired locations at a speed of ~0.4 nm/sec[2791] to build a meaningful pattern. It took 22 hours[2791] to make the entire logo, or ~38 min/atom. The experiment had to be carried out at 4 K (i.e., liquid helium temperatures) because the arrangement would have been unstable at room temperature. Numerous similar examples of "atomic graffiti"[775] followed the IBM experiment, including atoms patterned in the shape of a world map;[2792] the word "atom"[2895] and "nanoworld",[2897] spelled out with atoms, in Japanese; the word "Peace," Einstein's famous equation

Fig. 2.25. IBM logo spelled out using 35 xenon atoms arranged on a nickel surface by an STM (courtesy of IBM Research Division).

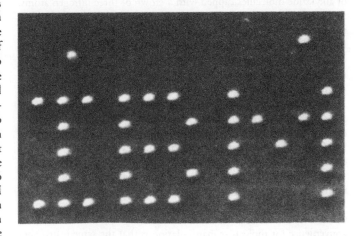

"$E=mc^2$," and even a reproduction of the well-known Einstein portrait with the scientist's tongue sticking out;[300] a sketch of a "molecule man" using 28 individual CO molecules on a platinum surface;[2792] gold nanoparticles spelling out "USC"[2793] and "Zyvex";[2794] and sulfur atoms removed from a surface to make letters 2 nm high.[2795] In 1996, Gimzewski's group[1735] used an STM tip to manipulate individual buckyballs along terraces on a grooved copper plate, making a "molecular abacus."

Some variant of an SPM would appear to be the most promising tool for direct molecular manipulation. Once a tip lies within ~1 nm of a surface, the potential barrier can be lowered sufficiently for atoms to be induced from the surface by field evaporation;[2796] an applied tip voltage ionizes the atom which can then be guided around by the tip. Depending on voltage and separation, atoms, atom clusters, or molecules can be pried out, pushed in, or nudged around on a surface. By 1998, techniques for direct atomic manipulation proceeded at room temperature and ~1000 times faster than the original IBM logo had been assembled. For example, the Nanomanipulator,[2716-2724] an interactive haptic control system created by a group at the University of North Carolina at Chapel Hill, allows near-real-time manipulation of individual gold atoms across a surface using a hand-held master-slave controller that drives an STM probe while the position of the atom is displayed on a monitoring screen visible to the user. Partially funded by NSF, Silicon Graphics, and TopoMetrix,[3156] the Nanomanipulator is a fully-integrated system that enables investigators to "feel" the interatomic forces as the user pushes atoms around on a surface.[2724] In one demonstration, a TV-watching user herded a gold atom, slipping and sliding, into a slot in the planar workplace in about 1 minute; when force feedback was turned off, movements tended to run wild. IBM Almaden has also experimented with removing individual atoms from metal surfaces using an STM hooked into a Virtual Reality Dataglove apparatus.

To manufacture atomically precise parts, it also will be necessary to manipulate covalent bonds at the probe tip. STMs have broken and created chemical bonds; ~1 volt pulses were used to pull atoms out of crystals, binding them to the tip, and then to re-insert them back into the crystal.[2749,2758] In 1995, the first demonstration of catalysis on a nanometer scale was reported by scientists at the Molecular Design Institute at LBL.[2797] They used an AFM modified to function like an ultrafine-point pen for catalytic calligraphy to change the chemical composition of a material surface one molecule at a time. A surface was prepared as a self-assembled monolayer (SAM) of alkylazide molecules capped with a crown of three nitrogen atoms, then platinum-coated chromium was deposited onto an AFM silicon tip just a few atoms wide. The SAM was soaked with a hydrogen-containing solvent, then scanned by the AFM over a 100 micron^2 area, with the platinum catalyzing a covalent bonding reaction in which hydrogen was added to the azides, transforming them into amines as revealed by selective fluorescent tags.

Tip technology is an important and fast-growing subspecialty of SPM research. In 1990, Drexler and Foster[217] suggested the use of custom-made, synthetic proteins to be mounted on the point of an SPM tip. Modified antibodies or specially designed proteins could serve as simple, first-generation "grippers" for binding and manipulating specific molecules, bringing them into position to react with other molecules in a precise and selective way. Functionalized SPM tips have been created to exploit antibody-antigen recognition[2798] and in the context of chemical force microscopy.[2755,2756] A major convenience for molecular manipulation is that the same instrument that does the chemistry and the molecular orienting can also be used to inspect the results.[322]

In 1996, Smalley's group at Rice University[2799] attached a single nanotube to the pyramidal silicon tip of an AFM and showed that it was quite robust and could image the bottom of deep trenches inaccessible to conventional tips. By 1998, progress had been made in functionalized carbon nanotubes for use on AFM tips. Most notably, Wong and colleagues[2800] prepared nanotube tips by oxidation in air at 700°C, burning off all but 2% of the original material and leaving the ends covered with carboxyl (-COOH) groups whose chemistry is rich and well-understood. Four different kinds of tips were created: (1) the original carboxyl tip, which is acidic; (2) an amine-terminated tip (made by forming an amide bond to one of the amine groups in ethylenediamine ($H_2NCH_2CH_2NH_2$)), which is basic; (3) a hydrocarbon-terminated tip (made by forming an amide bond to benzylamine ($C_6H_5CH_2NH_2$)), which is hydrophobic; and (4) a biotin-terminated tip (made by forming an amide bond to a biotin derivative), which shows specific binding to streptavidin. AFM contact forces between tips and selected substrates were shown to be sensitive to pH and to the chemical details of the substrate in ways consistent with the tips' intended chemistry.

Wong's tips had three closely related advantages over previous techniques. First, when a functional group is attached to the apex of an Si_3N_4 or SiO_2 tip, these groups usually adhere to the sides of the tip as well; upon using the tip as a tool, there is a constant hazard that contact with the sides of the tip will alter the workpiece in unwanted places. Unlike these tips built with bulk techniques, the ends of Wong's tips are very different from their sides—the carboxyl groups are attached only on the ends of the nanotube, not on the sides. Second, Wong's tips have lateral dimensions set by the nanoscale dimensions of nanotubes, not by top-down fabrication techniques. Note the authors: "...the small effective radius of nanotube tips significantly improves resolution beyond what can be achieved using commercial silicon tips....we have recently demonstrated that lateral resolution of <3 nm can be achieved by using COOH-terminated single-walled nanotubes tips".[2740-2742] Third, single-walled nanotube tips are much closer to yielding truly single atom tips with controlled chemistry than any other alternative. J. Soreff notes that a (10, 10) nanotube with a 1.4-nm diameter has just 20 atoms at an open end. Even given a statistical distribution of tubes with varying numbers of carboxyl groups attached to their ends, one should be able to build a ligand which covers the whole end of the tube, yielding a method for ensuring that just one molecule of known structure and orientation was present at the end of the probe.

Theoretical studies have employed molecular dynamics simulations and other techniques to investigate the behavior of mechanosynthetic tool tips.[10,2760,2761,2764,3250] For example, Drexler[10] proposed using an acetylene radical to perform selective abstractions of hydrogen from a diamond surface (Fig. 2.26A), and this proposal was further studied in Musgrave's ab initio quantum chemistry analysis[2762] and Sinnott's molecular dynamics modeling of the reaction at room temperature on a diamond {111} surface;[2763,2764] other H-abstraction studies have been done.[10,2907] One possible structure for a hydrogen abstraction tool might be similar to an anthracene whose end had been modified as shown in Figure 2.26B; prior to use, the structure must be activated by removal of the terminal hydrogen.[1199] Brenner and colleagues[2764] describe further work modeling the parallel abstraction of several hydrogen atoms from the diamond {111} surface. Such reactions are similar to those involved in the well-studied chemical

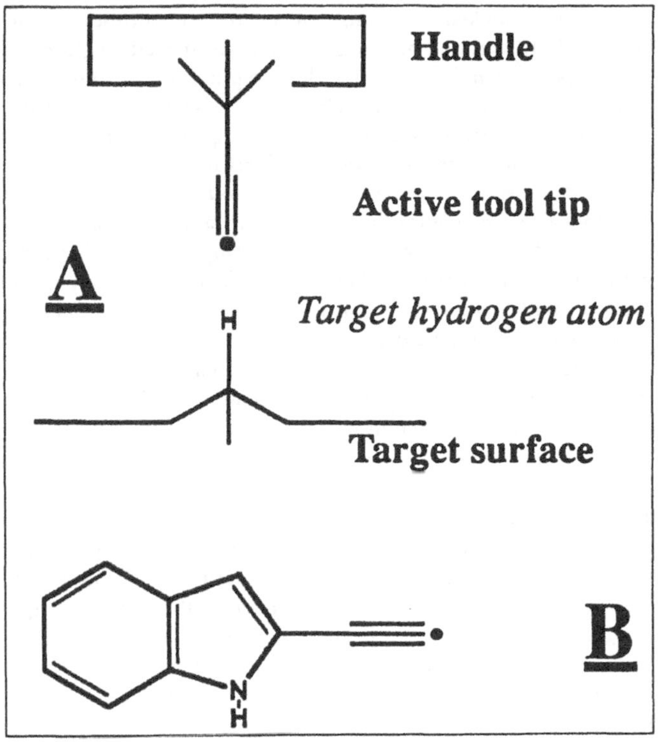

Fig. 2.26. Schematic of proposed hydrogen abstraction tool (redrawn from Merkle[1199]).

vapor deposition of diamond,[2765-2769] but adding only positional control and applied mechanical force; more detailed theoretical studies of diamond mechanosynthesis reactions have begun.[2770,3250]

R. Merkle[2602] has proposed a simple mechanosynthetic system capable of fabricating a large class of useful stiff hydrocarbons. Merkle's system includes positionally-controlled hydrogen abstraction and deposition tools (to remove or add hydrogen atoms to a workpiece), carbene and dimer deposition tools (to add one or two carbons to a workpiece), a silicon radical tool (to remove a carbon), and four other specialized tools. Each proposed tool has a molecular handle structure that could be permanently affixed to a suitably functionalized AFM tip (or other appropriate mechanosynthetic nanomanipulator). As each operation is performed on the butadiyne* (a.k.a diacetylene,[2801] C_4H_2) hydrocarbon feedstock in an inert (e.g., vacuum or noble gas) environment, one or more tools are brought to the workpiece at the necessary position and angle, and any necessary force is applied via the AFM. Interestingly, except for a small number of "vitamin parts"[115] involving transition metals, Merkle's system can in theory synthesize all of its own mechanosynthetic tools, thus establishing net positive production of system components and illustrating a limited subset-level "quantitative parts closure" as first defined in 1982 by Freitas and Gilbreath[115] in connection with self-replicating machine systems (Chapter 14). Merkle acknowledges that several of the proposed reactions involve the simultaneous coordinated action of two, three, or even four positionally controlled tools, but suggests that two 6-degree-of-freedom manipulators plus some combination of appropriate jigs and fixtures should be sufficient in a more parsimonious system. However, steric hindrance of multiple tools at one site also was not explicitly addressed. Another potential problem to be overcome is loss of positional registration as the various functionalized tool heads are changed out at the AFM tip; such tips might be paired with a second positionally-invariant metrology tip on each tool head, allowing precise calibration of workspace location before proceeding back to the workpiece.

Others have suggested fabricating nanoparts by building up structures by stacking layers of individual atoms, perhaps constrained by sacrificial joiners and scaffolding, and honed by differential etching operations.[2802]

Assuming that "nanoparts" can be fabricated to atomic precision, can SPMs also be used to assemble these nanoparts into working nanomachines? Some preliminary work has been accomplished. For instance, arrays of nanoscale holes have been synthesized that could serve as "workpiece holders." In one experiment, C_{60} buckyballs were scattered about on a prepared surface, then an AFM pushed the individual spheres into their own little holes, securely seating them pending further processing.[2630] The C_{60}-impregnated perforated film was so durable that the buckyballs remained trapped after several months of storage. Similarly, Jung and colleagues in Gimzewski's group[2803] synthesized 4-legged porphyrin-based[2804] molecular "nanoparts" that were specifically designed for easy positioning on a copper surface. Pushing with an STM at room temperature, the authors displaced the ~1.5-nm wide nanoparts in predefined directions and rotated the 4-legged molecules at will, arranging, for example, the parts into a precise hexagonal configuration on the copper surface. The STM has been used to induce, and to view, the rotation of an individual oxygen molecule trapped on a platinum surface, as it is intentionally and stably rotated into any one of three distinct orientations.[2805] The forces required to slide, or alternatively to roll, a carbon nanotube across a graphitic surface have been directly measured by AFM.[2717]

The first known instance of a crude but purely mechanical "nanopart" assembly operation was performed in 1995 by Paul E. Sheehan and Charles M. Lieber.[1737] Two nanoscale parts with rectangular slots and a third 50-nm rectangular sliding "latch" member were milled from a MoO_3 crystal using an AFM, then the rectangular "latch" member was slid repeatedly from one slot to the other using the same AFM, making a three-nanopart reversible mechanical latch. Noted the authors: "The lateral force needed to break the latch, 41 nN, was large considering the small latch contact area, which suggests that relatively robust assemblies can be created with such devices. Such a reversible latch could serve as the basis for mechanical logic gates....Our results...demonstrate the ability to machine complex shapes and to reversibly assemble these pieces into interlocking structures."

In 1998, manipulation of nanoscale parts in the vertical dimension (e.g., normal to the surface plane) had only just begun.[2743-2745] The first three-dimensional structure built out of single "nanoparts" was demonstrated in 1997 by Requicha's group at the USC Laboratory for Molecular Robotics. First, an AFM was used to push 5-nm gold nanoparticles in the third dimension up and over surface protrusions or obstructions—for example, a 5-nm gold particle was shoved up onto a 2-nm-high protrusion, then slid back off again onto the surface.[2806] In another series of experiments conducted in air at room temperature with 15-30 nm gold nanoparticles deposited on silicon previously coated with a silane layer, Requicha's group used an AFM to build a simple 3-D pyramidal structure by pushing one gold "nanopart" on top of two others, then off again; the group also used the AFM to rotate and translate a dimer unit formed by two linked "nanoparts".[2807]

**Experimentalists are warned that butadiyne, chemically distinct from the more common molecule butadiene (C_4H_6), can polymerize explosively under some conditions.[2801]*

Three-dimensional nanoassembly might perhaps be more readily achieved if nanoparts could assist in their own assembly process. R. Merkle [personal communication, 1998] suggests that an SPM could be used to position DNA-tagged molecular building blocks. A building block tagged with a specific single-stranded DNA should preferentially adhere to a surface covered with the complementary DNA. If the building block has a second single-stranded DNA tag which is complementary to single-stranded DNA on the tip of an SPM, and if it is initially attached to the SPM tip by this tag, then it could be positioned by the SPM and attached to the surface. The relative strength of attachments could be adjusted by changing the number of base pairs in the complementary region between the two strands.[1066] A related suggestion, due to G. Fahy,[322] is that SPM tips for assembly could be designed with more than one binding site. The existence of at least two binding sites could allow precise orientation of a nanopart, permitting the nanopart to be presented to a desired target site (or another nanopart, possibly attached to another manipulator) at exactly the location and in exactly the orientation desired, assuming that each nanopart can bind to each tip in only one possible orientation. A convenient post-assembly nanopart release mechanism is also required.

In 1997, the Avouris group[2750,2771] at IBM Yorktown Heights demonstrated that the tip of an atomic force microscope (AFM) could be used to control the shape and position of individual multiwalled carbon nanotubes dispersed on a surface. Nanotubes could be bent, straightened, translated, rotated, and (under certain conditions) cut.

In 1998, Zyvex LLC (a developmental engineering company whose goal is to create a molecular assembler capable of manufacturing atomically precise structures[2794]) demonstrated the ability to manipulate carbon nanotubes in three dimensions inside a scanning electron microscope (SEM) having ~6 nm resolution at near-video scan rates. Zyvex's custom piezoelectric vacuum manipulator achieved positional resolutions comparable to SPMs along with the ability to manipulate objects along one rotational and three linear degrees of freedom with 0.1 nm spatial resolution.[2808] This prototypical device could probe, select and handle limited classes of nanometer-scale objects such as carbon nanotubes under real-time SEM inspection. Carbon nanotubes were attached to commercial atomic force microscope (AFM) tips either by van der Waals forces alone or by "nanosoldering" by a concentrated electron beam from the SEM. Forces applied to the nanotubes could be measured from the cantilevers' deflections (spring constants 0.01-100 N/m; see also Neumister and Ducker[2809]). Sometimes nanotubes were transferred from tip to tip. The manipulator could function both as a research tool for investigating properties of carbon nanotubes and other nanoscale objects without surface restrictions, and as a rudimentary building device for larger nanotube assemblies. Zyvex believed that this capability to select and manipulate nanoscale components and to examine directly their suitability as construction materials during various phases of the construction process would play an important role in enabling the technology of assembling mechanical and electronic devices from prefabricated components. Most impressively, the Zyvex system allowed the simultaneous coordinated operation of three independently controlled AFM tips within the same workspace, at different orientations. (A four-tip system was expected to be operational by mid-1999 [Mark Dyer, personal communication, 1999].) Two-handed coordinated micromanipulation under the view of an SEM had previously been demonstrated by others.[2810]

Tuzun and colleagues[2811] calculated the requirements for coaxial docking of two nanotubes of different diameters to form a molecular bearing. They looked at bearings formed from nanotubes 11 rings long, with 10 carbons per ring in the shaft and either 30 or 34 carbons per ring in the sleeve. For the computer simulations, Tuzun placed the sleeve of the bearing along the z axis and gave the shaft a small initial velocity towards it. A perfectly aligned shaft falls straight into a potential well from the van der Waals attraction to the sleeve; displaced or mis-oriented shafts can bounce off the edge of the sleeve. The docking envelopes for the molecular dynamics calculations and for the rigid body calculations had essentially the same shape, but with slightly different sizes. For the atomistic calculation, a shaft aligned parallel to the sleeve (with a 30 carbon ring sleeve) can be displaced by 0.26 nm before it fails to dock, while in the rigid body calculation the displacement can only be 0.16 nm. The authors note that "if an end of the shaft points closely enough to the center of the sleeve, it will fall into the non-bonded potential energy well and the two nanotubes will dock." These calculations are important because they tell us what tolerances can be accepted during the manual assembly process. Note the authors: "A question just as important as how to design or operate nanomachines is how to assemble them".[2811] Interestingly, one of Zyvex's experiments[2808] produced a multiwalled carbon nanotube that thinned in three steps along its length, suggesting the most likely explanation that the inner shells had been pulled from the outer shells. This phenomenon has also been observed by others and is known as the "sword and sheath" failure[2812]—the exact inverse of the purposeful nanotube insertion operation investigated by Tuzun and colleagues.

In order to produce large numbers of nanoparts and nano-assemblies, massively parallel SPM arrays and microscale SPMs[2772-2774] would be most convenient. Force-sensing devices such as piezoelectric,[2813] piezoresistive,[2814] and capacitive[2815] micro-cantilevers made it possible to construct microscale AFMs on chips without an external deflection sensor. (We exclude fixed-tip arrays[2816] in the following discussion.) In 1995, Itoh and colleagues[2817] at the University of Tokyo fabricated an experimental piezoelectric ZnO_2-on-SiO_2 microcantilever array of ten tips on a single silicon chip. Each cantilever tip lay ~70 microns from its neighbor, and measured 150 microns long, 50 microns wide and 3.5 microns thick, or ~26,000 micron^3/device, and each of the devices could be operated independently in the z-axis (e.g., vertically) up to near their mechanical resonance frequencies of 145-147 KHz at an actuation sensitivity of ~20 nm/volt—for instance, 0.3-nm resolution at 125 KHz.

Parallel probe scanning and lithography has been achieved by Quate's group at Stanford, which has progressed from simple piezoresistive microcantilever arrays with 5 tips spaced 100 microns apart and 0.04-nm resolution at 1 KHz but only one z-axis actuator for the whole array,[2818] to arrays with integrated sensors and actuators that allow parallel imaging and lithography with feedback and independent control of each of up to 16 tips, with scanning speeds up to 3 mm/sec using a piezoresistive sensor.[2819,2820] By 1998, Quate's group had demonstrated[2821-2827,2829] arrays of 50-100 independently controllable AFM probe tips mounted in 2-D patterns with 60 KHz resonances, including a 10 x 10 cantilevered tip array fabricated in closely spaced rows using throughwafer interconnects on a single chip.

MacDonald's group at the Cornell Nanofabrication Facility has pursued similar goals. In 1991, the team fabricated their first submicron stylus, driven in the xy plane using interdigitating MEMS comb drives,[2830] including the first opposable tip pair (Fig. 2.27). By 1993, they had produced a 25-tip array on one xyz actuator,[2831,2832] and by 1995 a complete working micro-STM (including xy comb drives) measuring 200 microns on an edge and a micro-AFM measuring 2 mm on an edge including a 1-mm long cantilever with

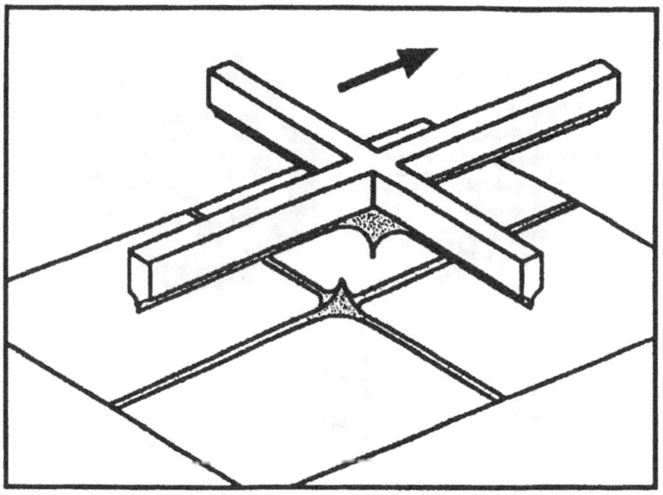

Fig. 2.27. Schematic of an opposable STM tip pair (redrawn from Yao, Arney and MacDonald[2830]).

a 20-nm diameter integrated tip on a 6-micron high by 1-micron diameter support shaft.[1749,1974] MacDonald's group demonstrated tip arrays with 5 micron spacings, exploiting the same process used to make the working micro-STM.[2833,2834] With the same technology tips or small arrays of tips could be spaced 25-50 microns apart and integrated with individual z-axis microactuators, so that one xy-axis manipulator could support many tips with each tip having a separate z actuator. By 1997, the group[2835] had built and tested an array of micro-STMs on the surface of an ordinary silicon chip, with each tip on a cantilever 150 microns long with 3-D sensing and control. The largest prototype array has 144 probes,[2836] arranged in a square consisting of 12 rows of 12 probes each, with individual probe needles about 200 microns apart. Further development was to focus on increasing the range of movement and on fitting more and smaller probes into the same space.

2.4 Molecular Components and Molecular Assemblers

Assuming that various elementary molecular parts fabrication and assembly operations can be performed for certain limited classes of structures, perhaps as described in Section 2.3, then what structures would be interesting and useful to build? This Section briefly describes a small set of possibly useful molecular mechanical components (Section 2.4.1) and then concludes with a discussion of the concept of the molecular assembler (Section 2.4.2).

2.4.1 Molecular Mechanical Components

In order to lay a foundation for molecular manufacturing, it is necessary to create and to analyze possible designs for nanoscale mechanical components that could, in principle, be manufactured. Because these components could not yet be built in 1998, such designs could not be subjected to rigorous experimental testing and validation. Designers were forced instead to rely upon ab initio structural analysis and computer studies including molecular dynamics simulations. Noted Drexler:[10] "Our ability to model molecular machines (systems and devices) of specific kinds, designed in part for ease of modeling, has far outrun our ability to make them. Design calculations and computational experiments enable the theoretical studies of these devices, independent of the technologies needed to implement them."

In nanoscale design, building materials do not change continuously as they are cut and shaped, but rather must be treated as being formed from discrete atoms.[2845] A nanoscale component is a supermolecule, not a finely divided solid. Any stray atoms or molecules within such a structure may act as dirt that can clog and disable the device, and the scaling of vibrations, electrical forces, thermal expansion, magnetic interaction and surface tension with size lead to dramatically different phenomena as system size shrinks from the macroscale to the nanoscale.[10]

Molecular bearings are perhaps the most convenient class of components to design because their structure and operation is fairly straightforward. One of the simplest examples is Drexler's overlap-repulsion bearing design,[10] shown with end views and exploded views in Figure 2.28 using both ball-and-stick and space-filling representations. This bearing has exactly 206 atoms including carbon, silicon, oxygen and hydrogen, and is comprised of a small shaft that rotates within a ring sleeve measuring 2.2 nm in diameter. The atoms of the shaft are arranged in a 6-fold symmetry, while the ring has 14-fold symmetry, a combination that provides low energy barriers to shaft rotation.* Figure 2.29 shows an exploded view of a 2808-atom strained-shell** sleeve bearing designed by Drexler and Merkle[10] using molecular mechanics force fields to ensure that bond lengths, bond angles, van der Waals distances, and strain energies are reasonable. This 4.8-nm diameter bearing features an interlocking-groove interface which derives from a modified diamond {100} surface. Ridges on the shaft interlock with ridges on the sleeve, making a very stiff structure. Attempts to bob the shaft up or down, or rock it from side to side, or displace it in any direction (except axial rotation, wherein displacement is extremely smooth) encounter a very strong resistance.[279] Whether these bearings would have to be assembled in unitary fashion, or instead could be assembled by inserting one part into the other without damaging either part, had not been extensively studied or modeled by 1998.

Molecular gears are another convenient component system for molecular manufacturing design-ahead. For example, Drexler and Merkle[10] designed a 3557-atom planetary gear, shown in side-, end-, and exploded views in Figure 2.30. The entire assembly has twelve moving parts and is 4.3 nm in diameter and 4.4 nm in length, with a molecular weight of 51,009.844 daltons and a molecular volume of 33.458 nm^3. An animation of the computer simulation shows

---

**At the atomic scale, the two opposing surfaces have periodic bumps and hollows, but the periods of these bumps are different for the two surfaces—that is, they are "incommensurate."[10,3243] Two incommensurate surfaces cannot lock up in any particular position, hence the barrier to free rotation is very low, on the order of ~0.001 kT (thermal noise at room temperature).[280]*

***Components of high rotational symmetry may consist of (a) intrinsically curved, (b) strained-shell, or (c) special-case structures.[10] In the case of (b), the bearing illustrated in Figure 2.29 has bond strains of around ~10% (~38 zJ/atom), and similar hydrocarbon bearings have been designed with bond strains of ~5% (~11 zJ/atom) [R. Merkle, personal communication, 1998]. For comparison, strain energies[1866,2615] are $\lesssim$ 3 zJ/atom for diamond lattice, ~25 zJ/atom in C_{240}, ~7-27 zJ/atom in the walls of infinite carbon nanotubes of diameter 0.7-1.3 nm, up to ~59 zJ (13% strain) for some bonds around a Lomer dislocation in diamond,[2861] ~70 zJ/atom in C_{60}, and at least ~80 zJ/atom for C_{36}. Fullerenes are among the most highly strained natural molecules ever isolated. For symmetrical diamondoid structures with negligible hoop stress, permissible bond strains may in theory be as large as ~140 zJ/atom producing a ~23% bond strain;[10] nanotube breaking strain is 20-30% for various chiral forms, and buckling strain is ~8% in axial compression. Bond strain in a simple strained-shell bearing can be lowered by making the bearing bigger, thereby reducing the curvature. Thus strained shell bearings are feasible, although in 1998 it remained unclear exactly how small they could be before becoming unstable.*

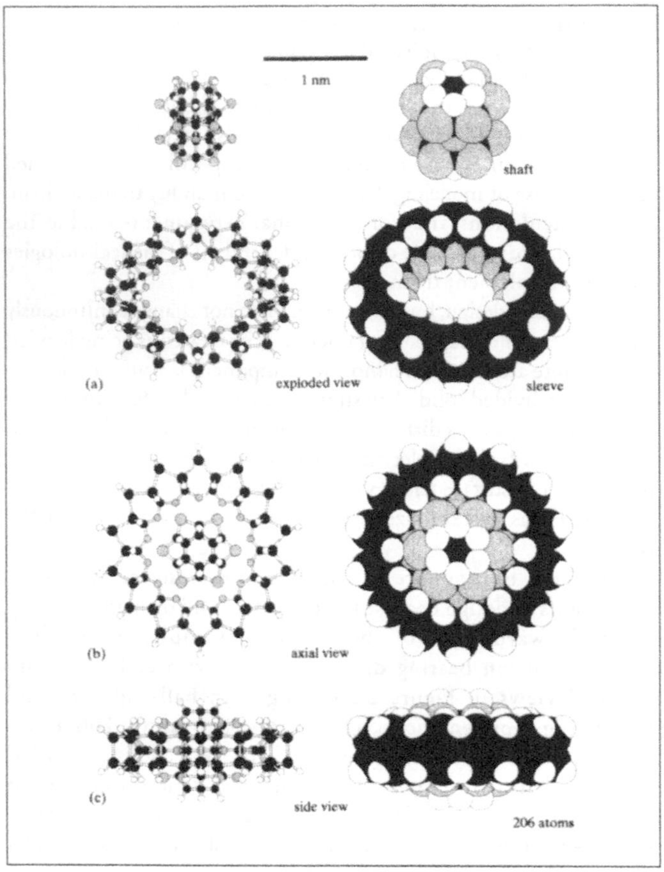

Fig. 2.28. End views and exploded views of a 206-atom overlap-repulsion bearing (courtesy of K.E. Drexler[10]).

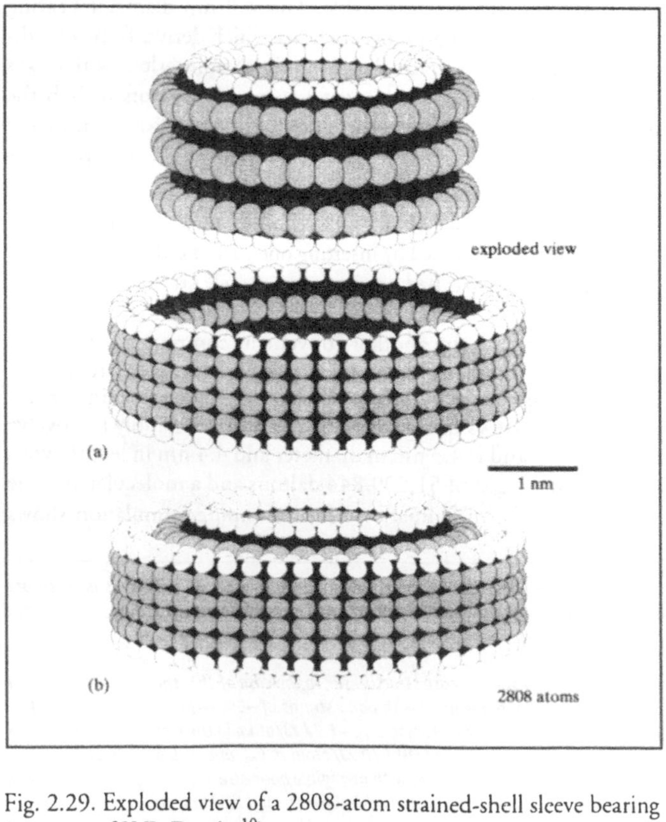

Fig. 2.29. Exploded view of a 2808-atom strained-shell sleeve bearing (courtesy of K.E. Drexler[10]).

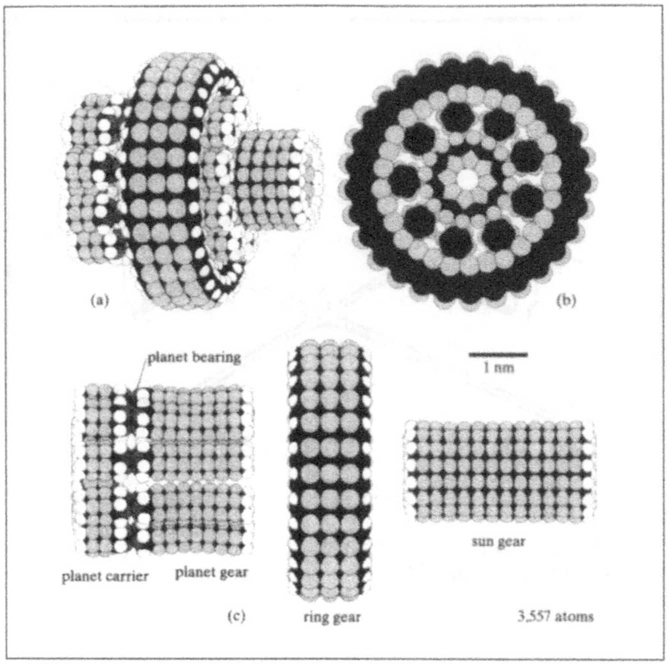

Fig. 2.30. End-, side- and exploded-view of a 3557-atom planetary gear (courtesy of K.E. Drexler[10]).

the central shaft rotating rapidly and the peripheral output shaft rotating slowly. The small planetary gears rotate around the central shaft, and they are surrounded by a ring gear that holds the planets in place and ensures that all of the components move in the proper fashion. The ring gear is a strained silicon shell with sulfur atom termination; the sun gear is a structure related to an oxygen-terminated diamond {100} surface; the planet gears resemble multiple hexasterane structures with oxygen rather than CH_2 bridges between the parallel rings; and the planet carrier is adapted from a Lomer-dislocation[2894] array created by R. Merkle and L. Balasubramaniam, and linked to the planet gears using C-C bonded bearings. View (c) retains the elastic deformations that are hidden in (a)—the gears are bowed. In the macroscale world, planetary gears are used in automobiles and other machines where it is necessary to transform the speeds of rotating shafts.

W. Goddard and colleagues at CalTech[2844,2845] performed a rotational impulse dynamics study of this "first-generation" planetary gear. At the normal operational rotation rates for which this component was designed (e.g., <1 GHz for <10 m/sec interfacial velocities), the gear worked as intended and did not overheat.[2844] Started from room temperature, the gear took a few cycles to engage, then rotated thermally stably at ~400 K. However, when the gear was driven to ~100 GHz, significant instabilities appeared although the device still did not self-destruct.[2844] One run at ~80 GHz showed excess kinetic energy causing gear temperature to oscillate up to 450 K above baseline.[2845] One animation of the simulation shows that the ring gear wiggles violently because it is rather thin. In an actual nanorobot incorporating numerous mechanical components, the ring gear would be part of a larger wall that would hold it solidly in place and would eliminate these convulsive motions which, in any case, are seen in the simulation only at unrealistically high operating frequencies.

Drexler and Merkle[2847] later proposed a "second-generation" planetary gear design (Fig. 2.31) with 4235 atoms, a molecular

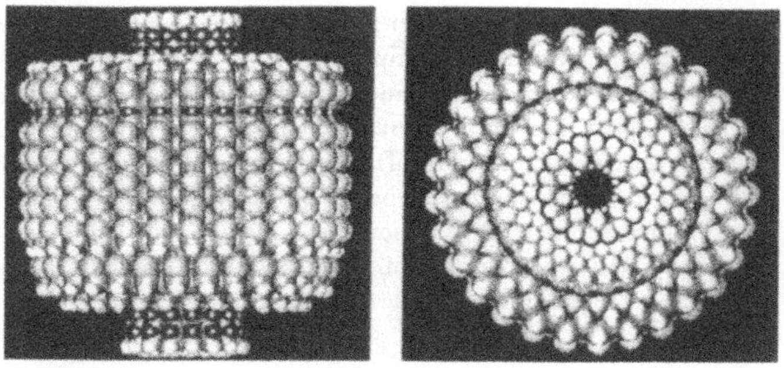

Fig. 2.31. Side and top views of a 4235-atom "second generation" planetary gear (courtesy of K.E. Drexler and R.C. Merkle[2847]).

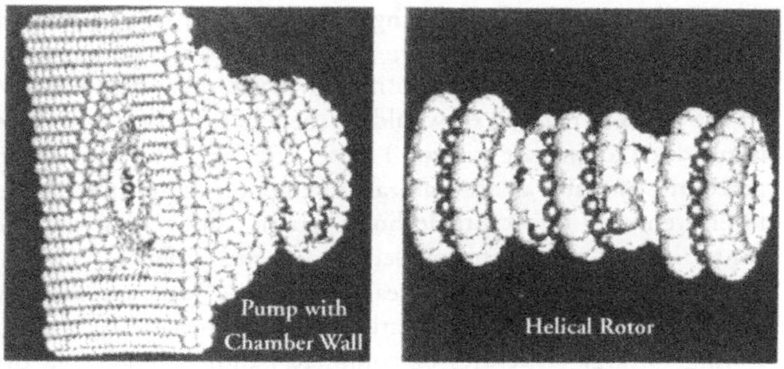

Fig. 2.32. Side views of a 6165-atom neon gas pump/motor (courtesy of K.E. Drexler and R.C. Merkle[2858]).

weight of 72,491.947 daltons and a molecular volume of 47.586 nm^3. This new version was indeed more stable but still had too much slip at the highest frequencies. Commenting on the ongoing design effort, Goddard[2845] suggested that an optimal configuration could have the functionality of a planetary gear but might have an appearance completely different from the macroscopic system, and offered an example: "Because a gear tooth in the xy plane cannot be atomically smooth in the z-direction, we may develop a Vee design so that the Vee shape of the gear tooth in the z-direction nestles within a Vee notch in the race to retain stability in the z-direction as the teeth contact in the xy plane. This design would make no sense for a macroscopic gear system since the gear could never be placed inside the race. However, for a molecular system one could imagine that the gear is constructed and that the race is constructed all except for a last joining unit. The parts could be assembled and then the final connections on the face made to complete the design" analogous to the ZARBI system of Rebek.[131]

Another class of nanodevice that has been designed is a gas-powered molecular motor or pump.[2858] The pump and chamber wall segment shown in Figure 2.32 contain 6165 atoms with a molecular weight of 88,190.813 daltons and a molecular volume of 63.984 nm^3. The device can serve either as a pump for neon gas atoms or (if run backwards) as a motor that can convert neon gas pressure into rotary power. The helical rotor has a grooved cylindrical bearing surface at each end, supporting a screw-threaded cylindrical segment in the middle. In operation, rotation of the shaft moves a helical groove past longitudinal grooves inside the pump housing. There is room enough for small gas molecules only where facing grooves cross, and these crossing points move from one side to the other as the shaft turns, moving the neon atoms along. Goddard[2845] reported that preliminary molecular dynamics simulations of the device showed that it could indeed function as a pump, although "structural deformations of the rotor can cause instabilities at low and high rotational frequencies. The forced translations show that at very low perpendicular forces due to pump action, the total energy rises significantly and again the structure deforms." Merkle acknowledged that the pump moves neon atoms at an energy cost of 185 Kcal/mole-Angstrom (12,900 zJ/atom-nm), which is not very energy-efficient. Further refinement of this crude design is clearly warranted.

Conveyor systems would also be useful. Employing a primitive molecular CAD software package called Crystal Sketchpad, G. Leach[2861] created a design for a 5-nanopart, ~2500-atom conveyor belt system comprised of two rollers, two axles, and a belt consisting of a strained thin-walled diamond sheet. The design has not been subjected to further computational analysis, either to minimize rotational energy barriers or to optimize rotational dynamics or operational stability.

Drexler and Merkle[2859] have also produced a preliminary design for a 2596-atom fine-motion controller (Fig. 2.33). A general-purpose molecular assembler arm must be able to move its "hand" by many atomic diameters, position it with fractional-atomic-diameter accuracy, and then execute finely-controlled motions, perhaps to transfer one or a few atoms in a guided chemical reaction. Human arms use large muscles and joints for large motions and more finely-controlled finger motions for precision; the device presented here can execute precise finger-like motions over several atomic diameters with associated 90-degree rotations. The core of the device consists of a shaft linking two hexagonal endplates, sandwiching a stack of eight rings, making a modified Stewart platform (Section 9.3.1.5). In a complete system, each ring would be rotated by a lever driven by a cam mechanism. Each ring supports a strut linked to a central platform (here shown raised,

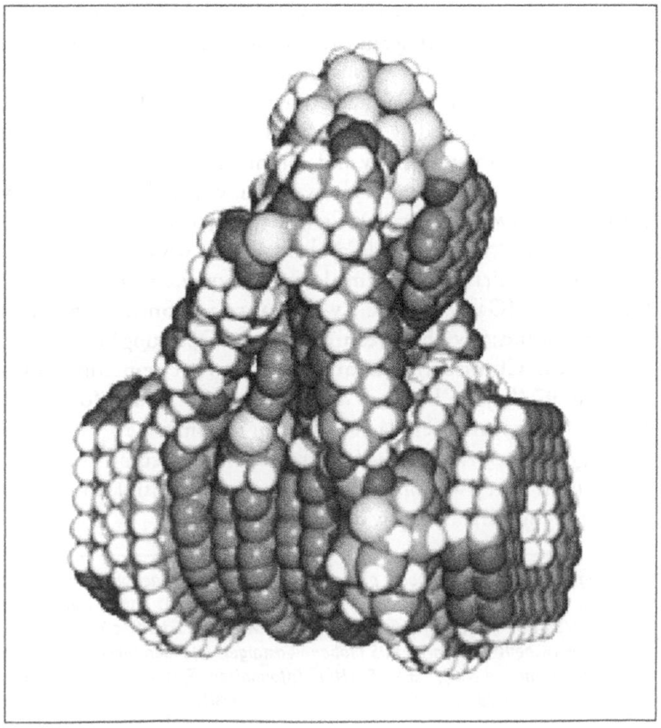

Fig. 2.33. Side view of a 2695-atom fine motion controller (courtesy of K.E. Drexler and R.C. Merkle[2859]).

displaced, and twisted). Rotating a ring moves a strut; moving a strut moves the platform; positioning all eight rings (over-)determines a platform position in x, y, z, roll, pitch, and yaw. (If the struts were rigid, six would do the job; here, two struts have been added to increase stiffness.) Notes Drexler: "The chief design problem is to enable an adequate range of motion without mechanical interference or unacceptable bond strains, and within the size constraints set by available modeling tools and patience."

Almost all current design research in molecular nanotechnology is restricted to computer simulation, which allows the design and testing of large structures or complete nanomachines, and the compilation of growing libraries of molecular designs. The work is relatively inexpensive and does not require the support of a large team. Of course, calculations of many-body systems are notoriously difficult, with many computer packages making a number of simplifying assumptions—e.g., nuclei as point masses, electrons treated as a continuous charge distribution, and 3-D potential energy functions derived semi-empirically from experimental data and treated as a classical field despite their true quantum mechanical character (for ease of computation). Notwithstanding these shortcuts, Tuzun and colleagues[2664] claim that classical simulations may over-estimate the rate of energy transfer between vibrational modes even at low energies, in which case "current designs for various nanocomponents [would] actually perform better and be more stable than recent molecular dynamics simulations suggest."

Goddard[2853] notes that future nanosystem simulations may require 1-100 million atoms to be considered explicitly, demanding major improvements in molecular dynamics methodologies. By 1998, new algorithms for parallel processing of massive molecular dynamics simulations were being developed,[2854] producing methods and optimized parallelized computer programs efficient for high capacity molecular dynamics simulations of 10,000-1,000,000 atoms for finite molecular structures.

Ultimately, Computer-Aided (Molecular) Design (CAD) systems[2861] will be needed to efficiently design and analyze molecular components and their higher-order assemblies. CAD systems are commonplace in macroscale engineering and architecture, as are Computer-Aided Manufacturing (CAM) systems in macroscale manufacturing. In the molecular realm, Computer Aided Synthesis Design (CASD)* has been avidly pursued by computational chemists since the 1980s, and by 1998 many university and commercial molecular modeling software packages were already well-known, including Alchemy (Tripos Inc.; www.tripos.com), Cerius2 (Molecular Simulations Inc.; www.msi.com), Chem3D (CambridgeSoft; www.camsoft.com), Conformer (Princeton Simulations; www.conformer.com), Gaussian94 (Gaussian Inc.; www.gaussian.com), Hyperchem (Hypercube Inc.; www.hyper.com), Molecular Operating Environment (Chemical Computing Group Inc.; www.chemcomp.com), MOPAC97 (Fujitsu Ltd.; www.winmopac.com), RealMol/CAVE/NAMD (Fraunhofer Institute for Computer Graphics; www.igd.fhg.de/www/igd-a4/research/chemie), Sculpt (Interactive Simulations Inc.; www.intsim.com/products/index.htm), and Spartan (Wavefunction Inc.; www.wavefun.com).

In 1998, the capacity of such systems to design and manipulate large nanoscale mechanical components was extremely limited. A few very primitive molecular nanotechnology design packages had been attempted, including Crystal Sketchpad,[2861] DiamondCAD (www.zyvex.com/diamond.html), Molecular Assembly Sequence Software (www.carol.com/mass.shtml), Molecular Modelling Toolkit (starship.python.net/crew/hinsen/mmtk.html), and NanoCAD (world.std.com/~wware/ncad.html). The possible design of molecules for specific purposes using genetic software techniques had also been investigated.[2955]

2.4.2 Molecular Assemblers

Drexler[8-10] has proposed the molecular assembler,** a device resembling an industrial robot which would be capable of holding and positioning reactive moieties in order to control the precise location at which chemical reactions take place. This general approach would allow the construction of large atomically precise objects by a sequence of precisely controlled chemical reactions. Much like the ribosome in biology (Section 2.3.1), an assembler would build various classes of useful molecular structures following a sequence of instructions. During this process, the assembler would provide three-dimensional positional and full orientational control over the molecular component (analogous to the individual amino acid in the ribosome model) that is being added to a growing complex molecular structure (analogous to the growing polypeptide in the ribosomal model). In one approach, a molecular assembler may be capable of forming any one of several different kinds of chemical bonds (e.g., by changing tool tips), not just a single kind such as the peptide bond that the ribosome makes. In bonding atoms or molecules to one another, the assembler would provide any needed energy (especially if the reaction happens not to be energetically favored) through physical force, thus performing mechanosynthesis (as opposed to the traditional means of chemical synthesis in solution). In another approach, a molecular assembler might be capable only of noncovalent assembly operations, wherein nanoparts are fabricated by other means and then presented to the assembler, which assembles the nanoparts into working nanomachines.

The first simple molecular assembler will almost certainly be a macroscale device, perhaps a modified SPM system as was being pursued by Zyvex[2794] in 1998. Multiple SPM heads could be equipped with a small number of nanoscale tool tips. In one scenario, nanoparts fabricated using bulk chemistry techniques would be inspected and selected by the SPM, then assembled one by one into working nanomachines (e.g., the desired useful nanoscale products). Such assembly operations will be very slow, because the placement of each new component may require simultaneous rotations and translations of large macroscale SPM components. Assembly time scales roughly linearly with assembler size[10] because smaller assembler components moving at a given velocity need to travel less distance to accomplish a given physical operation, hence consuming less time and energy per physical operation. An important early developmental goal thus will be to design and fabricate nanoscale molecular assemblers.

**Existing CASD software/database packages include CAMEO (reaction chemistry assistant; William L. Jorgensen, Yale Univ.; zarbi.chem.yale.edu/programs/cameo.html), CAS (reaction data base; www.cas.org/CASFILES/casreact.html)), Chiron (retrosynthetic analysis of chiral precursors; Steve Hanessian, Univ. of Montreal; www.netsci.org/Resources/Software/Cheminfo/chiron.html), CIARA (Vogel Scientific Software Inc.; www.vogelscientific.com), Crossfire (Computer Assisted Synthesis, Beilstein Information Systems; www.beilstein.com), EROS (Johann Gasteiger, Erlangen University; schiele.organik.uni-erlangen.de), LAHSA (retrosynthetic analysis; Alan Long, Harvard University; long@midas.harvard.edu), REACCS (MDL Information Systems Inc.; www.mdli.com), SYNGEN (Jim Hendrickson, Brandeis University; syngen2.chem.brandeis.edu/syngen.html), SYNLIB (W. Clark Still, Columbia University), and SYNTREE (Trinity Software Inc.; www.trinitysoftware.com/Trinity/orgchem/SYNTREE.HTM).*

***But not a "universal" assembler: "Though assemblers will be powerful (and could even be directed to expand their own toolkits by assembling new tools), they will not be able to build everything that could exist" (Drexler[8] at page 246). The term "universal assembler" appears only in a section heading in Drexler's popular work* Engines of Creation[8] *but not in the text; the term appears nowhere in Drexler's technical work* Nanosystems.[10]

At its most basic level, the simplest possible nanoscale molecular assembler may be comprised of one or more nanoscale manipulators (Section 9.3). For example, the diamondoid telescoping manipulator arm described in Section 9.3.1.4 (Figs. 9.8 and 9.9) has about 4 million atoms excluding the base and control and power structures; doubling the size to account for support structures gives a molecular weight per arm of ~100 megadaltons and a total molecular volume of ~140,000 nm^3. Designed for high strength and stiffness, this robot arm should be able to hold a molecular fragment stiffly enough to make it react with a chosen end of a carbon-carbon double bond with an error rate of only 10^{-15}.[10] The robot arm could guide chemical reactions with high reliability at room temperature in vacuo, with little need for sensing the positions of the molecules with which it is working.[279] Alternatively, with appropriate tool tips, such an arm could grasp and manipulate individual prefabricated nanoparts in solution phase. Assembly of nanoparts without fabrication may require only a very small tool set.

The manipulator arm must be driven by a detailed sequence of control signals, just as the ribosome needs mRNA to guide its actions. However, such detailed control signals can be provided by external acoustic, electrical, or chemical signals that are received by the robot arm via an onboard sensor or power transducer, using a simple "broadcast architecture"[10,280,2872] (Chapter 12), a technique which can also be used to import power (e.g., Section 6.3.3). Such transducers may be extremely small, on the order of $(\sim 10\ nm)^3$ each.[10] Interestingly, the biological cell may be regarded as an example of a broadcast architecture:[2872] the nucleus, located external to the cytoplasm, broadcasts mRNA chemical signals to millions of spatially diverse cytoplasmic ribosomes, thereby remotely controlling the construction of cellular proteins.

Thus a two-armed mechanical molecular assembler that receives power and instructions from some external agency may have a total molecular volume of ~300,000 nm^3 (a cube ~67 nm on an edge), containing ~16 million atoms with a molecular weight of ~200 megadaltons—very roughly the mass and scale of a medium-size virus particle, such as an adenovirus. For comparison, the average enzyme (a biochemical crimping tool) weighs about ~0.1 megadalton, while a typical ribosome (a primitive "protein assembler") weighs ~4.2 megadaltons. A simple mechanical assembler in the 10-100 megadalton range cannot be ruled out. However, such a device might have a very small set of tool tips and an extremely limited manufacturing repertoire.

Multiple nanoscale assemblers each capable of independent simultaneous actuation may require control signals more conveniently provided by an onboard nanocomputer (Section 10.2). This programmable nanocomputer must be able to accept stored instructions which are sequentially executed to direct the manipulator arm to place the correct moiety or nanopart in the desired position and orientation, thus giving precise control over the timing and locations of chemical reactions or assembly operations. The mechanical nanocomputer analyzed by Drexler[10] requires ~16 nm^3 per logic gate and ~40 nm^3 per data register. If such components could be used to construct the equivalent of the most primitive 4-bit Intel 4004 microprocessor, then the nanocomputer could process ~10^5 bits/sec (~25,000 ops/sec) at a ~1 KHz clock speed within a mechanism volume of ~36,000 nm^3 (Section 10.2.1), again neglecting power supply, I/O linkages, and the like. An additional ~160,000 nm^3 of rod logic registers (Section 10.2.1) adds ~1 kilobyte of onboard RAM memory or ~40 kilobytes of internal tape memory (conservatively assuming a tape storage density comparable to linear DNA). (A memory tape containing all bits needed for complete self-description (Table 2.1) may be considerably longer, even allowing for substantial data compression.) Doubling the total volume to account for support structure and other overhead gives a minimum mechanical nanocomputer molecular volume of ~400,000 nm^3, roughly 70 million atoms with a molecular weight of ~800 megadaltons. Thus the smallest nanocomputer-driven nanoscale molecular assembler with two manipulator arms may have a total molecular volume of ~700,000 nm^3 (a cube ~88 nm on an edge), containing ~86 million atoms with a molecular weight of ~1 gigadalton.

Table 2.1 Information Required to Describe Some Self-Replicating Systems

Self-Replicating System	# of Bits Needed to Specify System	References
Penrose ratcheting 2-blocks	0.238×10^3	2879
Rebek's self-replicating molecules	$\sim 1 \times 10^3$	131,2452
Human PrP protein (prion)	1.5×10^3	2877,2878
Ebola virus	25.4×10^3	2875
Penrose ratcheting 12-blocks	$\sim 49 \times 10^3$	2880,2881
Typical human ribosome	280×10^3	997
von Neuman's Universal Constructor	$\sim 500 \times 10^3$	280,1985
1988 Internet Worm	$\sim 500 \times 10^3$	280,2874
Pyrenomas salina (algae)	1.32×10^6	997
M. capricolum (mycoplasma)	$1.448\text{-}2.2 \times 10^6$	2876
E. coli (bacterium)	8.4×10^6	997
S. cerevisiae (yeast)	26×10^6	997
D. melanogaster (insect)	280×10^6	997
200-megadalton 2-arm nanoassembler	$\boldsymbol{384 \times 10^6}$	***Section 2.4.2***
1-gigadalton 2-arm nanoassembler	$\boldsymbol{2.32 \times 10^9}$	***Section 2.4.2***
G. domesticus (bird)	2.4×10^9	997
X. laevis (amphibian)	6.2×10^9	997
H. sapiens (human genome)	6.6×10^9	997
Various flowering plant species	$0.12\text{-}220 \times 10^9$	997
NASA Lunar Manufacturing Facility	272×10^9	115

By 1998, only a small amount of research targeted at actual assembler design had begun. Following Drexler's original discussions,[8-10] during 1991-1998 R. Merkle authored or co-authored a continuing series of papers discussing various operational aspects and specific components of assembler design, including mechanosynthetic positional control,[2761,2762] general design considerations for assemblers,[280,2868] the broadcast architecture,[2872] convergent assembly,[2869] binding sites,[1199] positioning devices,[1239] mechanosynthetic path sets,[2602] designs for a neon pump[2858] and a fine motion controller,[2859] and possible assembler casings.[2281] J.S. Hall has considered high-level designs for a nanoscale parts-fabrication and parts-assembly nanorobot.[2870] Zyvex,[2794] founded in 1996 by James von Ehr, has set itself the task of building the first programmable nanoassembler in a 5-10 year time frame (e.g., by ~2006). W. Goddard and colleagues[2853] have proposed a series of molecular dynamics simulations of simple assemblers, although by 1998 these studies evidently had not yet begun. According to Goddard's original proposal:

> *"Ultimately we need a programmable synthetic system to make a real device. Even though we may not have tools for all the chemical steps and may not have designs for all the pumps, engines, and transmissions needed, we propose to study the dynamics of simplified prototype assemblers. In these studies we anticipate having (1) a reservoir or supplies area for providing the various building units (atoms and fragments) required, (2) a work area in which we construct the nanomachine device (initially we will consider assembling the structure on top of a diamond surface), and (3) a molecular scale nano-hand which will extract the atoms from (1) and carry them to (2). We will then use extensions of our massive*

molecular dynamics program to operate the system: moving the tip from reservoir to work area, moving it to contact the appropriate surface site, moving it to regenerate the active tip, and then moving it back to add new atoms and molecules. This will include proper temperature effects, molecular vibrations, energy release upon the various chemical steps, etc. The ground rules here are that a realistic force field be used and that all pieces be treated at the atomic level (but some might be semi-rigid). This will use the force field developed for nanosynthesis. The purpose of these simulations is to examine issues of vibration caused by chemical forces as the tool picks up and delivers atoms to the growing surface. Also we want to consider the effect of energy release in the chemical steps on the thermal fluctuations in these systems (which may cause displacements and vibrations)."

Building mega-atom or giga-atom nanoproducts one at a time would be incredibly expensive and time consuming. For example, imagine that we wish to construct a simple medical nanorobot such as the 1-micron spherical respirocyte[1400] described in Chapter 22, which consists of ~18 billion atoms (dry structure). A factory employing a coordinated team of 100 macroscale SPM assemblers, each able to place ~1 atom/sec-SPM on a convergently-assembled workpiece achieves a pitiful manufacturing throughput rate of ~2 respirocytes per decade. Nanoscale assemblers with appendages ~10^6 times smaller than macroscale SPM assemblers might plausibly achieve net assembly rates of ~10^6 atoms/sec-nanoassembler, but even a production line employing ~300 such nanoassemblers (which the abovementioned 100-SPM factory team could build in ~1 year, assuming ~10^7 atoms/nanoassembler) can only manufacture ~1 respirocyte nanorobot per minute. At that rate, it would take ~2 million years to build the first ~1 cm^3 therapeutic dosage containing ~10^{12} respirocyte nanorobots.

The necessary solution to this mass-production bottleneck is to employ any of several massively parallel approaches to manufacturing, including such techniques as self-assembly (Sections 2.3.1 and 2.3.2), convergent assembly,[10,2869] or, most usefully, self-replication (Chapter 14). The basic advantage of self-replication is readily illustrated. Consider a single ~10^8-atom "seed" nanoassembler (having an onboard nanocomputer) that has been painstakingly built in ~10^6 sec using the abovementioned 100-SPM macroscale assembler team, working at ~1 atom/sec-SPM. The seed nanoassembler is first programmed to build a copy of itself, which it accomplishes (working at ~10^6 atoms/sec-nanoassembler) in ~100 sec. These two nanoassemblers then each build a copy of themselves in another ~100 sec; now there are four nanoassemblers. After ~48 generations, requiring a total of ~80 minutes to complete, there are ~3 x 10^{14} nanoassemblers.* These nanoassemblers are then reprogrammed for the manufacture of 18-billion-atom respirocytes and are fed the appropriate, presumably different, feedstock. This vastly expanded nanoassembler manufacturing system can now produce ~10^{12} respirocytes (~1 cm^3 therapeutic dose) per minute.

The design of machines able to make copies of themselves was first described by von Neumann.[1985] Many variations on this theme have been reviewed by Freitas and Gilbreath[115] and Sipper,[2871] and design for self-replication in the context of nanoscale assemblers has been considered by Drexler,[8-10] Merkle,[116,2868,2872,2873] and Hall.[2870] As Drexler[10] notes: "It may seem somehow paradoxical that a machine can contain all the instructions needed to make a copy of itself, including those selfsame complex instructions, but this is easily resolved. In the simplest approach, the machine reads the instructions twice: first as commands to be obeyed, and then as data to be copied. Adding more data does not increase the complexity of the data-copying process, hence the set of instructions can be made as complex as is necessary to specify the rest of the system. By the same token, the instructions transmitted in a replication cycle can specify the construction of an indefinitely large number of other artifacts."

The estimated information content of self-replicating systems—the length of the instruction tape—can be surprisingly small (Table 2.1). Von Neumann's original analysis[1985] concluded that perhaps twelve different kinds of units of unknown complexity could be required as building materials, and Haldane[2884] inferred that as many as ~10^5 individual parts might be needed to make a replicator. This inference was refuted just three years later with the arrival of the first in a stream of very simple but ingenious designs for mechanical self-replicating machines that were assembled and operated in the late 1950s. In the first example,[2879] a pair of joined ratchetlike blocks,[2886] when placed in a "sea" of left and right blocks and then physically agitated, replicated itself from this well-ordered input substrate, making more block-pairs until all the single blocks were used up, a process similar to chemical autocatalysis. More complex congeries of blocks, including clever four-block, eight-block, and 12-block replicators that could replicate themselves in a sea of blocks were presented by Penrose.[2880,2881] Jacobson[2882] demonstrated a 3-unit replicator consisting of toy train engines circulating on HO model railroad tracks, and Morowitz[2883] designed a simple two-unit device with one unit comprised of about a dozen components including switches, batteries and electromagnets, that could assemble copies of itself from parts floating on the water surface of a bathtub. In 1998, Lohn and colleagues[2885] gave two designs for simple self-replicating systems that could be constructed out of wood, batteries and electromagnets, with explicit analogies to nanoscale fabrication. Several important conclusions may be drawn from these examples:

First, replication is fundamentally so simple a task that machines capable of displaying this behavior pre-date most of the modern electronic computer era.

Second, assembly is an inherently simpler operation than fabrication. A complex part may embody hundreds or thousands of prior fabrication and assembly operations, yet may be installed within an assemblage in a single step. Hence nanopart assembly may be an easier candidate for early implementation in first-generation self-replicating molecular manufacturing systems than is molecular fabrication.

Third, and most important, the simplest nanoreplicator may require the ability to assemble, but not to (atomically) fabricate, in order to replicate itself. A nanomachine capable of assembly alone can replicate itself only from a very limited set of well-ordered input materials of relatively high complexity, but such a machine can be extremely simple both in structure and function. Certainly a nanomachine capable of both assembly and fabrication can replicate itself from a more diverse and disordered set of more elementary input materials—but only at the expense of far greater internal structural and functional complexity.

At least two distinct models of replication have been identified in replicating systems design.[115] The first model may be called the "unit replication" or organismic model (Fig. 2.34), in which the replicator is an independent unit which employs the surrounding substrate to directly produce an identical copy of itself; both the original and the copy remain fertile and may replicate again, thus

**Numerous complexities and limitations have been ignored here. For example, exponential growth cannot continue indefinitely in a finite environment with limited materials transport speeds—e.g., a 2-nm wide nanopart suspended in 310 K water diffuses only ~26 nm in 10^{-6} sec (Eqn. 3.1). Mechanical replicating systems designed purely for molecular manufacturing may be inflexible and brittle, employing limited energy resources and materials feedstocks not found outside of the immediate manufacturing environment.*

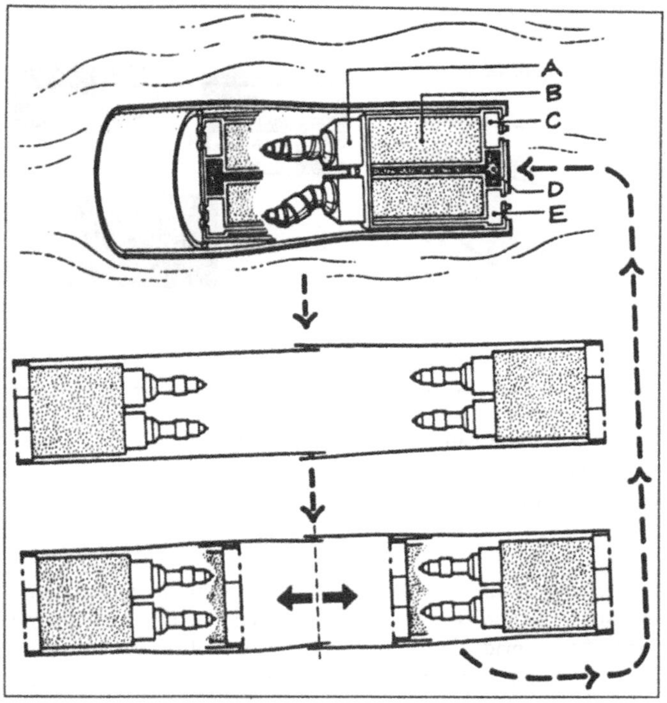

Fig. 2.34. Schematic example of unit replication (courtesy of K.E. Drexler, C. Peterson and G. Pergamit[9]). A) nanocomputer; B) stored instructions; C) fuel intake, power supply; D) motor; E) machinery for raw materials processing.

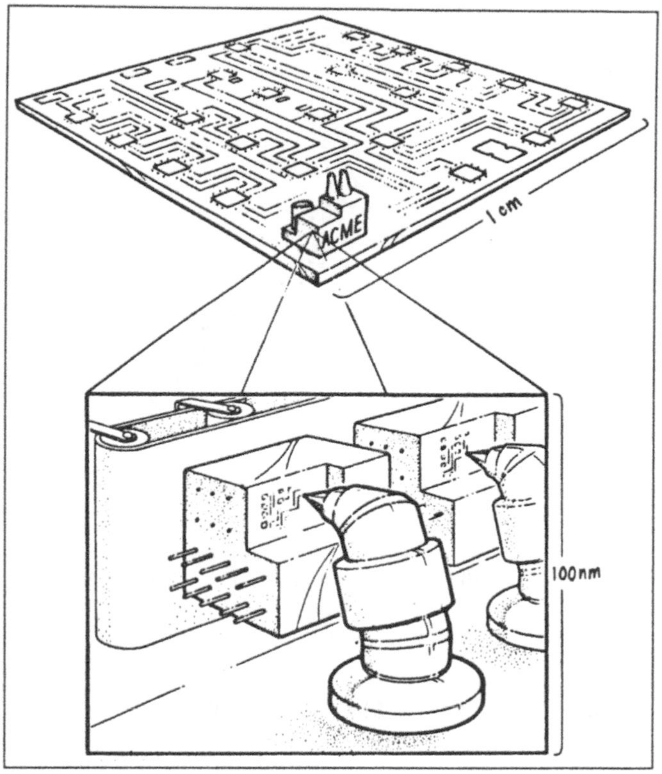

Fig. 2.35. Schematic example of unit growth: nanoassembler fabricating a nanocomputer in the factory model (courtesy of K.E. Drexler, C. Peterson and G. Pergamit[9]).

exponentiating their numbers. The second model may be called the "unit growth" or factory model (Fig. 2.35), in which a population of specialist devices, each one individually incapable of self-replication, can collectively fabricate and assemble all necessary components comprising all specialist devices within the system, hence the factory is capable of expanding its size (or of manufacturing duplicate factory systems) indefinitely in an appropriate environment. The factory model is sometimes called "bootstrapping," which is any production of more productive capacity, from less. T. McKendree [personal communication, 1999] likens the situation to an ant colony: "There necessarily is the line of reproducing queens, making a sufficient number of ants feasible; [however,] most of the queen's products are 'workers' that perform useful functions, but themselves are incapable of reproduction."

It cannot be emphasized too strongly that mechanical medical nanodevices will not self-replicate inside the human body, nor will they have any need for self-replication themselves (Section 1.3.3). Machines that perform medical tasks are fundamentally different from machines that manufacture other machines. As R. Merkle explains:[2873] "While self-replicating systems are the key to low cost [manufacture], there is no need (and little desire) to have such systems function in the outside world. Instead, in an artificial and controlled environment they can manufacture simpler and more rugged systems that can then be transferred to their final destination. Medical devices designed to operate in the human body don't have to self-replicate: we can manufacture them in a controlled environment and then inject them into the patient as needed. The resulting medical device will be simpler, smaller, more efficient and more precisely designed for the task at hand than a device designed to perform the same function and self-replicate. This conclusion should hold generally: optimize [product] device design for the desired function, manufacture the [product] device in an environment optimized for manufacturing, then transport the [product] device from the manufacturing environment to the environment for which it was designed. A single device able to do everything would be harder to design and less efficient."

In an effort to stimulate scientific and engineering interest in constructing the first nanoassembler, in November 1995 the Foresight Institute created the $250,000 Feynman Grand Prize,[2860] with funding contributed by Zyvex founder James von Ehr and St. Louis venture capitalist Marc Arnold. The prize will be awarded to the individual or group that first achieves both of two significant nanotechnology breakthroughs—first, the design and construction of a functional nanometer-scale robotic arm, and second, the design and construction of a functional 8-bit adder computing nanodevice. According to Grand Prize rules, the robotic nanomanipulator must fit entirely inside a 100-nm cube, carry out actions directed by input signals of specified types, be able to move to a directed sequence of positions anywhere within a 50-nm cube, complete all directed actions with a positioning accuracy of 0.1 nanometer or better, and perform at least 1,000 accurate, nanometer-scale positioning motions per second for at least 60 consecutive seconds. The adder must fit entirely within a 50-nm cube, and must be capable of adding accurately any pair of 8-bit binary numbers, discarding overflow, accepting input signals of specified types, and producing its output as a pattern of raised nanometer-scale bumps on an atomically precise and level surface. (J.S. Hall notes that a conventional 8-bit adder may be constructed using a total of 94 AND, OR, and NOT gates; using XOR gates, the total may be reduced to 37 gates.) Both devices may accept inputs from acoustic, electrical, optical, diffusive chemical, or mechanical means, although

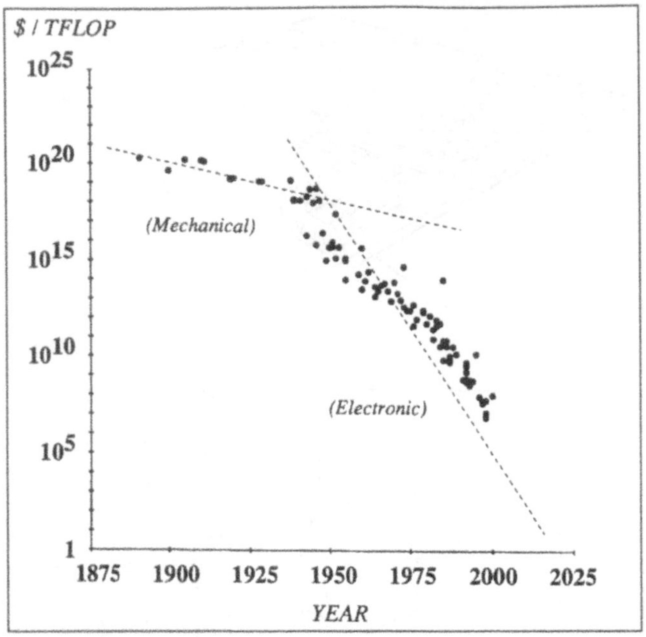

Fig. 2.36. Estimated cost of 1 TeraFLOP (~10^{14} bits/sec) of peak computing power (constant $1998 per TFLOP).

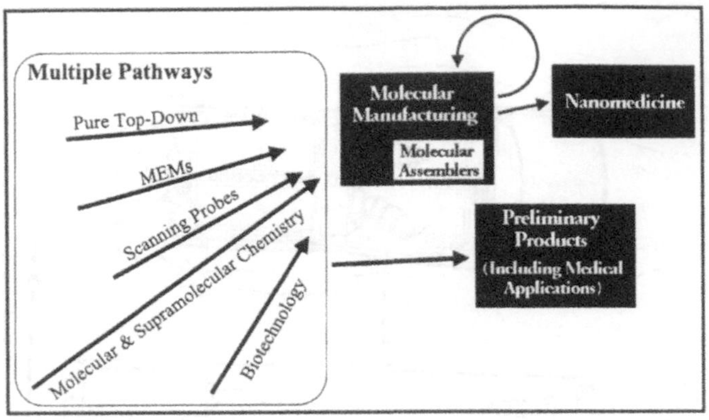

Fig. 2.37. Multiple pathways lead to molecular manufacturing, the self-supporting ability to design and build to atomic precision, which enables nanomedicine.

any mechanical driving mechanism used for input must be limited to a single linkage that either slides or rotates on a single axis. To demonstrate the capacity for mass-production, at least 32 copies of each device must be provided for analysis and destructive testing by judges.

Once nanoassemblers are available, the design of far more complex nanomachines each containing tens or hundreds of billions of precisely arranged atoms will require new molecular CAD (Section 2.4.1) tools and techniques, including automated hierarchical design decomposition of objects (that must be built up from an array of nanoparts) and a shape description language.[10] Nanosystem design compilers, conceptually similar to silicon compilers that generate a complex pattern of transistors and conductors from an abstract specification of the properties of a digital circuit, will also be required for efficient nanorobot design.[10] Given a fully specified design that meets all constraints necessary to physically permit assembly, all operations of the assembly process must be specified using an assembly-process compiler. Explains Drexler:[10] "The design of structures and assembly procedures by hierarchical decomposition directly generates a tree of assembly steps. If this tree has been chosen to generate parts of the appropriate sizes and numbers, then it can be mapped onto a manufacturing layout. The vast number of manipulator motions to be specified at the finest, earliest, and most-dispersed levels of the assembly process can be planned in parallel by identical software systems running almost independently on separate processors. The result of this parallel assembly-process compilation is a set of instructions that, when executed by the transportation system and manipulator controllers of a manufacturing mechanism, will result in the assembly of an object corresponding to the initial design." Scale-up to larger systems, including the control, coordination, and programming of large aggregates of cooperating nanorobots, is discussed in Volume II.

Since molecular manufacturing systems can be used to make more molecular manufacturing systems, it is believed that the capital costs of production can be quite low. Drexler[73] claims that an analysis of inputs, outputs, and productivity suggests the total cost of production can be in the range familiar in agriculture and in the production of industrial chemicals—on the order of tens of cents per pound. Merkle[262] has made similar assertions, for example: "Eventually (after amortization of possibly quite high development costs), the price of assemblers (and of the objects they build) should be no higher than the price of other complex structures made by self-replicating systems. Potatoes—which have a staggering design complexity involving tens of thousands of different genes and different proteins directed by many megabits of genetic information—cost well under a dollar per pound." Such analogies from conventional agriculture or industrial chemistry are not strictly applicable to the medical products and pharmaceutical areas, where structural precision, product repeatability, and intensive quality control are of supreme importance, and where most products are subject to rigorous government regulation—unlike potatoes, which vary widely in size, shape, and molecular constitution, and generally do not require stringent product liability insurance, multi-phase clinical trials, or FDA approval.

Still, it is likely that molecular manufacturing will eventually allow reasonably inexpensive production of large batches of designed medical nanorobots. As a very crude analogy, even in 1995 a typical mail-order bioscience vendor[2887] could manufacture 15 micromoles (~9×10^{18} product items) of customized oligonucleotides for $18/base up to at least 110 bases with a convenient 48-hour turnaround on orders; other online vendors offer similar or slightly higher prices up to 200-mer sequences with additional charges for necessary purifications.[2888] If a billion-base structure could be induced to self-assemble (Section 2.3.1) from 10 million different sets of 100-mer custom-built oligonucleotides (total ~20 billion atoms), forming a desired ~20-billion-atom nanomachine, then, optimistically assuming a ~100% yield, the cost would be ~$\$2 \times 10^{-9}$ per nanomachine or ~$2000 per ~1 cm^3 of product volume which would include 10^{12} finished nanomachines. In 1998, many specialty biotechnology-related drug treatments were comparably expensive. For example, treatments for multiple sclerosis using two closely related ~22.5 kilodalton interferons were administered in dosages of ~1 milligram/week at a treatment cost of ~$10,000/yr,[2950] which is equivalent to a treatment cost of ~$\$2 \times 10^{-9}$ (2 "nanodollars") per giga-atom. The famous HeLa (Henrietta Lacks) cell line[2890] is an example of a once tiny population of unique cancerous cells that were purposely replicated in vitro (~24-hour replication time) over many decades and are now widely available worldwide at very low cost (e.g., $216 per 1-$cm^3$ ampule of the ATCC CCL-2 HeLa cell line[2891]). Swallowable therapeutic pills containing bacteria (i.e., natural biological nanomachines) are already widely available over the counter for gastrointestinal refloration, as for example Salivarex™ which "contains a minimum of ~2.9 billion beneficial bacteria per capsule",[3048] and Alkadophilus™ which "contains 1.5 billion organisms per capsule",[3049] both at a 1998 price of ~$0.2 x 10^{-9} per bacterium.

Another useful analogic approach to cost estimation is suggested by the plunging price of computer power during the 20th century. Figure 2.36 shows the cost, in constant 1998 U.S. dollars, of a computer processing capability equivalent to ~1 TeraFLOP (10^{12} floating-point operations per second, ~10^{14} bits/sec assuming 64-bit words). The plotted data is from a compilation of 67 historical computers by Moravec[1] through 1989, with an additional 27 data points for other computers spanning 1973-1999 added by the author. The chart shows that the cost of 1 TFLOP has fallen from $2 x 10^{20} in 1908 (the mechanical Hollerith Tabulator) to just $6 x 10^6 in 1998 (the SGI/Cray T3E-1200E), a 90-year price decline of almost 14 orders of magnitude—on average, a halving every ~2 years, a century-long example of Moore's Law. This trend may give us some confidence that even if the first individual 1 micron^3 nanorobot costs ~$100,000 to assemble (much like the first Nippondenso microcar; Section 2.2), eventually the unit price may fall at least 14 orders of magnitude to below ~$$10^{-9}$ per nanorobot or <$1000 per ~1 cm^3 dosage (10^{12} nanorobots). Recycling or remanufacturing each nanomachine ~1000 times before final discard would then imply a net ~$1/cm^3 treatment cost. Of course, in 1998 all such estimates were mere guesswork, but the ultimate expectation of relatively low-cost nanomedical treatments was certainly rational, if not provable.

This Chapter has demonstrated that there are many different pathways leading toward molecular nanotechnology, each one of which provides incremental benefits to motivate further travel down the paths (Fig. 2.37). The likelihood of all the paths being blocked is low, even if we have little confidence that we can predict which approach will succeed first.[8,9] Progress along the many pathways will provide precursor products, including some early medical applications, but the ultimate achievement of molecular manufacturing will finally make nanomedicine feasible.

As Drexler concluded *Nanosystems*:[10] "Each step along [these pathways] will present great practical challenges, but each step will also bring valuable new capabilities. The long-term rewards, measured in terms of scientific and technological capabilities, appear large." This author agrees. For the remainder of the present work, we shall assume that a molecular manufacturing technology will someday exist that can economically manufacture macroscopic batches of microscopic machines comprised of atomically-precise nanoscale components. The medical applications and implications of such a technological capability are the principle subject of this three-volume book.

CHAPTER 3

Molecular Transport and Sortation

3.1 Human Body Chemical Composition

The human body consists of ~7 x 10^{27} atoms arranged in a highly aperiodic physical structure. Although 41 chemical elements are commonly found in the body's construction (Table 3.1), CHON comprises 99% of its atoms. Fully 87% of human body atoms are either hydrogen or oxygen.

Somatic atoms are generally present in combined form as molecules or ions, not individual atoms. The molecules of greatest nanomedical interest are incorporated into cells or circulate freely in blood plasma or the interstitial fluid. Table 3.2 summarizes the gross molecular contents of the typical human cell, which is 99.5% water and salts, by molecule count, and contains ~5000 different types of molecules. Appendix B lists 261 of the most common molecular and cellular constituents of human blood, and their normal concentrations in whole blood and plasma. This listing is far from complete. The human body is comprised of ~10^5 different molecular species, mostly proteins—a large but nonetheless finite molecular parts list. By 1998, at least ~10^4 of these proteins had been sequenced, ~10^3 had been spatially mapped, and ~7,000 structures (including proteins, peptides, viruses, protein/nucleic acid complexes, nucleic acids, and carbohydrates) had been registered in the Protein Data Bank which at that time was maintained at Brookhaven National Laboratory.[1144] Given the current accelerating pace of improving technology,[1145] it is likely that the sequences and 3-D or tertiary structures of all human proteins will have been determined by the second decade of the 21st century.

Table 3.1 Estimated Atomic Composition of the Lean 70-kg Male Human Body[749,751,752,817]

Element	Sym	# of Atoms	Element	Sym	# of Atoms
Hydrogen	H	4.22 x 10^{27}	Cadmium	Cd	3 x 10^{20}
Oxygen	O	1.61 x 10^{27}	Boron	B	2 x 10^{20}
Carbon	C	8.03 x 10^{26}	Manganese	Mn	1 x 10^{20}
Nitrogen	N	3.9 x 10^{25}	Nickel	Ni	1 x 10^{20}
Calcium	Ca	1.6 x 10^{25}	Lithium	Li	1 x 10^{20}
Phosphorus	P	9.6 x 10^{24}	Barium	Ba	8 x 10^{19}
Sulfur	S	2.6 x 10^{24}	Iodine	I	5 x 10^{19}
Sodium	Na	2.5 x 10^{24}	Tin	Sn	4 x 10^{19}
Potassium	K	2.2 x 10^{24}	Gold	Au	2 x 10^{19}
Chlorine	Cl	1.6 x 10^{24}	Zirconium	Zr	2 x 10^{19}
Magnesium	Mg	4.7 x 10^{23}	Cobalt	Co	2 x 10^{19}
Silicon	Si	3.9 x 10^{23}	Cesium	Cs	7 x 10^{18}
Fluorine	F	8.3 x 10^{22}	Mercury	Hg	6 x 10^{18}
Iron	Fe	4.5 x 10^{22}	Arsenic	As	6 x 10^{18}
Zinc	Zn	2.1 x 10^{22}	Chromium	Cr	6 x 10^{18}
Rubidium	Rb	2.2 x 10^{21}	Molybdenum	Mo	3 x 10^{18}
Strontium	Sr	2.2 x 10^{21}	Selenium	Se	3 x 10^{18}
Bromine	Br	2 x 10^{21}	Beryllium	Be	3 x 10^{18}
Aluminum	Al	1 x 10^{21}	Vanadium	V	8 x 10^{17}
Copper	Cu	7 x 10^{20}	Uranium	U	2 x 10^{17}
Lead	Pb	3 x 10^{20}	Radium	Ra	8 x 10^{10}
					Total: 6.71 x 10^{27}

Table 3.2 Estimated Gross Molecular Contents of a Typical 20-μm Human Cell[398,531,758-760,938]

Molecule	Mass %	MW (daltons)	# Molecules	Molecule %	Number of Molecular Types
Water	65	18	1.74 x 10^{14}	98.73	1
Other Inorganic	1.5	55	1.31 x 10^{12}	0.74	20
Lipid	12	700	8.4 x 10^{11}	0.475	50
Other Organic	0.4	250	7.7 x 10^{10}	0.044	~200
Protein	20	50,000	1.9 x 10^{10}	0.011	~5,000
RNA	1.0	1 x 10^6	5 x 10^7	3 x 10^{-5}	---
DNA	0.1	1 x 10^{11}	46	3 x 10^{-11}	---
TOTALS	*100%*	---	*1.76 x 10^{14}*	*100%*	---

Transporting and sorting such a broad range of essential molecular species will be an important basic capability of many nanomedical systems. The three principal methods for distinguishing and conveying molecules that are most useful in nanomedicine are diffusion transport (Section 3.2), membrane filtration (Section 3.3), and receptor-based transport (Section 3.4). The Chapter ends with a brief discussion of binding site engineering (Section 3.5).

3.2 Diffusion Transport

Fluidic transfer of material, known as convective-diffusive transport, can occur either by convection due to bulk flow or by diffusion due to Brownian motion. In convective transport, material is carried along fluid streamlines at the mean velocity of the fluid, with a velocity distribution such as that in Poiseuille flow (Section 9.4.1.5). Bulk flow is customarily regarded as the most important physiological transport mechanism in the human circulation. Only for the smallest molecules, such as water or glucose, does the time required to diffuse across the width of a capillary roughly equal the time taken by a fluid element to flow the same distance (~0.02 sec). Larger molecules such as fibrinogen take ~100 times longer (~2 sec) to diffuse across one capillary width.

However, bulk flow in the body is usually laminar. Transported materials travel parallel to (and thus cannot reach) fluid/solid interfaces such as the surfaces of blood vessels or membranes. Wall interactions are made possible by diffusion, a random process in which particles can move transversely to fluid streamlines in response to molecular-scale collisions.

Additionally, the movement of micron-scale devices within a bulk fluid flow is dominated by viscous, not inertial, forces (Section

9.4.2.1). Molecular transport to and from such nanodevices is governed by diffusion, not by bulk flow.

3.2.1 Brownian Motion

A particle suspended in a fluid is subjected to continuous collisions, from all directions, with the surrounding molecules. If the velocities of all molecules were the same all the time, the particle would experience no net movement. However, molecules do not have a single velocity at a given temperature, but rather have a distribution of velocities of varying degrees of probability. Thus from time to time, a suspended particle receives a finite momentum of unpredictable direction and magnitude. The velocity vector of the particle changes continuously, resulting in an observable random zigzag movement called Brownian motion.

Einstein[385] approximated the RMS (root mean square) displacement of a particle of radius R suspended in a fluid of absolute viscosity η and temperature T, after an observation period τ, as:

$$\Delta X = (kT\,\tau / 3\,\pi\,\eta\,R)^{1/2} \quad \text{(meters)} \qquad \text{\{Eqn. 3.1\}}$$

where k = 1.381 x 10^{-23} joule/kelvin (K) or 0.01381 zJ/K (Boltzmann's constant). Particles under bombardment also experience a rotational Brownian motion around randomly oriented axes, with the RMS angle of rotation:

$$\Delta\alpha = (kT\,\tau / 4\,\pi\,\eta\,R^3)^{1/2} \quad \text{(radians)} \qquad \text{\{Eqn. 3.2\}}$$

although for $\tau < \tau_{min} = M / 15\,\pi\,\eta\,R$, where M is particle mass (see below), rotation is ballistic.

In human blood plasma, with η = 1.1 centipoise (1.1 x 10^{-3} kg/m-sec) and T = 310 K, a spherical 1-micron diameter nanodevice (R = 0.5 micron) translates ~1 micron in 1 sec ($v_{brownian}$ ~ 10^{-6} m/sec) or ~8 microns (~the width of a capillary) after 77 sec ($v_{brownian}$ ~ 10^{-7} m/sec), and rotates once in ~16 sec (τ_{min} = 2 x 10^{-8} sec). In the same environment, a rigid 10-nm particle (roughly the diameter of a globular protein) would translate ~8 microns in one second ($v_{brownian}$ ~ 10^{-5} m/sec) while rotating ~250 times, due to Brownian motion (τ_{min} = 2 x 10^{-12} sec).

The instantaneous thermal velocity over one mean free path, the average distance between collisions, is much higher than the net Brownian translational velocity would suggest. For a particle of mass M = 4/3 $\pi\,\rho\,R^3$ with mean (working) density ρ, the mean thermal velocity is:

$$v_{thermal} = (3\,kT / M)^{1/2} \qquad \text{\{Eqn. 3.3\}}$$

At T = 310 K, a spherical 1-micron diameter nanodevice of normal density (e.g., taking $\rho \sim \rho_{H_2O}$ = 993.4 kg/m^3 to minimize ballasting requirements; Section 10.3.6) has $v_{thermal}$ ~ 5 x 10^{-3} m/sec; for a spherical 10-nm diameter protein with ρ ~ 1500 kg/m^3, $v_{thermal}$ ~ 4 m/sec.

3.2.2 Passive Diffusive Intake

Medical nanodevices will frequently be called upon to absorb some particular material from the external aqueous operating environment. Molecular diffusion presents a fundamental limit to the speed at which this absorption can occur. (Once a block of solution has passed into the interior of a nanodevice, it may be divergently subdivided and transported at ~0.01-1 m/sec along internal pathways of characteristic dimension ~1 micron far faster than the <1 mm/sec bulk diffusion velocity across 1 micron distances; Section 9.2.7.5.)

For a spherical nanodevice of radius R, the maximum diffusive intake current is:

$$J = 4\,\pi\,R\,D\,C \qquad \text{\{Eqn. 3.4\}}$$

where J is the number of molecules/sec presented to the entire surface of the device, assumed to be 100% absorbed (but see Section 4.2.5), D (m^2/sec) is the translational Brownian diffusion coefficient for the molecule to be absorbed, and C (molecules/m^3) is the steady-state concentration of the molecule far from the device.[337] (Blood concentrations in gm/cm^3 from Appendix B are converted to molecules/m^3 by multiplying Appendix B figures by (10^6 x N_A/MW), where N_A = 6.023 x 10^{23} molecules/mole (Avogadro's number) and MW = molecular weight in gm/mole or daltons.) For rigid spherical particles of radius R, where R >> R_{H_2O}, the Einstein-Stokes equation[363] gives:

$$D = kT / (6\,\pi\,\eta\,R) \qquad \text{\{Eqn. 3.5\}}$$

though this is only an approximation because D varies slightly with concentration, with departure from molecular sphericalness, and other factors.

Measured diffusion coefficients in water for various molecules of physiological interest, converted to 310 K, are in Table 3.3. Diffusion coefficient data for ionic salts such as NaCl and KCl, which dissociate in water and diffuse as independent ions, are for solvated electrolytes. A 1-micron (diameter) spherical nanodevice suspended in arterial blood plasma at 310 K, with C = 7.3 x 10^{22} molecules/m^3 of oxygen and D = 2.0 x 10^{-9} m^2/sec, encounters a flow rate of J = 9.2 x 10^8 molecules/sec of O_2 impinging upon its surface. (The same calculation applied to serum glucose yields J = 1.3 x 10^{10} molecules/sec.) The characteristic time for change mediated by diffusion in a region of size L scales as ~L^2/D (Eqn. 3.9, below). Across the diameter of an L = 1 micron nanodevice, small molecules such as glucose diffuse in ~0.001 sec, small proteins like hemoglobin in ~0.01 sec, and virus particles diffuse in ~0.1 sec. Diffusion coefficients of the same molecules in air at room temperature are a factor of ~60 higher, because η_{air} ~ 183 micropoise at 20°C.

In blood, the diffusivity of larger particles is significantly elevated because local fluid motions generated by individual red cell rotation lead to greater random excursions of the particles.[388] The effective diffusivity $D_e = D + D_r$, where the rotation-induced increase in diffusivity $D_r \sim 0.25\,R_{rbc}^2\,\dot{\gamma}$, with red cell radius R_{rbc} ~ 2.8 microns (taken for convenience as a spherical volume equivalent) and a typical blood shear rate (Section 9.4.1.1) $\dot{\gamma}$ ~ 500 sec^{-1}, giving D_r ~10^{-9} m^2/sec in normal whole blood. The elevation of diffusivity caused by red cell stirring is just 50% for O_2 molecules. However, for large proteins and viruses the effective diffusivity increases 10-100 times, and the effective diffusivity of particles the size of platelets is a factor of 10,000 higher than for Brownian molecular diffusion.

The diffusion current to the surface of a nanodevice can also be estimated for various nonspherical configurations.[337] For instance, the diffusion current to both sides of an isolated thin disk of radius R is given by J = 8 R D C. The two-sided current to a square thin plate of area L^2 is J = $(8/\pi^{1/2})$ L D C. The steady-state diffusion current to an isolated cylinder of length L_c and radius R is approximated by J = 2 π L_c DC / (ln ($2L_c$/R) - 1), for L_c >> R. The diffusion current through a circular hole of radius R in an impermeable wall separating regions of concentration c_1 and c_2 is J = 4 R D (c_1-c_2).

3.2.3 Active Diffusive Intake

Foraging nanodevices operating in aqueous environments may only modestly exceed the maximum rates of passive diffusive intake described in Section 3.2.2 by engaging in active physical movements designed to increase access to the desired molecules, as described quantitatively below.

Table 3.3 Translational Brownian Diffusion Coefficients for Physiologically Important Molecules Suspended in Water at 310 K *(most values converted from measured data at 20 °C).*[390,754,761-763]

Diffusing Particle in Water	Mol. Wt. (gm/mole)	Diff. Coeff. D (m^2/sec)
H_2	2	5.4×10^{-9}
H_2O	18	2.31×10^{-9}
O_2	32	2.0×10^{-9}
Methanol	32	1.5×10^{-9}
HCl	36.5	3.6×10^{-9}
CO_2	44	1.9×10^{-9}
NaCl	58.5	1.5×10^{-9}
Urea	60	1.3×10^{-9}
Glycine	75	1.0×10^{-9}
KCl	75	2.0×10^{-9}
α-Alanine isomer	89	9.5×10^{-10}
β-Alanine isomer	89	9.7×10^{-10}
Glycerol	92	8.8×10^{-10}
$CaCl_2$	111	1.2×10^{-9}
Glucose	180	7.1×10^{-10}
Mannitol	182	7.1×10^{-10}
Citric acid	192	6.9×10^{-10}
Sucrose	342	5.4×10^{-10}
Milk lipase	6,669	1.5×10^{-10}
Ribonuclease	13,683	1.3×10^{-10}
Insulin	24,430	7.7×10^{-11}
Scarlet fever toxin	27,000	1.0×10^{-10}
Somatotropin	27,100	9.4×10^{-11}
Carbonic anhydrase Y	30,640	1.1×10^{-10}
Plasma mucoprotein	44,070	5.6×10^{-11}
Ovalbumin	43,500	8.1×10^{-11}
Hemoglobin	68,000	7.3×10^{-11}
Serum albumin	68,460	6.5×10^{-11}
Transferrin	74,000	6.2×10^{-11}
Gonadotropin	98,630	4.7×10^{-11}
Collagenase	109,000	4.5×10^{-11}
Actin	130,000	5.3×10^{-11}
Plasminogen (profibrolysin)	143,000	3.1×10^{-11}
Ceruloplasmin	143,300	5.0×10^{-11}
γ-Globulin	153,100	4.2×10^{-11}
Immunoglobulin G (IgG)	158.500	4.2×10^{-11}
Hyaluronic acid	177,100	1.3×10^{-11}
Glucose dehydrogenase	190,000	3.6×10^{-11}
Fibrinogen	339,700	2.1×10^{-11}
Collagen	345,000	7.3×10^{-12}
Urease	482,700	3.7×10^{-11}
Cytochrome a	529,800	3.8×10^{-11}
α-Macroglobulin	820,000	2.5×10^{-11}
β-Lipoprotein	2,663,000	1.8×10^{-11}
Ribosome	4,200,000	1.3×10^{-11}
Viral DNA	6,000,000	1.4×10^{-12}
Urinary mucoprotein	7,000,000	3.4×10^{-12}
Tobacco mosaic virus	31,340,000	5.6×10^{-12}
T7 Bacteriophage	37,500,000	9.5×10^{-12}
Polyhedral silkworm virus	916,200,000	2.3×10^{-12}
1-μm spherical nanodevice	$\sim 8 \times 10^{11}$	4.1×10^{-13}
Platelet (~2.4 μm)	$\sim 4 \times 10^{12}$	1.6×10^{-13}
Red Blood Cell (~5.6 mm)	$\sim 6 \times 10^{13}$	6.8×10^{-14}

3.2.3.1 Diffusive Stirring

The first strategy for active diffusive intake is local stirring. For this, the nanodevice is equipped with suitable active appendages used to manipulate the fluid in its vicinity. Transport by stirring is characterized by a velocity v_a, the speed of the appendage, and by a length L_a, its distance of travel, which together define a characteristic stirring frequency $\nu_{stir} \sim v_a/L_a$ sec^{-1}. Movement of molecules over a distance L_a by diffusion alone is scaled by a characteristic time $\sim L_a^2/D$ (Section 3.2.2), which defines a characteristic diffusion frequency $\nu_{diff} \sim D / L_a^2$ sec^{-1}. Stirring will be more effective than diffusion only if $\nu_{stir} > \nu_{diff}$, that is, if $v_a > D / L_a$. For local stirring, L_a cannot be much larger than the size of the nanodevice itself. Assuming L_a = 1 micron and D = 10^{-9} m^2/sec for small molecules, then v_a > 1000 microns/sec, a faster motion than is exhibited by bacterial cells but quite modest for nanomechanical devices (Section 9.3.1). With D=10^{-11} m^2/sec for large proteins and virus particles, v_a > 10 microns/sec, well within the normal microbiological range.

The ratio of stirring time to diffusion time, or Sherwood number, is:

$$N_{Sh} = L_a \, v_a / D \qquad \text{\{Eqn. 3.6\}}$$

provides a dimensionless measure of the effectiveness of stirring vs. diffusion. For bacteria absorbing small molecules, $N_{Sh} \sim 10^{-2}$. Micron-scale nanodevices with 1-micron appendages capable of 0.01-1 m/sec movement can achieve $N_{Sh} \sim$ 10-1000 for small to large molecules, hence could be considerably more effective stirrers.

In a classic paper, Berg and Purcell[337] analyzed the viscous frictional energy cost of moving the stirring appendages so that the fluid surrounding a spherical object (e.g., a nanodevice) of radius R, out to some maximum stirring radius R_s, is maintained approximately uniform in concentration. The objective is to transfer fluid from a distant region of relatively high concentration to a place much closer to the nanodevice, thereby increasing the concentration gradient near the absorbing surface. To double the passive diffusion current by stirring, the minimum required power density is:

$$P_d \approx \frac{12\,\eta\,D^2}{R^4}\left(\frac{R_s + 2R}{R_s - 2R}\right)^3 \quad (\text{watts/m}^3) \qquad \text{\{Eqn. 3.7\}}$$

If $\eta = 1.1 \times 10^{-3}$ kg/m-sec, R = 0.5 micron, D = 10^{-9} m^2/sec for small molecules, and using a modest L_a = 1 micron stirring apparatus giving R_s = 3R, then $P_d \sim 3 \times 10^7$ watts/m^3. This greatly exceeds the 10^2-10^6 watts/m^3 power density commonly available to biological cells (Table 6.8) but lies well within the normal range for nanomechanical systems which typically operate at up to $\sim 10^9$ watts/m^3. (Nanomedically safe in vivo power densities are discussed at length in Sections 6.5.2 and 6.5.3.) For D $\sim 10^{-11}$ m^2/sec for large molecules, $P_d \sim 3 \times 10^3$ watts/m^3, which is reasonable even by biological standards. The maximum possible gain from stirring is $\sim R_s/R$, because the current is ultimately limited to what can diffuse into the stirred region.

Local heating due to stirring is minor. Given device volume V $\sim$1 micron^3, $P_d = 3 \times 10^7$ watts/m^3, mixing distance $L_{mix} \sim$ 5 microns, and thermal conductivity K_t = 0.623 watts/m-K for water, then $\Delta T \sim (P_d V / L_{mix} K_t)$ = 10 microkelvins; taking heat capacity $C_V = 4.19 \times 10^6$ J/m^3-K for water, thermal equilibration time $t_{EQ} \sim L_{mix}^2 C_V / K_t$ = 0.2 millisec.

3.2.3.2 Diffusive Swimming

The second strategy for active diffusive intake is by swimming. Again, the nanodevice is equipped with suitable active propulsion equipment (Section 9.4) which enables it to move so as to continuously encounter the highest possible concentration gradient near its surface. Consider a spherical motile nanorobot of radius R propelled at constant velocity v_{swim} through a fluid containing a desired molecule for which the surface of the device is essentially a perfect sink (Section 4.2.5). Applying the Stokes velocity field flow around the sphere to the standard diffusion equation, a numerical solution by Berg and Purcell[337] found that the fractional increase in the diffusion current due to swimming is proportional to v_{swim}^2 for $v_{swim} \ll D/R$, and to $v_{swim}^{1/3}$ for $v_{swim} \gg D/R$.

Diffusive intake is doubled at a swimming speed $v_{swim} = 2.5\ D/R$, which for 1-micron devices is ~5000 microns/sec when absorbing small molecules, ~50 microns/sec for large molecules. The viscous frictional energy cost to drive the nanodevice through the fluid, derived from Stokes' law (Eqn. 9.73), requires an onboard power density of:

$$P_d = 9\,\eta\, v_{swim}^2 / 2\,R^2 \qquad \text{\{Eqn. 3.8\}}$$

If η = 1.1 x 10^{-3} kg/m-sec, v_{swim} = 2.5 D/R, R = 0.5 micron, D = 10^{-9} m^2/sec for small molecules, then P_d ~ 5 x 10^5 watts/m^3. For large molecules with D = 10^{-11} m^2/sec, P_d ~ 50 watts/m^3. Thus the energy cost of diffusive swimming appears modest for nanomechanical systems; gains in diffusion by swimming for nanodevices will be restricted primarily by the maximum safe velocity that may be employed in vivo (Section 9.4.2.6).

In general, outswimming diffusion requires movement over a characteristic distance $L_s \sim D/v_{swim}$.[389] For bacteria moving at ~30 micron/sec and absorbing small molecules, then L_s ~ 30 microns, roughly the sprint distance exhibited by flagellar microbes such as *E. coli*. For micron-scale nanodevices moving at ~1 cm/sec (Section 9.4), L_s ~ 1-100 nm for large to small molecules.

3.2.4 Diffusion Cascade Sortation

Nanodevices may also use diffusion to sort molecules. One of the remarkable features of diffusive sortation is that an input sample consisting of a complex mixture of many different molecular species can sometimes be completely resolved into pure fractions without having any direct knowledge of the precise shapes or electrochemical characteristics of the molecules being sorted. This can be a tremendous advantage for nanodevices operating in environments containing a large number of unknown substances. Another major advantage is the ability to readily distinguish isomeric (though not chiral) molecules. As one example of many possible, molecules suspended in water will diffuse into an adjacent region of pure water at different speeds, giving rise to dissimilar time-dependent concentration gradients which may be exploited for sortation by interrupting the process before complete diffusive equilibrium is reached.

For simplicity, assume we wish to separate two molecular species initially present in solution in equal concentrations ($c_1 = c_2$), but having unequal diffusion coefficients ($D_1 < D_2$). Consider a separation apparatus with two chambers. Chamber A contains input sample concentrate. Chamber B contains pure water. A dilating gate (Section 3.3.2) separates the two chambers. The gate is opened for a time Δt approximated by:

$$\Delta t = \frac{(\Delta X)^2}{2\,D_2} \sim \frac{L^2}{2\,D_2} \qquad \text{\{Eqn. 3.9\}}$$

which relates the diffusion coefficient to the mean displacement ΔX, taken here as L, the length of Chamber B. Table 3.4 gives an estimate of the time required for diffusion to reach 90% completion for glycine, a typical small molecule, in aqueous solution.

After Δt has elapsed, the gate is closed. (A gate with 10-nm sliding segments moving at 10 cm/sec closes in 0.1 microsec.) The faster-diffusing component D_2 approaches diffusive equilibrium in Chamber B, but the slower-diffusing component does not; it is present only in smaller amounts. This gives a separation factor c_2/c_1 ~ D_2/D_1 for each diffusion sortation unit. If n units are connected in series, with each unit receiving as input the output of the previous unit, the net concentration achieved by the entire cascade is ~$(D_2/D_1)^n$. Such cascades are commonplace in gaseous diffusion isotope separation[875] and other applications.

Table 3.4 Estimated Time for Diffusion to Reach 90% Completion for Glycine in Aqueous Solution at 310 K.[397]

Diffusion Distance	Diffusion Time (sec)	Mean Velocity
1 nm	10^{-9}	1 m/sec
10 nm	10^{-7}	100 mm/sec
100 nm	10^{-5}	10 mm/sec
1 micron	10^{-3}	1 mm/sec
10 microns	10^{-1}	100 micron/sec
100 microns	10	10 micron/sec
1 mm	1000 (17 min)	1 micron/sec
1 cm	10^5 (28 hr)	0.1 micron/sec

Figure 3.1 shows a 2-dimensional representation of an efficient design for a simple diffusion unit that might be used in a sortation cascade. Each unit consists of 5 chambers of equal volume, 7 dilating gates, 3 flap valves, 3 pistons, and 2 sieves which pass only water (or smaller) molecules. Each chamber is roughly cubical with L ~ 35 nm along the inside edge; including full piston throws and drives, controls, interunit piping and other support structures, each unit measures ~125 nm x 100 nm x 80 nm or ~0.001 $micron^3$ with a mass of ~10^{-18} kg.

The following is a precise description of one complete cycle of operation for each unit:

1. The cycle begins with fluid to be sorted in Chamber A, Chambers B and W full of pure water with piston W all the way out, Chambers R and D empty with pistons R and D all the way in, and all valves and gates closed.
2. Gate AB is opened for a time Δt, then closed. For a small molecule such as urea (MW = 60 daltons), Δt= 1 microsec; for a large molecule such as the enzyme urease (MW = 482,700 daltons), Δt= 35 microsec.
3. Valves AI- and AI+, and gate AR, are opened. Piston R is drawn fully out, slowly to preserve laminar flow and to prevent mixing. Fluid in Chamber A is drawn into Chamber R. Fluid passing through the DO gate of the previous unit in the cascade enters Chamber A through valve AI-. Fluid passing through the RO valve of the subsequent unit in the cascade enters Chamber A through valve AI+. All valves and gates are closed. Chamber A is now ready for the next cycle.
4. Gates WB and BD are opened. Piston W is slowly pushed all the way in while piston D is slowly pulled all the way out. Concentrated solution in Chamber B is transferred into Chamber D as pure water in Chamber W is transferred into Chamber B, again preserving laminar flow. Both gates are closed; Chamber B is now ready for the next cycle.
5. Gates RW and DW are opened. Pistons R and D are slowly and simultaneously pushed halfway in while piston W is pulled all the way out. Forced at high pressure (~160 atm) through ~0.3 nm diameter sieve pores (Section 3.3.1), half of the solvent water present in Chambers R and D is pushed into Chamber W, filling Chamber W with water. (This design allows for easy backflushing if sieve pores become clogged.) Both gates are closed; Chamber W is now ready for the next cycle.

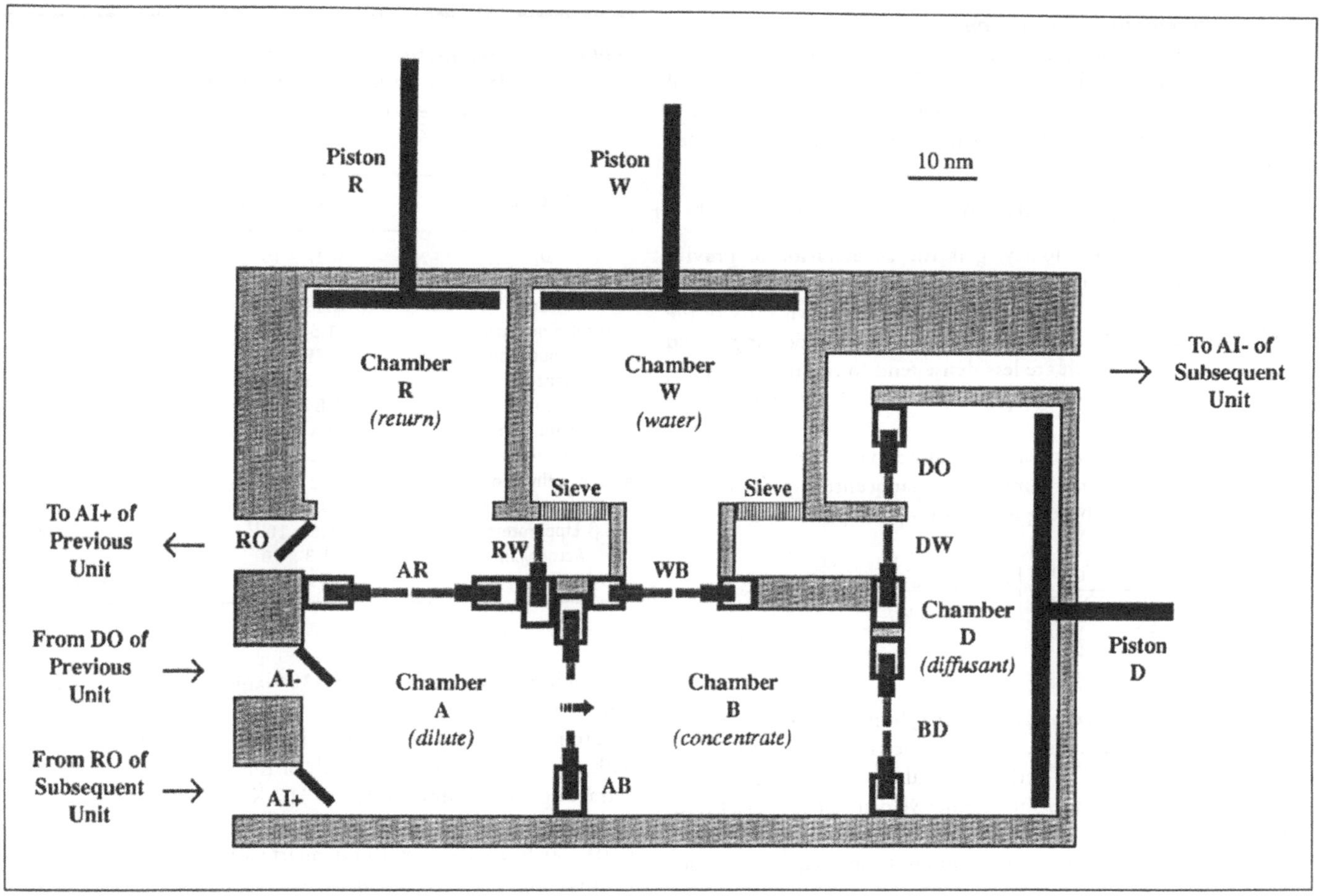

Fig. 3.1. Schematic of diffusion cascade sortation unit.

6. Valve RO and gate DO are opened. Pistons R and D are slowly and simultaneously pushed the rest of the way in. Concentrated return fluid passes through valve RO and back to the AI+ input port of the previous unit in the cascade for further extraction. Concentrated diffusant fluid passes through gate DO and on to the AI- input port of the subsequent unit in the cascade for further purification. The valve and gate are closed; Chambers R and D are now empty and ready for the next cycle.

7. Return to Step (1). Adjacent units operate in counterphase while previous and subsequent units operate in synchrony, in a two-phase system.

Increasingly purified sample passes through a multi-unit sortation cascade as described above. For small molecules, a cascade of n ~ 1000 units (total device volume ~ 1 micron^3) completely resolves two mixed molecular species with D_2/D_1 = 1.01. As a crude approximation, $D \sim 1 / MW^{1/3}$ for small spherical particles,[390] so this cascade separates small molecules differing by the mass of one hydrogen atom which should be sufficient for most purposes. Structural isomeric forms of the same molecule, such as α-alanine and β-alanine, often have slightly different diffusion coefficients, thus are also easily separable using a diffusion cascade. However, stereoisomeric (chiral) forms cannot be sorted by diffusion through an optically inactive solvent like water.

For large molecules, a 1 million-unit cascade (total device volume ~1000 micron^3) provides D_2/D_1 ~ 1.00001, sufficient to completely separate large molecules differing by the mass of a single carbon atom. The fidelity of such fine resolutions depends strongly upon the ability to hold constant the temperature of the chamber, since D varies directly with temperature (Eqn. 3.5). Device temperature stability will be determined by at least three factors: (1) the accuracy of onboard thermal sensors in measuring T ($\Delta T/T < 10^{-6}$; Section 4.6.1), (2) the rapidity with which the temperature measurement can be taken (10^{-9} to 10^{-6} sec; Section 4.6.1), and (3) the time that elapses between the temperature measurement and the end of the diffusive sortation process (which may be of the same order as the gate closing time, ~10^{-6} sec).

Most of the waste heat is generated in this device by forced water sieving (Section 3.3.1). To remain within biocompatible thermogenic limits (~10^9 watts/m^3), each unit may be cycled once every ~3 millisec, a 0.8% duty cycle of a ~23 microsec sieving stroke. Subject to this restriction, each unit would consume ~1 picowatt in continuous operation. A unit presented with a ~0.1 M concentration of small molecules processes ~10^6 molecules/sec (e.g., ~1 gm/hour of glucose using 1 cm^3 of n = 1000-unit cascades), or ~10^4 molecules/sec for a unit presented with large molecules at ~0.001 M, circulating ~10^9 molecules/sec of water as working fluid while running at 340 cycles/sec. Additional chamber segments on each unit, combined with more complex diffusion circuits among the many units in a cascade, should permit the simultaneous complete fractionation of the input feedstock even if hundreds of distinct molecular species are present.

By 1998, diffusion-based separation had been demonstrated in microfluidic devices.[2689]

3.2.5 Nanocentrifugal Sortation

Nanoscale centrifuges offer yet another method for rapid molecular sortation, by biasing diffusive forces with a strong external field. The well-known effect of gravitational acceleration on spherical particles suspended in a fluid is described by Stokes' Law for Sedimentation:

$$v_t = 2\, g\, R^2\, (\rho_{particle} - \rho_{fluid}) \,/\, 9\, \eta \qquad \text{\{Eqn. 3.10\}}$$

where v_t is terminal velocity, g is the acceleration of gravity (9.81 m/sec^2), R is particle radius, $\rho_{particle}$ and ρ_{fluid} are the particle and fluid densities (kg/m^3), and η is coefficient of viscosity of the fluid. Particles which are more dense than the suspending liquid tend to fall. Those which are less dense tend to rise ($\rho_{particle} / \rho_{fluid}$ ~0.8 for lipids, up to ~1.5 for proteins, and ~1.6 for carbohydrates in water).

This separation process may be greatly enhanced by rapidly spinning the mixed-molecule sample in a nanocentrifuge device. For ideal solutions (e.g., obeying Raoult's law) at equilibrium:[390]

$$c_2/c_1 = \exp\left[\left(\frac{MW_{kg}\,\omega^2}{2\,R_g\,T}\right)\left(1 - \frac{\rho_{fluid}}{\rho_{particle}}\right)\left(r_2^2 - r_1^2\right)\right] \qquad \text{\{Eqn. 3.11\}}$$

where c_2 is the concentration at distance r_2 from the axis of a spinning centrifuge (molecules/m^3), c_1 is the concentration at distance r_1 (nearer the axis), MW_{kg} is the molecular weight of the desired molecule in kg/mole, ω is the angular velocity of the vessel (rad/sec), T is temperature (K) and the universal gas constant R_g = 8.31 joule/mole-K. The approximate spinning time t required to reach equilibrium is

$$t_s = \ln(r_2/r_1) \,/\, (\omega^2\, S_d) \qquad \text{\{Eqn. 3.12\}}$$

where S_d is the sedimentation coefficient, usually given in units of 10^{-13} sec or svedbergs (Table 3.5). Research ultracentrifuges have reached accelerations of ~10^9 g's.

Consider a cylindrical diamondoid vessel of density ρ_{vessel} = 3510 kg/m^3, radius r_c = 200 nm, height h = 100 nm, and wall thickness x_{wall} = 10 nm, securely attached to an axial drive shaft of radius r_a = 50 nm (schematic in Fig. 3.2). A fluid sample containing desired molecules enters the vessel through a hollow conduit in the drive shaft, and the device is rapidly spun. If rim speed v_r = 1000 m/sec (max), then $\omega = v_r / r_c = 5 \times 10^9$ rad/sec ($\omega / 2\pi = 8 \times 10^8$ rev/sec). The maximum bursting force $F_b \sim 0.5\, \rho_{vessel}\, v_r^2 = 2 \times 10^9$ N/m^2, well below the 50×10^9 N/m^2 diamondoid tensile strength conservatively assumed by Drexler.[10] Since S_d ranges from 0.1-200 x 10^{-13} sec for most particles of nanomedical interest (Table 3.5), minimum separation time using acceleration $a_r / g = v_r^2 / g\, r_c = 5 \times 10^{11}$ g's, when $r_2 = r_c$ and $r_1 = r_a$, is t_s = 0.003-6.0 x 10^{-6} sec. Fluid sample components migrate at ~0.1 m/sec.

Maximum centrifugation energy per particle $E_c = (MW_{kg} / N_A)\, a_r\, (r_c - r_a)$ ~ 10,000 zJ/molecule, or ~10 zJ/bond for proteins, well below the 180-1800 zJ/bond range for covalent chemical bonds (Section 3.5.1). However, operating the nanocentrifuge at peak speed may disrupt the weakest noncovalent bonds (including hydrophobic, hydrogen, and van der Waals) which range from 4-50 zJ/bond. The nanocentrifuge has mass ~10^{-17} kg, requires ~3 picojoules to spin up to speed (bearing drag consumes ~10 nanowatts of power, and fluid drag through the internal plumbing contributes another ~5 nanowatts), completes each separation cycle in ~10^4 revs (~10^{-5} sec), and processes ~300 micron^3/sec which is ~10^{13} small molecules/sec (at 1% input concentration) or ~10^9 large molecules/sec (at 0.1% input concentration).

Table 3.5 Sedimentation Coefficients for Particles in Aqueous Suspension at 310 K *(1 svedberg = 10^{-13} sec; values converted from measured data at 20°C)*[390,754]

Particle	Sed. Coeff. (sec)	Mol. Wt.
O_2	0.12 x 10^{-13}	32
CO_2	0.07 x 10^{-13}	44
Glucose	0.18 x 10^{-13}	180
Insulin monomer	1.5 x 10^{-13}	6,000
Ribonuclease	1.75 x 10^{-13}	13,683
Lysozyme	2.03 x 10^{-13}	17,200
Insulin	1.84 x 10^{-13}	24,430
Ovalbumin	3.4 x 10^{-13}	43,500
Serum albumin	4.3 x 10^{-13}	68,460
Alcohol dehydrogenase	7.2 x 10^{-13}	150,000
Catalase	10.7 x 10^{-13}	250,000
β-Lipoprotein	5.6 x 10^{-13}	2,663,000
Actomycin	11.3 x 10^{-13}	3,900,000
TMV	175 x 10^{-13}	31,340,000

From Eqn. 3.11, the nanocentrifuge separates salt from seawater with c_2/c_1 ~ 300 across the width of the vessel ($r_c - r_a$ = 150 nm); extracting glucose from water at 310 K, c_2/c_1 ~10^5 over 150 nm. For proteins with $\rho_{particle}$ ~ 1500 kg/m^3, separation product removal ports may be spaced, say, 10 nm apart along the vessel radius while maintaining c_2/c_1 ~ 10^3 between each port. Vacuum isolation of the unit in an isothermal environment and operation in continuous-flow mode could permit exchange of contents while the vessel is still moving, sharply reducing remixing, vibrations, and thermal convection currents between product layers. A complete design specification of product removal ports, batch and continuous flow protocols, compression profiles, etc. is beyond the scope of this book.

Variable gradient density centrifugation may be used to trap molecules of a specific density in a specific zone for subsequent harvesting, allowing recovery of each molecular species from complex mixtures of substances that are close in density. The traditional method is a series of stratified layers of sucrose or cesium chloride solutions that increase in density from the top to the bottom of the tube. A continuous density gradient may also be used, with the

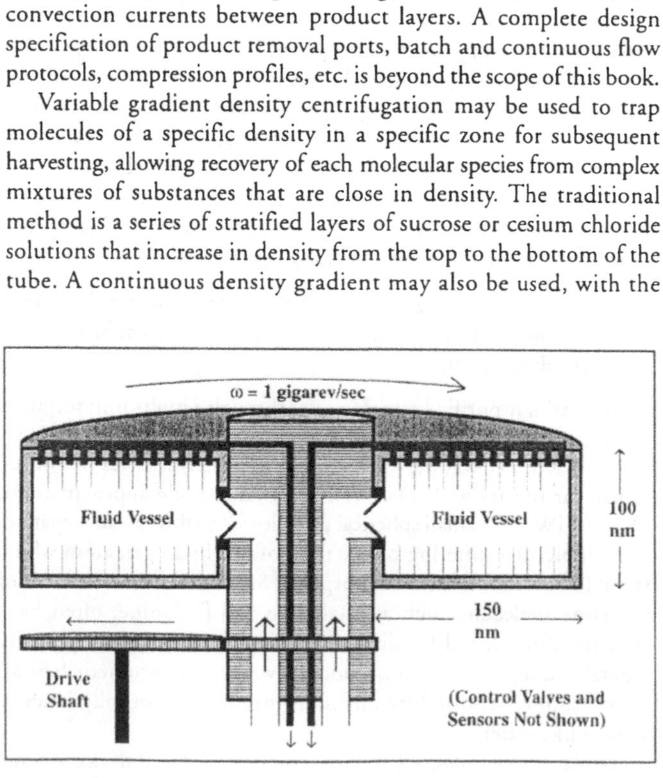

Fig. 3.2. Schematic of teragravity nanocentrifuge.

density of the suspension fluid calibrated by physical compression. For example, the coefficient of isothermal compressibility $\kappa = -(\Delta V_l/V_l) / \Delta P_l = (\Delta\rho_{fluid} / \rho_{fluid}) / \Delta P_l = 4.492 \times 10^{-5}$ atm^{-1} for water at 1 atm and 310 K (compressibility is pressure- and temperature-dependent). Applying P_l = 12,000 atm to the vessel raises fluid density to 1250 kg/m^3,[567] sufficient to partially regulate protein zoning. A multistage cascade (Section 3.2.4) may be necessary for complete compositional separation. Protein denaturation between 5000-15,000 atm[585] due to hydrogen bond disruption may limit nanocentrifugation rotational velocity. Protein compressibility may further reduce separability. The balance between the differential densities and the differential compressibilities will determine the equilibrium radius of the protein in the centrifuge; in the limiting case of equal compressibilities for a given target protein and water, there is no stable equilibrium radius.

The nanocentrifuge may also be useful in isotopic separations. For a D_2O/H_2O mixture, c_2/c_1 = 1.415 per pass through the device; $c_2/c_1 = 10^6$ is achieved in a 40-unit cascade. Tracer glycine containing one atom of C^{14} is separated from natural glycine using a 113-unit cascade, achieving $c_2/c_1 = 10^6$.

3.3 Membrane Filtration

Filtration through a permeable membrane is closely related to the process of diffusion, since in both cases random molecular motions help carry the process to completion. However, the presence of a membrane adds a new measure of control that is not exploited in simple diffusive transport. This control may be either passive or active, unidirectional or bidirectional, as described below.

3.3.1 Simple Nanosieving

Nanometer-scale isoporous molecular sieves (with ovoid, square, or hexagonal holes) are common in almost every taxonomic group of eubacteria and archaeobacteria.[525] Other well-known examples of nanoporous structures are the 6-nm pore arrays found in reverse osmosis and kidney dialysis membranes.

Likewise, it is possible for a nanodevice to sort molecules by simple sieving.[987,1177] In this process, a sample containing particles of various sizes suspended in water passes through a graduated series of filters perforated by progressively smaller holes of fixed size and shape. Between each filtration unit, the filtration residue consists almost exclusively of particles having a narrow range of sizes and shapes. For example, a series of n = 100 filtration units could reliably differentiate an input sample containing particles from 0.2-1.2 nm into 100 separate fractions, each fraction consisting predominantly of particles differing in mean diameter by ~0.01 nm. (In a practical system, several passes would be required to achieve complete discrimination; Section 3.2.4.) A ~0.01 nm difference in molecular diameter corresponds to the mean contribution of ~1 additional carbon atom to the size of a small molecule (MW ~ 100 daltons), or to the mean contribution of ~100 additional carbon atoms to the size of a large molecule (MW ~ 100,000 daltons, ~17,000 atoms). A nanomembrane might even permit the (slow, multi-pass) sieving of oxygen from air, since the molecular diameters of N_2 and O_2 differ by ~0.01 nm (Section 3.5.5).

Two opposing forces are at work when moving water and solutes through a membrane. One is the osmotic pressure established by the presence of nonpermeating solutes; the other is the hydraulic or fluid pressure. The velocity of material movement depends on the relative values of the osmotic and hydraulic forces, and on the size of the pores in the filter.

Osmotic pressure p_π is given by the Donnan-van't Hoff formula:[403]

$$p_\pi = \left(\frac{R_g\, T\, (c_2 - c_1)}{MW_{kg}}\right)\left(1 + \frac{Z^2\,(c_2 - c_1)}{c_s}\right) \quad (\text{N/m}^2)$$

{Eqn. 3.13}

where R_g = 8.31 joules/mole-K, T is temperature in kelvins (K), c_2 and c_1 are solute concentrations on either side of the membrane in kg/m^3 ($c_2 > c_1$), MW_{kg} is the molecular weight of the solute in kg/mole, and the Z^2 term (dependent upon polymer-polymer interactions) is a correction factor for highly concentrated solutions which for some solvents and temperatures may equal zero; Z = net solute charge number and c_s is the concentration in kg/m^3 of a second solute, as for example when the first solute is a protein and the second solute is salt, as in human serum. Water at 310 K dissolves a maximum of c_2 = 370 kg/m^3 of sodium chloride (a 37.0% solution, by weight), and MW_{kg} = 0.05844 kg/mole for NaCl, so for salt water solutions the theoretical maximum $p_\pi \sim 1.6 \times 10^7$ N/m^2 ~ 160 atm. Natural bloodstream concentrations of salt produce p_π ~ 3 atm. Since osmotic pressure depends on the number of molecules present, the contribution from large molecules is usually negligible. For instance, total protein concentration in human blood serum is c_2 ~ 73 kg/m^3, MW_{kg} ~ 50 kg/mole (~50,000 daltons), so p_π ~ 0.04 atm.

In theory, extremely large hydraulic counterforces up to 10^5 atm may be applied in nanomechanical systems, for example by a piston, to overcome osmotic backpressure. As a practical matter, however, rapidly pushing small molecules at high pressure through nanoscale holes is an effective method for generating significant amounts of waste heat; a design compromise is required.

Consider a simple sorting apparatus in which a square piston is used to compress solvent fluid (say, water) trapped in a chamber $h_{chamber}$ in length and $L_{chamber}^2$ in cross-sectional area, forcing the fluid to filter through pores of radius r_{pore} (~ target molecule radius) covering a fraction α_H (~50%) of the surface of a square nanoscale sieve of thickness h_{sieve} and area L_{sieve}^2. Solute which is dissolved or suspended in the solvent is sorted based on molecular size; a sequence of sieving runs using sieves having progressively smaller pore radii produces an ordered sequence of molecular size fractions. (In small molecules, adding the mass of one hydrogen atom increases the me n linear dimension of the molecule by 0.1-1%.)

The first design constraint on this system relates to its maximum operating pressure. If ΔP is applied pressure (N/m^2), then avoiding boiling the solvent water and denaturing proteins requires at least that $\Delta P_{max} < C_V\, \Delta T_{boil}$, where the heat capacity of water $C_V = 4.19 \times 10^6$ joules/m^3-K and ΔT_{boil} = 373 K - 310 K = 63 K give $\Delta P_{max} <$ 2600 atm. The designs presented below operate at 6% of this maximum (ΔT ~ 3 K) or less.

There are two major design constraints on the duration of the power stroke, or t_p:

1. *Molecular Rotation Constraint* — Flow through the sieve must be slow enough to allow molecules to align with the holes. Assuming round pores, the total number of pores in the sieve is $N_{pore} = \alpha_H\, L_{sieve}^2 / \pi r^2$. The volume processing rate (m^3/sec) of the sieve $\dot{V}_{sieve} = \dot{V}_{chamber} = h_{chamber}\, L_{chamber}^2/t_p$, hence the molecule processing rate is $\dot{N} = \dot{V}_{chamber}\, c_{target}$ (molecules/sec) where c_{target} is the concentration of target molecules (molecules/m^3). At any one time, each pore channel through the sieve can hold at most $N_{channel} = h_{sieve} / 2\, r_{pore}$ molecules in single file; during each power stroke, at most $N_{stack} = \dot{N}\, t_p / N_{pore}$ molecules pass through each pore. Hence the time available for molecular rotation $t_{rot} = t_p\, (N_{channel} / N_{stack})$, which assumes the layer of rotating target molecules in the vicinity of the pores approximates sieve thickness h_{sieve}, a reasonable assumption as long as the typical molecular diffusion time (across

a distance h_{sieve}) << t_{rot}. Taking $N_{rot} \sim 10$ as the mean number of molecular revolutions needed to ensure proper pore alignment with noncircular sieve holes (the most difficult case), then, from Eqn. 3.2, $\Delta\alpha = (kT\ t_{rot} / 4\pi\eta\ r_{pore}^3)^{1/2} \gtrsim 2\pi N_{rot}$, where η is solvent viscosity (1.1×10^{-3} kg/m-sec for plasma) at T = 310 K. Solving for minimum t_p gives:

$$t_p \geq \frac{32\pi^4 N_{rot}^2\ \eta\ c_{target}\ h_{chamber}\ r_{pore}^6}{kT\ \alpha_H\ h_{sieve}} \quad \text{(sec)} \quad \text{\{Eqn. 3.14\}}$$

2. *Pressure/Flow Constraint* — Flow through the sieve must be fast enough to establish a sufficient pressure to oppose osmotic backflows. From the Hagen-Poiseuille law (Section 9.2.5), the volume processing rate through each pore is $\dot{V}_{pore} = \pi\ r_{pore}^4\ \Delta P_{sieve} / 8\ \eta\ h_{sieve}$ and the volume processing rate through the entire sieve is $\dot{V}_{sieve} = N_{pore}\ \dot{V}_{pore} = \dot{V}_{chamber}$; solving for maximum t_p gives:

$$t_p \leq \frac{8\ \eta\ h_{chamber}\ h_{sieve}\ L_{chamber}^2}{\alpha_H\ \Delta P_{sieve}\ r_{pore}^2\ L_{sieve}^2} \text{(sec)} \quad \text{\{Eqn. 3.15\}}$$

Equating these two bracketing constraints, $h_{sieve} \gtrsim 150$ nm for large molecules ($r_{pore} \sim 5$ nm) but $h_{sieve} \gtrsim 1$ nm for small molecules ($r_{pore} \sim 0.32$ nm).

As a final constraint, power released by fluid flow through the chamber and sieve must not exceed safe thermogenic limits. Given the maximum safe power density for in vivo nanomachines given in Section 6.5.3 as $D_n = 10^9$ watts/m^3, then:

$$D_{device} = \frac{P_{device}}{(h_{chamber} + h_{sieve})\ L_{chamber}^2} \leq D_n \quad (\text{watts/m}^3) \quad \text{\{Eqn. 3.16\}}$$

where D_{device} = device power density (watts/m^3), total device power $P_{device} = P_{chamber} + P_{sieve}$ (watts), chamber fluid flow power $P_{chamber} = \pi\ L_{sieve}^4\ \Delta P_{chamber}^2 / 128\ h_{chamber}\ \eta$, sieve fluid flow power $P_{sieve} = \alpha_H\ L_{sieve}^2\ r_{pore}^2\ \Delta P_{sieve}^2 / 8\ h_{sieve}\ \eta$, and $\Delta P_{chamber} = 16\ \alpha_H\ h_{chamber}\ r_{pore}^2\ \Delta P_{sieve} / \pi\ L_{sieve}^2\ h_{sieve}$. For small molecules such as NaCl or glucose, $\Delta P_{sieve} \gtrsim 160$ atm to overcome maximum osmotic backpressure; for large molecules (e.g., ~50,000 dalton proteins), we assume $\Delta P_{sieve} \gtrsim 1$ atm to ensure sieving. The following designs are not optimized but illustrate the tradeoffs involved.

For small molecules ($r_{pore} \sim 0.32$ nm), an exemplar ~1 micron^3 device has $h_{chamber}$ = 1 micron, $L_{chamber} = L_{sieve}$ = 0.6 micron, h_{sieve} = 1.5 microns, t_p = 0.016 sec, ΔP_{sieve} = 160 atm, $\Delta P_{chamber}$ = 0.0001 atm. Piston velocity ~ 60 micron/sec and $\dot{V} = 2.5 \times 10^{-17}$ m^3/sec for a 0.1 M solution of target molecules, yielding a processing rate of 1.5×10^9 molecules/sec (1.5×10^{-16} kg/sec); the device processes its own mass every ~7 sec or every ~430 power strokes. Device power P_{device} = 400 pW and power density $D_{device} = 4 \times 10^8$ watts/m^3.

For large molecules ($r_{pore} \sim 5.0$ nm), an exemplar ~1 micron^3 device has $h_{chamber}$ = 1 micron, $L_{chamber} = L_{sieve}$ = 0.9 micron, h_{sieve} = 0.15 microns, t_p = 0.010 sec, ΔP_{sieve} = 1 atm, $\Delta P_{chamber}$ = 0.0004 atm. Piston velocity ~ 100 micron/sec and $\dot{V} = 9.8 \times 10^{-17}$ m^3/sec for a 0.001 M solution of target molecules, yielding a processing rate of 5.9×10^7 molecules/sec (4.9×10^{-15} kg/sec); the device processes its own mass every ~0.2 sec or every ~20 power strokes. Device power P_{device} = 80 pW and power density $D_{device} = 8 \times 10^7$ watts/m^3.

Sieve pores can become clogged by particles of radius R ~ r_{pore} if the applied hydraulic pressure ΔP_{clog} exceeds the thermal energy of the trapped particles, or:

$$\Delta P_{clog} > 9\ kT / 8\ \pi\ R^3 \quad (\text{N/m}^2) \quad \text{\{Eqn. 3.17\}}$$

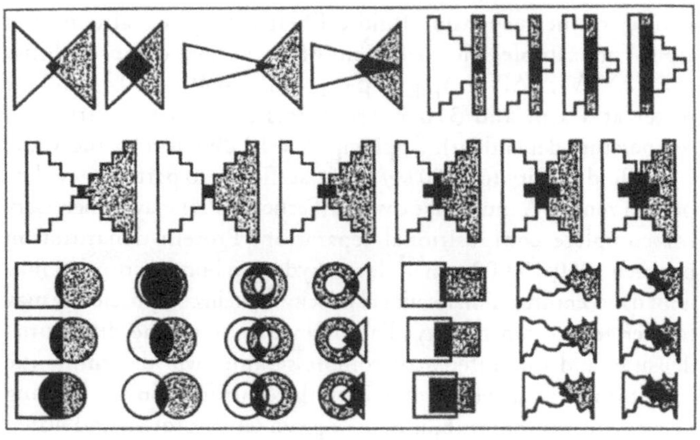

Fig. 3.3. Variable size/shape apertures using two nanoscale perforated sliding plates.

By this criterion, $\Delta P_{clog} > 500$ atm for small molecules and $\Delta P_{clog} > 0.1$ atm for large molecules. From the values of ΔP_{sieve} given above, clogging is unlikely for small molecules but is possible at the highest concentrations of large molecules. In 310 K water, large molecules diffuse ~3 nm and small molecules diffuse ~17 nm in ~10^{-7} sec, just far enough to clear the hole, so a ~10 MHz sawtooth pressure profile imposed on the power stroke may ensure sufficient backflushing action to avoid serious blockages. To reduce the possibility of clogging due to surface force adhesion (Section 9.2.3), as a design criterion the work of adhesion should be reduced to $W_{adhesion} < \Delta P_{sieve}\ r_{pore} \sim 5 \times 10^{-3}$ J/m^2 for small molecules and ~ 0.5×10^{-3} J/m^2 for large molecules likely to come into contact with sieve pore surfaces. Clogging due to long-term random polymerizations can be minimized by periodically exchanging the entire contents of the input chamber with fresh solution, by operating the device at reduced power density, or by periodically replacing the sieve.

3.3.2 Dynamic Pore Sizing

A more efficient nanosieve[3251] system can be designed if pore size and shape can be actively modified during device operation, as for example by exchanging filters (from a membrane library stocking various pore sizes) each half cycle. Better, if pores can be reliably dilated or constricted in place during a period of time $\Delta t << t_p$, then filtration cascades can be more rapidly reconfigured to match changing input feedstock characteristics or to extract varying selections of desired molecules at will. Additionally, fully differentiating sieving cascades can be collapsed into a single unit, providing more compact devices especially useful in chemical sensor systems requiring preconcentration of sample (Section 4.2.1). Control of pore shape should also provide finer discrimination among molecules of similar size but different shape, such as some isomers of nonchiral molecules.

Two or more overlapping surfaces containing regular arrays of perforations of fixed size and shape can conveniently generate a wide variety of pore geometries. Control of pore geometry is achieved by sliding or rotating one surface relative to the other surface by a small increment, as suggested schematically by the examples in Figure 3.3.

Circular dilating apertures can also be constructed using a matched set of overlapping segments, which may be driven either radially or tangentially to enlarge or contract the hole like an irising camera diaphragm (Fig. 3.4), consistent with Akey's model of the nuclear pore complex present on the cell nucleus surface.[1409] Diaphragming mechanisms may be vertically staggered to maximize areal hole density in filtration surfaces (at the cost of increased vertical rugosity). Filters constructed of hydrogen-passivated diamondoid can have pores with <0.1 nm feature sizes, although H-free fullerene materials might avoid any possibility of dehydrogenation shearing.

Methods of positioning surfaces to accuracies of ~0.01 atomic diameter (~0.001 nm) are discussed in Section 3.5.6. Assuming pore sizing blades require ~25 nm^2 of diamondoid contact surface per pore and each blade travels 25 nm at 0.01 meter/sec during one cycle, sliding friction[10] dissipates ~0.01 zJ/pore, or ~4 x 10^{-18} watts/pore during each 2.5 microsec resizing cycle. Since fluid friction approaches kT for nanometer-size holes changing size in ~10^{-9} sec, maximum blade speed is ~1 m/sec and the fastest resizing cycle is ~10^{-8} sec.

A single sieving unit with controllable pores can be moderately efficient. Consider a design similar to that described in Section 3.3.1, except for a separate chamber and piston on either side of the filter block. Suppose that the particles desired to be extracted are of radius r, and the next smallest possible pore size is r - Δr. The device operates in two phases. In the first phase, the sample is placed in the first chamber, pore size is set equal to r, then the first piston forces the fluid through the membrane. Particles larger than r remain behind and are flushed from the first chamber. The pores then contract to r - Δr, and the second piston pushes the remaining filtrate back into the first chamber. After this second phase, particles of radius ~(r ± Δr) remain in the second chamber at significantly higher concentration and may be removed for further use. Analogous double-sieve editing paradigms are commonplace in biological systems.[1520]

Other designs might work equally well, such as a 3-chamber flowthrough design using a variable pore membrane with pores of size r between the first and second chamber, a membrane with pores of size r - Δr between the second and third chamber, and a piston at either end (one pushing, one pulling), thus concentrating molecules of size r ± Δr in the central chamber. M. Krummenacker suggests fixed chambers with a moving sieve operated as a dragnet. Filtration processes may be most useful in performing complete separations of complex mixtures. But they are inefficient in the sense that the energy expended to orient molecules passing through pores is wasted if the molecules are allowed to randomize on the other side; a eutactic mill-like molecule handling system (Section 3.4.3) might preserve this order and greatly improve energy efficiency.

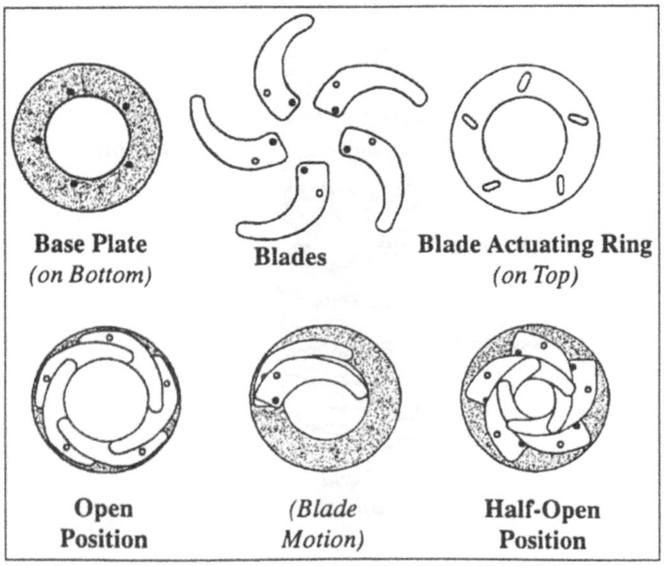

Fig. 3.4. Circular dilating "iris" diaphragm mechanism for dynamic nanopore sizing.

3.3.3 Gated Channels

Besides controlling nanopore size and shape, individual molecular transport channels can be gated either mechanically (e.g., ligand gating)[2348] or electrically (e.g., voltage gating).[1050] Either method might usefully be employed to control molecular transport through the surfaces of medical nanodevices in a process that could very loosely be described as molecular transistor gating.

A good example of mechanical gating in biology is the nicotinic acetylcholine receptor channel, probably the best understood ligand-gated channel.[391,396] Nerve impulses are communicated across neuromuscular junctions and autonomic ganglia via neurotransmitters such as acetylcholine. STM images[419] confirm that the receptor itself is cylindrical, a bundle of 5 rod-shaped polypeptide subunits arranged like barrel staves with outside diameter ~6.5 nm. The receptor protrudes 6 nm on the synaptic side of the membrane and 2 nm on the cytoplasmic side. The water-filled channel pore lies along the symmetry axis, lined by 5 α-helices, with a 2.2 nm wide mouth on the synaptic surface, a 0.65 nm waist where the structure dives through the cell membrane, and a 2 nm wide cytosolic exit.

Normally, the channel is closed and no ions may pass. In this closed state, the channel is occluded at the waist by a ridge of large residues forming a tight hydrophobic ring. Each subunit has a bulky leucine at the bend in the α-helix, a critical position. When two acetylcholine molecules bind to the receptor, these helices allosterically tilt, shifting the position of the ridges. The pore becomes open because it is now lined with small polar residues rather than by large hydrophobic ones. This conformational change allows 2.5 x 10^7 Na^+ ions/sec to flow through the channel, about 10% of the diffusion-limited rate. (Anions like Cl^- cannot enter the pore because they are repelled by rings of negatively charged residues positioned at either end of the receptor.)

Acetylcholine binding opens the gate in less than 100 microsec under physiologic conditions. Subsequent rapid destruction of acetylcholine by acetylcholinesterase, an enzyme tethered to the membrane surface by a covalently attached glycolipid group, closes the gate in ~1 millisec. Much faster gating action (~10^{-8} - 10^{-6} sec) could be achieved by nanodevices operating variable-scale nanopores (Section 3.3.2) in response to sensor data or other control signals. Such signals could drive the insertion or retraction of diamondoid rods, wedges, or trapdoors across the channel lumen to regulate the transmission of molecules having specific sizes, shapes, and charge distributions.

Transport channels through nanodevice surfaces may also be gated electrically.[392] In contrast to the acetylcholine receptor, which is relatively nondiscriminating and allows both inorganic and organic cations to pass, the voltage-gated calcium channel has a highly discriminating mechanism with a Ca^{++}:Na^+ permeation ratio on the order of 1000:1. (The high specificity of the voltage-gated Ca^{++} channel is a consequence of a single-file pore mechanism involving a pair of specific Ca^{++} ion binding sites. Selectivity is assured if either of the two sites is occupied by Ca^{++}, as monovalent ions do not bind strongly enough to the free site or generate sufficient electrostatic repulsion to push the first Ca^{++} ion through the channel.[395]) Potassium channels[1311,3435-3437] are 100 times more permeable to K^+ than to Na^+, and sodium channels favor the passage of Na^+ over K^+ by a factor of 12. All three of these voltage-gated channels are important in the generation and conduction of neural action potentials.

A nerve impulse is an electrical signal produced by the flow of ions across the plasma membrane of a neuron. Neuron interiors have high concentrations of K^+ and low concentrations of Na^+. The resting potential of a neuron is -60 mV. An action potential may be generated when the membrane potential is slightly depolarized to -40 mV. This opens the Na^+ voltage-gated channels, rapidly accelerating depolarization to a peak of +30 mV in ~1 millisec. Then Na^+ channels close and K^+ channels open, allowing K^+ ions to exit the cell, restoring the -60 mV resting potential. Only ~1 ion of every ~10^6 Na^+ and K^+ ions present in the local extracellular medium and the axoplasm participate in each such nerve impulse.

The sodium channel is a single polypeptide chain with four repeating units. Each repeating unit folds into six transmembrane alpha helices, including one that is positively charged called the S4 helix. The S4 helix is the voltage sensor that triggers the opening of the gate. Three positively charged residues on each S4 helix are paired at the resting membrane potential with negative charges on other transmembrane helices in a staircase geometry. The initial small depolarization event produces a spiral motion of each S4 accompanied by the net movement of one or two charges to the extracellular side of the membrane, essentially turning this left-handed hydrogen-bonded "molecular screw" through a ~60° rotation.[395] This outward 0.5-nm translation of the four S4 segments opens the sodium gate by removing a steric barrier to ion flow. The energy cost of moving ~6 electrical charges (~10^{-18} coul) from the cytosolic to the extracellular side of the membrane against a ~100 mV potential (thus opening the gate in ~75 microsec) is ~100 zJ. Quantum tunneling activation of sodium channels, taking 1-1000 microsec, has been analyzed by Chancey.[679]

Artificial ion-gated polymer membranes were reported in 1982,[393] protein engineering of switchable pore-forming proteins is well-known,[880] and "intelligent gels" are being developed that can change size and molecular porosity in response to chemical, electrical or thermal stimuli. In 1998, however, electroporation was a more commonly used method in biological research and a useful technique for "transfecting" cells in genetic studies. Electroporation employs a brief intense pulse of electricity to provide a force that opens cellular pores, enabling the insertion of macromolecules like DNA into cells of interest; laser pulses reduce cell loss to 10% by using a square-wave pulse to effect rapid and reversible pore formation.[1295] Artificial pH-gated 200-nm diameter nanopores[2335] and natural pH-gating of virion pores in the cowpea chlorotic mottle virus[2391] were demonstrated in 1998.

The first true voltage-gated nanomembrane was fabricated by Charles Martin and colleagues in 1995.[394] This membrane consists of cylindrical gold nanotubules with inside diameters as small as 1.6 nm. When the tubules are positively charged, cations are excluded and only negative ions are transported through the membrane. When the membrane receives a negative voltage, only positive ions are transported through the tubules. Nanodevices may combine voltage gating with pore size and electrosteric constraints to achieve precision transport control with moderate molecular specificity at diffusion-limited throughput rates. In 1997, an ion channel switch biosensor with sub-picomolar sensitivity and quantitative detection time of ~600 sec was demonstrated by an Australian research group.[3039,3040]

3.4 Receptor-Based Transport

The most efficient of all modes of molecular transport involves receptor sites capable of recognizing and selectively binding specific molecular species. Many receptors reliably bind only a single molecular type; others, such as sugar transporters, can recognize and transport several related sugar molecule types. In nanomechanical systems, artificial binding sites of almost arbitrary size, shape, and electronic charge may be created and employed in the construction of a variety of highly efficient molecular sortation and transport devices, described below. A discussion of binding sites and receptor engineering follows in Section 3.5.

3.4.1 Transporter Pumps

While gated channels enable ions to flow rapidly through membranes in a thermodynamically downhill direction, active pumps use a source of free energy to force an uphill transport of ions or molecules. In biology the energy supply is usually ATP or photons of light; medical nanomachines can make use of vastly more diverse energy sources (Chapter 6). Actually, the term "pump" may be something of a misnomer because the action is highly specific—only one or a very small number of molecular species are selectively transported.

Molecular pumps generally operate in a four-phase sequence: (1) recognition (and binding) by the transporter of the target molecule from a variety of molecules presented to the pump in the input substrate; (2) translocation of the target molecule through the membrane, inside the transporter mechanism; (3) release of the molecule by the transporter mechanism; and (4) return of the transporter to its original condition, so that it is ready to accept another target molecule. Such molecular transporters that rely on protein conformational changes are ubiquitous in biological systems, and are illustrated schematically in Figure 3.5.

The minimum energy required to pump molecules is the change in free energy ΔG in transporting the species from one environment having concentration c_1 to a second environment having concentration c_2, given by:

$$\Delta G = kT \ln(c_2 / c_1) + \frac{Z_e F \Delta V}{N_A} \qquad \text{\{Eqn. 3.18\}}$$

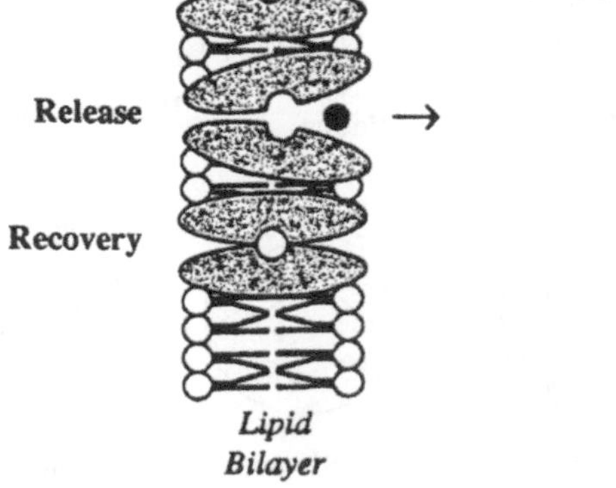

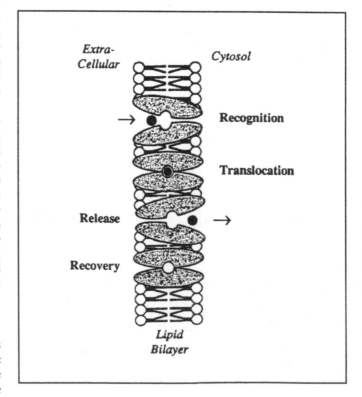

Fig. 3.5. Schematic of transporter molecular pump operation (uniport).

where k = 0.01381 zJ/K (Boltzmann constant), T = 310 K, Z_e is the number of charges per molecule transported (i.e., the valency), F = 9.65 x 10^4 coul/mole (Faraday constant), ΔV is the potential in volts across the membrane, and N_A is Avogadro's number. So for example, transport of an uncharged molecule across a $c_2/c_1 = 10^3$ gradient (typical in biology) costs ~30 zJ. An extremely aggressive $c_2/c_1 = 10^6$ concentration gradient costs ~60 zJ/molecule, plus another ~30 zJ/ion if we are moving Ca^{++} ions against a 100 mV potential. An artificial nanopump of dimension ~10 nm moving at a conservative ~1 cm/sec velocity operates at MHz frequencies, transporting ~10^6 molecules/sec for a continuous power consumption of ~0.03 pW at $c_2/c_1 = 10^3$. Such a pump has a mass ~10^{-21} kg.

Transporter pumps need not be limited to the movement of a single molecular species in a single direction, which biochemists call a uniport transport mechanism.[3649] Numerous well-known biological systems are capable of moving two molecules simultaneously in one direction (symport mechanisms), two molecules sequentially in opposite directions (antiport mechanisms),[3642-3648] and charged molecules in one direction only, thus building up an electrical charge on one side of the membrane (electrogenic mechanisms).[3633-3637,3643] Such pumps exist in nature for numerous ions, amino acids, sugars, and other small biomolecules.[398] Active drug efflux systems[400] and multidrug resistance[399] are made possible by the expression of bacterial genes coding for molecular pumps that are constantly evolving new specificities to increasing numbers of microbicidal drugs.

The action of the Na^+ - K^+ antiporter, a familiar ion pump present in all mammalian cells, is illustrated in Figure 3.6. Three Na^+ and two K^+ ions are transported per 10 millisec cycle, requiring the hydrolysis of one ATP molecule to ADP to drive the conformational changes. (More than one-third of the ATP consumed by a resting animal is used to pump these two ions.) Hydrolysis of ATP liberates ~80 zJ/molecule of free energy, so the antiporter is transporting Na^+ and K^+ at a cost of 16 zJ/ion at a 0.5 KHz frequency. Pump site density is ~1000/micron^2 of cell membrane in neural C fibers.[800] (The Na^+ - K^+ pump can also be operated in reverse to synthesize ATP from ADP by exposing the mechanism to steep ionic gradients.) By contrast, artificial nanomechanical antiporter and symporter devices will operate at MHz frequencies.[1177] They should be able to transport much larger molecules, and may also be fully reversible.

3.4.2 Sorting Rotors

Drexler's molecular sorting rotor[10] is a related class of nanomechanical device capable of selectively binding molecules from solution and then transporting these bound molecules against concentration gradients (Fig. 3.7). The archetypal sorting rotor is a disk with 12 binding site "pockets" along the rim exposed alternately to the external solution and interior chamber by axial rotation of the disk. (Other designs may have more, or fewer, pockets.) Each pocket selectively binds a specific molecule when exposed to the solution. Once the binding site (Section 3.5) rotates to expose it to the interior chamber, the bound molecules are forcibly ejected by rods thrust outward by the cam surface (or using some other means by which receptor affinity can be adjusted during the inbound transport process). In the case of protein molecules, the debinding geometry must be carefully designed to avoid denaturation during ejection. Also, the rotor in Figure 3.7 implicitly assumes that target molecules remain in the liquid or gaseous state after importation. M. Krummenacker observes that most bloodborne molecular species will precipitate as solids unless they are well-solvated; thus nanomedical sorting systems may require internal solvent or in some cases should be made completely eutactic (Section 3.4.3). The discovery of positionally disordered water molecules resident inside protein hydrophobic cavities[1047] suggests that good rotor designs may also need to include solvent drainage channels.

Molecular sorting rotors can be designed from about 10^5 atoms (including housing and pro rata share of the drive system), measuring roughly 7 nm x 14 nm x 14 nm in size with a mass of 2 x 10^{-21} kg. Rotors turn at ~86,000 rev/sec with a conservative rim speed of 2.7 mm/sec and an almost negligible drag power of ~10^{-16} watts against the fluid, sorting small molecules at a rate of 10^6 molecules/sec with laminar flow. From Eqn. 3.18, the energy cost of small-molecule sortation at 310 K ranges from ~10 zJ/molecule at low pressures ($c_2/c_1 = 10$) up to ~40 zJ/molecule when pumping against the highest head pressures ($c_2/c_1 = 10^4$, ~30,000 atm for natural bloodstream

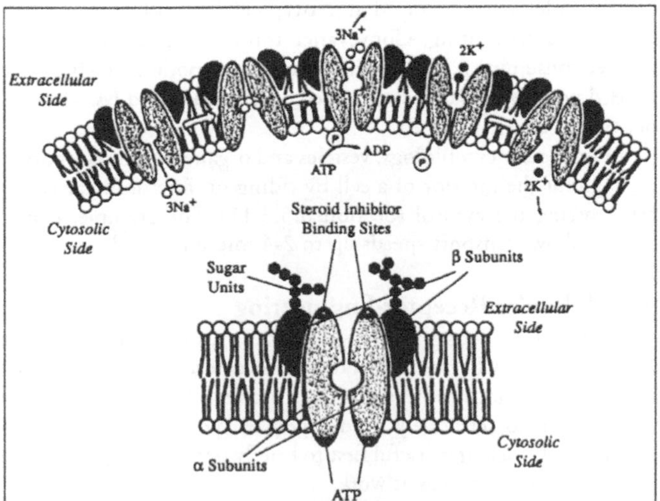

Fig. 3.6. Schematic of sodium-potassium antiporter ion pump operation.

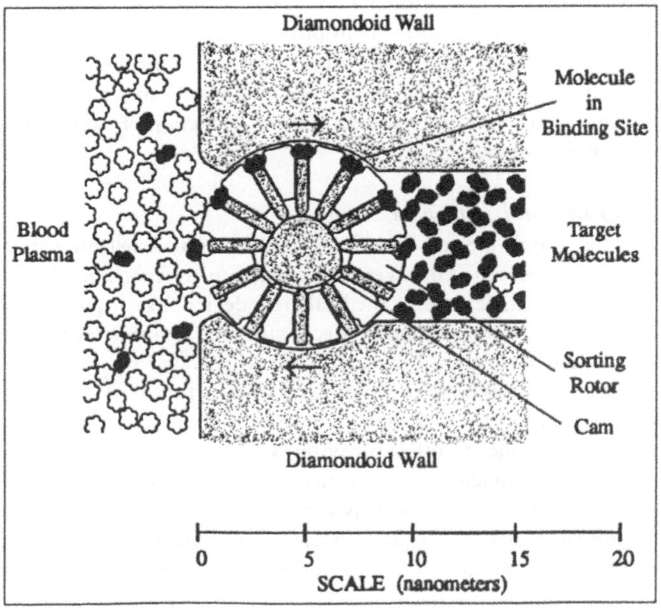

Fig. 3.7. Molecular sorting rotor (modified from Drexler[10]).

concentrations of salt with osmotic p_π ~ 3 atm), consuming 0.01-0.04 pW per device in continuous operation. Rotors are fully reversible, so they can be used to load or unload target molecules depending on the direction of rotor rotation. Cylindrical rotors with many receptor rows are somewhat more energy-efficient, and rotor lifetimes[10] should be $>10^6$ sec (Chapter 13).

Typical molecular concentrations in the blood for target molecules of nanomedical interest are ~10^{-11} – 10^{-3} molecules/nm^3, which should be sufficient to ensure ~99% occupancy of rotor binding sites (Section 3.5.2). Rotors targeting serum hormones and other low-concentration species at the parts-per-billion level must slow to <1 rev/sec to ensure complete receptor occupancy and to avoid exceeding diffusion limits.

Sorting of ionically charged species can use binding sites that display opposite charge, effectively increasing the affinity of the binding site for the charged species. Many ionic species dissolved in water are actually more complex than their symbolic representation would suggest. As an example, a naked proton (H^+) in water is always highly hydrated, usually as $H_5O_2^+$ or $H_7O_3^+$,[996] or even as $H_9O_4^+$ in strong acid solutions.[2337] Small ions from Li^+ to I^- are also found in solvent cages, bound with energies $\gtrsim$330 zJ relative to vacuum;[2338] for instance, Li^+ and I^- are coordinated to 4-6 water molecules.[1149,3235] As a result, the design of an appropriate binding site or filtration process for such ions can likewise become more complex. The existence of biological channels that show remarkable selectivity for specific ions (e.g., Na^+ channels that largely exclude K^+ ions, and vice versa; Section 3.4.1) provides one design approach for dealing with such species.

Drexler[10] has also proposed cascades of sorting rotors (Fig. 3.8) to achieve high fidelity purification and a contaminant fraction of $<10^{-15}$. However, since only ~10^{10} small molecules can be stored in 1 micron^3 volume (typical for nanomedical devices), 100% process purity requires a contaminant fraction of only $<10^{-10}$ which can be ensured in micron-scale nanosystems using at most 5 stages, starting from a dilute input substrate containing only 1 part per billion of the target molecule with each stage providing a concentration factor of ~10^4. For statistically pure extractions of more common molecules in blood and cytoplasm, a 3- or 4-stage cascade will usually suffice. Note that the optimal receptor structure may differ at different stages in a cascade,[10] and that each 12-arm outbound rotor can contain binding sites for 12 different impurity molecules. The first-stage receptor will likely pass only a relatively small number of different contaminant species, so the number of outbound rotors in the entire system can probably be reduced to a small fraction of the number of inbound rotors.

3.4.3 Internal Transport Streams

After pump mechanisms described above have reliably sorted externally-encountered target molecules into reservoirs filled with species of a single type, a medical nanodevice may require these molecules to be transported to specific internal locations for further processing. Bulk fluid flow or fluidized (solvated or suspended) transport through nanopipes may suffice for some purposes (Section 9.2.5). However, in many cases it will be necessary to present reagent molecules to other subsystems as a well-ordered stream of precisely positioned moieties transported in vacuo, especially for mechanochemical operations (Chapter 19).

For this purpose, Drexler[10] proposes molecular mills—eutactic systems of nanoscale belts moving over rollers, with reagent-binding devices mounted on the belt surface (Fig. 3.9). This class of device can be assembled into complex molecular transportation networks using conditional switching, crossed-axis belting, and transit speed/frequency multipliers,[10] and may also be employed to drive mechanosynthetic chemical reactions. The benchmark mechanism uses 10-nm diameter rollers to carry closely packed reagent devices measuring 4 nm x 4 nm x 2 nm, or 32 nm^3. A 20-roller mill mechanism 1 micron long has a ~2 micron long belt with 500 reagent devices and delivers 10^6 molecules/sec at a belt speed of 4 mm/sec. Total power dissipation is ~1.4×10^{-18} watts, a rate of ~0.001 zJ per moiety (or per reagent device) delivered or ~10^{-6} zJ/nm traveled per reagent device. Total mill mechanism mass is ~6×10^{-20} kg.

An alternative to roller/belt mill mechanisms is a non-connected stream of pallets pushed along tracks, also in vacuo. Such tracks may include merging junctions, distribution junctions, multi-plane crossings and switching stations, as well as straight and curved sections. Assuming each pallet is a 32 nm^3 reagent device held to the track by pins in grooves resembling cam followers, energy dissipation by phonon scattering[10] is given approximately by:

$$P_{drag} = \frac{4}{3} \frac{\varepsilon_p \, \omega_{therm} \, v^2}{v_{sound}} \qquad \text{\{Eqn. 3.19\}}$$

where $\varepsilon_p = 2 \times 10^8$ joules/m^3 (phonon energy density), σ_{therm} (a thermally-weighted scattering cross section) ~10^{-20} m^2 for reagent devices of mass $m = 10^{-22}$ kg assuming a sliding contact of stiffness ~30 N/m in a moderately stiff medium, v = 4 mm/sec sliding speed, and $v_{sound} = 10^4$ m/sec (~speed of sound in diamond), giving P_{drag} ~4×10^{-21} watts per reagent device, or P_{drag} / v ~ 10^{-6} zJ/nm traveled per reagent device (pallet). Note that volume containerization of pallet-transported molecules is least efficient at the smallest scales, where surface area per unit enclosed volume is highest, since energy usage is proportional to the surface area of the carrier. Containerization (Section 9.2.7.7) of n >> 1 molecules for large-pallet transport is more efficient.

A less energy-efficient, but far more versatile, internal molecular transport device is the 100-nm telescoping manipulator arm[10] described in Section 9.3.1.4. This flexible ~10^{-19} kg device employs a binding tip to pick and place small and large molecules alike, moving them at ~1 cm/sec with repeatable placement accuracy of 0.04 nm. Multiple devices can be used to establish an internal ciliary transport system (Section 9.3.4); standardized volume containerization of molecules permits rapid stereotypical handoff motions and efficient parcel routing. Conveyance through a 100-nm arc takes 10^{-5} sec consuming 0.1 pW while the arm is in motion, or ~10 zJ/nm traveled per reagent molecule or per container transported (vs. ~1000 zJ per typical covalent bond).

In molecular cytobiology, vesicles and organelles are transported throughout the interior of a cell by riding on microtubular cables crisscrossing the cytosol (Section 8.5.3.11). For example, neural vesicles show transport speeds up to 2-4 microns/sec.[938]

3.5 Molecular Receptor Engineering

Molecular recognition requires a detailed surface complementarity between the target molecule and its receptor. The interplay of various molecular forces between ligand and receptor causes them to selectively bind together, typically engineered to occur in ~10^{-6} sec. It is useful first to briefly review and quantify the principal physical forces at work.

3.5.1 Physical Forces in Molecular Recognition

Covalent bonds, which occur when atoms share electrons, are the strongest bonds. Aside from metals and salts, most material objects are made of atoms held together by covalent bonds. The atoms comprising biological molecules like proteins, nucleic acids

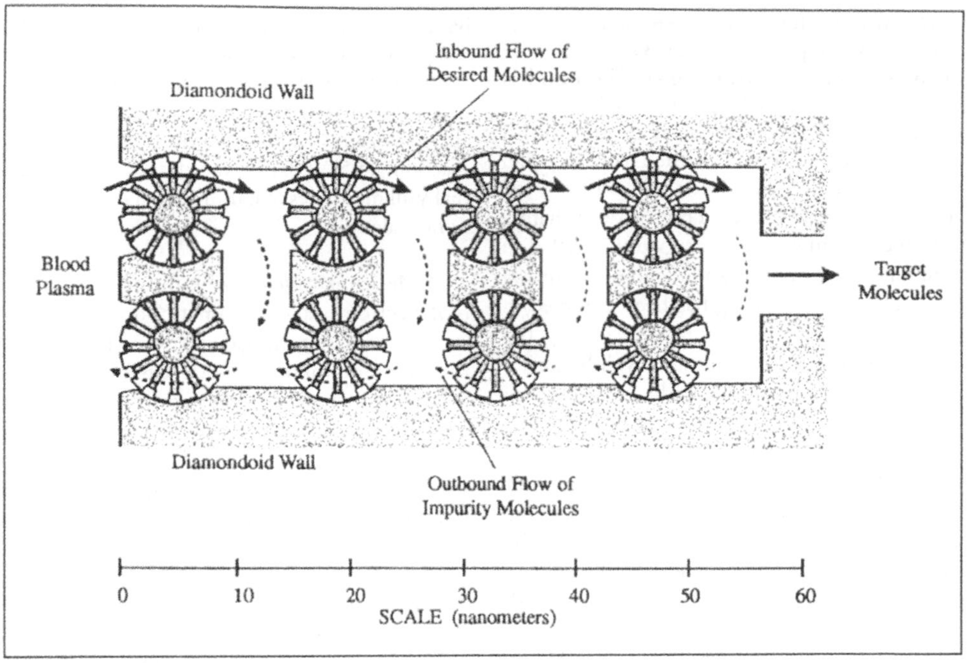

Fig. 3.8. Sorting rotor cascade (modified from Drexler[10]).

and lipids are strung together mostly by single, double, or triple covalent bonds, as are receptors and diamondoid nanomechanical structures. Interatomic bond strengths range from 181 zJ/bond for O-F up to 1785 zJ/bond for C-O.[763] Covalent bond lengths range from 0.10-0.16 nm within CHON-atom molecules, giving a typical covalent bond rupture force of ~10 nN/bond.

But as Jean-Marie Lehn[765] points out, "there is a chemistry beyond the molecule"—noncovalent supramolecular chemistry (Section 2.3.2). The bonds employed in molecular recognition are weak noncovalent bonds. Noncovalent bonds are largely responsible for the secondary and higher order structure of macromolecules. On a per-bond basis, noncovalent bonds are 1-3 orders of magnitude weaker than covalent bonds. However, the possibility of combining within a limited area a great number of noncovalent bonds having complementary elements allows the formation of a large specific association whose affinity may be of the same order of magnitude as a covalent bond.[401] The high combinatorial diversity provided by many complementary elements allows numerous orthogonal specific associations, enabling self-assembly of many components; by comparison, covalent chemistry offers a poor diversity of reactivities. An additional advantage is that the formation of noncovalent bonds often is not hindered by high energy barriers. At least five types of noncovalent bonds may be distinguished: electrostatic, hydrogen, van der Waals, π aromatic, and hydrophobic.

1. *Electrostatic Bond* — The electrostatic bond between two charged particles (e.g., the "salt bridge" in proteins) is a dipole interaction whose energy E_e is given by Coulomb's law as:

$$E_e = \left(\frac{e^2}{4\pi\, \varepsilon_0}\right)\left(\frac{Z_1 Z_2}{\kappa_e r}\right) \exp(-K_{dh} r) \quad \text{(joules)} \qquad \text{\{Eqn. 3.20\}}$$

where e = 1.60 x 10^{-19} coul (elementary charge), ε_0 = 8.85 x 10^{-12} farad/m (permittivity constant), Z_1 and Z_2 are the numbers of

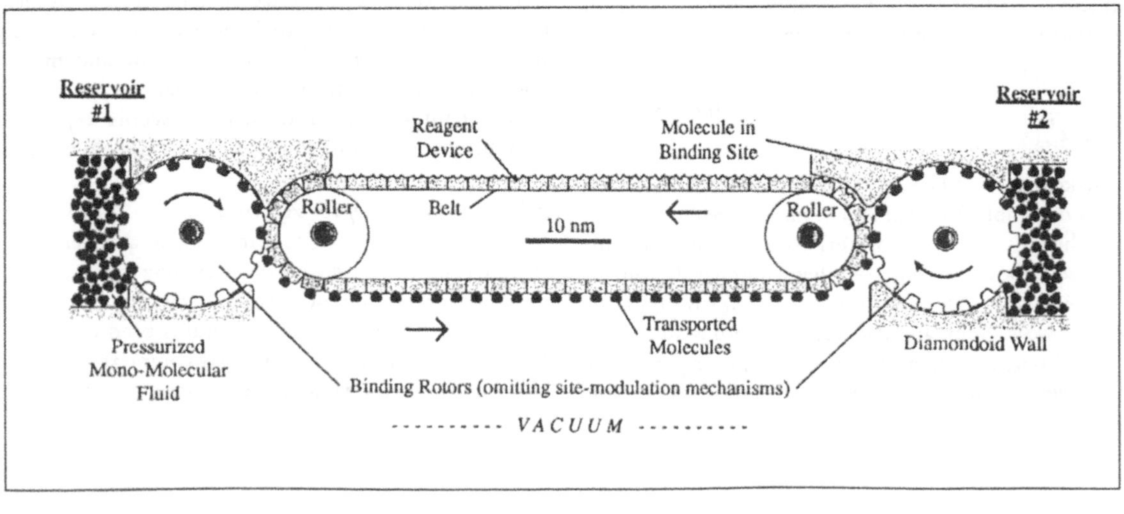

Fig. 3.9. Molecular mills for internal transport: simple transfer between two reservoirs.

attractant charges, r is the distance between the charges, and κ_e is the dielectric constant (74.3 for pure water at 310 K, usually reduced to ~40 in a hydrophobic environment). The bond is strengthened if the charges are in a hydrophobic environment. Conversely, the presence of electrolytes weakens the bond energy due to a shielding effect, given by K_{dh}, the Debye-Huckel reciprocal length parameter, which has a value of 1.25 nm^{-1} for 0.15 M NaCl (~1% solution, ~human blood). Thus two unit charges separated by 0.3 nm produce an interaction energy of E_e = 19 zJ in a hydrophobic environment, 10 zJ in pure water, and 6.3 zJ in 1% salt water. Long-range electrostatic trapping has been observed in single-protein molecules at liquid-solid interfaces, raising the implication that the interaction of protein molecules with biological cell surfaces may be much more efficient than predicted by random diffusion.[2144]

Most isolated amino acids in neutral solution are zwitterionic—the molecule has no overall charge but carries both a negatively charged group (carboxyl, CO_2^-) and a positively charged group (amino, NH_3^+). In proteins the individual amino acids are polymerized, giving a peptide backbone which is electrically neutral except for the ends of the chain. Most of the standard amino acids found in proteins have uncharged side chains, although histidine, lysine and arginine each have a positive charge at neutral pH and both glutamic and aspartic acids normally carry a negative charge.

2. *Hydrogen Bond* — A second important noncovalent interaction is the hydrogen bond, a dipole formed when a hydrogen atom covalently bonded to an electronegative atom is shared with a second electronegative atom (typically an oxygen, nitrogen or fluorine atom), such that the proton may be approached very closely by an unshared pair of electrons. Hydrogen bonds are largely responsible for the unusual thermodynamic properties of water and ice, and the DNA double-helical and protein α-helical and β-structure conformations are extensively hydrogen bonded. Highest bonding energies occur when donor and acceptor atoms are 0.26-0.31 nm apart. Typical hydrogen bond strengths in proteins are 7-50 zJ.

3. *Van der Waals Interaction* — A third important noncovalent force is van der Waals interactions (London dispersion forces).[1149] There is an attractive component due to the induction of complementary partial charges or dipoles in the electron density of adjacent atoms when the electron orbitals of two atoms approach to a close distance. There is also a strongly repulsive component at shorter distances, when the electron orbitals of the adjacent atoms begin to overlap, commonly called steric hindrance. The van der Waals attractive bonding energy between two parallel plates of area A and separation z_{sep} is approximated by:

$$E_{vdW} = \frac{H\,A}{12\,\pi\,z_{sep}^2} \qquad \text{\{Eqn. 3.21\}}$$

where the Hamaker constant H = 37 zJ for water, 66 zJ for glycerol, 340 zJ for diamond (Table 9.1). For A = 0.4 nm^2 (small molecule), z_{sep} = 0.3 nm, then E_{vdW} = 4 zJ (water) to 8 zJ (small organic molecules)—close to the mean energy of a thermally excited harmonic oscillator, kT ~ 4.3 zJ at 310 K. While van der Waals bonds are individually very weak, they are also very numerous since they involve all pairs of neighboring atoms. For example, experimental analysis of an antigen molecule trapped in the anti-hen egg-white lysozyme monoclonal antibody Fv active binding site found 86 distinct interatomic contact points with antigen-antibody separations ranging from 0.25-0.46 nm, averaging 0.36 nm.[416] Since intermolecular dispersion forces act on all molecules, there are probably no ligands with MW > 400 daltons which cannot be receptored (Section 3.5.5). That is, van der Waals interactions ensure that virtually all molecules of nanomedical interest are theoretically bindable noncovalently.

4. *Aromatic π Bonds* — A fourth type of interaction (π electron to π electron), called "aromatic" or "π" bonding, occurs when two aromatic rings (conjugated π systems) approach each other with the plane of their aromatic rings overlapping, with successive π-bonded systems stacked like layers in a cake. This results in a noncovalent attractive force with a bond strength of ~40-50 zJ. (That is, the planes of conjugated π systems attract each other when superimposed.) π bond stacking forces contribute to nucleic acid stability at least as much as the hydrogen bonds between bases.[401]

5. *Hydrophobic Forces* — Finally, there are the strong hydrophobic forces, due entirely to solvent entropy changes. When two nonpolar residues approach each other, the surface area exposed to solvent is reduced, increasing the entropy of all the water present and decreasing the entropy of the residues, adding to the binding energy a hydrophobic free energy of ~17 zJ/nm^2 of contact surface area that was formerly exposed to water.[413]

In designing an artificial binding site, the above forces may be combined to achieve the desired level of affinity and specificity for a given ligand. All forces are not equally useful in this regard, however. For example, hydrophobicity is the major factor in stabilizing protein-protein associations.[402] But hydrophobicity is almost entirely nonspecific, hence contributes little to ligand discrimination. By contrast, the proper formation of hydrogen bonds and van der Waals contacts require complementarity of the surfaces involved. Such surfaces must be able to pack closely together, creating many contact points, and charged atoms must be properly positioned to make electrostatic bonds. Thus van der Waals and polar interactions may contribute little to the dynamic stability of the ligand-receptor complex, but they do determine which molecular structures may recognize each other.[402] Other design elements of binding sites, such as directed channeling of substrates into the receptor,[2017] may also prove useful.

In analyzing molecular forces, note that at the nanoscale level, surface/surface, molecule/surface, and molecule/molecule interactions may feature very complicated behaviors. Nanodevices performing work may generate both thermodynamic and mechanical local nonequilibrium conditions, so calculations based on the general forms of interactions and on macroscopic expressions valid at equilibrium conditions should be taken only as basic estimates.

3.5.2 Ligand-Receptor Affinity

For a ligand binding to a receptor in a solvent, there will be a characteristic frequency with which existing ligand-receptor complexes dissociate as a result of thermal excitation, and a characteristic frequency with which empty receptors bind ligands as a result of Brownian encounters, forming new complexes, with the frequency of binding proportional to the concentration of the ligand in solution,

c_{ligand} (molecules/nm^3).[10] For simple processes, the equilibrium constant K_d, taken in the direction of dissociation, is:

$$K_d = k_d / k_a \text{ (molecules/nm}^3) \quad \text{\{Eqn. 3.22\}}$$

where k_d is the dissociation rate constant (sec^{-1}) and k_a is the association rate constant (nm^3/molecule-sec). The k_a rate constant reflects mainly the molecular weight of the ligand, and thus varies little among antibody, enzyme, or other receptor systems. For example, Delaage[401] notes that changing the solution pH for growth hormone from 7.5 to 4.0 increases K_d by a factor of 3000, due to k_d increasing by a factor of 1600 but k_a decreasing only by a factor of 1.7. Hence it is the rate constant of dissociation, k_d, which accounts for the vast bulk of affinity in receptor systems.

Thus receptor affinity is usually taken as the inverse of the dissociation rate constant, which may be placed in the context of the half-life of the ligand-receptor complex approximated[401] by:

$$t_{1/2} \sim \ln(2) / k_d \text{ (sec)} \quad \text{\{Eqn. 3.23\}}$$

Observed half-lives range from <0.1 microsec ($k_d \sim 10^7$ sec^{-1}) for the enzyme catalase to a few months ($k_d \sim 10^{-7}$ sec^{-1}) for enzyme inhibitors such as the Kunitz inhibitor of trypsin[406] and for avidin-biotin binding.[407] The smaller the k_d (or the K_d), the greater the affinity and so the more firmly the receptor grasps the ligand.

The probability $P_{occupied}$ that a receptor will be occupied[10] is given by:

$$P_{occupied} = \left(\frac{c_{ligand}}{K_d}\right) P_{unoccupied} \quad \text{\{Eqn. 3.24\}}$$

where $P_{unoccupied} = 1 - P_{occupied}$. To ensure $P_{occupied}$ = 99% receptor occupancy, K_d must ~ c_{ligand} / 100. For target molecules present at the 10^{-3} - 10^{-11} gm/cm^3 concentrations typically found in human blood (Appendix B), $c_{ligand} = 3 \times 10^{-3}$ molecules/nm^3 for glucose to $c_{ligand} \sim 10^{-11}$ molecules/nm^3 for female serum testosterone, giving a range of $K_d \sim 10^{-4}$ - 10^{-13} molecules/nm^3 to achieve 99% occupancy.

How much binding energy per receptor will this require? The free energy of dissociation ΔG_d of a ligand-receptor complex is related to its equilibrium dissociation constant K_d by:

$$\Delta G_d = - kT \ln(K_d / K_0) \quad \text{\{Eqn. 3.25\}}$$

which refers to a standard reference state where all chemical species are 1 M (i.e., $K_0 \sim 0.6$ molecules/nm^3) and attributes a free energy of zero to a complex with a dissociation constant of 1 M.[402]

For T = 310 K, the range of required K_d gives a range for ΔG_d of 39.4 zJ for glucose (at typical serum concentrations) to 128 zJ for female serum testosterone.

However, when ligand and receptor associate there is a loss of three degrees of freedom in each of translational and rotational entropy, which may be estimated using the classical Sackur-Tetrode equations, giving an entropic free energy range (for translation and rotation combined) of ΔG_s = 80 zJ for very small molecules (MW ~10 daltons), to 120 zJ (MW ~10^2 daltons), 200 zJ (MW ~10^4 daltons), and 280 zJ for large molecules (MW ~10^6 daltons).[427]

Thus to form a ligand-receptor complex with a dissociation constant K_d, the receptor design must provide a free energy of binding of at least:

$$\Delta G_{total} = \Delta G_d + \Delta G_s \quad \text{\{Eqn. 3.26\}}$$

or 120-410 zJ/molecule for designed receptors achieving 99% occupancy operating over the likely range of physiological concentrations and temperatures. This is consistent with Drexler's estimate of 161 zJ binding energy required to ensure reliable receptor occupancy for small plentiful molecules.[10]

3.5.3 Ligand-Receptor Specificity

While affinity measures the strength of the binding of a ligand to a receptor, specificity defines the degree to which a receptor can distinguish between similar ligands. That is, the affinity of the target molecule for the receptor must be greater than the affinity of any other ligand in the environment that is competing for that same receptor, by some threshold multiple.

How much greater is enough? In natural dynamic cellular systems, the threshold multiple appears to be a factor of ~10^2-10^3. For example, the carrier which expels Ca^{++} from erythrocytes presents a variation in K_d of 10^{-6} to 10^{-3} in going from the interior to the exterior of the cell.[404] The active transport of amino acids by hepatocytes normally involves $K_d \sim 10^{-1}$, but under conditions of deprivation a high affinity carrier with $K_d \sim 10^{-3}$ comes into play.[405]

However, the key to assessing specificity in the nanomedical context would be to tally all the competing molecules in the in vivo environment, determine which are the nearest competitors, and then design to avoid them by imposing appropriate energy barriers. By 1998, only a very few competitive ligand-receptor binding analyses had been performed.[1078] Until a complete molecular inventory of the human body becomes available, the following crude estimate of nearest-neighbor differences must suffice.

The human body contains a minimum of $N_{prot} \sim 10^5$ distinguishable proteins (Section 3.1). The maximum number of distinguishable proteins in the biosphere was given by Kauffman[766] who estimates a useful biological catalytic task space of $N_{prot} \sim 10^8$ distinct protein forms, a tiny subset of the ~20^{500} possible 500-residue protein sequences. If the average protein is constructed from $N_{residue} \sim 500$ amino acids (MW ~50,000 daltons), then the average protein may differ from its most similar neighbor by $n_{var} \sim \log(N_{prot})/\log(N_{residue})$ = 1.9-3.0 residues. (The precise magnitudes of N_{prot} and $N_{residue}$ are not crucial to our conclusion.) Most proteins are confined to cells containing $N_{prot} \sim 5000$ different protein types each (Table 3.2); given that evolution has probably optimized local specificity to ensure that closely competing crucial ligands rarely appear in the same cell, it seems reasonable to assume that the average closest-neighbor ligand may differ from the average target ligand by at least $n_{var} \sim 1$ residue.

How much is receptor affinity reduced when binding molecules differing by $n_{var} \sim 1$ residue from the target ligand on receptor-accessible surfaces—the minimum threshold required to ensure specificity within a cell? In one experiment the relative affinity of an antibody constructed for succinylglycinamide-linked histamine (histamine-SGA), which was the target molecule, and the same molecule but with one methyl group or one carboxylic group removed and replaced with a hydrogen, was 1.45×10^4 or 2.5×10^5, respectively, due to steric hindrance.[401] Similar investigations with antibodies for SGA-linked serotonin produced relative affinities of 500-1000,[408] and with antibodies for single alanine substitutions in Human Growth Hormone (HGH), ~1000.[418] The relative affinity of a particular RNA oligomer for theophylline and caffeine, two ligands which differ by only a single methyl group, was measured experimentally as 10,900.[1078] Computational receptor experiments in which CH replaces N suggest a decline in relative affinity of ~5×10^4.[10] Indeed, the change of a single hydrogen atom on a ligand is usually sufficient to destroy its specificity for, or activity within, a particular enzyme. The single-residue affinity reduction at a receptor-accessible surface appears to be of order ~10^3 - 10^5.

Each increase of ~10 zJ in bonding energy causes the reaction equilibrium constant to decline (hence receptor affinity to rise) by a factor of ~10 (Eqn. 3.25). If a difference in affinities of ~10^3-10^5 between the target molecule and its nearest competitor likely to be present in the environment provides sufficient receptor specificity for nanomedical purposes, this requirement corresponds to a binding energy differential affinity of ~30-50 zJ at 310 K between target and closest-neighbor ligands.

3.5.4 Ligand-Receptor Dynamics

Diamondoid structures can exhibit a stiffness and rigidity one or two orders of magnitude greater than that available in protein structures. In general, stiffer structures permit greater specificity because they enhance exclusion of non-target ligands based on van der Waals overlap forces (called steric hindrance) and allow narrower tolerances in distinguishing acceptable ligands.

In less-stiff protein-based receptors, each of the atoms is engaged in relatively large, rapid jiggling movements. Experimental and theoretical work has been done on the atomic fluctuations within the basic pancreatic trypsin molecule, a small enzyme with 58 amino acids and 454 heavy (non-hydrogen) atoms. This work established that fluctuations increase with distance from the center of the molecule, with the magnitude of RMS fluctuations ranging from ~0.04 nm for backbone atoms to ~0.15 nm for the ends of long side chains (roughly one atomic diameter), and an average of 0.069-0.076 nm per atom over the entire molecule.[409] A similar experimental analysis of reduced cytochrome c, a common metabolic enzyme, shows that RMS fluctuations of each of the 103 amino acid residues in the molecule averages ~0.11 nm with lattice disorder (~0.05 nm) included, and fluctuations range from 0.09-0.16 nm (Fig. 3.10). Antibody core domain movements display RMS fluctuations of 0.04-0.19 nm.[412] Hence it appears that the average atom within the typical protein receptor oscillates ~0.1 nm every ~10^{-12} sec, although frequently residues with long side chains (e.g., arg, lys) have much higher RMS deviations than average.

By contrast, in stiff diamondoid-based receptors each of the atoms is locked in a rigid crystalline structure and thus is subject to thermal displacements approximately 10 times smaller. The RMS displacement for a quantum mechanical harmonic oscillator[10] is given by:

$$\Delta X = \left[\left(\frac{\hbar\omega}{k_s}\right)\left(\frac{1}{2}+\frac{1}{e^{\hbar\omega/kT}-1}\right)\right]^{1/2} \qquad \text{\{Eqn. 3.27\}}$$

where $\hbar$ = 1.055 x 10^{-34} joule-sec, kT = 4.28 zJ at T = 310 K, and angular frequency $\omega = (k_s/\mu_{red})^{1/2}$ rad/sec where k_s is mechanical stiffness and μ_{red} is the reduced mass = $m_1m_2/(m_1 + m_2)$. For C-C atoms (e.g., in the receptor body), k_s = 440 N/m, $m_1 = m_2 = 2\times10^{-26}$ kg, thus ω = 2.1 x 10^{14} rad/sec, so the RMS displacement of each atom is only ~0.005 nm every ~3 x 10^{-14} sec. For C-H atoms (e.g., on the hydrogen passivated receptor surface), k_s = 460 N/m, m_1 = 2 x 10^{-26} kg (C), and m_2 = 1.673 x 10^{-27} kg (H), thus ω = 5.5 x 10^{14} rad/sec, so the RMS displacement of each atom is ~0.008 nm every ~1 x 10^{-14} sec. Similarly, at 310 K the RMS thermal displacement of a 1-nm wide, 10-nm long diamondoid rod is ~0.01 nm, including elastic and entropic contributions.[10]

The ratio of RMS displacements for protein/diamondoid receptors is ~10:1, so the minimum addressable volume (hence inverse maximum specificity) of a diamondoid receptor should be ~10^3 smaller than for protein receptors, a ~30 zJ binding energy advantage for diamondoid receptors.

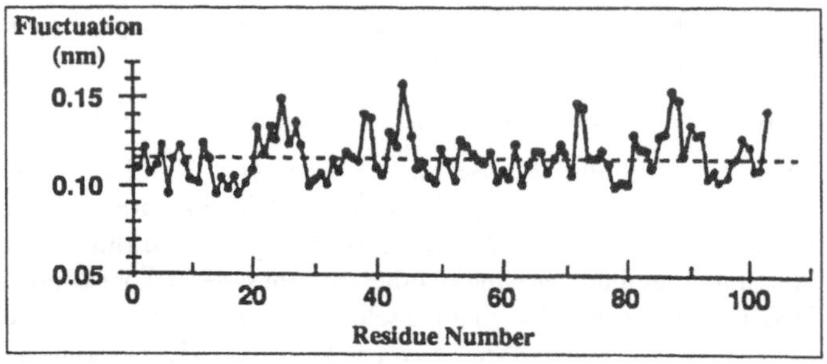

Fig. 3.10. Experimental RMS fluctuations in ferrocytochrome C (residue averages shown as function of residue number; redrawn from Karplus and McCammon[409]).

3.5.5 Diamondoid Receptor Design

Natural enzymes and antibodies are proteins folded into highly organized, preformed shapes that present a ready-made "keyhole" into which a target ligand will fit. The enzyme is folded in such a way as to create a region that has the correct molecular dimensions, the appropriate topology, and the optimal alignment of counterionic groups and hydrophobic regions to bind a specific target molecule. Tolerances in the active sites can be narrow enough to exclude one isomer of a diastereomeric pair. For example, D-amino acid oxidase will bind only D-amino acids, not L-amino acids.

These "keyholes" are extremely floppy, yet still achieve fair specificity. This is a consequence of "induced fit" in protein binding sites. That is, the interaction of the target molecule with an enzyme induces a conformational change in the enzyme, resulting in the formation of a strongly binding site and the repositioning of the appropriate amino acids to form the active site. The receptor flexes, balloons, hinges, or contracts by 0.05-1.0 nm in just the right places to maximize specificity as the selected ligand enters the site. In some cases such as O_2 and CO binding by myoglobin, ligands enter the receptor through a series of temporary voids that appear and disappear in the receptor as ~10 picosec dynamic structural fluctuations.[409] Induced fit can reduce receptivity to undesired proteins that exploit relative geometry by bonding enough to bring portions of their surfaces into alignment with the same receptor sites that bind desired proteins. Folding transitions appear to be the most prevalent and to possess the most possibilities for adaptability or induced fit.[1068]

For smaller molecules, it is likely that recognition processes will be relatively inefficient, time-consuming, and more difficult to engineer if they involve a good deal of rearrangement of the receptor's shape.[382] Thus there is considerable interest among chemists in designing artificial receptors that have their cavities already formed into the shape appropriate for the intended substrate.[1057] For instance, rigid-cavity "spherand" receptors are exceptionally efficient at binding metal ions.[410] Bowl-shaped molecules such as cryptaspherands, calixarenes, and carcerands can be lined with chemical groups along their walls and with charged groups along their rims to achieve high binding specificity.[410,411,1262] Self-assembling capsules or "container molecules" made of hydrogen-bonded subunits, capable of limited molecular recognition, have been synthesized.[2143,2336] A designed receptor for creatinine was demonstrated in 1995,[222] and in 1998, K. Suslick and colleagues[2714] designed metalloporphyrin-dendrimeric artificial receptors that can bind straight, skinny molecules but block out bent or fat molecules. Container molecules with 0.2-0.4 nm portals control entry to their interiors using "French door" and "sliding door" gates[417] and

Table 3.6 Maximum Binding Energy Available in a Dispersion-Force Receptor with 0.3-nm Contact Boundary for CHON Target Molecules of Various Sizes

Mean # of Atoms in Target Molecule	Approx. Molecular Weight (daltons)	Spherical Surface Area of Target Molecule	Spherical Surface Area of Receptor	Spherical Receptor Cavity Volume	Maximum vdW Binding Energy Theoretically Available
10	60	0.80 nm^2	2.6 nm^2	0.39 nm^3	16 zJ
10^2	600	3.7 nm^2	6.9 nm^2	1.7 nm^3	72 zJ
10^3	6,000	17 nm^2	24 nm^2	11 nm^3	330 zJ
10^4	60,000	80 nm^2	93 nm^2	84 nm^3	1600 zJ
10^5	600,000	370 nm^2	400 nm^2	740 nm^3	7200 zJ

hinges.[2548] Active binding sites for small simple molecules such as NO,[2912,2913] CO,[3228] and C_2H_4[2914] are well-known.

Ultimately, receptors will be designed to nanoscale precision and may be constructed using diamondoid materials.[1199] Electrostatic, hydrophobic, and hydrogen-bond forces will add immensely to artificial receptor specificity and are essential for binding small molecules. For example, using a 0.2-nm range in a saline environment, 10-40 charge contacts would be required to bind molecules of various sizes and concentrations using electrostatic force alone, which is ~0.5 charge/nm^2 over the entire surface of a 60,000 dalton globular protein (vs. ~1 charge/nm^2 for the surface of an isolated zwitterionic amino acid). Or, a 7 nm^2 hydrophobic cavity having the exact folded shape of the target ligand generates ~120 zJ binding energy as the molecule stuffs itself into the cavity to exclude its surface from solvent water.

But consider a theoretical receptor that employs van der Waals dispersion forces alone. Atoms comprising the typical protein or CHON target molecule in the human body have an average atomic mass of ~6 amu/atom and an average density of 1500 kg/m^3, giving a mean molecular volume of ~6.7 x 10^{-30} m^3 per atom in the target molecule. Assume for simplicity a spherical receptor surface that forms a negative image of the surface of the target molecule. The receptor surface lies ~1.5 x (minimum van der Waals contact distance) ~0.3 nm from the perimeter atoms of the target molecule, and completely encloses the target molecule (thus requiring at least one moving part). Table 3.6 shows that the theoretically available maximum binding energy E_{vdW}, using only dispersion forces (from Eqn. 3.21), should be sufficient to adequately bind all but the smallest target molecules according to the criteria set forth in Section 3.5.2. (Proteins are actually ellipsoidal with a much larger surface area A_p = 0.111 $MW^{2/3}$ nm^2,[413] than if they were spherical*, so Table 3.6 figures are conservative for protein binding; proteins typically have a ~60%-85% interior packing density.[3211]) Dispersion forces alone can provide the minimum required binding energy of ~120 zJ with A_p ~6 nm^2 of contact surface (MW > 400 daltons) at 0.3 nm mean range, and dispersion-force receptors can offer exceptionally high affinities for molecules >1000 atoms.

What about specificity? Given the ability to design diamondoid binding sites to at least localized <0.01 nm tolerances, chirality is readily detected and (purely as a design exercise) it may even be possible to distinguish diatomic nitrogen and oxygen on the basis of size alone. The molecular lengths (major axis) of N_2 and O_2 are 0.250 nm and 0.253 nm, but the molecular widths (minor axis) are 0.140 nm and 0.132 nm, respectively. (Diatomic molecules get longer and narrower at higher molecular weight.) Thus N_2 is distinguishable from O_2 on the basis of width (~0.01 nm). With a van der Waals energy well depth of 1.1-1.4 zJ for N_2 and O_2, in a tight receptor these gases are bound at an energy density corresponding to 3000-4000 atm of pressure.

3.5.6 Minimum Feature Size and Positioning Accuracy

Maximum displacement measurement accuracy in nanoscale devices is ~0.01 nm (Section 4.3.1), and RMS thermal displacement in diamondoid bonds is ~0.01 nm at 310 K (Section 3.5.4). Thermal displacements in 10-nm long diamondoid rods are ~0.01 nm at a 1-nm rod width, ~0.02 nm at 0.5-nm width, and ~0.10 nm at 0.3-nm width.[10] However, it is possible to construct components to even narrower tolerances.

For instance, a single C-O bond inserted into a diamondoid rod in a collinear carbon chain extends rod length by 0.1402 nm, the C-O bond length. An adjacent rod into which an N-N bond is similarly inserted is extended by 0.1381 nm, the N-N bond length. By bonding these rods (aligned at one end) it is possible to build diamondoid structures having 0.002-nm features** (at the other end), which at 310 K will nonetheless suffer thermal displacements of ~0.01 nm or more. Similarly tiny displacements can be induced in binding cavity surfaces by inserting a foreign atom deep inside the bulk diamondoid structure, causing dislocation strains that decline in magnitude at greater distances from the compositional disturbance.***

**The formula for A_p is valid for small and medium size monomeric proteins (50-320 residues). The ratio of actual protein surface area to the surface area of a smooth ellipsoid of equal volume increases with molecular weight, since larger proteins are more highly textured and aspherical in shape. For oligomers whose monomers have 330-840 residues, surface areas ~MW and are 20%-50% greater than those given by A_p.*

***For even finer feature control, the ground state atomic radius R_a depends on nuclear mass (m_n), proton mass (m_p) and electron mass (m_e) through the reduced mass of the electron $\mu_e = m_e m_n / (m_e + m_n) \sim m_e (1 - (1836 A_{mass})^{-1})$, or $R_a \sim 1/\mu_e$, where A_{mass} is nucleus mass number and $m_p/m_e = 1836$. Thus, a 25-nm rod consisting of 162 planes of C^{12} atoms is ~0.1 picometer (pm) longer than a 162-plane rod of C^{13} atoms; a single ground-state deuterium atom is measured as ~0.4 pm smaller than a hydrogen atom. SQUIDs and x-ray interferometers have been used to measure displacements of 10^{-7} nm, or ~1% of the nuclear diameter.[445]*

****J. Soreff points out that such strain fields have components at various spatial frequencies, and that at high spatial frequencies there is much design freedom but the effects decay exponentially with a short characteristic length, hence design choices are not spread uniformly throughout the constraint space but rather are clustered. As a result, it may not be possible to achieve a 0.01-nm designed receptor topography simultaneously everywhere across an entire binding surface, nor may it be possible via surface binding alone to distinguish molecules which differ only deep in their interiors.*

It is also possible to translate diamondoid components through a picometer step size,[433] much smaller than the unavoidable RMS thermal displacements, using any of several methods; for example:

A. *Levers* — Consider a 10-nm lever joined to a fixed bar by a pivot at one end, and driven axially by a ratchet interposed between lever and bar at the other end. Ratchet movements translate to smaller displacements at positions along the lever distant from the ratchet. Thus a follower rod attached to the lever 1 nm from the pivot and driven by a ratchet with 0.01-nm steps moves ~0.001 nm per ratchet step.

B. *Screws* — Consider a 3-nm diameter cylindrical screw with a 1-nm pitch. Rotating the screw through a 0.01-nm circumferential displacement causes the screw to move laterally by ~0.001 nm, which may be transmitted elsewhere in the machine by an attached follower rod. Of course, nanoscale screws or gears are sensitive to the precise cancellation of the potentials and hence cannot be perfectly smooth and circular, producing some unavoidable "knobbiness" under load.

C. *Gear Trains* — Consider a 32-nm diameter worm gear with 1-nm teeth. One rotation of the gear requires 100 rotations of the worm; hence a 0.1 nm displacement applied to the worm produces a 0.001 nm displacement in the gear. More efficient (and coaxial) compound planetary gear trains commonly employed in transmissions achieve displacement ratios up to 10,000:1, a hundred times better than the above example.

D. *Hydraulics* — Consider a sealed, fluid-filled, tapered pipe. A piston 1000 nm^2 in area is mounted at one end; another piston 10 nm^2 in area lies at the other end. A displacement of 0.1 nm applied to the smaller piston produces a 0.001 nm displacement in the larger piston. (Here again the finite size of molecules may produce "knobby" performance as fluid particles slip from one stable configuration to the next.)

E. *Compression* — Consider a rod upon which a compressive force of 100 nN/nm^2 (near the maximum diamondoid strength) has been imposed. Affixed to the rod are two crossbars spaced 4 nm apart. If the force on the rod is increased to 101 nN/nm^2, the gap between the crossbars compresses by ~0.001 nm.

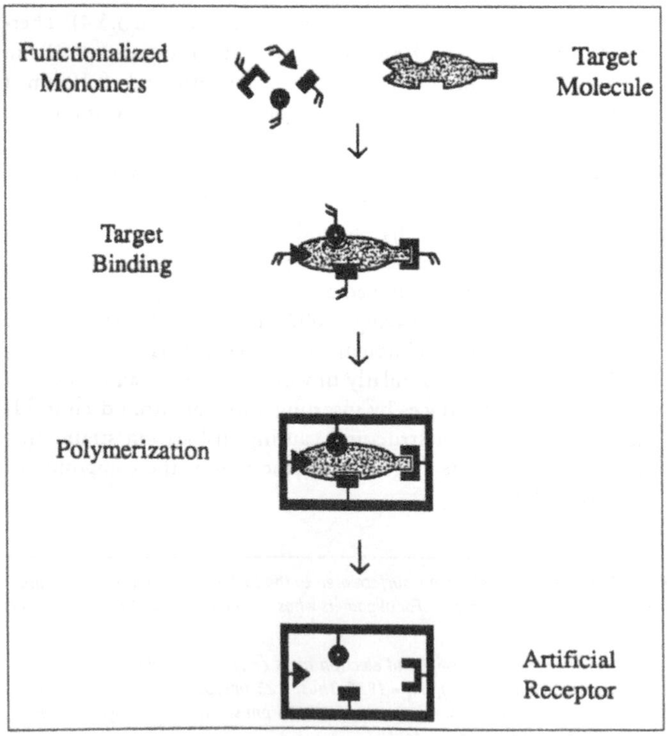

Fig. 3.11. Imprint model for creating artificial molecular receptors (redrawn from Ansell, Ramstrom and Mosbach[422]).

3.5.7 Receptor Configurations

Many different useful receptor configurations may be readily envisioned, of which the following brief descriptions are but a small sample. Note that most large target molecules of nanomedical interest are proteins which are probably floppy enough to permit entry into reasonably open multiply-concave rigid receptor structures; if not, hinges are easily added to the receptor design.

3.5.7.1 Imprint Model

Molecular imprinting[421,422] is an existing technique in which a cocktail of functionalized monomers interacts reversibly with a target molecule using only noncovalent forces. The complex is then cross-linked and polymerized in a casting procedure, leaving behind a polymer with recognition sites complementary to the target molecule in both shape and functionality (Fig. 3.11). Each such site constitutes an induced molecular "memory," capable of selectively binding the target species. In one experiment involving an amino acid derivative target, one artificial binding site per $(3.8\ nm)^3$ polymer block was created, only slightly larger than the $(2.7\ nm)^3$ sorting rotor receptors described by Drexler[10] (Section 3.4.2). Chiral separations, enzymatic transition state activity, and high receptor affinities up to $K_d \sim 10^{-7}$ have been demonstrated, with specificity against closely competing ligands up to $\Delta K_d \sim 10^{-2}$ (~20 zJ).

Several difficulties with this approach from a diamondoid engineering perspective include:

1. A sample of the target molecule is required to make each mold.
2. It is currently unknown how to prepare diamondoid castings.
3. Once the imprint has been taken, the site cannot easily be further modified.

3.5.7.2 Solid Mosaic Model

In the solid mosaic receptor model, the precise shape and charge distribution of the target molecule is already known. Working from this information, a set of diamondoid components could be fabricated which, when fitted together like a Chinese puzzle box, create a solid object having a cavity in the precise shape of the optimum negative image of the target molecule (Fig. 3.12A). The mosaic may contain point charges, voids, stressed surfaces, or dislocations to achieve fine positional control. Mosaic components may be as small as individual atoms, so this model is conceptually similar to 3D printing or raster-scan techniques in which the desired cavity formation is constructed atom by atom inside a nanofactory (Fig. 3.12B; Chapter 19). This model, like the imprint model, cannot easily be reconfigured once it has been constructed because each of the many unique parts may contribute to the entire structure. The construction of receptors from parts of fixed size and shape is crudely analogous to members of the heterodimer receptor class (a two-component receptor) such as $GABA_B$.[2687]

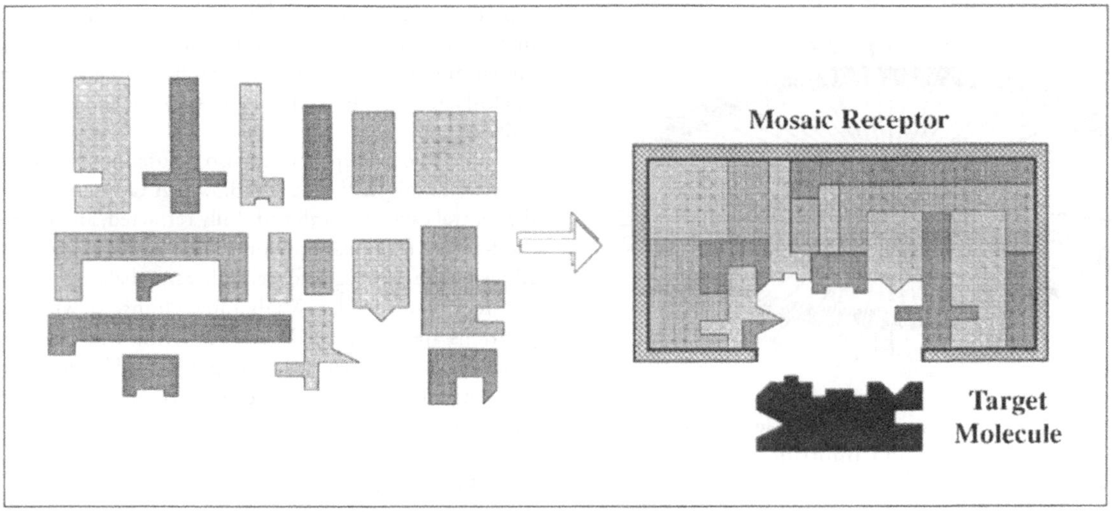

Fig. 3.12A. 2-D schematic representation of a 3-D solid mosaic model artificial receptor: Multiform block design.

M. Reza Ghadiri has designed a protein mosaic model using cyclic peptides that assemble spontaneously into nanotubes of predefined diameter; incorporation of hydrophobic amino acid side chains on the outside of these tubes leads to spontaneous insertion into bilayers, allowing the tubes to function as transmembrane ion channels.[2440] Other examples of mosaic model receptors are mesoporous silica filters with functionalized organic monolayers forming 3-6 nm sieve-like pores,[693,1522] and zeolites and zeolite-like molecular sieves. Zeolites are artificial crystal structures with precise and uniform 0.4-1.5 nm internal void arrays which can also be used as shape-selective catalysts able to favor one product over another that differs in size by as little as 0.03 nm, such as p-xylene and o-xylene.[430] By 1998, rational de novo computational design of artificial zeolite templates[431,432,934] and crystal engineering[695,948] had begun.

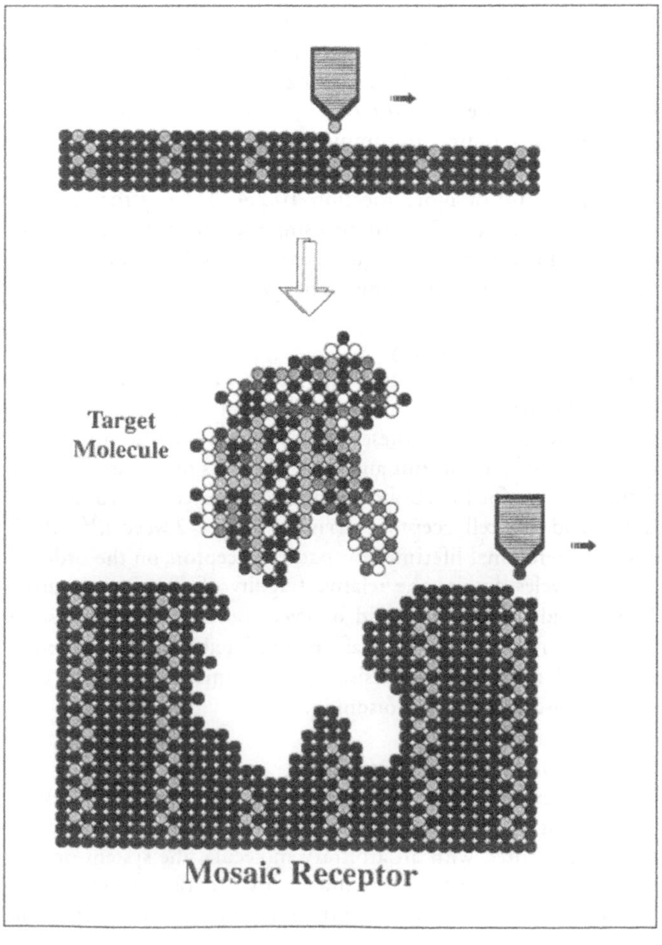

Fig. 3.12B. 2-D schematic representation of a 3-D solid mosaic model artificial receptor: raster scan design.

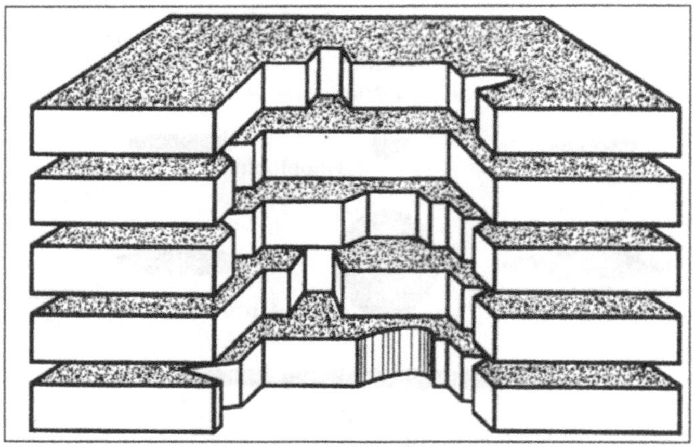

Fig. 3.13. Schematic representation of tomographic model for a reconfigurable artificial molecular receptor.

3.5.7.3 Tomographic Model

In the tomographic receptor model, the receptor engineer again starts with a known target molecule topography and designs a series of thin planar sections which, when stacked together in the correct order (using positionally-coded docking pins) and bonded, create a solid object containing the desired optimum binding cavity (Fig. 3.13). As in the mosaic model, point charges or dislocations in each planar segment can be used to manipulate cavity features and dimensions to precise tolerances. Unlike the mosaic model, a tomographic receptor can be reconfigured by partial disassembly and replacement

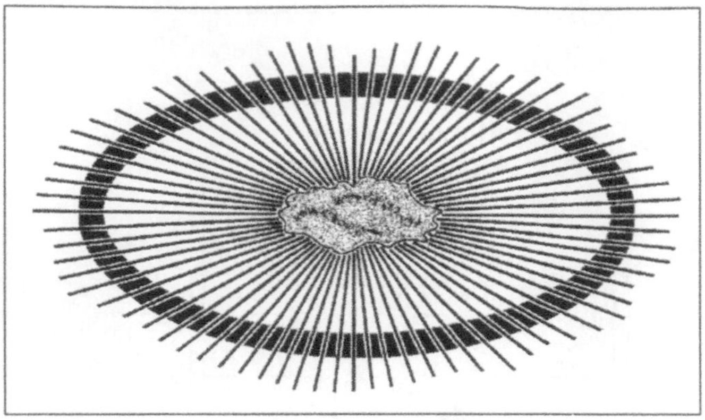

Fig. 3.14. Pin cushion model for a reconfigurable artificial molecular receptor (planar cutaway section omitting sensors and drive mechanisms).

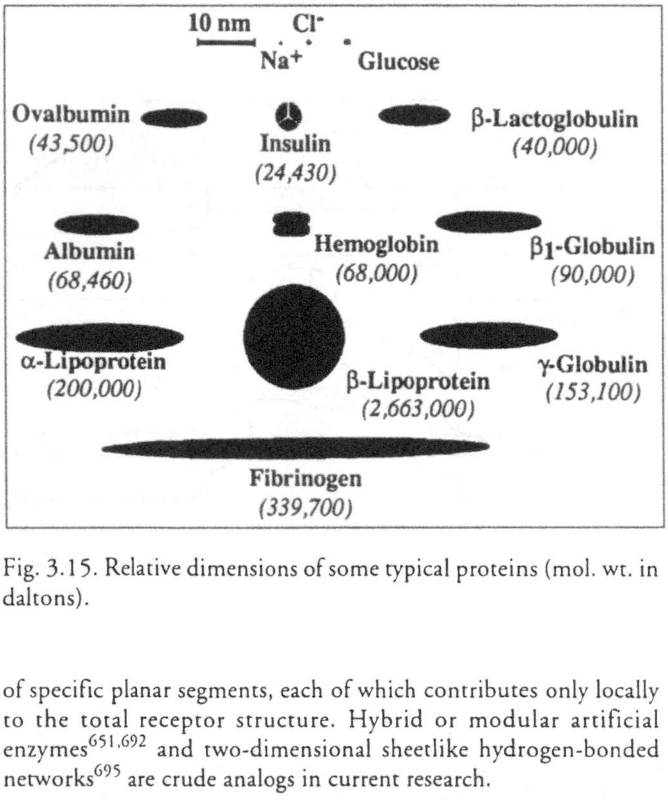

Fig. 3.15. Relative dimensions of some typical proteins (mol. wt. in daltons).

of specific planar segments, each of which contributes only locally to the total receptor structure. Hybrid or modular artificial enzymes[651,692] and two-dimensional sheetlike hydrogen-bonded networks[695] are crude analogs in current research.

3.5.7.4 Pin Cushion Model

The pin cushion receptor, suggested independently by K.E. Drexler [personal communication, 1996], is a hemispheroidal or hemiellipsoidal shell through which a number of rods protrude, each of which may be moved radially (Fig. 3.14). When inserted through the shell to varying depths, the endpoints of the rods define a negative image surface which may be made to mirror the topography and charge distribution of a known target molecule. Rods may be tipped with positive, negative or no charge, or they may terminate in any number of functionalized surface segments designed to optimally match parts of the target molecule shape. Other configurations such as a rectangular box, hinged plates with protruding rods, counterrotating rollers, or time-varying rod positioners are readily conceivable. Pin cushion receptors are easily reconfigured to bind different target molecules, hence may be regarded as fully programmable "universal" binding sites. The principal difficulty with the pin cushion receptor is its excessive size (compared to other receptor models) and its greater complexity (since each rod may be controllable individually).

Pin cushion receptors can also be used to discover the shapes of unknown molecules (Section 3.5.8): A target molecule is placed in the central cavity with all rods fully retracted, and the rods are slowly slid forward using nanopistons with force reflection feedback, until all pistons register zero force, indicating balance between attractive and repulsive van der Waals interactions, at which point all rod positions are recorded. Rods of differing end tip charge may then be tested for additional attractive potential. The final result is a precise mapping of the target molecule, which data may be stored or transmitted elsewhere for future use.

3.5.7.5 Construction Costs

The active binding site of a receptor consisting of $(2.7\ nm)^3$ ~19 nm^3 of structural atoms and constructed with 0.001-nm feature sizes in theory requires information from 2×10^{10} voxels (volume pixels) for complete description. However, there are only N_{atom} ~1000 atoms involved in the structure and their locations cannot be arbitrarily chosen. Atomic scale (~0.1 nm) resolution would require ~19,000 voxels; each voxel minimally requires an index number (~$\log_2(19{,}000)$ ~14 bits), an atomic identifier (~$\log_2(92)$ ~7 bits), and a charge identifier (~$\log_2(3)$ ~2 bits), for a total of 23 bits/voxel which gives 4×10^5 bits/receptor at atomic scale resolution. Drexler[10] estimates the number of configurational options per atom N_{opt} ~ 150; hence a description of the receptor could require as few as $N_{atom} \log_2(N_{opt})$ ~ 7×10^3 bits.* Assuming energy dissipation of ~3 zJ/bit for rod logic register reading[10] or ~kT ln (2) (Eqn. 7.1), then each time the receptor description is retrieved, stored or processed may require a minimum energy dissipation of ~10^4-10^6 zJ. Reversible computing may reduce this energy requirement by a factor of 10-100 or more (Section 10.2.4.1). Construction of a receptor containing ~1000 atoms using the nanomanipulator arm mentioned in Section 3.4.3 requires ~10^{-2} sec and consumes ~0.001 picojoule (~10^6 zJ) of mechanical energy.

3.5.7.6 Receptor Durability

Receptor durability is difficult to estimate ab initio. Molecularly imprinted polymer sites can be stored at least several years without loss of performance, but these receptors have only been tested to $\gtrsim$100 cycles of use without any detectable loss of memory.[422] The lifetime in vivo for metabolic enzymes often exceeds ~10^5 sec (~1 day),[172] and taste cell receptors survive ~10^6 sec (~2 weeks),[423] which suggests operational lifetimes for natural receptors on the order of 10^7-10^{12} cycles despite the relative fragility of protein structures. Diamondoid structures should be even more durable because of their superior physical strength, affirmative forcible ejection of bound ligands each cycle, and high resistance to chemical degradation thus reducing susceptibility to poisoning.

3.5.8 Ligand-Receptor Mapping

To achieve a fully general-purpose receptor capability in nanomedical systems, two classes of analytic function are essential.

First, presented with an arbitrary molecule, the system or user must be able to infer from the molecule's structure the shape and electronic configuration of an optimal receptor geometry that will

**Higher level descriptions may allow considerable additional information compaction, as for instance where a 30-bit word indexes a single receptor structure stored in a library containing perhaps 10^9 distinct designs.*

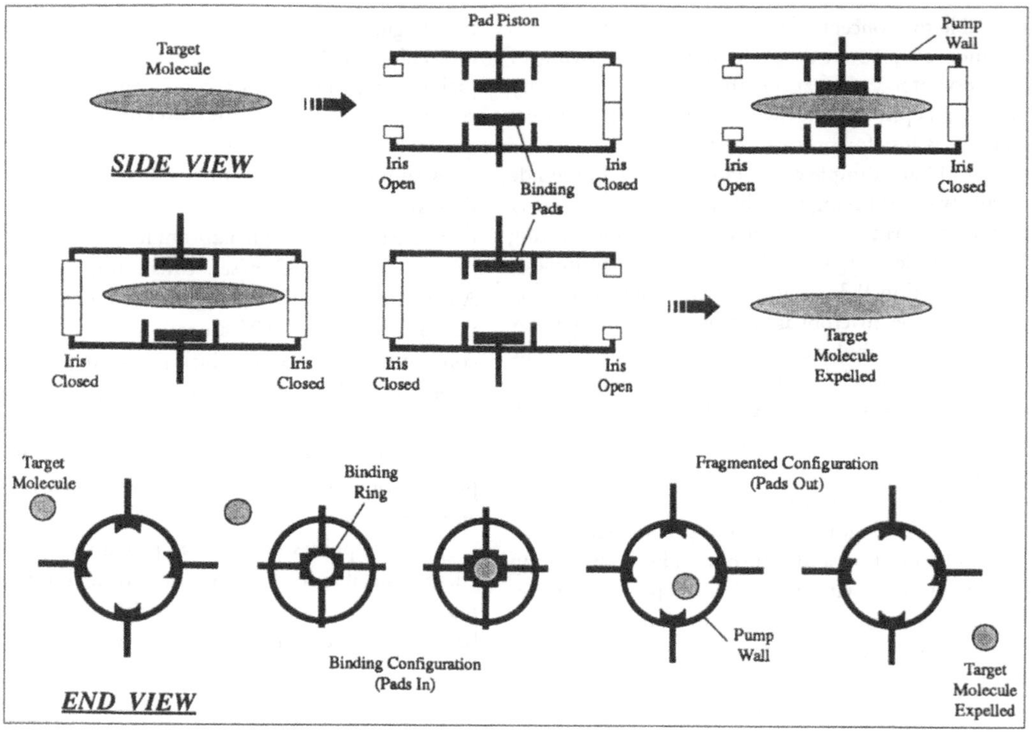

Fig. 3.16. Schematic of large-molecule shuttle pump using fragmentable binding ring and iris diaphragms.

efficiently bind it, with a particular affinity and specificity (as a design specification). This discovery procedure may involve a process akin to molecular imprinting (Section 3.5.7.1), fluorescent dye affinity matching on testing chips (Chapter 20), Structure-Activity Relationships (SAR) by NMR techniques,[424] or pin cushion receptor mapping (Section 3.5.7.4).

Second, presented with an arbitrary protein-built binding site embedded in living tissue, the system or user must be able to infer the molecule(s) which the given receptor could bind, and to compute the affinity and specificity of that activity. This capability may require a rather diverse steric toolkit. Biological receptors are constructed in one of ~500-1000 distinct shapes or "domains," such as the well-known Y-shaped antibody immunoglobulin domain (~100 residues) and other assorted clefts, folds, kringles and coils. Several hundred distinct fold families are known, though it is believed there are only ~20 major domain types,[414] and Chothia[2604] believes that "the large majority of proteins come from no more than one thousand families."

One mapping technique would employ a series of rodlike probes inserted into the receptor cavity like a pick gun or other lockpicking tool. After physically securing the receptor, the first crude probes quickly map the cavity to nanometer scale. Based on this preliminary information, subsequent probes having ever-finer discrimination chart smaller features as well as charge distributions by inserting a predetermined set of test rods with functionalized tips in a standard sequence, to rapidly prune the huge configurational space down to a single unique electrophysical shape using the minimum possible number of tests. (A 1 nm^3 volume of multi-element diamondoid receptor structure has ~10^{148} possible distinct configurations, by one conservative estimate,[10] requiring at least 492 binary tests to eliminate all but one configuration. Antibody domains contain ~10^{50} possible configurations, requiring 166 binary tests.) Cavity Stuffer, a software package comprising an experimental design tool to investigate automated cram-packing of predefined cavities using randomly branched polymers, is a preliminary effort in this general direction,[425] although the algorithmic task of discovering an unknown receptor contour may be considerably more challenging.

Another approach to receptor mapping would be the reversible chemical or mechanical denaturation of the receptor protein followed by precise nondestructive amino acid sequencing (Chapter 20), from which tertiary structure and activity could then be computationally inferred. Algorithms to perform such computations are the subject of intense current research interest.[952] Even imperfect tertiary structure predictions should greatly reduce the search space, so that only a partial residue sequencing may be necessary for unambiguous identification from a library of possible proteins. Once the target ligand structure has been inferred, the subsequent design and manufacture of receptor-specific agonists and antagonists, including catalysts and cofactors, activators and inhibitors, promoters and repressors, should be comparatively easy.

3.5.9 Large Molecule Binding, Sorting and Transport

Is there any size limit for target molecules to be transported? Natural receptors have already been found for large molecules including low-density lipoproteins (LDLs) > 1,000,000 daltons[426] and high-density lipoproteins (HDLs).[1038]

The methods described in earlier Sections can be adapted for binding large molecules (>1000 atoms; Fig. 3.15), including molecules far wider than the binding device itself (e.g., ~200-nm diameter virus particles and larger). Making a binding site for a large molecule should be physically easier (albeit computationally more challenging) than making a binding site for a small molecule because of the greatly increased area of interaction. For example, a binding energy of 400 zJ may be realized by creating a dispersion-force binding area covering only ~25% of the surface of a 10,000-atom target molecule (Table 3.6) or a mere ~0.02% of a 200-nm virus particle.

This makes possible the concept of binding pads—small surfaces with dimples (concave or convex), each dimple consisting of precisely-placed nanometer-scale features that are complementary to specific patches (e.g., epitopes) on the surface of the large target molecule. (Specificity is lost for portions of the molecule outside the particular patches.) Each dimple could effectively grasp the side of the large molecule without having to fully enclose it—a capability useful in nanorobot foot pads during cell walking and anchoring (Section 9.4.3), in handles for nanociliary or nanomanipulator transport functions (Section 9.3.2), and for chemotactic sensing (Section 4.2.6). (For example, macrophage receptors for LDLs employ a "pad" consisting of three globular cysteine-rich domains.[426]) The large compliance of target protein molecule subunits should prove curative for any misalignment problems caused by cumulative small errors in bond lengths across large diamondoid receptor structures.

Rather than using sorting rotors, which become unwieldy when large molecule binding pockets must be used, the shuttle pump illustrated schematically in Figure 3.16 may provide reasonably efficient large molecule sortation and transport. The shuttle pump consists of a diamondoid tube within which a receptor ring moves between iris diaphragms at either end (shuttling mechanism not shown). The receptor ring is constructed as two or more binding pad segments. For molecule pickup, the ring is pressed together, forming an annular binding region for the target large molecule, which binds and is shuttled to the other side. The receptor ring is then fragmented, destroying binding affinity and unlocking the target molecule, which escapes via diffusion. The shuttle returns to the pickup side, the receptor is pressed together again, and the cycle repeats. A biocompatible solvent environment is maintained during large-protein manipulation tasks.

Assuming a roughly spherical large molecule and laminar fluid flow at 1 atm forcing pressure (Section 9.2.7), a 10-nm diameter molecule moves through a 20-nm long pump (~10^{-20} kg, ~10^{6} atoms) in ~10^{-6} sec at ~0.02 m/sec, consuming ~0.02 pW during transfer. A 200-nm virus-size target molecule moves through a 400-nm long pump (~10^{-17} kg, ~10^{9} atoms) in ~10^{-2} sec at ~60 microns/sec, consuming ~10^{-16} watts during transfer; at ~0.0002 atm, release time is diffusion limited. The transfer force exerted on a 10-nm molecule is ~1 pN, ~600 pN on a 200-nm virion; a binding energy of 400 zJ at a 0.2-nm contact distance gives a binding force of ~2300 pN, sufficient to hold a particle of either size firmly during transport and release.

J. Soreff points out that as protein size increases, so does the energy available for local minima in the binding. Desired proteins may become stuck in incorrect positions, or undesired proteins may become partially adhered to a receptor. Besides designing to minimize these possibilities, using a multireceptor cascade with different combinations of binding patches at each stage should allow complete exclusion of undesired large-molecule species.

CHAPTER 4

Nanosensors and Nanoscale Scanning

4.1 Nanosensor Technology

Medical nanorobots need to acquire information from their environment to properly execute their assigned tasks. Such acquisition is achieved using onboard nanoscale sensors, or nanosensors, of various types. Nanosensors allow for medical nanodevices to monitor environmental states at three different operational levels:

1. Internal nanorobot states,
2. Local and global somatic states (inside the human body), and
3. Extrasomatic states (sensory data originating outside the human body).

The general physical limits to sensory perception are reviewed by Block[810] and Bialek.[811]

The specific nanosensor technologies required include sensors to detect chemical substances (Section 4.2), displacement and motion (Section 4.3), force and mass (Section 4.4), and acoustic (Section 4.5), thermal (Section 4.6), and electromagnetic (Section 4.7) stimuli. Typical sensor device mass, volume, and sensitivity limits are summarized in each Section. In vivo bioscanning is briefly described in Section 4.8, followed by external macrosensing in Section 4.9. Methods of getting sensors in and out of the body are explained in Chapter 16, and methods of getting sensor information out of the body are described in Chapter 7. A discussion of sensor biocompatibility is deferred to Chapter 15.[3234]

4.2 Chemical and Molecular Nanosensors

The area of chemical microsensors is well developed, and there is increasing research interest in nanoscale chemical sensors,[438] "chemosensors"[1226] and "biosensors".[989] The most common nanomedical application of chemical sensors will be to measure the concentration of specific molecules and biopolymers in aqueous solvent—whether in blood serum, interstitial fluid, or cytosol. This may be accomplished using ordered arrays of receptors or by using sorting rotors to directly count molecular populations in known sample volumes. Spatial and temporal concentration gradient sensing is also essential in navigation, communications, and in mediating rapid response to environmental stimuli. Chemotactic sensors may be used to sample the chemical composition of surfaces.

4.2.1 Broadband Receptor Arrays

One simple broadband concentration sensor, shown schematically[10] in Figure 4.1, consists of a graduated series of receptors having uniformly high specificity but engineered with progressively greater affinities (successively smaller equilibrium dissociation constants K_d (molecules/nm^3); Section 3.5.2) for the target molecule, which is present in the test sample at concentration c_{ligand}. Exposure of the receptor array to the test sample for a time t_{EQ} necessary to reach diffusion-driven equilibrium gives a probability of receptor occupancy $P_{occ} \sim 0.91$ in a receptor with $K_d \sim 0.1 c_{ligand}$, $P_{occ} \sim 0.50$ in a receptor with $K_d \sim c_{ligand}$, and $P_{occ} \sim 0.09$ in a receptor with $K_d \sim 10 c_{ligand}$.

During each measurement cycle, all steric probes are simultaneously extended into their associated receptor volumes at a time t_{EQ} after presentation of sample to the array. Probes which reach full extension register an empty receptor; those which cannot fully extend register an occupied receptor. After registration, the probes are retracted and ejection rods are thrust into all receptors (typically requiring ~1 nanonewton (nN) of force for occupied receptors) to empty them while the test chamber is flushed clear in preparation for the next cycle to begin. Ideally, the probe rod pushing into the binding site should push the bound molecule further into the binding site to avoid complications that may arise due to competing kinetic barriers, and ejection rods should push molecules far enough to ensure that the next resample is independent.

Consider a series of N steric probe units as proposed by Drexler.[10] Each probe measures 8 nm x $(2.5\ nm)^2 \sim 50\ nm^3$ and has mass ~ 2×10^{-22} kg. The ratio of the dissociation constants of adjacent units is $\kappa = K_{d_i} / K_{d_{i+1}} > 1$, with $K_{d_1} \sim 10^{-4}$ molecules/nm^3 and $K_{d_N} \sim 10^{-13}$ molecules/nm^3 typically in the human body, and so $N = 1 + \{\log_{10}(K_{d_1}/K_{d_N}) / \log_{10}(\kappa)\}$.

Minimum measurement error occurs when c_{ligand} exactly matches the K_d of a probe unit, that is, when $c_{ligand} = K_{d_i}$ (i.e., $P_{occupied_i} = 0.5$). Maximum measurement error occurs when c_{ligand} lies exactly midway between two probes such that $K_{d_i} > c_{ligand} > K_{d_{i+1}}$, or, more specifically, at the geometric midpoint $c_{ligand} = (K_{d_i} K_{d_{i+1}})^{1/2} = K_{d_i} \kappa^{-1/2}$. In this case, Eqn. 3.24 becomes

$$P_{occupied_i} = \left(\frac{c_{ligand}}{K_{d_i}\ \kappa^{-1/2}} \right) P_{unoccupied_i} \qquad \text{\{Eqn. 4.1\}}$$

where $P_{unoccupied_i} = 1 - P_{occupied_i}$. Additionally, sampling error is $\sim N_m^{-1/2}$ when N_m independent measurements are taken (i.e., N_m measurement cycles employing all N probe units during each cycle), for $N_m >> 1$, establishing an error bound on the probability of receptor occupancy of $P_{occupied_i} \pm N_m^{-1/2}$. If two concentrations $c_1 = P_{occupied_i} / (1 - P_{occupied_i})$ and $c_2 = (P_{occupied_i} + N_m^{-1/2}) / (1 - (P_{occupied_i} + N_m^{-1/2}))$ may be distinguished, where $P_{occupied_i}$ is given by Eqn. 4.1, then the minimum detectable concentration differential $\Delta c / c$ is

$$\Delta c/c = [c_2/c_1] - 1 = \frac{\left(1+\kappa^{-1/2}\right) N_m^{-1/2}}{1 - \left(1+\kappa^{-1/2}\right)^{-1} - N_m^{-1/2}} - 1 \qquad \text{\{Eqn. 4.2\}}$$

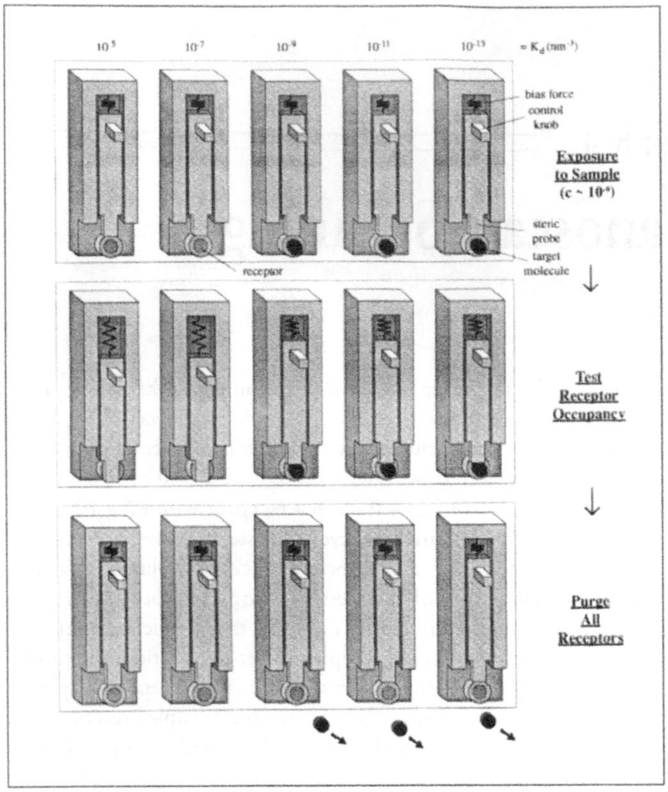

Fig. 4.1. Schematic of broadband chemical concentration sensor array using 5 receptor units with steric probes.

For $\kappa >> 1$, Eqn. 4.2 reduces to: $(\Delta c / c)_{large} \sim (1 + \kappa^{1/2}) / N_m^{1/2}$. In the limit as κ approaches 1 and $N_m >> 1$, Eqn. 4.2 reduces to: $(\Delta c / c)_{small} \sim \kappa^{-1/2} (\Delta c / c)_{large}$.

For $\kappa = 10$ (an N = 10-probe sensor, sufficient to span the entire $K_d = 10^{-4}$ to 10^{-13} molecules/nm^3 range using one probe per decade), $\Delta c / c = 0.94$ (94%) at $N_m = 100$, 0.20 (20%) at $N_m = 1000$, (0.06) 6% at $N_m = 10{,}000$, and 0.006 (0.6%) at $N_m = 10^6$ measurement cycles. Little additional discrimination is obtained by using more than N ~ 10 probes in the sensor. For $N_m = 1000$, $\Delta c / c = 0.89$ (89%) at $\kappa = 178$ (N = 5 probes), 0.20 (20%) at $\kappa = 10$ (N = 10 probes), 0.136 (13.6%) at $\kappa = 1.23$ (N = 100 probes), and 0.135 (13.5%) at $\kappa = 1.0021$ (N = 10,000 probes). Note that $\Delta c / c = 0.20$ (20%) is equivalent to detecting a pH variation of ~0.08 (e.g., $10^{(0.08)} - 1 \sim 0.20$).

Sensor cycle time ~t_{EQ} may be crudely approximated by the number of random ligand-receptor encounters ($N_{encounters} \sim 100$; Drexler[10]) necessary to ensure binding divided by the number of ligands striking the receptor surface per second,[434] or

$$t_{EQ} \sim \left(\frac{N_{encounters}}{A\, c_{ligand}}\right)\left(\frac{\pi\, MW_{kg}}{2\, kT\, N_A}\right)^{1/2} \text{(sec/cycle)} \qquad \text{\{Eqn. 4.3\}}$$

where A = active receptor cross-sectional area ~0.1 nm^2 for small molecule (MW ~100 gm/mole) receptors to ~10 nm^2 for large molecule (MW ~10^5 gm/mole) receptors; $c_{ligand} = 10^{-2}$ nm^{-3} for the most common molecules to 10^{-12} nm^{-3} for rare molecules in the human body; MW_{kg} = target ligand molecular weight in kg/mole, k = 0.01381 zJ/K (Boltzmann constant), T = 310 K (human body temperature), and $N_A = 6.023 \times 10^{23}$ molecules/mole (Avogadro's number).

For common small molecules, $t_{EQ} \sim 10^{-6}$ sec; for common large molecules, $t_{EQ} \sim 0.2 \times 10^{-6}$ sec, but a sample chamber ~(25 nm)^3 in size is diffusion-limited to a minimum $t_{EQ} \sim 10^{-5}$ sec for $c_{ligand} \gtrsim 10^{-4}$ nm^{-3}. For the rarest small molecules in the human body, $t_{EQ} \sim 800$ sec, ~200 sec for rare large molecules, and a larger chamber may also be required. Preconcentration of the test sample by dehydration using sorting rotors (Section 3.4.2) to rapidly remove water from the sample chamber reduces t_{EQ} to 10-40 sec for very rare molecules.

Steric probes using a driving force[10] of ~100 pN, over 2 nm of motion per cycle require 200 zJ/measurement. If 1000 measurement cycles of a 10-probe sensor suffice to determine concentration to ~2 significant figures, this information costs ~0.002 pJ to acquire, a power consumption of from ~10 pW for large common molecules to ~10^{-9} pW (~0.6 kT/sec) for small rare molecules while the sensor is working. Power dissipation may run up to ~10 times higher, depending upon the number of occupied receptors that must be cleared via ejection rods during each cycle.

4.2.2 Narrowband Receptor Arrays

If the concentration of the target ligand varies only slightly within known limits, similar results may be obtained using a narrowband sensor that employs a repeating array of a single receptor type tuned to the maximum expected concentration c_{max} of the target ligand (Fig. 4.2). If the sensor consists of N_r receptors, choosing $K_d \gtrsim c_{max} N_r^{-1} / (1 - N_r^{-1})$ ensures that all receptors are occupied at $c = c_{max}$, thus avoiding array saturation at concentrations below c_{max}. At minimum sensitivity, $K_d \sim c_{min} (1 - N_r^{-1}) / N_r^{-1}$, and so $(1 + (\Delta c / c)) = (c_{max} / c_{min})^{(N_r^{-1})}$ for the entire array. Thus the minimum detectable concentration differential $\Delta c / c$ for the array is

$$\Delta c/c = \left(N_r - 1\right)^{(2/N_r)} - 1 \qquad \text{\{Eqn. 4.4\}}$$

If A = receptor unit active area (~50 nm^2), L = receptor unit length (~10 nm), and receptor arrays are packed in parallel sheets with separation Δx (~10 nm, for small-molecule diffusion in ~10^{-6} sec) to allow sample access, sensor volume $V_s = A L N_r (1 + (\Delta x / L))$ and sensor scale ~ $V_s^{1/3}$. Thus a sensor with $N_r = 100$ receptor units achieves $\Delta c / c = 0.10$ (10%) with a (46 nm)^3 sensor; $N_r = 1400$ receptor units achieves $\Delta c / c = 0.01$ (1%) with a (112 nm)^3 sensor. A dedicated micron-scale nanodevice employing a (1.44 micron)^3 sensor array having 3 million receptor cells could at best distinguish 0.001% concentration differentials in ~ 3 sec (from Eqn. 4.6) for common molecules like serum glucose.

The ion channel switch (ICS) biosensor (aka. the "Australian sensor") can detect small-molecule concentrations as low as ~10^{-14} nm^{-3} in a ~600 sec measurement time.[3039,3040]

4.2.3 Counting Rotors

Concentration may be determined by varying exposure time to the sample. One energy-efficient design (Fig. 4.3) uses an input sorting rotor running at varying speeds (according to target concentration) synchronized with a counting rotor (linked by rods and ratchets to a data storage register device) to assay the number of molecules of the desired type that are present in a known volume of fluid. The counting rotor uses a steric probe, moved up and down in synchrony with the arrival of a binding site under the test probe, to count the number of molecules transferred by the sorting rotor. The fluid sample is drawn from the environment into a 4000 nm^3 reservoir ($L_{reservoir} \sim 16$ nm) with the equivalent of 10^4 refills/sec on a flow-through basis, using paddlewheel pumps or reciprocating

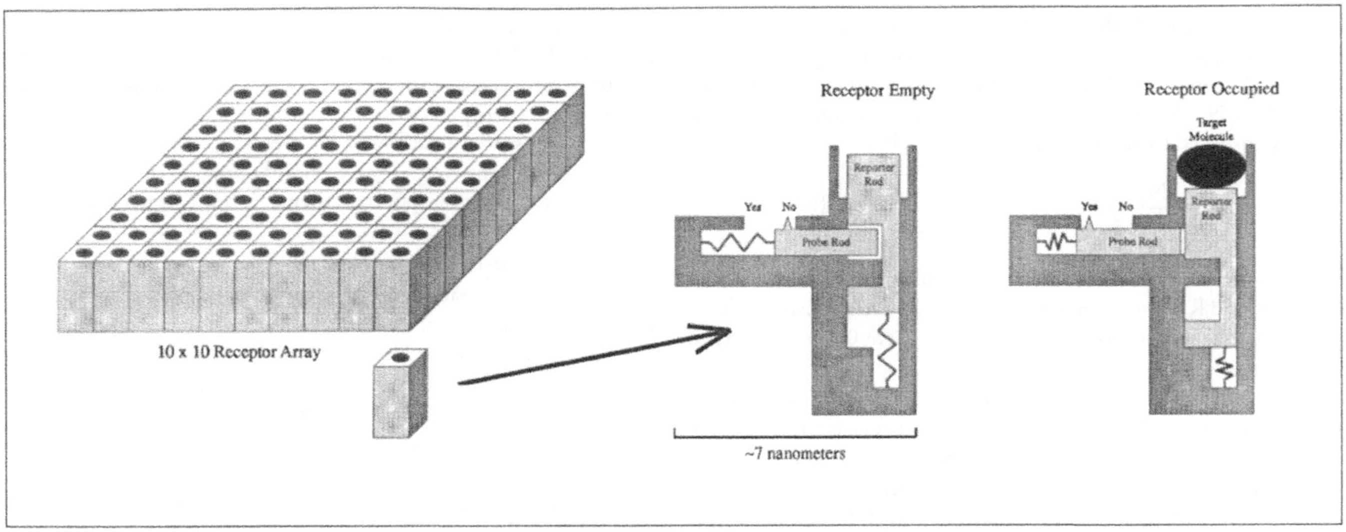

Fig. 4.2. Schematic of narrowband chemical concentration nanosensor array using receptors of a single type.

pistons (Section 9.2.7; not shown) operated slowly enough to avoid damaging molecules in the sample volume. This sensor, which measures 45 nm x 45 nm x 10 nm comprising ~500,000 atoms (~10^{-20} kg), should count $\dot{N}$ ~ 10^4 - 10^5 molecules/sec of small common molecules present at typical human serum concentrations of 10^{-3} - 10^{-2} nm^{-3}, such as glucose, with the rotor spinning at ~1% of normal speed (Section 3.4.2). Clogging of intake apertures in vivo is addressed in Sections 3.3.1 and 9.2.3, and in Chapter 15.

For rare molecules with c ~ 10^{-11} nm^{-3}, the count rate for a single sensing rotor falls to $\dot{N}$ ~ 10^{-4} molecules/sec. However, a (340 nm)^3 reservoir (a ~10^4 larger chamber volume) serviced by a bank of 10^4 rotors (4 x 10^{-18} kg additional mass) improves the count rate for rare molecules to $\dot{N}$ ~ 1 molecule/sec; that is,

$$\dot{N} \sim 2500\, c_{ligand}\, L^3_{reservoir} \quad \text{(molecules/sec)} \qquad \text{\{Eqn. 4.5\}}$$

Sample preconcentration may allow further improvement by a factor of up to 10-100. Energy requirements are comparable to those for sorting rotors (Section 3.4.2) except for the need to retrieve ~all target molecules from a known sample volume, which slows the sorting process, requiring ~10 zJ/count for common molecules and ~100 zJ/count for the rarest molecules in the human body. Large-molecule concentrations may be measured using a shuttle pump (Section 3.5.9) and a counting device.

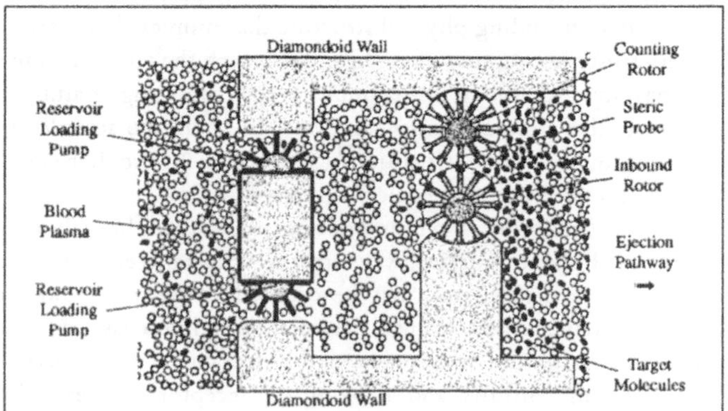

Fig. 4.3. Chemical concentration sensor using counting rotors.

4.2.4 Chemical Assay

It may also be useful to design a sensor that is capable of detecting as many different chemical species as possible, in contrast to detecting the precise concentration of a single species, for use in chemomessaging (Section 7.4.2.4), chemonavigation (Section 8.4.3), cellular diagnosis (Chapter 21), and other in vivo assay work. Counting rotors may be used for this purpose. Each 12-receptor sorting rotor/counting rotor pair has a minimum 400 nm^3 volume.[10] Allowing an additional ~800 nm^3 per pair to account for power, control, mechanical attachments and housings, which includes ~300 nm^3 per pair for sample chamber volume and sample access, requires ~100 nm^3 per receptor, roughly the same as for the steric probe units described in Section 4.2.1. A dedicated 1 micron^3 chemical assay nanorobot, which includes ~0.25 micron^3 sample volume, with ~10^7 pairs (receptors) could thus continuously scan for as many as ~10^7 different chemical species, counting $\dot{N}$ ~ 1 large molecule/sec at concentrations of c_{ligand} ~ 10^{-10} molecules/nm^3.

4.2.5 Chemical Nanosensor Theoretical Limits

Berg and Purcell[337] estimated that an ideal concentration sensor, limited only by diffusion constraints and drawing through a spherical boundary surface of radius r_s, provides a minimum detectable concentration differential Δc / c of

$$\Delta c / c = (1.61\, \Delta t\, D\, c\, r_s)^{-1/2} \qquad \text{\{Eqn. 4.6\}}$$

where Δt = time (sec), D is diffusion coefficient ~10^{-9} m^2/sec for small molecules (Table 3.3), and c = concentration (molecules/m^3). Using a sample chamber with r_s = 10 nm, a concentration of c = 3 x 10^{-3} nm^{-3} for serum glucose could be measured with 1% uncertainty in Δt ~ 260 microsec, or with 0.01% uncertainty in 2.6 sec. A dedicated micron-scale nanodevice using a 10-sec sampling time could at best distinguish a 0.0005% concentration differential for small common molecules like serum glucose but only a 27% concentration differential for large rare serum molecules like somatotropin.

Berg and Purcell[337] also found that the capture of small molecules at nanorobot surfaces can be surprisingly efficient. Specifically, for a spherical nanodevice of radius R, across whose surface are uniformly distributed N_r receptor spots of radius r_r, the maximum diffusion current absorbed by the receptor array, J_{array}, is

$$J_{array} = J\left(\frac{N_r\, r_r}{N_r\, r_r + \pi R}\right) \qquad \text{\{Eqn. 4.7\}}$$

where J = maximum diffusive intake current, given by Eqn. 3.4. For r_r = 1 nm and R = 1 micron, the J_{array} is fully 50% of J using only N_r = 3100 surface receptors, which occupy a mere 0.1% of the total device surface area.

For a purely sensory spherical nanodevice, a uniform distribution of a relatively small number of chemoreceptors confers optimal sensitivity. However, in applications where sensors (which attract and then release) are in competition with pumps (which strongly attract and then remove) for the same target molecules at the nanodevice surface, greater sensing efficiency may be achieved by clustering the sensors, as in a "nose" organ.[437]

Proteins may be modified as they age within biological cells. For instance, under steady state conditions, ~10% of protein molecules may exhibit carbonyl (oxidation) modifications,[2138] glycosylation (non-enzymatic), and dysfunctional proteins may be ubiquitinized (Chapter 13) and phosphorylated under enzyme control. Heat shock also modifies proteins. Chemosensor receptors must be carefully designed to accommodate changes in target ligand structures or sites that are likely to be subject to such alterations.

4.2.6 Spatial Concentration Gradients

Medical nanodevices can detect both extremely steep and extremely shallow spatial concentration gradients. For example, a receptor array sensor (Section 4.2.1) consisting of 10 steric probe units has a total volume of ~1000 nm^3 including its prorated share of drive systems, housings, etc. In just a few measurement cycles, adjacent sensors can detect a maximum concentration change from 10^{-2} nm^{-3} to 10^{-11} nm^{-3} across a mean nanosensor separation of 10 nm on a nanodevice surface, a steep chemical spatial gradient of ~10^{10}% per nanometer. J. Soreff points out that maintaining a steep concentration gradient of a freely diffusing species implies a power dissipation of ~kT per molecule per time to diffuse a concentration-halving distance. For a common, small, tethered molecule with c_{ligand} ~ 3 x 10^{-3} molecules/nm^3 that diffuses ~1 nm in t_{diff} ~ 1 nanosec, implied power density D_{mol} ~ kT c_{ligand} / t_{diff} ~ 10^{13} watts/m^3, a power density that might possibly be encountered in the vicinity of chemoelectric transducers (Section 6.3.4.5). (Such high power densities never occur on macroscale dimensions, and heat rapidly diffuses at nanoscale dimensions; Sections 4.6.1.)

Similarly, counting rotor sensors (Section 4.2.3) for small common serum molecules like glucose deployed at opposite ends of a 1-micron nanodevice can detect a concentration differential of ~10^{-4} over a ~1 sec measurement period, a shallow chemical spatial gradient of only ~10^{-5} % per nanometer. Even lower gradients may be detected by communication (Chapter 7) between physically separated cooperating nanodevices.

4.2.7 Temporal Concentration Gradients

Koshland and Macnab[435] have shown that bacteria possess a mechanism for sensing small temporal concentration gradients. A bacterium detects a spatial gradient of attractant not by comparing the concentration at its head and tail, but rather by traveling through space and comparing its observations over time. *E. coli* can measure a ~0.01% gradient[436] during the time it travels one body length (~2 microns) at top speed (20-40 microns/sec), a minimum temporal gradient of 0.1% per second. This appears very efficient, since the counting rotor sensor proposed in Section 4.2.3 is not much better, achieving ~0.01% per second. As for peak gradients, the 10-probe receptor array sensor described in Section 4.2.1 can detect a maximum concentration change (e.g., from an already-known rare concentration) in ~10^{-4} sec, a peak temporal gradient of ~10^{15} % per second.

4.2.8 Chemotactic Sensor Pads

Besides concentration sensing, chemical sensors may be used to determine the chemical characteristics of surfaces. A binding pad coated with an array of reversible, possibly reconfigurable, artificial receptors (Section 3.5.9) may be pressed against test surfaces such as cell membranes, or the perimeters of very large molecules, in order to detect the presence of specific chemical ligands. If pad receptor specificity is high for the target ligand, then the degree of pad "stickiness" to the test surface is a good measure of the population of target ligands on that surface. Probing two-dimensional surfaces with receptors may be constrained by orientation effects, since binding may require a specific relative orientation of ligand and receptor. Compliant pad receptors can reduce this problem but may impair lateral resolution—there is a three-way tradeoff among angular tolerance, lateral resolution, and multioriented multicopy receptors. A physical contact sensor prevents confusion of surface-bound and free-solvated ligands of the same species. The selective and reversible stickiness of such pads can also be exploited for locomotion (Section 9.4.3.1).

Molecular adhesion experiments in chemical force microscopy[440,1066] and interfacial force microscopy[441] using AFM probes with functionalized tips (Section 2.3.3) typically detect maximum adhesive noncovalent force differentials of 40-160 piconewton (pN)/ligand for competing ligands at a peak-force distance of ~0.2 nm. Forces >10 pN are readily measured by nanosensors (Section 4.4.1), so binding pad sensors should give an exact count of the number of target ligands present per unit area of test surface if (receptor areal number density) > (ligand areal number density) > (1 ligand / pad area), and if contact time is adequate. Receptors for many different ligands can be mounted on moving rotors or belts, or employed as interchangeable tool tips (Section 9.3.2), thus allowing a single sensor pad to reconfigure its specificity or sensitivity under external control.

4.2.9 Receptor Sensors

Ligand mimics may also be used to allow a medical nanodevice to detect a particular receptor in its environment. Each such "receptor sensor" is a protruding physical structure that mimics all or part of the electrosteric structure of the ligand to which the target receptor has maximum specificity. For example, probes consisting of artificial structures that simulate antigen peptides (8-15 amino acids long) bound in an MHC-like structure[439] (Section 8.5.2.1) could be used to sense the presence of specific T-cell receptors.

Sensing pads displaying ligand mimic structures are brought into contact with the test surface. Any target receptors present will bind to a mimic structure, thus may be counted as the sensor sweeps slowly across the surface. Immediately after recognition has occurred, the mimic structure may be reversibly fragmented, destroying receptor/mimic affinity and allowing the receptor to release the mimic. Mimics are mounted on the sensor pad with an appropriately elastic compliance to prevent structure detachment during a measurement scan.

Receptor sensing is most useful in detecting receptors for large molecules. In the case of receptors for small molecules, there may sometimes be insufficient space in the target molecular volume to match the surface electrosteric structure, to accommodate ligand fragmentation control rods or cables, or to build internal boundaries sufficient to permit ligand fragmentation without creating undesirable reactive species. Some of these problems with small-molecule receptors may be partially overcome by employing an annular repulsive ring through which a mimic ligand may be forcibly retracted without fragmentation, but receptor orientation effects will present additional constraints.

4.3 Displacement and Motion Sensors

The ability to precisely measure position and displacement, velocity and acceleration, rotation and orientation are essential requirements for nanoscale locomotion, physical manipulation, and navigation. A comprehensive analysis is beyond the scope of this book, but the following approximations should prove useful in nanomedical design.

4.3.1 Displacement Sensors

Diamondoid parts may contain features, or be positioned, in picometer (1 pm = 10^{-12} m) steps, much smaller than the unavoidable RMS thermal vibrations (Section 3.5.6). The nanomanipulator robot arm described in Section 9.3.1.4 may be moved in picometer increments, and the RMS thermal longitudinal displacements at the tip of a 20-nm long, 10-nm wide diamondoid lever is ~1 pm.[10] Displacement sensitivity of 10 pm is routinely achieved in STMs. It is claimed this can be improved down to the ~1 pm level;[433] STM resolution of 2 pm has been demonstrated experimentally.[1260] A C_{60} molecule used as the active element in an electromechanical amplifier transmits ~100 times more electrical current when physically compressed by 100 pm,[561] suggesting a minimum deformation detection limit of a few picometers. (A strain gauge and a vibration sensor using a (17,0) carbon nanotube (~2000 atoms) has been proposed.[2908])

Thermally-induced positional uncertainty in the displacement of nanoscale components is approximated[10] by the classical value

$$\Delta x \sim (kT / k_s)^{1/2} \qquad \text{\{Eqn. 4.8\}}$$

where T is temperature (K) and k_s is the Hooke's law spring constant, or restoring force stiffness (N/m). At 310 K, this classical approximation is accurate to within $\lesssim$10% of the quantum mechanical treatment for harmonic oscillators with RMS displacements $\Delta x \gtrsim 10$ pm.[10] Spring stiffness k_s is ~0.1 N/m for nonbonded (noncovalent) interatomic interactions, ~30 N/m for covalent bond angle bending, ~400 N/m for covalent bond stretching, and ~1000 N/m for solid 1 nm^3 diamondoid blocks.[10] At 310 K, springs of such stiffness produce minimum displacement uncertainties of 200 pm, 10 pm, 3 pm and 2 pm, respectively.

The log ratio of detection energy to noise energy, the signal/noise ratio (SNR), for a displacement sensor is derived from the harmonic potential (1/2) $k_s x^2$ as

$$\text{SNR} \sim \ln\left(\frac{\text{signal energy}}{\text{noise energy}}\right) \sim \ln\left(\frac{k_s\,\Delta x^2}{2\,kT}\right) \qquad \text{\{Eqn. 4.9\}}$$

Assuming a very stiff k_s = 600 N/m, a minimal SNR = 1 gives a minimum detectable displacement of 6 pm, or 10 pm at a more reasonable SNR = 2 (20 dB). The conservative conclusion is that Δx_{min} ~ 10 pm displacements should be reliably detectable by medical nanosensors in vivo, in a measurement time t_{meas} ~ 10^{-9} sec (Section 4.3.2). This compares favorably with the stereocilia of the inner ear, which can only detect 100 pm displacements in 10^{-5} sec.[446]

4.3.2 Velocity and Flow Rate Sensors

Typical thermal velocities of nanoscale diamondoid components at 310 K, from Eqn. 3.3, are ~60 m/sec for 1 nm^3 objects, ~2 m/sec for $(10\ nm)^3$ objects, 0.06 m/sec for $(100\ nm)^3$ objects, and 0.02 m/sec for 1 $micron^3$ objects. These thermal motions are in degrees of freedom whose range of motion is largely confined, by design, to sub-nanometer distances (Section 4.3.1) within nanoscale measuring devices. However, objects of nanomedical interest may have velocities ranging from ~10^{-9} m/sec (Section 9.4.4.2) to ~10^3 m/sec (e.g., the speed of sound in water), and may include biological elements in the environment or internal machine components. Thus it is useful to explore the fundamental limitations involved in measuring the full range of this physical variable.

There are at least two simple ways to determine a velocity. First, velocity may be measured by transferring the kinetic energy of a moving object or fluid volume to a sensor element. The movement of the sensor element is then clocked as it traverses a known distance. Second, and more efficiently, the passage of the moving object may sequentially trip two latches located a known distance apart, again revealing the moving object's velocity; alternatively, detecting the presence or absence of a protruding feature on a passing body using probe rods (e.g., Fig. 4.5) can determine velocity without any requirement for large kinetic energy transfers. The need for physical gating movements by sensor components and computational register-shift operations using diamondoid rods moving at ~GHz clocking speeds[10] suggests a conservative minimum stable sensor cycle time of ~10^{-9} sec (Section 10.1).

The two principal restrictions on the maximum detectable velocity v_{max} are the maximum linear dimension of the sensor element, or L_{sensor}, and the minimum event time that may be accurately discriminated, or Δt_{min}. For a sensor element with thermal noise energy ΔE ~ 10 kT = 43 zJ at 310 K, the quantum mechanical limit is $\Delta t_{min} \gtrsim \hbar / (2\,\Delta E)$ ~ 10^{-15} sec. Δt_{min} is also limited by the thermal variation in length of the individual latches. If the minimum detectable latch displacement is Δx ~ 10 pm (Section 4.3.1), and the maximum speed of latch displacement is approximately the speed of sound in the latch material (e.g., v_{sound} ~ 17,300 m/sec for diamond), then Δt ~ $\Delta x / v_{sound}$ ~ 10^{-15} sec, near the quantum mechanical limit. Δt is further restricted by the minimum detectable phase variance between latches located at either end of the sensor. An acoustically-transmitted clock pulse emitted from a centrally-located source that is Δx closer to one of the two latches can discriminate a phase variance of $\gtrsim \Delta x / L_{sensor}$ ~ 10^{-5} taking L_{sensor} ~ 1 micron, so the minimum discriminable time is again Δt_{min} ~ $10^{-5}\,L_{sensor} / v_{sound}$ ~ 10^{-15} sec; hence v_{max} ~ $L_{sensor} / \Delta t_{min}$ ~ 10^9 m/sec ~ c (= 3×10^8 m/sec, the speed of light).

However, unlike photons, physical objects moving in an aqueous medium are normally limited to the speed of sound in that medium,* e.g., v_{sound} ~ 1500 m/sec in water at 310 K (Table 6.7). If v_{max} is taken as ~10^3 m/sec, then for a sensor of size L_{sensor} ~ 1 micron the required time discrimination is only Δt_{min} ~ L_{sensor} / v_{max} ~ 10^{-9} sec.

The minimum detectable velocity v_{min} is limited by the minimum measurable linear displacement Δx ~ 10 pm and the limits of our patience in making the measurement. For a maximum measurement time of t_{meas} ~ 1 sec, v_{min} ~ $\Delta x / t_{meas}$ ~ 0.01 nm/sec in vacuo. In a nanomedically-relevant aqueous medium, the systematic

**Crystal dislocations,[3042] high-speed bullets, detonation waves and other nanomedically-relevant phenomena can exceed the local speed of sound, but supersonic operations are hardly conservative and a turbulent medium adds additional sources of error to the measurement.*

motion of a free-floating (untethered) object of radius R is masked by added Brownian noise as defined in Eqn 3.1, giving the limiting $v_{brownian} = \Delta X / \tau \gtrsim 260$ nm/sec for R = 10 micron and $v_{brownian} \gtrsim 2.6$ micron/sec for R = 100 nm, where $\tau = t_{meas} = 1$ sec. The thermal motions of tethered objects moving along surfaces (e.g., vesicles transported along microtubules by kinesin motors; Section 9.4.6) are more restricted, hence Brownian velocity masking is reduced.

Modest accuracy may be achieved using acoustic reflection in a Doppler velocimeter. Employing acoustic waves of frequency ν, the minimum measurable velocity change $\Delta v = v_{sound} / (\nu\ t_{meas}) = 150$ microns/sec in an aqueous medium at 310 K with $v_{sound} = 1500$ m/sec, $\nu \sim 10$ MHz, and $t_{meas} = 1$ sec, corresponding to the shifted frequency $\nu\ (1 + (\Delta v / v_{sound}))$ having enough time to make one extra cycle during t_{meas}. Even at such long wavelengths (~150 microns), significant backscattering of ultrasound from ~7.82-micron red cells is observed experimentally.[3044]

Velocity sensors may also be used to estimate volumetric flow rates in fluidic channels[442] and blood vessels[443] by measuring the speed at which fluid passes a nanodevice resting on the vessel wall. The parabolic velocity profile of v is a function of radial distance r from the center of a cylindrical vessel of radius R for Hagen-Poiseuille flow[361] (Section 9.2.5):

$$v = \frac{\left(R^2 - r^2\right)\Delta P}{4\,\eta\,L_v} \qquad \text{\{Eqn. 4.10\}}$$

where absolute viscosity $\eta = 1.1$ centipoise (1.1×10^{-3} kg/m-sec) for plasma at 310 K and ΔP is the pressure change along the length of a vessel of length L_v. A 1-micron nanodevice obtains measurements of v at various distances from the vessel wall, then fits these data to Eqn. 4.10 to find the choice of R that minimizes the variation in estimated $\Delta P / L_v$, which should be roughly constant under nonaccelerative conditions. Once R is determined, $\Delta P / L_v$ is known as well as the cross-sectional area (πR^2) of the vessel lumen, and a simple integration of the radial velocity distribution provides the flow rate in m^3/sec. Unfortunately, the usefulness of this technique is limited by boundary layer effects (Section 9.4.2.6).

4.3.3 Acceleration Sensors

Accelerations inside nanoscale devices are often measured in the trillions of g's ($g = 9.81$ m/sec^2). For example, an L = 1 nm diamondoid block ($m = 3.5 \times 10^{-24}$ kg) with thermal energy ~kT experiences random thermal accelerations of $a_{therm} \sim kT / g\, m\, L = 10^{11}$ g's; a 10-nm logic rod with vibrational energy ~kT experiences ~10^{12} g oscillations; a 200-nm wide hoop spinning axially with 1000 m/sec rim speed has rotational acceleration of a ~ 10^{12} g's.

4.3.3.1 Box-Spring Accelerometers

As one member of a class of devices, a simple nanoscale omnidirectional accelerometer is conceptualized as a reaction mass suspended by three pairs of reaction springs (one pair per orthogonal directional axis) with each spring connected to the walls of an evacuated box (Fig. 4.4). Acceleration in any direction extends some springs and compresses others, which is measured by force or

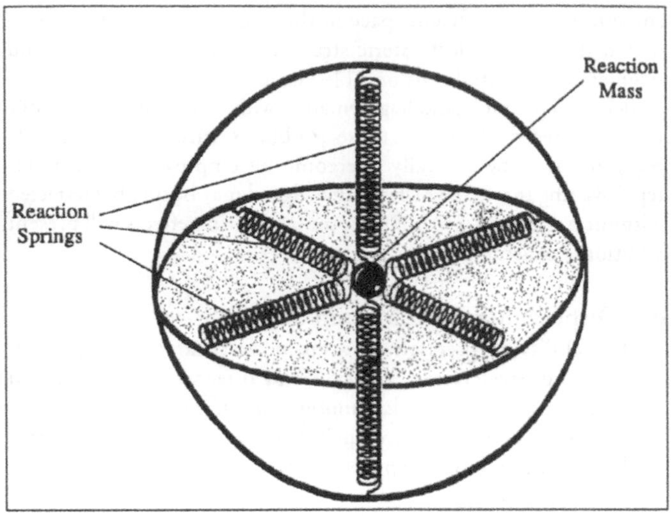

Fig. 4.4. Schematic of box-spring omnidirectional accelerometer.

displacement sensors attached to each spring. The signal/noise ratio for this sensor is

$$SNR = \ln\left(\frac{E_{spring}}{E_{noise}}\right) = \ln\left(\frac{m^2\, a^2}{2\, kT\, k_s}\right) \qquad \text{\{Eqn. 4.11\}}$$

For a sensor mass $m = 10^{-17}$ kg (~78 nm-wide platinum* or ~140 nm-wide diamond cube) suspended with $k_s = 1$ N/m floppy springs at T = 310 K, the minimum detectable acceleration $a_{min} = 1.6 \times 10^6$ g's for SNR = 1 and 2.6×10^6 g's for SNR = 2 (undamped resonant acceleration ~ L k_s/m ~ 10^9 g's for L=100 nm). Undamped resonance frequency $\omega_{res} = (k_s/m)^{1/2} = 3 \times 10^8$ radians/sec, which is measurable (Section 4.3.4.3).

Sensor mass exchanges reciprocally with acceleration sensitivity in Eqn. 4.11, so the lower limit even for a dedicated micron-scale platinum-core box-spring accelerometer is a_{min} ~1000 g's at SNR ~ 2 (undamped resonant acceleration ~ 10^6 g's for L = 2 microns). The maximum detectable acceleration requires m ~ 10^{-23} kg (~1.4 nm diamond cube) and k_s ~ 1000 N/m, giving a_{max} ~5×10^{13} g's at SNR = 1.

If the accelerometer depicted in Figure 4.4 is installed near the center of mass of a nanorobot, the sensor may avoid confusing centrifugal and translation forces. Otherwise, information from multiple sensors must be combined to obtain an unambiguous measurement. Multiple measurements can improve the SNR for constant accelerations of long duration.

In 1998, ~100-nm vibrating-beam silicon accelerometers were under development by Analog Devices and Daimler-Benz. Tunneling accelerometers had been fabricated with ~10^{-6} g resolution at a 350 Hz bandwidth or ~10^{-8} g/Hz$^{1/2}$.[3041] Silicon-based capacitive accelerometers (5-1000 g full scale) manufactured by Silicon Designs (Issaquah, WA) were widely used in automotive airbag safety systems; in 1998, Motorola shipped its ten-millionth accelerometer, and the global market for automotive silicon accelerometers was expected to reach $463 million by 2002.

**Platinum is probably the ideal choice for medical nanodevice components requiring maximum density. Depleted uranium, a relatively abundant element, is more common in macroscale nonmedical devices. However, pure U^{238} has a density of 19,050 kg/m^3, somewhat lower than the density of Pt (21,450 kg/m^3) or even gold (19,320 kg/m^3). Uranium and its compounds are highly toxic, and finely divided (e.g., micron-scale) uranium metal is pyrophoric (spontaneously combustible) in air. By comparison, Pt metal is almost completely inert in air and in the body, thus is nontoxic, and is mechanically ~50 times stronger than gold (Table 9.3). Only two elements have higher density than Pt: Os (22,480 kg/m^3) and Ir (22,420 kg/m^3). Osmium is brittle even at high temperatures and the powdered metal oxidizes in air, giving off osmium tetroxide which has a strong smell and is highly toxic (as little as 100 nanograms per m^3 of air causes lung congestion, skin and eye damage). Iridium metal is also very brittle and, like osmium, is at least five times less abundant than Pt.[691,763]*

4.3.3.2 Displacement Accelerometers

Formed elements in the human bloodstream (e.g., red cells, white cells, platelets) typically are buffeted by much smaller accelerations. For example at 310 K, instantaneous random thermal accelerations of $a_{thermal} \sim 500$ g's are experienced by a 0.2-micron virus particle, ~0.05 g's by a 2-micron platelet, ~10^{-4} g's by a 10-micron neutrophil—and ~0.4 g's by a 1 micron^3 spherical nanorobot. Force-based sensors cannot easily detect such low accelerations, since the smaller the sensor, the larger the a_{min} for a given SNR (Eqn. 4.11). An alternative approach uses displacement sensors to determine an object's velocity twice in rapid sequence, allowing acceleration to be computed from the difference.

Consider a constantly accelerating object that triggers three clocking latches at positions x_1, x_2, and x_3, in sequence. Time and position of the object are measured as (x_1, t_1), (x_2, t_2), and (x_3, t_3). The measured constant acceleration is then given by

$$a = \frac{v_{32} - v_{21}}{t_{32} - t_{21}} \quad (\text{m/sec}^2) \qquad \{\text{Eqn. } 4.12\}$$

where $v_{32} = (x_3 - x_2) / (t_3 - t_2)$, $v_{21} = (x_2 - x_1) / (t_2 - t_1)$, $t_{32} = (t_3 + t_2) / 2$ and $t_{21} = (t_2 + t_1) / 2$. If adjacent latches are an equal distance x_{latch} apart so that $x_{latch} = (x_3 - x_2) = (x_2 - x_1)$, and taking $t_1 = 0$, then Eqn. 4.12 reduces to

$$a = \frac{2\, x_{latch}(2t_2 - t_3)}{t_3\, t_2 (t_3 - t_2)} \quad (\text{m/sec}^2) \qquad \{\text{Eqn. } 4.13\}$$

Assume that a slowly accelerating external object passes three clocking latches that are fixed to the exterior of a nanorobot of radius R. Measurements of the object's velocity incur an unavoidable error due to nanorobot thermal motion. The object is observed to pass between latch pairs during a measurement time ~t_{meas}. During this same interval, from Eqn. 3.1 the nanorobot translates a distance $\Delta X = (kT\, t_{meas} / 3\, \pi\, \eta\, R)^{1/2}$, incurring a maximum velocity measurement error of ~$\Delta X / t_{meas}$, and thus from Eqn. 4.12 a maximum acceleration measurement error of ~$2\, \Delta X / t_{meas}^2$ if $(t_3 - t_2) \sim (t_2 - t_1) \sim t_{meas}$. Thus the minimum detectable acceleration is

$$a_{min} \sim \left(\frac{4\, kT}{3\, \pi\, \eta\, R\, t_{meas}^3} \right)^{1/2} \quad (\text{m/sec}^2) \qquad \{\text{Eqn. } 4.14\}$$

Taking T = 310 K, η = 1.1 x 10^{-3} kg/m-sec and R = 1 micron, then $a_{min} \sim 10^{-7}$ g's for t_{meas} = 1 sec; $a_{min} \sim 0.004$ g's for a more reasonable $t_{meas} = 10^{-3}$ sec measurement time in the in vivo environment. Onboard reference oscillators with the requisite accuracy are described in Section 10.1.

4.3.3.3 Fluid Acceleration Sensors

Biological fluid accelerations may also be inferred from measurements of spatial pressure gradients. Ignoring frictional and gravitational forces and assuming laminar flow, fluid acceleration a_{fluid} is given by

$$a_{fluid} = -\frac{\Delta P}{\rho\, \Delta x} \quad (\text{m/sec}^2) \qquad \{\text{Eqn. } 4.15\}$$

where ρ = fluid density (e.g., blood plasma is an almost incompressible Newtonian fluid, with $\rho \sim 1025$ kg/m^3 at 310 K) and ΔP is the measured change in pressure over a distance Δx. The mitral and aortic valves in the heart ($\Delta P / \Delta x \sim 10^5$ N/m^3, $a_{fluid} \sim 10$ g's,[474] $\Delta x \sim$ a few cm), as well as valves in the veins and lymphatics, operate as bistable analog decelerometers employing this principle.[444] Micron-scale medical nanorobots traveling across blood vessel surfaces could use pressure sensors capable of 10^{-6} atm resolution (Section 4.5.1) to infer local blood flow accelerations to an accuracy of ± 0.01 g from sequential measurements taken 1 mm apart.

4.3.3.4 Pivoted Gyroscopic Accelerometers

Consider a cylindrical gyroscope spinning at an angular velocity ω (radians/sec), with radius r and thickness h, whose center of gravity lies a distance L_p from a frictionless pivot point along the rotational axis. The pivot point defines the center of a spherical sensor grid of radius $R \geq (r^2 + 4h^2)^{1/2}$ having distinguishable grid elements located a distance $\Delta x \sim 1$ nm apart. Under uniform acceleration a, the gyroscope precesses around its spin axis at an angular velocity $\omega_p = 2\, a\, L_p / \omega\, r^2 = \Delta x / R\, t_{meas}$, where t_{meas} is measurement duration. Hence the minimum detectable acceleration is

$$a_{min} = \frac{\Delta x\, r^2\, \omega}{2\, L_p\, R\, t_{meas}} \quad (\text{m/sec}^2) \qquad \{\text{Eqn. } 4.16\}$$

by comparing precessional motion against the grid.

In choosing an ω with which to measure a_{min}, there is an upper and a lower limit. The upper bound is the bursting strength condition

$$\omega = \omega_{max} < \left(\frac{2\, \sigma_w}{\rho\, r^2} \right)^{1/2} \quad (\text{rad/sec}) \qquad \{\text{Eqn. } 4.17\}$$

where σ_w is a safe working stress = 10^{10} N/m^2 (~0.2 tensile strength) for diamond[10] and ρ is the density of the gyroscope material (~3510 kg/m^3 for diamond). The lower bound is the minimum spin angular velocity below which the pivoted gyroscope cannot spin stably about the vertical axis and begins to wobble,[448] thus ruining the measurement. The lower bound is given by

$$\omega = \omega_{min} = \left(\frac{4\, a_{min}\, L_p \left(r^2 + \frac{1}{3} h^2 \right)}{\pi\, h\, \rho\, r^6} \right)^{1/2} \qquad \{\text{Eqn. } 4.18\}$$

If $\omega_{max} / \omega_{min} > 1$, then nonwobbling spin velocities are available below the bursting speed of the gyroscope cylinder. Since this ratio scales with R, there is a minimum sensor size R_{min} below which no useful spin velocities are available. Combining Eqns. 4.16 and 4.18 and solving the quadratic in ω gives

$$R_{min} = \frac{2\, \Delta x \left(r^2 + \frac{1}{3} h^2 \right)}{\pi\, h\, t_{meas}\, r^3 (2 \sigma_w\, \rho)^{1/2}} \qquad \{\text{Eqn. } 4.19\}$$

For $t_{meas} = 10^{-3}$ sec, $R_{min} \gtrsim 69$ microns (optimum r = 48 microns, h = 25 microns); for t_{meas} = 1 sec, $R_{min} \gtrsim 6.9$ microns (optimum r = 4.8 microns, h = 2.5 microns). Thus it appears that pivoted gyroscopic accelerometers likely will be employed only in devices >> 10 microns in size (but see Section 4.3.4.1). Microscale gyroscopes implemented in silicon have been discussed by Greiff[1383] and others.[447]

4.3.3.5 Accelerative Onset

Aside from pure acceleration, the rate of accelerative onset—sometimes called jolt, surge, or jerk—can produce additional damaging effects on macroscale mechanical and biological structures. For example, the effects of accelerative onset ($\dot{a}$) on the human body were studied by Col. John Paul Stapp[1714] in a series of aggressive rocket sled experiments conducted during the 1950s.[1714-1716] For human subjects, cardiovascular shock was entirely absent for $\dot{a} \lesssim$ 500-600 g/sec but began to appear at $\dot{a} \gtrsim$ 1100-1400 g/sec, at 1-40 g accelerations. Human tolerance to linear decelerative force is determined both by rate of onset and peak acceleration; the endurance limit for well-restrained healthy young males has been given as $\lesssim$500 g/sec and $\lesssim$50 g for $\lesssim$0.2 sec durations.[1717]

By 1998, the effects of accelerative onset on nanomechanical structures had not been extensively studied, but similar limits might apply to nanomachines. For example, a diamond rod of length L_{rod} = 1 micron, cross-sectional area S_{rod} = 0.01 micron^2, mass m_{rod} = 3.5 x 10^{-17} kg, and working strength W_{rod} ~ 5 x 10^{10} N/m^2 (Table 9.3) fails when subjected to a static acceleration $a_{fail} \gtrsim W_{rod} S_{rod} / m_{rod}$ ~ 10^{12} g. But accelerative shocks can produce dynamic amplification in the response spectrum of elastic systems. Dynamic stress rises to a peak of roughly twice the corresponding static value when $\dot{a}_{peak} \gtrsim 4 \nu_{res} a_{max}$ for a trapezoidal pulse shape, where ν_{res} is the frequency of natural vibration of the system,[363] because the stresses from the free oscillations of the system, induced by the changes in the acceleration of the system, can add to the static stresses from the acceleration, with damage done by the total stress. Taking k_s ~ 1 N/m for the rod described above, then ν_{res} ~ 30 MHz (Section 4.3.3.1) and $\dot{a}_{peak}$ ~ 10^{20} g/sec at a_{max} ~ 10^{12} g. For comparison, the teragravity nanocentrifuge (Section 3.2.5) has mass m ~ 10^{-17} kg and is spun up to a_{max} = 5 x 10^{11} g's in $\gtrsim 10^{-6}$ sec, giving $\dot{a} \lesssim 5 \times 10^{17}$ g/sec << $\dot{a}_{peak}$.

4.3.4 Angular Displacement

There are circumstances in which it is necessary for a medical nanodevice to measure, establish or maintain a preferred orientation, as for example nanorobots with a clearly defined "top" and "bottom" or nanodevices performing lengthy intracellular operations requiring precision stationkeeping. Measurement of rotation rates may also be required.

4.3.4.1 Gimballed Nanogyroscopes

Pivoted gyroscopes of the type described in Section 4.3.3.4 are impractical for orientational sensing in all but the largest medical nanodevices. Setting ω_{max} (Eqn. 4.17) equal to ω_{min} (Eqn. 4.18), taking a_{min} = g = 9.81 m/sec^2 (gravitational acceleration), and optimizing for minimum sensor size gives a critical nonwobbling nonbursting spin velocity ω_{crit} ~ 6.8 x 10^7 radians/sec at a minimum device radius of ~35 microns. If a pivoted gyroscope is smaller than this minimum radius, then spinning it slower than ω_{crit} causes the gyro to tumble helplessly, while spinning it faster than ω_{crit} tears the gyro apart.

However, a triaxially gimballed nanogyroscope may be regarded as having its pivot point near its center of mass, so L_p becomes very small and ω_{min} becomes very slow, making nanogyroscopes feasible in medical nanorobots. Taking h = 1 micron, r = 0.5 micron, ρ = 3510 kg/m^3 and a_{min} = g in Eqn. 4.18, then if the gimbals are aligned such that L_p = 1 nm between the pivot point and the effective center of gravity along the rotation axis, then ω_{min} ~ 400 rad/sec. If gimbal tolerances are improved to L_p = 0.1 nm, then ω_{min} ~ 125 rad/sec.

How stable is a nanogyroscopic orientation standard? There are two principal considerations.

First, Brownian thermal rotation in all three angular degrees of freedom (θ, φ and ψ) gives rise to a small nutation around the nanogyroscopic precession axis of magnitude $\Delta\theta_{nutate} \sim p_\varphi / p_\psi$, where p_φ and p_ψ are angular momenta of the gyro.[448] The minimum value for p_φ is approximated by (1/2) kT ~ (1/2) p_φ^2 / I_1, where I_1 = (1/4) m r^2 + (1/12) m h^2, the moment of inertia around φ, and m = $\pi r^2 h \rho$. The maximum value for p_ψ is given by the burst-strength condition $\omega < \omega_{max}$ (Eqn. 4.17) as $p_\psi \sim I_3 \omega$, where I_3 = (1/2) m r^2, the moment of inertia around ψ. Hence:

$$\Delta\theta_{nutate} \sim \left(\frac{kT\left(r^2 + \frac{1}{3}h^2\right)}{2\pi\sigma_w h r^4} \right)^{1/2} \quad \text{(radians)} \qquad \text{\{Eqn. 4.20\}}$$

For T = 310 K, r = 0.5 micron, h = 1 micron, σ_w ~ 10^{10} N/m^2, $\Delta\theta_{nutate}$ ~ 0.8 microradian.

Second, the gimbal bearings have small frictional losses, exerting small torques on the gyro and causing a small precession away from the original orientation. The angular velocity of precession $\omega_{precess}$ ~ $T_{gimbal} / (I_3 \omega)$ (rad/sec) where T_{gimbal} is the frictional torque caused by an imperfect gimbal bearing. Assume that the gimbal is driven by external forces to oscillate at some frequency ν_{gimbal}, and that a gimbal bearing dissipates power at the rate of P_{gimbal} (watts), so that each oscillatory motion of the gimbal dissipates $E_{gimbal} = P_{gimbal}/\nu_{gimbal}$ (joules). If the angular amplitude of the gimbal motion is α_{gimbal} (radians) and the gimbal radius is r_{gimbal}, then the gimbal bearing travels $X_{gimbal} = \alpha_{gimbal} r_{gimbal}$ (meters) per gimbal oscillation and the force applied in dissipating an energy E_{gimbal} is $F_{gimbal} = E_{gimbal}/X_{gimbal}$. Thus, the torque applied by each gimbal oscillation event is $T_{gimbal} = F_{gimbal} r_{gimbal} = P_{gimbal} / (\nu_{gimbal} \alpha_{gimbal})$; $P_{gimbal} = k_p v_{gimbal}^2$ (see Drexler[10]), where $v_{gimbal} = \alpha_{gimbal} \nu_{gimbal} r_{gimbal}$ is the sliding speed of the gimbal bearing surfaces during movement and k_p is a constant that depends solely on the geometry of the bearing.

The change in orientation angle caused by each gimbal oscillation event is $\Delta\theta_{osc} = \omega_{precess} / \nu_{gimbal}$. The number of gimbal oscillations N = t ν_{gimbal}, where t is elapsed time since the gyro was last calibrated. If gimbal oscillations are independent and randomly distributed, then the total change in orientation angle is very roughly $\Delta\theta_{precess} \sim \Delta\theta_{osc} N^{1/2}$; assuming r_{gimbal} ~ r, then:

$$\Delta\theta_{precess} \sim \frac{2 k_p \alpha_{gimbal} \left(t \nu_{gimbal}\right)^{1/2}}{\pi r^2 h \rho \omega} \quad \text{(radians)} \qquad \text{\{Eqn. 4.21\}}$$

From Drexler[10], k_p = 2.7 x 10^{-14} watt-sec^2/m^2 as a conservative value for a small (~2 nm) stiff bearing. Random hydrodynamic flows induced by thermal fluctuations inside biological cells have a characteristic duration t_{fluct} ~ 10 millisec,[1069] which suggests α_{gimbal} ~ 0.06 radians (~3°) from Eqn. 3.2 for an R ~ 1 micron in cyto nanorobot. Taking r = 0.5 micron, h = 1 micron, ρ = 3510 kg/m^3 for diamond (giving m ~ 3 x 10^{-15} kg), ω = 1 x 10^9 rad/sec (just below the ω_{max} ~ 4.8 x 10^9 rad/sec bursting speed), and assuming $\nu_{gimbal} \sim t_{fluct}^{-1}$ = 100 Hz (to which the results are not terribly sensitive), then $\Delta\theta_{precess}$ ~ 10^{-8} t$^{1/2}$ (radians). Thus a $\theta_{precess}$ ~ 1 microradian orientation shift takes ~1 hour; a $\theta_{precess}$ ~ 4 microradian shift takes ~1 day; and a $\theta_{precess}$ ~ 70 microradian (~10 arcsec) shift takes ~1 year. (Total angular error $\Delta\theta_{total} = \Delta\theta_{precess} + \Delta\theta_{nutate}$.) Thus a gimballed nanogyroscope may be sufficiently stable to serve as a readily storable, easily transportable, and highly accurate onboard orientation standard.

4.3.4.2 Nanopendulum Orientation Sensing

A nanopendulum may also be employed for orientational sensing. As one example of a large class of related devices, consider a simple rigid spherical nanopendulum of radius r and mass m, with a large hemispherical bob free to swing through the entire solid angle about a central pivot point (Fig. 4.5), with a gimballed housing to allow active avoidance of the pivot support beam. The nanopendulum bob moves along a spherical surface located far enough from a

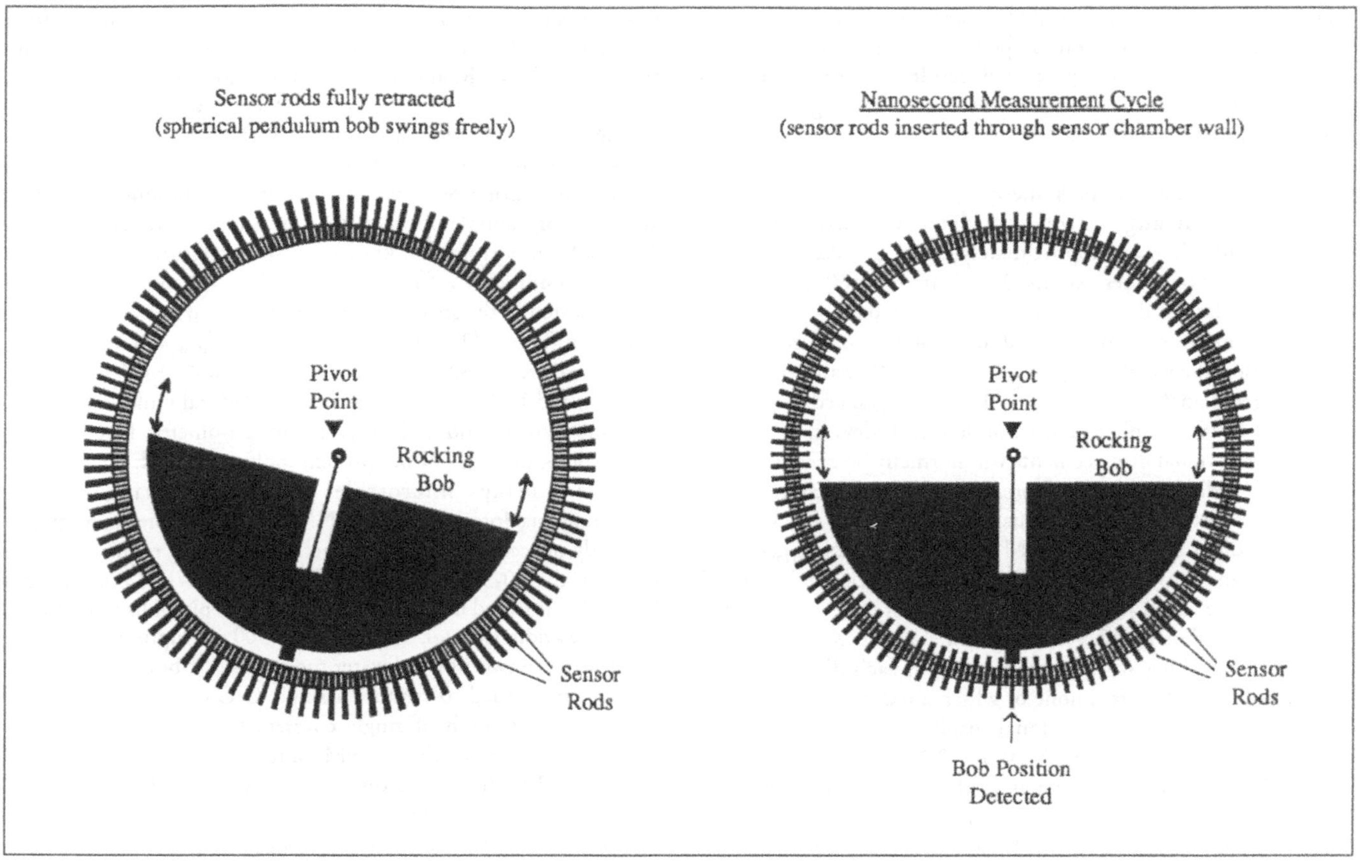

Fig. 4.5. Spherical nanopendulum sensor for angular displacement and rotational velocity.

concentric spherical sensor grid of radius $R = r + z_{sep}$ to minimize van der Waals interactions (Sections 3.5.1 and 9.2), with bob and sensor surfaces electrically neutral or uniformly mutually repulsive. Much like the pin cushion receptor model (Section 3.5.7.4), the sensor grid consists of a spherical array of diamondoid sensor rods $\Delta x \sim 1$ nm wide that are rapidly and simultaneously extended into the evacuated sensor cavity to determine bob position during a measurement cycle of duration t_{meas}. Radial sensor rod velocity should exceed typical tangential bob velocity by at least 1-2 orders of magnitude. For the example given below, a sensor stud on a 500-nm bob that is turning at $v_{turn} \sim v_{thermal} = 3.6$ mm/sec passes a ~1 nm sensor rod in ~280 nanosec; a sensor rod displacing ~1 nm in the radial direction in ~1 nanosec travels at $v_{rod} \sim 1$ m/sec. This nanopendulum may serve both as an orientation sensor and as a rotation rate sensor, using principles similar to vestibular (semicircular canal) mechanics.[449]

If a simple nanopendulum spherical sensor housing with bob initially at rest in a uniform vertical gravity field g is rotated through the smallest detectable angle θ_{min} (radians) around the center pivot, then ignoring friction, the bob's position over the sensor grid moves a distance Δx, hence

$$\Delta\theta_{min} = \Delta x / r \qquad \text{\{Eqn. 4.22\}}$$

For $\Delta x = 1$ nm and $r = 500$ nm, $\Delta\theta_{min} \sim 2$ milliradians (~0.1 deg). For a practical sliding interface (e.g., between bob and sensor surface) of contact area S and turning velocity v_{turn}, Drexler[10] estimates frictional dissipation, primarily driven by shear-reflection drag and band-stiffness scattering, as $P_{drag} \sim k_1 v_{turn}^2 S$, where $k_1 \sim 400$ kg/m^2-sec, hence the energy dissipated between the bob and the nearest sensor rod (the one interacting with the bob) is $E_{drag} \sim k_1 v_{turn} S \Delta x$. Bob gravitational energy $E_{bob} = m\,g\,r \sin\Delta\theta_{min} \sim m\,g\,r\,\Delta\theta_{min}$ for small displacements. The bob swings freely at the minimum displacement if $E_{bob}/E_{drag} > 1$. If $m = 10^{-15}$ kg, $r = 500$ nm, and $S = 1$ nm^2, then $v_{turn} < 2.5$ m/sec or $\omega < 49$ megaradians/sec for the bob to swing freely (vs. $v_{thermal} = 3.6$ mm/sec (Eqn. 3.3) and $\omega_{res} \sim 9900$ rad/sec for this pendulum).

The bob-up/bob-down energy differential is ~2 m g r = 9.8 zJ ~ 2.3 kT for $m = 10^{-15}$ kg and r = 500 nm. To distinguish opposite orientations ($\Delta\theta \sim \pi$) requires $N_{meas} \sim (kT / 2\,m\,g\,r)^2 \sim 1$ measurement for this sensor. To distinguish $\Delta\theta_{min} \sim 2$ milliradians requires averaging $N_{meas} \sim (kT / E_{bob})^2 \sim 190{,}000$ independent measurements (of ~0.002 kT/measurement) or $t_{meas} \sim 190$ microsec using a sensor rod clock cycle of ~1 nanosec. Thus, after subtracting out the effects of translation displacements as determined by linear accelerometers (Section 4.3.3), a nanodevice can measure angular displacements in its orientation to within $\pm\Delta\theta_{min}$ in a measurement time $t_{meas} \sim 10^{-4}$ sec. With sensor rods moving at ~1 m/sec, energy dissipation for each rod sliding in its housing is ~0.01 zJ/cycle (Section 10.2.1). If only ~100 test rods need be triggered to continuously track the moving stud, then a sensor rod clock cycle of ~1 nanosec implies a continuous nanopendulum power dissipation of ~1 pW; additional drag power loss between stud and contacting rod is only P_{drag} ~0.0004 pW.

Many other configurations of this basic device are readily conceived and may be more volume-efficient, including nested spheres or ovoids, two-dimensional rocking disk sections for in-plane rotational measurements (three devices required for monitoring all angular degrees of freedom in a rigid rotator), and multiaxial circumferential tracks or tubes containing rolling balls or sliding plugs. J. Logajan suggests that a pair of linear three-dimensional translation accelerometers should be able to unambiguously extract the 3 translation and 3 rotation components of all possible acceleration vectors. Rotation about any axis will result in distinctly different mass displacements while accelerated translation along any axis will result in identical displacements.

4.3.4.3 Nanopendulum Tachometry

The smallest angular velocity detectable using a simple nanopendulum is given approximately by $\omega_{min} \sim \Delta x / r\ t_{meas} = 2$ milliradian/sec (~0.1 deg/sec) for $\Delta x = 1$ nm, r = 500 nm, and $t_{meas} = 1$ sec. The largest detectable angular velocity $\omega_{max} \sim 2\pi / t_{meas}$ if t_{meas} is the minimum time required to count one complete rotation of the sensor; the smallest $t_{meas} \sim 2\pi / \omega_{max} \sim 100$ nanosec for $\omega_{max} \sim 49$ megaradians/sec—or ~5% of the bursting speed (Eqn. 4.17) for an r = 1 micron spherical diamondoid nanodevice.

What rotational displacements will normally be encountered by an in vivo medical nanorobot? From Equation 3.2, a 1-micron device experiences instantaneous Brownian rotations of $\omega_B = (kT / 4\pi\eta R^3 \tau)^{1/2}$ radians/sec, where $\tau = (MW_{kg} / 32\pi kT N_A c_{H_2O} R^4)^{1/2}$, the mean time between molecular collisions with the device (mostly by water molecules), from Equation 4.3, where $c_{H_2O} \sim 3.3 \times 10^{28}$ molecules/m^3. For R = 0.5 microns and T = 310 K, $\tau \sim 6 \times 10^{-20}$ sec/collision and $\omega_B \sim 7 \times 10^9$ rad/sec, with each displacement of $\sim \tau\ \omega_B = 4 \times 10^{-10}$ radian, none of which are detectable. However, the net of all Brownian rotational displacements is one rotation every 16 sec, ~0.4 radian/sec (Section 3.2.1).

The largest measurable angular displacements in vivo are caused by tumbling due to differential shear forces in the bloodstream. Normal vessel wall shear rates in physiological bloodflow range from 100-1400 radians/sec in the larger arteries to 500-4000 radians/sec in the smaller arteries and capillaries.[386] The measured rolling velocity of white cells during vascular "tank tread" locomotion (Section 9.4.3.6) on venule walls is ~40 micron/sec, or ~8 radians/sec, which may be encountered by nanodevices employing cytocarriage (Section 9.4.7). The human vestibular mechanism has a frequency response range of 0.048-260 radians/sec.[449]

Thus, the maximum range of physiologically relevant rotation rates is 10^{-2} to 10^4 radians/sec. Since the natural harmonic frequency of a simple nanopendulum is $\omega_{res} = (g/r)^{1/2} = 4400$ radians/sec for r = 500 nm, the possibility of forced oscillations and resonance need be faced only when measuring the highest likely physiological rotation rates, in which case the addition of a damping force $F_{damp} \sim m\ v_{turn}\ \omega_{res}$ during resonance events should eliminate the problem. F_{damp} for critical damping peaks at ~mg ~ 0.01 pN for the $m = 10^{-15}$ kg, r = 500 nm case ($v_{turn} \sim 2$ mm/sec).

4.4 Force Nanosensors

Piconewton forces may be applied and must be detected by medical nanodevices. Pendulum- and cantilever-based sensors may be used to probe nanoscale forces, to monitor the ambient gravitational field, to measure molecular-scale masses to single-proton accuracy, and to discriminate among molecules having different isotopic composition.

4.4.1 Minimum Detectable Force

Extremely small forces have been measured using macroscale instrumentation, particularly the atomic force microscope (AFM). In 1998, experimental forces of 1 nN in the contact regime and 1 pN in the noncontact regime were routinely measured.[450] In 1994, D. Rugar achieved a force sensitivity of 5×10^{-16} N using an AFM with a 90-nm thick cantilever at room temperature,[489] and in 1998 Rugar reported a force resolution of 7×10^{-18} N using a magnetic resonance force microscope (MRFM) with a 230-micron long, 60-nm thick, silicon cantilever.[3256] The theoretical limit on the force sensitivity of the AFM has been estimated as 10^{-18} - 10^{-19} N for temperatures near absolute zero[445,489] using fiber optic interferometry or other techniques. However, many of these methods are impractical or impossible to employ in medical nanodevices.

What is the minimum force F_{min} likely to be detectable by nanorobot sensors? Several lines of reasoning produce consistent answers. For example, force may be measured by the displacement Δx of a beam against the known resistive pressure provided by a spring of minimum stiffness k_s; that is, $F_{min} \sim k_s \Delta x$. However, the energy stored in the spring must exceed thermal noise energy, with SNR ~ ln $(k_s \Delta x^2 / 2 kT)$ (Eqn. 4.9), giving $F_{min} = 2kT e^{SNR} / \Delta x$. For T = 310 K and SNR = 2, $F_{min} = 100$ pN at $\Delta x = 0.6$ nm, 10 pN at 6 nm, and 1 pN at 60 nm. Indeed, the natural molecular motors (kinesin, dynein, and actin-myosin) have isometric force outputs on the order of 1-14 pN per protein molecule, which are routinely observed using microscale cantilever spring sensors measuring total forces of 10-100 pN.[452-455,1058,1247] Breaking antigen-antibody or receptor-ligand interactions generally requires rupture forces in the 50-300 pN range.[3200] A force of ~160 pN separates biotin that is seated in its avidin receptor; ~85 pN pulls iminobiotin out of the avidin receptor.[1075] A force of ~300 pN ruptures a hydrogen bond between two isolated water molecules,[1030] but >3000 pN are likely to be needed to rupture a single C-C covalent bond.[10,1131] The rupture strength of single covalent bonds has been directly measured experimentally by AFM as, for instance, 2000 ± 300 pN for Si-C (528 zJ/molecule dissociation enthalpy, 0.185 nm bond length) and 1400 ± 300 pN for Au-S.[3193]

Force sensing may also require using measurement devices that involve sliding interfaces of two mutually inert periodic surfaces. This motion may be characterized by the potential energy of interaction, ~0.1-1 zJ as determined by Monte Carlo simulations of typical diamondoid material at 0.2-0.5 nm separations.[10] Assuming a minimum 0.5 zJ energy barrier, for small sliding contacts the typical force amplitude $F_{min} \sim 1.7 \times 10^{10}\ \Delta V_{barrier} \sim 8.5$ pN.[10]

A force of 10 piconewtons across a small-molecule receptor (0.3 nm)^3 of surface area 0.09 nm^2 represents an energy density of $\sim 10^8$ J/m^3 x 0.027 nm^3 = 2.7 zJ ~ 0.6 kT. And the nanorobotic manipulator arm described in Section 9.3.1.4 is capable of ~picometer step sizes, representing a minimum applicable force of $F_{min} \sim 10$ pN assuming 0.04 m/N compliance[10] for the entire mechanism. Thus as a conservative estimate, the smallest force that is reliably detectable (and applicable) by nanodevices is probably ~10 pN.

Finally, a nanosensor of dimension L able to distinguish two forces differing by ΔF newtons has a probability of erroneous measurement[10] of

$$P_{err} \sim \exp(-L\ \Delta F / 4\ kT) \qquad \{\text{Eqn. } 4.23\}$$

For $\Delta F = 10$ pN and T = 310 K, $P_{err} = 1\%$ for L = 8 nm, or 0.01% for L = 16 nm, so reliable nanoscale picoforce sensors may be ~10-20 nm in size.

4.4.2 Nanogravimeters

Research in space medicine has discovered that micron-scale elements of the immune system have extraordinary sensitivity to gravity. One study found that bone marrow-derived (B6MP102) macrophage single cells respond after 8 seconds to exposure to a 10^{-2} g hypogravity environment as indicated by increased cell spreading,[468] a well-known marker of cell activation. Individual immune system cells placed in microgravity exhibit enhanced growth but depressed differentiation,[468] decreased activation by concanavalin

A,[470] a 20% reduction in glucose metabolism, increased resistance to antibiotics, increased number of pseudopodia on monocytes, and changes in cytoplasmic streaming velocity and frequency.[469]

As of 1998, the exact mechanism by which the leukocyte "gravity sensor" operates remained unknown. It has been speculated that differences in densities of several organelles, such as the nucleolus, the ribosomes, and the centrioles, could generate detectable pressures on the structure of the cytoskeleton under gravitational loading[469,471] mediated through mechanosensitive stretch-activated ion channels or the extracellular matrix.[468] While indirect gravitational effects that modify the cellular environment (such as reduced sedimentation or decreased thermal convection due to hypogravity) could also be responsible, a direct interaction of the gravitational force with cellular structures[472,473] appears to be the most likely sensor mechanism. For instance, if a change in gravitational loading equivalent to the force generated by a natural molecular motor (F ~ 1 pN; Section 4.4.1) is detectable by the cytoskeleton, and this force is applied to the entire mass of a (10 micron)^3 cell (m ~ 10^{-12} kg), then the minimum detectable gravitational acceleration is g ~ F/m ~ 1 m/sec^2 = 0.1 g, which should be adequate to detect the onset of hypogravity.

A nanomechanical gravity sensor of similar size to a macrophage cell may be at least 100,000 times more sensitive. For example, the energy of a tethered mass swinging freely in a uniform gravity field is approximately $E_g \sim m\ g\ \Delta h$, where Δh is the maximum vertical amplitude of the motion. To be detectable, oscillator energy must exceed thermal noise energy, so SNR ~ $\ln(m\ g\ \Delta h\ N_{meas}^{1/2} / kT)$, giving $g_{min} = kT\ e^{SNR} / m\ \Delta h\ N_{meas}^{1/2} \sim kT\ e^{SNR} / \rho\ L^4\ N_{meas}^{1/2}$ for a bob mass of density ρ and size L^3, N_{meas} independent measurements, and assuming $\Delta h \sim L$. If T = 310 K, SNR = 2, N_{meas} = 1, and ρ = 21,450 kg/m^3 (Pt), then g_{min} = 0.1 g for L ~ 1 micron, 0.01 g for L ~ 2 microns, 10^{-5} g for L ~ 11 microns, and 10^{-6} g for L = 20 microns, the size of the average human tissue cell (Section 8.5.1).

Regarding nanogravimeter design, for a pendulum of length L in a gravity field g ~ 9.81 m/sec^2 (1 g), the resonant period of the motion $T_{res} = 2\pi\ (L/g)^{1/2} = 2 \times 10^{-3}$ sec for L = 1 micron, 9×10^{-3} sec for L = 20 microns. If Δt_{min} = 1 nanosec is the minimum detectable decrease in resonant period caused by an increase in gravity from g to g + Δg, then the minimum detectable change in gravitation force is

$$\Delta g / g = 1 - \left(\frac{L}{g\,k_g^2} \right) \sim \frac{10^{-9}}{L^{1/2}} \qquad \text{\{Eqn. 4.24\}}$$

for a medical nanorobot, where $k_g = (\Delta t_{min} / 2\pi) + (L/g)^{1/2}$. For L = 1 micron, $\Delta g / g \sim 10^{-6}$; for L = 20 microns, $\Delta g / g \sim 2 \times 10^{-7}$.

4.4.3 Single-Proton Massometer

A nanopendulum may also be used to measure molecular-scale masses. Torsion, helical spring, and vibrating rod mechanisms all will work, but one of the most efficient designs for weighing the smallest masses may be the coiled suspension-spring cantilever massometer illustrated schematically in Figure 4.6, which is analogous in principle to the traditional quartz crystal microbalance.[2896] In this design, a beam of length L_{beam} and circular cross-sectional radius R_{beam} is hinged at one end and carries a sample holder of solid volume V_{sample} at the other end. The beam is supported (a variable distance L_{spring} from the hinge) by a spring consisting of a movable suspension rod of total length l_{rod}, circular cross-sectional radius r_{rod}, and spring constant $k_s \sim \pi^2\ r_{rod}^4\ E\ G / (G\ l_{rod}^3 + E\ \pi\ r_{rod}^2\ l_{rod})$ using spring (rod) material of density ρ, Young's modulus E, and shear modulus G.* The natural resonance period for this unloaded system is $T_0 = (2\pi\ L_{beam}/L_{spring})\ (m_0/k_s)^{1/2} = Z\ m_0^{1/2}$, where $Z = (2\ L_{beam} / L_{spring}\ r_{rod}^2)\ ((G\ l_{rod}^3 + E\ \pi\ r_{rod}^2\ l_{rod}) / E\ G)^{1/2}$ and $m_0 = \rho\ (V_{sample} + \pi\ L_{beam}\ R_{beam}^2 + \pi\ l_{rod}\ r_{rod}^2)$. Gravitational loading is negligible for suspension system mass m << $(k_s\ L_{spring}^2 / g\ L_{beam}^2)$ ~ 10^{-15} kg; m ~ 10^{-20} kg in the exemplar system.

After adding a test mass Δm to the sample holder, the resonance period increases to $T_m = Z\ (m_0 + \Delta m)^{1/2}$, which may be detected if $T_m - T_0 \geq \Delta t_{min}$ ~ 1 nanosec, the minimum convenient time interval (Section 10.1). Hence the minimum detectable molecular weight ΔMW, expressed in proton masses ($m_p = 1.67 \times 10^{-27}$ kg), is

$$\Delta MW = \Delta m / m_p = m_p^{-1} \left[\left(m_0^{1/2} + \Delta t_{min}/Z \right)^2 - m_0 \right] \quad \text{(protons)} \qquad \text{\{Eqn. 4.25\}}$$

In Figure 4.6, beam and rod are coiled in two dimensions (although three-dimensional coiling, more difficult to depict, provides maximum compactness). L_{beam} and l_{rod} are chosen to minimize total coil area $A_{coil} = 2\ R_{beam}\ L_{beam} + 2\ r_{rod}\ l_{rod}$. Using aluminum for the rod and beam (E = 6.9×10^{10} N/m^2, G = 2.6×10^{10} N/m^2, ρ = 2700 kg/m^3), L_{beam} = 1200 nm, l_{rod} = 1920 nm, r_{rod} = 0.5 nm, V_{sample} = 1 nm^3, and $\Delta t_{min} = 10^{-9}$ sec, then ΔMW ~ 1 proton for L_{spring} = 1 nm >> Δx_{min} = 0.01 nm, the minimum measurable displacement (Section 4.3.1). (For L_{spring} > 1 nm, physiological ~1 g accelerative loads on a ~1 micron nanorobot in which the sensor is embedded produce undetectable accelerative beam displacements < Δx_{min}.)

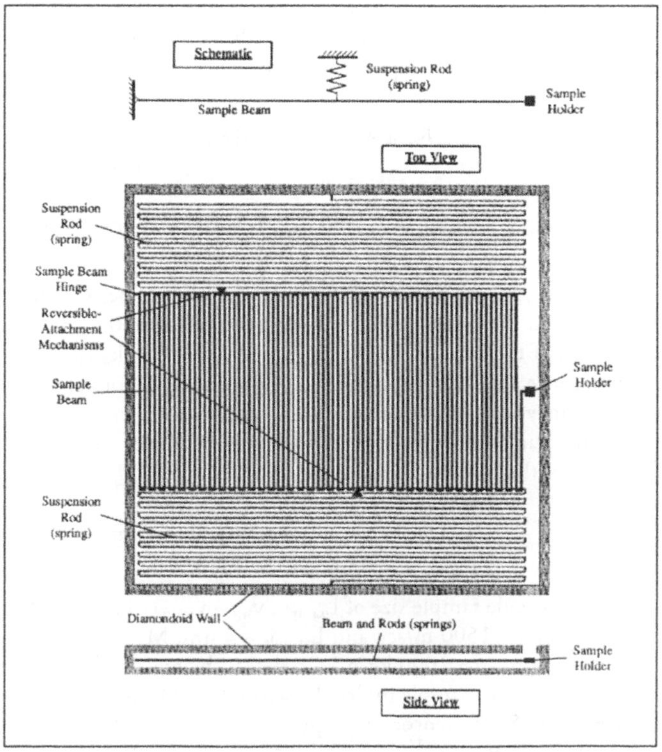

Fig. 4.6. Single-proton massometer sensor using coiled suspension-spring cantilever.

**The l_{rod}^3 dependence of k_s is not strictly valid for a folded structure because the forces at the end of a folded spring have a smaller mechanical advantage, so the structure acts somewhat stiffer. Further investigation is warranted. However, a large number of alternative low-stiffness structures are available including van der Waals contacts with low loading, gas springs, diamagnetic traps and actively controlled electrostatic traps [J. Soreff, personal communication, 1997].*

Moving the suspension rod closer to the sample holder reduces device sensitivity. For $L_{spring} = L_{beam}$, minimum $\Delta MW \sim 1200$ protons, permitting moderately large molecules to be weighed in minimum time ($\sim 10^{-6}$ sec). Using a very thin sensor configuration ($h_{sensor} \sim 20$ nm) and coils occupying ~50% of sensor cavity space, sensor dimensions are $(79\ nm)^2 \times 20$ nm giving a massometer volume $\sim 10^5\ nm^3$ or ~0.01% of the total volume of a 1 $micron^3$ nanorobot. Sensor mass is $\sim 3 \times 10^{-19}$ kg, including diamondoid housing and prorated share of support mechanisms. If one measurement cycle including sample loading/unloading operations can be completed every ~10 microsec, then the device processes its own mass of glucose molecules in ~10 sec. Note that biological molecules weighed in air or in vacuo may lose water of hydration, whereas weighing in water presents other complications that merit further investigation.

J. Soreff points out that for a molecule on a spring, the precision of the measurement is linked to the sharpness of the resonance, which is optimized to the degree the vibrational frequency of the spring/molecular mass system is kept well below the vibrational resonance frequencies of the molecule itself. The following discussion reports the results of a simple lumped-element analysis of the effects of internal vibration on the massometer completed for the author by J. Soreff, which confirms the previously described performance estimates for the massometer.

Suppose that it is desired to weigh some mass M to a precision ΔM by attaching it to a weak measuring spring (spring constant k_{weak}) and measuring the shift in resonant frequency. The shift in frequency due to coupling to an internal mode of the sample must be less than $(1/2)\ (\Delta M\ /\ M)\ (1\ /\ 2\ \pi)\ (k_{weak}/M)^{1/2}$. If the sample has some lowest internal mode frequency ν_{int}, then approximating the sample as two M/2 masses separated by x_{strong} connected by a strong spring (k_{strong}) gives $\nu_{int} = (1/\pi)\ (k_{strong}/M)^{1/2}$. If this sample is attached to a weak measuring spring of length x_{weak}, which is in turn attached to a rigid support, then the equations of motion are:

$$(M/2)\, x''_{strong} = -\, k_{weak}\, x_{weak} + k_{strong}\left(x_{strong} - x_{weak}\right) \quad \text{\{Eqn. 4.26\}}$$

$$(M/2)\, x''_{strong} = k_{strong}\left(x_{weak} - x_{strong}\right) \quad \text{\{Eqn. 4.27\}}$$

Setting $x_{weak} = e^{st}$ and $x_{strong} = R\ e^{st}$ where t = time, s = time constant, and $R = -(1 + (2\ k_{weak}\ /\ M\ s^2))$, and since the angular frequencies of the two springs are $\omega_{strong} = 2\ \pi\ \nu_{int} = 2\ (k_{strong}/M)^{1/2}$ and $\omega_{weak} = (k_{weak}/M)^{1/2}$, then the lower frequency solution for $\omega_{weak} << \omega_{strong}$ may be approximated by $s = i\ \omega_{weak}\ (1 - \omega_{weak}^2\ /\ 2\ \omega_{strong}^2)$ and so the (undesired) fractional change in frequency due to the flexibility of the object to be weighed is

$$\omega_{weak}/\omega_{strong} < \left(\Delta M/M\right)^{1/2} \quad \text{\{Eqn. 4.28\}}$$

For a molecule sample size of L_{sample}, $\nu_{int} \sim \nu_{sound}\ /\ L_{sample} \sim 500$ GHz for $\nu_{sound} \sim 1500$ m/sec and $L_{sample} \sim 3$ nm; $M = \rho\ L_{sample}^3 = 2.7 \times 10^{-23}$ kg for $\rho = 1000\ kg/m^3$. To detect the mass difference of a single proton in a sample molecule, sensor $Q = M\ /\ m_p = 16{,}000$; from Eqn. 4.28, the sensor may operate at a factor of $Q^{1/2}$ below ν_{int}, or $\nu_{spring} \sim \nu_{int}\ /\ Q^{1/2} \sim 4$ GHz. A period of 0.25 nanosec is slightly too short to allow a phase shift of $\Delta t_{min} \sim 1$ nanosec, since the period is only one-quarter of this. However, a phase shift of π radians should accumulate in $t_{meas} = Q\ /\ 2\ \nu_{spring} \sim 2$ microsec and should be detectable by looking at magnitudes of forces. Interestingly, an SPM microprobe of circular cross-section and exponential profile with a 0.1 nm^2 tip has been proposed that could also reach ~proton mass detection sensitivity at room temperature and 1 atm pressure with an eigenmode frequency of 10 GHz;[1195] an electrically-driven carbon nanotube-based resonant-beam balance demonstrated $\sim 10^{-17}$ kg ($\sim 10^{10}$ proton or ~0.01 $micron^3$ mass) sensitivity in 1999.[3023]

Existing surface acoustic wave (SAW) devices[458] are chemical sensors that can measure areal mass densities as small as 80 picogram/cm^2, or 0.01 N_2 molecule per nm^2 of surface, though current devices are limited to ~$micron^2$ areas. A proposed quartz microresonator microbalance could detect a 10^{-6} molecular monolayer,[459] the equivalent of 5×10^{-9} molecule per nm^2. Detection of ~400 million protons using an MRFM vibrating rod ~60 nm thick was demonstrated by Rugar[3256] in 1998.

4.4.4 Isotope Discrimination

It will often be useful in nanomedicine to distinguish molecules containing different isotopes of the same chemical elements, for example to count the number of organic molecules in a sample that contain radioactive C^{14} atoms in place of stable C^{12} atoms or to make direct assays of heavy radiometal-contaminated tissues. Nanodevices may also sort isotopically heteronuclear molecules into homonuclear fractions, for example to separate deuterochemicals from hydrochemicals or to acquire isotopically pure materials with which to construct:

a. small, high-speed rotors with precisely balanced mass distributions;[10]

b. components with extremely fine size differences (Section 3.5.6);

c. nanostructures with maximum thermal conductivity (Table 4.1), or mixed isotopes to reduce thermal conductivity (Section 6.3.4.4 (D)); or

d. long-lived isotopically pure structures that generate no internal radioactivity, thus promoting longer device lifetimes (Chapter 13).

The most reliable sensor for discriminating among isotopes within target molecules is the single-proton massometer (Section 4.4.3). Isotopes of any chemical element differ in mass by at least ~1 neutron (~protonic) increments. Thus a massometer with single-proton resolution can resolve all isotopes starting from chemically pure samples. Isobars (atoms having the same mass number) and isotones (atoms having the same number of neutrons) may be finally resolved chemically; nuclear isomers differing in mass by ~0.001 amu cannot be resolved. Teragravity centrifugation (Section 3.2.5) and time-of-flight particle-beam deflection techniques (Section 4.7.1) may also prove useful.

Isotopes vary in many subtle ways due to their mass differences, although it is not yet clear how a potential isotope nanosensor might exploit some or all of these distinctions:

A. *Line Shifts* — The electronic energy states of atoms or molecules depend on the reduced nuclear mass, causing a spectral line shift of ~1.0005 between hydrogen and deuterium, less among heavier isotopes, detectable spectroscopically.

B. *Hyperfine Structure* — Isotopes differ in electrical quadrupole moment, nuclear spin and magnetic moment, giving rise to hyperfine structure in the optical spectra, especially in the heavier elements. For example, the magnetic moments of hydrogen and deuterium (2.79268 and 0.857387 nuclear magnetons, respectively) are distinguishable via NMR (Section 4.8.3). The NMR frequency in a 10 kilogauss magnetic field is 42.5759 MHz for H, 6.53566 MHz for D. Of course, not all isotopes are NMR sensitive.

Table 4.1 Isotopic Variation in Bulk Properties Possibly Useful in Nanomedicine[390,475,476,763,1309,2325,2690,2703,2962-2964]

Bulk Property	Units	Common Isotope	Rarer Isotope	Comments
Absolute density	kg/m^3	997.044 (H_2O)	1104.45 (D_2O)	at 25°C
Critical density	kg/m^3	325 (H_2O)	363 (D_2O)	
Critical pressure	atm	218.5 (H_2O)	218.6 (D_2O)	
Critical temperature	°C	374.2 (H_2O)	371.5 (D_2O)	
Temperature of maximum density	°C	3.98 (H_2O)	11.2 (D_2O)	
Freezing point	°C	0 (H_2O)	3.82 (D_2O)	
Boiling point	°C	100 (H_2O)	101.42 (D_2O)	
Triple point (solid/liquid/vapor)	K	13.96 (H_2)	18.73 (D_2)	
Triple point (Ice I/Ice III/liquid)	K	251.2 (H_2O)	254.4 (D_2O)	at 2054/2181 atm (H_2O/D_2O)
Heat of fusion	kcal/mole	0.028 (H_2)	0.047(D_2)	at triple point
Heat of vaporization	kcal/mole	9.70 (H_2O)	9.96 (D_2O)	
Heat of formation	kcal/mole	-68.32 (H_2O)	-70.41 (D_2O)	liquids at 25°C
Formation rection equilibrium constant	---	41.553 (H_2O)	42.664 (D_2O)	logarithm at 25°C, liquid state
Electrochemical reaction potential	volts	0 ($2H^+ + 2e = H_2$)	-0.044 ($2D^+ + 2e = D_2$)	at 25°C
Thermodynamic entropy	cal/K	16.72 (H_2O)	18.16 (D_2O)	liquids at 25°C
Lower limit of inflammability	% conc.	4.65% (H_2)	5.0% (D_2)	combustion in O_2 at 1 atm
Upper limit of inflammability	% conc.	93.9% (H_2)	95.0% (D_2)	combustion in O_2 at 1 atm
Surface tension	joule/m^2	0.07275 (H_2O)	0.0678 (D_2O)	at 20°C
Absolute viscosity	kg/m-sec	0.001002 (H_2O)	0.00126 (D_2O)	at 20°C
Dielectric constant	---	80.36 (H_2O)	79.755 (D_2O)	at 20°C
Refractive index	---	1.33300 (H_2O)	1.32844 (D_2O)	
Solubilities	gm NaCl/liter	359 (H_2O)	305 (D_2O)	at 20°C
Aqueous dissociation constant	---	1.79×10^{-5} (NH_4OH)	1.10×10^{-5} (ND_4OH)	K_b, 25°C, 0.1-0.01N
Thermal conductivity	watts/m-K	~3000 (pure C^{12})	2000 (1% C^{13})	diamond at room temperature
Thermal diffusivity	cm^2/sec	18.5 (0.1% C^{13})	12.3 (1% C^{13})	diamond at room temperature
Isothermal compressibility	kg/m^3	1250 (H_2O)	1390 (D_2O)	at 12,000 atm, 37°C
Ionization energy	---	13.9965(H_2O)	14.869 (D_2O)	logarithm at 25°C
Ion mobilities	(mole/liter)^2	1.008×10^{-14} (H_2O)	1.54×10^{-15} (D_2O)	ion product at 25°C
Molar magnetic susceptibility	cm^3/mole	-12.97×10^{-6} (H_2O)	-12.76×10^{-6} (D_2O)	liquids at 20°C
Superfluidity transition temperature	K	2.12 (He^4)	0.003 (He^3)	near absolute zero
Superconductivity transition temperature	K	9 (PdH)	10 (PdD)	
Reversible glass/liq. transition, Ice Ih	K	129 (H_2O)	134 (D_2O)	
Acoustic wave speed	m/sec	1284 (H_2)	890 (D_2)	at STP
Acoustic wave speed temp. dependence	m/sec-K	+2.2 (H_2)	+1.6 (D_2)	at 1 atm
Isotope-exchange chemical reaction rates	m^6/sec	6.05×10^{-46} ($O^{16}+O^{32}{}_2$)	9.26×10^{-46} ($O^{16}+O^{36}{}_2$)	ozone formation
Relative crystal lattice constant	---	1 (natural Ge)	1.00002 (Ge^{76})	at 27°C
Tunneling vibrational voltage	millivolts	358 (C_2H_2)	266 (C_2D_2)	at 8 K

C. *Vibrations and Rotations* — Molecular spectra are especially sensitive to isotopic changes, since the quanta of vibrational and rotational energies are directly dependent upon the masses of the atoms involved, and there are also some subtle effects from differences in nuclear spin. Separations are commonly achieved by laser excitation.

D. *Cross-Sections* — Isotopes have different thermal neutron capture cross sections; for instance, the cross-section of C^{12} is 3.7×10^{-3} barns (1 barn = 10^{-24} cm^2) compared to 9×10^{-4} barns for C^{13} and $<10^{-6}$ barns for C^{14}. (Electron scattering might be better, since the electron is less likely to cause the nucleus to fission and it is generally difficult to use neutrons to probe samples on the molecular scale.) Similarly, the neutron cross-section for H_2O is 0.6 barns compared to 9.2×10^{-4} barns for D_2O.

E. *Other Properties* — Isotopes differ slightly in various bulk properties, many of which could be measured in submicron-scale aliquots by nanosensors. The ability of both large mammals and micron-size photosynthetic plant cells to preferentially concentrate C^{12} or C^{13} in organic matter,[1094] and the predicted ability of carbon nanotubes to selectively extract tritium from low-concentration H_2-T_2 mixtures,[3046] constitute proofs of principle that at least some of the bulk properties listed in Table 4.1 may become useful in achieving nanoscale isotopic separation orpurification.

4.5 Pressure Sensing

This Section describes the ability of medical nanodevices to detect and measure fluid pressure variations while functioning inside the human body. Generation of acoustic signals for power transmission (Section 6.3.2), communication (Section 7.2.1), and navigation (Section 8.3.3) are considered elsewhere. Acoustic macrosensing is described in Section 4.9.1.

4.5.1 Minimum Detectable Pressure

A change in the ambient pressure in a fluid environment (ΔP) may be determined by measuring the change in volume (ΔV) of a fixed quantity of gas at constant temperature, relative to a known sensor volume at a known reference pressure. (Thermal sensors elsewhere in the nanorobot provide readings by which corrections can be made for temperature variations.) If the sensor volume consists of a cylinder of fixed cross-sectional area, the change in volume is converted into a linear displacement of a piston located at the interface between gas and fluid environment. The change in Gibbs free energy[10] is $\Delta G = \Delta P\ \Delta V$, while thermal noise ~kT. Pressure sensor signal/noise ratio SNR ~ ln ($\Delta P\ \Delta V$ / kT), so at the minimum ΔG the minimum detectable pressure ΔP_{min} is measured at the maximum possible volume change, or V_{sensor} (the sensor volume), given approximately by

$$\Delta P_{min} \sim kT\ e^{SNR} / V_{sensor} \qquad \text{\{Eqn. 4.29\}}$$

using the classical ideal gas formulation. At SNR = 2, a $(22\ nm)^3 = 10^4\ nm^3$ sensor (~5×10^5 atoms or ~10^{-20} kg for a cube with 1 nm thick walls) can detect a minimum pressure change ΔP_{min} ~ 0.03 atm; a $(680\ nm)^3 = 0.3\ micron^3$ sensor (~3×10^9 atoms, ~6×10^{-17} kg) detects $\Delta P_{min} \sim 10^{-6}$ atm, probably near the practical limit for mobile in vivo medical nanodevices. Note that ΔP_{min} scales approximately as the inverse cube of mean sensor dimension, and immunity to thermal noise scales exponentially with sensor volume. Current silicon micromachined pressure sensors are ~1 mm^3 with 10^{-3} atm sensitivity,[456,457] a factor of ~10^{12} poorer sensitivity than the theoretical minimum for their size. (A field-effect chemical sensor with an active sensing volume of 0.1 mm^3 that measures pressure indirectly has detected a 10^{-11} atm step in hydrogen gas with t_{meas} ~ 3 sec,[458] only a factor of 1000 above the theoretical minimum for a sensor of that size.) The human ear can detect pressure waves as small as 2×10^{-10} atm.

A less sensitive approach relies on the observation that a change in pressure P alters both density and bulk modulus of a compressed fluid, variations that may be detected by measuring the change in the speed of sound v_s in the working fluid, given by

$$v_s = (B/\rho)^{1/2} \qquad \text{\{Eqn. 4.30\}}$$

where B is bulk modulus of the fluid and ρ is fluid density. $(dB/dP)/B$ may be up to several times larger than $(d\rho/dP)/\rho$ for molecular fluids, but there is some $(dv_s/dP)/v_s$ for each fluid. Differentiating Eqn. 4.30 with respect to P and using $d\rho/dP = \rho/B$, then $dv_s/dP = (dB/dP - 1) / 2\rho^{1/2} B^{1/2}$. For water at 1 atm, dB/dP ~ 8.4 atm/atm,[567] ρ ~1000 kg/m^3 and B = 22,000 atm, giving dv_s/dP ~ 0.25 m/sec-atm. If Δv_s is the measured change in acoustic speed, then:

$$\Delta P_{min} = \Delta v_s / (dv_s/dP) \qquad \text{\{Eqn. 4.31\}}$$

Velocity can be measured to ~0.1 mm/sec accuracy using a micron-scale velocity sensor and t_{meas} ~ 1 sec (Section 4.3.2), so a minimum Δv_s ~ 0.1 mm/sec implies ΔP_{min} ~ 0.0004 atm.

4.5.2 Spatial Pressure Gradients

Two 0.3-micron^3 pressure sensors located at either end of a 1-micron nanorobot could detect pressure changes as small as 10^{-6} atm per micron, a ~1 atm/m spatial gradient. The maximum detectable gradient would involve adjacent measurements of minimum (10^{-6} atm) and maximum (~10^4 atm) absolute pressure, a theoretical peak spatial gradient of ~10^{16} atm/m, though a practical device could not survive exposure to such extreme shear force.

4.5.3 Temporal Pressure Gradients

Driving the sensor at a frequency near ν_{res} may cause large amplitude excursions unless the motion is heavily damped. The lowest possible undamped resonance frequency ν_{res} for piston-type acoustic sensors of size ~ L with minimum spring constant $k_s \sim 2\ kT / L^2$ for a maximally sensitive spring having an energy of ~kT when stretched by L, and piston mass m, is

$$\nu_{res} = \left(\frac{1}{2\pi}\right)\left(\frac{k_s}{m}\right)^{1/2} \qquad \text{\{Eqn. 4.32\}}$$

where $m = \rho L^2 h$ for a piston of area L^2, height h, and density ρ. Assuming h/L = 0.1 and ρ ~ 1000 kg/m^3, ν_{res} = 21 MHz for an L = 22 nm sensor ($k_s = 1.8 \times 10^{-5}$ N/m) and ν_{res} = 4 KHz for an L = 680 nm sensor ($k_s = 1.9 \times 10^{-8}$ N/m). Resonance frequency may be adjusted by selecting appropriate k_s and m. In practical devices resonance will occur at a slightly lower frequency than ν_{res} and with some broadening of the peak, because m should also include the masses of the shank of the piston plus a time-varying portion of the fluid mass occupying the piston's chamber (depending upon the time-varying position of the piston).

Consider the surface of a piston of height h, area L^2 and mass m to which a pressure spike of amplitude P (N/m^2) and frequency ν_{driven} is applied, producing a stroke length X_{stroke}. The solution for the equation of motion of an undamped forced harmonic oscillator has a maximum amplitude of $X_{stroke} = F_{spike} / \text{abs}(\ m\ (\omega_{driven}^2 - \omega_{res}^2))$ where $\omega = 2\pi\nu$, $F_{spike} = P L^2$ and m is defined above. The driving frequency that produces stroke length X_{stroke} = L is given by:

$$\nu_{driven} = \left(\frac{1}{2\pi}\right)\left[\left(\frac{P}{\rho L h}\right) - 4\pi^2 \nu_{res}^2\right]^{1/2} \qquad \text{\{Eqn. 4.33\}}$$

For an L = 22 nm sensor driven to full throw by a minimum detectable ΔP_{min} = 0.03 atm pressure spike (again taking h/L = 0.1 and ρ ~ 1000 kg/m^3), ν_{driven} = 34 MHz; ν_{driven} = 45 GHz when the sensor is driven to full throw by the maximum possible pressure spike P_{max} = 39,000 atm consistent with water remaining in the liquid state (see below). The piston may be driven at these frequencies, or slower, using triangular-wave pulse trains of pressure spikes of these magnitudes.

For an L = 680 nm sensor driven to full throw by a minimum detectable $\Delta P_{min} = 10^{-6}$ atm pressure spike, ν_{driven} = 6 KHz; ν_{driven} = 1.5 GHz when the sensor is driven to full throw by the maximum pressure spike P_{max} = 39,000 atm.

What is the maximum tolerable pressure spike in aqueous media? The requirement of subsonic piston motion in water gives the highest maximum: $P_{max} < (1/2)\ \rho\ v_{sound}^2$ (N/m^2), if ρ = 3510 kg/m^3 for a solid diamondoid piston and the speed of sound v_s ~ 1450 m/sec in water (Eqn. 4.30) for bulk modulus $B_{water} = 2.2 \times 10^9$ N/m^2, ρ_{water} = 1000 kg/m^3, giving P_{max} < 39,000 atm. However, rapid dissipative pressure spikes P_{max} > 26,000 atm add sufficient energy to boil 310 K water, and isothermal static compression of pure water at 310 K causes crystallization into Ice VI near ~11,500 atm. Additional restrictions on (and features of) high-frequency pressure transducers are described in Sections 6.3.3, 6.4.1, and 7.2.2.

4.5.4 Ullage Sensors

It will often be necessary to determine the degree to which a fluid storage tank is full or empty. In most circumstances, an ullage sensor may consist of a simple static pressure sensor embedded in the tank wall, with readout calibrated according to the van der Waals equation for gases and liquids (Section 10.3.2). A fractal network of chemical sensors permeating the internal volume of the tank could provide continuous readouts of local concentration which could be integrated to estimate total storage in the tank. The force required to rotate a paddle inside the tank would increase as a tank was filled, due to the increase in net viscosity of the contents (Section 9.4.1.1). Transmission time of thermal or acoustic pulses might also give some measure of fluid concentration and physical phase. C. Phoenix suggests storing liquids in a piston, allowing direct and precise molecular volume readout, in designs where this is convenient; in theory, a piston that slides the minimum measurable distance of ~10 pm (Section 4.3.1) within the 2-nm-diameter throat of a water-filled cylinder could detect the removal of a single water molecule from the column.

4.6 Thermal Nanosensors

The ability of medical nanodevices to measure both absolute temperature and changes in temperature is crucial for monitoring in vivo physiological thermoregulatory mechanisms and intracellular energy transactions. Precision thermal sensing is also important within nanoscale devices to provide corrective input for pressure, chemical, and displacement sensors, and to improve the stability of onboard clocks. General limits of thermal sensing are considered in Section 4.6.1, followed by several proposals for specific implementations.

4.6.1 Minimum Detectable Temperature Change

A sensor system consisting of N atoms has (3N-6) internal coordinates and thus ~(3N-6) oscillators, each with an average energy of ~kT assuming no modes are high enough to be frozen out. However, the standard deviation of the energy of the oscillators around the mean energy is ~kT, and these energy fluctuations are uncorrelated (ignoring coupling between the oscillators), so (3N-6) of them will have an average fluctuation of kT $(3N\text{-}6)^{1/2}$. (By comparison, the energy in one 10-micron infrared photon is ~5 kT.) As a result, an instantaneous measurement of the total energy of all N atoms gives a minimum detectable temperature change ΔT_{min} of

$$\Delta T_{min} / T = (3N-6)^{-1/2} \sim (3N_{meas}\, n_d\, V_{sensor})^{-1/2}$$

{Eqn. 4.34}

for a set of N_{meas} independent temperature measurements using a sensor of volume V_{sensor} constructed with material of atomic number density n_d, which might be maximized using diamond (n_d = 1.76 x 10^{29} carbon atoms/m^3).

Thermal equilibration time $t_{EQ} \sim L^2 C_V / K_t$ (Eqn. 10.24) for a sensor of size L, of heat capacity C_V (1.8 x 10^6 joules/m^3-K for diamond) and of thermal conductivity K_t (2000 watts/m-K for diamond[460]). Thus, $t_{EQ} \sim 10^{-13}$ sec for a sensor of size L = 10 nm, 10^{-11} sec for L = 100 nm, and 10^{-9} sec for L = 1 micron, so thermal sensors up to 1 micron in size should easily achieve thermal equilibration within a typical measurement cycle time $\Delta t_{min} \sim 10^{-9}$ sec. Sensor measurement time $t_{meas} = N_{meas} \Delta t_{min}$.

A (57 nm)^3 sensor can detect $\Delta T_{min} / T = 10^{-4}$ (~31 millikelvins at 310 K) in a single measurement (N_{meas} = 1), with measurement time t_{meas} ~ 1 nanosec. A sensitivity of $\Delta T_{min} / T = 10^{-6}$ (~310 microkelvins at 310 K) may be achieved using either a ~1 micron^3 sensor with a single measurement (N_{meas} = 1, t_{meas} = 1 nanosec) or a (124 nm)^3 sensor with N_{meas} = 1000 independent measurement cycles and t_{meas} = 1 microsec. Finally, a 1 micron^3 sensor can detect $\Delta T_{min} / T = 3 \times 10^{-9}$ (~1 microkelvin at 310 K) with N_{meas} = 100,000 independent sensor cycles, giving a measurement time t_{meas} ~ 100 microsec.

These figures are confirmed by experimental estimates of detector noise temperature, such as $\Delta T_{min} / T = (k / L^3 C_V)^{1/2} \sim 10^{-6}$ for a silicon nitride detector[678] with C_V = 5.2 x 10^6 joules/m^3-K and L ~ 1 micron. It has been calculated that sensitivity of ~1 microkelvin is theoretically possible using quartz electronic microresonators as precision thermometers.[462,1699] Thermocouple probes with 100 nm tips have already shown ~100 microkelvin sensitivity,[463] tunneling thermometers capable of measuring thermoelectric potential localized to atomic-scale dimensions have been proposed,[464] and experiments leading toward "yoctocalorimetry" were being pursued in 1998.[2928]

For comparison, heat sensors in human skin have $\Delta T_{min} / T \sim 3$ x 10^{-4} (~90 millikelvins), and the infrared sensor pit of the rattlesnake is sensitive to an energy intensity of ~0.8 pJ/micron^2 in a measurement time t_{meas} ~35 millisec and achieves $\Delta T_{min} / T \sim 3$ x 10^{-6};[701,826] mosquitos register $\Delta T_{min} / T \sim 6$ x 10^{-6} at a distance of ~1 cm.

4.6.2 Piston-Based Temperature Sensors

Consider a coiled cylinder of cross-sectional area A filled with gas at pressure P, with a piston at one end whose movement is resisted by a constant-force spring (Fig. 4.7). Increasing gas temperature from the coldest temperature at which the sensor will operate (piston at maximum ingress), T_0, to some warmer temperature T_1 causes the piston to move from position x_0 to position x_1 while the spring holds pressure constant at P inside the cylinder during the measurement. If Δx is the smallest measurable piston displacement and $\Delta T = T_1 - T_0$, then the poorest accuracy is

$$\Delta T / T_0 = \frac{x_1 - x_0}{x_0} = \frac{\Delta x}{x_0} = N_{meas}^{-1/2} (N+1)^{-1/2} \qquad \text{\{Eqn. 4.35\}}$$

because Δx has a thermal noise component as well,[10] and the number of gas molecules $N = n_d V_{sensor}$ where $n_d \sim 10^{28}$ gas molecules/m^3 at P = 1000 atm (Table 10.2). Sensitivity is maximized at the largest feasible x_0; for $\Delta T / T_0 = 10^{-6}$ (~300 microkelvins at 310 K) and $\Delta x = \Delta x_{min}$ = 1 nm (Section 4.2.1), then x_0 = 1000 microns, N = 10^9 gas molecules at 1000 atm (using the van der Waals equation of state) and 310 K taking N_{meas} = 1000, giving $V_{sensor} = 10^{-19}$ m^3 and thus a cylinder cross-sectional area of $A = V_{sensor} / x_0$ = (10 nm)^2. There are ~1000 gas molecules per nanometer of cylinder length, each traveling with mean thermal velocity v_t ~ 500 m/sec (Eqn. 3.3). Tightly coiled into a cubical volume, the folded sensor size is $L_{sensor} \sim V_{sensor}^{1/3} \sim$ (464 nm)^3 and measurement time $t_{meas} = N_{meas} \Delta t_{min}$ ~ 1 microsec. Sensor mass is ~10^{-16} kg.

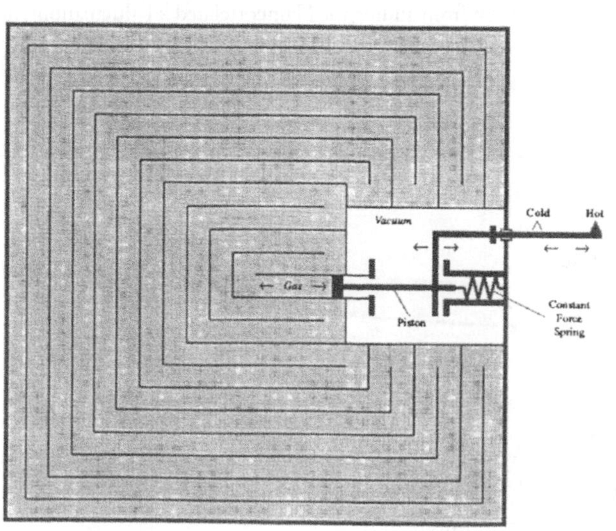

Fig. 4.7. Two-dimensional representation of a three-dimensional micro-kelvin piston-based coiled-cylinder temperature sensor.

The coiled tube design, though not strictly necessary, is nonetheless convenient because it allows a continuous sensor element to be arbitrarily distributed through the nanorobot volume, to be concentrated in multiple specific interior regions, or to be placed inside nanorobot components that will be required to flex such as metamorphic protuberances. If instead the working gas is placed in a cubical box of side L_{box} with a sensor piston of area A_p, any change in temperature causes the piston to move a distance $\Delta x = (L_{box}^3/A_p)(\Delta T / T_0) \sim (k T_0 / k_s)^{1/2}$, where $k_s = (A_p/L_{box}^2)(N kT_0 / L_{box}^2)$, from Drexler;[10] hence

$$\Delta T / T_0 \sim \left(A_p / N L_{box}^2\right)^{1/2} \qquad \text{\{Eqn. 4.36\}}$$

which argues for a small piston, a large box, and a high operating pressure to achieve maximum sensitivity. For A_p = 100 nm², N = 10^9 molecules, and L_{box} = 464 nm, $\Delta T / T \sim 10^{-6}$.

4.6.3 Thermal-Expansion Temperature Sensors

Consider a thin rod of length x and width w, constructed as a sandwich of two dissimilar materials each of thickness h, having coefficients of linear expansion α_1 and α_2, respectively (Fig. 4.8). When heated, the two materials expand differentially to lengths of $x(1 + \alpha_i \Delta T)$ (neglecting the quadratic and higher-order terms in α_i), producing a cantilever deflection of $\theta_t = (x/h)(\alpha_1 - \alpha_2)$ (radians) from simple geometry. The minimum detectable temperature change $\Delta T_{min} = 2 \pi \Delta x_{min} / x \theta_t$ or

$$\Delta T_{min} = \frac{8 \pi h^3 w^2 \Delta x_{min}}{(\alpha_1 - \alpha_2) V_{rod}^2} \qquad \text{\{Eqn. 4.37\}}$$

where volume of the sandwich rod V_{rod} = 2 h w x. Taking Δx_{min} = 10 pm, $\alpha_1 = 2.38 \times 10^{-5}$ /K for aluminum,[460] $\alpha_2 = 8 \times 10^{-7}$ /K for diamond at 310 K,[460] h = w = 5 nm, and assuming sensor volume $V_{sensor} \sim 2 V_{rod}$ in a tightly packed three-dimensional coil configuration, ΔT_{min} = 1 microkelvin for an $L^3 \sim (227\ \text{nm})^3$ sensor ~ 1% of the volume of a 1-micron nanorobot. Use of a suitable negative-coefficient material for α_2, such as the ceramics zirconium tungstate[1025] and cordierite, can further reduce L by 5%-10%.

Measuring the volume of the sensor is essentially like taking an inventory of total stored thermal energy, which has a $kT N^{1/2}$ fluctuation term from adding the N uncorrelated kT fluctuations; hence

$$\Delta T / T_0 \sim \left(N_{meas}\, n_d\, V_{sensor}\right)^{-1/2} \qquad \text{\{Eqn. 4.38\}}$$

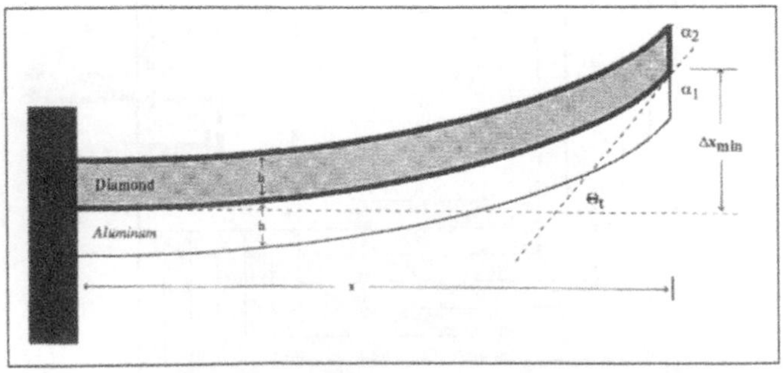

Fig. 4.8. Thermal expansion temperature sensor (schematic representation only).

Hence, to achieve $\Delta T \sim 1$ microkelvin at T_0 = 310 K with this sensor may require $N_{meas} \sim 47$ million independent measurements of Δt_{min} = 1 nanosec each, or $t_{meas} \sim 47$ millisec.

Micromechanical silicon cantilever heat sensors (microcalorimeters) of ~20,000 micron³ volume have already achieved ΔT_{min} = 10 microkelvins at room temperature ($\Delta T_{min} / T \sim 3 \times 10^{-8}$), responding to ~1 pJ of heat in a measurement time $t_{meas} \sim 1$ millisec.[461] Thermal-expansion nanosensors might also exploit the temperature sensitivity of viscoelastic materials (e.g., modulus of relaxation).

4.6.4 Mechanochemical Temperature Sensors

Since binding rates are temperature sensitive, a chemical concentration sensor using steric probes immersed in a sample containing a precisely known concentration of target ligands can be used as a temperature sensor. Similarly, enzyme reaction rates increase with a change in temperature according to

$$\Delta T = \frac{10 \ln(k_2/k_1)}{\ln(Q_{10})} \qquad \text{\{Eqn. 4.39\}}$$

where $\Delta T = T_2 - T_1$, k_1 and k_2 are the reaction rate constants at temperatures T_1 and T_2, and Q_{10} is the well-known temperature coefficient—the ratio of the rates of reaction measured at two temperatures 10°C apart. $Q_{10} \sim 2$ for most enzymes, but may range up to 4 for some enzymes that catalyze reactions with unusually high activation energies. Assuming $Q_{10} \sim 4$, the (112 nm)³ sensor with $\Delta c / c$ = 0.01(1%) from Section 4.2.2 can distinguish temperatures 0.07 K apart; the huge (1.44 micron)³ sensor with $\Delta c / c = 10^{-5}$ (0.001%) resolves $\Delta T \sim 72$ microkelvins. Because of their relative volumetric inefficiency, such sensors are best used in large ΔT applications. Similar considerations apply to thermal sensors based on the temperature sensitivity of protein folding (as in heat shock protein mediators of cellular responses to a 5 K change[465,466]), protein thermal contraction,[1261] and thermal conformation rate constants for protein α helices that typically coil in $\sim 10^{-6}$ sec.[467,2324] The quantum tunneling transmission coefficient for ion channels is also exquisitely temperature-sensitive[679] and thus could serve as the basis of a nanoscale thermal sensor.

4.6.5 Spatial Thermal Gradients

Two (200-400 nm)³ thermal sensors located at either end of a 1-micron nanorobot can detect temperature changes as small as 10^{-6} K per micron, a ~1 kelvin/m spatial gradient. The maximum detectable gradient in nanomedical systems would involve adjacent measurements differing by ~100°C, a peak spatial gradient of ~10^8 kelvins/m. The detection event must be completed before the two sensors can thermally equilibrate, e.g., $t_{meas} < t_{EQ} = L^2 C_V / K_t$ (Eqn. 10.24). If the material between the sensors is mostly diamondoid, then $t_{EQ} \sim 10^{-9}$ sec; if mostly water, then $t_{EQ} \sim 10^{-5}$ sec, for L = 1 micron.

4.6.6 Temporal Thermal Gradients

On the timescale of nanomachine operations, typically 10^{-9} - 10^{-6} sec, the human body provides an essentially isothermal operating regime. However, medical nanorobots circulating in the bloodstream may encounter ΔT of ~3 K during one circulation time ~60 sec under normal circumstances (Section 8.4.1), a temporal thermal gradient of ~0.1 kelvin/sec, or >10 kelvin/sec at 1 mm tissue depth for a fingertip placed on a 600 K stove. Thermal nanosensors can take independent measurements differing by as much as ~100°C in ~10^{-9} sec (e.g., Section 4.6.2), giving a maximum detectable thermal gradient of 10^{11} kelvins/sec, far in excess of physiological rates.* Detection of the minimum ~1 microkelvin change between two measurements taken 1 sec apart probably represents the minimum practical temperature gradient, ~1 microkelvin/sec. For comparison, the record-holder in the insect world is the eyeless cave beetle *Speophyes lucidulus*, whose antennae can detect thermal change rates as small as ~3000 microkelvins/sec.[812]

The extraordinary thermal conductivity of diamond ensures that endogenous nanorobot waste heat is rapidly conducted to the surrounding aqueous medium. For example, a 1 micron^3 diamondoid nanorobot generating 10 picowatts of onboard power at its core experiences a temperature differential of ~10^{-8} K between core and perimeter (using thermal conductivity K_t = 2000 watts/m-K for diamond[460]), well below minimum detectable limits.

4.7 Electric and Magnetic Sensing

4.7.1 Electric Fields

The electric field E (volts/m) caused by a single point charge q (e.g., an electron or singly-charged ion) is given by Coulomb's law as

$$E = \frac{q_e}{4 \pi \varepsilon_0 \kappa_e r^2} \qquad \text{\{Eqn. 4.40\}}$$

where $q_e = 1.60 \times 10^{-19}$ coul (one charge), $\varepsilon_0 = 8.85 \times 10^{-12}$ farad/m (permittivity constant), κ_e = dielectric constant of the matter traversed by the electric field (κ_e = 74.31 for pure water at 310 K, 5.7 for diamond, 1 for vacuum or air), and r = distance from the charge, in meters. The field at a distance of 1 nm from a point charge is ~10^9 volts/m in air, 2 x 10^7 volts/m in water. The force between two unit charges F = q_e E = 230 pN in air, 3 pN in water, at 1-nm separation.

What is the magnitude of electric fields likely to be encountered in nanomedical situations? Electric fields in the human body may be generated from internal or external sources. Internally, ions and individual molecules may carry static electric fields. For example, the surface of an isolated charged amino acid (Section 3.5.5) has ~1 charge/nm^2. Debye-Huckel shielding due to counterion flow in salty fluids (as are found in the human body) reduces these fields very rapidly with distance. From Eqn. 3.20, the static field from a single charged amino acid floating in human plasma falls from ~6 x 10^6 volts/m at a range of 1 nm to 0.7 volts/m at r = 10 nm. In plant cells, photosynthetic "receivers" detect gradients in the electrochemical potential of the order of 1 eV across distances on the order of 1 nm, an instantaneous ~10^9 volts/m.

The most important internal electrical sources are the electrochemical gradients caused by gated channel and transporter molecular pump operations at the intracellular level; muscular, membrane, digestive, and neural activity at the intercellular and organ level (see also Section 4.9.3.1); and piezoelectric fields generated by movement of collagenous tissues (e.g., tendon and elastin), bones, and many other biological materials.[1939-1942,3089-3095] Typically these sources generate potentials of 10-100 millivolts over distances of 0.01-10 microns, producing local fields in the range of 10^3-10^7 volts/m. For example, the 50 millivolt transmembrane potential necessary to open a sodium channel corresponds to an electric field of 5 x 10^6 volts/m. (See also Section 4.8.7.) Interestingly, implanted electrical devices such as pacemakers may produce up to 600 volts/m one millimeter from the casing.

External sources may also contribute to detectable nanomedical electric fields within the human body, though usually to a lesser degree. Placing a hand flat between two plates charged to E_p = 3 x 10^6 volts/m (near the breakdown voltage for air) induces an instantaneous field of E ~ E_p / κ_{water} = 42,000 volts/m transversely through the limb. (A DC field induces ion current flows which accumulate surface charge and cancel out the internal field after ~one RC time.) Electric fields directly beneath high-tension power lines are 2,000-11,000 volts/m, or 50-1000 volts/m at a lateral displacement of 25 meters along the ground.[477] Household appliances produce 200-300 volt/m fields;[477] 20 amperes flowing through standard Romex copper wiring in the walls of a house produces 100-600 volts/m in the middle of a room, up to 24,000 volts/m at the wall (E = B / $\mu_0 \varepsilon_0$ c; c = the speed of light, B from Eqn. 4.44); static sparks from carpet walking are ~10,000 volts/m, and ~10^5 volts/m makes hair stand on end. Quiescent atmospheric charge is ~100 volts/m, rising to 5000 volts/m during severe thunder-storms oscillating from positive to negative over a ~10,000 volt/m range. Lightning bolts (~20 coul 0.002-sec discharge) produce 60,000 volt/m spikes at a distance of 10 meters from the strike, 600 volts/m at a range of 1 kilometer. Electron-hole avalanches in semiconductors are initiated by fields $\gtrsim$ 5 x 10^7 volts/m.[129] Penal electrocutions use ~1500 volts/m. (See also Section 7.2.3.)

Direct force sensing of these electric fields is ineffective; from Eqn. 4.40, the minimum detectable field $E_{min} = F_{min} / q$ = 6 x 10^7 volts/m using F_{min} = 10 pN (Section 4.4.1) and a single-charge sensor. Particle deflection seems more efficient. Consider a collimated stream of singly-charged particles, each of mass m and initial velocity V_0 entering an evacuated test chamber of length L and experiencing a uniform electric field E, causing a lateral displacement $\Delta x = q E L^2 / 2 m V_0^2$ measured by the sensor. For this measurement, SNR ~ ln ($m V_0^2$ / 2 kT), so the minimum detectable electric field is

$$E_{min} = \frac{4 kT \Delta x_{min} e^{SNR}}{q L^2} \quad \text{(volts/m)} \qquad \text{\{Eqn. 4.41\}}$$

For Δx_{min} = 10 pm (Section 4.3.1), T = 310 K and SNR = 2, E_{min} = 10,000 volts/m for a sensor of size L = 28 nm, or 100 volts/m for L = 280 nm, allowing measurement of all nanomedically relevant fields that are homogeneous across the entire device. Using the larger 280-nm sensor, time of flight is ~10^{-12} sec for electrons or ~10^{-9} sec for U^{238} ions, permitting t_{meas} ~ 10^{-9} sec and dissipating at least ~30 pW waste heat (due to kinetic impact) in continuous operation. Time-varying electric fields can be measured up to t_{meas}^{-1} ~ GHz frequencies, and electric current may be determined using standard techniques because current density is scale-invariant.[10] Care must be taken to eliminate measurement error due to exogenous magnetic fields. Piezoelectric or other electromechanical transducers can convert electricity into mechanical signals (Section 6.3.5) appropriate for all-mechanical computation and control systems.

Another class of electric field detector of similar size and sensitivity is the electrosensitive gel sensor. For example, the negatively charged heparan sulfate proteoglycan network found in the secretory granule matrix expands 50% in volume within milliseconds of exposure to a ~2 volt/micron field, and the response appears linear with voltage.[498] Thus the length of a 400-nm long gel-filled sensor of fixed cross-sectional area should expand a minimally-detectable 10 pm (= Δx_{min}) in a 100 volt/m field. Similar sensitivities to small periodic fields, analogous to shark electroreceptors (maximum sensitivity ~10^{-7} volts/m,[813]), are found in ion-channel embedded

*Heating and cooling rates during ultrasonic cavitation in water exceed ~10^9 kelvins/sec.[625]

artificial membranes that selectively amplify electric signals in noisy environments via stochastic resonance.[514] Stochastic resonance in neurons permits detection of electric fields as weak as 10 volts/m.[566]

The theoretical limits have been analyzed by Weaver and Astumian[814] and by Block,[810] who conclude that the minimum detectable static field for a hollow spherical sensor of radius r_{sen} and shell membrane thickness d_{mem} (capacitance $C_e = 4 \pi \varepsilon_0 \kappa_e r_{sen}^2 / d_{mem}$) is

$$E_{minDC} = \left(\frac{2}{3 r_{sen}^2}\right)\left(\frac{kT d_{mem}}{4 \pi \varepsilon_0 \kappa_e}\right)^{1/2} \quad \text{(volts/m)} \qquad \text{\{Eqn. 4.42\}}$$

Using κ_e = 74.31 for water at T = 310 K, r_{sen} = 0.5 micron and d_{mem} = 10 nm gives E_{minDC} = 200 volt/m. Increasing r_{sen} to 5 microns reduces E_{min} to ~2 volts/m. To detect a periodic field of frequency ν_e by sampling over ($\nu_e t_{meas}$) cycles for a measurement time t_{meas}, Block[810] gives

$$E_{minAC} = \frac{E_{minDC}}{\left(\nu_e t_{meas}\right)^{1/2}} \quad \text{(volts/m)} \qquad \text{\{Eqn. 4.43\}}$$

Using ν_e = 1 MHz and t_{meas} = 1 sec gives E_{minAC} = 0.2 volt/m. Cylindrical sensors are 10-100 times more sensitive, and sensitivity may possibly be further enhanced by coupling the periodic electric potential to a Michaelis-Menten type enzyme or a similar nanomechanism embedded in the sensor shell to achieve tuning.[814] Fields as small as ~10^{-4} volts/m may be detectable by ~20-micron mammalian living cells;[814] such detection may trigger biochemical observables which may be monitored or eavesdropped by resident nanomedical devices. Submicron-scale electrometers capable of ~0.1 electrons/$Hz^{1/2}$ (charge per unit bandwidth) have been demonstrated experimentally, and also single-electron transistors (SETs) to 10^{-4} electron/$Hz^{1/2}$, with the potential to reach 10^{-6} electron/$Hz^{1/2}$.[2926] Galvanotropic bacteria have been reported in the literature.[3351]

Radiofrequency receivers for power transmission and communication in vivo are described in Sections 6.4.2 and 7.2.3. Antenna radiation patterns may also be useful in diagnostics and macrosensing applications (Section 7.2.3). Piezoelectric macrosensing of bone loads is briefly described in Section 4.9.3.3.

4.7.2 Magnetic Fields

The most significant source of biomagnetic fields, generated by electric charges moving as currents through the body, is neural impulses. The magnetic field generated by these currents is given by Ampere's law as

$$B = \frac{\mu_0 \kappa_m i}{2 \pi r} \qquad \text{\{Eqn. 4.44\}}$$

where B is magnetic flux density (teslas), μ_0 is the permeability constant (~$4\pi \times 10^{-7}$ henry/m), relative permeability κ_m = 1 for most biological materials and in vacuo, i is electric current (~0.2 microamperes for human nerve impulses), and r = distance from the current-carrying conductor. Hence B ~ 0.04 microtesla for r = 1 micron, adjacent to an axonal conductor. For comparison, magnetic fields directly beneath high-tension power lines are 10-40 microtesla, or 2-8 microtesla at a lateral displacement of 25 meters along the ground.[477] Household appliances produce 1-1000 microtesla at a distance of 3 cm and 0.01-2 microtesla at a 1-meter range[477] (electric shavers produce 0.4-60 microtesla at a range of 15 cm[1294]). 20-amp Romex wiring in the walls of a house can produce 2 microtesla in mid-room, up to 80 microtesla at the wall, though in 1998 the average strength in 98% of U.S. homes from artificial sources was 0.05-0.09 microtesla, typical exposures throughout the day were 0.1-1 microtesla, and the federal workplace standard was a maximum of 100 microtesla.[1099] Magnetotactic marsh bacteria,[501] birds and insects[502,503,1089] can detect the geomagnetic field vector (identifying Earth's magnetic poles), which is 30-70 microtesla, depending on geographic position. Behavioral thresholds have been measured as 0.005-0.02 microtesla for pigeons and 0.001-0.01 microtesla for honeybees,[815,816] and no more than 1000-2000 microteslas for human subjects.[1130] Some biochemical changes have been observed in human cells exposed to ~10-100 microtesla 60 Hz fields,[477,1099] although the data are controversial; it appears the fields pump iron atoms through cell membranes, potentially causing peroxidation or other damage to occur. In 1998, transcranial magnetic stimulation was used to expedite recovery of motor skills for stroke patients, and was being explored as a treatment for depression and a means of altering patient mood. Lightning bolts (i ~ 10,000 amp/discharge) produce 200 microtesla spikes at a distance of 10 meters from the strike, 2 microtesla at a range of 1 kilometer.

Computer simulations of a fully heterogeneous human body divided into 37,000 $(1.31 \text{ cm})^3$ voxels produced a maximum induced current of 8.84 amp/m^2 (average ~1 amp/m^2) when the body was exposed to a uniform 60 Hz 1-tesla magnetic field.[930] Patients undergoing Echo-Planar MRI scanning report "tickling" and "pain" when exposed to field changes exceeding 60 tesla/sec; ventricular fibrillation may result from myocardial current densities of 4 amp/m^2, which is induced at 250 tesla/sec.[490]

The simplest magnetosensor is a freely pivoting permanent magnet that experiences a restoring force when the magnet's axis is not aligned with the external field. This "compass effect" is also employed by magnetotactic bacteria, which have ~0.1 micron ferromagnets in magnetosomes in their cells that allow them to detect and track the geomagnetic field vector.[501,2330] Permanent magnets of cross-sectional area A_{magnet} and length l_{magnet} made of Alnico or Alcomax (ρ ~ 8000 kg/m^3) can provide B_{magnet} ~ 1.4 tesla. (In 1998, the record flux density was 13.5 tesla for dipole magnets,[697] ~27 tesla for resistive magnets.[1026]) The force on such a magnet immersed in an external field of flux B is $F = B B_{magnet} A_{magnet} / \mu_0$, so the minimum detectable flux B_{min} is

$$B_{min} = \frac{\mu_0 \kappa_m F_{min}}{B_{magnet} A_{magnet}} \qquad \text{\{Eqn. 4.45\}}$$

If the minimum detectable force is F_{min} = 10 pN (Section 4.4.1), B_{min} = 50 microtesla for A_{magnet} = 0.4 micron^2, about right for magnetotactic bacteria, and B_{min} = 2 microtesla for A_{magnet} = 2 micron^2.

The limitations of force sensing may be avoided by suspending the bar magnet from its center of mass and allowing it to oscillate in vacuo about its stable equilibrium position in the external field B, making a simple harmonic oscillator with period

$$t_{magnet} = 2\pi\left(\frac{\mu_0 \kappa_m I_{mag}}{B B_{magnet} A_{magnet} l_{magnet}}\right)^{1/2} \qquad \text{\{Eqn. 4.46\}}$$

where the moment of inertia $I_{mag} = m_{magnet} ((A_{magnet}/4) + (l_{magnet}^2/12))$. Oscillator energy $E_m \sim B\ B_{magnet}\ A_{magnet}\ l_{magnet}\ /\ \mu_0\ \kappa_m$, so the minimum detectable external field is

$$B_{min} = \frac{\mu_0\ \kappa_m\ kT\ e^{SNR}}{B_{magnet}\ A_{magnet}\ l_{magnet}} \qquad \text{\{Eqn. 4.47\}}$$

For B_{magnet} = 1.4 tesla, $A_{magnet} = (660\ nm)^2$, l_{magnet} = 660 nm, T = 310 K and SNR = 2, then B_{min} = 0.1 microtesla and $t_{magnet} = 6 \times 10^{-4}$ sec ($\sim t_{meas}$), allowing a ~KHz sampling frequency. Magnet mass $m_{magnet} \sim 2 \times 10^{-15}$ kg. Several classes of molecular magnets have been described in the literature.[2598-2600]

Another class of magnetosensor detects the change in dimensions when a magnetic body is magnetized, which is called magnetostriction. For instance, iron-cobalt ferrite expands by $\Delta L\ /\ L \sim 7.5 \times 10^{-4}$ at saturation magnetostriction in a ~1 tesla field, permitting detection of ~10 millitesla field changes using a 1 micron sensor and $\Delta x_{min} \sim 10$ pm. Small magnetostrictive volume changes make possible a sensor of even greater sensitivity. A field of ~0.2 tesla causes a fractional volume increase of $\sim 10^{-6}$ in iron and up to 40×10^{-6} in some iron-nickel (~30% Ni) alloys. A $(370\ nm)^3$ magnetostriction sensor monitored by stretch sensors with displacement sensitivity Δx_{min} = 0.1 nm (~1 atomic radius) can in theory detect $B_{min} \sim 0.1$ microtesla. Magnetostriction is nonlinear with applied field, and there are significant hysteresis effects which may confuse data interpretation. However, multisensor arrays combining positive- and negative-magnetostriction materials should enhance signal extraction. Since the change in volume is small, temperature compensation may be required.

Hall effect probe microscopes have demonstrated 10 microtesla sensitivity with 350 nm spatial resolution,[478] and alternative nanoscale magnetic detectors such as direct-current SQUID (superconducting quantum interference device) magnetometers, stray field devices, and magnetic spin sensors are being developed.[450] In 1999, microSQUID could measure magnetic moments as small as $\sim 10^4$ Bohr magnetons[3274] or $\sim 10^{-19}$ J/tesla, roughly 7×10^6 protons or a 14-nm iron cube. Magnetoencephalographs using SQUID magnetometers to measure external electromagnetic fields produced by neural traffic in the brain can register 10^{-6} - 10^{-3} microtesla signals.[810] Other biomagnetic measurement techniques have helped to investigate electrophysiological disturbances in heart muscle and in the brain.[479] By 1998, microcoils as small as 100 microns in diameter had been constructed using microcontact printing of 25 micron wide silver wires, producing magnetic flux densities >0.4 tesla with a 10 milliamp current, switchable in $<10^{-3}$ sec.[1196]

4.7.3 Optical Sensing

In biosystems and nanosystems alike, the detection of an optical photon is a high-energy event. A single photon of red light at λ = 700 nm carries an energy of 280 zJ, a blue photon at 400 nm conveys 500 zJ, and an ultraviolet (UV) photon at 200 nm transmits 1000 zJ to its receptor. These energies, ranging from 65-234 kT, exceed thermal noise by a wide margin, hence are all easily detectable reliably by suitable nanosensors. Note that optical photon detection does not require a nanosensor the size of one wavelength or larger—for example, 1-nm chlorophyll molecules have no difficulty absorbing 660-nm photons.

Biological systems provide numerous examples of single-photon transducers, including photopigment molecules such as chlorophyll and rhodopsin which mediate electron transfers in $\lesssim$1 picosecond by undergoing conformational changes,[1692] triggering a series of biochemical events. An estimated 100-500 cell membrane channels are affected by the detection of a single optical photon. The first documented case of a physiological role for chlorophyll in animals has been found in the fish *Malacosteus niger*, which uses a chlorophyll derivative to see far-infrared light.[1528] Mammalian cells also act as indirect UV sensors (e.g., see Section 10.4.2.3), as for instance when energy absorption induces perturbations of membrane structure or a conformational change in membrane proteins, activating the JNK cascade below 300 pJ/micron^2,[481] and centrosomes may serve as cellular directional IR sensors in single fibroblast cells.[1960] Integration times for photon sensors are briefly treated in Section 4.9.4.

Artificial "bioelectronic" cyanine-quinone chromophore molecules ~1 nm in size can detect optical photons of wavelengths λ = 580-630 nm, and can trigger and reset in 1-3 picosec (governed by the tunneling times associated with reformation of the zwitterionic states of the inputs[21,480]), in theory permitting ~100 GHz modulations to be received. Exciton-generating poly(p-phenylene vinylene) polymer switches have the potential to achieve ~THz switching speed;[733] a birefringent Kerr medium also switches in a few picoseconds. Chalcogenide glass has viscosity $>10^{13}$ kg/m-sec in darkness, but $\sim 5 \times 10^{11}$ kg/m-sec under illumination.[1306] Proposals for specific implementations of photoergic transducers (Section 6.3.6) and optical cables (Sections 6.4.3.2 and 7.2.5.2) are elsewhere.

4.7.4 Particulate and High-Energy Radiation

High energy photons including x-rays ($\lambda \sim 2$ nm, $\sim 10^5$ zJ or 0.0001 picojoule) and gamma rays ($\lambda \sim 0.002$ nm, ~0.1 picojoule), and ejecta from the decay of radioactive nuclei such as α-particles (helium nuclei, ~1 picojoule) and β-particles (free electrons, 0.01-0.1 picojoule) may be extremely destructive to nanomechanical systems (Chapter 13) and are difficult to reliably measure quantitatively. For example, a charged particle with 0.01 pJ of kinetic energy (K.E.) traversing a decelerative electrostatic field of 10^9 volts/m requires K.E./qE ~ 60 microns to slow to a halt. However, particle-induced visual sensations have been observed by dark-adapted astronauts in space,[504] and Ruderfer[702] has suggested that even solar neutrinos may be detectable by the human brain (though most physicists would find this implausible). The nucleoelectric transducer described in Section 6.3.7.1 could be adapted to serve as a directional α particle sensor.

4.8 Cellular Bioscanning

The goal of cellular bioscanning is the noninvasive and non-destructive in vivo examination of interior biological structures. One of the most common nanomedical sensor tasks is the scanning of cellular and subcellular structures. Such tasks may include localization and examination of cytoplasmic and nuclear membranes, as well as the identification and diagnostic measurement of cellular contents including organelles and other natural molecular devices, cytoskeletal structures, biochemical composition and the kinetics of the cytoplasm.

The precision and speed of medical nanodevices is so great that they can provide a surfeit of detailed diagnostic information well beyond that which is normally needed in classical medicine for a complete analysis of somatic status. Except in the most subtle cases a malfunction in any one component of the cellular machinery (Section 8.5) normally provokes a cascade of pathological observables in many other subsystems. Detection of any one of these cascade observables, if sufficiently unique and well-defined, may provide adequate diagnostic information (see Chapter 18) to plan a proper reparative procedure.

DNA is one of the few cellular components that is regularly inspected and repaired. Most homeostatic systems adopt a more simple philosophy of periodic replacement of components regardless of functionality. Nanomedicine allows the philosophy of inspection and repair to be extended to all cellular components (Chapters 13 and 21). The following discussion briefly describes a few of the sensory techniques that may be useful in achieving this objective.

4.8.1 Cellular Topographics

Tactile topographic scanning provides the most direct means for examining cellular structures in vivo.[484-486,2723-2727] For example, ex vivo live cell scanning in air by commercially available atomic force microscopy (AFM; Section 2.3.3) using a 20-40 nm radius tip allows nondestructive feature resolutions of ~50 nm across the top 10 nm of the cell. Investigators have used the scanning tip to punch a hole in the cell, then pull back and scan the breach, observing the membrane heal itself via self-assembly in real time. Up to ~KHz scanning frequencies are possible, with up to 1024 data points per scan line. The nanomechanical manipulator arm described in Section 9.3.1.4 achieves comparable tip velocities and positional accuracies.

Assuming a scan rate of ~10^6 pixels/sec, a micron-scale nanodevice, once securely anchored (Section 9.4.3.3) to the surface of a (~20 micron)^3 human cell, could employ a tactile scanning probe to image the 0.1% of plasma membrane lying within its (1.4 micron)^2 vicinity in ~2 sec to ~1 nm^2 resolution (~1 mm/sec tip velocity), or ~50 sec to ~0.2 nm (e.g., atomic) resolution (~0.2 mm/sec tip velocity). Inside the cell, and again post-anchoring, an entire 6 micron^2 mitochondrial surface could be imaged to atomic resolution in ~100 sec; the surface of a 100-nm length of 25-nm diameter microtubule could be atomically resolved in 0.2 sec—though of course in a living cell these structures may be changing dynamically during the scanning process. From Eqn. 5.5, continuous power dissipation of a (0.1 micron)^2 scan head moving at 1 mm/sec through water is ~0.002 pW (~kT/pixel at ~10^6 pixels/sec), though of course the energy cost of sensing, recording, and processing each pixel must be at least ~10 kT/pixel (ignoring the possibility of pre-computational image compression), so the total scanner power draw could be as high as 0.02-0.1 pW in continuous operation. Special scanning tips and techniques should allow topographic, roughness, elastic, adhesive, chemical, electrostatic (charge density), conductance, capacitance, magnetic, or thermal surface properties to be measured.

For large (~0.1-1 micron) cellular components, identification and preliminary diagnosis of improper structure may be possible using measured surface characteristics which may be matched to entries in an extensive onboard library, perhaps combined with dynamic monitoring of anomalies in cross-membrane molecular traffic using chemical nanosensors. Most membranes are self-sealing, so it should also be possible to gently insert a telescoping member into the target organelle (Section 9.4.5), which member then slowly reticulates and extrudes smaller probes with sensory tips in a fixed pattern and step size, allowing the acquisition of detailed internal structural and compositional information.

Small (~1-10 nm) protein-based components of the cell such as enzymes, MHC carriers, and ribosomes are self-assembling or require only modest assistance (e.g., molecular chaperones) to self-assemble. Reversible mechanical denaturation of these smaller proteins, using diamondoid probe structure to displace water molecules (thus reducing hydrophobic forces) and by using specialized handling tools akin to functionalized AFM tips and molecular clamps, may be followed by precise nondestructive amino acid sequencing (Chapter 20) to allow identification and diagnostic compositional analysis. Afterward, the protein molecule may be refolded back into its original minimum-energy conformation, possibly with the assistance of chaperone-like structures in some cases.[3045]

4.8.2 Transcellular Acoustic Microscopy

Acoustic microscopy is another noninvasive scanning technique that can provide nanomedically useful spatial resolutions. Frequencies are in the GHz range, far exceeding the relaxation time of the protoplasm. A cryogenic acoustic microscope operated at 8 GHz has demonstrated 20 nm lateral resolution in liquid helium.[482] By 1998, the best resolution achieved with water as the coupling fluid has been 240 nm at a frequency of 4.4 GHz.[488] Operated in water at 310 K, a nanomechanical 1.5 GHz acoustic microscope would achieve a far-field minimum lateral resolution $\lambda/2$ ~ 500 nm, ~10^5 voxels per human cell, sufficient to locate and count all major organelles and a few intermediate-scale structures. Scanning acoustic microscopes (SAM) operated at 2 GHz in reflection mode (which allows detection of interference effects) achieve 30-50 nm resolution in the direction of the acoustical axis, and the Subtraction SAM approach reveals topographical deviations of 7.5 nm at 1 GHz.[483] It has been proposed that picosecond ultrasonics could be used to obtain an image of the cytoskeleton with detail comparable to that of conventional x-ray images of a human skeleton.[1022]

Power requirements are a significant constraint on acoustic reflection microscopy (echolocation). In the simplest case, consider an acoustic emitter of radius r_E which converts an input power of P_{in} into acoustic power of intensity $I_E \le I_{max}$ = 1000 watts/m^2 (Section 6.4.1) with efficiency e%, conservatively taken here to be 0.50 (50%). The emitter produces a train of omnidirectional pressure pulses of amplitude $A_p = (2\ \rho\ v_{sound}\ I_E)^{1/2}$ (N/m^2) (Eqn. 4.53) and frequency ν which travels a distance X_{path} to a target of radius r_T. As the signal reaches the target, its amplitude has been reduced by (r_E / X_{path}) due to the $1/r^2$ dependence of intensity in spherical waves (Section 4.9.1.5) and by $e^{-\alpha_{tiss}\ \nu\ X_{path}}$ by attenuation (Eqn. 4.52) with $\alpha_{tiss} = 8.3 \times 10^{-6}$ sec/m for soft tissue.

Upon reaching the target, a fraction $f_{reflect}$ of the signal is reflected as a point source echo; if the target surface has an acoustic impedance similar to liver tissue and the medium is similar to water, then from Eqn. 4.54 and Table 4.3, $f_{reflect}$ ~ 0.05 (5%). The echo then travels a distance X_{path} back to a receiver (which may or may not be located near the emitter), the amplitude again losing (r_T / X_{path}) by geometry and $e^{-\alpha_{tiss}\ \nu\ X_{path}}$ by attenuation. The echo is finally detected by the receiver which can measure a pulse of minimum pressure amplitude ΔP_{min} ~ 10^{-6} atm (Section 4.5.1).

Combining these relations gives the following result:

$$P_{in} \gtrsim \frac{\pi\ \Delta P_{min}^2\ X_{path}^4}{2\ \rho\ v_{sound}\ e\%\ f_{reflect}^2\ r_T^2\ e^{-4\ \alpha_{tiss}\ \nu\ X_{path}}} \quad \text{(watts)}$$

{Eqn. 4.48}

To scan the entire interior of a (20 micron)^3 cell, whether from within or without, requires $X_{path} \gtrsim$ 20 microns. A frequency of ν = 1.5 GHz allows v_{sound}/ν ~ 1 micron spatial resolution. The fastest possible pulse repetition time is X_{path}/v_{sound} ~ 13 nanosec. Assuming r_E = r_T = 0.5 micron, P_{in} ~ 7 pW or ~5 watts/m^2, well within the safe intensity range for acoustic radiation (Section 6.4.1). At maximum safe transmitter intensity I_{max}, the longest scannable path length at 1.5 GHz is X_{path} ~ 46 microns.

Power constraints are somewhat less severe in the case of acoustic transmission microscopy (acoustic tomography), a technique which requires a minimum of two physically separated components (e.g., a transmitter and a receiver). Consider an acoustic emitter radiating a series of omnidirectional pressure pulses of frequency ν which travel across a tissue cell of width X_{path}, to be detected by a receiver on the other side after a signal transit time $t_{cell} \sim X_{path} / v_{cell}$, where v_{cell} is the speed of sound in the cytosol. In the simplest case, assume that the cytosol is clear except for one target of interest along the path (e.g., an organelle) in which the speed of sound is $v_{target} \neq v_{cell}$. The minimum detectable difference in travel times between a signal that passes through the target and one that does not is Δt ($\sim 10^{-9}$ sec for diamondoid systems), so the minimum resolvable target size is $r_{min} \sim v_{target} v_{cell} \Delta t / 2 \text{ abs}(v_{target} - v_{cell})$ when $r_{min} \gtrsim v_{cell} / \nu$. For soft tissue targets in water at 1.5 GHz, $r_{min} \sim 30$ microns; for tooth enamel in water (see Table 6.7), $r_{min} \sim 1$ micron. However, the use of sampling gates will permit the detection of phase shifts that are much less than the characteristic time constant of the system in incoming waves, hence the minimum thickness of objects in theory detectable by acoustic tomography can be far smaller than the values for r_{min} estimated above.

Computing acoustic tomographic power requirement P_{in} in a similar manner as for echolocation, except that the transmitted signal rather than the echo is detected and assuming the signals are of approximately equal strength regardless of the path taken, gives:

$$P_{in} \gtrsim \frac{\pi \, \Delta P_{min}^2 \, X_{path}^4}{2 \, \rho \, v_{cell} \, e\% \, r_T^2 \, e^{-2\alpha_{tiss} \nu X_{path}}} \quad \text{(watts)} \qquad \text{\{Eqn. 4.49\}}$$

Using the same values as the previous example, $P_{in} = 1$ pW for $X_{path} \sim 45$ microns; for $X_{path} \sim 140$ microns, $P_{in} = 1000$ pW, near I_{max}.

In either mode of operation, data gathering is accelerated by positioning more than one receiver around the target. Sensitivity is boosted by increasing emitter size, taking multiple measurements, or by illuminating the target with some large external source located elsewhere in the tissue or even outside of the organ. However, cells and body tissues are mesoscopic "junkyards"—highly heterogeneous media which may produce large numbers of nontarget scattering events, thus increasing the difficulty of extracting signal from noise. Additional complications arise due to:

1. scattering on rough surfaces;
2. rapid pressure variations with range in the Fresnel zone or near field of the transmitted signal;
3. cytoplasmic viscosity inhomogeneities due to the asymmetric arrangement of cytoskeletal structure, granules, vacuoles, and the endomembrane system; and
4. variation in cytoplasmic Young's modulus due to time-varying tensions in semirandomly-distributed cytosolic fibrillar elements (e.g., a relaxed or contracted state) which alter elasticity and thus the local speed of sound.

4.8.3 Magnetic Resonance Cytotomography

Electrostatic scanning is largely ineffective because of Debye-Huckel shielding (Section 4.7.1). Magnetic stray field probes allow resolution of 10 nm physical features, but only for materials with substantial magnetic domains—which most biological substances lack. But nuclear magnetic resonance (NMR) imaging[2181] may allow cellular tomography by creating 3-D proton (hydrogen atom) density maps.[451,489] Atomic density maps of other biologically important elements with nonzero nuclear magnetic moments (including D, Li^6, B^{10}, B^{11}, C^{13}, N^{14}, N^{15}, O^{17}, F^{19}, Na^{23}, Mg^{25}, P^{31}, Cl^{35}, K^{39}, Fe^{57}, Cu^{63} and Cu^{65})[396,3257] may also be compiled. For example, sodium imaging is already used clinically to assess brain damage in patients with strokes, epilepsy, and tumors.

In a hypothetical NMR cytotomographic nanoinstrument, a large permanent magnet is positioned near the surface of the cell or organelle to be examined. This creates a large static background magnetic field that polarizes the protons. The spatial gradient of this field establishes a unique resonant frequency, called the Larmor frequency, within each isomagnetic surface throughout the test volume. A second time-varying magnetic driver field (e.g., vibrating permanent magnet or weak rf field) is then scanned through the full range of resonant frequencies, exciting into resonance the protons (nuclear spins) in each isomagnetic surface, in turn. Depending on the sensor implementation chosen, each resonance detected may cause absorption of driver field energy, an increase in measured impedance, or even a return echo of magnetic energy (if the driver field is operated in pulse echo mode) as the excited protons relax to equilibrium in ~1 sec.[490] The large polarizing magnet is then rotated to a new orientation, moving the isomagnetic surfaces to new positions within the test volume, and the scan is repeated. A 3-D map of the spatial proton distribution may be computed after several scan cycles.

Only those regions within a linewidth of resonance ΔB will generate an appreciable signal, and the expected spatial resolution (say, along the z-axis) $\Delta z = \Delta B / (dB/dz)$, where dB/dz is the spatial flux gradient of B. For a polarizing field B = 1.4 tesla placed adjacent to a (20 micron)^3 cell, the cross-cell gradient $dB/dz \sim 7 \times 10^4$ tesla/m; placed next to a (1 micron)^3 organelle, $dB/dz \sim 1.4 \times 10^6$ tesla/m. Assuming an effective NMR linewidth ~ 0.002 tesla,[489] minimum spatial resolutions are 29 nm and 1.4 nm, respectively.

Unfortunately, the smallest reliably detectable energy in the sensor element is $\sim kT \, e^{SNR}$. The energy required to flip a single proton is $E_{flip} = 4 \pi \nu_L L_{proton}$, where $L_{proton} = 5.28 \times 10^{-35}$ joule-sec (the quantized spin angular momentum of the proton) and the Larmor resonance frequency $\nu_L = \gamma_{proton} B$; γ_{proton} is the gyromagnetic ratio (4.26×10^7 Hz/tesla for protons) and B is the polarizing magnetic flux. However, the population difference between spin-up and spin-down nuclei in NMR is very small. For small energy differences, the Boltzmann distribution only allows a fraction $E_{flip} / 2 kT$ to be flipped before the upper and lower state populations are made equal and the absorption disappears. In order to flip $N_{flip} \sim kT \, e^{SNR} / 4 \pi \nu_L L_{proton}$ protons, the sample volume must include at least:

$$N_{min} \sim 2 \, e^{SNR} \left(\frac{kT}{4 \pi \nu_L L_{proton}} \right)^2 \quad \text{(protons)} \qquad \text{\{Eqn. 4.50\}}$$

For T = 310 K, SNR = 2 and B = 1.4 tesla, $n_L = 60$ MHz and $N_{min} \sim 1.7 \times 10^{11}$ protons.

When scanning a cell or organelle, the vast majority of the protons present are in water molecules (Table 3.2). Water at 310 K has a proton density $n_{water} = 6.7 \times 10^{28}$ protons/m^3, compared to $n_{fat} \sim 6.4 \times 10^{28}$ protons/m^3 (palmitic acid). Distinguishing fat from water thus requires a minimum sample volume of $N_{min} / (n_{water} - n_{fat}) \sim 55$ micron^3.

Proteins range from 4.4×10^{28} protons/m^3 (aspartic acid minus one water) to 7.6×10^{28} protons/m^3 (leucine minus one water), average $n_{protein} \sim 5.6 \times 10^{28}$ protons/m^3; $n_{carbohydrate} \sim 5.8 \times 10^{28}$ protons/m^3 (glucose minus one water), allowing NMR cellular tomography to resolve minimum feature sizes of 2-4 microns (5 - 60 micron^3). This resolution may include intracellular structures such as the endoplasmic reticulum (rough ER ~1100 micron^3, smooth ER ~400 micron^3), the Golgi complex (~500 micron^3), the nucleus (~270 micron^3), possibly the nucleolus (~50 micron^3) (Table 8.17), and even large localized ferritin granule concentrations.

In 1998, the minimum sample size for microcoil (~470 micron diameter) NMR scanning was ~10,000 micron^3 or ~10^{16} protons for a 1-minute measurement cycle.[1061] Individual T-cell vacuoles ~1 micron in diameter labeled with dextran-coated iron oxide particles have been imaged by MRI.[2317]

4.8.4 Near-Field Optical Nanoimaging

Electromagnetic waves of optical wavelength λ that interact with an object are diffracted into two components, called "far-field" and "near-field." The propagation of electromagnetic radiation over distances z > λ acts as a spatial filter of finite bandwidth, resulting in the familiar diffraction-limited resolution ~λ/2.[492] Classical optics is concerned with this far-field regime with low spatial frequencies < 2/λ, and conventional optical imaging will be difficult at the cellular level in vivo (Section 4.9.4). (Short-wave x-rays will damage living biological cells.) Information about the high spatial frequency components of the diffracted waves is lost in the far-field regime, so information about sub-wavelength features of the object cannot be retrieved in classical microscopy.

However, for propagation over distances z << λ, far higher spatial frequencies can be detected because their amplitudes are then of the same order as the sample (z = 0). This second diffraction component is the "near-field" evanescent waves with high spatial frequencies > 2/λ. Evanescent waves are confined to subwavelength distances from the object. Thus a localized optical probe, such as a subwavelength aperture in an opaque screen, can be scanned raster fashion in this regime to generate an image with a resolution on the order of the probe size.

The original Near-field Scanning Optical Microscope (NSOM) surpassed the classical diffraction limit by operating an optical probe at close proximity to the object. The NSOM probe uses an aluminum-coated "light funnel" scanned over the sample. Visible light emanates from the narrow end (~20 nm in diameter) of the light funnel and either reflects off the sample or travels through the sample into a detector, producing a visible light image of the surface with ~12 nm resolution at λ = 514.5 nm[492] provided the distance between light source and sample is very short, about 5 nm, with signal intensities up to 10^{11} photons/sec (~50 nanowatts). This represents a resolution of ~λ/40. The near-field acoustic equivalent is found in the medical stethoscope, which exhibits a resolution of ~λ/100.[576]

Applications include dynamical studies at video scanning rates, low-noise high-resolution spectroscopy, and differential absorption measurements. Optical imaging of individual dye molecules has already been demonstrated,[3195,3196] with the ability to determine the orientation and depth of each target molecule located within ~30 nm of the scanned surface.[493] Molecules with nanometer-scale packing densities have been resolved to ~0.4-nm diameters using STMs to create photon emission maps[494] (an electric current generates photons in the sample), and laser interferometric NSOMs have produced clear optical images of dispersed oil drops on mica to ~1 nm resolution.[495] Live specimen 250-nm optical sectioning for three-dimensional dynamic imaging has also been demonstrated.[496]

Submicron laser emitters have been available since the late 1980s.[497] It should be possible to use NSOM-like nanoprobes to optically scan the surfaces of cells or organelles to ≲1 nm resolution, mapping their topography and spectroscopic characteristics to depths of tens of nanometers without penetrating the surface. However, a proper membrane-sealing invasive light funnel ~20 nm in diameter might not seriously disrupt some cellular or organelle membranes and thus could be inserted into the interiors of these bodies or through the cytoskeletal interstices to permit deeper volumetric scanning. The thermal conductivity of water at 310 K is 0.623 watts/m-K and the energy per 500-nm photon is 400 zJ, so for 1 micron^3 of watery tissue the maximum scan rate is ~35 micron^3/sec-K, if e^{SNR} photons are used to image each 1 nm^3 voxel with SNR = 2. Thus a 1-sec volumetric optical scan of an aqueous ~1-micron^3 sample volume to 1 nm^3 resolution requires a ~1 nanowatt scanner running at ~GHz bit rates, raising sample volume temperature by ~0.03 K.

NSOM permits the determination of five of the six degrees of freedom for each molecule, lacking only the optically inactive rotation around the dipole axis.[493] In principle, it should be possible to produce ≲ 1 nm resolution near-field optical scans of in situ protein molecules, since with atomically precise fabrication and single lines of atoms as conductors a minimum light guide (metal-dielectric-metal) is 3 atoms wide. Given a molecular laser[990] and adequate collimation, photons passing through folded proteins will scatter according to the molecular structure. Detection of sufficient photons comprising these scattering patterns should allow the noninvasive determination of protein structure; polarized photons provide information on chirality. Absorption and fluorescent signals will be visible from phenyl rings, tryptophan, and bound cofactors such as ATP and adenine (which is fluorescent). Positions of monoclonal antibodies on virus surfaces are now identifiable experimentally using NSOM;[1258] it should be possible to map binding sites on virus and cell surfaces using fluorescently labelled antibodies. Single molecule detection has been proposed as a tool for rapid base-sequencing of DNA[991,992] (Chapter 20).

Other optically-based cellular imaging techniques must be distinguished. Optical Coherence Tomography (OCT) uses Michelson interferometry to achieve ~10 micron spatial resolutions over tissue depths of 2-3 mm in nontransparent tissue in the near infrared.[736] However, OCT requires numerous physical components not easily implemented on a micron-size detector (e.g., beam splitter, lens-grating pair, galvanometer mirror, optical prism), femtosecond pulse shaping, and illumination power levels of ~10^7 watts/m^2 >> 100 watts/m^2 "safe" continuous limit in tissue (Section 6.4.2). Bioluminescence techniques in which the light source is placed inside the tissue (e.g., a transgenic mouse with a luciferase gene in every cell of its body) has a spatial resolution limited to ~10% of the depth, or ~10 microns resolution at a ~100 micron depth.[737] Coherent anti-Stokes Raman scattering (CARS) already permits organelle imaging in living cells and can in theory create a point-by-point chemical map of a cell using two intersecting lasers.[3239]

Three-dimensional observation of microscopic biological non-living structures by means of x-ray holography requires a high degree of spatial coherence and good contrast between target and surroundings. Good contrast may be achieved in the wavelength range between the K absorption edges of carbon (λ = 4.37 nm) and oxygen (λ = 2.33 nm), the "water window" where carbon-containing biological objects absorb radiation efficiently but water is relatively transparent.[988] A 50-micron diameter emitter has been tested that uses near-IR 5-femtosecond laser pulses impinging upon a helium gas target to create a well-collimated (<1 milliradian) beam of coherent soft x-rays at a 1 KHz repetition rate producing a brightness of 5×10^8 photons/mm^2-milliradian^2-sec, a peak x-ray intensity of >10^{10} watts/m^2 on the propagation axis behind the He target.[988]

4.8.5 Cell Volume Sensing

Many cellular parameters need not be measured directly in order to be detected by a medical nanodevice. Cell volume sensing is a case in point.[1198] An intracellular nanodevice can indirectly monitor changes in the volume of the cell in which it resides by one of two methods. First, measurements of the mechanical deformation of the cellular membrane, stretch-activated channels, or cytoskeletal strains and structural changes are quite sensitive to alterations in total cell volume. Second, concentration or dilution of the cytoplasmic environment through cell shrinkage or swelling leads to the activation of various volume-regulation responses which may be detected by the nanorobot. Changes in the concentration of soluble cytosolic proteins may nonspecifically affect enzyme activity via "macromolecular crowding"[491] (and see Section 8.5.3.3). Minor changes in cell volume can cause severalfold changes in ion transport. Cellular signalling entities that have been linked to the transduction and amplification of the primary volume signal include Ca^{++} transients, phosphoinositide turnover, eicosanoid metabolism, kinase/phosphatase systems such as JNK and p38, cAMP, and G-proteins.[491] These signal amplification pathways may be monitored using chemical concentration sensors aboard the medical nanodevice, allowing the nanorobot to eavesdrop (Section 7.4.5.2) on the natural sensory channel traffic of the cell.

4.8.6 Noninvasive Neuroelectric Monitoring

In many ways the neuron is the most nanomedically important class of cell in the human body. Nanomedical applications regarding neurons and the brain are addressed in Chapter 25. The following is a brief summary of noninvasive (i.e., no axonal membrane penetration) nanotechnological methods for monitoring the electrical traffic of individual neurons. Noninvasive measurement of axonal traffic within nerve bundles will require multiple sensors and greater sensitivity to compensate for shielding by the perineurium, a tight resistive sheath enclosing the bundle ~20 microns thick with resistivity ~4000 ohm-cm.

4.8.6.1 Electric Field Neurosensing

The "typical" ~20 micron human neuron discharges 5-100 times per second, moving from -60 mV potential to +30 mV potential in $\sim 10^{-3}$ sec. Thus the variation in electric field at the axonal surface is ± 4500 volts/m. Since electric field sensors can detect 100 volt/m fields up to GHz frequencies (Section 4.7.1), an electric sensor attached by circumaxonal cuff or pressed against the axonal surface (possibly at the node of Ranvier) should readily detect each action potential discharge. (The diameter of human nerve axons is 0.1-20 microns.[799]) By 1998 silicon-to-neuron extracellular junctions already permitted direct stimulation of individual nerve cells in vitro without killing the cells,[513] and extracellular electrodes were commonly used to detect neuronal electrical activity noninvasively, both in vivo[573] and in vitro.[572,574,575] Artificial electric fields may also be employed to trigger or moderate neural signals (Section 7.4.5.6). Cell membrane capacitance is typically ~0.01 picofarads/micron^2,[2288] and varies with the state of the health of the cell.[2289,2290]

4.8.6.2 Magnetic Field Neurosensing

The magnetic flux density caused by a single action potential discharge is ~0.1 microtesla at the axonal surface, which may be detected by a "compass oscillator" type magnetosensor with a ~KHz maximum sampling rate (Section 4.7.2).

It might be possible for artificial magnetic fields to directly influence neural transmissions. Even a static 65 millitesla field has been shown to reduce frog skin Na^+ transport by 10-30%.[500] Each neuronal discharge develops an electrical energy of ~20 picojoule ($\sim 10^{10}$ kT), far smaller than the magnetic energy stored in a B = 1.4 tesla field of a permanent micromagnet traversing an $L^3 = (20 \text{ micron})^3$ volume which from Eqn. 6.9 is $B^2 L^3 / 2 \mu_0 \sim 6000$ pJ. If properly manipulated, such a field may be sufficient to enhance, modulate, or extinguish a passing neural signal.

4.8.6.3 Neurothermal Sensing

While neurons come in many shapes and sizes (Chapter 25), our "exemplar" ~14,000-micron^3 neuron discharging ~90 mV into an input impedance of ~500 Kohms produces ~0.2 microampere current per pulse and generates a continuous (average) 100-300 pW of waste heat as measured experimentally (Table 6.8). The discharge rate of 5-100 Hz can produce brief surges up to ~2000 pW during a high-frequency train, but the duty cycle of such trains is far less than 100%, reducing time-averaged dissipation to the observed 100-300 pW range.

Single impulses are measured experimentally to produce 2-7 microkelvin temperature spikes in cold or room-temperature mammalian non-myelinated nerve fibers[801] and ~23 microkelvins in non-myelinated garfish olfactory nerve fibers[3482] at an energy density ranging from 270-1670 joules/m^3-impulse from 0-20°C.[3483-3485] In non-myelinated fibers the initial heat occurs in two temperature-dependent phases: a burst of positive heat, followed by rapid heat reabsorption (called the negative heat).[3484] The positive heat derives from the dissipation of free energy stored in the membrane capacity, and from the decrease in entropy of the membrane dielectric with depolarization.[3483,3484] An L ~ 20-micron neuron in good thermal contact with an aqueous heat sink at 310 K has thermal conductance L $K_t \sim 10^{-5}$ watts/K, so trains of 5-100 Hz impulses lasting 1 second should raise cellular temperature by 10-30 microkelvins; up to ~200 microkelvin thermal spikes from such trains have been observed experimentally.[801] These events are easily detectable by nanoscale thermal sensors capable of ~1 microkelvin sensitivity up to ~1 KHz (Section 4.6.3). The ~microkelvin heat signature of individual impulses or very short pulse trains can probably be temporally resolved because the minimum pulse repetition time is ~10 millisec (at 100 Hz) which is much longer than the thermal time constant for an L ~ 20-micron neuron (thermal conductivity K_t = 0.528 watts/m-K and heat capacity $C_V = 3.86 \times 10^6$ joules/m^3-K for brain tissue; Table 8.12) which is $t_{EQ} \sim L^2 C_V / K_t \sim 3$ millisec.

4.8.6.4 Direct Synaptic Monitoring

The synaptic cleft between the axonal presynaptic terminal and the dendritic postsynaptic membrane is 10-20 nm in most synapses, although in the vertebrate myoneural junction it may be as large as 100 nm. Contact area per bouton is ~1 micron^2, giving a total gap volume of $\sim 10^7$-10^8 nm^3. The density of acetylcholine receptors is highest in muscles along the crests and upper thirds of the junctional folds (~10,000/micron^2), and is lowest in the extrasynaptic regions (~5/micron^2).[802] (Other neurotransmitters exist; Table 7.2 and Section 7.4.5.6.) Each action potential discharge triggers the release of $\sim 10^4$-10^5 molecules of acetylcholine into the gap volume of an active neuromuscular junction (diffusion time ~1 microsec), raising c_{ligand} from near zero to $\sim 3 \times 10^{-4}$ molecules/nm^3 (~0.0005 M)[531] in ~1 millisec, followed by near-complete hydrolyzation by acetylcholinesterase during the 1-2 millisec refractory period. Into the gap volume may easily be inserted a $\sim 10^5$ nm^3 neurotransmitter concentration sensor (Section 4.2.3) able to measure ~100 acetylcholine molecules in ~1 millisec (Eqn. 4.5), thus detecting pulses at the fastest discharge rate. A similar device could be used to precisely regulate neuro-transmitter concentration at the junction, and hence the neural signal itself, under nanodevice control (Section 7.4.5.6). Simple electrochemical and mechanochemical artificial synapses have been demonstrated.[499]

4.8.6.5 Other Neurosensing Techniques

Many other noninvasive neurosensing techniques are readily conceivable. For instance, counting rotors (Section 3.4.2) or sodium magnetic resonance imaging (Section 4.8.3) could detect changes in the ionic composition (e.g., Na^+, K^+) of the periaxonal fluid before, during, and after discharge.

4.8.7 Cellular RF and Microwave Oscillations

Starting in 1968, H. Frohlich, observing that millivolt electrical potentials maintained across cell membranes ~10 nm thick give rise to huge fields ~10^7 volts/m (Section 4.7.1) possibly producing an electret state, theorized that membrane molecules must be highly electrically polarized and thus could interact to produce coherent surface acoustic vibrational modes in the 10-100 GHz (microwave) frequency range;[680,681] the longest wavelength is about twice the membrane thickness. Interestingly, this frequency span is very close to the maximum trigger/reset frequency for bioelectronic molecules (Section 4.7.3). Note that (~100 mV) (1.6 x 10^{-19} coul) ~ 4 kT, so a membrane molecule with a single charge on either end should be reliably reoriented by a depolarization wave, coupling pressure waves and electrostatic field fluctuations. However, the direct detection of 10-100 GHz millimeter radiation by non-nanotechnological means is experimentally difficult and controversial because the tests must be performed in vivo in close proximity to an actively metabolizing cell in water—and water strongly absorbs microwaves over macroscale ranges (e.g., ~99% absorption in 3 mm at 100 GHz).

Nevertheless, active cells have shown enhanced Raman anti-Stokes scattering, an effect ascribed to the converse of the Frohlich oscillations. In one study, the normalized growth rate of yeast cultures was enhanced or inhibited when irradiated by CW microwave fields of ~30 watts/m^2 of various frequencies; growth rate data spanning 62 separate runs revealed a repeatable frequency-dependent spectral fine structure with six distinct peaks of width ~10 MHz near 42 GHz.[682] Investigations of related phenomena are ongoing and voluminous; the interested reader should peruse *Bioelectromagnetics*, the archival journal of this field.

From Eqn. 6.32, 100 GHz waves attenuate only ~1% after passing through ~3 microns of soft tissue. A single electron injected into an integral membrane protein could act as an oscillating dipole, making a 300 volt/m signal 10 nm from the protein antenna with an energy transfer of ~0.004 kT per cycle;[686] ~1000 oscillating electrons could produce a measurable field. A 20-micron diameter cell modeled as a nonuniform spherical dipole layer with transmembrane dipoles located 10 nm apart and embedded in a dissipative medium could produce 10^2-10^5 volt/m microwave fields 1-10 microns from the cell surface.[687]

Thus, a variety of rf and microwave electromagnetic emanations may in theory be detectable both within and nearby living cells which could prove diagnostic of numerous internal states. Such states may include cytoskeletal dynamics,[684] metabolic rates,[682] plasmon-type excitations due to the collective motion of ions freed in chemical reactions,[688] positional, rotational or conformational changes in biological macromolecules and membranes,[680,721] internal movements of organelles and nerve traffic conduction,[685] cellular pinocytosis,[1938] cellular reproduction events,[683] cell membrane identity (e.g., distinguishing erythrocyte, Gram-positive and Gram-negative cell coat conductivities at 10 KHz[728]), and cell-cell interactions.[687,688]

4.9 Macrosensing

Macrosensing is the detection of global somatic states (inside the human body) and extrasomatic states (sensory data originating outside the human body). While the treatment here is necessarily incomplete, the discussion nevertheless gives a good feel for the kinds of environmental variables that internally-situated nanodevices could sense. Not all capabilities outlined here need be available on every nanorobot, since injection of a cocktail of numerous distinct but mutually cooperative machine species allows designers to take full advantage of the benefits of functional specialization. In many cases, a given environmental variable can be measured by several different classes of sensor device. However, since these devices are microscopic it is in theory possible to operationalize almost all of the macrosensing capabilities described below in one patient using just a billion devices (~10 mm^{-3} whole-body deployment density), a total volume of ~1 mm^3 of nanorobots or ~0.1% of the typical ~1 cm^3 therapeutic dose[1400] (Chapter 19).

A general discussion of methods for communicating macrosensory information to the human user is in Section 7.4.6, and is mentioned briefly in Section 4.9.5 below.

4.9.1 Acoustic Macrosensing

4.9.1.1 Cyto-Auscultation

Can sounds generated by a single cell be detected, and thus be useful for diagnosis? Probably not, given that low frequency acoustic radiators are notoriously inefficient (Section 7.2.2.1). For example, mitochondrion organelles of the giant amoeba *Reticulomyxa* are shuttled back and forth by 1-4 cytoplasmic dynein motors while riding on the outside of a bundle of 1-6 microtubules.[453] Each dynein motor generates 2.6 pN of force and drives the mitochondria at up to ~10 micron/sec, developing 0.3-1.0 x 10^{-16} watts of mechanical power within each 320-nm diameter organelle. Taking each organelle as a cylindrical acoustic radiator with a mechanical input power of P_{in} ~ 10^{-16} watts at ν ~ 1000 Hz, the output acoustic pressure at the organelle surface is only ~10^{-9} atm (Eqn. 7.6), an acoustic power intensity I ~ 10^{-15} watts/m^2 (Eqn. 4.53) which is not detectable by micron-sized nanorobots. Nevertheless, cells and intracellular elements are capable of vibrating in a dynamic manner with complex harmonics that can be altered by growth factors and by the process of carcinogenesis,[1201] so the possibility cannot be completely ruled out.

4.9.1.2 Blood Pressure and Pulse Detection

Blood pressure ranges from 0.1-0.2 atm in the arteries to as low as 0.005 atm in the veins. The systolic/diastolic differential ranges from 0.05-0.07 atm in the aorta and 0.01-0.02 atm in the pulmonary artery, falling to 0.001-0.003 atm in the microvessels, or 0.003-0.005 atm if the precapillary sphincter is dilated.[361,363] In venous vessels, pulse fluctuations are 0.002-0.010 atm in the superior vena cava, 0.004-0.006 atm in the subclavian vein, ~0.004 atm in venules generally, and ~0.0005 atm in the brachial vein.[361] There is also a ~0.05 Hz random fluctuation in the microvessels with amplitude on the order of 0.004-0.007 atm.[363] Both blood pressure and pulse rate can be reliably monitored by a medical nanodevice virtually anywhere in the vascular system using a (68 nm)^3 pressure sensor with ~0.001 atm sensitivity (Section 4.5.1). (See also Section 8.4.2.)

Pulse propagation through body tissue is somewhat muted due to absorption in compressible fatty membranes, but most cells lie within 1-3 cell-widths of a capillary so the cardiac acoustic signal should still be measurable using more sensitive detectors. The time-averaged interstitial pressure in subcutaneous tissue is 0.001-0.004 atm.[363]

Arterial pulse waves (vascular oscillations) carry subtle messages about the health of internal organs and the arterial tree. The idea of using pulse waves for diagnosis has a long history dating back 2000 years in China. For example, in the *Book on Pulse Waves* by Wang Shu-He (201-285 AD), waves detected by manual probing are classified using such subjective and qualitative descriptors as floating, deep, hidden, rapid, slow, moderate, feeble, replete, full, thready, faint, weak, soft, slippery, hesitant, hollow, firm, long, short, swift, running, intermittent, uneven, taut, string-tight, gigantic, or tremulous.[361] Abnormal waves were empirically related to disease states. Wave data gathered by nanodevices could make possible a theoretically sound, quantitative system of noninvasive observation, classification, and diagnosis as a supplement to other nanomedical tools.

4.9.1.3 Respiratory Audition

The variation of mechanical pressure over a complete respiratory cycle is ~0.003 atm in the pleura, ~0.002 atm at the alveoli, detectable by nanomedical pressure sensors positioned in the vicinity of the respiratory organs. Holding a deep breath further stretches the pulmonary elastic tissue, up to 0.02 atm.

However, turbulent flows at Reynolds number $N_R > 2300$ in the trachea, main bronchus and lobar bronchus produce a whooshing noise that may be the loudest noncardiac sound in the human torso during conventional auscultation. The energy dissipation for turbulent flow in a tube is

$$P_{turb} = P_{lam} Z = 8 \pi \eta_{air} v^2 L Z \quad \text{(watts)} \qquad \text{\{Eqn. 4.51\}}$$

where P_{lam} is the dissipation for laminar (Poiseuillean) flow in a long circular cylindrical tube of length L, v is the mean flow velocity, and turbulence factor $Z = 0.005 (N_R^{3/4} - (2300)^{3/4})$, a well-known empirical formula.[363] For $\eta_{air} = 1.83 \times 10^{-5}$ kg/m-sec for room-temperature air (20°C), $P_{turb} = 0.87$ milliwatts for the trachea (L = 0.12 m, v = 3.93 m/sec and $N_R = 4350$ at 1 liter/sec volume flow; Table 8.7); $P_{turb} = 0.66$ milliwatts for the main bronchus (L = 0.167 m, v = 4.27 m/sec and $N_R = 3210$); and $P_{turb} = 0.09$ milliwatts for the lobar bronchus (L = 0.186 m, v = 4.62 m/sec and $N_R = 2390$), totalling ~1.6 milliwatts acoustic emission from a ~120 cm^3 upper tracheobroncheal volume. This is a power density of 13 watts/m^3 corresponding to a pressure of 4×10^{-5} atm assuming a 300 millisecond measurement window at the maximum respiration rate.

The amplitude of an acoustic plane wave propagating through tissue attenuates exponentially with distance due to absorption, scattering and reflection. The amplitude is given approximately by

$$A_x = A_0 e^{-\alpha F x} \qquad \text{\{Eqn. 4.52\}}$$

where A_0 is the initial wave amplitude in atm, A_x is the amplitude a distance x from the source, and α is the amplitude absorption coefficient. The function F expresses the frequency dependence of the attenuation. For pure liquids, $F = F_{liq} = \nu^2$ (Hz^2); for example, $\alpha_{liq} = 2.5 \times 10^{-14}$ sec^2/m for water at room temperature. However, for soft tissues, $F = F_{tiss} \sim \nu$ (Hz).[505]* Values for α_{tiss} (in sec/m) are in Table 4.2; the value for diamond was estimated from the acoustic line discussion in Section 7.2.5.3. Assuming <10 KHz bronchial turbulence noise of initial amplitude $A_0 = 4 \times 10^{-5}$ atm, $A_x \sim 3.7 \times 10^{-5}$ atm through 1 meter of typical soft tissue; $A_x \sim 3.4 \times 10^{-5}$ atm even if 0.1 meter of bone is interposed in the acoustic path. Either A_x is reliably detected from anywhere in the body using a >(210 nm)^3 pressure sensor (Eqn 4.29).

Table 4.2 Amplitude Absorption Coefficients for Acoustic Waves in Human Body Tissue[628,629,730]

Body Tissue	Coefficient α (sec/m)	Body Tissue	Coefficient α (sec/m)
For α_{liq} (sec^2/m):		Fat	7.0×10^{-6}
Water	2.5×10^{-14}	Soft tissue (avg)	8.3×10^{-6}
Castor oil	1.2×10^{-11}	Liver	1.0×10^{-5}
Air (STP)	1.4×10^{-10}	Nerves	1.0×10^{-5}
For α_{tiss} (sec/m):		Brain (adult)	1.1×10^{-5}
Diamond (est.)	$\sim 2 \times 10^{-15}$	Kidney	1.2×10^{-5}
Aqueous humor	1.1×10^{-6}	Muscle	2.3×10^{-5}
Vitreous humor	1.2×10^{-6}	Eye lens	2.6×10^{-5}
Blood	2.1×10^{-6}	Polythene (plastic)	5.8×10^{-5}
Brain (infant)	3.4×10^{-6}	Bone	1.6×10^{-4}
Abdomen	5.9×10^{-6}	Lung	4.7×10^{-4}

4.9.1.4 Mechanical Body Noises

Many other mechanical body noises should be globally audible to properly instrumented medical nanodevices. If normal chewing motions (of hard foods) release 1-10 milliwatts in a ~100 cm^3 oral volume with a ~1 sec jawstroke, power density is ~10 watts/m^3 or ~10^{-4} atm of tooth-crunching noise. A stomach growl registering 45 dB (vs. 30 dB whisper, 60 dB normal conversation) at 2 meters has a source power of 160 milliwatts; released from a 10 cm^3 gastric sphincter volume gives a ~2×10^{-6} atm acoustic wave, detectable throughout the body. Walking and running releases 20-100 joules/footfall for a 70 kg man; assuming the energy is absorbed within a ~1 cm thickness or within ~1 second by the sole of the foot, Eqn. 4.53 implies an upward-moving planar compression wave of 0.4-2.0 atm, easily detectable by acoustically instrumented nanodevices body-wide. (Shoe insoles dissipate energy and alter the shock wave pulse shape.)[3493,3494] Hand-clapping generates 0.02-0.2 atm pulses, also easily detectable.

Lesser noises including ~30 millisec hiccups at (4-60)/min,[2122] intestinal and ureteral peristalsis, sloshing of liquid stomach contents, heart murmurs, a tap on the shoulder by a friend, nasal sniffling and swallowing, clicks from picking or drumming fingernails, crepitations, manustuprations and ejaculations, the rustling noise of clothing against the skin, flapping eyelids, anal towelling, bruits (including murmurs and thrills) due to vascular lesions, dermal impact of water while showering, copulatory noises, urethral flow turbulence during urination, transmitted vibrations from musical instruments, creaking joints, and squeaking muscles can be detected locally if not globally. Implantation of significant interconnected in vivo diamondoid structures may produce increased sensitivity to internal noises, due to the extremely low acoustic absorption coefficient of diamond (Table 4.2).

4.9.1.5 Vocalizations

Average source power for conversational speech in air is ~10 microwatts at the vocal cords (60 dB), up to ~1000 microwatts for shouting (90 dB) and as little as 0.1 microwatts (30 dB) for whispering.[3511] Vocal cord surface area ~1 cm^2, giving an acoustic intensity I ~ 0.001-10 watts/m^2. (Using the decibel notation, dB = 10 $\log_{10}$ (I/I_0), where $I_0 \sim 5 \times 10^{-13}$ watts/m^2 in air, $I_0 \sim 1 \times 10^{-16}$ watts/m^2 in water.) In a planar traveling wave, pressure amplitude A_p (N/m^2) is related to power intensity I by

$$A_p = (2 \rho v_{sound} I)^{1/2} \quad (N/m^2) \qquad \text{\{Eqn. 4.53\}}$$

For water at 310 K, $\rho = 993.4$ kg/m^3 and $v_{sound} = 1500$ m/sec, therefore $A_p = 0.0005$-0.05 atm for speech, detectable by nanodevices throughout the body due to minimal attenuation at audible frequencies (Section 4.9.1.3). Other easily detectable vocalizations include whistling, humming, coughing, sneezing, rales, wheezing,

**Most medical ultrasound textbooks assume a ~ν dependency of attenuation in soft tissues; apparently, the actual dependency[730] is ~$\nu^{1.1}$.*

Table 4.3 Acoustic Impedance for Specular Reflection by Acoustic Waves Crossing a Material Interface[536,628,629,730,763]

Body Tissue	Impedance (kg/m^2-sec)	Body Tissue	Impedance (kg/m^2-sec)
Air	400	Liver (25°C)	1.65×10^6
Lung	1.80×10^5	Blood	1.65×10^6
Fat	1.39×10^6	Nerve (optic)	1.68×10^6
Aqueous humor	1.51×10^6	Muscle	1.73×10^6
Water	1.52×10^6	Lens of eye	1.84×10^6
Brain (25°C)	1.57×10^6	Nylon	2.9×10^6
Skin	1.6×10^6	Skull bone	7.80×10^6
Soft tissue (avg.)	1.63×10^6	Enamel	1.71×10^7
Kidney	1.63×10^6	Diamond	6.3×10^7

expectorating, eructations, flatus, vomiting, hawking and noseblowing.

In the case of spherical waves diverging from an omnidirectional transmitter of radius r at a distance X from the transmitter, average intensity declines inversely as the square of the distance and so I in Eqn. 4.53 must be replaced by $(I\, r^2 / X^2)$.

4.9.1.6 Environmental Sources

Can in vivo nanodevices directly detect sounds emanating from the environment outside of the body, such as other people talking in the same room or a door slamming? The waves from an external acoustic source of power P_R watts travel through the air and, upon arriving at the air/skin interface a distance x_R from the source with amplitude $A_{incident}$, are transmitted through the interface with amplitude $A_{transmit}$. For a specular reflector—interface dimensions (human body ~ 2 m) > acoustic wavelength (~0.03-3.0 m for typical audible sounds in air)—with acoustic impedance Z_1 and Z_2 on either side of the interface and perpendicular incidence,[506,628]

$$A_{transmit} = A_{incident}\left[1 - \mathrm{abs}\left(\frac{Z_1 - Z_2}{Z_1 + Z_2}\right)\right] \qquad \text{\{Eqn. 4.54\}}$$

Acoustic impedance, like the speed of sound, is essentially frequency-independent over the nanomedically-relevant range of ultrasonic frequencies. For Z_{air} = 400 kg/m^2-sec and assuming Z_{skin} ~ 1.6×10^6 kg/m^2-sec from Table 4.3, then $A_{transmit} = (5 \times 10^{-4})\, A_{incident}$. In other words, there is ~99.95% reflection from the air-skin interface, which is why coupling mediums like gels and oils are commonly employed in ultrasound imaging. If an immediately subdermal nanodevice can detect a minimum $A_{transmit}$ ~ 10^{-6} atm, then from Eqn. 4.53 and simple geometry:

$$P_R = \frac{2\,\pi\, x_R^2\, A_{incident}^2}{\rho\, v_{sound}} \qquad \text{\{Eqn. 4.55\}}$$

For STP (1 atm, 0°C) air, ρ = 1.29 kg/m^3 and v_{sound} = 331 m/sec. If the minimum detectable pressure ~10^{-6} atm (Section 4.5.1) ~ $A_{transmit}$, then at a distance of x_R = 2 meters the acoustic source must have a power of ~2000 watts, far exceeding the ~1 milliwatt output of a person loudly shouting. To hear normal conversation at x_R = 2 m, minimum nanodevice detector sensitivity falls to 7×10^{-11} atm requiring a subdermal pressure nanosensor ~(17 micron)^3 in size (Eqn. 4.29), roughly the dimensions of a single human cell; other methods may prove more efficient (Sections 4.9.5 and 7.4.6.3).

Of course, an ex vivo acoustic nanosensor may receive sound that has passed through no interface, hence may detect pressure waves ~3 orders of magnitude lower in amplitude. Assuming $A_{transmit} = A_{incident}$, P_R ~ 600 microwatts, so ex vivo nanorobots with a 0.3 micron^3 sensor could hear people shouting at x_R = 2 meters. To hear talking (~10 microwatt source) requires a 2.4 micron^3 ex vivo pressure sensor (limit ~10^{-7} atm), from Eqn. 4.29.

Optimally positioned and calibrated nanomedical pressure sensors could directly measure changes in the ambient barometric pressure to within $\pm 10^{-6}$ atm. Normal atmospheric variation due to weather ranges from 0.94-1.05 atm; such slow moving changes are readily monitored. Very near the Earth's surface, the air pressure P at altitude h above sea level is approximated by $P = e^{-k_p h}$ (atm), where $k_p = 1.16 \times 10^{-4}\ m^{-1}$ at 20°C; at sea level, a 10^{-6} atm change in pressure reflects a change in altitude of only ~1 cm. However, the opening or closing of a door inside a (~5 m)^3 room that displaces >125 cm^3 of air also causes a minimally detectable >10^{-6} atm pressure pulse. Other sources of environmental pressure variation such as infrasonic (~0.2 Hz) microbaroms from offshore ocean storms,[1526] wind entering through open windows, forced-air currents from central heating or A/C systems, or even the movements of nearby people and pets may be detectable and thus may further confuse the measurement, reducing absolute accuracy unless suitable corrections are made.

4.9.2 Proprioceptive Macrosensing

4.9.2.1 Kinesthetic Macrosensing

Using a navigational transponder network (Section 8.3.3), a population of ~10^{11} nanodevices each spaced an average ~100 microns apart throughout the body tissues can determine relative location to a positional accuracy of ~3 microns and an angular accuracy of ~2 milliradian, with the data updatable once every millisecond. Thus dispersed, the network can continuously monitor and record the relative positions of all limbs with worst-case (cumulative error) ~0.8 mm accuracy over a 2-meter span (Section 8.3.3). These devices can prepare high-resolution dynamic maps of body position, velocity, acceleration and rotation, allowing precise real-time digital kinesthesia during sports or artistic activities such as gymnastics, pole vaulting, or ballet; during transportative activities such as driving cars around hairpin turns, roller-coaster rides, military aircraft maneuvers and space launches; during precision tool-using such as needle-threading, antique watch repair, or while using the fingers as measurement calipers; during self-defense activities requiring complex motions such as karate or judo; and during emergency situations such as automobile crashes and tumbling motions during falls from great heights. All such sensory data is readily outmessaged to the patient or user in real time (Section 7.4).

Nanorobots could assist in path integration or the reconstruction of experienced limb trajectories.[1040] Given the ability to determine rotation rates and to measure applied forces and torques, the network should also be able to forecast the anticipated future positions of limbs. By comparing these projections to actual results, the network can then infer the viscosity of the medium in which the activity is taking place (e.g., air or water), whether the environment is stable or is translating or rotating in some direction, and whether the human user is physically supported or in free-fall. Internal nanodevices can directly measure if a body is sitting, standing, laying prone, inverted, falling, floating or diving, and then communicate that information directly to the human user (Section 7.4). Detection of patient activity states—e.g., the patient is sitting, standing, or walking—can be used to control nanorobot behaviors (Chapter 12), activate or deactivate outmessaging displays (Section 7.4.6), and so forth. A simple macroscale wearable tactile "compass belt" that would convey desired geographical directions has already been proposed.[2994]

4.9.2.2 Orientational Macrosensing

Since nanopendular sensors can reliably determine the direction of the local gravity field vector to within ~2 milliradians in ~10^{-4} sec (Section 4.3.4.2), the navigational network can poll its members and arrive at an accurate consensus on which direction is up. Nanodevices affixed to relatively stable hard body parts will exhibit more consistent orientational readings. Measurement of the gravity vector allows the vertical orientation of the rest of the body to be precisely fixed in space, especially useful for gymnasts, trapeze artists, underwater divers in murky lakes, and vestibular-impaired individuals, to whom this information may be outmessaged directly (Section 7.4).

The gravitational vector may also be indirectly measured, albeit more slowly and less accurately, by monitoring the body's natural reactions to changes in the axis of gravitational loading. For instance, the variation in head-to-toe hydrostatic pressure for a 1.7 m tall, 70 kg human standing in a 1-g gravity field is ~0.17 atm; the ability to measure a systematic cross-body differential of 10^{-6} atm allows the detection of a ~10^{-5} g change along the lengthwise aspect, or ~10^{-4} g change along the transverse aspect. Thus a continuously updated whole-body barostatic map allows the human body to serve as a three-dimensional gravity/orientation sensor.

4.9.2.3 Body Weight Measurement

A network of nanodevices can inventory the volume and density of each of the body's ~10^8 $(1\ mm)^3$ voxels using a combination of acoustic ranging, somatic mapping, and flowmetry. Each voxel is identified as fat, muscle tissue, bone mass, interstitial fluid, and so forth. These measurements allow the body's weight to be precisely computed as volume times density, rather than the usual method of determining weight using gravitational force data. The existence of a natural physiological "ponderostat," a crudely analogous humoral body-mass detector, has been proposed[507]; indeed, the insulin-leptin system[3265] has been found to serve a related purpose, and is easily eavesdropped by medical nanorobots.

4.9.2.4 Gravitational Geographic Macrosensing

Medical nanodevices can measure variations in the gravity field to ~10^{-6} g's for L = 20 micron gravimeters in a measurement time t_{meas} = 2-9 millisec (Section 4.4.2). This implies that in vivo nanodevices can take precise measurements of their latitude and altitude relative to sea level ~100 times every second. Gravity increases toward the poles and at lower altitudes. Specifically, using the formula of Cassinis (accounting for rotational and polar flattening effects on the Earth) with the Bouguer correction to the free air variation by altitude (assuming flat topography), measured gravity g_{meas} is given approximately by

$$g_{meas} = g_0\left[1 + k_1 \sin^2(\theta_L) - k_2 \sin^2(2\,\theta_L)\right] - k_3\,h + k_4\,h\,\rho_{earth}$$

{Eqn. 4.56}

where θ_L = terrestrial latitude (equator = 0°), h = height above sea level in meters, g_0 = 9.78039 m/sec^2 (equatorial sea-level value of g), k_1 = 5.2884 x 10^{-3}, k_2 = 5.9 x 10^{-6}, k_3 = 3.086 x 10^{-6} sec^{-2}, k_4 = 4.185 x 10^{-7}, and ρ_{earth} = 5522 kg/m^3.

Since sea-level g varies from 9.78039 m/sec^2 at the equator to 9.83217 m/sec^2 at the north pole, a 20-micron gravimeter ($\Delta g = 10^{-6}$ g) detects a change in position of 1 arcmin of latitude or ~1900 meters north/south along the Earth's surface. Similarly, since at 45° latitude g varies from 9.806 m/sec^2 at sea level to 9.803 m/sec^2 at 1000 meters altitude, a 20-micron gravimeter detects a change in altitude of ~3.3 meters (e.g., upstairs vs. downstairs in a house). For comparison, in 1998 high-quality commercial gravity gradiometers measured gradients of ~10^{-9} g/meter and allowed the compilation of micro-g (~1 milligal) resolution aerial gravity maps;[1527] atom interferometers measured the gravitational acceleration of atoms to a precision of 10^{-10}.

To achieve such phenomenal positional accuracies, the nanodevice must be able to computationally resolve several complicating factors. First, localized mass concentrations representing nonuniformities in crustal density produce residuals of up to ±0.0006 m/sec^2, which may be removed from the data using a standard map of known terrestrial isostatic variations and anomalies. Indeed, matching observations to such a map could provide useful longitudinal information as well. Another complication is the variation in gravity due to tidal forces amounting to ~3 x 10^{-7} g's, twice daily, which lies at the limits of detectability for a 20-micron gravimeter. Other minor geodesic and terrain-related corrections, too complicated for discussion here, may also need to be applied in certain circumstances. Note that the presence of nearby heavy objects does not influence measurement accuracy: a 100-ton building 10 meters away adds a lateral acceleration of only 7 x 10^{-9} g's to a human body.

One final complication is that patient movements create kinematic accelerations that must be distinguished from the gravitational accelerations. Gravity readings can be corrected by taking derivatives of the signals from kinesthetic monitoring to give gravity in the reference frame of the patient's room, and many individual measurements may be averaged to improve accuracy since the gravity vector normally changes only very slowly.

4.9.3 Electric/Magnetic Macrosensing

4.9.3.1 Vascular-Interstitial Closed Electric Circuits

In vivo studies of the electric properties of blood vessels shows that the walls of veins and arteries present a specific electric resistance ~200 times greater than the conductive medium of blood (plasma)—roughly 200 ohm-m vs. 0.7 ohm-m. Thus blood vessels are properly regarded as relatively insulated conducting cables which can electrically connect an injured tissue with surrounding noninjured tissue. Capillaries form an electric junction with the interstitial fluid, so the electric gradient can be canceled by ionic transport. Cell membranes are insulating dielectrics with resistance and capacitance, penetrated by ionic channels or gates for ionic transport. Additionally, in 1941 Szent-Gyorgyi suggested the possibility of semi-conduction in proteins, a theory which has since been elaborated by many investigators.[690]

B. Nordenstrom[689,690,3489] has proposed that the above schema represents a system for selective electrogenous mass transport of material between blood and tissue which he calls Vascular-Interstitial Closed (electric) Circuits (VICCs)—in effect, an additional electro-circulatory system operating in parallel with the well-known diffusive, osmotic, and hydrodynamic mechanisms of regular bloodstream materials transport. As long as ions can leak through open pores and migrate through ion channels, long distance transport cannot take place and the VICC system remains primarily a local (e.g., within tissues), not global, electrical circuit. Connections also exist with conductive media including cerebrospinal fluid, bile, and urine.[3490]

Nanorobots capable of monitoring the status of local VICCs may rapidly and efficiently acquire a wealth of systemic information without the need for direct inspection of the affected tissues. For example, when a working muscle produces catabolic products such as lactic acid, an electrochemical potential gradient develops between the muscle and surrounding tissue in a known manner.[3491] Injured tissues become polarized in relation to surrounding tissue, as initial catabolic degradation products acidify the tissue. Malignant neoplasms, benign neoplasms, and internally necrotic granulomas all may polarize electrically in relation to surrounding tissue; a vascular thrombus also contains ionized material. Large deflections in the diffusion potential of blood occur if blood is deoxygenated or is infected with Gram-negative bacteria. Blood changes its electric potential from +500 mV to +1000 mV during spontaneous coagulation, and the spontaneous electric potential at the site of a crush injury of the iliac crest in rats oscillated several times between +190 mV and -60 mV over a four day experimental trial.[690]

Nordenstrom proposes that in vivo electrophoresis via the VICC system may also play a role in mediating leukotaxis. When tissue is artificially polarized by electrodes, accumulation of granulocytes with margination and development of pseudopods is the result. In one experiment, exposure of a mesenterial membrane to a 1 microampere 1 volt field for 30 minutes stimulated diapedetic bleeding near the anode. At higher power, the arterio-capillaries contracted, narrowed, and emptied of blood cells, while the veno-capillaries and venules widened and filled with granulocytes. Monitoring such actions of local VICCs experiencing natural voltage fluctuations could alert medical nanorobots to the presence of local injuries, tissue changes, or pathologies that otherwise might go unnoticed for a considerable time.

4.9.3.2 Electric/Magnetic Geographic Macrosensing

Detection of electric fields to ~100 volts/m (Section 4.7.1), the normal vertical atmospheric gradient, in theory might allow determination of aboveground altitude to ~1 m accuracy if the time between recalibrations is very brief. However, a human body (which is a good conductor), standing on level ground, acquires a slight negative surface charge and becomes "part of the ground" electrically. This distorts upward the equipotentials that usually run parallel to the ground, thoroughly corrupting an altitude measurement. Nearby lightning hits and storms are detectable, which is useful.

However, medical nanodevices with appropriate magnetometers can measure variations in magnetic field to ~0.1 microtesla using a (660 nm)^3 permanent magnet sensor, in a measurement time t_{meas} ~ 0.6 millisec (Section 4.7.2). Geomagnetic field maps of the Earth's surface are highly nonisotropic in both latitudinal and longitudinal directions; knowledge of the field plus the absolute direction of true north (e.g., using a nanogyroscope; Section 4.3.4.1) gives longitude information from the separation of the planetary magnetic and spin poles. This implies that properly equipped in vivo nanodevices can establish their latitude and longitude on Earth's surface ~1000 times every second by this means. In particular, the horizontal component of the geomagnetic field vector ranges from 0-41 microtesla from magnetic pole to magnetic equator; the independent vertical field component ranges from 0-70 microtesla. Thus a 0.1-microtesla sensor should resolve each component to an accuracy of ~11 arcmin or ~20 km in both latitude or longitude. Terrestrial surface magnetic anomalies (e.g., iron deposits) produce local variations of 0.03-30 microtesla and are thus detectable. Additional complications to these measurements include artificial magnetic field sources, the 0.01-0.1 microtesla solar daily variation, occasional magnetic storms producing erratic geomagnetic fluctuations of 0.01-5 microtesla, sudden-commencement ionospheric electrojets up to 0.3 microtesla, and various long-term secular variations in the geomagnetic field.

Radio, television, and direct broadcast satellite signals probably are not detectable by individual nanodevices (Section 7.2.3), but such detection may be indirectly achieved in vivo using nanorobot-accessible dedicated macroscale antennas implanted in the body (Section 7.3.4).

4.9.3.3 Piezoelectric Stress Macrosensing

The piezoelectric effect (Sections 6.3.2 and 6.3.5) is "the production of electrical polarization in a material by the application of mechanical stress".[3089] Many materials in the human body are piezoelectric, including tendon and elastin, dentin and bone.[1939-1942,3089-3095] This polarization, or surface charge, varies as the physical stress imposed on the material changes over time. Thus, measurement of the piezoelectric effect in bone or tendon can provide information on the physical loads that are being carried by these materials. For example, a shear stress applied along the long axis of a bone alters the polarization voltage that appears on a surface at right angles to the axis.[3089] In another experiment,[3093] piezoelectric surface charges on a loaded human femur were measured to range from -131 to +207 picocoulombs/cm^2 (-8 to +13 charges/micron^2) from one end of the bone to the other end, depending upon position along the shaft. Real-time monitoring of this data would permit specific inferences as to the amount of load the bone was carrying and from what direction, including bending, shearing, and twisting forces, from which whole-body activity states could subsequently be inferred. Knowledge of these surface charge variations might also be exploited in osteographic (Section 8.2.4) or functional (Section 8.4) navigation.

4.9.4 Optical Macrosensing

In vivo medical nanodevices can gather little useful optical information from the external environment. Here's why.

In biological soft tissues, scattering dominates absorption except in the pigmented layers of the epidermis and stratum corneum. Thus the propagation of light in tissues may be regarded as occurring in two steps.[509,510]

In the first step, optical photons of intensity I_0 falling perpendicularly on skin are transmitted according to Beer's law through tissue to a depth z with a transmitted intensity of

$$I_z = I_0 \left(1 - r_{sp}\right) e^{-\sigma_t z} \quad \left(\text{watts/m}^2\right) \qquad \{\text{Eqn. 4.57}\}$$

where r_{sp} = specular reflection coefficient for visible light (Fresnel reflection at the air-tissue surface) ~ 4%-7%,[508] or 0% if the original light source lies within the body; and the transmission coefficient $\sigma_t = \sigma_a$ (absorption coefficient ~ 300 m^{-1}) + σ_s (scattering coefficient ~ 30,000 m^{-1}) for various human soft tissues at optical wavelengths.[510] (Coefficient values for the most heavily pigmented skin layers may be 5-7 times higher.)[508] Typical values for σ_t ~ 10,000-100,000 m^{-1}, average ~30,000 m^{-1} for soft tissue, although exceptionally clear tissues with σ_t = 1000 m^{-1} have been reported.[510,729] Thus the mean free path of an optical photon in human soft tissue is 10-100 microns, average ~ 30 microns (~1.5 tissue cell-widths), up to an extreme maximum of ~1 mm for the most transparent tissues known. For σ_t ~ 30,000 m^{-1}, at z = 150 microns, I_z / I_0 ~ 0.01 and ~99% of all photons have been scattered at least once from their initial path.

In the second step, in an unbounded medium the patch of fully scattered photons continues to propagate through the tissue via diffusion until all photons are absorbed. The complicated governing diffusion equation has not yet been been completely solved analytically,[510] but the asymptotic diffusive fluence is given roughly by

$$I_d \sim I_i \, e^{-\sigma_d z} \quad \left(\text{watts/m}^2\right) \qquad \{\text{Eqn. 4.58}\}$$

where σ_d is the diffusion exponent or effective attenuation coefficient (averaging ~900 m^{-1} for typical soft tissues but with an extremely wide range reported over the ultraviolet, visible, and near-infrared wavelengths, from 10-1,000,000 m^{-1}.)[729] As a crude approximation, the initial intensity of the fully scattered photon patch $I_i \sim I_0 (1 - r_{sp})\, a_{scat}$, where $a_{scat} = \sigma_s / (\sigma_s + \sigma_a) \sim 0.987$ is the albedo for single particle scattering.

Over the optical band from 400-700 nm, incident intensity I_0 = 100-400 watts/m^2 when standing in direct sunlight; artificial lighting in homes and offices is typically 0.1-10 watts/m^2; moonlight provides only $I_0 \sim 10^{-4}$ watts/m^2; and the absolute threshold for human vision is ~10^{-8} watts/m^2.[585] For $\sigma_d \sim 900$ m^{-1}, the intensity ratio of transmitted/incident visible light falls to $I_d / I_0 = 0.1$ at z = 2.5 mm depth (~eyelids), ~10^{-4} at z = 1 cm depth, and ~10^{-11} at z = 2.8 cm—a depth at which the tissue would be completely dark to the human eye even under direct sunlight illumination at the outermost skin surface.

An optical nanosensor with N_{sensor} receiver elements, with each receiver element having an area A_e = 1 nm^2 and capable of single-photon detection, requires an integration time for reliable detection of e^{SNR} photons given by

$$t_{meas} \sim \frac{h\, \nu\, e^{SNR}}{I_d\, N_{sensor}\, A_e} \quad \text{(sec)} \qquad \text{\{Eqn. 4.59\}}$$

where h = 6.63 x 10^{-34} joule-sec and ν = 4.3-7.5 x 10^{14} Hz for optical photons. Let us assume that a patient is standing in $I_0 \sim 400$ watt/m^2 direct unfiltered sunlight, and that t_{meas} = 1 sec, SNR = 2, N_{sensor} = 25,000 elements giving a nanorobot eyespot of $A_e N_{sensor}$ = 0.025 $micron^2$, and that σ_d = 900 m^{-1}. Then from Eqns. 4.58 and 4.59 the maximum tissue depth for optical photon detection is $z_{max} \sim 17$ mm ($I_d \sim 10^{-4}$ watt/m^2) which includes a volume of tissue comprising up to ~30% of total body volume. Changes in illumination at the minimum indoor artificial level of ~0.1 watts/m^2 are visible to $z_{max} \sim 7$ mm depth. This eyespot, if exposed to air on the outermost surface of the skin, is just sensitive enough to detect full moonlight.

Our general conclusion is that variations in normal indoor lighting may be directly measurable by nanorobots stationed within the outermost ~1 cm of body tissues. Imaging, as opposed to the simple illumination detection system described here, is a much more difficult design challenge (Chapter 30). Direct stimulation of retina-resident nanosensors is described in Section 7.4.6.5 (D).

4.9.5 Neural Macrosensing

The ability to detect individual neural cell electrical discharges noninvasively in many different ways (Section 4.8.6), coupled with the abilities (A) to recognize and identify specific desired target nerve cells (Section 8.5.2, Chapter 25) and (B) to pool data gathered independently by spatially separated nanodevices in real time (Section 7.3), offers the possibility of indirect neural macrosensing of complex environmental stimuli by eavesdropping on the body's own regular sensory signal traffic.

For example, facultatively mobile nanodevices may swim into the spiral artery of the ear and down through its bifurcations to reach the cochlear canal, then position themselves as neural monitors in the vicinity of the spiral nerve fibers and the nerves entering the epithelium of the organ of Corti (cochlear or auditory nerves) within the spiral ganglion (Figure 7.4). These monitors can detect, record, or rebroadcast to other nanodevices in the communications network all auditory neural traffic perceived by the human ear. Advanced speech recognition systems (Section 7.4.2.3) may permit recovery of spoken words and identification of individual speakers (including vocalizations by the user), recognition of background noises, reception and validation of cues or commands spoken directly to in vivo nanosystems by authorized medical personnel, and so forth. Since properly configured monitors can also modulate or stimulate nerve impulses (Sections 4.8.6 and 7.4.5.6), these devices may add audible signals to the audio traffic, thus may be employed as hearing aids (using feedback loops), real-time language translation mechanisms, continuous vocalization/audition recorders, voice-stress analyzers, or nanodevice-user communications links (Section 7.4).

Nanomonitors positioned at the afferent nerve endings emanating from hair cells located in the otolithic membrane of the utricle and saccule and in the cristae ampullaris of the semicircular canals allow medical nanodevices to directly record, amplify, attenuate, or modulate the body's own sensations of gravity, rotation, and acceleration, although kinesthetic sensory management might also be required for complete control. Motor neurons likewise can be monitored to keep track of limb motions and positions, or specific muscle activities, and even to exert control (Section 7.4.6.2). Neuron-resident nanorobots may detect auditory effects induced in the brain by pulsed microwaves from external sources.[3473] Feline cochlear neurons sensitive to audible frequencies of >300 Hz respond to single microwave pulses at a threshold-specific absorption rate of 6-11 watts/kg-pulse,[3479,3480] while in humans the threshold for effect, which depends on energy per pulse, may be as low as ~0.02 joule/m^2-pulse for people with low hearing threshold.[3481]

Olfactory and gustatory sensory neural traffic similarly may be eavesdropped by nanosensory instruments (Section 7.4). Nerve taps in the medulla oblongata or at the phrenic nerve that drives the diaphragmatic muscles allow direct monitoring of respiratory activity. Pain signals may be recorded or modified as required, as can mechanical and temperature nerve impulses from other receptors located in the skin. Even psychological variables such as emotionality, vigilance, and mental workload may be directly monitored by measuring ANS activity in sympathetic efferent fibers outside of the brain.[512]

The most complex and difficult challenge in neural macrosensing will be optic nerve taps. The retina is thoroughly vascularized, permitting ready access to both photoreceptor (rod, cone, bipolar and ganglion) and integrator (horizontal, amacrine, and centrifugal bipolar) neurons. However, the optic nerve bundle itself has ~10^6 tightly bunched individual nerve fibers, a 10-100 MHz signal bandwidth, and significant natural data compression techniques which all must be untangled in real time. Developing algorithms capable of interpreting raw optical nerve traffic,[3018-3021] say, to recognize a specific human face or a specific scene in the vision field, would prove a significant research challenge. (Direct monitoring of photoreceptors or retinal membrane potentials and other techniques (Section 7.4.6.5) may simplify untangling of the signal compression.) Rapid visual field identification using artificial neural nets is also a subject of much current research interest. Eyeball rotations (e.g., via resident intradevice nanogyroscopes; Section 4.3.4.1), eyelid position, pupil aperture, and lens accommodation under ciliary muscle control must be monitored to supplement the vision field analysis.

4.9.6 Other Macrosensing

We have only scratched the surface of the potential for nanorobot macrosensing. Medical nanodevices can quantitatively monitor variables not normally accessible to human consciousness, such as:

1. hormone and neurotransmitter levels;
2. gastroelectric oscillations and skin conductivity;

3. pupil dilations;
4. drug and alcohol (and breakdown product) concentrations in the blood;
5. internal organ damage or malfunction;
6. digital real-time performance data on vital organs or limbs (e.g., continuous kidney volume throughput, pancreatic insulin output, cholesterol metabolism in the liver, or lactic acid production in specific muscles during exercise); and
7. continuous mapping of thermoregulatory isotherms from which the temperature and heat capacity of the external medium (e.g., swimming pool water, cool night air) and the presence of sunlight or shade on the skin (via dermal thermal differentials) may be inferred (Section 8.4.1.3).

Various chemical substances cyclically increase and decrease in serum concentration with time of day, permitting crude temporal macrosensing (Section 10.1.1). Other substances (e.g., aldosterone; Appendix B) significantly vary in serum concentration depending upon whether the patient is supine or standing, thus permitting limited biochemical postural macrosensing.

If nanorobots can leave and re-enter the body (Section 8.6; Chapter 16), then macrosensing may include direct sampling of the external environment upon demand and the possibilities for remote data acquisition become virtually limitless.

CHAPTER 5
Shapes and Metamorphic Surfaces

5.1 Flexible Form and Function

It has been asserted that nanomechanical systems fundamentally differ from systems of biological molecular machinery in their basic architecture—specifically, that nanomechanical components are supported and constrained by stiff housings, while biological components often can move freely with respect to one another.[10] As regards medical nanodevices, this may be a somewhat artificial distinction. The likelihood that most nanoscale components will be connected in rigid arrays does not imply that the nanomachines themselves must be entirely rigid in shape, nor does it rule out the possibility that some major nanomachine components may be designed to allow periodic reconfiguration and repositioning.

Why might a flexible shape be useful in nanomedicine? While cell membranes are self-sealing, large wall breaches during cell repair operations can be problematical. A flexible shape makes it easier for a cell repair nanodevice to enter the cytoplasm with minimum disruption, for instance by elongating and narrowing so as to present the narrowest possible aspect during plasma membrane and cytoskeletal penetration (Section 9.4.5). When navigating through narrow passages in hard biological substances such as bone or enamel, a nanorobot with a rigid shape is more likely to scrape or jam than is a more flexibly-shaped device. Extensible volumes allow the projection of compliant mechanical pseudopods of various sizes and shapes from the nanomachine surface. Deformable bumpers make it easier to establish and maintain reliable multidevice linkages in large-scale cooperative nanorobotic architectures.

Flexibility expands the options available for nanodevice mobility to include amoeboid and pulsatile peristaltic locomotion (Section 9.4.3), surface deformation natation (Section 9.4.2.5.1), and circumvascular tissue diving or nanorobot diapedesis (Section 9.4.4). Fluidlike surfaces are ubiquitous among motile microorganisms. Malleable nanodevices situated on a cardiac or arterial luminal surface can adopt minimum fluid drag configurations.

Microhydrodynamic stability is another factor. For example, when placed in a bloodflow of constant speed in a tubular vessel, a rigid sphere, rod, or disk will tumble as it travels, due to the differential axial velocity field. But external fluid stresses distort a deformable object like an emulsion droplet from its original spherical shape into an ellipsoid oriented at a constant angle to the direction of flow. The fluid stresses are transmitted across the droplet interface; the surface and interior fluid circulates about the particle center in a tank tread motion.[386] Shape changes can also be employed for steering and orientational control during active nanorobot swimming (Section 9.4.2.5): Hard-shelled particles without active mobility don't marginate laterally in blood vessels; deformable surfaces can radially migrate.[362] Flexible surfaces may also be used to minimize the increment to blood viscosity caused by the presence of bloodborne nanorobots (Section 9.4.1.4).

A flexible or "metamorphic" surface is a nanodevice exterior surface comprised of independently controllable elements that can translate or rotate their relative positions, thus enlarging or contracting total surface area of the device, or changing its shape, with or without altering the membership of elements in the surface, with or without altering the enclosed volume of the entire nanomachine, while maintaining continuous structural integrity and nonpermeability of the surface. The range of possible designs is enormous. Metamorphic surfaces may include integument systems with semirigid components; hinged elements with fixed relative position and area, allowing variable volume; partially mobile surfaces having unit elements of fixed size but variable position relative to their neighbors, allowing control of surface area as well as volume; and even fully metamorphic surfaces with surface elements free to rotate, alter shape or orientation, slide, or even change membership, permitting maximum surface/volume flexibility.

Device shape is driven by task requirements which may or may not demand surface flexibility, as described in Section 5.2. Section 5.3 presents a number of design alternatives for metamorphic surfaces and manipulators, and briefly considers the impact of surface flexibility on internal configurational design. Section 5.4 examines the challenges of metamorphic bumpers which serve as interdevice fasteners and junctions. Discussion of the biocompatibility of nanodevice surfaces[3234] is deferred to Chapter 15.

5.2 Optimum Nanorobot Shape

The optimum nanorobot shape varies according to the function the device is designed to perform and the environment in which the device must operate.[3582] A consideration of the many different functions that medical nanodevices are asked to perform suggests several general classes of tasks requiring specific group geometries which drive the choice of optimum individual nanodevice geometry for each task class. For comparison, microscopic unicellular bacteria generally take three basic forms: spherical or ellipsoidal (the cocci), cylindrical or rod-shaped (the bacilli), and curved rod, spiral, or comma-shaped (the spirilla), though there is at least one example of a square bacterium.[2028]

5.2.1 Free-Floating Solitary Nanodevices

Free-floating simple nanorobots intended solely as materials delivery or storage devices, or used as omnidirectional communications, navigational or control transponders operating independently in vivo, have no preferred orientation. Thus these nanorobots may be spherically symmetric with rigid surfaces. Spherical particles produce the smallest possible increment in blood viscosity as they tumble, in part because spheres offer the smallest possible interaction surface per unit volume of any geometrical shape. Such simple nanomachines are the kind most likely to be deployed in the greatest numbers, and their reduced surface area minimizes potential biocompatibility problems.

These free-floating nanodevices must have ready access to all tissues via blood vessels. Since they are nonmotile machines, to avoid getting stuck they must not physically extend wider across their longest axis than the width of human capillaries, which average 8 microns in diameter but may be as narrow as 4 microns (Section 8.2.1.2).

Consider a nanodevice of fixed surface area A_n, total volume V_n, and longest transdevice diameter L_n. Then:

A. For a spherical device of radius r, then $L_n = 2\,r$, $A_n = 4\,\pi\,r^2$, and $V_n = (4/3)\,\pi\,r^3$.

B. For a prolate spheroidal (football-shaped) device of length 2a, width 2b, and eccentricity $e = (a^2 - b^2)^{1/2} / a$, then $A_n = 2\,\pi\,b^2 + 2\,\pi\,a\,b\,(\arcsin(e)\,/\,e)$ and $V_n = (4/3)\,\pi\,a\,b^2$. For an oblate spheroidal device, $A_n = 2\,\pi\,a^2 + \pi\,b^2\,(\ln(\{1+e\}/\{1-e\})\,/\,e)$ and $V_n = (4/3)\,\pi\,a^2\,b$. In both cases, $L_n = 2a$ and the maximum enclosed volume per unit area occurs at a = b (e.g., a sphere).

C. For a right circular disk or cylindrical device of radius r and height h, then $L_n = (h^2 + 4r^2)^{1/2}$, $A_n = 2\,\pi\,r\,(h + r)$, and $V_n = \pi\,r^2\,h$. Maximum enclosed volume per unit area occurs at $h = 2^{1/2}\,r$.

D. For a right circular conical device of radius r and height h, then $L_n = 2r$ for $h \leq 3^{1/2}\,r$ (but $L_n = (h^2 + r^2)^{1/2}$ if $h > 3^{1/2}\,r$), $A_n = \pi\,(r^2 + r\,(h^2 + r^2)^{1/2})$, and $V_n = \pi\,r^2\,h\,/\,3$. Maximum enclosed volume per unit area occurs at $h = 3^{1/2}\,r$.

E. For a right triangular prismatic device (Fig. 5.4) with three equal sides of length s and height h, then $L_n = (h^2 + s^2)^{1/2}$, $A_n = 3\,h\,s + 3^{1/2}\,s^2/\,2$, and $V_n = 3^{1/2}\,s^2\,h\,/\,4$. Maximum enclosed volume per unit area occurs at $h = s\,/\,2^{1/2}$.

F. For a cubical device with three equal sides of length s, then $L_n = (3^{1/2})\,s$, $A_n = 6\,s^2$, and $V_n = s^3$.

G. For a right square prismatic device with two equal sides of length s and height h, then $L_n = (h^2 + 2\,s^2)^{1/2}$, $A_n = 2\,s^2 + 4\,h\,s$, and $V_n = h\,s^2$. Maximum enclosed volume per unit area occurs at h = s.

H. For a right hexagonal prismatic device (Fig. 5.4) with six equal sides of length s and height h, then $L_n = (h^2 + 4\,s^2)^{1/2}$, $A_n = 6\,s\,(h + 3^{1/2}\,s\,/\,2)$, and $V_n = 27^{1/2}\,s^2\,h\,/\,2$. Maximum enclosed volume per unit area occurs at $h = 2^{1/2}\,s$.

I. For a truncated octahedral device (Fig. 5.5) of edge s, then $L_n = (10^{1/2})\,s$, $A_n = (6 + 432^{1/2})\,s^2$, and $V_n = (128^{1/2})\,s^3$.

J. For a rhombic dodecahedron[1101] (Fig. 5.6) of edge s, then $L_n = (48^{1/2}\,/\,3)\,s$, $A_n \sim (11.3137)\,s^2$, and $V_n \sim (3.0792)\,s^3$.

K. For a nonregular octahedron (Fig. 5.8) of equatorial edge s and vertex edge $(3^{1/2}\,/\,2)\,s$, then $L_n = (2^{1/2})\,s$, $A_n = (8^{1/2})\,s^2$, and $V_n = (1/3)\,s^3$.

L. For a regular octahedron[1101] (Fig. 5.9) of edge s, then $L_n = (2^{1/2})\,s$, $A_n = (12^{1/2})s^2$, and $V_n = (2^{1/2}\,/\,3)\,s^3$.

Table 5.1, computed using the above relations, confirms that spheres offer the greatest storage volume per unit surface area and thus are the most efficient shape for this application.

5.2.2 Actively Swimming Nanodevices

Nanodevices of another class may swim rapidly through the bloodstream. It should be possible to navigate even the fastest-moving arterial flows if desired. This locomotive capability is risky to the patient if employed by large numbers of devices simultaneously (Section 9.4.1), and may not be necessary for many of the applications proposed in this book.

Bloodstream swimming by nanorobots is qualitatively dissimilar to surface swimming or to a submarine moving through the ocean at depth. Unlike these macroscale analogs where inertial forces prevail, in the microscale environment viscous forces dominate. Inertial and gravitational forces are almost irrelevant. Bloodstream swimming by simple reciprocal motions is not possible (Section 9.4.2.5). Rather, it is necessary to use deformation, helical, or other drive systems, all of which involve either a tubular shape to allow propulsed fluids to pass through the center of the device, or an axially symmetric form such as a conical-, egg- or teardrop-shaped spiral to minimize viscous drag while "drilling" through the fluid during locomotion. Red blood cells assume a biconcave shape only when in static equilibrium. In a flowing condition, lone erythrocytes deform into the shape of a bullet or slipper in the capillary blood vessels;[362] at lower shear rates in the arteries, multiple cells aggregate into cylindrical rouleaux oriented roughly in the direction of flow (Section 9.4.1.2). Metamorphic surfaces may allow a nanodevice to configure all fluid contact planes to achieve minimum drag for every velocity vector employed and every fluid traversed.

Are conventional streamlined shapes necessary or useful for micron-scale swimmers? In the macroscopic world, a body traveling through water experiences the least resistance to forward motion (drag) if it is rounded in the front and tapers to a rear point in the familiar shape of a tuna or whale—the animal thus shaped meets little drag, ~10 times less than would a sphere or a person of the same size.[2022] However, streamlining and special hydrofoil shapes serve mainly

A. to reduce induced drag, which largely disappears in nonturbulent microscale flows; and

B. to reduce pressure drag, an inertial force which also becomes relatively unimportant at the microscale.

For example, the ratio of viscous drag to pressure drag may be computed from Eqns. 9.89 and 9.90 as $F_{viscous}/F_{inertial} = (12\,\eta_{fluid}\,/\,C_D\,\rho_{fluid})\,(1\,/\,R_{nano}\,v_{nano}) \sim 10^{-5}\,/\,(R_{nano}\,v_{nano})$ in 310 K water. Given that the highest likely nanorobot swimming speed in vivo is $v_{nano} \sim 1$ cm/sec (Section 9.4.2.6), then $F_{viscous}/F_{inertial} \gtrsim 100$ for $R_{nano} \lesssim 10$ micron. Thus at the microscale, viscous forces predominate. Viscous forces are determined by total surface area in contact with fluid, so the lowest drag on a moving mass is produced (all else being equal) by a shape that presents the minimum possible surface area to the fluid, that is, approximating a sphere. The drag even on extremely pointed shapes differs little whether the object is moving forward or sideways. For instance, experiments show that the most extreme needle-shaped bodies fall about half as fast sideways as they do end-on.[1378] Note that natural micron-scale swimmers such as bacteria and small metazoans are typically ovoid or cylindrical, rather than fishlike, in shape.

An examination of 218 genera of free-floating and free-swimming bacteria[3582] revealed that motile genera are less likely to be spherical and have larger axial ratios (typically 3:1) than nonmotile genera. Spherical shapes were found to produce the largest random dispersal by Brownian motion, and oblate spheroids were rare, possibly due to the increased surface area. Prolate spheroids provided a reduced sinking speed; elongation slightly favored swimming speed, but strongly improved the temporal detection of chemical stimulus gradients by any of three different mechanisms—the probable explanation for the popularity of rod-like shapes in motile bacteria (though others[3615] have been proposed).

Table 5.1 Geometrical Factors for Bloodstream-Traversing Nanorobots of Maximum Volume with Largest Transdevice Diameter L_n = 4 μm

Nanodevice Geometrical Type	r	h	s	Enclosed Volume	Surface Area	Volume/ Surface	Shown in Figure:
Spherical/Spheroidal	2.00 μm	---	---	33.51 μm^3	50.27 μm^2	0.6667 μm	---
Truncated octahedron	---	---	1.26 μm	22.90 μm^3	42.85 μm^2	0.5343 μm	Fig. 5.5
Disk/Cylindrical	1.63 μm	2.31 μm	---	19.35 μm^3	40.46 μm^2	0.4783 μm	---
Rhombic dodecahedron	---	---	1.73 μm	16.00 μm^3	33.94 μm^2	0.4714 μm	Fig. 5.6
Hexagonal prism	---	2.31 μm	1.63 μm	16.00 μm^3	36.48 μm^2	0.4386 μm	Fig. 5.4
Cubic/Square prism	---	---	2.31 μm	12.32 μm^3	32.00 μm^2	0.3850 μm	Fig. 5.4
Circular conical	2.00 μm	3.46 μm	---	14.51 μm^3	37.70 μm^2	0.3849 μm	---
Regular octahedron	---	---	2.83 μm	10.67 μm^3	27.71 μm^2	0.3849 μm	Fig. 5.9
Triangular prism	---	2.31 μm	3.27 μm	10.67 μm^3	31.86 μm^2	0.3349 μm	Fig. 5.4
Non-Regular octahedron	---	---	2.83 μm	7.54 μm^3	22.63 μm^2	0.3333 μm	Fig. 5.8

5.2.3 Intracellular Nanodevices

Nanodevices intended to perform tasks inside human tissues by leaving the bloodstream and entering the cell or nucleus will require a physical configuration consistent with the particular mission and the specialized tools required (Chapter 21). Metamorphic surfaces may assist in cyto devices in achieving nondisruptive membrane penetrations (Section 9.4.5), deployment and manipulation of flexible mechanical pseudopods or motive appendages (Sections 5.3.1 and 9.3.1.6), and reconfiguration of sensors or other subsystems (Section 5.3.5). Cell repair nanorobots could adopt one configuration to seek the target cell, a second to penetrate the membrane, and yet a third while operating within the cytosol.

Basic device shape will not be driven by hydrodynamic considerations because cell repair nanorobots spend the bulk of their operational time on site, not in transit, and need move only relatively slowly when they travel between worksites (Chapter 21). Nor will device shape be governed by tessellation rules (Section 5.2.4), since these machines will normally spend most of their time in solitary activity or at least out of direct physical contact with other nanorobots working nearby (Chapter 21). Thus the strongest purely geometric influence on these most complex of nanodevices may be volume storage efficiency. A spherical shape or near-spherical icosahedral shape (as in many viruses) can contain the largest possible mass of nanocomputers, mass memory, power supplies, repair consumables, specialized tools, communications and navigational equipment, and so forth.

However, cellular repair machines may also need to dock with other nanomachines at irregular intervals to receive supplemental materials, fuel, or information, so it would be convenient to use a shape with a large number of planar faces across which such transfers might readily be effected. A space-filling shape (Section 5.2.5) also allows ready aggregation of operational units in vivo for ad hoc conferencing plus efficient storage of unused units. A truncated octahedron with a total of 14 hexagonal and square faces (Section 5.2.5) is the space-filling polygonal shape with the highest volume/surface ratio, closest to the sphere (Table 5.1).

5.2.4 Tessellating Nanodevice Aggregates: Nanotissues

Some of the most important applications of medical nanodevices involve cooperative activity by millions or billions of nanorobots in close physical proximity with each other. In such cases it may be essential that individual machines fit together snugly in a mosaic pattern, or periodic tessellation, across a surface to achieve an air-tight or watertight seal. The most important additional complication is that biological surfaces are usually in motion. To accommodate such motion, nanorobots may use inflatable or expansible perimeter "bumpers" to achieve a continuously tight fit. Metamorphic surfaces are used to construct these bumpers (Section 5.4).

This Section discusses nanodevice aggregates whose tasks require them to completely occupy stationary or moving surfaces. Section 5.2.5 discusses optimum shapes for aggregated nanodevices whose tasks require them to uniformly fill volumes with nanomachinery.

5.2.4.1 Tiling Nondeforming Surfaces

If the surface to be covered by a nanorobot aggregate has constant area, such as the exterior of a bone, tooth, or fingernail, or the inner surface of a passive sinus or duct, or the skull and meninges, or certain components of the eyeball (cornea, sclera, etc.), then the question is how to completely tile a fixed surface using prismatic units of a particular shape, a familiar problem in spatial geometry.[519,520] Orthogonally-arrayed unit circles achieve a packing density of only 78.54%, while hexagonal packing of unit circles achieves 90.70% coverage. However, as is well-known, triangles, squares, or hexagons are the only regular polygonal prismatic solids that can completely tile a plane by themselves, achieving 100% packing density (Fig. 5.1). There are also an infinite number of irregular planar polygonal tessellations using a wide variety of tile shapes (Fig. 5.2), although nanorobots with these shapes would suffer extraordinarily low volume/surface ratios—an extremely inefficient use of space.

Triangles, rectangles, or regular hexagons (e.g., a roll of chicken wire) can be used alone to tile a cylindrical surface. The deformation of nanorobot bumpers into curved wedge segments allows tiling of

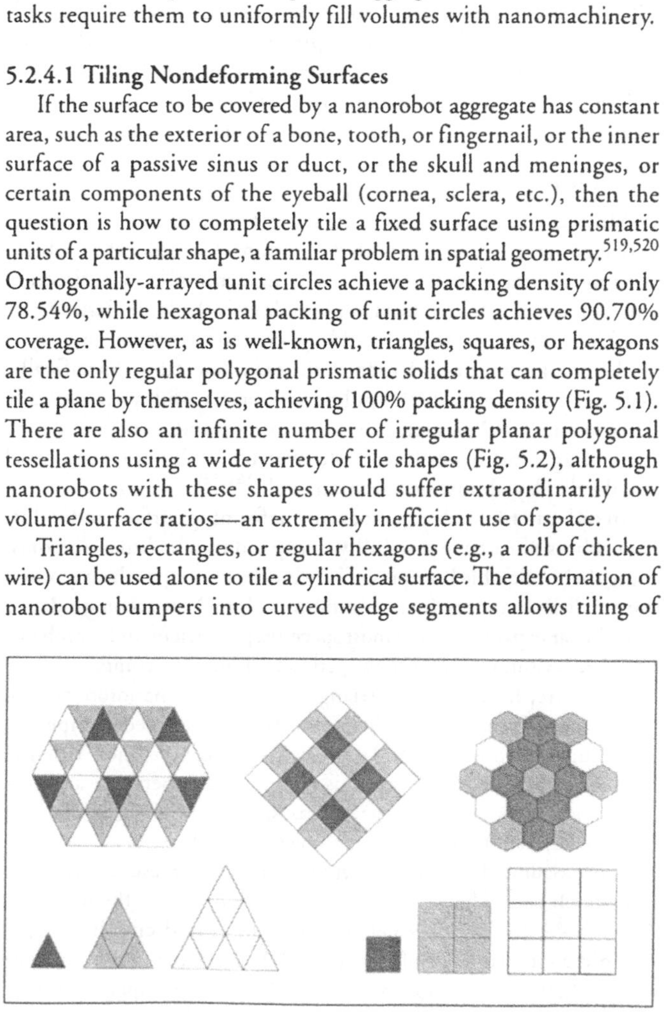

Fig. 5.1. Regular tessellations that fill a plane using only one kind of polygon.

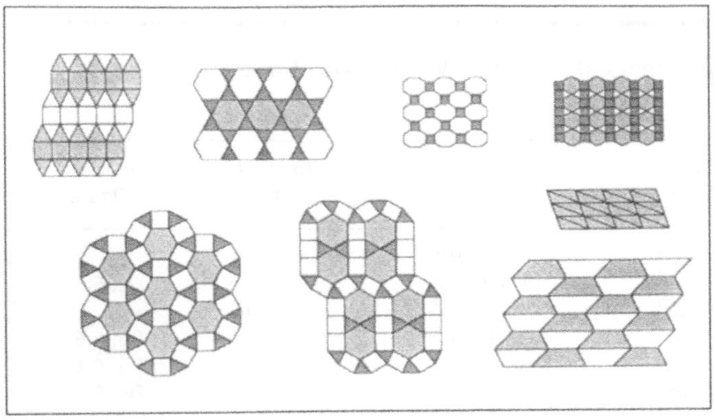

Fig. 5.2. Semiregular and nonuniform periodic (using more than one kind of polygon) tessellations.

ellipsoidal or other randomly curved surfaces provided the minimum radius of curvature r_{curve} is relatively large (e.g., $r_{curve} >> L_n$). For areas containing smaller radii of curvature ($r_{curve} > L_n$), a combination of three regular polygonal prisms may be used to completely tile any arbitrarily curved surface: hexagonal prisms for flat sections, mixed with pentagonal prisms to add positive curvature (e.g., convexity, like a sphere) and heptagonal prisms to add negative curvature (permitting concave surface deformations). Artificial fullerene and natural radiolarian structures illustrate this approach (Fig. 2.19).[522,523,1308] Triangular prisms can also be used to tile arbitrarily curved surfaces; for example, some geodesic domes[539] and the polio virus are symmetrical spherical arrangements of alternating triangles.[384] (Many viruses are regular icosahedra.)

5.2.4.2 Tiling Deforming Surfaces

Most physiological surfaces are subject to periodic deformation, or stretching, along one or both dimensions. Consider the problem of tiling a surface that is periodically deforming in one direction only. A good example in human physiology is the large elastic arteries which circumferentially distend and contract as they absorb ~50% of the stroke volume of each ventricular ejection. Specifically, diameter oscillations in the pulmonary artery and aorta typically range from 9%-12%, averaging 11% for men and women under 35 years of age and 6.5% for people over 65.[521] By contrast, vessel lengths display almost no variation at all.[361,521]

In order to tile such a monoaxially deforming surface, individual nanorobots must have the ability to expand in one dimension only, using their inflatable bumpers. The nanodevice shape which requires the smallest bumpers (i.e., minimum volume) to accommodate a given linear expansion is the most space-usage efficient and is probably preferred. Assuming continuous perimeter bumpers, compare a series of N square, hexagonal, or triangular prismatic nanorobots with equal sides of length s, height h, and fully contracted bumpers of minimum depth b (Fig. 5.3). The center-to-center linear distance between adjacent square units is $L_0 = s + 2b$; between adjacent hexagonal units along the stretch axis, $L_0 = 3s/2 + 3b/3^{1/2}$; and between adjacent triangular units along the stretch axis, $L_0 = s + 3^{1/2}\,b$.

Now assume the center-to-center distance increases by ΔL along the stretch axis. The increase in bumper volume for the squares is $\Delta V_s = h\,\Delta L\,L_0\,(N-1)/N$ per square. (For closed circuits such as complete circular rings of tiles, the (N-1)/N factor drops out.) The useful interior nanorobot volume (in which nonbumper machinery may be present) is $U_s = h\,s^2 = h\,(L_0 - 2b)^2$. For the hexagons, $\Delta V_h = h\,\Delta L\,L_0\,3^{1/2} / 3$ per hexagon, and $U_h = h\,s^2\,27^{1/2} / 2$ where $s = 2((L_0/3^{1/2}) - b) / 3^{1/2}$. For the triangles, $\Delta V_t = (3^{1/2} / 2)\,h\,\Delta L\,(L_0 + 3^{1/2}\,b)\,(N-1)/N$ per triangle, and $U_t = (3^{1/2} / 4)\,h\,s^2$ where $s = L_0 - 3^{1/2}\,b$.

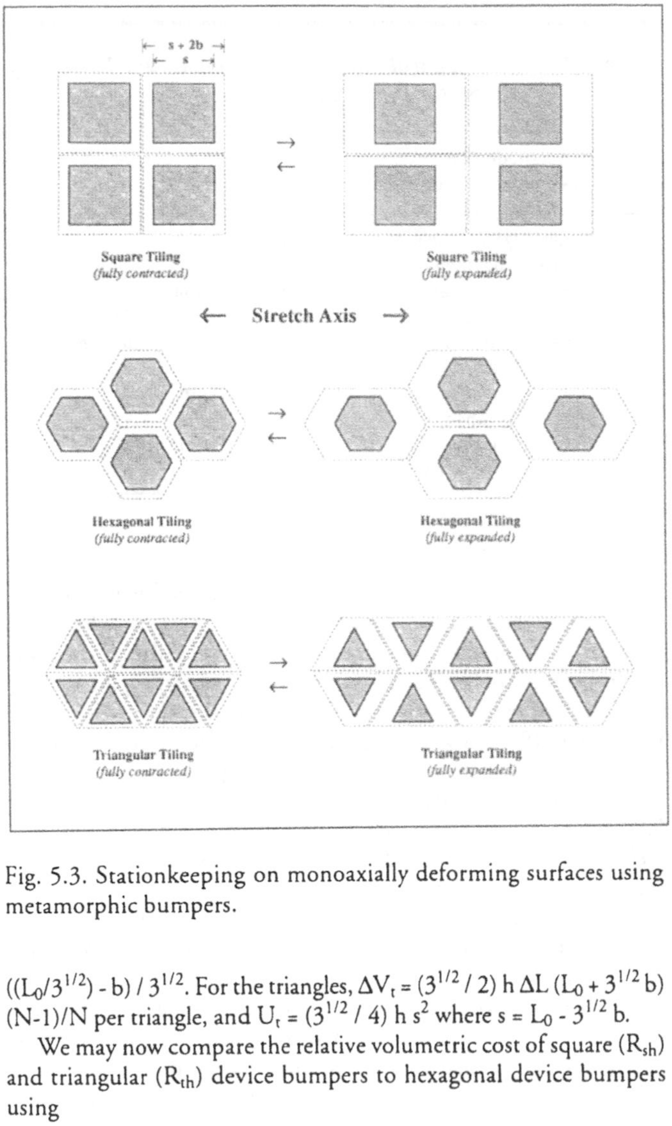

Fig. 5.3. Stationkeeping on monoaxially deforming surfaces using metamorphic bumpers.

We may now compare the relative volumetric cost of square (R_{sh}) and triangular (R_{th}) device bumpers to hexagonal device bumpers using

$$R_{sh} = \frac{\Delta V_s/U_s}{\Delta V_h/U_h} = \left(\frac{27^{1/2}(N-1)}{N}\right)\left(\frac{(L_0/3^{1/2})-b}{L_0-2b}\right)^2 \qquad \text{\{Eqn. 5.1\}}$$

$$R_{th} = \frac{\Delta V_t/U_t}{\Delta V_h/U_h} = \left(\frac{2\,(N-1)}{N}\right)\left[3^{1/2} + (3b/L_0)\right] \qquad \text{\{Eqn. 5.2\}}$$

For any choice of $(b/L_0) \geq 0$, then $R_{sh} > 1$ for all $N > 2$ and $R_{th} > 1$ for all $N > 0$. That is, bumpers on square or triangular devices inevitably require a larger percentage change in nanorobot volume to effect a given linear adjustment, hence the hexagonal prism is always the more space-efficient shape for tasks requiring monoaxial deformations. (Squares are more efficient than triangles except for $0.43\,L_0 < b < 0.52\,L_0$.)

Similar results follow from an analysis of tiling a surface that is simultaneously deforming in both dimensions. Most moving biological surfaces stretch along both axes at once, often at different rates and phases. Examples include the skin (which can stretch up to 100% before permanent damage is observed[521]), the abdominal diaphragm, cardiac chamber walls (papillary muscles thicken while shortening 7-20% during an isometric contraction[362]), alimentary surfaces, and various bladders, glands and sacs. Tendons typically stretch 5% (up to 10% in the human psoas tendon[521]) while contracting slightly in width. Apparently hexagonal prisms are also the most efficient shape for tessellating nanorobots aggregating on biaxially deforming surfaces; the intuitive rationale is that the most efficient shape is closest to a circle, with minimal perimeter length enclosing maximal area. In nature, epidermal squamous cells are arranged in hexagonal columns and onion skin cells also form neat arrays of hexagons. Hexagonal territorial partitioning is common among surface-feeding bird and fish species.[2029,2030]

5.2.5 Space-Filling Nanodevice Aggregates: Nano-Organs

In specialized structures such as synthetic bones or artificial organs constructed as aggregates of millions or billions of nanorobots, it may be necessary for nanodevices to completely occupy specific three-dimensional volumes. This is the familiar problem of space-filling polyhedra in spatial geometry.

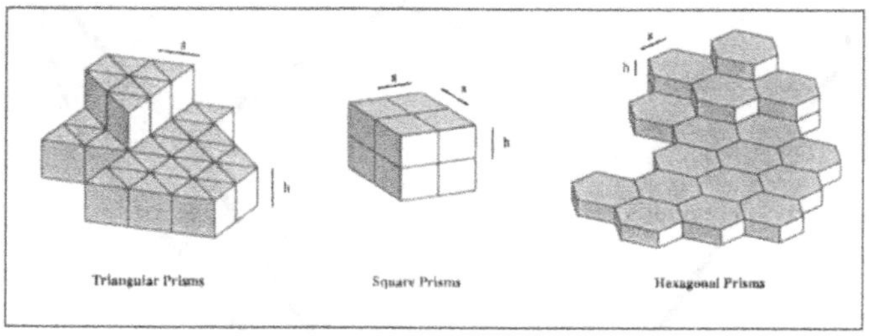

Fig. 5.4. Uniform space filling using one kind of polyhedron: triangular, square and hexagonal prisms.

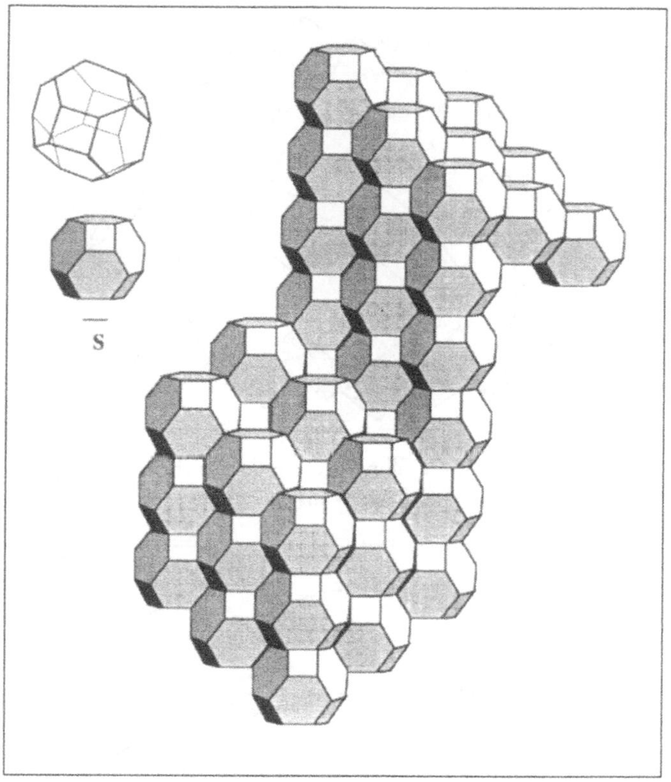

Fig. 5.5. Uniform space filling using only the truncated octahedron.

The volumetric packing factor of closely-packed spheres of equal radius is only $(3\pi^2 / 64)^{1/2} \sim 0.68017$;[519] by comparison, protein-interior packing densities are ~60%-85%.[3211] The simplest way to completely fill a volume (e.g., packing factor = 1) is to use a prism having a horizontal cross-section of a shape that will tile surfaces, as previously described (Section 5.2.4.1). Multiple planar fully-tiled surfaces can then be stacked vertically to fill the volume. Space-filling forms include triangular, square, and hexagonal prisms (Fig. 5.4). Of these, the hexagonal prism has the highest volume/area ratio and appears to be the most efficient prismatic form.

Only five other shapes can uniformly fill volumes by themselves and thus may be candidates for space-filling nanorobots. The most important of these is the truncated octahedron, similar to the tetrakaidecahedron,[1101] which can fill space all by itself (Fig. 5.5). The truncated octahedron is formed by cutting the 6 corners off a regular octahedron (which has 8 faces, all triangles; Fig. 5.9), making a 14-hedron consisting of 6 small squares and 8 large hexagons, with 24 vertices and 36 edges. A truncated octahedron surrounded by 14 identical polyhedra contacting and matching each of its faces forms a solid unit in space resembling the original unit—that is, very close to spherical. Such an aggregate with many planar facial contacts permits easy docking, fastening, and transmission of forces in all directions. Weyl,[524] following Lord Kelvin,[520] long ago recognized that this 14-hedron has the highest volume/area ratio of all the space-filling polyhedra (Table 5.1) and is a close mathematical model of soap bubble froth.

Four other single-species space-filling polyhedra are known. The first is the garnet-shaped rhombic dodecahedron, which has 12 faces, all of which are rhombuses (Fig. 5.6). The volume/area ratio of this 12-hedron is intermediate between the 14-hedron and the hexagonal prism; the shape is found in back-to-back formations in the planar hexagonal honeycomb cell of the bee.[519] The second is the closely related rhombo-hexagonal dodecahedron (Fig. 5.7), which is also self-packing. The third is the non-regular octahedron (8 faces, all triangles; Fig. 5.8), which results from truncating a cube such that all eight vertices are replaced by triangular faces with the new vertices coinciding with the intersection of the face diagonals of the original cube.[519] Hence the equatorial edges are all the same but the vertex edges are half the length of a circumscribed cube's interior diagonal, as distinct from the regular octahedron (Fig. 5.9) with all sides equal,

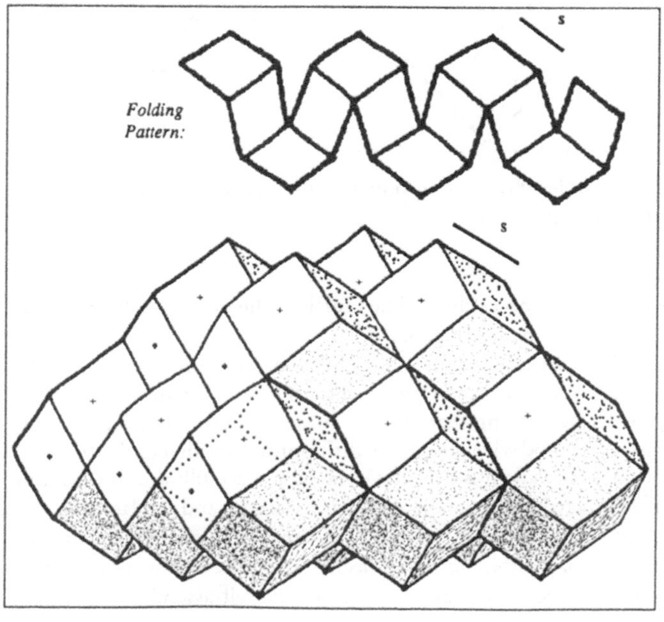

Fig. 5.6. Uniform space filling using only the rhombic dodecahedron (modified from Williams[1101]).

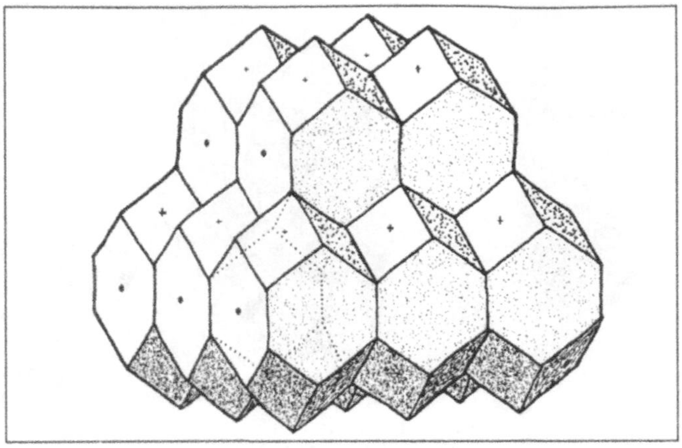

Fig. 5.7. Uniform space filling using only the rhombo-hexagonal dodecahedron (modified from Williams[1101]).

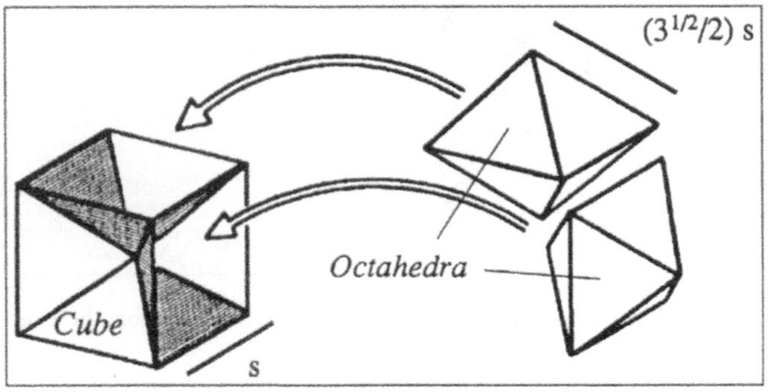

Fig. 5.8. Uniform spacing filling using only the non-regular octahedron (modified from Gasson[519]).

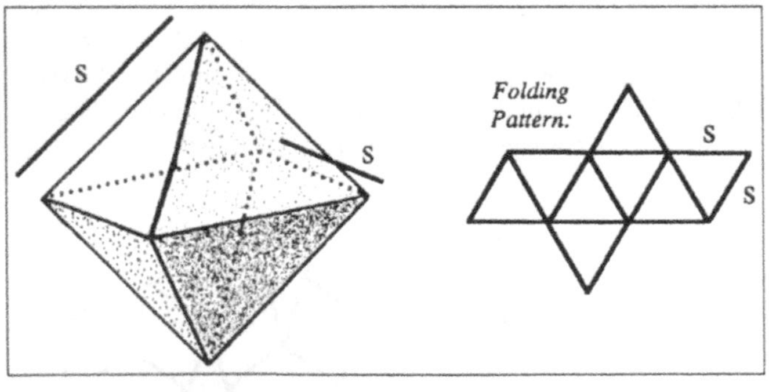

Fig. 5.9. Solid and folding geometry of the regular octahedron (modified from Williams[1101]).

which is not space-filling. The fourth of the rare space-filling solids is the trapezohedra (Fig. 5.10).[518]

There are also an infinite number of nonuniform space-filling systems in which two or more kinds of polyhedra are combined.[518] Nanodevices filling space by this means would require at least two distinct nanodevice species of the appropriate shapes. Perhaps the best-known variant is the octet element, a space-filling unit consisting of an ordered combination of regular tetrahedra and regular octahedra. Unique interlocking interfacial or other features can ensure that major subassemblies of the collective structure can only fit together in one correct way as an aid in automatic self-assembly and quality assurance.

Finally, many biological solids are so thoroughly perforated with holes and tubes that they are more properly regarded as porous rather than completely filled solids. These forms are simulated using open packings of polyhedra arrays[518] that may be employed to form near-arbitrary networks[2843] of interior voids and channels in artificial organs, as required. Zeolites and other molecular sieves provide excellent models of this configuration.[382,2468,2469]

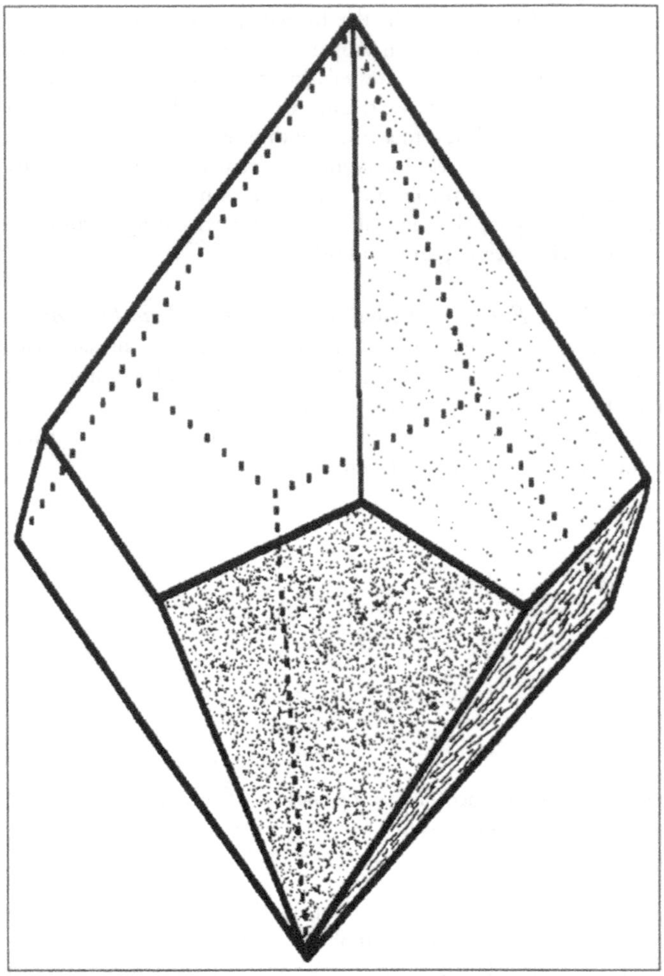

Fig. 5.10. Solid geometry of the space filling trapezohedron (modified from Williams[1101]).

5.3 Metamorphic Surfaces

Metamorphic surfaces are ubiquitous throughout the animal kingdom. The best known examples are the skins of dolphins[2034,2035] and sharks,[2036,2037] which may actively manipulate the contours of their rubbery integuments in real time to reduce or eliminate skin turbulence and thus maintain near-perfect streamlines to maximize swimming speed (though some have questioned this interpretation).[2022,2038]

A precise control of the skin may seem foreign to us because, aside from eyebrow-raising, humans have lost volitional local dermal mobility in most areas of the body. Many lower animals can exercise precise control because they possess a well developed layer of cutaneous striped muscle, the paniculus carnosus, of which only vestigial remnants remain in the subdermal tissues of human beings. In man, the skin is more or less firmly attached to relatively inelastic and immobile fascia, which in turn is attached to major musculature, bone, or other underlying structures, particularly on the extremities and anterior chest wall.

An ability to control a nanorobot surface has many interesting applications and implications. This Section describes basic design considerations, specific configurations, and other useful aspects of nanoscale metamorphic surfaces.

5.3.1 General Design Considerations

Basic design for any metamorphic surface includes a consideration of minimum feature size, linear extensibility, volumetric limits, areal expansion limits, and maximum distension speed. Other design considerations include tensile and compressive strength along all likely stress vectors at both minimum and maximum surface extensions, and the resistance of surfaces to cuts and tears.

5.3.1.1 Dimple Size

The smallest possible feature, or "dimple size," on a metamorphic surface is defined by the minimum turning radius of the surface. In most designs, this radius is determined by the minimum lateral extent of the component blocks of which the surface is comprised. Considerations of radiation-induced structural failure in diamondoid materials and components[10] suggest a minimum unit size L ~ 10 nm (Chapter 13), roughly the thickness of the cellular lipid bilayer membrane. A single 180° turn requires a minimum of two linear segments; the minimum structural turning radius is $r_{min} = L / 2^{1/2} \sim$ 7 nm at a 90° joint angle, giving a minimum metamorphic feature diameter of ~14 nm. In most practical systems, power and control access requirements necessitate turning radii several times larger than this theoretical minimum, perhaps ~40-50 nm. Such larger structures should still be able to physically manipulate even the theoretically smallest biological cells (which are ~40-50 nm in diameter[527]).

5.3.1.2 Keyhole Passage

The minimum aperture through which a longitudinally stretched but laterally compressed nanodevice may pass is determined mainly by the minimum size of its internal incompressible components, not the minimum turning radius of its skin. The smallest working complex nanomachines of the human body, the ribosomes, are ~25 nm in diameter; the minimum size of a ~100 pW mechanochemical power supply is ~50 nm (Section 6.5.3). Add to this the width of the integument component blocks and it is difficult to imagine even the most flexible artificial nanodevice squeezing through a keyhole less than 50 nm in diameter—roughly the maximum dimension of the intercellular contact space.[526] A design limit of 100 nm would be more conservative.

In the macroscopic world, the octopus can stretch itself quite thin, passing rubberlike through small holes and narrow crevasses less than 10% of its size; arms, eyes, and even head can alter shape and elongate when necessary, with keyhole passage limited by its beak, the only hard part in its body.[3133]

5.3.1.3 Extensibility

The most useful property of a flexible metamorphic surface is its extensibility, defined here as the percentage length increase of a fully stretched material relative to its length at zero stretch. Maximum values for natural materials used to construct the human body include 7% for cartilage, 10% for collagen, 30% for muscle, 60%-100% for skin, and up to 170% for arterial wall material if muscles are artificially relaxed.[364] Linear elasticities of ~1000% are commonplace in artificial gels,[528] rubbers, and other elastic materials, corresponding to ~1000-fold enclosed-volumetric changes. The El Tor strain of the *Vibrio cholerae* microbe shrinks 300-fold to the size of a large virus when plunged suddenly into cold salt water and remains viable in that state.[384]

If the shape of a metamorphic surface can be controlled to $\sim r_{min}$ (Section 5.3.1.1), then nanodevices may extrude these surfaces to define useful working subvolumes such as manipulatory appendages (e.g., prehensile fingers; see below), locomotive appendages (e.g., nanopseudopods; Section 9.3.1.6), large exterior hydrodynamic features (e.g., stabilizing fins), tools (e.g., a screw-shaped prow for easier cell penetration; Section 9.4.5.2), reconfigurable mechanical data arrays (e.g., Braille-like surface texturing), engulf formations (Section 5.3.4), perimeter contact bumpers (Section 5.4), or even entire second skins (see below). In theory, such extrusions can be quite large relative to device size.

For example, consider a nanodevice of volume V_n with an onboard pocket of volume $V_f = f\,V_n$ containing $N_b = f\,V_n / L_b^3$ metamorphic unit surface blocks each L_b^3 in size. This is sufficient metamorphic material to extend a hollow cylindrical (hemisphere-capped) finger of diameter d_f out a total length $l_f = f\,V_n / \pi\, d_f\, L_b$. For f = 0.01(1%), V_n = 1 micron^3, L_b = 10 nm, and d_f = 100 nm ($\pi\, d_f / L_b \sim 31$ blocks per circumference), $N_b = 10^4$ blocks in the pocket and l_f = 3 microns maximum linear extension. Thus in theory, a finger which can extend three times the body length of the entire nanorobot can be stored in a (215 nm)^3 pocket at the nanodevice surface. Ten such fingers, functionally equivalent to two microsized human hands, would occupy only $(10/6)\ f^{2/3} \sim 0.08$(8%) of total nanodevice surface area and $10f \sim 0.10$(10%) of nanodevice volume.

Note also that a volume V_f of metamorphic blocks could be used to construct an enlarged second skin surrounding the entire nanodevice, enclosing an expanded volume $V_e = (V_f / 6\, L_b)^{3/2}$ if the shell is of thickness L_b. For V_n = 1 micron^3 and L_b = 10 nm, nanorobot volume may double (V_e/V_n = 2) if 9.5% of device volume is metamorphic blocks; nanorobot volume may expand up to tenfold if ~28% of its volume is in controllable metamorphic blocks.

There are two limiting cases of extensibility. The first case is isoareal expansion, in which total surface area remains constant while volume increases dramatically. An example is the erythrocyte, which under osmotic stress expands from its normal disk shape into a sphere due to the influx of water. Volume rises from 94 micron^3 to a high of 164 micron^3 when spherized, a 74% increase, but surface area rises from 135 micron^2 to just 145 micron^2, a mere 7% increase.

The second limiting case is isovolemic extension, wherein surface area expands at constant volume, a transition of perhaps more relevance to nanodevices containing an irreducible fixed volume of onboard nanomachinery. For instance, if a spherical device of radius r_s morphs into a disk of equal volume with height h_d and radius $r_d = \alpha\, r_s$, surface area increases by a factor of:

$$e_{area} = \frac{3\alpha^3 + 4}{6\alpha} - 1 \qquad \text{\{Eqn. 5.3\}}$$

For α = 4.7, $h_d \sim r_s / 17$ and areal extensibility e_{area} = 10.2 (1020%) while enclosed volume remains unchanged.

5.3.1.4 Reactivity

Another important parameter of nanorobot metamorphic surfaces is their reactivity—the speed with which they can execute a full-range structural modification. Energy requirements are key, given a power budget of P_m (watts) for morphing. In particular, metamorphic block velocity is limited both by the sliding power dissipation due to sliding block surfaces of area S that are sliding at a velocity v_{slide}, or

$$v_{slide} = \left(\frac{P_m}{k_l\, S} \right)^{1/2} \qquad \text{\{Eqn. 5.4\}}$$

where k_l = 400 kg/m^2-sec (Section 4.3.4.2), and by the drag power dissipated in driving a circular surface of radius r through a 310 K aqueous (plasma, interstitial or cytosolic) environment of viscosity η = 1.1 x 10^{-3} kg/m-sec at a velocity v_{drag}, given[337] by

$$v_{drag} = \left(\frac{P_m}{6 \pi \eta r} \right)^{1/2} \qquad \text{\{Eqn. 5.5\}}$$

Assuming we wish to restrict total morphing energy dissipation to a budget of P_m = 0.1 pW for a 1 micron^3 nanorobot, then for S = 6 micron^2 of sliding surfaces and r ~ 0.5 micron, v_{drag} ~ 0.3 cm/sec (< v_{slide} = 0.6 cm/sec in vacuo). Using 0.3 cm/sec, the full-range morphing action to, say, double the nanorobot diameter (~0.5 micron of radial motion) requires ~0.2 millisec for the surface of the entire nanorobot to complete the motion.

The 10-finger manipulator described in Section 5.3.1.3 may also extend at v_{drag} ~ 0.3 cm/sec while remaining within the 0.1 pW energy budget, although a single individual finger may extend at v_{drag} ~ 1 cm/sec (<< v_{slide} = 1.6 m/sec in vacuo) allowing maximum deployment within the cytosol in ~0.3 millisec. Thus metamorphic surfaces in vivo can exhibit ~KHz frequency large-motion oscillations. By comparison, deformed erythrocytes when released from micropipette suction recover their normal biconcave shape in ~100 millisec.[371] Contractile gel fibers ~1 micron thick can shrink to 4% of their initial volume in ~1 millisec when triggered by an electrochemical reaction or an applied voltage of ~5000 volts/m.[357]

5.3.2 Metamorphic Surface Configurations

At least five classes of metamorphic surface configurations are readily discernible. Undoubtedly, many more may be conceived. The structural models briefly described below are not intended as specific design proposals but rather as geometrical representations of alternative design pathways that could provide the desired capability.

5.3.2.1 Accordion Model

The Accordion Model is characterized by a surface folded in a repeating-W pattern, as in a Japanese fan or butterfly wing pleating; photographic and accordion bellows use what is known in origami* as a "basic fold." Point/line vertices may employ rigid hinges or flexural members.[1251] Fold geometry may be double-triangular, triangular-square, or double-square; may consist of segments of varying lengths; or may consist of a series of hinged blocks (Fig. 5.11). This surface remains flexible even near full distension, provided that obtuse angles may be continuously accessed. The main drawback of this model is its likely propensity to surface fouling in vivo due to the large number of concave pockets formed during flexure.

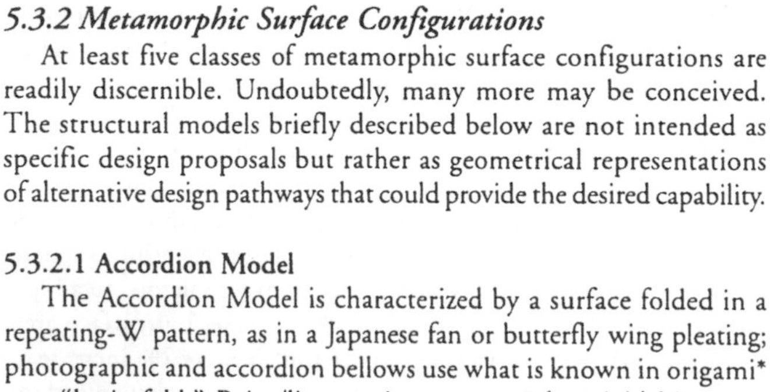

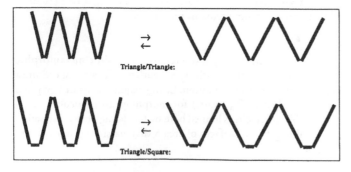

Fig. 5.11. Accordion model.

Folding or unfolding may require no sliding surfaces. Treating the model as a simple spherical surface expanding into a watery medium, from Section 5.3.1.4 a radial distension velocity of v_{drag} ~ 0.3 cm/sec may be expected for a 1-micron nanodevice with a 0.1 pW metamorphic power budget. If $N_{segment}$ is the total number of segments in a maximally extended surface of area A_{max}, then for square segments of area L^2 and thickness H, $N_{segment} = A_{max} / L^2$ and the fully folded surface has area $A_{min} = L\,H\,N_{segment}$. For L = 10 nm, H = 1 nm, and A_{max} = 10 micron^2 ($N_{segment} = 10^5$), then A_{min} = 1 micron^2 and a 0.1-pW power budget allows one full-range motion from A_{min} to A_{max} in $t_{motion} = (A_{max}^{1/2} - A_{min}^{1/2}) / (2 \pi^{1/2} v_{drag})$ ~ 0.2 millisec. For the accordion model, areal extensibility e_{area} ~ (L - H) / H = 9.00(900%) in this example.

5.3.2.2 Parasol Model

In the Parasol Model, the metamorphic surface consists of a series of overlapping plates pressed snugly together in the vertical dimension, but free to slide in the horizontal plane (Fig. 5.12). Each plate has at least one orthogonal stabilizing keel or "handle" through which the segment is connected to subsurface control (Section 5.3.3) or rigidification mechanisms. The minimum number of plate planes is two, which allows both one-dimensional and (limited) two-dimensional extensions. In the two-dimensional case, the lower plates are allowed to rotate codirectionally under a torsion-spring restoring force applied in the plane of the lower surface, keeping all edges tight under the upper plates to maintain leakproofness. A modest areal expansibility of e_{area} ~ 0.28(28%) is depicted. The maximum number of plate planes is limited by nanodevice radius (hence maximum stack depth) and operating specifications such as surface rigidity, rugosity, reactivity and controllability. Self-scraping plates produce a fouling-resistant dysopsonic design—the device simply "shrugs" in all directions, neatly guillotining any biological adherents from their attachment points on the diamondoid surface. Vertical spring tensions are adjusted to keep plates pressed tightly together, ensuring watertightness even while in motion. Corrugation features can be added to the underside of each plate to increase contact area and watertightness during plate tipping in curved configurations. Related crudely analogous structures include systems of fixed scales (e.g., lizard or snake skins) and roof tile shingle patterns on houses.

Consider an annular cylindrical section of diameter D comprised of a two-plane (p = 2) parasol surface with square top plates of area L^2 and rectangular bottom plates of area L(L-h) where h is the width of the handle and also the minimum overlap of adjacent plates at full extension. Then $A_{min} = N_{plates} L^2 = \pi\, D\, L$ and $A_{max} = A_{min} + (N_{plates} - 1)(L^2 - 3hL)$, hence areal extensibility $e_{area} = (A_{max} - A_{min}) / A_{min} = (N_{plates} - 1 / N_{plates})(1 - 3h/L)$. For N_{plates} >> 1 and h << L, the theoretical limit for a 2-plane parasol is e_{area} ~ 1.00(100%).

Extensibility is greatly improved by using additional plate planes. In the compact configuration of Figure 5.13, for p >> 1, $A_{min} = N_{plates} L^2$, $A_{max} \sim N_{plates}\, L\, (pL - p^2 h + h)$ and areal extensibility $e_{area} = p - 1 - (h/L)(p^2 - 1)$, with maximum e_{area} occurring at p = L/2h. Hence for L = 10 nm and h = 1 nm, h/L = 0.1 and maximum e_{area} = 1.60(160%) using p = 5 plate planes; the minimum plausible h/L ~ 0.01, which gives maximum extensibility e_{area} = 24.00(2400%) using p = 50 plate planes, giving a maximum surface rugosity of ~98 nm at full distension if h = 2 nm.

If an external mechanical pressure is applied perpendicular to a parasol surface, the degree of deformation will depend strongly on various details of design. Given the extensive cabling and spring-loading of plates a surface stiffness of k_s ~ 10 N/m should be

*The ancient practice of origami (the art of folding three-dimensional objects out of paper without cutting or pasting) has systematically explored the geometries of folded flat sheets;[1102-1105] the mathematics of origami is well-studied.[1106-1111]

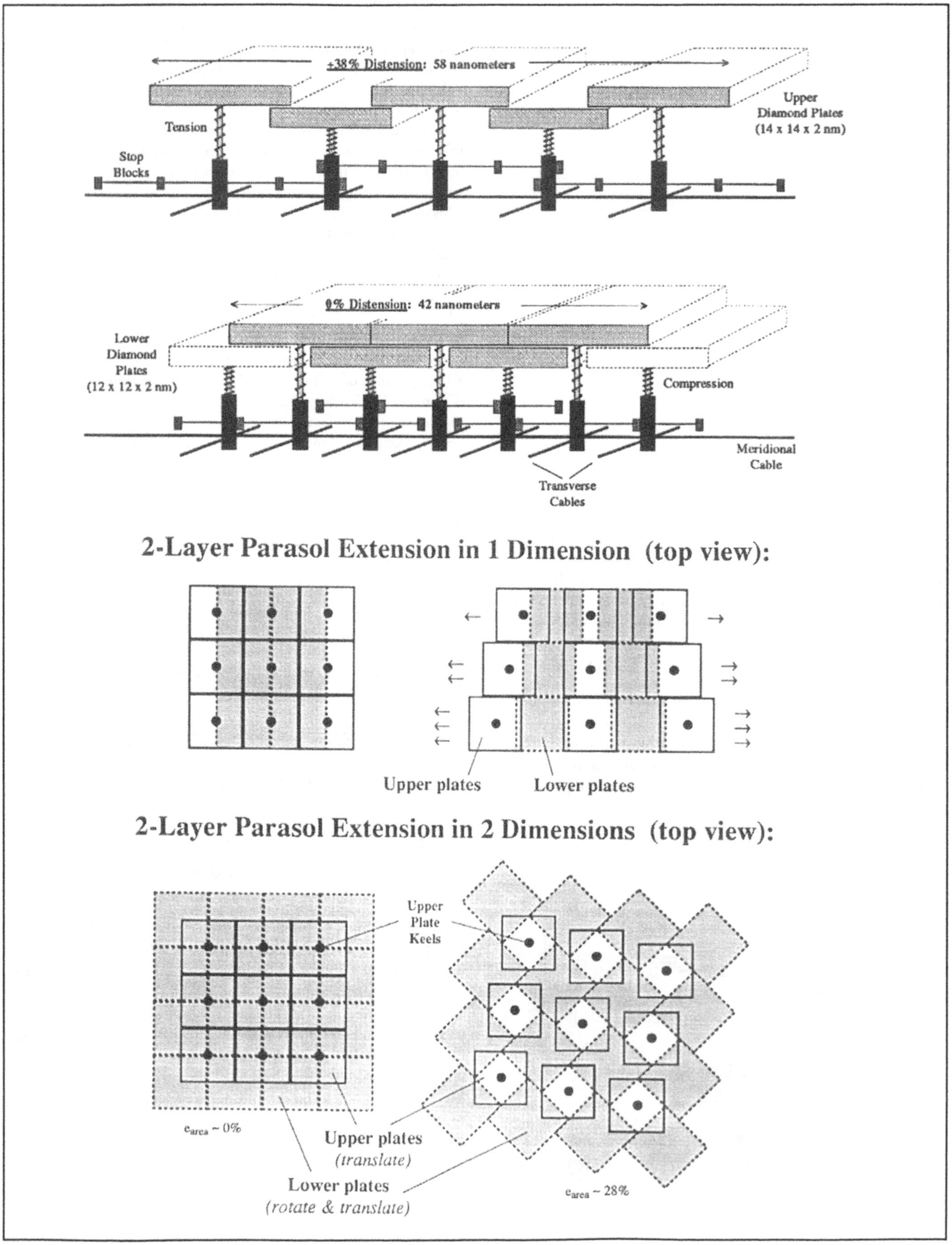

Fig. 5.12. Schematic of parasol model.

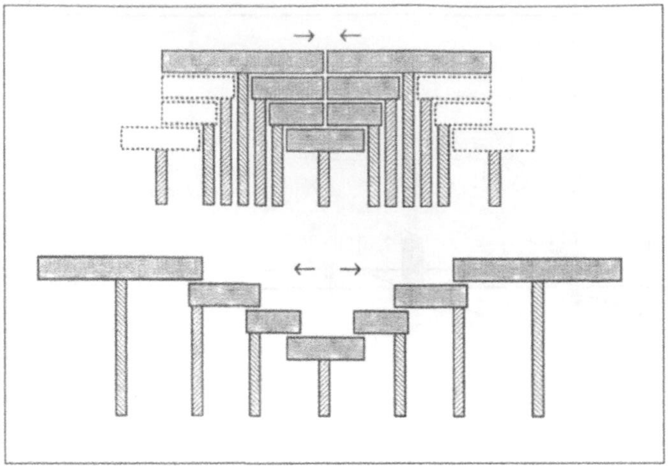

Fig. 5.13. Schematic of multiplane parasol configuration (tension/compression springs and control cables omitted).

achievable, in which case a point force of 1 nN deforms the parasol surface by ~0.1 nm.

5.3.2.3 Telescoping Model

Metamorphic surfaces using the Telescoping Model (Fig. 5.14) consist of nested, tight-fitting congruent shapes or blocks under tension fitted tightly into sleeves. The surface expands as progressively smaller segments telescope out from the main body. Typical configurations might include nested annular cylinders, sliding "dominoes" (tethered blocks), the "trombone" (sleeved blocks), or even a multisegment approach. In nature, centipedes, worms, and wasps with extended thoraxes use tubular segments to achieve flexible surfaces.

Given the many sliding interfaces and higher pressures involved, telescoping surfaces should be carefully designed to preclude possible surface oxidation. At high enough pressures sliding diamondoid plates may strip each other's passivating hydrogens, allowing newly exposed carbon atoms in the contacting surfaces to weld the plates tight; unpassivated graphene sheets (Section 5.3.2.4) may be optimal for this configuration.

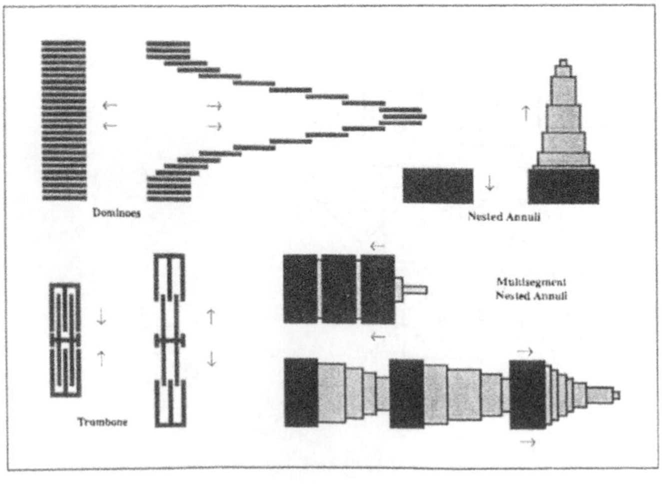

Fig. 5.14. Telescoping model: various configurations (control cables and screw drive mechanisms omitted).

5.3.2.4 Flexible Fabric Model

Two properties of metamorphic surfaces are most useful: flexibility and extensibility. The graphene sheet (of which fullerene tubes and ellipsoids are made; Section 2.3.2) is probably the ideal example of a flexible but nonextensible isoareal nanofabric that could be used to wrap a nanorobot exterior with any continuous shape having turning radii as small as 1.1 nm. The graphene sheet is a one-atom thick purely carbon surface (no hydrogen passivation yet chemically inert) arranged in a mostly hexagonal array of atoms with an occasional pentagon or heptagon for curvature (Section 5.2.4.1). This sheet has the highest tensile strength of any known 2-dimensional network, about 50 times the strength of high-carbon steel and 1.5 times the strength of crystalline diamond (Table 9.3). It has a higher packing density (atoms/nm^2) than any other network made of any other atoms in the periodic table—even a 2-D slice of diamond. The graphene sheet is effectively impermeable under normal chemical conditions—naked carbon atoms or small carbon cluster radicals will not readily bond with it, and even helium atoms up to 5 eV (~40,000 K) just bounce off. The material is probably extremely bioinactive (Chapter 15). Graphene is also an excellent conductor of heat (as good as diamond) and electricity (better than copper if appropriately doped) along the plane of the sheet, but is a poor cross-plane conductor.

The ultimate flexible and extensible volume in common experience is the rubber balloon, which readily distends its volume by several orders of magnitude with an areal extensibility of ~15,000%. Rubber is a linear polymer of isoprene $(C_5H_8)_n$ with individual molecules of n = 1000-5000 heavily cross-linked during vulcanization with 1-2% sulfur, somewhat resembling a network of coiled springs that is easily stretched. Although isoprene surfaces are porous and bioactive, hence inappropriate for nanorobot exteriors, Drexler[10] has proposed an analogous coiled pleat configuration (Fig. 5.15) that could probably be implemented using graphene sheets embedded with reciprocal non-zero-curvature elements to provide the needed countertension. The

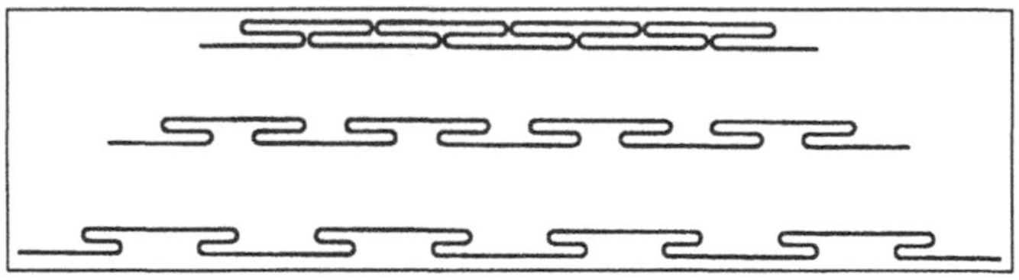

Fig. 5.15. Flexible fabric model: coiled pleat configuration.

triple-pleat configuration shown has areal extensibility e_{area} ~ 8.00(800%). As with the Accordion Model, a drawback of this design is a propensity for surface fouling in vivo due to the presence of numerous trapping pockets.

Other more dynamic configurations of flexible fabrics may be imagined. Graphene sheets may be unfurled from interior storage, like a spring-roller window shade, a rolled-up sleeping bag, or a serpentin or pito (coiled "party blowouts"). For example, R.C. Merkle[2281] notes that the minimum gas pressure differential needed to uncoil and inflate a collapsed, tightly-coiled graphene tube of radius R is given by:

$$p_{inflate} \gtrsim 2\ E_v\ /\ R \qquad \text{\{Eqn. 5.6\}}$$

where E_v is the energy of two graphite sheets held together by the van der Waals forces between them. Merkle estimates E_v ~ 0.25 J/m^2 from computer simulations, in line with Kelly's experimental value[2280] of E_v = 0.234 J/m^2. Thus a coiled tube with R = 100 nm requires at least $p_{inflate} \gtrsim 50$ atm to inflate; larger diameter tubes require less pressure differential to uncoil.

Fabrics may be comprised of tightly-woven 1.1-nm fullerene tubes with the length of each such "thread" individually controlled by winding or unwinding from numerous internal spools. In biology, various species of worms achieve linear extensibilities of up to 800% by changing the relative pitch angles of helically wound inextensible collagen fibers.[529] A dynamically reconfigurable support trusswork sheathed in flexible surface materials also permits ready shape-changing; the octet truss geometry is one of the strongest known [P. Salsbury, personal communication, 1997].

5.3.2.5 Block Exchange Model

The most difficult surface to construct is also the most volume-efficient and indefinitely extensible configuration—a surface consisting entirely of replaceable blocks or prisms of fixed geometry. In this model, surface blocks connected by snap-together interfaces are disconnected, rotated, exchanged, moved, and reconnected by subsurface block-moving mechanisms which may include manipulator arms (Section 9.3.1), conveyor systems (Section 3.4.3), and the like. Cytoskeletal components (e.g., subsurface actin microfilaments; Section 8.5.3.11) are similarly lengthened or shortened by adding or subtracting monomeric units during movement and various intracellular transport processes. Blocks combining at least one pentagonal, hexagonal, and heptagonal face can be removed, rotated to expose a new face, then refastened in a new relationship to their neighbors to alter surface concavity or convexity at will. Design constraints include a requirement that each edge of the surface faces must be of the same length, and that blocks should have angles ≤ 90° on all edges of the face that will form the surface, so that the face can be flush with adjacent faces [C. Phoenix, personal communication, 1999]. Blocks containing different "letters" from a pattern "alphabet" on various faces (e.g., different Braille-like dots on each surface, like spots on dice cubes) can also be used to post tactile-readable information mechanically on the nanorobot surface, or individual rods in rod arrays can be selectively extended or retracted from the surface to create tactile-readable displays similar to refreshable Braille displays used by the deafblind (Section 7.4.6.1).

Block-built tubular members or protrusions of any other shape may be extruded, lengthened, rotated, or reabsorbed, as required. Internal block exchange allows periodic antifouling maintenance to be performed, eliminating biomatter contamination of the external nanorobot surface. Careful design should permit a waterproof boundary to be maintained throughout the reconfiguration process (Fig. 5.16). The extensibility and reactivity of efficient block exchange models has already been explored in Section 5.3.1.

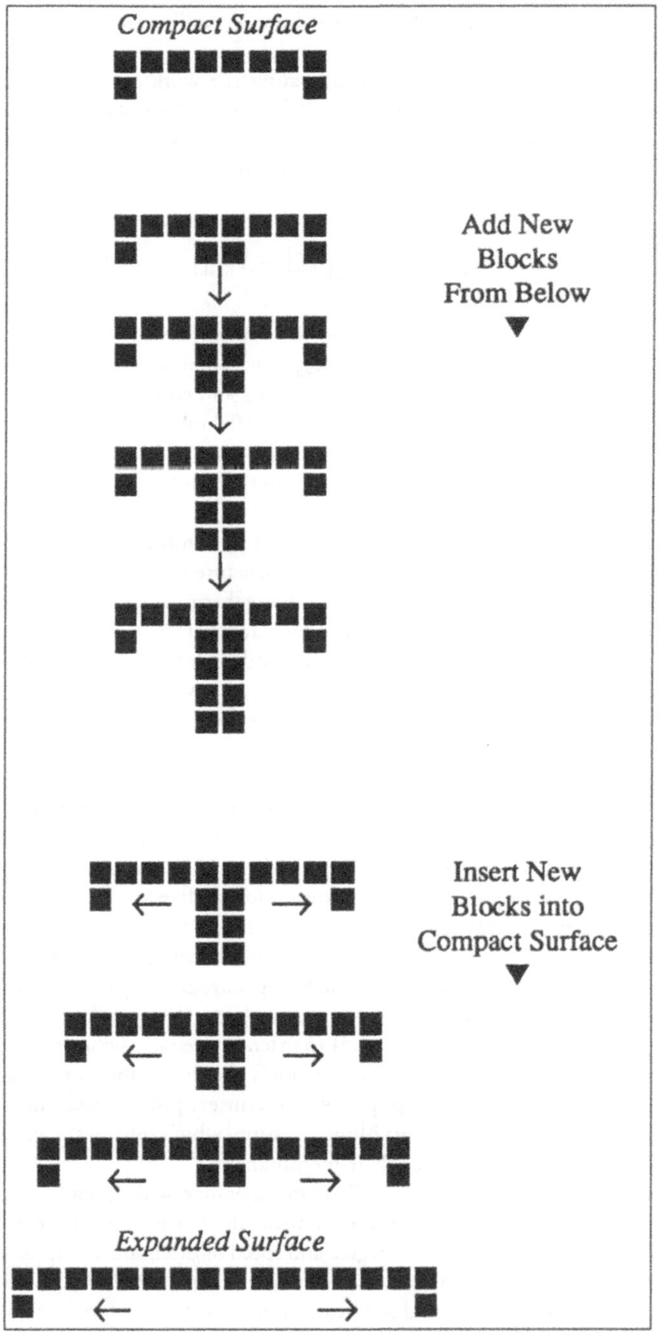

Fig. 5.16. Block exchange model (block motive and control components omitted).

5.3.3 Metamorphic Power and Control

The power required to control a given section of metamorphic surface may be provided by two simple counterbalancing mechanisms. First, the space between an interior hard shell and the distensible outer surface is pressurized using a working fluid such as gas or water. Second, the pressurization force is resisted by a gridwork of independently controllable nanoscale cables each attached to specific sets of metamorphic surface units (e.g., Fig. 5.12). Applying tension to a cable causes the units to which it is attached to selectively retract; releasing tension allows those same units to distend. This system is crudely analogous to the system of circular and longitudinal muscle fibers found in the intestines, and to the hydrostatic skeleton found in small marine organisms such as earthworms, nematodes, and to a lesser extent in echinoderms, some molluscs, caterpillars and spiders.[364] A counterbalanced surface reverts to its compact shape in the event of a physical breach with escape of working fluid, an important fail-safe design element.

Fully inflating one of the 3-micron long metamorphic fingers described in Section 5.3.1.3 requires filling its 0.015 micron^3 interior volume with ~700,000 molecules of N_2 gas at a 2-atm working pressure, accomplished in 70 millisec within a 0.1 pW power budget using a bank of 10 sorting rotors (Section 3.4.2). This gas may be stored onboard in a (41 nm)^3 (~0.00007 micron^3) pressure vessel at 1000 atm (Table 10.2). If energy efficiency is the primary concern, it should be possible to recover most of the compressive sorting power using a generator subsystem to charge an energy storage buffer as the gas passes from the high to the low pressure regime. If distension speed is the primary design goal, gas may be rapidly vented from the pressure vessel into the finger volume in milliseconds, bypassing the generator subsystem.

Of course, such rapid venting causes the working gas to cool. Ignoring the normally relatively small amount of work done on the external medium, the temperature change during free expansion of a van der Waals gas (Section 10.3.2) is simply:

$$\Delta T_{expand} = -\left(\frac{A_{vdW}\ \mu_{gas}}{C_{V_{gas}}}\right)\left(V_{init}^{-1} - V_{final}^{-1}\right) \qquad \{Eqn. 5.7\}$$

where A_{vdW} = van der Waals gas constant for intermolecular attraction, μ_{gas} is the moles of gas present, $C_{V_{gas}}$ is volumetric heat capacity of the gas, and V_{init} and V_{final} are the starting and ending gas volumes, respectively.[1031] Taking A_{vdW} = 1.390 x 10^{-6} m^6-atm/mole^2 (Table 10.1) and $C_{V_{gas}}$ = 20.8 J/mole-K for N_2 gas, and from the above example μ_{gas} = 1.2 x 10^{-18} moles (~700,000 molecules N_2), V_{init} = 6.9 x 10^{-23} m^3, and V_{final} = 1.5 x 10^{-20} m^3, then ΔT_{expand} = -120 K. However, this temperature change is rapidly conducted throughout a micron-scale diamondoid nanorobot structure in ~10^{-9} sec (Section 4.6.1), since diamond is ~3200 times more thermally conductive than water. The maximum instantaneous temperature decline in a $V_{nanorobot}$ ~ 1 micron^3 block of diamond with $C_{V_{diamond}}$ = 1.82 x 10^6 joules/m^3-K is only $\Delta T_{cool} = \Delta T_{expand}\ C_V\ \mu_{gas}\ /\ V_{nanorobot}\ C_{V_{diamond}}$ = 0.0016 K, below biologically detectable limits (Section 4.6.1).

Controlled power transmission may also be achieved by dividing the extensible surface into compartments, then pressurizing or decompressing adjacent compartments to produce differential movement, or triggering contractile gels in various compartments; by manipulating tension to tendon bundles affixed to the end of a lengthy protuberance to control tip position (Section 9.3.1.2); by mechanically rotating an internal ribcage consisting of noncoplanar ovate sections; by acoustically triggering a progression of locks and ratchets; or by using telescoping screw drives (Section 9.3.1.4) or electrostatic drives (Section 6.3.5) to extend or retract specific surface segments. In biology, butterflies exemplify the first of these methods. Upon emerging from its pupal skin, the insect pulls its abdominal segments inward to raise its blood pressure, which inflates the veins of the wings and expands their membranes.[2022]

The dexterity of a controlled protuberance will depend upon the fineness of the control mechanism, the stiffness of the metamorphic configuration, the degree and speed of extension, the applied tip load, special jointing and numerous other factors; ~0.1-1 nm positioning accuracy and application of nanonewton forces at the tip should be feasible. Pressure-driven ratchets may transduce acoustic power/control pulses transmitted internally to sensors or end effectors located at the tip.

5.3.4 Engulf Formations

Flexible nanomachines may adopt special physical configurations optimally suited for the defense of the human body. Cytocidal mechanisms are discussed in Section 10.4, but consider here a metamorphic spherical nanorobot of radius r_s which reshapes itself into a thin disk of equal volume, thickness h_d, and radius $r_d = (4\ r_s^3\ /\ 3\ h_d)^{1/2}$. This accomplished, the nanodevice next folds itself into a hollow ball, enclosing a spherical cavity of radius $r = r_d\ /\ 2$. Areal extensibility e_{area} required to complete the first transformation, the principal source of surface stretching, is given by Eqn. 5.3.

Thus a spherical nanorobot 4 microns in diameter (r_s = 2 microns), after first flattening itself into a pancake that is h_d ~ 0.1 micron thick with e_{area} ~ 12.00(1200%), can then curl into a hollow ball and completely surround a spherical biomass ~8 microns in diameter. This is large enough to engulf virus particles, most known bacteria, most in vivo nanodevices, and most of the formed elements in human blood including platelets, erythrocytes, and lymphocytes.

5.3.5 Reconfiguring Surface-Penetrating Elements

The ability to reshape a nanodevice surface implies that some configurational flexibility of external components is required. It must be possible to add, remove, or reposition stable nanodevice elements whose function requires penetrating the metamorphic surface, including sensors (Chapter 4), manipulators (Section 9.3), sorting rotor banks (Section 3.4.2), antigen semaphores (Section 5.3.6), and bulk material intake and outlet ports. A schematic of the process for removing such an element from the surface while maintaining watertightness is shown in Figure 5.17; to install an element, the process is reversed.

Some limited configurational flexibility of internal nanorobot components may also be useful but should be restricted to nonessential or insensitive systems to avoid unnecessarily multiplying system complexity. Any movable trusswork should rotate around a configurationally stable core. Storage areas, nanofactory work volumes, pressure vessels, fluid/tool transfer pathways, and voids are the easiest internal elements to compress or reshape during a nanodevice reconfiguration event. Internal transfer stream mechanisms like conveyor belts may be designed modularly to permit limited modifications of device functionality. A few special purpose internal subsystems may tolerate positional or rotational uncertainty. For example, a clocking subsystem emitting a synchronizing periodic omnidirectional acoustic click may lie in any orientation within the

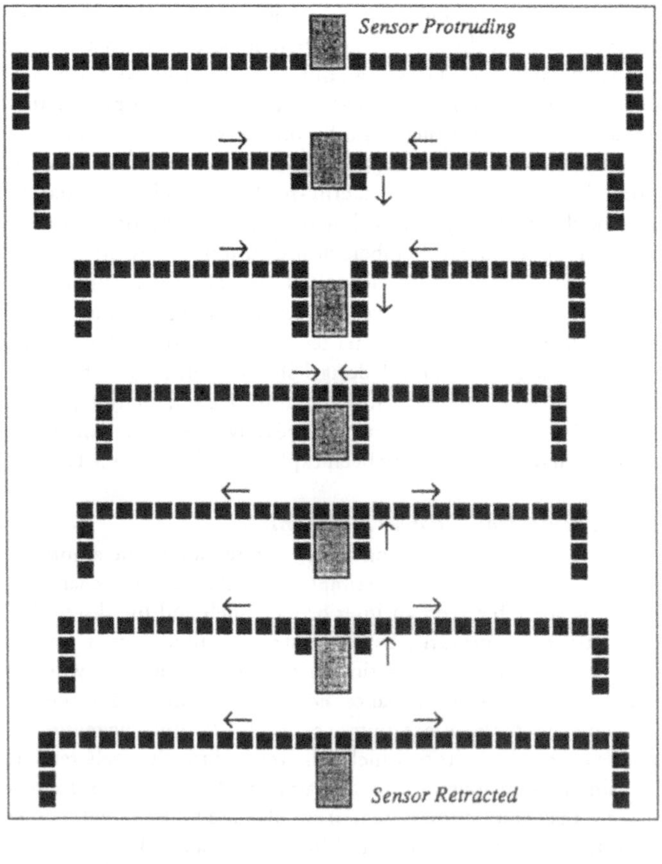

Fig. 5.17. Schematic representation of a watertight block surface reconfiguration: removing an embedded sensor element (block motive and control components omitted).

nanorobot; acoustic transit time across a 1-micron diamondoid nanorobot is ~10^{-10} sec < Δt_{min} (~10^{-9} sec; Section 10.1), thus the clock may be positionally insensitive as well.

5.3.6 Presentation Semaphores

It will often be necessary to modify nanorobot surface biochemical characteristics, as for example to present self-antigen to ensure biocompatibility (Chapter 15), to present targeted non-self-antigens to facilitate cytocarriage (Section 9.4.7) or elimination from the body (Chapter 16), or to create a traveling solvation wave (e.g., hydrophilic, lipophilic) on the nanorobot exterior surface to facilitate cytopenetration (Section 9.4.5.3). At concentrations of 1-10 nanomolar, there are 10^4-10^5 MHC Class I plasma membrane molecules per typical tissue cell, or ~10 MHC proteins/micron^2 at the cell surface (Section 8.5.2.1).*

The MHC Class I molecule (Section 8.5.2.1) consists of a ~45,000 dalton glycosylated polypeptide chain crudely shaped like a "hand" which is noncovalently grasping a 12,000 dalton nonglycosylated peptide microglobulin (Fig. 8.33). Eliminating anchor and attachment components which do not participate in recognition leaves an active antigen "semaphore" component measuring roughly 3 nm x 6 nm x 8 nm that must protrude from the cell surface.

To present this semaphore to the external environment at a nanorobot surface, a device roughly analogous to the manipulator arm described in Section 9.3.1.4 may be used. The manipulator arm includes a 7-nm diameter internal tool transport channel which can allow presentation and exchange of MHC-like molecules mounted on diamondoid jigs to the ~700 nm^2 device tip, where they may be locked into position for temporary display. Total presentation mechanism volume is ~10^5 nm^3, plus ~200 nm^3 per antigen stored on board. Staggered arrays of presentation ligands mounted on pistons can create nanorobot surfaces with controlled spatially structured chemical characteristics (Fig. 5.18).

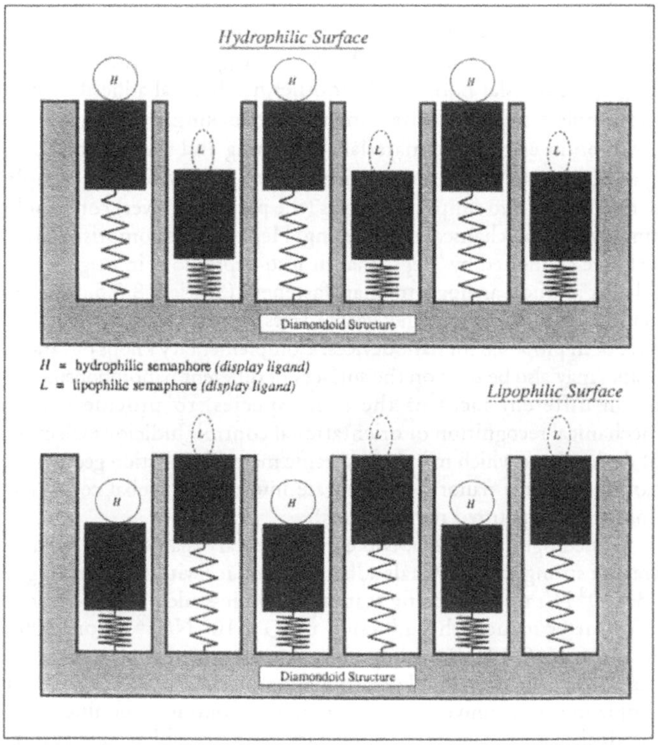

Fig. 5.18. Schematic of presentation semaphore mechanism.

An alternative method involves a two-roller mill-type device using a continuous conveyor belt 80 nm in length with 10 antigen-binding jigs mounted on the belt spaced ~5 nm apart. An opening at one end allows exposure of one antigen at a time to the external environment. Each of the 10 antigens, all of which may be different, are rotated into place as required, under computer control. As with the previous system, existing bound antigens may be exchanged internally using mill-like mechanisms. The core of the device measures 10 nm x 30 nm x 50 nm ~ 15,000 nm^3, or ~50,000 nm^3 including drive and control mechanisms and housing, with a ~300 nm^2 presentation face. Assuming a ~10^5 watt/m^3 power requirement (Section 6.5.6), power dissipation is ~10^{-17} watts per semaphore or ~0.03 pW/micron^2.

Either semaphore device has an external presentation surface area <1000 nm^2. Providing the requisite ~10 antigens/micron^2 requires at most ~1% of nanorobot surface committed to semaphores, or ~0.1% of the volume of a 1 micron^3 nanorobot for all semaphore devices, excluding antigen storage.

5.3.7 Chromatic Modification

The external surface color of nanodevices and their macroscopic aggregates is also subject to design and operational control, which may be useful in some special applications. Pure diamondoid in the flawless crystalline form will be clear and largely colorless; impurities commonly found in commercial and investment gemstones that impart bluish (~0.1% B substituted for C), yellowish (~0.1% N substituted for C), or other (e.g., blood-red, kelly green)[3524] hues are unlikely in nanomanufactured materials, as are graphitic deposits that produce black streaking or onyxlike coloration.[2641] Perception of chromaticity is limited by such factors as the minimum spatial resolution of the human eye (~ 0.5 arcmin or ~30 microns at closest focus of 10 cm), the maximum wavelength of visible light (~0.7 micron), and the degree of physical proximity of individual colored nanodevices when aggregated.

The simplest method for imparting a specific surface color is to add a thick coating of engineered corundum. Pure corundum (aluminum oxide) is colorless and has a hardness and chemical inertness only slightly inferior to diamond. Sapphire is the best-known crystalline form. Sapphire can be manufactured in a full spectrum of blues, pinks, yellows, oranges, teals, lavenders, greens, grays, whites, and all intermediate hues. More colors with greater intensity exist with sapphires than with any other gemstone. The broad color palette is achieved by replacing aluminum atoms with ~0.1% iron atoms and ~0.01% titanium atoms. Rubies, also corundum crystals, achieve their vivid reds by replacing a few aluminum atoms with atoms of chromium. The biocompatiblity of sapphire and ruby coatings is largely unexplored. If this should present a problem, a thin overcoating of transparent diamond preserves the color effects while presenting a potentially bioinactive interface[3234] (Chapter 15) to the external environment. Given the differences in crystal structures and atomic lattice sizes between diamond and sapphire, there may be some sacrifices in materials properties at such interfaces; D.W. Brenner [personal communication, 1999] is

**As few as 210-340 MHC Class II/peptide complexes per antigen-presenting cell (~0.1 molecules/micron^2) are needed to stimulate T cell interleukin-2 production[3456] and a minimum of ~0.2 molecules/micron^2 of agonist MHC/peptide complex can trigger proliferation and immunological synapse formation,[3453] although a threshold density of ≳ 60 molecules/micron^2 of accumulated MHC-peptide complexes are required for full T cell activation.[3453]*

unaware of any computational modeling studies having been performed on the atomically-bonded diamond-corundum interface as of 1998.

In larger devices or in macroscopic aggregates, color may be created and dynamically manipulated by embedding micron-scale light-emitting solid-state lasers in the surface. For a surface to appear a certain color, embedded monochromatic optical lasers must emit light of sufficient brightness to compete with other illuminated surfaces that may be present in the visual field. The required intensity is probably ~1 watt/m^2 (Section 4.9.4) or ~1 pW/micron^2—a feasible energy emission budget for micron-scale nanorobots. For example, Shen[732] has constructed 0.86-micron thick three-color electrically-tunable organic light-emitting devices[2560] which generate ~0.5 pW/micron^2 with ~1% energy efficiency; red-only LEDs have achieved efficiencies up to 16%,[1054] and larger diode lasers have achieved up to 60%-66% efficiencies.[3144,3145] Organic light-emitting devices (OLEDs) using small organic molecules can have high brightness (2-4 pW/micron^2), half-lifetimes of >4000 hours, and can be made with a wide range of emission colors in a ~300 nm thick sandwich.[3188] White-light organic electroluminescent devices ~100 nm thick have produced ~3 pW/micron^2 at 15 volts;[1048] 0.1-1% energy efficiency is typical.[1049] (Commercially available LEDs like Hewlett-Packard's gallium arsenide VCSEL blue-light laser chip have active layers ~10 microns thick and ~11% energy efficiency. LED chips typically have lifetimes ~10^8 sec, and other microcavity lasers are well-known.[3255]

If surface color is a serious design objective, arrays of frequency-selective absorbers or emitters such as rhodopsin, fluorescein, carotenoids, luciferins, or engineered porphyrins can be placed below a thin transparent diamondoid window. Active manipulation of covershades to block or expose these windows could permit rapid modulation of chromatic surface characteristics (e.g., polychromatic sparkling). Diverse surface pattern morphologies are theoretically available;[1051,3447] dynamic texture arrays can produce marked changes in color and other optical properties.[1041] Coherent modulation of the optical characteristics of aggregated nanorobots over large areas allows the creation and control of optical patterns visible to the human eye (e.g., epidermal displays; Section 7.4.6.7) with ~micron resolution at frequencies up to ~10 KHz consistent with a conservative ~1 cm/sec covershade speed. The visibility of subdermal chromomorphic devices is greatly reduced by photon scattering and absorption processes at greater depths in tissue (Section 4.9.4). Pure suspensions of spherical nanorobots in clear fluid will partake of the nanorobot surface color; suspensions of nonspherical, irregularly-shaped devices will appear milky due to scattering effects. Another design consideration is photochemical stability, especially for nanodevices that must operate in open sunlight or near other sources of ultraviolet (UV) radiation. To avoid photochemical damage, such devices may require a UV-opaque surface or components purposely designed for photochemical stability[10] (see Chapter 13).

5.4 Metamorphic Bumpers

Nanorobots may use circumferential metamorphic bumpers to achieve a continuously tight fit to neighboring devices while laboring cooperatively in nanotissues overlaying moving biological surfaces (e.g., see Chapter 22). Bumpers are crudely analogous to the cell-cell adherens junction found in human epithelial sheet cells.[531] In this junction, a continuous adhesion belt (the zonula adherens or belt desmosome) surrounds each of the interacting cells in the sheet, resulting in a narrow adhesive zone mediated by Ca^{++}-dependent transmembrane linker glycoproteins. Within each cell, a contractile bundle of actin filaments runs adjacent to the adhesion belt and parallel to the cellular membrane, serving as control cables for this biological junctional "bumper" system. Oriented contraction of the actin filaments causes specific localized movement of the sheet, as for example the rolling of epithelial tissue into a closed tube. Nanorobots linked by narrow equatorial-band or wide whole-wall bumpers into nanotissues may perform similar feats, under continuous computer control.

The other principal class of anchoring junction is the spot desmosome, a buttonlike point of intercellular contact that rivets together certain types of epithelial tissue cells. Each desmosome is a spoon-shaped molecule about 30 nm long, spaced at ~8 nm intervals across the cell surface, with the straight tail of each spoon firmly embedded in a subsurface cytoskeletal plaque and the head of the spoon protruding ~10 nm outside of the cellular lipid bilayer membrane.[312,531] Matching spot desmosome heads on neighboring cells adhere, gluing the cells together while maintaining a 10-20 nm intercellular gap.

Tighter junctions (~2 nm) called occluding junctions form nearly watertight seals in certain critical areas such as between the cells lining the digestive system. Blood platelets are also intensely reactive cells that respond to a variety of stimuli to undergo shape change, adhesion, primary and secondary aggregation, and a process known as viscous metamorphosis in which membrane fusion occurs between adjacent platelets with the loss of membrane integrity.[530]

5.4.1 *Nanojunction Mechanisms*

Neighboring nanorobots must be able to reliably identify the presence of others and then join together tightly into cohesive nanotissues, forming planar or three-dimensional arrays. In nanodevices, a broad array of fastening technologies from both the biological[533] and the engineering[1614] worlds is available for design inspiration.

For simple adhesion, micromechanical velcro,[532] sticky tethers,[535] magnetic latches (F_{min} ~ 1600 nN for A_{magnet} = 1 micron^2, B = B_{magnet} = 1.4 tesla; Eqn. 4.45), or other mechanical adhesives offer the simplest means of attachment. Interlocking mechanisms are common in engineered materials (e.g., plug and socket, hook and eye, distension bulbs or dilators)—many of which are simple derivations of two simple machines (the plane and lever) commonly employed in mechanical engineering. Hepatic cells comprising liver walls are connected by "pegs" that fit into depressions in neighboring cells in a crude analogy to snap fasteners (Section 8.2.5, and see below); similar knobbed adhesive interfaces[10] and docking envelopes[1614] have been proposed for nanodevices. Complementary knobs of various shapes may also be used on the surfaces of different nanorobot species, or on different faces of the same species, to provide simple mechanical recognition or orientational control. Judicious selection of device shape which mandates specific mateable junction geometries can force a large nanorobot aggregate into desired global configurations (e.g., structured nano-organs).

Pressed tightly together, two complementary diamondoid surfaces create a strong van der Waals adhesive interface with tensile strength ~3 x 10^9 N/m^2; interposing scattered atomic-scale bumps ~0.2 nm in diameter reduces this adhesion to ~3 x 10^8 N/m^2,[10] or ~3000 atm (Section 9.2.1). Providing each metamorphic nanorobot species with complementary Braille-like adhesion plates may provide either a simple means of universal attachment or a unique recognition and interlock pattern of great complexity. Adherent plates are readily detached by inserting corrugated wedge mechanisms or by deforming the adhesive pattern. For comparison, adhesion between biological cells (as determined by measurements of the force required for detachment of ~20-micron tissue cells by micromanipulation, shear, or jets of fluid) is typically ~1-100 nN/micron^2.[1454,1455,1458,1459]

Reversible adhesion may also be achieved using surface-mounted matched nanomechanical manipulator arms (Section 9.3.1) which can grasp or release their counterpart in an adjacent cell, under computer control.

5.4.2 Transbumper Communication

Besides occluding and anchor junctions, mutually attached biological cells use gap junctions[2922] or "communicating junctions" to exchange inorganic ions and other small water-soluble molecules like sugar and ATP. Connexons are hexagonal transmembrane proteins with tiny pores; when connexons in the membranes of two cells are aligned, they form a continuous aqueous channel linking the two cell interiors that can open and close in a way similar to the acetylcholine receptor channel described in Section 3.3.3. When the calcium level of a cell rises—often a signal that the cell is sick or compromised—connexons close and quarantine the unhealthy neighbor.[312] A force of 6-10 pN is required to physically pry apart each connexin-32 hepatic cell gap junction unit, each unit a combined pair of hexagonal cylinders ~7.5 nm in height and 7 nm in diameter with a 2-nm pore through the center.[1223] Another communicative adhesive mechanism is provided by bacterial sex pili,[1588,3549] filamentous surface adhesive organelles that are long thin hollow protein tubes (typically ~300 per cell) with sticky receptors on their ends that bind to recipient cell walls, allowing DNA to pass from cell to cell.[2328] Integrins (Section 8.5.2.2) mediate cell binding to extracellular matrix and anchorage-dependence mechanical signals.[718]

Similar mechanisms may be employed in metamorphic bumper walls to establish stable physical conduits among neighboring nanorobots in an array. Such conduits may transmit information, materials, nanoscale components, power (acoustic or hydraulic), or even structural forces (including tension, compression or torsion) to provide stability or movement of the entire nanotissue assemblage. Hinges[534] and related mechanisms allow contact to be maintained as the metamorphic surface expands, contracts, twists or translates.

5.4.3 Bumper Mechanics

Methods of inflation and deflation of metamorphic volumes have been described in Section 5.3.3. Interbumper connection forces may be 10^7-10^9 N/m^2, easily exceeding potentially disruptive forces typically encountered inside the human body. Consistent with available power resources and likely operating environments, metamorphic bumpers may be driven at frequencies of 10-1000 Hz at full-range amplitude, or faster in cases of limited-range amplitude oscillations. This response rate matches or exceeds the speeds of all important mechanical tissue movements found in the human body including respiration (0.1-1 Hz), pulse (1-2 Hz), muscle contractions during violent exercise (1-10 Hz) or tetanic contractions (15-60 Hz), and even nerve cell discharge events (5-100 Hz). The fastest known animal muscle speeds[739] are found in the ~90 Hz rattle-shaker of the western diamondback rattlesnake;[1245] the ~90 Hz hummingbird wingbeat; the ~200 Hz toadfish swim bladder;[1245] the synchronous muscle contractions of the katydid, *Neoconocephalus robustus*, at 212 Hz,[3161] and the cicada, *Chlorocysta viridis*, at 224 Hz;[3162] and finally the record 1046-2200 Hz wingbeat of the tiny midge *Forcipomyia*.[739,2033]

CHAPTER 6
Power

6.1 Nanodevice Energy Resources

Device energetics may represent the most serious limitation in nanorobot design. Almost all medical nanodevices will be actively powered. Mechanical motions, pumping, chemical transformations and the like all require the expenditure of energy, measured in joules. Even a drug molecule interaction with a biological receptor site reduces free energy by ~50 kT (Section 3.5.2) or ~210 zJ (1 zeptojoule (zJ) = 10^{-21} joule) at 310 K. Heat dissipation is also a major consideration in nanomachine design, particularly when large numbers of nanomachines are deployed. Power, of course, is the rate of energy consumption or production, measured in joules/sec or watts.

Energy, like money, has both a storage and a transactional character. Section 6.2 reviews the various forms of stored energy that may be accessible to working nanodevices in vivo. Section 6.3 describes how one form of energy can be converted into another form, while Section 6.4 discusses how energy may be transmitted from one place to another—both representing the transactional aspect of energy use. Section 6.5 closes the Chapter with an enumeration of issues and techniques useful in assessing energy requirements and performance restrictions in medical nanodevice design.

6.2 Energy Storage

For medical nanorobots, onboard volume is a precious and limited commodity. Viscous forces dominate inertial and gravitational forces, so mass is almost irrelevant. Hence energy stored per unit volume (joules/m^3) is an appropriate figure of merit for nanoscale energy storage devices.

Energy storage devices may be required to maintain temporary power during subsystem failures, metamorphic transitions, or during temporary unavailability of environmental energy resources; to provide supplementary supplies during brief periods of overcapacity consumption; or to buffer normal energy usage among subsystems generating large fluctuations. Stored energy may also be used to power short-lived medical nanodevices on missions of limited duration. For example, a 1 micron^3 storage device with storage density of 2 kT/nm^3 (~10^7 joules/m^3) contains sufficient energy to power a 10 picowatt (pW) nanorobot for ~1 second. Chemical storage devices (providing up to 10^{11} joules/m^3; Section 6.2.3) may extend this duration to 10^4 sec (~3 hours).

6.2.1 Gravitational Energy Storage

Not surprisingly, the gravitational field offers one of the weakest forms of energy storage available to nanodevices. The energy density attainable using a storage device of density ρ and size L (height) in a gravity field g is

$$E_{storage} = \rho \, g \, L \quad (\text{joules/m}^3) \qquad \{\text{Eqn. 6.1}\}$$

For ρ = 2000 kg/m^3, g = 9.81 m/sec^2 and L = 1 micron, $E_{storage}$ = 2 x 10^{-2} joules/m^3.

6.2.2 Mechanical Energy Storage

6.2.2.1 Pendulums and Springs

Energy may also be stored in mechanical systems. A gravitational pendulum of cord length r with a bob of density ρ and characteristic diameter L that is tangentially displaced a distance Δx has potential energy ~$\rho \, L^3$ g stored in a volume of order ~r L Δx for small Δx, hence energy density is approximately:

$$E_{storage} \sim \rho \, g \, L^2 / r \quad (\text{joules/m}^3) \qquad \{\text{Eqn. 6.2}\}$$

Taking ρ = 2000 kg/m^3, g = 9.81 m/sec^2 and L = r = 1 micron, then $E_{storage}$ = 2 x 10^{-2} joules/m^3, the same as Eqn. 6.1, as expected.

Stretched springs provide significantly greater energy storage capacity. For example, a diamondoid spring of size ~L and stretching stiffness k_s has harmonic potential (1/2) $k_s \, x^2$ for a displacement x and volume L^3, with energy density:

$$E_{storage} = \frac{k_s \, x^2}{2 \, L^3} = \left(\frac{E}{2}\right)\left(\frac{x}{L}\right)^2 \qquad \{\text{Eqn. 6.3}\}$$

where (x/L) = strain and E = Young's modulus. Conservatively taking strain = 5% and E = 1.05 x 10^{12} N/m^2 for diamond, then $E_{storage}$ = 1.3 x 10^9 joules/m^3. However, strains may be applied in three dimensions as well as in tension, shear, or torsion, so total energy storage may be somewhat higher. The fracture surface energy of the weakest {111} diamond plane E_f = 5.3 joules/m^2, and the distance between {111} planes is L_{plane} ~ 0.24 nm given that there are ~1.8 x 10^{19} bonds/m^2,[10] so the theoretical maximum mechanical energy storage density in a diamond block is $E_{storage}$ ~ E_f / L_{plane} = 2 x 10^{10} joules/m^3.

6.2.2.2 Flywheels

The maximum energy that can be stored in an axially spinning flywheel is E_{fly} = (1/2) $I_{fly} \, \omega_{max}^2$, where ω_{max} is the maximum angular velocity (bursting speed) given by Eqn. 4.17 and I_{fly} = (1/2) mr^2 is the rotational inertia of a disk of radius r, height h, and mass m = $\pi \, r^2$ h ρ. Dividing by disk volume, all geometric variables drop out giving maximum $E_{storage}$ = (1/2) σ_w for flywheels of any size. Adopting a fairly aggressive working stress σ_w = 10^{11} N/m^2, $E_{storage}$ ~ 5 x 10^{10} joules/m^3, an excellent power density. In 1998, commercially available electric micromotors already achieved energy storage densities of ~10^5-10^6 joules/m^3.[556]

More intuitively, J. Sidles points out that the energy that can be stored in a compact flywheel is of the order of either:

1. the chemical binding energy per atom, times the number of atoms in the flywheel (~same as chemical energy storage), or
2. the yield stress of the material comprising the flywheel, times the volume.

Both methods give estimates that agree to within an order of magnitude. Thus flywheels offer little advantage over chemical fuels in terms of stored energy density (Section 6.2.3), regardless of their size or material composition.

If high-velocity flywheels must ride on bearings of large stiffness, this may cause sufficient frictional drag to render flywheel energy storage impractical even for vacuum-isolated systems. Consider a cylindrical sleeve bearing of radius r_{bear} and length l_{bear} axially supporting the flywheel described in the previous paragraph with axial bearing stiffness of k_s = 1000 N/m and bearing surface velocity $v_{bear} = v_{fly}\,(r_{bear} / r)$ and flywheel rim velocity $v_{fly} = (4\,E_{storage} / \rho)^{1/2}$. According to Drexler,[10] the drag power for a nanoscale bearing is dominated by band-stiffness scattering as:

$$P_{drag} = \frac{\left(1.42 \times 10^{-31}\right) k_s^{1.7}\, v_{bear}^2}{\left(l_{bear}\, r_{bear}\right)^{0.7}} \quad \text{(watts)} \qquad \text{\{Eqn. 6.4\}}$$

The energy initially stored in the flywheel is:

$$E_{fly} = \left(\frac{\pi}{4}\right) r^2\, h\, \rho\, v_{fly}^2 \qquad \text{\{Eqn. 6.5\}}$$

so the time required for the flywheel to lose half of its energy due to drag friction, its "energy half-life" or $\tau_{1/2}$, is:

$$\tau_{1/2} \sim \left(\frac{E_{fly}}{P_{drag}}\right) \ln(2) \qquad \text{\{Eqn. 6.6\}}$$

Thus a flywheel of radius r = 200 nm and thickness h = 20 nm (m ~ 9 x 10^{-18} kg for diamond) supported by a bearing of radius r_{bear} ~ h/2 = 10 nm and length l_{bear} ~ h = 20 nm with maximum flywheel energy density $E_{storage}$ = 5 x 10^9 joules/m^3 has v_{fly} = 2400 m/sec, v_{bear} = 120 m/sec, E_{fly} = 13 picojoules (pJ), P_{drag} = 25 pW, so $\tau_{1/2}$ = 0.35 sec and the flywheel loses 99% of its energy in just 2.3 sec. A much larger ~1 micron^3 flywheel of radius r = 500 nm, thickness h = 1300 nm and r_{bear} = 50 nm loses 99% of its energy in just 140 sec.

On the other hand, it may be possible to substantially improve the energy storage time if a bearing with much lower drag is available. R. Merkle points out that a spinning, perfectly symmetric diamondoid disk made of isotopically pure carbon and supported by two coaxial carbyne rods on either side should exhibit negligible bearing losses and no vibration. The carbyne rod is one dimensional, and the electron cloud along the rod is rotationally symmetric (for single and triple bonds), so the disk cannot readily interact with its rod supports. The major source of energy loss is off-axis rotation during spin-up which could induce vibration in the carbyne support, so spinning the disk up to speed may require larger bearings which could be disengaged after spin-up.

A lateral velocity sufficient to destroy the C-C carbyne bonds ($E_{lateral}$ ~ 550 zJ/bond) is $v_{destroy} \sim (2\,E_{lateral} / m)^{1/2}$ = 0.4 m/sec for r = 200 nm and h = 20 nm—much larger than the flywheel thermal velocity $v_{thermal}$ ~ 0.04 m/sec (Eqn. 3.3). Since F ~ 30 nN of force will break a C-C bond (Section 4.4.1), a lateral acceleration sufficient to destroy the support rods requires F/m ~ 0.3 x 10^9 g's, far in excess of the ~0.4 g's typically anticipated for 1-micron spherical nanorobots in vivo (Section 4.3.3.2). Thermal noise will cause the flywheel housing and supports to jiggle, but the phonons will be transmitted along a one-dimensional pathway (the carbyne rod) which cannot couple to the disk rotation. Energy losses due to rotational resistance (as the nanorobot constantly rotates to new spatial orientations) can be made negligible using a nanogyroscopic gimballed housing (Section 4.3.4.1). Safety issues must also be addressed, such as providing energy-absorbing device housings that are highly explosion-resistant.

6.2.2.3 Pressurized Fluids

Compressed fluids can store mechanical energy limited only by the tensile strength and aspect ratio of their container (Section 10.3.1) and the rupture strength of their valving system. A "conservative" working stress for diamondoid pressure containers is σ_w ~ 10^{10} joules/m^3 (~100,000 atm). Gases or liquids, either of which are compressible, may be used as the working fluid depending on energy density and design buoyancy requirements (Section 10.3.6). For example, cycling between 1-1000 atm of pressure at 310 K the density of compressed water varies from 993.4-1038.0 kg/m^3 while the density of compressed oxygen varies from 1.26-670 kg/m^3 (Table 10.2). The energy stored in a compressed fluid is ~$\int P dV$; thus at the ~1000 atm cycle limit, the compressed water stores ~2 x 10^6 J/m^3 and the compressed gas stores ~1 x 10^8 J/m^3. (Materials are thermodynamically forbidden to have negative volume compressibilities. However, lanthanum niobate and a few other crystals exhibit negative linear compressibilities; such materials may be used to fabricate porous solids that either expand in all directions when hydrostatically compressed with a penetrating fluid or behave as if they are incompressible.[1297])

For safety reasons, fluid pressures in excess of 1000 atm (10^8 joules/m^3) should rarely be used in nanomedical systems (Chapter 17). Any mechanical energy storage system with readily accessible catastrophic energy release modes that is operated near maximum capacity (e.g., fluids >10^5 atm) in vivo risks causing significant damage to nearby tissue cells in the event of device malfunction or rupture.

6.2.3 Chemical Energy Storage

Chemical energy storage offers an ideal combination of high storage density, abundant physiological resources, and superior safety in the event a device is physically compromised. As shown in Table 6.1 (values computed from stoichiometric reaction formulas), chemical energy storage density (fuel only*) ranges from 10^8 joules/m^3 to 10^{11} joules/m^3, as compared to 10^6-10^9 joules/m^3 for mechanical media and 10^6-10^8 joules/m^3 for electric/magnetic storage (Section 6.2.4). Electrochemical batteries typically achieve 10^7-10^{10} joules/m^3 (e.g., 5-micron thick rechargeable lithium microbatteries have energy density ~2 x 10^9 joules/m^3,[588] and tin-lithium material can reach ~8 x 10^9 joules/m^3).[715] As of 1998, prototype ~4000 nm^3 Cu/Ag nanobatteries had demonstrated ~7 x 10^7 joules/m^3 or ~2 x 10^4 watts/m^3 power density.[589]

Table 6.1 offers many interesting revelations:

1. Assuming "safe" ~1,000 atm storage, a pressurized hydrogen/oxygen mixture has the greatest energy per unit mass (excluding the mass of the containment vessel) but has almost the lowest energy per unit volume, hence is too inefficient for

*Not all fuels require oxidizer, e.g., ATP. For fuels that require oxidizer, taking oxidizer volume into account (e.g., O_2 at 1000 atm) reduces overall energy storage density to ~7% of fuel-only density for diamond, ~25% for most organics, and ~65% for hydrogen. Also, note that $E_{avail} = E_{storage} - E_{activation}$, where E_{avail} is available energy and $E_{activation}$ is the net unrecoverable activation energy required to release the stored chemical energy.)

Table 6.1 Energy Storage Density for Various Chemical Fuels (fuel only)

Energy Storage Fuel	Storage Density (joules/m³)	(joules/kg)
ATP	1.4×10^8	1.0×10^5
H_2 @ 10^3 atm (*g*)	4.9×10^9	1.2×10^8
Nitroglycerine	1.0×10^{10}	6.3×10^6
Glycine (amino acid)	1.0×10^{10}	6.5×10^6
Wood	1.1×10^{10}	1.9×10^7
Urea	1.4×10^{10}	1.1×10^7
Methanol	1.8×10^{10}	2.2×10^7
Vegetable protein	2.3×10^{10}	1.7×10^7
Acetone	2.4×10^{10}	3.1×10^7
Glucose	2.4×10^{10}	1.6×10^7
Glycogen (starch)	2.5×10^{10}	1.8×10^7
Animal protein	2.5×10^{10}	1.8×10^7
Carbohydrate	2.6×10^{10}	1.7×10^7
Gasoline	2.8×10^{10}	4.4×10^7
Butane	3.0×10^{10}	4.9×10^7
Fat	3.3×10^{10}	3.9×10^7
Palmitic acid (lipid)	3.3×10^{10}	3.9×10^7
Palmitin (lipid)	3.4×10^{10}	4.0×10^7
Leucine (amino acid)	3.5×10^{10}	2.7×10^7
Cholesterol (lipid)	4.2×10^{10}	3.9×10^7
H_2 @ 10^5 atm (*s*)	7.2×10^{10}	1.2×10^8
Diamond	1.2×10^{11}	3.3×10^7

free-swimming medical nanorobots where interior volume is a scarce commodity.

2. The classic explosive, nitroglycerine (included solely for comparison), ranks poorly on either measure of energy density.

3. ATP, sometimes proposed as an alternate energy source for in cyto operations,[261,1259] has the lowest energy density on the list, though its use cannot be excluded in the earliest-generation medical nanodevices for metering out small energy packets of known magnitude.

4. Lipids and fats generally store more energy per unit volume than carbohydrates, proteins, or even hydrogen.

5. Cholesterol, twice as plentiful as serum glucose on a gm/cm³ basis (Appendix B), is in theory the most favored biochemical energy storage molecule with nearly double the storage density of glucose.

6. Diamond has the highest known oxidative chemical storage density, possibly surpassed only by fullerene materials, probably because it also has the highest atomic number density per unit volume.

7. Hydrogen stored in solid form (H_2 solidifies at ~57,000 atm at room temperature, making 600 kg/m³ crystals[568]), yields an extraordinarily high chemical energy density, second only to diamond.

Combining the values for molecular energy density given in Table 6.1 with the bloodstream concentrations given in Appendix B reveals that the chemical energy content of blood plasma (~ 3 liters in adult males) includes ~3×10^8 joules/m³ for all lipids (~8×10^7 joules/m³ from total cholesterol alone), ~2×10^7 joules/m³ for serum glucose, ~1×10^6 joules/m³ for each of the common amino acids, and even ~4×10^6 joules/m³ for urea. Cytoplasmic chemical energy content is of similar magnitude, with the addition of ~6×10^4 joules/m³ for ATP. (See Table 6.4 for related data.)

The question naturally arises whether some biocompatible artificial energy molecule could be added to the human bloodstream to provide a supplementary chemical energy source for a working in vivo nanorobot population. To this end, an injection of ~0.7 cm³ of diamond colloid (the most energy-dense chemical fuel known—it has been used as rocket fuel) encapsulated in trillions of suitable submicron-scale biocompatible carrier devices provides an energy resource equal in size to the entire serum glucose supply, a negligible ~0.01% addition to whole blood volume. Ten trillion 0.1-micron³ passive carriers would have a mean separation of ~10 microns in the blood.

6.2.4 Electric and Magnetic Energy Storage

The energy density in a static electric field of strength E traversing a material of dielectric constant κ_e is given by:

$$E_{storage} = \frac{1}{2} \varepsilon_0 \kappa_e E^2 \qquad \text{\{Eqn. 6.7\}}$$

where $\varepsilon_0 = 8.85 \times 10^{-12}$ farad/m (permittivity constant) and dielectric constant $\kappa_e = 5.7$ for diamond. Electrostatic motors (Section 6.3.5) in nanomechanical systems may exhibit an electric field strength of ~0.2×10^9 volts/m.[10] However, the maximum field that may be employed in an electrostatic energy storage device is limited by the dielectric strength or breakdown voltage $E = 2 \times 10^9$ volts/m for diamond[537] (about the highest known for any material), giving a maximum electric storage density of 1.0×10^8 joules/m³.

What about magnetic storage density? Since isolated magnetic poles (analogous to the electron) are not known to exist, magnetic field energy can be stored only in an array of aligned atomic dipoles. The energy density of the static magnetic field of a permanent magnet comprised of atoms with dipole moment M_{dipole} and number density N_{dipole} producing a flux density B at 100% saturation is given by:

$$E_{storage} \sim M_{dipole} N_{dipole} B \qquad \text{\{Eqn. 6.8\}}$$

For iron atoms with bulk density 7860 kg/m³, then $N_{dipole} = 8.5 \times 10^{28}$ atoms/m³ and $M_{dipole} = 1.8 \times 10^{-23}$ ampere-m²,[1662] giving $E_{storage} = 2.1 \times 10^6$ joules/m³.

Only a negligible amount of magnetic energy is stored in a magnetic field created by a permanent current loop in a nanoscale ring of superconducting material. For a wire loop of radius R_{loop} and thickness d_{wire} carrying current I, and following the notation of Eqn. 4.44, peak magnetic flux density is $B = \mu_0 I / 2 R_{loop}$ at the center of the loop,[1662] so the peak energy density is given by:

$$E_{storage} = \frac{B^2}{2 \mu_0} = \frac{\mu_0 I^2}{8 R_{loop}^2} \qquad \text{\{Eqn. 6.9\}}$$

Aluminum conductors in integrated circuits are limited to I_d ~3×10^9 ampere/m² due to electromigration; thin-film high-temperature superconductors[550] have achieved $I_d > 3 \times 10^{10}$ ampere/m². Taking $I = (I_d \sim 10^{10}$ ampere/m²$) \{\pi (d_{wire}/2)^2\} \sim 10^{-4}$ amperes for $d_{wire} = 100$ nm, $\mu_0 = 1.26 \times 10^{-6}$ henry/m, and $R_{loop} = 0.5$ micron, then $E_{storage} = 6.3 \times 10^{-3}$ joules/m³.

Electromagnetic waveguides, radiator cavities and fiberoptic closed loops are too lossy or of inappropriate scale to permit direct nanodevice photonic energy storage. Energy stored in excited or partially ionized molecular or atomic states, coherent (lasing) and fluorescing media, and enzymatic activated complexes (e.g., at peak activation energy) generally also lack sufficient duration or stability to be useful, although the metastable excited electronic 2^3S state of solid He^4 at 19.8 eV has a 2.3-hour lifetime and thus a theoretical storage density of 5×10^{11} joules/m^3 for 100% electronically excited solid helium.[661]

6.2.5 Nuclear Energy Storage

By nanotechnological standards, the energy stored in atomic nuclei is huge. For instance, the energy density of an un-ionized radioactive atom of U^{235} is 1.5×10^{18} joules/m^3, counting the kinetic energy of all fissile decay products in the total. Hydrogen that undergoes fusion into helium actually provides a much poorer volumetric energy storage density than for fission, ~4.4×10^{16} joules/m^3 (again assuming storage of fuel as molecules), largely due to the comparatively high atomic number density of fissionable heavy metals. The highest practical energy density would be achieved by storing some theorized form of matter-friendly stabilized antimatter perhaps converted to a two-phase hypergolic (self-igniting) fuel,[565] up to a maximum of ~2×10^{21} joules/m^3 (fuel only) for platinum/antiplatinum annihilation. The difficulty, of course, is accessing this potential resource in a controlled and well-shielded fashion (Section 6.3.7).

6.3 Power Conversion

Almost all energy available to biological processes on Earth originates in the consumption of the highest naturally-available energy density resource—nuclear fuels in the Sun. After transfer across space via high-energy photons, this energy is absorbed via photosynthesis by plant life on Earth and converted into chemical energy stores of moderate energy density. These chemical energy stores are then consumed by animal life and converted into mechanical or electric energy stores of lower energy density, or are completely degraded to heat.

Medical nanodevices join this energy ecology by consuming onboard energy stores (Section 6.2) or by absorbing fresh energy resources from the environment, converting these resources into other forms to accomplish useful work and possibly recovering for reuse a portion of this energy via reversible or regenerative processes, then finally releasing heat as the ultimate outcome of irreversible processes. Clearly the key to medical nanorobot power supply is the efficient conversion of energy from one form to another.

The energy conversion matrix in Table 6.2 provides a convenient conceptual framework with which to organize and guide our discussion. Representative technologies are listed for each cell in the matrix. An exhaustive discussion of every matrix element is beyond the scope of this book. Instead, a selection of the most important categories are illustrated with one or two specific examples. Serial chains of multiple conversion processes may in some cases provide increased efficiency over competing pathways, conserve volume or mass, provide faster conversion (e.g., permit higher power density), allow partial energy regeneration, or serve other specific design objectives.

A note on nomenclature: In this book, energy conversion processes are named using the source energy first, followed by the resultant energy form. Thus a device which converts chemical energy into acoustic energy employs a "chemoacoustic" process, and so forth.

6.3.1 Thermal Energy Conversion Processes

The second law of thermodynamics says that it is impossible to to convert heat into useful work if the heat reservoir and the device are both at the same temperature, as demonstrated by Feynman's classical example of the Brownian motor using an isothermal ratchet and pawl machine,[2611] although nonequilibrium fluctuations, whether generated by macroscale electric fields or chemical reactions far from equilibrium, can drive a Brownian motor.[696] It has also been suggested that reversible-energy-fluctuation converters can obtain useful electrical work from thermal Nyquist noise, up to power densities of 10^{15}-10^{16} watts/m^3 at ~300 K.[1606,1607]

Of course, a reversible Carnot-cycle heat engine can extract useful work from even a small temperature differential with a Carnot efficiency of e% = ΔT / T. For example, a nanorobot circulating with the blood between core and peripheral tissues may experience a temperature variation up to several kelvins during each vascular circuit of duration t_{circ} ~ 60 sec (Section 8.4.1). From this small temperature differential an ideal biothermal thermomechanical engine may extract a maximum power:

$$P_n = \frac{V_n\, C_V\, \Delta T\, e\%}{t_{circ}} = \frac{V_n\, C_V (T_2 - T_1)^2}{T_2\, t_{circ}} \qquad \text{\{Eqn. 6.10\}}$$

where nanorobot thermal storage volume is V_n = 1 micron^3, heat capacity $C_V = 4.19 \times 10^6$ joules/m^3-K for a device filled with water, T_2 = 310 K at the human body core and T_1 = 307 K at the periphery. The thermal store, vacuum-isolated to prevent heat loss (see below), is equilibrated in the hotter core environment to T_2, which heat is then stored until the device reaches the cooler peripheral environment at T_1. From Eqn. 6.10, this temperature differential yields at most P_n ~ 0.002 pW with efficiency e% = $(T_2 - T_1) / T_2$ ~ 0.01(1%) and a peak (accessible) energy density of $P_n\, t_{circ} / V_n$ ~ 10^5 joules/m^3. The change in temperature can be made to cause gas in a three-dimensional coiled piston to slowly expand or contract, driving a rod back and forth thus providing a cyclical linear mechanical output, a Stirling engine configuration. The gas expansion is isobaric and reversible because thermal equilibration time $t_{EQ} \sim V_n C_V / h K_t = 10^{-5}$ sec for a conduction layer of thickness h ~ 0.5 micron and thermal conductivity K_t = 0.623 watt/m-K for water at 310 K, so $t_{EQ} \ll t_{circ}$. (Exploiting the diurnal variation in mean body temperature, typically ranging from 309.3 K in early morning to 310.4 K in the evening, produces at most ~2×10^{-7} pW of power.) A nanorobot resting on the epidermal surface may exploit the temperature differential between skin and air, up to 8-13 K (Section 8.4.1.1) giving a maximum Carnot efficiency e% ~ 0.04 (4%); for classical radiative transfer (see below), the nanorobot develops a net power through an L^2 = 10 micron^2 epidermal contact surface of $P_n \sim \sigma (T_2^4 - T_1^4) L^2 e\%$ = 0.04 pW.

Nakajima[541] has built and operated a 50 mm^3 Stirling engine working at 10 Hz between 273-373 K producing 10^{-2} watts (power density 2×10^5 watts/m^3), and has demonstrated the theoretical engineering feasibility of microscale Stirling engines. In 1993 Jeff Sniedowski of Sandia National Laboratories constructed a 50-micron steam engine on a silicon chip producing forces ~100 times higher than those of electrostatic motors of similar size.[3486] (The steam was produced electrically.) Computer simulations of a molecular-scale steam engine have been performed by Donald W. Noid at Oak Ridge National Laboratory.[3488] A conservative and practical upper limit to nanorobot Carnot efficiency is probably ~50% (T_2 = 620 K).

Table 6.2 Energy Conversion Matrix: Power Transduction Technologies that Convert One Form of Energy into Another

OUTPUT / INPUT	Thermal	Mechanical	Acoustical	Chemical	Electrical/ Magnetic	Photonic	Nuclear
Thermal	• Thermal Conduction • Heat Exchangers	• Biothermal Heat Engine • Shape Memory Alloy Motor • Steam Engine • Stirling Engine	• Whistling Teakettle	• Phase-Change Cooling • Endothermic Chemical Reaction	• Thermocouple • Pyroelectricity • Thermophoto-voltaics	• Thermo-Luminescence • Blackbody Cavity Radiator	• Thermionic Emission
Mechanical	• Pulled Rubber Band Gets Hot • Frictional Heating	• Self-Winding Watch • Axle Bearing • Gear Train • Windmill	• Pressure Actuator • Clapping Hands • Siren	• Mechano-Chemical Synthesis • Piezo-Chemistry	• Piezocrystals • Electrostatic DC Generator • Wind Electric	• Piezo-Luminescence • Tribo-Luminescence	• Fracto-Fusion • Pressure-Sensitive Radioactivity
Acoustical	• Acoustic Heating • Thermo-Acoustic Refrigeration	• Pressure Actuator • Edison's Phonograph (to record)	• Pneumatic Tube • Hydraulics	• Sonochemistry	• Electrical Audio Microphone	• Sono-Luminescence • Acousto-Optical Modulators	• (Explosive) Compression of Fissile Bomb Core
Chemical	• Exothermic Chemical Reaction	• Internal Combustion Engine • Glucose Engine • Flagellar Motor • Actin-Myosin Motor	• Alka Seltzer Dissolving • Chemical Explosion	• Cellular Metabolism (Lipids, Glucose, ATP)	• Fuel Cell • Chemical Battery	• Bio-/Chemi-Luminescence • Chemical Lasers	• Chemically-Modulated Electron Capture in Be^7
Electrical/ Magnetic	• Joule Heating • Peltier Cooling	• Electrostatic DC Motor • Dielectric Actuator • Piezoceramics • Electroscope	• Stereo Speaker • Piezoelectric Crystal	• Electrolysis • Voltage-Gated Ion Channels and Nano-Membranes	• Eletrical Transformer • Induced Currents	• Quantum Laser • LED/Lightbulb • UV Arc Lamp • Electro-Luminescence • Klystron	• Particle Accelerator-Manufactured Radioisotopes
Photonic	• Optical Refrigerator • Dielectric Heating	• Laser-Heated Gas Actuator • Optical Tweezers • Solar Light • Chalcogenides	• Opto-Pneumatic Actuator	• Photography • Photo-synthesis • Light-Driven Proton Pumps	• Photovoltaic Cell • CCD/Charge-Coupled Device • RF Loop Antenna	• Fluorescence • Microwave Waveguides • Photo-Luminescence	• Laser Pellet Fusion • Photonuclear Emission
Nuclear	• Nuclear Bomb • Conventional Nuclear Power Plant	• Nuclear Bomb • Project Orion Propulsion System	• Nuclear Bomb • Geiger Counter (indirectly)	• Nuclear Bomb • Radiation-Driven DNA Mutation • Radiation Chemistry	• Nuclear Bomb • Radioactive Thermoelectric Generator (RTG) • Betavoltaics	• Nuclear Bomb • Cerenkov Radiation Counter • Cathodo-Luminescence	• Nuclear Bomb • Moderated Fissile Chain Reaction • Matter/Anti-matter Annihil.

A heat engine may exploit the temperature difference between the largely isothermal human body acting as a sink and a hot, high-capacity source of stored heat energy. Because the rate of conductive heat loss is scale-dependent, such exploitation is not feasible in nanodevices relying on stored heat sources unless a vacuum isolation suspension is employed (Section 6.3.4.4). As a simple demonstration, consider a vacuum-isolated spherical thermos bottle of inside radius r, coated with a material of total emissivity e_r and filled with a hot working fluid of heat capacity C_V at initial temperature T_2. Conduction and convection are eliminated; heat loss in vacuo occurs only by radiative transfer. In the classical macroscopic formulation, radiated power $P_r = 4 \pi r^2 e_r \sigma (T_2^4 - T_1^4)$ (watts), where $\sigma = 5.67 \times 10^{-8}$ watts/m^2-K^4 (Stefan-Boltzmann constant). The thermal energy contained in the hot material is $H_r = (4/3) \pi r^3 C_V (T_2 - T_1)$ (joules); hence the time required for half of the energy to radiate away is:

$$\tau_{1/2} \sim \left(\frac{H_r}{P_r}\right) \ln(2) = \frac{\ln(2)\, r\, C_V (T_2 - T_1)}{3\, e_r\, \sigma \left(T_2^4 - T_1^4\right)} \qquad \text{\{Eqn. 6.11\}}$$

For r = 1 micron, $C_V = 4.2 \times 10^6$ joules/m^3-K for water, $e_r = 0.02$ for polished silver, $T_1 = 310$ K inside the human body, and $T_2 = 350$ K up to 647 K (~critical temperature of water at 218 atm pressure), $\tau_{1/2} \lesssim 6$ sec (at $T_2 \gtrsim 350$ K) starting from an initial (accessible) energy density of ~10^8 joules/m^3; $H_r = 1.5$ nanojoule for a 1-micron core at 647 K. Almost the entire thermal energy store (~99%) leaks away in just 40 sec (at $T_2 = 350$ K). Smaller thermos bottles leak even faster, due to the ~r dependence of $\tau_{1/2}$.

Radiators lying within <1 micron of a lower-temperature material surface exhibit near-field anomalous radiative transfer (Section 6.3.4.4 (E)) and thus exhibit different cooling characteristics than Eqn. 6.11 predicts. Taking $P_r = P_{anomalous}$ from Eqn. 6.21 for spherical surfaces <200 nm apart, then $\tau_{1/2} \sim 0.01\ (h^2 c^2 / k^3)\ (r\, C_V / \sigma_{cond}\, T_2^2)$ (seconds); for $T_2 = 647$ K and r = 1 micron, $\tau_{1/2} \sim 10$ sec using a germanium shell but ~10^5 sec using a boron shell.

Other thermomechanical transducers include sandwich cantilevers (Section 4.6.3) made of composite materials with high coefficients of linear expansion (e.g., heated metal bimorphs[547]), Nitinol or other temperature-sensitive shape-memory alloys,[548] thermally-driven phase-change microactuators,[545] thermally-powered contraction turbines,[597] and thermally-driven contractile proteins.[1261] Thermochemical transducers that make use of thermal energy stored as a phase change of a refrigerant can display energy densities of ~10^8 joules/m^3,[1197] and a thermoacoustic Stirling engine with no moving parts has been demonstrated.[3267]

A thermoelectric transducer may be constructed from a crystal with piezoelectric properties. When such a crystal is heated or cooled, charges are produced on its surfaces (called pyro-electricity[553] or heat electricity) setting up mechanical strains in the crystal that produce the same electrical effect as the application of external forces in piezo-electricity.[551] Both bone and tendon exhibit the pyro-electric effect;[3088] all pyroelectric materials are piezoelectric, though the converse is not true.[3089] Thermocouples are another example of direct thermoelectric energy transduction, and thermophotovoltaic generators are well-known.[1983]

A high emissivity blackbody radiator provides thermooptical transduction at temperatures >650 K, increasing in efficiency up to ~6000 K.

6.3.2 Mechanical Energy Conversion Processes

It has been suggested[540] that "simple physical shaking" may be sufficient to provide power to nanorobots, much like a self-winding watch that employs mechanical rectification. Material moves through human lymphatic vessels (Section 8.2.1.3) in this manner: The lymphatics have no direct musculature (or cilia) of their own, but depend upon external physiological motion sources such as blood vessel contractions and skeletal movements to induce periodic pressures on the lymphatic vessels, moving material along via one-way valving. Experiments using respiratory chambers found that spontaneous physical activity or "fidgeting" consumed an average of 348 Kcal/day (range 100-700 Kcal/day) or ~17 watts of power[2935] and could be a major cause of individual differences in 24-hour energy expenditure.[2936,2937] In a nanorobot, a mechanomechanical transducer would convert environmental motion into mechanical energy for internal storage or immediate utilization.

Consider a medical nanodevice embedded in the hand of a human being who is waving his arm back and forth in a perfect sinusoidal motion of lateral amplitude X_{move} meters and period t_{move} seconds per cycle (t_{move}^{-1} Hz). If the mechanomechanical transducer consists of a spring-loaded bob mass of density ρ_{trans}, volume V_{trans} and mass m_{trans} whose motion is rectified using a ratchet and pawl mechanism, the maximum velocity of the mass is $4\,X_{move} / t_{move}$ at the centerpoint of the armswing, the acceleration profile crudely resembles a square wave of amplitude $A_{move} = 16\,X_{move} / t_{move}^2$, and the maximum extractable nanorobot power P_n is:

$$P_n \sim \frac{8\,\rho_{trans}\,V_{trans}\,X_{move}^2}{t_{move}^3} - \frac{kT}{t_{move}} \sim \frac{m_{trans}\,A_{move}\,X_{move} - 2\,kT}{2\,t_{move}}$$

(watts) {Eqn. 6.12}

For ρ_{trans} = 21,450 kg/m^3 (platinum bob), V_{trans} = 1 $micron^3$, T = 310 K inside the human body, and k = 0.01381 zJ/K (Boltzmann constant), the constant microtwitching of human muscles of ~0.1 mm amplitude and ~10 Hz provides a mechanical energy of ~kT, hence P_n ~ 0 from this source. Ignoring the 10 g, 1-second accelerative impulse due to passage through the beating heart, each ~1 meter circulation of the blood involving a ~60 sec passage from an aortal velocity of ~1 m/sec to a capillary velocity of ~1 mm/sec, provides only P_n ~ 10^{-6} pW. The twice per circuit passage through the beating heart raises the full-circuit total to P_n ~ 10^{-3} pW; that is, most of the mechanical energy in each circuit is localized in the heart. Nanorobots with a 1 $micron^3$ transducer resident in the diaphragm during normal respiration can obtain P_n ~ 3 x 10^{-6} pW assuming X_{move} ~ 2 cm, t_{move} ~ 3 sec. In normal walking with X_{move} ~ 0.6 m and t_{move} ~ 1 sec, P_n ~ 0.06 pW; for the most violent handwaving exercise with X_{move} = 0.3 m and t_{move} = 0.2 sec (5 Hz), P_n = 2 pW. All of these figures optimistically assume 100% mechanical efficiency.

Nanorobots resident in the chest walls experience cyclical displacements of X_{move} ~ 2.5 cm and t_{move} ~ 3.3 sec (0.3 Hz) for normal shallow breathing at 10/min, up to X_{move} ~ 5 cm and t_{move} = 1 sec (1 Hz) for deep breathing during heavy exertion (Section 8.2.2), a chest velocity range of v_{move} = 2-10 cm/sec, giving P_n = 3-400 x 10^{-6} pW (Eqn. 6.12) for a pendulum transducer. Another alternative in the chest is a simple spring-loaded stretch transducer. If the diaphragm and chest wall muscles cost P_{chest} = 1-25 watts to operate depending upon exertion level, then the applied force F_{chest} = P_{chest} / v_{move} = 50-250 N; an X = 5 cm displacement for a 90-cm circumference chest cavity gives a δ ~ 5% distension. Thus a two-phase L = 100 nm stretch transducer produces $P_n = 2\,\delta\,L\,e\%\,F_{chest} / t_{move}$ = 150-2500 pW, conservatively taking mechanical efficiency e% = 0.001(0.1%) to account for poor coupling and a highly nonisotropic tissue stress tensor. Similar power levels are available in contractile cardiac tissues, near joints that flex during normal arm or leg motions, and in the pedal dermis during walking.

Another example of mechanomechanical transduction is a simple gear train, which transmits mechanical rotational power from one location to another. In one example given by Drexler,[10] a 17 nm^3 steric gear pair transmits 1 nanowatt of mechanical power, giving a power density of 6 x 10^{16} watts/m^3 with a mechanical efficiency of 99.997%. Complex hectomicron-scale gear trains have been fabricated.[558] Sandia's Microelectronics Development Laboratory mass-produces 100-micron motors and gears.[1259] Properly designed molecular bearings will have lifetimes that are not limited by wear but only by the static lifetime of the bearing (e.g., due to radiation damage).

In 1998, there was at least one unconfirmed experimental report of direct mechanochemical energy transduction,[2924] in which the mechanical energy of stirring of water over a catalyst bed of powdered cuprous oxide was alleged to produce H_2 and O_2 gas effluent.

Mechanoacoustic transduction may be achieved by operating the pressure-driven actuators described in Section 6.3.3 in reverse, using an oscillating mechanical energy input such as a reciprocating rod to drive the piston. See Section 7.2.2.1 for a more complete treatment of the vibrating piston acoustic radiator.

Mechanoelectric transduction is commonplace in atomic force microscope (AFM) sensors using piezoresistive cantilevers that produce a varying electrical potential in response to changing mechanical loads. Typical coupling constants (e.g., mechanoelectric efficiency) are 11% for polyvinylidene fluoride (PVDF), and 35-59% for lead zirconate titanate (PZT).[993] Transduction of mechanical to electrical signals can also be achieved by mechanically modulating a tunneling contact junction as a mechanically controlled electrical switch, as occurs at the tip of a scanning tunneling microscope (STM) in response to varying physical loads. Fullerene molecules also change their electrical resistance in response to mechanically-applied loads, providing mechanoelectrical switching (Section 10.2.2). Alternatively, operating the nanoscale electrostatic DC motor[10] described in Section 6.3.5 in reverse converts it into a mechanoelectric generator, transforming rotational mechanical energy into electrical current at high efficiency. Cochlear outer hair cells are capable of both mechanoelectrical and electromechanical transduction.[3597]

Cardiac mechanoelectric transducers have also been proposed or tested.[593,722,723,3513-3517] In 1966, Ko[633] fabricated a mechanical converter that converted heart movement into the vibration of a piezoelectric rod to generate AC electric power that was rectified and used to power a pacemaker; such devices were installed on dogs' hearts and generated 30 microwatts for several months. Electropaced skeletal muscles (latissimus dorsi) have been used to compress an implanted plastic balloon counterpulsation device to produce pulmonary artery diastolic pressure augmentation.[3519-3521] There are proposals to use piezoelectric bimorphs to transform the mechanical energy of diaphragm motions during breathing[592,3516] and of the circumferential movements of the aorta and other elastic arteries during each pulse cycle[593,3522] into electrical energy, but transducer fatigue and biocompatibility issues were problematical.[590,3517,3518] Piezoelectric fields developed in moving bones[3090-3095] and collagenous tissues[1939-1942] possibly could be tapped. Indeed, many biological materials have been found to be piezoelectric, including tendon, elastin, silk, dentin, ivory, wood, aorta, trachea, intestine, and even nucleic acids.[3089] A gait-powered battery-charging system exploited ground reaction forces associated with the heel-strike and toe-off phases to convert the autologous mechanical energy of walking into electrical energy using a piezoelectric array embedded in the midsole of a shoe.[3523] Shoe manufacturers have already put LEDs in sneakers (LED flashing is powered by footfall energy), and hand-cranked power supplies for laptop computers were being developed by Freeplay Power Group in 1999.[3185] Keyboard typing produces 0.1-30 milliwatts/finger (Section 7.4.2.1).

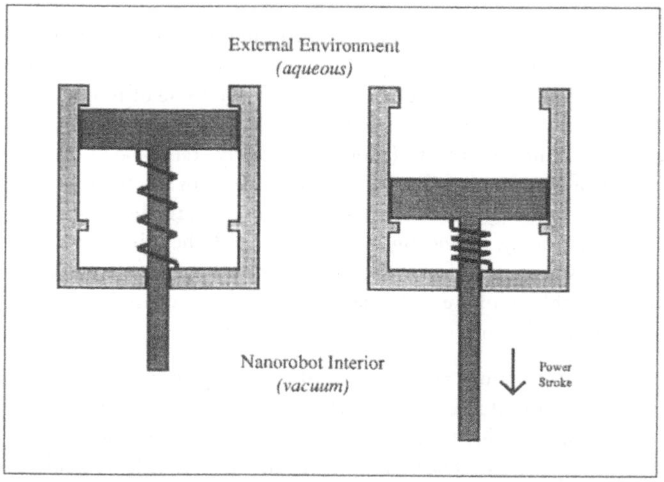

Fig. 6.1. Pressure-driven actuators for acoustomechanical power transduction.

Piezoluminescent crystals provide mechanooptical power transduction, and micromachined optical shutters[546] have demonstrated mechanical switching of optical signals.

6.3.3 Acoustic Energy Conversion Processes

Most clearly useful for medical nanorobots are acoustomechanical transducers (Section 4.5.1) that can directly apply motive power to internal nanomechanical manipulator and computational systems. Drexler[10] has described a simple transducer that can function as a pressure-driven actuator, which is abstractly modeled as a constant-force spring that resists the motion of a piston moving between two limit stops (Fig. 6.1). Such a device which experiences a cyclical volumetric change of ΔV in response to above-ambient pressure pulses of amplitude ΔP at a frequency ν_p converts acoustic pulse energy into the mechanical energy of piston motion with almost 100% thermodynamic efficiency when the expansion is isothermal and reversible (e.g., when thermal equilibration time $t_{EQ} << \nu_p^{-1}$, which should always hold for $\nu_p \lesssim 1$ GHz).

Recognition of four additional restrictions on the net mechanical power (P_n) available from a piston-type transducer produces a very conservative power estimate:

$$P_n \sim \nu_p \left(\Delta P\, \Delta V - E_{friction} - E_{inertia} - E_{drag} - E_{heat}\right) \quad \{\text{Eqn. 6.13}\}$$

The product of ΔP, the change in pressure during a stroke, and ΔV, the change in piston volume, is the change in Gibbs free energy per cycle.[10] The piston energy lost to friction may be estimated from Eqn. 6.4 using the observation that interface velocity $v \sim 2\, \nu_p\, L$ for a piston of dimension $\sim L^3$, thus $E_{friction} \sim 10^{-25}\, \nu_p\, L^{0.6}$; for $E_{friction} < kT$, $L < 0.05$ micron for $\nu_p = 1$ GHz, $L < 5000$ microns for $\nu_p = 1$ MHz. The energy lost in overcoming piston inertia $\sim 1/2\, mv^2$ where $m = \rho_p L^3$, so $E_{inertia} \sim 2\, \rho_p\, \nu_p^2\, L^5$ for a piston of density ρ_p; for $E_{inertia} < kT$, $L < 4$ nm for $\nu_p = 1$ GHz, $L < 60$ nm for $\nu_p = 1$ MHz. Fluid viscous drag occurs when the piston must push itself through a viscous external aqueous medium in which the pressure pulses are traveling. However, if $L << \lambda = v_{sound}/\nu_p$ then the range of piston motion is far smaller than one wavelength and $E_{drag} \sim 0$ for submicron transducers: at $\nu_p = 1$ GHz, $\lambda = 1.5$ microns in water at 310 K. Finally, $E_{heat} \sim kT$ because useful work may not be extracted from an isothermal medium. L_{min} is the size of the receiver piston for which $P_n \leq 0$.

Of course, this is a very conservative approach because much depends upon how predictable the acoustic source is. J. Soreff notes that in the case of externally supplied, constant frequency, constant amplitude pressure waves, both $E_{inertia}$ and E_{heat} are negligible because the capture of energy from the piston can be phase locked to the incoming waves, and the piston spring constant can be tailored to put the kinetic energy of the piston into a potential energy store at the end of its travel. Phase locking still requires an energy expenditure of kT for sensing, but this sensing could be spread over many cycles, given a source with a long coherence time.

Table 6.3, with values computed using Eqn. 6.13 and acoustic pressure estimates from Section 4.9.1, shows that a modest amount of acoustic energy is available from normal physiological processes within the human body, which are assumed to generate planar traveling waves. Path length is not important here because of the weak attenuation at such low frequencies (Section 4.9.1.3). For a single ($\sim$1 micron)^3 transducer, usable received acoustic power up to $P_n \sim 0.004$ pW is regularly available from continuous sources. Intermittent or sporadic usable power sources up to $P_n \sim 5$ pW are also available. In many cases these sources would be in phase with the biothermal transducer described in Section 6.3.1.

Large epidermally-placed nanorobots may convert the force of wind resistance into usable energy. In theory, nanorobots may receive $P_n = (1/2)\, e\%\, \rho_{air}\, A\, v_{run}^3 \sim 1$ pW for efficiency $e\% = 0.30(30\%)$, STP air density $\rho_{air} = 1.29$ kg/m^3, and transducer area $A = 1$ micron^2 for a person walking or running at $v_{run} = 1.8$ m/sec ($\sim$4 mph). However, as a practical matter much less power is available to micron-size nanorobots because there is a near-skin boundary layer of relatively still air.

External sources of acoustic energy can also be employed (Section 6.4.1). Power pulse cycling depends on sensor design. For example, to avoid damaging the aforementioned acoustic sensor devices with large acoustic pulses intended to provide power, power pulses should be shaped with a slow initial amplitude rise sufficient to gently "peg" all sensor pistons to their distal stops, followed by a sharp upramp to peak amplitude, then a shallow decline sufficient to gently return sensor pistons to their proximal stops, followed by a sharp decline

Table 6.3 Estimated Acoustic Energy Available from Physiological Sources within the Human Body

Physiological Acoustic Energy Source Within the Human Body	Maximum Pressure Change	Typical Frequency	Minimum Transducer Size	Continuously Available Power (picowatts) (Averaged Over One Complete Cycle) L = 1000 nm	L = 200 nm	L = 100 nm
	(ΔP)	(ν_p)	(L_{min})	(P_n)	(P_n)	(P_n)
Vocalization/Shouting	0.05 atm	1000 Hz	10 nm	5	0.04	0.005
Footfall impacts/Running	2.0 atm	4 Hz	4 nm	0.8	0.006	0.0008
Vocalization/Talking	0.005 atm	1000 Hz	20 nm	0.5	0.004	0.0005
Vocalization/Whispering	0.0005 atm	1000 Hz	45 nm	0.05	0.0004	0.00005
Footfall impacts/Walking	0.4 atm	1 Hz	10 nm	0.04	0.0003	0.00004
Clapping hands (vigorously)	0.2 atm	2 Hz	10 nm	0.04	0.0003	0.00004
Chewing crunchy food	0.0001 atm	1000 Hz	76 nm	0.01	0.00008	0.000006
Clapping hands (softly)	0.02 atm	2 Hz	22 nm	0.004	0.00003	0.000004
Respiratory airflow turbulence	0.00004 atm	1000 Hz	103 nm	0.004	0.00003	0
Arterial pulse	0.02 atm	1 Hz	27 nm	0.002	0.00002	0.000002
Subcutaneous interstitial cycles	0.003 atm	1 Hz	50 nm	0.0003	0.000002	0.0000003
Arteriovenous transit cycle	0.14 atm	0.02 Hz	49 nm	0.0002	0.000002	0.0000002
Capillary pulse	0.002 atm	1 Hz	57 nm	0.0002	0.000002	0.0000002

in pulse amplitude, thus safely completing the power cycle. An acoustic-powered legged microrobot ~1 mm in size with resonant actuators has been fabricated and tested.[352,559]

The Space Thermoacoustic Refrigerator (STAR) developed by Steven L. Garrett for NASA in the early 1990s uses 160 dB sound waves in a confined space to create a spatial thermal gradient in a working fluid, an example of acoustothermal energy conversion.[3446] Sonoluminescence caused by focused high-frequency sound waves in water provides an example of acoustophotonic power transduction.[543,716] Acoustochemical processes are well-known in the field of sonochemistry,[625,1084,1085,1523] including ultrasonic depolymerization. Acoustomechanical fluid-driven microturbines ~250 microns in diameter have been fabricated and operated at ~KHz frequency with lifetimes of ~10^8 revolutions.[1218]

6.3.4 Chemical Energy Conversion Processes

The following Section describes possible energy sources for chemically-powered foraging nanorobots. Chemically-powered tethered or stored-energy nanorobots may have different constraints (see Sections 6.4.3.5, 6.5.3, and 6.5.4).

6.3.4.1 Human Chemical Energy Resources

The first step in evaluating chemical power transduction alternatives for medical nanorobots is to assess the chemical energy resources readily available within the human body. A complete inventory is beyond the scope of this book, but a few broad conclusions may be drawn.

Table 6.4 summarizes major representative chemical energy resources available within typical individual human tissue cells, within the human blood volume, and within an entire 70 kg adult human body. Burning a protein or carbohydrate in oxygen releases ~4.1 Kcal/gm (17 x 10^6 joules/kg); burning lipids in oxygen releases ~9.3 Kcal/gm (39 x 10^6 joules/kg). In theory, proteins represent the most plentiful energy resource in blood and cells, but extensively accessing this source may require disassembly of essential cellular structures, considerable preprocessing (e.g., denaturation and lysis), and disposal of nitrogen-containing waste products.* Free amino acids and short peptides are too dilute to be of much value. ATP, usually available only inside cells with a high turnover rate, is also of very limited utility (though it is fairly stable—one can buy bottles of powdered ATP and store it for years in the freezer).

Fats potentially offer the most plentiful natural energy source in the human body, providing over 80% of body heat in the absence of carbohydrates. Unfortunately, high energy density serum lipids such as cholesterol are not freely available but instead are present only in three bound forms that ensure solubility:

1. chylomicrons and other plasma lipoprotein carriers (protein-coated lipid droplets <0.5 microns in diameter), to transport lipids throughout the body from the intestine after absorption of dietary fat, or from the liver after lipid synthesis to storage in adipose tissue or for utilization elsewhere in the body;[3525]
2. fatty acids bound to serum albumin, to transport fat from adipose tissue to elsewhere in the body; and
3. ketone bodies (acetoacetate and beta-hydroxybutyrate) to transport lipids processed by or synthesized in the liver.

Anhydrous lipid droplets 0.2-5 microns in diameter are often found in the cytosol. Excepting operations inside adipocytes (wherein triglyceride droplets occupy nearly the entire cytosol), fat utilization by medical nanomachines would probably require some physical nanopipetting or other preprocessing to dislodge the lipid from its carrier, and different energy extraction pathways may be required depending on whether the fatty molecules thus liberated are saturated or unsaturated, etc.

Carbohydrates are soluble in water and thus exist in free form throughout the body. Large individual molecules of glycogen (10-40 nm in diameter) float freely as granules in the cytosol, usually coated with a ~5 nm thick monolayer of digestive enzymes (Section

*The human body secretes urea because it lacks the necessary enzymes to further process the nitrogen. Nanorobots could make use of bacterial enzymatic or other chemical processes to obtain energy from nitrogenous wastes—for example, by exploiting the ammonia oxidation reaction: $4NH_3\ (g) + 3O_2\ (g) \rightarrow 2N_2\ (g) + 6H_2O\ (g) + 2105\ zJ$.

Table 6.4 Estimated Chemical Energy Resources in the Human Body

Chemical Fuel	Energy Available in 70 kg Human Body (joules)	Energy Available in 5.4 Liters of Whole Blood (joules)	Energy Available in Typical 20-μm Cell (joules)
ATP	$2.2\text{-}4.1 \times 10^4$	$1.7\text{-}3.1 \times 10^2$	$0.6\text{-}1.0 \times 10^{-9}$
Glycine (amino acid)	$3.5\text{-}4.8 \times 10^4$	$2.8\text{-}6.0 \times 10^2$	$0.9\text{-}1.2 \times 10^{-9}$
Leucine (amino acid)	$1.2\text{-}1.7 \times 10^5$	$2.0\text{-}2.9 \times 10^3$	$3.0\text{-}4.3 \times 10^{-9}$
Lactate	$0.6\text{-}2.6 \times 10^5$	$0.4\text{-}1.6 \times 10^4$	$0.5\text{-}2.4 \times 10^{-8}$
Glucosamine	$0.5\text{-}1.1 \times 10^6$	$3.6\text{-}7.7 \times 10^4$	$0.5\text{-}1.1 \times 10^{-7}$
Urea	$0.7\text{-}1.4 \times 10^6$	$1.2\text{-}2.4 \times 10^4$	$1.8\text{-}3.5 \times 10^{-8}$
Glucose, free	$3.3\text{-}4.9 \times 10^6$	$5.6\text{-}8.2 \times 10^4$	$0.8\text{-}1.2 \times 10^{-7}$
Glycogen (starch), granules	$4.2\text{-}6.3 \times 10^6$	$0.1\text{-}1.6 \times 10^4$	$1.3\text{-}80 \times 10^{-7}$
Cholesterol (lipid)	$1.4\text{-}2.8 \times 10^7$	$2.4\text{-}4.7 \times 10^5$	$3.6\text{-}7.0 \times 10^{-7}$
Total carbohydrate	$3.3\text{-}5.4 \times 10^7$	$0.6\text{-}1.1 \times 10^5$	$0.8\text{-}9.0 \times 10^{-6}$
Total protein	$1.3\text{-}2.5 \times 10^8$	$1.9\text{-}2.0 \times 10^7$	$1.4\text{-}2.9 \times 10^{-5}$
Total fat (lipid)	$1.6\text{-}9.8 \times 10^8$	$0.9\text{-}1.3 \times 10^6$	$6.2\text{-}9.4 \times 10^{-6}$

8.5.3.7). Glucose is the preferred human body fuel—a nearly constant bloodstream inventory of ~5 grams is maintained homeostatically from a buffer supply of ~350 grams of glycogen stored mainly in the liver and muscles. Glucose transporters maintain[3649-3654] cytosolic concentrations at comparable levels to the blood. Nerve cells can only metabolize glucose and ketones; sperm cells are surrounded by a fructose bath, from which they absorb chemical energy to power flagellar engines during their short-lived locomotion (Section 6.3.4.2).

Because of its abundance, high energy density, and relative ease of use (e.g., high solubility), glucose is probably the ideal fuel for most in vivo nanomedical applications. A 1 micron^3 onboard store of glucose fuel powers a 10 pW nanorobot for 2400 sec of operation without further refueling. The equilibrium free glucose mass in a typical human tissue cell provides ~10^4 sec of power for a 10 pW nanodevice; during strenuous exercise, a typical tissue cell can normally replace its entire glucose store in <10^3 sec via membrane glucose transporters, providing a continuous fuel supply for at least ~100 pW of nanorobot demand.* If this is still insufficient for the intended application, artificial lipophilic oxyglucose transporter structures may be inserted through the cellular membrane to provide supplementary power levels up to the diffusion limit (Section 6.5.3). (An additional 100-8000 nanojoules of polymerized glucose, present as glycogen granules, may be available in some cells.) For a (20 micron)^3 tissue cell, from Eqn. 3.4 the maximum diffusion-limited glucose current is J_{glu} = 6-30 x 10^{10} glucose molecules/sec. Assuming ~50% absorption efficiency at the cell surface (Section 4.2.5), ~50% energy conversion efficiency (see below), and that the local extracellular space has sufficient fluid volume to supply adjacent cells at peak rates, then the maximum theoretical total continuous power draw in cyto is 70,000-300,000 pW for foraging glucose-consuming nanodevices with unlimited access to oxygen (e.g., onboard storage). If oxygen supplies were restricted to that which could passively diffuse through cell walls, the comparable in cyto diffusion-limited total oxygen current would be J_{O_2} = 2 x 10^{10} O_2 molecules/sec, a ~4000 pW power limit. (For comparison, the basal power consumption of a typical 20-micron human cell is ~30 pW; Table 6.8.)

The following Sections include brief technical sketches of several possible approaches to chemoergic power transduction. The methods outlined are rather crude. An ideal design might involve complex nanomachinery that has yet to be designed, which may perhaps more closely resemble in efficiency and function the enzymatic and "proton pump" biological nanomachines that are found in nature, or the natural chemophotonic transducers employed in bioluminescence.[3564]

6.3.4.2 Biological Chemomechanical Power Conversion

Many examples of direct chemomechanical power transduction are found in nature. Perhaps the most familiar is the mechanism of muscle contraction mediated by the sliding of interdigitating myosin and actin filaments—the actomyosin molecular motor.[1246] Myosin is constructed of domains joined by hinges and is powered by ATP. The globular head domain of the myosin motor, called myosin subfragment-1 or "S1", is a whale-shaped molecular device ~5 nm wide at the head and ~20 nm long, containing ~50,000 atoms (~500 nm^3). When the ATP molecule binds to an open ATPase pocket on S1, this action causes a conformational change in the S1 protein, which releases its hold on the associated actin filament. The pocket can then close further, clipping the terminal phosphate from the ATP (making ADP) and powering yet another conformational change which increases affinity for actin. The phosphate is released as S1 again binds to actin, pulling the pocket open wider and triggering a ~2 millisec power stroke as the spent ADP molecule is ejected.[578] During each 0.05-sec cycle, the myosin motor advances 10 nm along the actin filament (~5 micron/sec velocity) pulling with a force of ~5 pN, a mechanical energy output of ~50 zJ, or ~10^{-6} pW (power density ~ 2 x 10^6 watts/m^3). The energy released in converting one ATP molecule to ADP is ~83 zJ, so the motor is ~60% efficient. A typical macroscale muscle may contain ~10^{11} individual actomyosin motors. The net energy efficiency of a muscle is at most 25%, doing the greatest work when it shortens by only ~10% of its length.[2022] In 1998, the myosin superfamily of protein motors contained 15 different classes, and ~30 different myosin species were known.[2279]

Other molecular motors similarly transduce chemical energy into mechanical motion to drive the beating of cilia (dynein; Section 9.3.1.1) and to drive the transport of vesicles and organelles along tracks within cells (kinesin; Section 9.4.6). In each case, the binding of ATP (or GTP) induces conformational transitions in the ~12 nm

**If 624 micromoles/min of glucose are transported per milligram of purified glucose transporter protein molecules of molecular weight ~100,000 daltons,[3656] then the mean glucose transport rate is ~1000 glucose molecules/sec-transporter which is equivalent to ~0.0025 pW/transporter assuming 50% metabolic utilization efficiency, supplying ~250 pW/cell for a 20-micron tissue cell embedded with ~10^5 transmembrane glucose transporters (membrane surface density ~40 transporters/micron^2).*

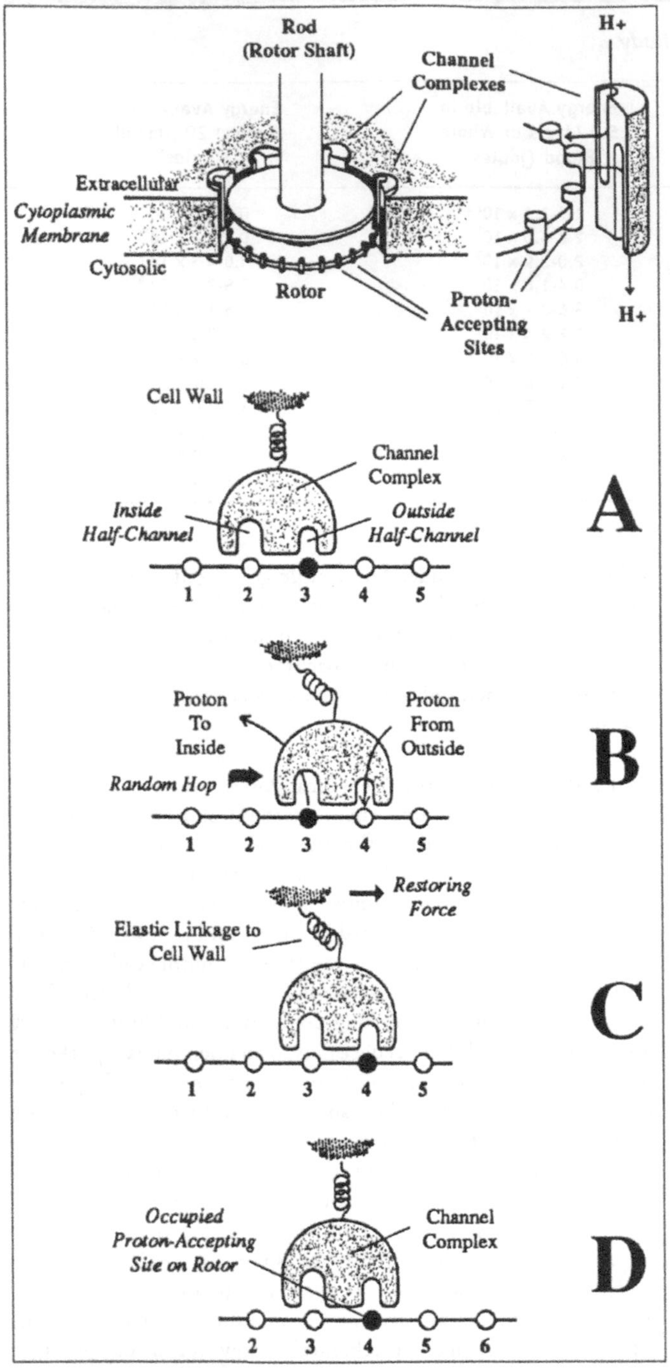

Fig. 6.2. Bacterial flagellar proton gradient chemomechanical motor.

motor proteins, which are reversed by the hydrolysis of bound ATP and release of ADP and phosphate, advancing the motor protein along the tubulin track and pulling with a force of ~2 pN.[1247] Another example is a component of the mitochondrial enzyme ATP synthase: F_1-ATPase, a ~1 nm rotor spinning in a ~12 nm barrel, the smallest rotary motor known, producing forces >100 pN and a rotary torque of ~40-80 pN-nm under high load,[1234,3198] and a calculated no-load rotational frequency of ~17 Hz with ~100% energy conversion efficiency.[2278,3198] Another strong molecular motor is RNA polymerase, which pulls with a stall force of ~25 pN at a 12-40% efficiency. Each human tissue cell probably contains ~50 different kinds of biological motors. A different type of chemomechanical motor protein—an enzyme called lambda exonuclease found in a bacteriophage virus—chews up one of DNA's double helix strands, leaving behind a single strand; the motor pulls >5 pN while moving along the strand, and is powered directly by the energy liberated from DNA's broken bonds.[3194]

In human mitochondria, the combined TCA (tricarboxylic acid) cycle (aka. Krebs cycle[892]) and cytochrome chain oxidative-phosphorylation convert 39 molecules of ADP to higher-energy ATP during the net metabolism of one glucose molecule, a chemochemical energy conversion efficiency of ~65%.[526] Combining this metabolic process with the myosin motor described earlier would yield a glucose-powered chemomechanical transducer that is ~39% efficient.

While all known eukaryotic motors are powered by ATP or GTP, neither is required for bacterial flagellar rotation. Rather, the flagellar ionic motor is a rotary device[1381] driven by the pH differential between the cytosolic and extracellular sides of the device. This ~5 x 10^6 atom, 50,000 nm^3 motor consists of a shaft attached to a rotor that spins up to 300 Hz (15 Hz at high load) inside a fixed stator ~30 nm in diameter attached to the peptidoglycan layer, driven by the flow of ~1000 protons (H^+ ions) per revolution. Stator and rotor surfaces lie ~0.5 nm apart.

Figure 6.2 illustrates how this proton-gradient driven machine works. The rotor has a set of ~100 proton-accepting sites around its periphery which interact with 8 channel complexes embedded in the stator. Each channel complex has two half-channels, one accessible from the (relatively alkaline) cytosol, the other from the (relatively acidic) extracellular space. A proton is transferred from a half-channel to an acceptor site on the rotor, but cannot be donated to the other half-channel unless the rotor rotates.[396] Referring to the Figure to trace one cycle, in the geometry shown in (A), site 2 is empty and site 3 is filled, so the complex can move right but not left. If random motion carries the complex one step to the right (B), the proton on site 3 can move into the cytosol and a new proton can move into the adjacent empty site 4 (C). The rotor then rotates counterclockwise a distance equal to the spacing between acceptor sites, to relieve the spring tension (D).[579] Reversing the geometry (which takes ~1 millisec, controlled by a protein switch) allows the motor to run backwards; this occurs naturally every few seconds in the absence of any environmental stimulus.[531] The motor develops ~10^{-4} pW with a power density of ~2 x 10^6 watts/m^3. Motor efficiency is <5% at low load, 50%-99%+ at high load.[581]

Flagellar ionic motors that run on sodium ions rather than protons have been found in some bacteria;[580] no doubt other alternatives could be employed in chemomechanically powered medical nanorobots. Drexler[10] estimates from first principles that chemically-driven engines can be designed to operate at >99% efficiency at a power density of ~10^9 watts/m^3.

Other natural chemomechanical engines involve fluid movements, including evaporative-driven ascent of sap in plants,[2031] hydrophilic- and hygroscopic-driven expansion due to water absorption, and osmotic pumps in cells, leaves, and plant roots.

6.3.4.3 Artificial Chemomechanical Power Conversion

Chemomechanical gel actuators have been reviewed by Tatara,[587] who describes a variety of polyelectrolyte gels and ion-exchange resins used to make centimeter-scale "mechanochemical pistons" and 100-micron polyelectrolyte fibers used to make chemomechanical "finger" actuators; unfortunately, these electrically-stimulated transducers may fatigue after only ~500 cycles. More interesting is the Sussmann-Katchalsky chemomechanical turbine (Fig. 6.3)—a continuous collagen fiber contracts as it enters a 10M LiBr solution, producing a contractile force that is converted into a torque to rotate the shaft of the output pulley.[597] The device has been patented, built, and operated with an energy conversion efficiency of ~40%. While it would be difficult to scale down this turbine to submicron dimensions, it nonetheless constitutes another useful proof of principle that direct chemomechanical power transduction may need only surprisingly simple mechanisms.

Astumian[696] has examined the use of nonequilibrium chemical drivers for micron and submicron Brownian motors. For instance, when ATP (negatively charged in solution) binds to a protein, it changes the protein's net charge. Thus two proteins that react with ATP at different rates would feel different electrostatic forces; this force differential can drive a motor. Astumian estimates that even a crudely designed chemically-driven Brownian motor could move in 10-nm steps at ~3 microns/sec, developing ~0.5 pN of force, ~3×10^{-6} pW of power, and a power density of ~10^6 watts/m^3. Many types of cellular protrusions such as filopodia, lamellipodia, and acrosomal extension do not involve molecular motors but rather the transduction of chemical bond energy into mechanical energy using Brownian ratchets to rectify random thermal motions by expending chemical energy in actin or tubulin polymerization.[1203]

6.3.4.4 Glucose Engines

There are many pathways for glucose oxidation in the human body, some which directly involve molecular oxygen. For instance, the glucose-6-phosphate dehydrogenase and the 6-phosphogluconic dehydrogenase enzymes both employ molecular oxygen directly to oxidize a glucose derivative. Although evolution has largely replaced pathways involving direct combination with oxygen, there are still a number of organisms (molds, some bacteria) which have retained these primitive pathways and a few can even be found in mammalian tissues. For example, enzymes in the liver use the reactions:

$$\text{Glucose} + O_2 \xrightarrow[\text{glucose oxidase}]{} \text{Gluconic acid} + H_2O_2 + 131\ \text{zJ} \qquad \{\text{Eqn. 6.14}\}$$

with

$$H_2O_2 \xrightarrow[\text{catalase}]{} H_2O + \frac{1}{2}O_2 + 166\ \text{zJ} \qquad \{\text{Eqn. 6.15}\}$$

One very crude approach for medical nanorobots is to use mechanochemistry techniques to force an exothermic chemical reaction, making a change in volume or generating heat which is subsequently exploited to produce mechanical motion. Given that glucose may be the preferred chemical fuel for nanomedical systems (Section 6.3.4.1), we concentrate our attention on the high-energy exothermic oxyglucose combustion reaction

$$C_6H_{12}O_6 + 6O_2(g) \rightarrow 6CO_2(g) + 6H_2O(g) + E_{glu}\ (= 4{,}765\ \text{zJ}) \qquad \{\text{Eqn. 6.16}\}$$

The kinetic model for the glucose oxidation reaction has not been extensively studied experimentally at pressures >30 atm, so it has not yet been proven that an oxyglucose mixture can be ignited at high pressure near human body temperature at 310 K (37°C). Such a model could have a complex structure, such as the well-studied stoichiometric H_2/O_2 mixture which shows a minimum ignition temperature of only ~380 K (107°C) at ~2500 atm.[582]

Pure sugar in air is not ignited by open flame (e.g., bunsen burner, matchstick), but readily burns if a catalyst such as ash is added.[3120] Exposed to moist air below 323 K (50°C), each molecule of anhydrous glucose hygroscopically absorbs a single molecule of noncovalently-bound water, yielding the monohydrate. Heated above 323 K, anhydrous glucose "caramelizes" when it reaches ~433 K (160°C). Caramelization is not oxidation, but rather is an endothermic decomposition process involving successive dehydration, condensation, and polymerization reactions, that includes the making and breaking of covalent bonds, resulting in brown melanines[3109-3111] and possibly some carbonization.[3087] At 433 K the total translational kinetic energy of the 7 oxyglucose reactant molecules would be 7(3/2)(kT) ~ 63 zJ.

What is the minimum ignition pressure ($P_{ignition}$) of glucose? Pressures of 5,000-15,000 atm deactivate antibodies, enzymes, and proteins (Table 10.3), and ignition temperatures normally fall with rising pressure in combustion reactions.[583,584] In food science, the well-known Maillard reaction ("browning")[3109-3111] between amino acids from protein (mainly lysine) and reducing sugars (glucose and lactose) involves a potpourri of Amadori rearrangements, Schiff's base formations, and Strecker degradations, and occurs during heating (cooking) and pressurization (e.g., the glucose-lysine system at 6000 atm),[3108] and even occurs slowly at body temperature, producing insoluble melanoids and glycosylating proteins during aging (Chapter 29). Initiating the Maillard reaction apparently requires 108-174 zJ/molecule (15.5-25 Kcal/mole),[3110] the rate increasing 2-3 times with each 10 K temperature rise.[3111] Pressure-induced peroxidation of lipids has been shown,[3113] with browning greatly accelerated by pressurized oxygen.[3218] It is also well-known that the hydrocarbons found in oils and greases, and many other organic compounds, will "ignite almost spontaneously" in oxygen stored in compressed tanks at ~150 atm.[3114] Upon contact with liquid oxygen (LOX), paper, textiles, asphalt, tar, kerosene, wood, stainless steel, teflon, and silicones are combustion hazards, and pulverized organic materials such as sawdust, polystyrene and charcoal,[3119] and powdered magnesium, can spontaneously ignite or explode:[3115-3118] "when saturated with LOX these materials have exploded after an impact as slight as a footstep".[3116] The density of oxygen molecules trapped in a mechanochemical binding site at 1000 atm is 12.6 molecules/nm^3, not much below the ~21.5 molecules/nm^3 density in LOX (Table 10.2).

Lacking firm experimental data, we provisionally approximate $P_{ignition}$ as the minimum ~63 zJ activation energy (required to induce covalent bond modification during caramelization), divided by the total reactant volume at 310 K computed by summing the volumes of one glucose (1.91×10^{-28} m^3/molecule) plus 6 molecular oxygens (8.85×10^{-29} m^3/molecule at 860 atm using van der Waals' equation; Section 10.3.2). The required energy density is 8.7×10^7 joules/m^3, which can be supplied to the reactants by applying a

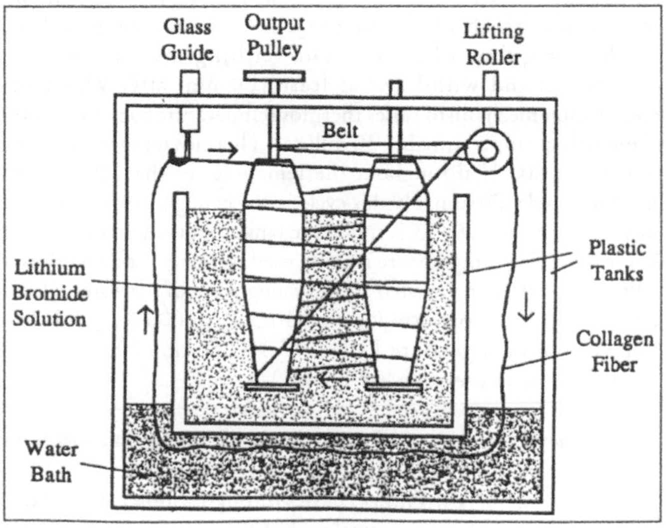

Fig. 6.3. Sussmann-Katchalsky chemomechanical turbine.

mechanical pressure of $P_{ignition}$ ~ 860 atm. Operating the glucose engine at $P_{ignition}$ ~ 1000 atm, possibly including durable catalysts to accelerate the reaction, thus would ensure complete and reliable combustion. (Note that biology already achieves full stepwise glucose oxidation at 310 K, constituting a general proof of principle.)

J. Soreff suggests several interesting design alternatives:

1. Convert glucose to a more stable fuel such as methane (which will not caramelize), possibly by biochemical means, incurring some loss in efficiency;
2. precompress the fuel/oxidizer mixture in a single tank to subignition pressures, then trigger the reaction purely thermally or possibly by adding free radical initiators such as benzoyl peroxide to the tank; or
3. nitrate the glucose hydroxyls, producing combustion and evolution of N_2 which must then be recycled back to HNO_3 via nitrogen fixation (Chapter 19) to nitrate the next batch of fuel.

Once oxyglucose combustion has taken place, the energy thus released may be converted to mechanical energy by various means. In the ideal case of an isothermal expansion at constant (P = 1000 atm) pressure, $P \Delta V = E_{glu}$ would imply a volume change ΔV ~ 47 nm^3, producing a ~5 nm power stroke on a piston of area ~10 nm^2 and a ~1 nN applied force. Vacuum isolation of the combustion chamber assembly (see below) helps prevent rapid energy dissipation via thermal conduction to the external medium. Burning 10^6 sec^{-1} glucose molecules in a ~500,000 nm^3 combustion/engine device (which includes a generous volumetric allowance for support structure) generates ~5 pW with a theoretical power density of ~10^{10} watts/m^3. Note that while the oxyglucose reaction products occupy 0.047 nm^3 more volume than the reactants, relying upon this volume change only allows a highly inefficient (~0.1%) extraction of ~5 zJ per glucose molecule at 1000 atm operating pressure.

A complete design for a working nanoscale glucose engine is beyond the scope of this book. However, as a concept demonstration without regard to maximizing efficiency, one simplistic implementation might employ a combustion chamber at the center of a vacuum-isolated "thermos bottle." A series of combustion events maintains the isolated heat source at a high operating temperature, thus providing a sizable temperature differential against the external medium. This differential can subsequently be used to drive a microscale Stirling engine to produce a mechanical power output,[541] or to stimulate mechanical motion by differential expansion of dissimilar materials (Section 4.6.3), or even to energize an electrical microthermocouple or pyroelectric nanocrystal (Section 6.3.1).

A key component of the glucose engine is a stable heat source, which requires at least five critical design elements:

A. *Combustion Mechanism*—Figure 6.4A shows a heat-generating mechanism which employs two opposed sorting rotors. These rotors contain binding sites which must be exceptionally robust and damage-resistant. Each rotor is a cylinder 40 nm tall with ten staggered rings of opposed binding sites (Fig. 6.4B). The left rotor has binding sites which accept one glucose molecule at a time from the aqueous fuel solution, simultaneously applying sufficient force to strip off the associated water of hydration. The right rotor has binding sites each of which accepts oxygen molecules, six at a time. During operation, these "crushing rotors" compress paired reactant packets into the activation volume required for the oxyglucose combustion reaction to occur. This reaction volume may change shape during the compression cycle, perhaps employing a judicious series of insertions and retractions of binding pocket rods in order

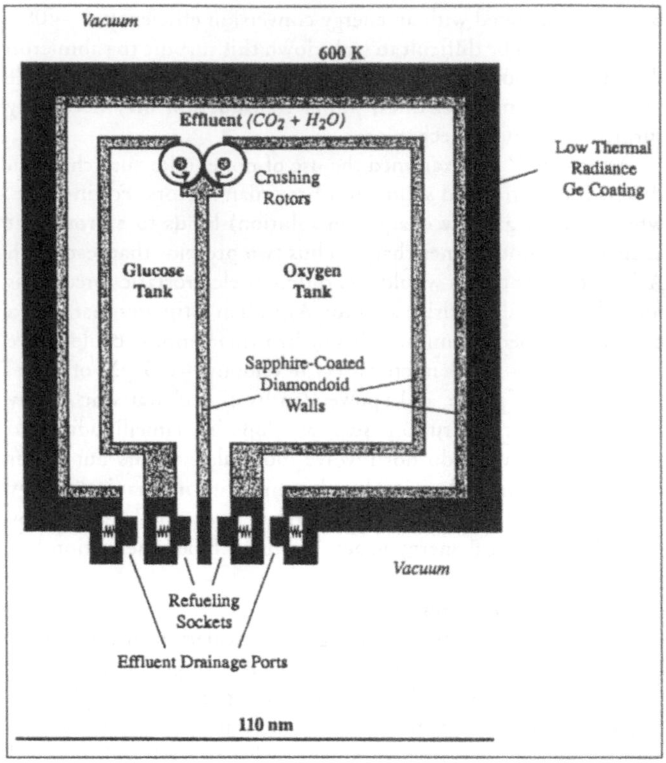

Fig. 6.4A. Glucose engine combustion chamber (top cutaway).

to accommodate intermediate reaction products and multistep reaction events. The end result is to force a complete combustion at the rate of 3 x 10^6 glucose molecules per second (~7 pW). Effluent molecules are ejected into the outer jacket, transferring their heat to the thermally-conductive structure in <10^{-9} sec (Section 4.6.1). The glucose solvation water discharge pathway is not shown in the Figure.

B. *Fuel Tanks*—The combustion mechanism has fuel tanks sized to stoichiometric requirements from which combustion reactants are drawn during each 100 millisec discharge cycle. Tanks are refilled once during each discharge cycle with a saturated 70% glucose (aqueous) solution and O_2 at >1000 atm pressure. During refueling, the thermos structure equilibrates to 310 K in ~10^{-9} sec by thermal conduction through the refilling mechanism, which physically plugs into the refueling sockets. Refilling requires <10^{-7} sec. The refilling mechanism then disconnects and withdraws at least 100 nm, after which the combustion mechanism raises thermos temperature back to the 600 K operating temperature in ~30 millisec. Thermos temperature then remains at 600 K throughout the remainder of the 100 millisec discharge cycle. Presumably this cycle is fast enough to avoid glucose fuel caramelization at 433 K inside the tank; if not, a faster cycle or a lower operating temperature may be used, forcing a somehat lower efficiency on the entire design. (The boiling point of the water solvent exceeds 433 K at >6.4 atm (Section 10.3.2); at 600 K, well below water's critical temperature T_{crit} = 647.3 K (Section 10.3.2), water remains liquid at pressures $\gtrsim$140 atm.)

C. *Rotor Drive Source*—Stacked above the 40-nm tall fuel/rotor complex is a second O_2 storage tank (~15 nm tall) at >2000 atm pressure (Figure 6.4B). This gas passes through a simple ducted turbine mechanism which is coaxial with the two rotors, driving rotor rotation. Spent drive gas passes into the main O_2 storage tank and

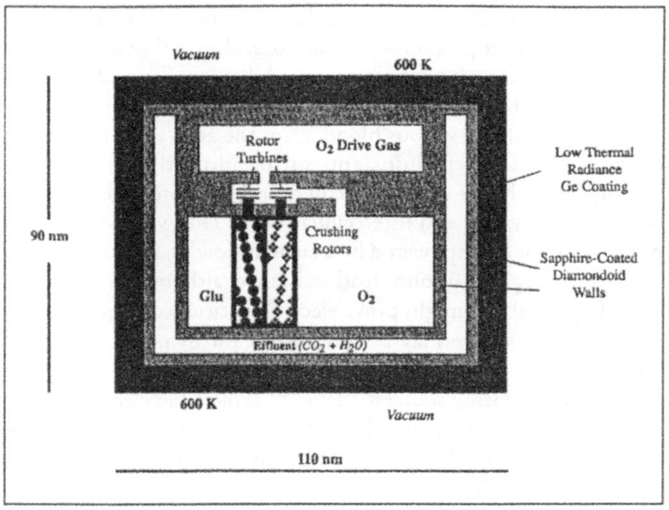

Fig. 6.4B. Glucose engine combustion chamber (side cutaway).

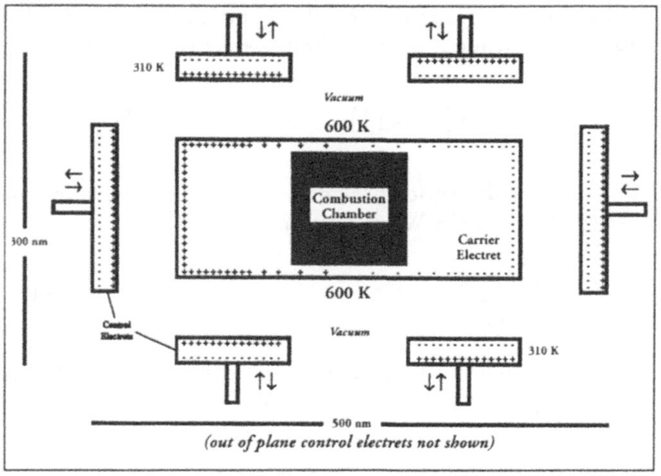

Fig. 6.4C. Glucose engine 3-D electrodynamic suspension (2-D schematic).

is later used as combustion reactant. Drive gas is recharged, and effluent gases are drained off, each process taking ~10^{-7} sec, once every 100 millisec discharge cycle.

D. *Electrodynamic Suspension*—It is crucial to avoid any thermally conductive physical pathways until the cycling Stirling engine (or other intentional energy transfer mechanism) calls for heat. Even the best thermal insulators such as wood, plastic and glass have conductivities K_t = 0.01-1 watts/m-K (Table 8.12, Appendix A), so a 10-nm cube of such material straddling a ΔT = 290 K temperature differential conducts away the entire energy store of E_{store} ~ 1 pJ in ~0.1-10 microsec. Using N_{rod} = 6 carbyne rod supports, each of cross-sectional area A_{rod} ~ $(0.2\ nm)^2$, length L_{rod} = 100 nm, and K_t = 2000 W/m-K for diamond, the thermal leakaway time is:

$$t_{leak} = \frac{E_{store}\, L_{rod}}{N_{rod}\, A_{rod}\, K_t\, \Delta T} = 0.7 \text{ microsec} \qquad \text{\{Eqn. 6.17\}}$$

still much too fast. (J. Soreff notes that glasslike disorder in molecular chains may be obtained by placing C^{12} and C^{13} atoms randomly throughout the carbyne structure, rendering local most of the high spatial and temporal frequency modes and possibly significantly reducing thermal conduction. For somewhat weaker strands, N/CH or O/NH/CH_2 units might be intermixed with similar effect.) Fortunately, vacuum non-contact isolation of the entire combustion assembly also is possible via electric levitation.

Earnshaw's theorem[2172] states that static levitation against gravity is not possible in classical physics using any combination of fixed magnets or electric charges. However, stable levitation may be achieved by using quantum effects (Section 9.2), diamagnetic suspension materials,[2173,2174] rotation of the suspended object as in the levitron,[2175] oscillating magnetic fields,[2176] or dynamic feedback control mechanisms. Three-dimensional electro-dynamic confinement of charged micron-sized aluminum particles was demonstrated experimentally in the late 1950s.[654] From the formulas given, a 100-nm particle with 10 surface charges (charge/mass ~ 1) can be stably confined to a 200-nm volume in a circular Lissajous pattern using a ~1 volt hyperbolic quadrupole AC field at a ~10 MHz resonance frequency plus a ~10 mV DC field to neutralize gravity. A stiffer confinement field on micron-scale particles has been produced inside a spherical void electrodynamic levitator constructed as two joined hemispheres,[655] and more complex configurations have been designed.[658,659] Electric suspension bearings for micromotors using a resonant circuit driven by radio frequency AC voltage can achieve stable levitation of charged objects without requiring feedback signals or sensors,[656,657] and stable passive trapping may also be achieved using cylindrically symmetric dielectrophoretic levitation electrode structures.[660] Translational and rotational motions may be imposed on the suspended object by applying appropriate DC or oscillating fields.

Levitation is particularly effective at the smallest scales. Electrically levitating an object of thickness t, density ρ, and dielectric strength $\kappa\, \varepsilon_0$, against a gravitational acceleration g requires an electric field:[656]

$$E_{lev} = \left(\frac{8\, \rho\, g\, t}{\kappa\, \varepsilon_0} \right)^{1/2} \qquad \text{\{Eqn. 6.18\}}$$

If r = 1000 kg/m^3, g = 9.81 m/sec^2, t = 100 nm, κ = 2.1 (e.g., Teflon), ε_0 = 8.85 x 10^{-12} farad/m, then E_{lev} = 20,000 volts/m or 20 mV across a 1 micron gap (~typical in biological cells). Two unit charges separated by 100 nm in vacuo feel a mutual repulsion of ~0.1 pN, sufficient to resist an external acceleration of ~10^4 g's on a $(100\ nm)^3$ block of density ρ = 1000 kg/m^3; 10^4 g's is the largest natural acceleration imposed on objects of this size inside the human body (Section 4.3.3.2) and is near the maximum safe acceleration for human cells (Chapter 11).

One possible stable open-loop levitation configuration is shown schematically in Figure 6.4C, wherein the combustion assembly is affixed to a simple permanently-polarized dipole electret carrier which is itself electrodynamically levitated by same-sign control electrets positioned at either end. Thermal electrets (electric field applied across heated material[727,2177]) may be made of wax, Teflon, or Mylar; several polymer electrets have extrapolated lifetimes of several thousand years at room temperature.[727] Homocharge electrets (electron beam-embedded charges[2177]) may have longer lifetimes at higher temperatures, or other thermostable electret materials with designed nanoscale charge patterns may be found.[3099]

E. *Thermal Insulation.* The combustion assembly shown in Figures 6.4A and 6.4B measures $(110\ nm)^2$ x 90 nm. For an isolated hot surface in proximity to a cooler surface, both surfaces of area A and separated by vacuum, the rate of heat transfer is given by:

$$P_{classical} = A\, e_r\, \sigma \left(T_2^4 - T_1^4\right) \qquad \text{\{Eqn. 6.19\}}$$

with variables as defined for P_r in Eqn. 6.11; the peak vacuum emission wavelength is given by Wien's relation as:

$$\lambda_{max} = \frac{0.2\, h\, c}{k\, T_2} \qquad \text{\{Eqn. 6.20\}}$$

which, for h = 6.63 x 10^{-34} joule-sec, c = 3 x 10^8 m/sec, k = 0.01381 zJ/K, and T_2 = 310 K, gives λ_{max} = 9.3 microns; at T_2 = 540 K, λ_{max} = 5.3 microns.

At planar separations $d \gtrsim \lambda_{max}$, radiative power is independent of separation distance. However, at smaller separations $d < \lambda_{max}$, radiative heat transfer may be greatly enhanced due to near-field coupling of nonradiative electromagnetic modes in the surfaces.[652,653] In particular, surfaces at temperatures between 300-600 K transfer heat approximately as $\sim(\sigma_{cond}\, d^4)^{-1}$ for 0.2 micron $\lesssim d \lesssim$ 2 microns, where σ_{cond} is electrical conductivity. Surfaces with 10 nm $\lesssim d \lesssim$ 200 nm again exchange energy independent of d, but according to:

$$P_{anomalous} \sim 0.574\, A \left(\frac{4\,\pi^2\, k^3}{h^2\, c^2}\right) \sigma_{cond}\, T_2^2 (T_2 - T_1) \quad \text{(watts)}$$

{Eqn. 6.21}

The basic energy exchange relation for d < 200 nm is simply $P_{glu} = P_{anomalous} + P_{ext}$, where the combustion power $P_{glu} = n_{glu}\, E_{glu} / t_{glu}$, n_{glu} = number of glucose molecules oxidized per cycle (e.g., 3 x 10^5), t_{glu} = combustion cycle time (e.g., 100 millisec), and P_{ext} is the working power extracted by the Stirling engine. Assuming d = 100 nm, a highly conductive silver or aluminum surface with σ_{cond} ~4-7 x 10^{18} sec^{-1} results in a negligible temperature differential ($T_2 - T_1$) ~ 0.0001 K. However, a germanium surface (melting point 1211 K) with σ_{cond} ~10^{11} sec^{-1} could allow a useful operating temperature T_2 > 600 K, giving a maximum Carnot efficiency ($T_2 - T_1$) / T_2 = 0.48(48%) (vs. ~25% for gasoline internal combustion engines). With device volume ~0.02 $micron^3$, power density would be ~10^9 $watts/m^3$. A boron surface (m.p. 2573 K) with σ_{cond} ~ 10^7 sec^{-1} might provide even better vacuum insulation properties. More research is required on the mechanisms of anomalous radiative heat transfer in order to fully assess the feasibility of this approach.

6.3.4.5 Chemoelectric Cells

The human body provides a renewable source of chemoelectric energy that may be tapped by various means. As long ago as 1959, Pinneo and Kesselman[595] reported powering an FM transmitter by simply inserting two steel electrodes into the brain of a cat, generating 0.5 microamperes at 40 millivolts. In another experiment by Reynolds[596] in 1963, electrodes inserted subcutaneously and abdominally into an anesthetized rat produced 400 millivolts and ~10 microwatts, powering an oscillator circuit for 8 hours with no sign of decline.* Since then, three classes of bioelectric energy have been distinguished: ionic concentration, biogalvanic, and biofuel cells.

The ionic concentration cell may exploit differences in chemical concentration by placing two similar electrodes in different compartments of the body having different chemical composition, generating a voltage proportional to the logarithm of the concentration ratio. By this means, it has been proposed that power could be drawn from the differences in oxygen and hydrogen ion concentration between arterial and venous blood,[590] or the acid-alkali differences between the stomach fluids and surrounding tissue. Similarly, trans-cytomembrane electrodes could develop potentials of 1-100 mV between cytosol and intercellular fluid. This would allow a 10 pW nanorobot to be powered by a current flow of 10 nanoamperes at 1 mV through a 10^5 ohm load resistance, although power draws exceeding ~100 pW might prove electrokinetically disruptive to the cell. Also, this source may be less reliable for dying or challenged human tissue.

Biogalvanic energy sources[590,3527-3530] exploit the electrochemical potential between metallic electrodes (the fuel) in an electrolyte solution. Two broad classes of galvanic pairs which generate electrical energy have been investigated for medical use: those in which both anode and cathode are consumed and go into solution, and those in which the cathode is inert. In the first group, zinc (anode) and silver chloride (cathode) electrodes have been implanted in human test subjects for up to two years. The Zn goes into solution as Zn^{++}; the AgCl cathode is converted into Ag and the Cl^- ion goes into solution. This chemoelectric source generates steady currents of ~0.2 picoamperes/$micron^2$ at ~1 volt or ~10 pW/50 $microns^2$ of electrode surface at 70%-90% efficiency, an energy density of 10^7 $watts/m^3$ assuming 20-nm thick electrodes. Similar output is obtained from galvanic pairs in the second group, of which the best studied is a zinc anode coupled with a palladium or platinum-black cathode; molecular oxygen combines with water at the cathode producing OH^- and H^+ ions. Unfortunately, galvanic sources provoke a significant host reaction, including formation of layers of necrotic debris, free neutrophils, granulation tissue and complete fibrous connective tissue encapsulation of long-term implants.[590,3512]

The biofuel cell[590,3526,3527] relies upon redox reactions in which neither anode nor cathode is consumed but merely act as catalysts, potentially a great advantage in nanomedical applications. The biofuel cell that has received the most attention for nanomedicine is the oxyglucose cell, which could rely upon an electrochemical process in which glucose is oxidized at the anode and molecular oxygen is reduced at the cathode according to the following equations:

$$C_6H_{12}O_6 + 6H_2O \rightarrow 6CO_2 + 24H^+ + 24e^- \quad \text{(anode)}$$

{Eqn. 6.22}

$$6O_2 + 12H_2O + 24e^- \rightarrow 24OH^- \quad \text{(cathode)} \qquad \text{\{Eqn. 6.23\}}$$

Decades-old experiments using platinum black electrodes[594] produced ~0.6 picoamps per $micron^2$ of electrode surface at ~0.3 volts, with power levels of 0.2 pW/$micron^2$ in vitro (declining over time due to the formation and absorption of gluconic acid at the anode), but only 0.004 pW/$micron^2$ in vivo (when implanted in rat or rabbit test animals) in part due to poisoning of the catalytic anode action by proteins. Complete electrochemical oxidation of glucose has not yet been demonstrated experimentally.[1015] Controlled-permeability membranes may eliminate these problems in nanomedical applications, but even using the aforementioned electrodes might allow a continuous power density of 10^7 $watts/m^3$ for a 10 pW oxyglucose biofuel cell using 50 $micron^2$ of electrodes 20-nm thick. Since gluconic acid can also be oxidized at potentials

Interestingly, when the rat was finally administered an instantly lethal intracardial injection of Nembutal the voltage required 75 minutes, after death, to fall to zero.

which oxidize glucose, gluconate may not be the only byproduct, thus appropriate means of disposing of any potentially undesirable byproducts must be included in a practical design. The addition of specific catalysts (e.g., ruthenium) to the electrodes could be helpful.

Ethanol fuel cells, though inefficient, are already in wide commercial use. For example, the Lion alcolmeter fuel cell alcohol sensor[2428] employs catalytic platinum electrodes (supported on a ~1 cm^3 PVC matrix disk assembly impregnated with acidic electrolyte) to produce electron flow by oxidizing ethanol to acetic acid (producing two free electrons per alcohol molecule) at the anode and reducing atmospheric oxygen at the cathode. Normal alcohol working concentrations are 5-900 parts per million typically producing up to ~10 microamps at ~5 millivolts across a 390 ohm load, or ~50 nanowatts (power density at most ~0.1 watt/m^3). The Lion fuel cell can also produce energy from all primary and secondary aliphatic alcohols but not from aldehydes, ketones, ether, esters, hydrocarbons or carboxylic acids. Other manufacturers of electrochemical fuel cells for alcohol sensing include PAS Systems, Guth Laboratories, and Intoximeter.[2429] Direct methanol fuel cells also were under development in 1998.

The following analysis was prompted by R. Merkle's suggestion that an oxyglucose biofuel cell using nanoscale membranes might achieve significantly higher power densities than indicated by past experiments (Fig. 6.5). Consider a proton (H^+) exchange nanomembrane consisting of a 1 nm thick diamondoid sheet containing a number of very narrow pores each lined with atoms of oxygen, fluorine or nitrogen, creating negatively charged channels with high proton affinity. A channel narrow enough to admit only protons but nothing else (~0.1 nm, excluding even helium atoms) and surrounded by a ~3 atom thick support wall makes a ~1 nm^3 pore structure ~1 nm wide.

The power generated by each pore due to proton flow is $P_{pore} = q \dot{N} V_p$, taking $q = 1.6 \times 10^{-19}$ joule/proton-volt, $\dot{N}$ is the proton flow rate in protons/sec, and V_p is the electrical potential through which the charges fall. Experimental observations suggest V_p may reach 0.75 volt at zero load, but averages 0.3-0.6 volts at moderate loads;[594] for this analysis, V_p will be taken as ~0.5 volt.[1017] As for $\dot{N}$, the nicotinic acetylcholine receptor channel (Section 3.3.3) has a 0.65-2.2 nm inside diameter and allows 2.5×10^7 Na^+ ions/sec to pass while the channel is open, comparable to the transport rate of artificial transmembrane peptide nanotube ion channels.[1177] Taking this flow rate as representative for $\dot{N}$, then $P_{pore} \sim 2$ pW/pore.

Redox fuel cells using transition metal catalysts typically achieve $n_{cat} \sim 10$ catalytic events/sec/catalytic atom.[1017] Oxidation of each glucose molecule produces 24 protons, so the required catalytic rate is $\dot{N}/24 \sim 10^6$ glucose molecules/sec per pore which in turn requires $\dot{N} / (24\, n_{cat}) \sim 10^5$ metal catalyst atoms per pore. Taking Pt atoms as representative, 10^5 Pt catalyst atoms have a volume of ~1500 nm^3. Including the 1 nm^3 pore structure and doubling the volume to allow for catalyst dispersal, fluid access and structural overhead gives a 3000 nm^3 single-pore catalytic unit generating 2 pW, or a power density of ~7×10^{11} watts/m^3. (Assumed catalyst atom usage is ~10^{17} atoms/watt; in 1999, the best Pt-catalyzed proton exchange membranes required ~10^{18} atoms/watt.[3264]) The current flow of 4 picoamps through each $(0.1\ nm)^2$ pore gives a current density of 4×10^8 amps/m^2, well below the ~10^{10} amp/m^2 maximum current density in bulk aluminum (Section 6.4.3.1). Since ~10^6 glucose molecules/sec are consumed per pore and each glucose molecule represents 4765 zJ of free energy, then total energy available is ~4.8 pW/pore. Thus it appears the device may be 2 pW / 4.8 pW ~ 40% efficient, though this figure is highly voltage-dependent.

J. Soreff notes that the oxyglucose biofuel cell can in theory operate near the thermodynamic limit but may require the design of a complex sequence of catalytic reactions, not unlike microbial metabolism.[2427] The glucose/gluconic acid source may have lower efficiency due to incomplete oxidation but could be useful in early systems because it requires optimization of catalytic sites for just one reaction. On the other hand, the production of protons and electrons from complete oxidation of glucose potentially encompasses a lengthy biochemical chain which possibly may be implemented using sets of immobilized enzymes in the manner of mitochondrial respiration. (Mitochondrial power density is 10^5-10^6 watts/m^3.)[781,786]

There are limits to efficiency set by mismatches between redox potentials at various steps in a respiratory chain. Given a single anodic chamber with a common electric potential and pH, concentrations of intermediates must be unequal to compensate for the redox potential mismatches at various steps. If these concentrations are too unequal, then the lowest concentration in the chain becomes the rate-limiting intermediate for the entire process. Throughput may be optimized by careful choice of intermediates, couplings between reactions, and catalyst design. To oxidize glucose, in biology, glycolysis requires ~18 enzymes, the TCA cycle ~9 enzymes, and the pentose phosphate pathway ~9 enzymes.[526] Soreff suggests that a slightly different strategy is to have separate oxidation/proton chambers for each stage in the catalytic pipeline, allowing intermediates to diffuse through semipermeable membranes or to be transported via molecular sorting rotors. This transfers the problem of matching redox potentials into the electrical domain where it is more easily resolved.

Oxyhydrogen fuel cells are another possibility, though probably at much lower power density because hydrogen must first be produced from the glucose fuel. This occurs naturally in the energy-generating hydrogenosomes of the trichomonads (which use the enzymes pyruvate:ferredoxin oxidoreductase and hydrogenase) and in the laboratory using related enzymes (from bacteria that live near hot underwater vents) to convert glucose into hydrogen gas and water. In a modern 350 K oxyhydrogen fuel cell, O_2 and H_2 are fed into adjacent chambers separated by a proton exchange membrane. This membrane allows only H^+ ions to flow to the O_2 side, making water as the sole waste product and establishing a net negative charge on the H_2 anode and a net positive charge on the O_2 cathode, an electrical potential of ~0.6 volts under load. This chemoelectric process is at least ~50% efficient but typically achieves only 10^4-10^6 watts/m^3 partly due to hydrogen's low volumetric energy density and partly due to the crude membranes currently in commercial use. Bacterium-based biofuel cells have also been investigated.[2427,3531]

6.3.5 Electrical Energy Conversion Processes

Microscale electrostatic motors have been fabricated since the late 1980s and are the subject of great current research interest.[556,557] Commercially available micromachined rotors ~1 micron thick and ~100 microns in radius respond to electric field intensities $>10^8$ volts/m producing motive torques of ~10 pN-m by converting electrical to mechanical energy, achieving power densities in the 10^4-10^5 watts/m^3 range with device lifetimes approaching 10^7 rotations.[556]

Drexler[10] has described a class of submicron direct-current (DC) electrostatic motors capable of converting between mechanical and electrical power in either direction at a power density of ~4×10^{14} watts/m^3 and an estimated efficiency >99%. (Typical macroscale brush DC motors can have 55%-75% efficiencies, while DC brushless motors can have efficiencies as high as 95%.)

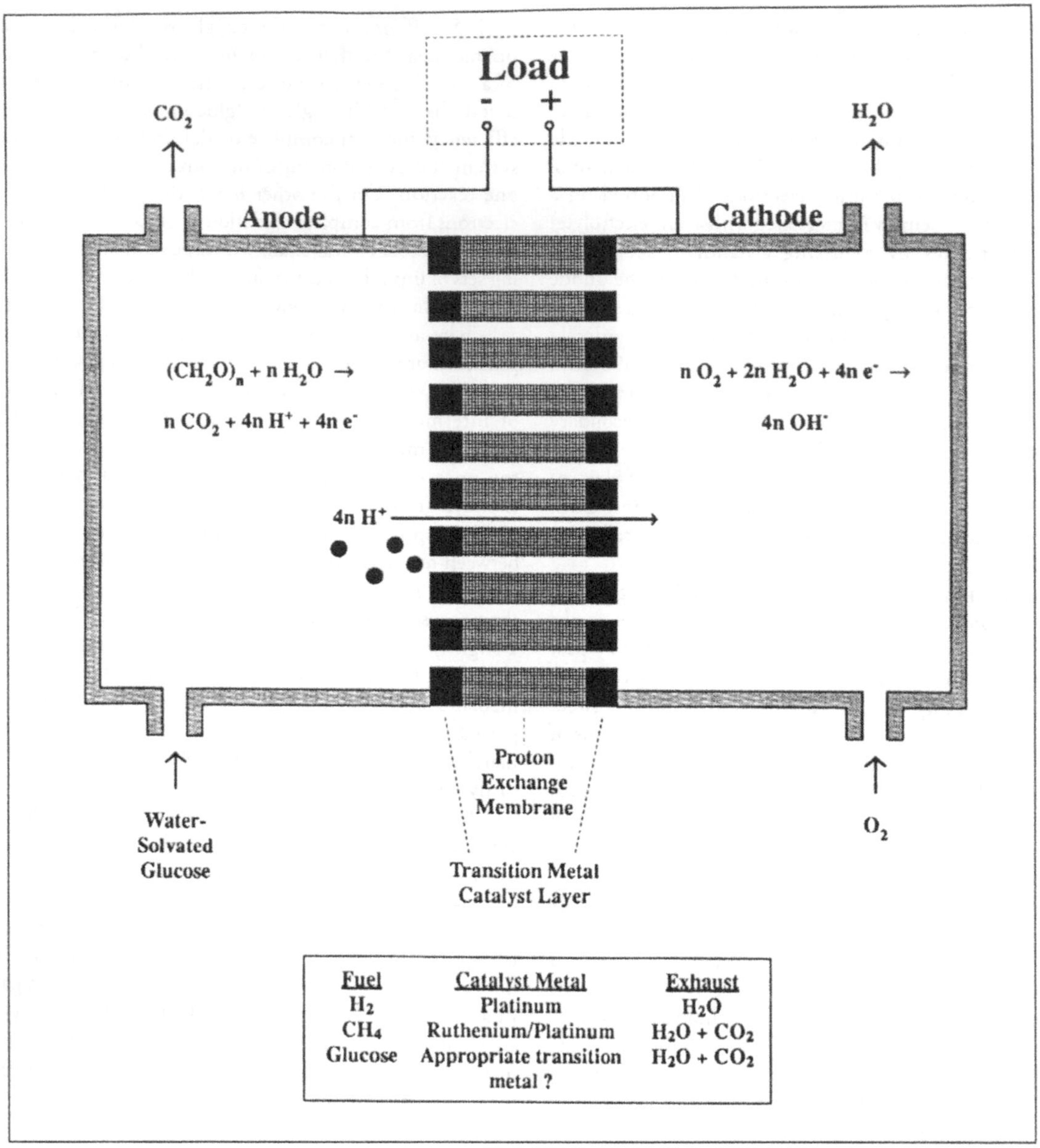

Fig. 6.5. Schematic of oxyglucose biofuel cell with proton exchange nanomembranes.

In one implementation (Fig. 6.6), electric charge is placed on the rim of a rotor as the rim passes within a dee electrode. This charge is then transported across a ~3 nm gap to the interior of the opposite dee electrode, where it is removed and replaced by a charge of opposite sign. Applying a voltage of proper sign across the dees causes the charges in transit to apply a torque to the rotor (like a Van de Graff generator operating in reverse), converting electrical into mechanical power.[10] As a specific example, a motor 390 nm in diameter and 25 nm thick driven by a electric field strength of ~0.2 x 10^9 volts/m spins with a near-maximum rim velocity of ~1000 m/sec; a current of ~110 nanoamperes and an electric potential of ~10 volts yields a power output of ~1.1 microwatts. Single electron-transfer events at nanometer electrodes have been generated and measured experimentally,[878] and macroscale "Dirod" electrostatic generators have been operated as electrostatic motors in a student laboratory.[3098]

Electrical energy is also converted into mechanical energy via the inverse piezoelectric effect.[553] Piezoelectric materials such as lead-zirconate-titanate ceramics (PZT) and natural mechanical resonators such as quartz, when subjected to an electric field, expand or contract depending on the orientation of the field to the piezoelectric polarization. For example, applying 100 volts across a 750 micron thick piezoelectric crystal causes it to deform by ~37 nm, or ~0.4 nm/volt.[628] There are also piezoelectric rotary actuators, with rotations measured in ~arcsec. The feasibility of fabricating ~1 micron thick quartz resonators by etching techniques was demonstrated decades ago.[554,555] PZT crystals are commonly used to provide movement of samples being examined in scanning probe microscopes such as STMs and AFMs.[1093] Piezoelectric drivers used in bimorph configurations as electromechanical transducers can produce large mechanical displacements but relatively small forces.[545] Dielectric induction micromotors 2 microns thick and 100 microns in diameter operating in water can be driven at 250 rev/sec at 110 volts applied potential, converting electrical to mechanical motion and producing a torque of 0.3 pN-m.[552] Electroactive polymers (EAPs)[3013,3124] and electrostrictive polymers such as i-PMMA are being investigated for use in "artificial muscles";[1301] an exceptionally high electrostrictive response (~4%) has been observed in electron-irradiated P(VDF-TrFE) copolymer.[1594] Electromechanical actuators based on sheets of single-walled carbon nanotubes have been described.[3238] Even bone can be made into an electret.[1941]

Electrostatic actuators can produce substantial mechanical forces. One electromechanical transducer described by Drexler[10] is a capacitor with one plate fixed and connected to a signal source, with the other plate grounded via a tunneling junction, leaving it free to move within a small range of displacements. One design with a 1-nm stroke length and a $(12 \text{ nm})^2$ plate area transduces an electrical voltage varying from 0-5 volts into a mechanical signal ranging from 0-1 nN.

A similar implementation for electromechanical transduction involves drawing a dielectric slab of area A_{slab} and dielectric constant κ_{slab} into a gap d_{gap} between the plates of a charged capacitor at voltage V_{cap} producing a field-dependent force, making a simple mechanical dielectric drive. Applying a time-varying input voltage of frequency ν_d (Hz) produces a mechanical output power of:

$$P_n = \left(\frac{\varepsilon_0 A_{slab}}{2\, d_{gap}}\right)\left(1 - \frac{1}{\kappa_{slab}}\right) \nu_d V_{cap}^2 \qquad \text{\{Eqn. 6.24\}}$$

For $\varepsilon_0 = 8.85 \times 10^{-12}$ coul/N-m^2 (vacuum permittivity constant), $A_{slab} = 100$ nm^2, $d_{gap} = 2$ nm, $V_{cap} = 1$ volt, $\kappa_{slab} = 5.7$ for diamond at 300 K, and $\nu_d = 5000$ Hz, $P_n = 0.001$ pW (power density 5×10^9 watts/m^3) and the force applied on the slab during $\Delta x = 1$ nm displacements is $P_n / (\Delta x\, \nu_p) \sim 1$ nN.

Electrothermal energy conversion occurs during simple joule heating, or during Seebeck effect or Peltier effect cooling, when current passes through a bimetallic junction causing one side to get hot and the other side cold.[1034,1035]

Electrochemical transduction may occur in enzymes with electric field-sensitive conformational states,[814] in voltage-gated ion channels and nanomembranes (Section 3.3.3), and in electrolytic cells which are chemoelectric cells (Section 6.3.4.5) operated in reverse.

Quantum-well nanostructures can be useful in fabricating electrooptical transducers such as light-emitting diodes, electroluminescent displays and submicron-scale solid-state lasers (Section 5.3.7), and electrochromic glass with voltage-dependent transmittance permits optical gating. Electric current sent through carbon nanotubes causes both field emission and luminescence, about one photon per 10^6 electrons—even a single nanotube makes a faint but visible glow,[1995] another case of electrooptical energy transduction.

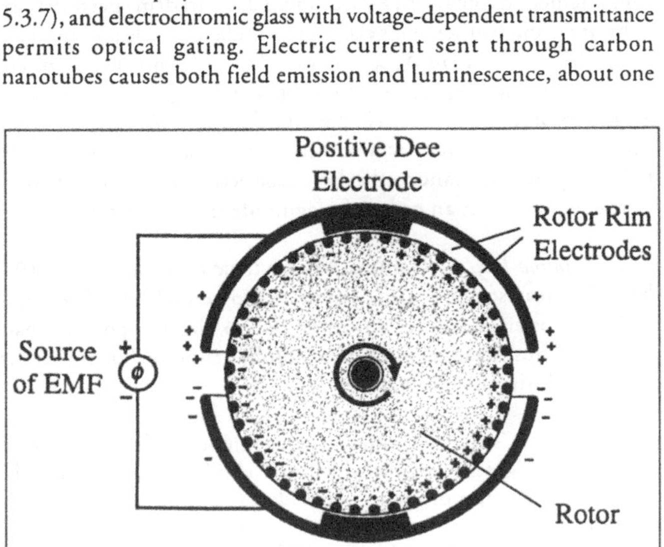

Fig. 6.6. Submicron direct-current electrostatic motor (schematic only, not to scale; redrawn from Drexler[10]).

Magnetomechanical transduction has also been employed to remotely power centimeter-size simple legged robots using magnetostrictive alloys as magnetic field-driven actuators in an 80 Hz 1-tesla field,[564] but this approach may find only limited utility in nanomedical systems because molecular-scale drives suffer from the adverse scaling properties of electromagnet fields.[10] Magnetic sensors (Section 4.7.2), perhaps using molecular magnets,[2598-2600] possibly could be employed as power transducers.

6.3.6 Photonic Energy Conversion Processes

Visible light falling on a blackened surface is quickly absorbed and thermalized, the simplest example of photothermal transduction. Such transduction is reversed in solid-state optical refrigerators, which achieve cooling with 2% energy efficiency by flooding a sample with infrared photons of a particular frequency that will dampen molecular vibrations, then allowing the object to shed energy as higher-energy fluorescent light.[549]

Optomechanical transduction has been demonstrated by using low-power laser light impinging upon an optofluidic convertor to create a pressure pulse of sufficient magnitude to operate a pneumatic actuator in a push-pull mode,[544] and an optical thermal "Brownian ratchet" uses rotating laser light to rectify the Brownian motion of a micron-scale plastic bead.[1043] Laser-heated gas micro-actuators have been studied,[560,640] and scattering forces from optical tweezers have been used to rotate small particles and thus may provide a means to power nanomachines by nonmechanical means.[775] Photoacoustic transduction has been induced directly in piezoelectric indium gallium arsenide optical signal delay devices[714] and in "photostriction" materials such as PLZT,[1065] and indirectly in aqueous suspensions of 30-nm carbon particles illuminated by a pulsed laser.[1056] A 200-micron long, 600-nm thick silicon nitride beam with a 250-nm thick coating of a glassy material made of arsenic and selenium (chalcogenide) contracts ~1 nm when illuminated by photons polarized along the length of the beam, and expands ~1 nm when illuminated by photons polarized across the width of the beam.[877] A ~300-micron optomechanical motor with diffraction grating developed for the DARPA MOEMS program operates at 20 volts and spins up to ~80 Hz.[1663]

Light-driven proton pumps achieve optochemical transduction when optical photons shining on a photosensitive minicell activate a proton pump that pumps hydrogen ions across a membrane, thus building up a large ionic charge differential across the membrane and chemically storing the energy of the incident light. Experimental photoelectrolysis cells producing hydrogen and oxygen from sunlight and water with 12.5% energy efficiency have been built.[1519] Green plants are optochemical transducers, but only 1-3% of the photonic energy falling upon a green plant is converted to chemical energy because most of the incident radiation is lost by reflection, transmission, or absorption by non-chloroplast pigments. Of the photons falling directly upon active photosynthetic pigments, up to ~35% is converted to chemical energy. Certain bacteria also employ photochemical transduction. Activation of unimolecular chemical reactions by ambient blackbody radiation has been demonstrated,[1122] and 10-100 GHz rotation in nanotube gears with dipole charges using laser-generated alternating electric fields has been simulated computationally.[1235,1236]

Photoelectric cells are a well-known technology for converting optical to electrical energy. Commercial solar panel arrays[3047] currently achieve ~10^5 watts/m^3, although polymer thin-film

(100-200 nm) photovoltaic cells may reach ~10^6 watts/m^3 at only 5.5% efficiency.[1059] Multilayer multi-band-gap photovoltaic cells can convert solar energy to electrical energy with efficiencies >30%,[562] and photocells and various natural photoreceptors such as the LH2 (light harvester) molecular complex of the *Rhodopseudomonas acidophila* bacterium can achieve efficiencies of 60%-90% at selected monochromatic wavelengths.[3532,3533] Photoelectric dendrimeric light-harvesting molecular antennas have been designed and synthesized.[2586-2591]

In the 400-700 nm optical band only, direct (cloudless noontime) sunlight energy flux is 100-400 watts/m^2. Taking the 100 watts/m^2 figure and applying a 30% conversion efficiency, power supply P_n to a nanodevice of circular cross-section of radius R is P_n ~ 100 (30%) πR^2 watts in direct sunlight requiring a circular collector spot ~0.7 microns in diameter to power a 10-pW nanorobot. Fullerene sheets exhibit interesting opto-electronic effects: high-intensity light shined on one side of a sheet induces an electrical voltage potential on the other face. Progress is also being made in developing optically pumped (optophotonic) molecular lasers.[990]

Low-frequency photons such as radiofrequency signals are readily converted into electrical current using millimeter-scale loop antennas (Section 6.4.2). For example, a 2-mm x 10-mm device implanted subdermally with a hypodermic needle electrically stimulates muscle using rf telemetry for control and power, in order to restore human motor functions.[563]

6.3.7 Nuclear Energy Conversion Processes

The concept of using nuclear energy as a power source for nanorobots has not been widely discussed or explored[3294], in part for sociocultural reasons. This Section describes a feasible radionuclide power system which emits essentially no radiation into the surrounding tissue. This is followed by a brief examination of the challenges in harnessing fission and fusion in medical nanodevices, and a few other somewhat speculative possibilities.

6.3.7.1 Radionuclides

The most common mode of fissile energy release occurs when an unstable radioactive atomic nucleus emits a small particle such as an electron (β^- decay), a positron (β^+ decay), a helium nucleus (alpha decay), or a high-energy photon (gamma decay), often transforming the nucleus into another element. Selection of an optimum radioactive fuel is guided primarily by safety criteria:

A. *Penetration Range* — The mass of the α-particle is ~7000 times greater than that of an electron, so the velocity and hence the range of α-particles in matter is considerably less than for β-particles of equal energy. Consequently the optimum radionuclide for medical nanorobots is predominantly an α emitter. A simple "stopping power" approximation[567] for the range of 1-10 MeV α-particles is:

$$R_\alpha \text{ (microns)} \sim 430\ E_{MeV}^{1.3}\ \rho_{absorb}^{-0.6} \qquad \text{\{Eqn. 6.25\}}$$

where E_{MeV} = energy per α decay (MeV) and ρ_{absorb} = absorber density (21,450 kg/m^3 for Pt). Thus a 3 MeV α-particle (initially traveling at ~0.04c) has a range of ~2 cm in air, ~30 microns in water, ~10 microns in germanium, and ~5 microns in platinum, with a fairly sharp cutoff and only ~1% straggling (fluctuation of particle range around mean range). By contrast, as a crude approximation the range of β-particles of equal energy (initially traveling at ~0.99c) is ~10^2 R_α and the range of γ photons and fast neutrons of equal energy is ~10^4 R_α, although "range" for these particles is imprecisely defined because beam intensity is never truly reduced to zero but rather decays exponentially with increased shielding. Partly because of the heavy shielding required, $_{61}Pm^{147}$-powered betavoltaic batteries developed in the 1970s achieved only ~30 watts/m^3,[603] while $_{94}Pu^{238}$-powered thermoelectric batteries produced up to ~58 watts/m^3;[631] over 2300 nuclear-powered cardiac pacemakers were implanted without mishap during 1970-76,[633] but new implantations apparently ceased in 1983.[3492]

The absorption of α-particles in matter results almost entirely from collisions with electrons, or ionization reactions, which create 10^5-10^6 ion pairs per ~MeV α-particle (depending upon absorber material), slowing the particle almost to a halt. For some light-nucleus absorbers, there may also be an extremely small contribution from direct interactions with the nucleus. Alpha-particles with energies as low as 4.8 MeV (e.g., from $_{88}Ra^{226}$) were observed to transmute atoms of all elements from $_5B$ up to $_{19}K$ (except for $_6C$ and $_8O$) with the emission of protons.[1007] Low-energy α-particles can also occasionally transmute light-atom nuclei to produce neutrons—one of the strongest such reactions involves 4.6 MeV α-particles emanating from $_{86}Rn^{222}$ striking a $_4Be^9$ absorber, wherein one α-particle out of every 5000 enters the beryllium nucleus and sends out a neutron (with a much longer range than an α-particle of equal energy), a 0.02% reaction probability.[1008] Thus the worst case (e.g., shield materials are poorly chosen) is one low-energy proton or neutron emitted per 10^9 - 10^{10} ion pairs generated (e.g., ~1 every 2000 sec at an α-particle current of 1 picoamp), though most such secondary reactions have far lower probabilities.

However, naturally emitted α-particles generally cannot penetrate the nuclei of heavier elements and therefore generally cannot create significant secondary radiation in heavy-nucleus absorbers, hence shielding should be made from heavier elements. To first order, overcoming Coulomb repulsion and entering the nucleus requires an α-particle energy $E_{repulse} > 2 Z e^2 / 4 \pi \varepsilon_0 r_{nucl}$ (joules),[1005] where Z is atomic number (nuclear charge number), e = 1.60 x 10^{-19} coul (elementary charge), ε_0 = 8.85 x 10^{-12} farad/m (permittivity constant), and Rutherford's classical formula for nuclear radius r_{nucl} ~ $\rho_{nucl} Z^{1/3}$,[1006] where ρ_{nucl} ~ 1.6 x 10^{-15} m.* Thus for example, using a $_{78}Pt$ absorber, r_{nucl} ~ 7 x 10^{-15} m and $E_{repulse}$ > 33 MeV; with a $_{32}Ge$ absorber, r_{nucl} ~ 5 x 10^{-15} m and $E_{repulse}$ > 18 MeV. In either case, the 2-4 MeV low-energy natural-emission alpha particles likely to be employed in nanomedical nucleoelectric systems (Table 6.5) have energies about an order of magnitude smaller than $E_{repulse}$.

B. *Gamma Rays* — Gamma rays are toxic to most biomaterials, have the greatest penetrating power, dissipate useful fissile energy, and may foster erosion of shielding due to electron-positron pair creation. Thus the ideal medical nanorobot radionuclide fuel emits no γ-rays during disintegration.

C. *Decay Chain* — Radioactive elements typically decay to progressively lighter elements which may also be radioactive. Ideally, each of the daughter products of the ideal radionuclide should meet the above criteria for the entire decay chain down to stable nuclei.

Since each decay event produces a fixed amount of energy, power density P_{rad} of a radionuclide of density ρ is proportional to the number of disintegrations per second, or inversely proportional to half-life, as:

*Some exotic artificial nuclei such as Li^{11} do not obey the classical $Z^{1/3}$ rule.[1128]

$$P_{rad} = \frac{k_{rad}\,\rho\,E_{MeV}}{AW\,t_{1/2}} \quad (\text{watts/m}^3) \qquad \{\text{Eqn. 6.26}\}$$

where AW = atomic weight (gm/mole), $t_{1/2}$ = half-life (sec), and $k_{rad} = 10^9 \ln(2)\, N_A\, E_{eV}$ where $N_A = 6.023 \times 10^{23}$ atoms/mole (Avogadro's number) and E_{eV} = 160 zJ/eV. To be useful in medical nanorobots, $t_{1/2}$ should be at least 10 days (~10^6 sec) or longer for convenience of storage and use—ideally, commensurate with the anticipated mission duration to preclude the need for potentially hazardous refueling operations in vivo. Table 6.5 gives power densities P_{rad} for several candidates and data for a few other benchmark radionuclides.[763,764]

Among all gamma-free alpha-only emitters with $t_{1/2} > 10^6$ sec, the highest volumetric power density is available using Gd^{148} (gadolinium) which α-decays directly to Sm^{144} (samarium), a stable rare-earth isotope. A solid sphere of pure Gd^{148} (~7900 kg/m³) of radius r = 95 microns surrounded by a 5-micron thick platinum shield (total device radius R = 100 microns) and a thin polished silver coating of emissivity e_r = 0.02 suspended in vacuo would initially maintain a constant temperature T_2 (far from a surface held at T_1 = 310 K) of:

$$T_2 = \left(T_1^4 + \frac{P_{rad}\, r^3}{3\, e_r\, \sigma\, R^2} \right)^{1/4} \sim 600\text{K} \qquad \{\text{Eqn. 6.27}\}$$

with a 75-year half-life, initially generating 17 microwatts of thermal power which can be converted to 8 microwatts of mechanical power by a Stirling engine operating at ~50% efficiency. (Smaller spheres of Gd^{148} run cooler.) While probably too large for most individual nanorobot designs, such spheres could be an ideal long-term energy source for a swallowable or implantable "power pill" (Chapter 26) or dedicated energy organ (Section 6.4.4). A ~0.2 kg block of pure Gd^{148} (~1 inch³) initially yields ~120 watts, sufficient in theory to meet the complete basal power needs of an entire human body for ~1 century (given suitable nucleochemical energy conversion and load buffering mechanisms, and a sufficiently well-divided structure). Nuclear powered energy organs are discussed further in Section 6.4.4.

A 1 micron³ block of radioactive gadolinium yields a useful ~3 pW of thermal power. However, a minimum of 5 microns of Pt shielding is still required, so the minimum possible diameter of a zero-emissions Gd^{148}-powered nanorobot is ~11 microns,* reducing power density to ~10^4 watts/m³.** The low energy density would produce a surface temperature of 320 K, allowing only ~3% thermal conversion efficiency.** Higher efficiencies may be achieved using semiconductor junction α-particle nucleoelectric transducers that convert the linear ionization trail of electron-hole pairs directly into electrical current in ~10^{-9} sec (Fig. 6.7). Such ionization in silicon and germanium is well-studied: the average energy loss per ion pair produced by a passing α-particle is 3.6 eV (580 zJ) for Si, 3.0 eV (480 zJ) for Ge;[567] an 11-micron thick Ge wall is required to stop the 3.18 MeV α-particles. A (1 micron)³ cube of Gd^{148} produces ~5 α-particles/sec, yielding an output current of ~1 picoampere at ~3 volts (e.g., ~3 pW). Unlike most nanomachinery for which a

Table 6.5 Volumetric Radioactive Power Density of Various Radionuclides[763]

Radionuclide	Half-Life (sec)	Alpha Emissions (MeV)	Beta Emissions (MeV)	Gamma Emissions (MeV)	Other Emissions	Volumetric Power Density (watts/m³)
$_{58}Ce^{142}$	1.6×10^{23}	1.50	---	---	---	3.0×10^{-8}
$_{92}U^{235}$	2.2×10^{16}	4.35	---	0.074-0.385	SF	1.1
$_{83}Bi^{210m}$	8.2×10^{13}	4.90	---	---	---	1.9×10^{2}
$_{64}Gd^{150}$	9.4×10^{12}	2.70	---	---	---	1.0×10^{3}
$_{6}C^{14}$	1.8×10^{11}	---	0.156	---	---	1.5×10^{4}
$_{88}Ra^{226}$	5.1×10^{10}	4.77	---	0.187-0.64	---	1.4×10^{5}
$_{64}Gd^{148}$	2.4×10^{9}	3.18	---	---	---	4.8×10^{6}
$_{61}Pm^{147}$	8.3×10^{7}	---	0.225	---	---	8.7×10^{6}
$_{94}Pu^{238}$	2.8×10^{9}	5.48	---	0.0436-0.875	SF	1.1×10^{7}
$_{96}Cm^{244}$	5.5×10^{8}	5.79	---	0.043-0.15	SF	2.0×10^{7}
$_{98}Cf^{250}$	3.1×10^{8}	6.02	---	0.043	SF	3.6×10^{7}
$_{16}S^{35}$	7.5×10^{6}	---	0.167	---	---	8.8×10^{7}
$_{98}Cf^{252}$	8.0×10^{7}	6.11	---	0.043-0.10	SF	1.4×10^{8}
$_{98}Cf^{248}$	3.0×10^{7}	6.23	---	0.045	SF	3.9×10^{8}
$_{96}Cm^{242}$	1.4×10^{7}	6.10	---	0.04409	SF	8.4×10^{8}
$_{84}Po^{210}$	1.2×10^{7}	5.30	---	0.79	---	1.3×10^{9}
$_{96}Cm^{240}$	2.3×10^{6}	6.26	---	---	SF	5.3×10^{9}
$_{15}P^{32}$	1.2×10^{6}	---	1.71	---	---	6.5×10^{9}
$_{98}Cf^{244}$	1.5×10^{3}	7.17	---	---	SF	9.2×10^{12}
$_{84}Po^{212}$	3.0×10^{-7}	8.78	---	---	---	8.6×10^{22}

SF = Spontaneous Fission

**The orbit radius r_{orbit} of an α-particle of mass $m = 6.68 \times 10^{-27}$ kg, charge $q = 2 \times (1.6 \times 10^{-19})$ coul and energy E_{MeV} = 3.18 MeV circling in a uniform magnetic field B = 1 tesla in vacuo is $r_{orbit} = (k_a E_{MeV}\, m / q^2 B^2)^{1/2}$ = 0.3 meter ($k_a = 3.2 \times 10^{-13}$), about as wide as a human body, so more compact in vivo nanocyclotronic storage of α-particle emissions to allow a controlled energy release is not feasible.*

***Plutonium dioxide radioactive thermal generator (RTG) systems developed by NASA and DOE in the 1980s produced thermal power of ~10^5 watts/m³ and electrical power of ~10^4 watts/m³, a ~10% conversion efficiency. Conventional large nuclear power plants average ~32% conversion efficiency, according to U.S. Federal Energy Information Agency statistics.*

single-point failure would ordinarily be fatal to machine function[10] (Chapter 13), the design presented here should be extremely resistant to such failures. The C-C bond energy is also ~3.4 eV, so direct nucleochemical transduction of α-particle energy into chemical form is theoretically possible — conversion of carbonaceous material to diamond crystal by fission fragment irradiation has been reported.[1029]

Are Gd^{148}-powered nanorobots safe? Yes, if their shielding remains intact. There are no β or γ emissions, and given adequate shielding, no α-particles can escape. Significant shield erosion is unlikely because:

1. almost all α-particle interactions are with orbital electrons, not nuclei, of shield atoms;
2. α-particle emission rates are low (e.g., ~5/sec);
3. radioactive impurities need not be present in nanomanufactured structures; and
4. background radiation is not a major reliability issue for homogeneous components larger than ~10 nm (Chapter 13).[10]

In the extremely unlikely event of complete shield removal, maximum range of α-particles in water or soft tissues is ~30 microns or ~one cell width. The radiation from the radioactive cores of ~1 billion Gd^{148}-powered nanorobots, if all their shielding was destroyed, would deliver a ~500 rad lifetime lethal radiation dose in ~1 day; an unshielded ~0.2 kg block of Gd^{148} (~100 watt output) delivers an LD50 (see below) dose in ~10 seconds. Gd^{148} is a non-fissionable material, hence fissile chain reactions or explosions are not possible. Indeed, gadolinium has the highest neutron absorption cross-section of any known element and is more useful in control rods or as a nuclear shield. As for chemical toxicity in the event of a breach, ionic Gd is rapidly converted to colloidal hydroxide and phosphates in the blood, which is then rapidly taken up by the reticuloendothelial system mostly in the liver and spleen;[598] half-time in the lung is ~2 hours.[600] In macrophages, the rare earths localize in lysosomes as insoluble phosphates.[599] Rare earths such as Gd or Sm are not particularly toxic—LD50 is typically 0.5-5 grams/kg body weight,[601] or 35-350 gm for a 70 kg human adult. No chemical carcinogenicity or mutagenicity has been found.[601] In 1998, Gd^{148} could be purchased from Los Alamos National Laboratory for $0.50/micron^3.[2315] This cost must be significantly reduced for Gd^{148}-powered nanorobots to become economically feasible.

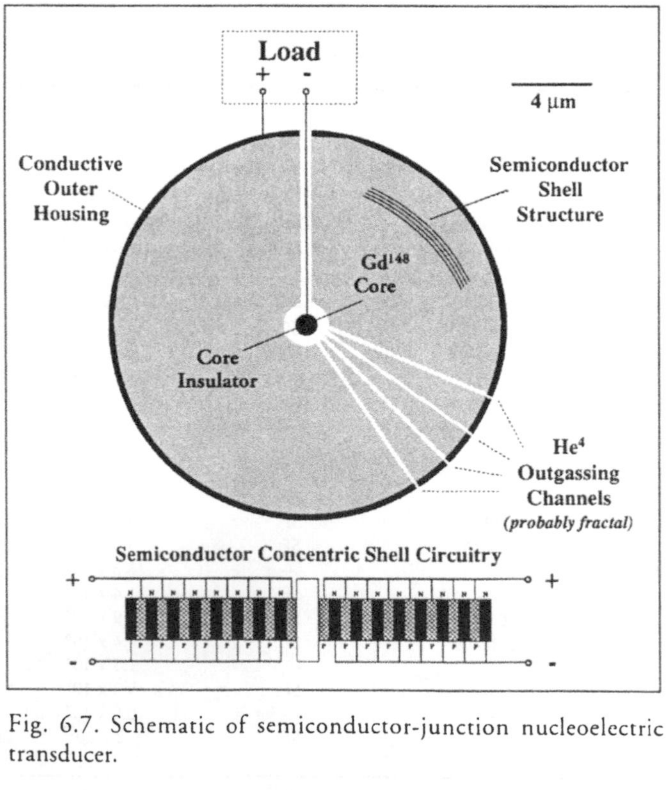

Fig. 6.7. Schematic of semiconductor-junction nucleoelectric transducer.

If greater operating power densities are required, radionuclide-powered nanorobots with power cores that are hotter or are smaller than ~1 micron^3 (but with shielded diameters still >11 microns) will require switching to a less-safe material of higher energy density, such as Po^{210}, which decays to stable Pb^{206} with a 5-month half life. For example, a Po^{210} spherical power core of radius 100 nm has a surface temperature of ~600 K and produces ~6 pW which may be tapped via heat engine as described earlier. However, such a heat source also produces one 0.79 MeV gamma photon every ~10^4 sec; unshielded, ~300 such photons represent a lethal dose (~500 rad or ~5 joules/kg soft tissue) to a single mammalian cell, giving a dose rate of ~10 millirad/hour vs. ~5 millirad/hour for the early implantable Pu^{238} nuclear thermoelectric batteries.[724] Thus the lifetime exposure* of any cell visited by Po^{210}-powered nanorobots is restricted for safety to at most ~1 nanorobot-month, which may be acceptable in many short-duration applications. No such restriction would apply to the Gd^{148} device, discussed earlier.

Larger amounts of energy (up to ~0.1% of rest mass) may be released by the fission of a heavy atomic nucleus into nuclei of two lighter elements of roughly equal mass, followed by any of ~50 distinct decay chains down to stable nuclei for the unstable fission fragments, as for example:

$$U^{235} \rightarrow \text{mixed fission products} + 200 \text{ MeV } (3.2 \times 10^{10} \text{ zJ}) \qquad \{\text{Eqn. } 6.28\}$$

which achieves ~0.091% mass conversion to energy. During fission, typically one neutron is absorbed by a nucleus but 1-3 neutrons are emitted, making possible a chain reaction. In effect, neutrons act as fission catalysts. Nuclear species which may support a net-energy-producing fissile chain reaction include U^{232}, U^{233}, U^{235} (critical mass ~ 3.6 kg), Pu^{239}, Am^{241} and Am^{242} (thermal or fast neutrons) and Th^{232}, Pa^{231} and U^{238} (fast neutrons only). From a

*The rad is the standard unit of absorbed dose, defined as 1 rad = 0.01 joule/kg. LD50 is the absorbed dose that produces lethality in 50% of all exposures, typically 400-500 rads for human tissue. The traditional LD50 for a 70-kg human body (~500 rads) thus requires the absorption of ~350 joules. For a single ~10 nanogram human liver cell, assuming the traditional LD50 (~500 rads) would require the absorption of ~50 pJ of ionizing radiation energy. To rigorously assess the safety of radiation emitted from nanorobots, the effects of the particular radiation on specific cells or organs must be evaluated.[3075-3078] There are large differences in organ sensitivity, ion-mass sensitivity, and environmental sensitivities such as variations in iron, Vitamin C, or melatonin levels. Lethality of cells is at one end of a continuum which also includes lower-dose effects (e.g., cancer transformation rates) that disturb the cell's function without killing it, thus harming the body the cell is serving. The availability of cellular repair devices vastly increases both LD50 and traditional "lifetime exposure" radiation limits that may be tolerated by humans (Chapter 24). Substantial genomic, biotechnological, and nanotechnological engineering to increase the radiation tolerance of cells (Chapter 24) also could help to minimize cancer risks and birth defects, and to allow human beings to more easily live and work in space. Nevertheless, a fundamental nanomedical design principle is to avoid using devices whose normal behavior causes additional damage to the body (Chapter 11).

nanomedical perspective, the minimum size of a neutron-mediated fission power plant is restricted primarily by the shielding requirement for γ-rays totalling ~5 MeV per reaction, which apparently precludes microscale in vivo medical fission reactors. For instance, ~8 cm of solid Pt shielding (e.g., a cantaloupe-sized ball, weighing ~46 kg) only reduces γ-ray intensity to 1% of its incident value. High γ fluxes are also very damaging to nanomachinery.

6.3.7.2 Nuclear Fusion

Still larger energies (up to ~1% of rest mass) are available from nuclear reactions in which light nuclei fuse to form heavier nuclei, although it appears that conventional nuclear fusion is unlikely to be practical for in vivo nanomedical applications. The deuterium-tritium (D-T) fusion reaction requires the lowest temperature to ignite—141 million K, which is 12.1 KeV or 1.94×10^{-15} joules per nuclei—and achieves 0.38% mass conversion to energy:

$$D^2 + T^3 \xrightarrow[12.1\ \text{KeV}]{} He^4 (3.5\ \text{MeV}) + n\ (14.1\ \text{MeV}) \qquad \text{\{Eqn. 6.29\}}$$

A D-T atom pair has volume ~10^{-3} nm^3; maximum diamondoid piston (controlled) compression at 10^5 atm puts 10^{-20} joules into this volume, too low by a factor of ~10^6. However, target bombardment may allow micron-scale fusion ignition. Although magnetic cyclotronic confinement of 12.1 KeV particles at B = 1 tesla requires a storage ring of radius r_{orbit} ~ 3 cm (Section 6.3.7.1), the length of a linear particle accelerator scales as ~K.E./qE (Section 4.7.4) so a 10^9 volt/m electric field requires only ~12 microns to accelerate an ionized triton or deuteron to the ignition temperature.

The first major problem with the D-T reaction from a nanomedical standpoint is the dangerously high flux of 14.1 MeV fast neutrons, which in human tissue interact with hydrogen to produce deuterium plus a 2.2 MeV γ-ray, and with nitrogen to produce radioactive C^{14} plus a 0.6 MeV proton. Neutrons, like γ-rays, are highly penetrating radiation, so using the D-T reaction will require much thicker shielding (see below). One alternative is to switch to a cleaner-burning (aneutronic fusion) but slightly hotter process such as the classical Cockcroft-Walton reaction involving proton bombardment of lithium which achieves 0.23% mass conversion to energy:

$$Li^7 + p \xrightarrow[125-1600\ \text{KeV}]{} 2He^4 + 16.73\ \text{MeV} \qquad \text{\{Eqn. 6.30\}}$$

(A competing neutron-emitting reaction ($Li^7 + p \rightarrow Be^7 + n$) occurs only at incident proton energies >1.6 MeV, and radiative absorption of the proton, producing a radiated γ-ray, occurs as a sharp resonance absorption at a proton bombardment energy of 440 KeV.[2463]) A ~10^9 volt/m linear accelerator ~125 microns in length can produce 125 KeV protons, and from Eqn. 6.25 a platinum shield ~18 microns thick absorbs ~100% of the 8.36 MeV α-particles produced, thermalizing the energy.

The second major problem with micron-scale fusion is its low reaction cross-section. Cross-section is a measure of the probability that a given nuclear reaction will take place. If I_0 incident protons/sec provoke I_r reactions/sec in a sample of thickness x with nuclear cross-section σ_n barns (1 barn = 10^{-24} cm^2) and target density N_{target} (atoms/cm^3) = $\rho\ N_A$ / AW, then

$$\frac{I_r}{I_0} = 1 - e^{-N_{target}\,\sigma_n\,x} \qquad \text{\{Eqn. 6.31\}}$$

To get more energy out of the fusion reaction than is put into the protons (e.g., energy breakeven), the reaction probability (I_r/I_0) > (125 KeV / 16.73 MeV) ~ 0.7%. For Li^7, AW = 7 and ρ = 0.534 gm/cm^3 so N_{target} = 4.6×10^{22} atoms/cm^3; with σ_n ~ 0.01-0.001 barns for the reaction over this energy range,[662] then to achieve energy breakeven the lithium target must be at least x > 16-160 cm thick. However, the range of 125 KeV protons in lithium is only ~0.0003 cm,[567] so energy breakeven cannot be achieved. As for the D-T reaction, one calculation for laser compression of D-T fuel pellets indicated that the minimum pellet diameter to achieve (explosive) ignition is ~4.2 mm and requires a total incident energy of 11.2 megajoules[602] in a ~nanosecond pulse. Smaller pellets could not achieve energy breakeven.* It is estimated that the minimum dimension of a high-temperature fusion reactor may be on the order of centimeters.[1023] But even if a ~10^{11} joule/m^3 energy density can be obtained with diamondoid materials allowing the reactor core to be as small as (5 cm)^3, a 2.3-cm thick Pt shield for the 14.1 MeV neutrons only reduces the incident intensity by half. Thus the smallest medically safe D-T fusion reactor is probably at least ~1 meter in diameter (e.g., to reduce incident fast neutron intensity by ~10^{-6} upon exit).

D-D fusion produces either neutrons or radioactive tritium effluent, only 3-4 MeV per reaction, and achieves only ~0.1% mass conversion to energy. The D-He^3 reaction produces 0.39% mass conversion with H and He^4 effluent (both particles charged, hence field-manipulable), but is harder to ignite (~60 KeV). There are always unavoidable neutron-producing reactions due to D-D reactions in the primary fuel and D-T reactions between the primary deuterium and the secondary tritium, although Petrie[2462] noted that neutron reactions can be less than ~5% of the D-He^3 reactions. He^3 is also very rare on Earth. The H-B^{11} reaction may produce C^{12} and is probably exoergic, but γ-rays are emitted.[1006,3534]

6.3.7.3 Exothermal Nuclear Catalysis

One solution to low nuclear reaction probability and a poor energy balance is to employ a nuclear catalyst. A number of possibilities have been investigated, as described below.

In principle, the two deuterons in a deuterium molecule can spontaneously fuse to form tritium + proton or He^3 + neutron, liberating 4 Mev of energy. The two electrons in the D_2 molecule act as a catalyst, holding the deuterons together so they can react. According to quantum mechanics, the deuterons can tunnel toward each other through the classically forbidden region of repulsion until they get so close (~2×10^{-15} m) that the strong force dominates and fusion occurs.[605]

In practice the rate of this reaction is very small, ~10^{-74} molecule^{-1} sec^{-1}.[609] But if an electron of mass M_e is replaced by a heavier negatively charged particle such as a muon (M_{muon} ~ 207 M_e), forming a muonic molecule, the required tunneling distance shortens by the ratio of the masses—in this case, from 5×10^{-11} m to 2×10^{-13} m, making penetration of the barrier much more likely and dramatically raising the reaction rate to ~10^6 molecule^{-1} sec^{-1}.[607]

Muon catalysis of the proton-deuteron reaction, initially proposed theoretically by Frank in 1947,[606] was first observed experimentally in 1957 by Alvarez.[604] It has since been shown to be an effective means of rapidly inducing fusion reactions in low-temperature

**More recent hydrodynamic simulations of a 10-micron D_2O-vapor-doped D_2 gas bubble compressed to 0.38 micron in 0.5 microsec using a 5-atm triangular spike superimposed on a 1-atm 27.6 KHz oscillating driving pressure produces a 2.2 KeV peak central temperature ~11 picosec before the bubble reaches minimum radius, which should be hot enough to generate at least a small number of thermonuclear D-D fusion reactions in the bubble.[933]*

(<1200 K) mixtures of hydrogen isotopes, with D-T reaction rates of ~10^9 sec^{-1}.[608,610,611] The field has had its own technical journal, *Muon Catalyzed Fusion*, since 1987, and there are excellent recent review articles.[663,664] But muon catalysis has long been considered impractical for large-scale fusion reactors because the muon is relatively short-lived (2 microsec) and is quickly captured by a helium nucleus formed in a fusion reaction.**[605] Typically the number of fusions catalyzed by a muon during its lifetime is ~150 in liquid D_2/T_2, but ~1000 are needed to achieve energy breakeven given the energy cost of artificial muon production.[664] More than 70% of the cosmic ray flux at Earth's surface consists of positive and negative muons, but the cosmic-ray induced fusion rate is still impractically low, ~10^{-26} watts/micron^3 in liquid deuterium targets.[665]

It has also been demonstrated experimentally that various changes in chemical composition, pressure, or electric fields can also act as nuclear catalysts, increasing the rates of nuclear transformations:

A. *Chemical Composition* — The rate of electron capture for Be^7 is 0.08% greater in BeF_2 than in metallic Be.[390]

B. *Mechanical Pressure* — The electron capture (EC) decay rates of Tc^{99} and Ba^{131} are measurably altered at a pressure of 100,000 atm.[612] At 230,000 atm there is a 0.35% increase in the electron density at the nucleus of the free Be atom; the observed increase in the EC decay constant of Be^7 oxide with pressure is so linear that it may be used as a method of pressure measurement in diamond anvil experiments in which optical access is impossible.[612] It has been suggested that very high pressures could induce fusion.[609,933] One experiment in which Pd and Ti immersed in D_2O were bombarded with intense ultrasound apparently produced above-background levels of He^4, an expected endproduct of D-D fusion processes.[1289]

C. *Fracture Deformations* — Fracto-fusion[621] experiments have detected neutron emission when a crystal of lithium deuteride or heavy ice is mechanically fractured, believed to be the consequence of deuteron acceleration by >10 KeV electric fields generated by a propagating crack in the crystal, consistent with D-D fusion.[614,620,1009] Heating, cooling, or fracturing metal specimens exposed to high-pressure D_2 (e.g., deuterated titanium) frequently produces statistically significant bursts of neutrons and emission of charged particles, rf signals and photons. It is proposed that crack growth results in charge separation on the newly formed crack surfaces, accelerating D^+ ions in the electric field across the crack tip to energies >10 KeV sufficient to significantly raise the D-D fusion probability.[618] Neutrons are reportedly generated when fragments of titanium are crushed with steel balls in a bath of heavy water.[619] It has also been speculated that the core of the spherical acoustic shock wave generated during sonoluminescence, if it remains stable to a 10-nm radius, might reach temperatures appropriate to fusion $\gtrsim 10^6$ K.[716,933]

D. *Electric Fields* — Claytor et al at Los Alamos National Laboratory passed a current of 2.5 amperes at 2000 volts through 200-micron diameter palladium wires in a glow discharge tube of D_2 gas at 0.3 atm for ~100 hours apparently producing ~10 nanocuries of tritium, with great care being taken to eliminate possible sources of contamination.[613] Deuterium-saturated $LiTaO_3$ crystals in a 75 KV/cm AC field exhibit elevated neutron emission attributed to D-D fusion.[2344] Wires of LiD exploded by high current pulses also emit fusion neutrons.[622]

E. *Metallic Deuterides* — Most controversial is the speculative possibility of metallic deuteride catalyzed fusion at temperatures between 300 K–1100 K,[615-617,624,740,3438] first reported (then later partially retracted!) in the years 1926-27.[666] Positive results are reported for a comprehensive series of experiments conducted at SRI International for the Electric Power Research Institute (EPRI) during 1989-94,[676,677] and for another comprehensive series of experiments conducted by the U.S. Naval Air Warfare Center at China Lake during 1989-96,[1275] and U.S. patents have been issued for such devices (e.g., Patterson and Cravens, U.S. #5,607,563 on 4 March 1997). In another class of experiments [Edmund Storms, personal communication, 1996], a hydrogenophilic metal such as palladium is loaded with deuterium at effective pressures ~10-100 atm, giving molecular loadings of D/Pd = 85%-95%. Palladium deuteride normally exists either as Pd_2D or PdD, but it is believed that the highest loadings[1610-1612] may give rise to significant concentrations of PdD_x (x=1-2), asserted to be the "nuclear active phase." Superstoichiometric palladium hydride (x = 1.33) at ~50,000 atm has been observed experimentally in x-ray diffraction studies,[667] although preliminary molecular simulation studies of deuterium-entrained metal lattices have given pessimistic results.[668]

Upon applying a current of ~1 nanoampere/micron^2 at ~1-10 volts to a superstoichiometric metallic deuteride, significant heat energy in excess of the electrical input is said to be developed as the deuterium is consumed, on the order of 10^6-10^9 watts/m^3. He^4 is claimed to be produced at the expected rate of ~10^{11} He^4 atoms/sec-watt,[1275] with neutrons, tritons (tritium nuclei), γ-rays and X-rays missing or detected in amounts far too small to account for the excess energy, which is asserted to be evidence of a catalyzed D-D aneutronic process at work. If the results of these experiments were confirmed, it might become possible to use diamondoid pistons to maintain continuously high deuterium loadings in an active catalytic crystal and thus to develop 1-1000 pW of aneutronic thermal energy in a precisely nanomanufactured porous 1 micron^3 metal-deuteride reactor with He^4 (23.85 MeV) as the principal (and benign) effluent, achieving storage densities >10^{16} joules/m^3 which would allow a completely self-contained >10 year fuel supply to be carried aboard a 10 pW nanorobot in a ~1 micron^3 fuel tank.

6.4 Power Transmission

Power may be stored in, and converted among, many different forms, but the ultimate energy resource must be received from some external source by medical nanodevices (e.g., chemical energy from ingested food). The following discussion concentrates on acoustic (Section 6.4.1), electromagnetic (Section 6.4.2), and tethered (Section 6.4.3) power transmission, and closes with a brief description of dedicated energy organs (Section 6.4.4).

6.4.1 Acoustic Power Transmission

Acoustically powered medical nanorobots may derive their energy either from sources indigenous to the human body (Section 6.3.3 and Table 6.3) or from artificial sources placed in or on the human body. Large arrays of microscale acoustic radiators could create focused coherent sonic beams. Such artificial sources are likely to involve ultrasonic frequencies designed to minimize any aural

*In 1975 an even heavier negatively-charged lepton was discovered, the tauon. The internuclear tunneling distance for a hypothetical tauonic deuterium molecule (M_{tauon} ~ 3500 M_e) is only ~10^{-14} m, which should catalyze fusion almost instantaneously. Unfortunately the tauon is shorter-lived than the muon (~10^{-11} sec), a lifetime much closer to the typical nuclear reaction time range of 10^{-13}–10^{-21} sec.

discomfort to the user. According to the official statement issued by the American Institute of Ultrasound in Medicine (AIUM) in 1978,[626] no significant biological effects have been reliably observed in mammalian tissues exposed in vivo to unfocused ~MHz ultrasound with intensities of 1000 watts/m^2 or less, although the onset of continuous-wave ultrasound-induced lysis of human erythrocytes has occasionally been detected experimentally at intensities as low as 60 watts/m^2 at 1.6 MHz when micron-size gas bubbles are also present.[3043] There are also no significant biological effects observed after continuous exposures exceeding 1 second in duration for total energy transfers of 500 kilojoule/m^2 or less. (The comparable hazard threshold for UV excimer laser light is ~0.5 kilojoule/m^2.[645]) Exposures of any duration >500 kilowatts/m^2 may cause cavitation and other harmful effects in biological tissue (see below). On the basis of additional experimental results, the AIUM in 1988 slightly revised its statement[627] to allow intensities as high as 10,000 watts/m^2 for exposures to highly focused sound beams, which is about the highest that human volunteers can tolerate.[505] (In 1985 the FDA allowed ultrasound intensities up to 7300 watts/m^2 for cardiac use, 15,000 watts/m^2 for peripheral vessels, and 1800 watts/m^2 for fetal, abdominal, intraoperative, pediatric, cephalic, and small-organ (breast, thyroid, testes) imaging.[628]) Figure 6.8 summarizes current standards in simplified graphical form.

Deleterious biological effects may occur in at least five ways:

1. *Transient Cavitation* — Transient bubbles which implode produce temperature increases of ~10^3 K and pressure spikes of ~10^3 atm localized in regions of a few microns in radius. Normal or transient cavitation requires ~10^5 watts/m^2 (~5.4 atm) at 30 KHz or ~10^6 watts/m^2 (~17 atm) at 1 MHz to form in water.[628] Intensities less than ~10^4 watts/m^2 will not produce transient cavitation in any tissue.[629]

2. *Stable Cavitation* — Small pre-existing bubbles surrounded by water resonate in synchrony with the acoustic field, with the liquid acting as the oscillating mass and the gas serving as the compliant component. For an air bubble of radius r_{bubble} (meters) in water, resonant frequency $\nu_{res} \sim 0.33 / r_{bubble}$ (Hz) for hard-shell-less bubbles up to ~1 MHz;[647] thus a 6-micron bubble resonates at ~60 KHz. Resonating bubbles have been reported in therapeutic beams at power intensities as low as 6800 watts/m^2 at 750 KHz.[628]

3. *Heating* — Dissipation of vibrational energy can initially heat tissues ~1 K/minute if applied at, say, 50,000 watts/m^2 at 3 MHz, in the hazard zone of Figure 6.8. Continuous exposure to 2000-6000 watts/m^2 at 0.1-10 MHz raises human tissue temperature by 1 K at equilibrium, which is considered safe.[629] Ultrasound intensities of ~2 x 10^7 watts/m^2 at the point of action are used to cauterize liver tissue after surgery.[158]

4. *Acoustic Torque and Fluid Streaming* — Physical fluid motions are driven by ultrasonic radiation pressure, typically ~0.001 N/watt, or ~1 pN/micron^2 at 1000 watts/m^2. Forces of this magnitude or larger can cause damaging shear stresses in molecules or cells and may give rise to small voltages in bone via the piezoelectric effect.[628]

5. *Shock Wave Formation* — Shock waves most easily form in liquids having low attenuation such as urine in the bladder or amniotic fluid. A 3-MHz 10-atm pulse shows a shock waveform after passing through 5 cm of water.[628]

Consider a micron-scale nanorobot located somewhere deep within the human body that wishes to receive acoustic power from an artificial external source. A "safe" I_{power} = 1000 watt/m^2 source pressed against the skin suffers three major reductions in intensity before its emanations reach the nanorobot. First, the power transferred to the entire body is reduced by a geometrical power reduction factor (PRF) which may be approximated as the ratio of the area of the transmitter in contact with the skin to the largest planar section through the torso, ~1500 cm^2. Second, after conversion of incident power intensity to pressure amplitude using Eqn. 4.53, transmitted amplitude is reduced by reflection losses (Eqn. 4.54), which may range from a 90% loss for a poorly-coupled source to just 10% loss for a well-coupled transmitter. Third, the pressure amplitude of the power signal is attenuated by absorption, reflection, and scattering as it passes through human tissue, as described by Eqn. 4.52.

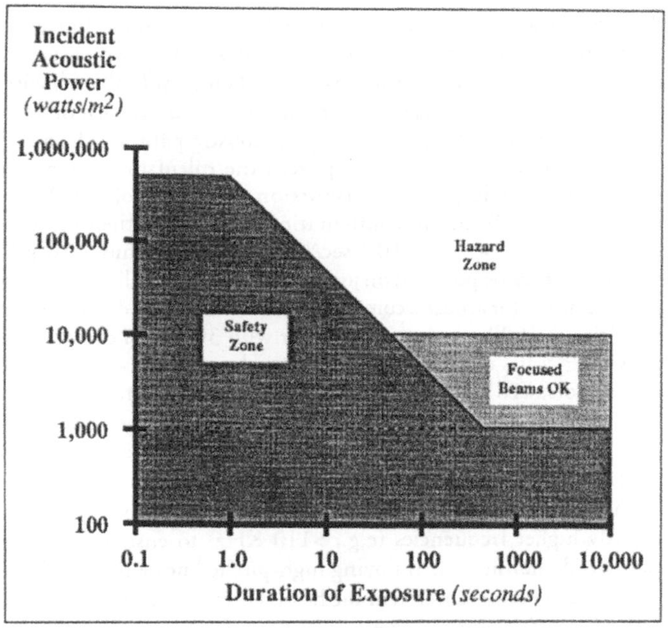

Fig. 6.8. Safety zone for human exposure to ultrasound.

Thus attenuated, the power signal finally reaches the nanorobot and is converted to mechanical power using a piston-type transducer as described by Eqn. 6.13. Combining all the above factors gives received power P_n which is a cubic and exponential function of acoustic frequency ν_p and an exponential function of acoustic path length X_{path}, which factors interact to produce an optimum acoustic power transmission frequency for various path lengths as shown in Figure 6.9. P_n is given by Eqn. 6.13, with $\Delta V = L^3$ and $\Delta P = (1 - R_{loss})(2\, \rho\, v_{sound}\, I_{power}\, PRF)^{1/2}\, e^{(-\alpha_{tiss} \nu_p X_{path})}$, where ρ = 993.4 kg/m^3, v_{sound} = 1500 m/sec in water at 310 K (Eqn. 4.53), and $R_{loss} = 1 - A_{transmit}/A_{incident}$ from Eqn. 4.54.

In operating table scenarios wherein acoustic transmissions from the table may reach all parts of the body within a very short path length (~10-30 cm) and the 1000 watt/m^2 transmitter may be well-coupled to ~40% of the patient's body surface giving PRF >1.00(100%), the power available to a ~0.3 micron^3 nanorobot receiver may be quite large, on the order of ~10^4 pW or greater even at sub-MHz frequencies at the 1000 watts/m^2 incidence level. Similar power levels might also be achieved using carefully-designed permanently-implanted acoustic radiator organs which are themselves powered by some external source such as induced emf, backpack batteries or even tethered household electrical current.

The greatest engineering challenge arises when whole-body acoustic power is to be supplied by some small extradermal source the size of a wristwatch, wallet, belt buckle, ankle bracelet, headband*, or amulet worn around the neck. The power curves in Figure 6.9 assume a wristwatch-band-sized radiator (~30 cm^2) with a PRF of 2% and a single 0.3 $micron^3$ receiver on the nanorobot. For a conservative design the longest acoustic path length in the human body (~200 cm) would govern the calculation, giving an optimum acoustic power transmission frequency of ~60 KHz, providing >40 pW in this configuration for a path entirely through soft tissue (α_{tiss} ~ 8.3 x 10^{-6} sec/m; Table 4.2). Thus a 10-pW nanorobot may be powered on just a ~25% duty cycle, allowing plenty of "quiet time" for acoustic communications, sensing, and navigational activities. A 1000 watt/m^2 transmitter with 30 cm^2 of contact area provides 3 watts of acoustic power, enough to supply ~10^{11} 10-pW nanorobots; ~10^{13} 10-pW nanorobots could be supported in the operating table scenario. For comparison, typical average power outputs of medical ultrasound scanners are 1-70 milliwatts at 0.5-20 MHz.[506,628]

As a practical matter, acoustic power transmission may require slightly higher frequencies (e.g., >110 KHz) to ensure that some patients do not hear an annoying high-pitched noise that would be perceived as being centered in the head. Ultrasonic hearing via bone or body-fluid conduction has been reported at least up to 108 KHz in humans, probably mediated by the saccule, an otolithic organ that normally responds to acceleration and gravity.[1372] Physical discomfort,[3536] intra-articular pain,[3537] and a lowering of electrical pain sensation threshold[3538] due to ultrasound exposure have also been reported in humans.

Figure 6.10 quantifies the effects of transdermal power reflection and receiver size, neither of which significantly influence the choice of optimum acoustic frequency although larger receivers have a steeper frequency cutoff due to rapidly rising piston inertia losses with frequency (Section 6.3.3).

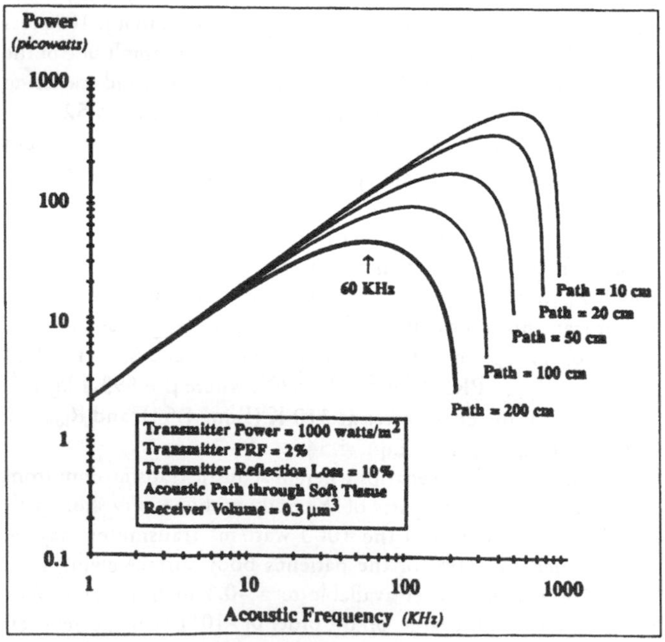

Fig. 6.9. Received acoustic power vs. acoustic frequency for various path lengths in the human body.

Net power received by medical nanorobots is also strongly influenced by the type of tissue lying across the acoustic path because of the exponential dependence of received power on the absorption coefficient α_{tiss} (Fig. 6.11). Similarly, Table 6.6 shows that very highly absorbent tissues such as bone, organs containing gas bubbles such as the stomach or bowel, and especially the air-filled lungs efficiently scatter and reflect large amounts of acoustic energy. Nanorobots positioned such that these highly attenuative tissues lie between them and the source should still receive adequate power due to internal acoustic reflection, since 99.95% of the acoustic amplitude reaching the skin-air interface from inside the body is reflected back into the body (Eqn. 4.54).

Available power declines rapidly for nanodevices located inside bone, bowel, or lung tissue, creating an "energy shadow". Fortunately the path lengths are sufficiently short within these regions of the body that such losses should not become severe. For example, a 1 $micron^3$ receiver located 200 cm from a 1000 watt/m^2 transmitter at 60 KHz with PRF = 2% and reflection loss = 10% at the skin receives 153 pW if the acoustic path passes through soft tissues only, 46 pW if the 200 cm acoustic path includes 1 cm of bone (with a 66% reflection loss at the tissue-bone interface), or 7 pW if the path length includes 5 cm of lung tissue (with an 80% reflection loss at the tissue-lung interface). If two or more acoustic power sources are simultaneously employed, destructive interference might occur within spatially periodic regions of smallest width on the order of one wavelength, or $\gtrsim v_{sound}/\nu_p$ ~ 1 cm (>>r_{nano}) for 150 KHz waves in water at 310 K, reducing locally available power.

Energy concentration, the opposite of energy shadowing, can also occur. If all nanorobot activity is confined to a specific organ or other small volume, a concave focusing transducer can shape pulse waves so that they arrive at a specific focal point within the body at high intensity. Spheroidally shaped regions in which the speed of sound is slower than in the surrounding medium (e.g., lower bulk modulus, or higher density or elasticity, as for instance a fat globule inside an organ; Eqn. 4.30 and Table 6.7) will tend to concentrate acoustic energy towards the center by refractive focusing.[928] Sound waves also bend toward the cold side of a thermal gradient, the low-pressure side of a pressure gradient, and the low-concentration side of a salinity gradient. Large tubular tissue systems with areal cross-sections >(~λ)^2 can act as acoustic waveguides; e.g., for 60 KHz waves in water, λ ~ 2.5 cm, roughly the diameter of the human aorta.

In general, liquids within the body are only weakly absorbing, allowing maximum transmission. Common sonolucent fluids include urine, aqueous humor, vitreous humor, amniotic and cystic fluids. In medical ultrasound, water immersion scanning is commonplace (99.77% transmission at water-tissue interface; Table 6.6) and a full bladder is a standard technique for obtaining an ultrasound window into the uterus. Muscle tissue acoustic absorption is anisotropic; a difference of a factor of 2.5 has been reported between the attenuation across and along its fibers.[628]

6.4.2 Inductive and Radiofrequency Power Transmission

Electrically-powered nanorobots may tap natural electric fields already present in the body (Section 4.7.1) or may seek to acquire electromagnetic power from external sources. Transdermal magnetic induction and radiofrequency energy transfer has been employed in radio tracking and biomedical telemetry since at least the

*The maximum acoustic threshold of pain for the human ear in air is ~100 watts/m^2 or ~140 dB, roughly independent of frequency within the audible range, for experienced habituated listeners.[628,1016] Animals may also take notice—maximum audible frequencies via air conduction are 20 KHz (humans), 33 KHz (monkeys), 40 KHz (dogs, pigs, rats), 45 KHz (cats, katydids), 95 KHz (deer mice), 98 KHz (bats), and up to ~250 KHz (dolphins), while birds and fish are generally limited to <12 KHz.[585]

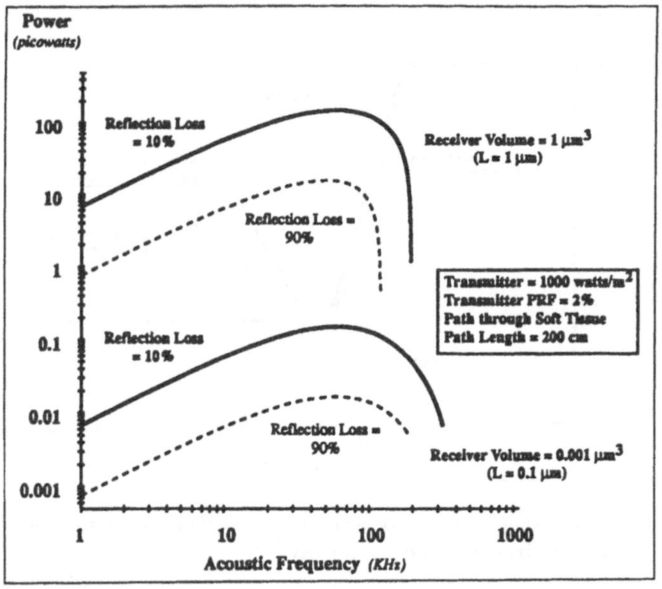

Fig. 6.10. Received acoustic power vs. acoustic frequency for various receiver volumes and reflection losses.

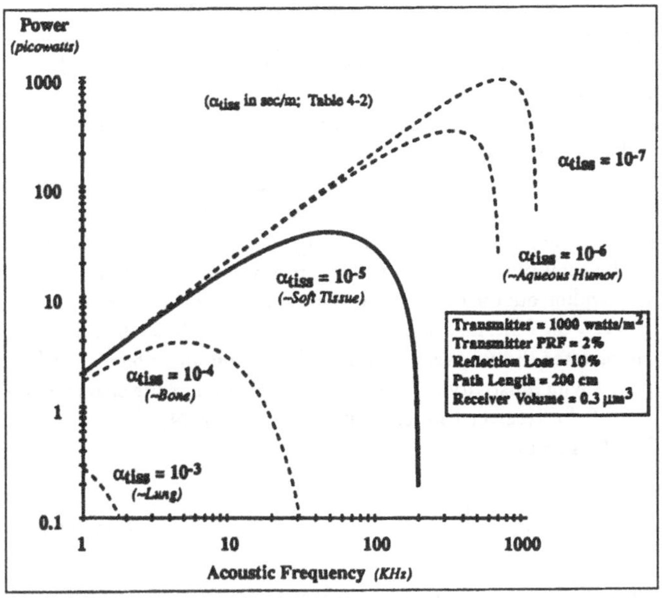

Fig. 6.11. Received acoustic power vs. acoustic frequency for various absorption coefficients in human tissue.

Table 6.6 Acoustic Energy Reflected and Transmitted at Various Tissue Interfaces[506,628]

Tissue Interface	Energy Reflected	Energy Transmitted
Kidney/Liver	0.0036%	99.9964%
Liver/Muscle	0.032%	99.968%
Muscle/Blood	0.07%	99.93%
Soft tissue/Water	0.23%	99.77%
Fat/Kidney	0.64%	99.36%
Lens/Vitreous humor	0.91%	99.09%
Fat/Liver	1.00%	99.00%
Lens/Aqueous humor	1.04%	98.96%
Fat/Muscle	1.08%	98.92%
Bone/Muscle	41.23%	58.77%
Soft tissue/Bone	43.50%	56.50%
Bone/Fat	48.91%	51.09%
Soft tissue/Lung	63.64%	36.36%
Diamond/Water	90.80%	9.20%
Muscle/Air	98.01%	1.99%
Water/Air	99.89%	0.11%
Soft tissue/Air	99.90%	0.10%
Diamond/Air	99.997%	0.0025%

Table 6.7 Velocity of Sound in Various Organs and Biological Materials at 310 K[363,506,628,730]

Biological Material	Velocity of Sound (m/sec)
Air bubbles*	20
Lung (collapsed)**	320
Dry air	353
Lung (normal)	630
Silastics	950
Ethanol	1160
Fat	1470
Water	1500
Aqueous humor	1510
Castor oil	1520
Vitreous humor	1540
Soft tissue (avg)	1540
Brain	1550
Liver	1565
Whole blood	1570
Kidney	1575
Muscle	1600
Optic nerve	1615
Lens of eye	1630
Glycerol	1880
Collagen (across axis)	2940
Bone (typical)	3550
Collagen (along axis)	3640
Skull bone	4090
Enamel (tooth)	5800
Diamond	~17,300

* 45% by volume in water
** pneumonitis

1920s,[634,635,637,638,3510] and commercially available miniaturized implantable transmitters are now commonplace in laboratory work,[639] but using this technique to power submillimeter devices is a relatively recent concept.[630]

The biological effects of radio waves, microwaves, and infrared rays are usually equivalent to the effects of heating, although non-thermal rf-induced vasodilation, possibly due to Ca^{++} flow manipulation, apparently has been observed in frogs.[3328] Radio waves mainly induce thermal agitation of molecules and excitation of molecular rotations, while infrared rays excite vibrational modes of large molecules and may release fluorescent emission as well as heat. Both types of radiation are preferentially absorbed by unsaturated fats. In the United States the maximum permissible continuous occupational exposure level to microwave radiation has been 50 watts/m^2 for the testes and 100 watts/m^2 for the whole body—essentially double the thermal radiance of a 100-watt (~2000 Kcal/day) ~2 m^2 human body, e.g., ~50 watts/m^2 across the skin, or roughly the intensity of direct sunlight on the skin (Section 4.9.4). Figure 6.12 compares several generally accepted international occupational and population exposure limits that have been adopted.[824] Michaelson[823] carried out extensive investigations and found no evidence for hazard at 100 watts/m^2, though there is conclusive evidence of potentially hazardous effects at levels above 1000 watts/m^2.

Single exposures to levels up to ~100 times these values may be briefly tolerated without injury, as for example photosetting dental fillings which require ~20 sec exposures to visible intensities of ~10^5 watts/m^2. Optical tweezers also demonstrate that monochromatic exposures of ~10^{11} watts/m^2 are tolerated by biological macromolecules immersed in an optically transparent aqueous medium due to fast thermal equilibrium at the micron scale.[1630,1631] On the other hand, the threshold of pain for ink-blackened human skin exposed to a radiant heat stimulus is ~10,000 watts/m^2 for 3-second exposures.[585]

An electromagnetic wave passing through the human body declines in intensity as it heats tissues and is attenuated approximately according to:

$$I = I_0 e^{(-2 \alpha_E d_x)} \quad (\text{watts/m}^2) \qquad \text{\{Eqn. 6.32\}}$$

where I = power per unit area transmitted through the tissue, $I_0 \le 100$ watts/m^2 (maximum safe incident intensity), d_x is depth of tissue penetration (meters), and α_E (meter^{-1}) is the total attenuation factor including scattering and absorption, the inverse of the mean free path. For radio frequency and microwave radiation, $\alpha_E = \alpha_e \nu_E^{1/2}$, where ν_E is incident frequency (Hz) and α_e ranges from 2 x 10^{-3} sec$^{1/2}$ m^{-1} for muscle to 10 x 10^{-3} sec$^{1/2}$ m^{-1} for vitreous humor but averages ~5 x 10^{-3} sec$^{1/2}$ m^{-1} for soft tissue.[635] At 100 MHz, 99% of incident power is removed in a 5-cm path length of soft tissue; at 1000 MHz (microwaves), 99% attenuation occurs within ~15 mm; at 10^6 MHz (far infrared), ~0.5 mm of tissue removes 99% of the energy. On the other hand, 53% of the incident energy at 0.1 MHz passes through a 20-cm thick human body unscattered and unabsorbed, thus remains available for utilization by medical nanodevices seeking electrical power. The dependence of α_E on ν_E varies significantly across the electromagnetic spectrum;[509,567,727] additionally, α_E for different tissues may deviate by up to a factor of 10 from the average values shown in Figure 6.13, especially in the IR-UV region.

Heetderks[630] has analyzed the feasibility of transmitting electrical power into the body using submillimeter receiver coils—a magnetic transcutaneous link, which is preferred when large power-transfer rates are required. In one of several designs, Heetderks starts with a 14-cm diameter transmitter coil (~diameter of the neck) with 11 turns (~40 microhenries inductance) and a 10 volt peak driving voltage at a frequency of 2 MHz delivering 4 watts RMS into the coil, a high but probably acceptable incident intensity of ~260 watts/m^2 at the skin. Inside the body, Heetderks uses a 400 micron diameter ferrite-core receiver coil with 60 turns spaced 50 microns apart, making a total receiver solenoid length of 3000 microns with ~0.89 microhenries inductance and Q = 40 for both transmitter and receiver, giving a fractional energy loss per cycle of $2\pi / Q \sim 16\%$. The receiver produces 1.1 volts and 320 microwatts in the ideal case where the receiver lies coplanar within the circumference of the transmitter coil. Large noncoplanar displacements may produce significant performance declines.

Each of Heetderks' receivers develops a power density of ~10^6 watts/m^3. Up to 600 receivers may be present within the volume of operation of each transmitter, collectively drawing up to 10% of unloaded transmitter coil power consistent with maintaining Q ~40. In a nanomedical application, each receiver could act as a microscopic power station, absorbing the externally supplied electromagnetic energy and then transducing it into other forms of energy which may more directly be tapped by in vivo medical nanorobots. In theory, a 100 watt/m^2 flux imposed on the entire ~2 m^2 human

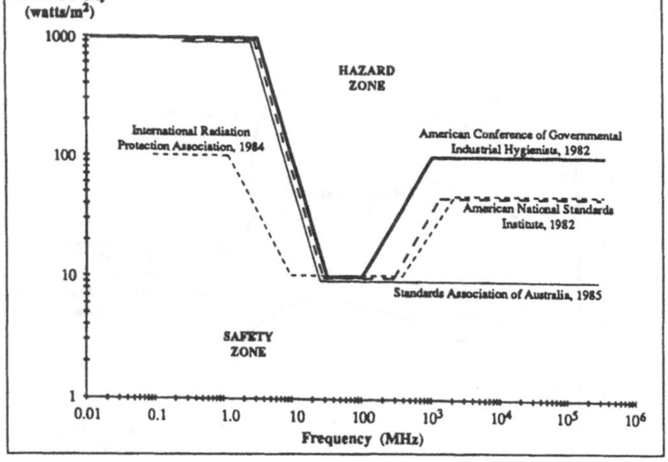

Fig. 6.12. Occupational exposure limits to electromagnetic radiation as equivalent plane-wave power density.[824]

body surface should allow the transdermal importation of ~20 watts, enough to support a population of ~10^{12} 10-pW nanorobots assuming 50% energy transduction efficiency among the widely dispersed "power stations".

How much smaller could Heetderk's receivers be made? A detailed design analysis is beyond the scope of this book, but a simple scaling estimate may be made as follows. For a receiver coil of magnetic inductance L_m (henries), resistance R_c (ohms), and rf waves of angular frequency ω_E (rad/sec), a coupling coefficient ($k_{coupling}$) between transmitter and receiver coils may be crudely approximated as the ratio of the power stored in the magnetic field of the LR oscillator to the total power delivered to the receiver coil by the transmitter, or (dividing out the terms for current) $k_{coupling} \sim \omega_E L_m / (R_c + \omega_E L_m)$. For $\nu_E = \omega_E / 2\pi$, $\mu_0 = 1.26 \times 10^{-6}$ henry/m, $\mu_f \sim 5$ (a self-inductance factor when the receiver coil of N_{coil} loops contains a ferrite core[630]), ρ_{wire} = wire resistivity ($\sim 3 \times 10^{-8}$ ohm-m), and L is the characteristic size of the receiver (meters), then $L_m \sim \mu_0 \mu_f N_{coil}^2 L^3$, $R \sim \rho_{wire} N_{coil}^2 / L$, and

$$k_{coupling}^{-1} \sim 1 + \frac{k_m}{\nu_E L^4} \qquad \text{\{Eqn. 6.33\}}$$

where $k_m = \rho_{wire} / 2\pi \mu_0 \mu_f \sim 10^{-3}$. For discrete-component (macroscopic) radios that receive broadcast signals, L ~ 1 cm and ν_E = 1-100 MHz, giving $k_{coupling}$ = 0.9-0.999, which is very good. For Heetderks' submillimeter receiver designs, $k_{coupling} = 10^{-3} - 10^{-5}$; for example, the receiver described above has L ~ 700 microns, ν_E = 2 MHz, giving $k_{coupling} \sim 5 \times 10^{-4}$, which is very poor. With such poor coupling, very large transmitter intensities are required to induce very small receiver power levels. Troyk and Schwan[636] have suggested that printed thin-film coils integrated directly with sensor circuitry driven by a special transmitter coil topology could provide adequate amounts of power to implanted coils having coupling coefficients up to two orders of magnitude lower than Heetderks' designs. However, even $k_{coupling} \sim 10^{-7}$ at 2 MHz only reduces receiver size to L ~ 500 microns, which is not much improvement. The L^4 scaling of $k_{coupling}$ suggests that magnetic transcutaneous power receivers smaller than ~500 microns may be impractical, given the negligible amounts of magnetic field energy that can be stored in nanoscale volumes (Section 6.2.4) and the likelihood that small AC circuits will be heavily damped.[10] (See also Section 7.2.3.)

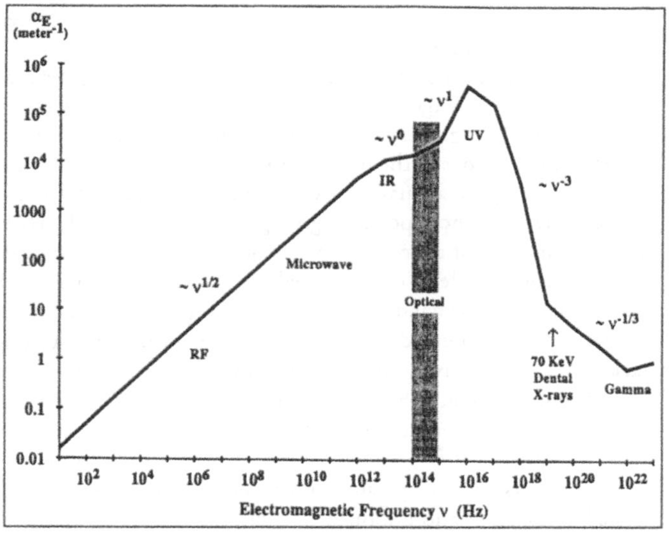

Fig. 6.13. Estimated total attentuation factor α_E (scattering + absorption) for electromagnetic radiation passing through human tissue.

However, efficient micron-scale MHz-frequency rf antennas may still be feasible for individual nanorobots, as suggested by the following simplistic analysis. Consider a simple spring pendulum with a bob of mass m_{bob}, density ρ (~diamondoid), thickness h_{bob}, and face area L^2, with n_q charges and total charge $Q_{bob} = n_q q_e = L^2 C_q$ (coul) permanently embedded on the bob surface, where C_q is bob surface charge density. An oscillating rf field of strength E_e (volts/m) and frequency ν_E drives the charges with a force $F = E_e Q_{bob} = m_{bob} a_{bob}$ at an acceleration a_{bob} (m/sec^2). The bob mass accelerates for a half-cycle of duration $t = (2 \nu_E)^{-1}$, periodically displacing a distance $x_{bob} = (1/2)\, a\, t^2 = Q_{bob} E_e / 8\, m_{bob} \nu_E^2$ and traveling at a mean velocity $v_{bob} \sim 2\, x_{bob} \nu_E$. The local energy density produced by the transmitter field is $D_E = (1/2)\, \kappa_e \varepsilon_0 E_e^2$ (joules/m^3) (variables defined in Section 4.7.1, for water), with transmitter power intensity $I_t = c\, D_E / n$ (watts/m^2) where $c = 3 \times 10^8$ m/sec (speed of light) and $n = \kappa_e^{1/2}$ is the refractive index for a nonmagnetic material at low frequency; hence $E_e = (2\, I_t / \kappa_e^{1/2} \varepsilon_0 c)^{1/2}$ (volts/m). At the end of each half-cycle the bob receives an energy $E_{1/2} = (1/2)\, m_{bob} v_{bob}^2$. Assuming mechanical rectification, a lever arm connected to the charged bob in the receiver transmits to the nanorobot a received power of $P_n \sim 2\, E_{1/2} \nu_E$ (watts); making the appropriate substitutions we have:

$$P_n = \frac{I_t\, L^2\, C_q^2}{8\, \rho\, h_{bob}\, \nu_E\, \kappa_e^{1/2}\, \varepsilon_0\, c} \quad \text{(watts)} \qquad \{\text{Eqn. 6.34}\}$$

An additional constraint is that bob travel x_{bob} must not exceed the space available within a receiver housing of depth L_{trav}. The bob travels slower but farther at lower rf frequencies, and the lowest possible operating frequency minimizes attenuation in tissues. Taking $x_{bob} \lesssim n_\# h_{bob} = L_{trav}$ as a limit establishes a minimum operating frequency that will not peg the bob against its stops, given by:

$$\nu_E \geq \left(\frac{I_t\, C_q^2}{32\, \rho^2\, h_{bob}^4\, n_\#^2\, \kappa_e^{1/2}\, \varepsilon_0\, c} \right)^{1/4} \quad \text{(Hz)} \qquad \{\text{Eqn. 6.35}\}$$

We require a high charge density and thus assume $C_q = 0.1$ coul/m^2 (~0.6 charge/nm^2), somewhat less than the ~0.16 coul/m^2 for charged amino acid molecules and the ~0.3 coul/m^2 for a "fully ionized surface",[1149] but well above the 0.005-0.02 coul/m^2 recorded experimentally for SiO_2 on mica,[1154] the 2×10^{-3} coul/m^2 for the electrodes in the electrostatic motor (Section 6.3.5) designed by Drexler,[10] and the 2×10^{-4} coul/m^2 figure given by Lowell and Rose-Innes[1151] cited as typical for "highly charged surfaces." For a water-immersed bob, the DC surface field from this 0.1 coul/m^2 charge density is a sustainable $E_{DC} = C_q / 2\, \kappa_e \varepsilon_0 = 76$ megavolts/meter.

Signal attenuation is minimal below ~1 MHz (Eqn. 6.32). Taking $I_t = 100$ watts/m^2, $L = 1$ micron, $\rho = 2000$ kg/m^3, $h_{bob} = 20$ nm, $n_\# = L_{trav} / h_{bob} = 50$ for $L_{trav} = L$, $\kappa_e = 74.31$ for 310 K water, and $\varepsilon_0 = 8.85 \times 10^{-12}$ farad/m, then minimum $\nu_E = 0.17$ MHz giving $P_n \sim 0.8$ pW delivered to the nanorobot producing a power density within the housing of $D_n = P_n / L_{trav} L^2 \sim 10^6$ watts/m^3. In a practical system, these receivers must be aligned precisely with the incident field to maximize energy coupling, possibly requiring dynamic orientation control of each onboard receiver. Resonating beam structures 8-30 microns in size that can serve as rf filtering and oscillator elements have been demonstrated experimentally at ~15 MHz.[879] High-frequency sub-micron electrometers with charge per unit bandwidth sensitivity of ~0.1 electron/Hz$^{1/2}$ have been demonstrated,[2926] and submicron rf mechanical resonators have been discussed by Cleland and Roukes.[2927]

In 1999, Pharma Seq[3432] was developing laser-photon-powered cubic ~250-micron rf microtransponders for use with oligonucleotide probes in DNA assays; suspended in slurry, each device had an integrated circuit storing the sequence of the oligo attached to it, and emitted a coded signal (the probe's serial number) to a nearby receiver when a fluorophore-labeled target DNA molecule binded to a complementary probe. However, direct visible-spectrum photonic powering of medical nanorobots in vivo is not promising except within a few millimeters of the unclothed epidermis and only in the presence of direct sunlight or strong artificial sources of illumination (>10-100 watts/m^2) near maximum safe exposure limits, due to the poor detection efficiency (low photon count rate sec^{-1} m^{-2}) and rapid attenuation of photons in human tissue (Section 4.9.4).

6.4.3 Tethered Power Transmission

Energy may be transferred to in vivo medical nanorobots via physical tethers. Virtually all forms of power may be transmitted in this fashion, including electrical, electromagnetic, acoustic, mechanical, and chemical energy. A general discussion of various factors and scenarios that favor or disfavor the use of tethers, as compared to other methods of energy transmission, is in Section 6.4.3.6.

6.4.3.1 Electrical Tethers

One of the most obvious methods for providing energy to nanodevices is simply to attach a power cord to each machine. The bending moment of a wire is proportional to its radius to the fourth power,[642] so molecular nanowires[1740,2866] are much more flexible than macroscopic wires. These power cables could be made of traditional metallic conductors (15-nm thick gold wires have been fabricated on a Si substrate) or doped polyacetylene chains (Section 10.2.3.3) and other organic conductors which have been used to make LEDs and polymer batteries.[382]

For an uninsulated single conductor of length L, square cross-sectional area A_w, surface area A (~ $4\, L\, A_w^{1/2}$ for $L >> A_w^{1/2}$), resistivity ρ_e, and surface emissivity e_r, carrying a steady current I (amps) across a potential V (volts) and a resistance R (ohms), developing power P (watts), transmitted power intensity P_{A_w} (watts/m^2), and volumetric power density D (watts/m^3), which heats the wire from ambient temperature T_0 up to the maximum desired operating temperature T_{max}, then from the standard electrical formulas and Eqn. 6.19:

$$R = \frac{\rho_e L}{A_W} \qquad \text{\{Eqn. 6.36\}}$$

$$I = \frac{V}{R} = \left(\frac{P}{R}\right)^{1/2} \sim \left(\frac{4\, e_r\, \sigma\, A_W^{3/2} \left(T_{max}^4 - T_0^4\right)}{\rho_e}\right)^{1/2} \qquad \text{\{Eqn. 6.37\}}$$

$$V = IR = (PR)^{1/2} \sim \left(\frac{4\, e_r\, \sigma\, \rho_e\, L^2 \left(T_{max}^4 - T_0^4\right)}{A_W^{1/2}}\right)^{1/2} \qquad \text{\{Eqn. 6.38\}}$$

$$P = I^2 R \sim 4\, e_r\, \sigma\, L\, A_W^{1/2} \left(T_{max}^4 - T_0^4\right) \qquad \text{\{Eqn. 6.39\}}$$

$$P_{A_W} = \frac{P}{A_W} \sim \frac{4\, e_r\, \sigma\, L \left(T_{max}^4 - T_0^4\right)}{A_W^{1/2}} \qquad \text{\{Eqn. 6.40\}}$$

$$D = \frac{\rho_e I^2}{A_W^2} \sim \frac{4\, e_r\, \sigma \left(T_{max}^4 - T_0^4\right)}{A_W^{1/2}} \qquad \text{\{Eqn. 6.41\}}$$

where σ = 5.67 x 10^{-8} watt/m^2-K^4 (Stefan-Boltzmann constant). Thus for a silver wire 1 micron in diameter and 1 meter long, with ρ_e = 1.6 x 10^{-8} ohm-m, e_r = 0.02 for polished silver, T_{max} = 373 K (boiling point of water) and T_0 = 310 K (body temperature), then R = 16,000 ohms, I = 50 microamps (current density I_d ~ 5 x 10^7 amps/m^2), A_w = 1 micron^2, A ~ 4 mm^2, V = 0.9 volt, P = 50 microwatts (sufficient power to operate a load of ~45 electrostatic motors ~390 nm in diameter, as described in Section 6.3.5), and D = 5 x 10^7 watts/m^3. Note that the minimum quantum unit of resistance in atomic- or molecular-scale wires is ~$h/2e^2$ ~ 13,000 ohms, where h = 6.63 x 10^{-34} joule-sec (Planck's constant) and e = 1.6 x 10^{-19} joule/eV, due to quantized conductance (e.g., Coulomb blockade) in narrow channels whose characteristic transverse dimension approaches the electronic wavelength.[1740] By 1998, metallic wires down to ~20 nm in width had been fabricated.[1517]

Wires with electrical and thermal insulation can safely carry higher currents in vivo (Section 6.5.5). If the wire in the preceding example is wrapped with a thermal insulator of thickness d_{insul} and thermal conductivity K_t, then the maximum current increases to:

$$I = \left(\frac{K_t \left(T_{max} - T_0\right) A_W\, d_{insul}}{L\, \rho_e}\right)^{1/2} \qquad \text{\{Eqn. 6.42\}}$$

Using water as the thermal insulator (K_t = 0.623 watt/m-K at 310 K), a d_{insul} = 1 micron layer allows the wire to rise to 373 K while the outside of the insulating jacket remains near 310 K. A 100-micron thick water jacket allows electrical current and voltage to safely rise by a factor of 10, thus power to rise by a factor of 100.

Another possibility is the fullerene (pure carbon) conductors (Section 10.2.2.1). For example, 7-12 nm nanotube ropes 200-500 nm in length at ~310 K conduct ~50 nanoamperes at ~1 millivolt, transmitting a total power of ~50 pW.[641] Boron nitride coated carbon nanotube wires should be highly oxidation-resistant.[1308] Field emission from room-temperature carbon atomic wires has been measured as 0.1-1 microamperes at 80 volts, or ~10 microwatts.[643] Nanowires a few nm wide and hundreds of microns long have already been fabricated, and continuous meter-length threads (and longer) have been proposed; current densities >10^{14} amps/m^2 have been pulled through a single chain of carbon atoms.[643]

If fullerene nanowires are doped with metal atoms, adding electrons or holes so that the charge carrier density is high, electrical conductivity may be precisely engineered from semiconductor levels up to equal or better than copper in the plane of the graphene sheet. Multitube cables may display a quantum confinement effect that sharply reduces the resistance, possibly giving an electrical conductivity 10-100 times that of copper at room temperatures, and may provide shielding comparable to coax. Doped electron-rich conductors are easily oxidized on the nanometer scale, but wrapping such conductors in a second concentric undoped outer nanotube provides an insulating jacket that is effectively chemically impermeable under normal conditions. By 1998, coaxial nanocables ~30 nm in diameter had been fabricated in lengths up to 50 microns.[2016] Boron-nitrogen (BN) equivalents of fullerene nanotubes are physically strong and good insulators. Low-temperature superconductivity has been demonstrated in doped[644] and undoped[3240] fullerenes.

An interesting alternative is a conveyor belt system for direct mechanical charge transport, crudely analogous to the charging system of a Van de Graff generator. Nanoscale conveyor belts (Section 3.4.3) could transport ~10^6 electrons/sec at a belt speed of 4 mm/sec, comparable to the ~1 cm/sec drift speed of electrons flowing in macroscale wires (Section 6.5.5). This gives a 0.2 picoampere current through a device with cross-sectional area ~(10 nm)^2, a modest current density of ~10^3 amperes/m^2 and electrostatic belt stress of ~1 atm between adjacent charges spaced ~4 nm apart. If a much smaller belt can be designed of a scale comparable to the 150-micron long computer data storage tape (Section 7.2.6) described by Drexler,[10] a belt speed of ~10 m/sec and charge density of ~1 electron/nm^2 (~amino acid density) on a 1 nm^2 belt gives a current of ~2 nanoamperes and a current density of ~10^9 amperes/m^2, comparable to the electromigration-limited ~10^{10} amperes/m^2 maximum current density in bulk aluminum,* with an electrostatic belt stress of ~3600 atm. Net belt mechanical energy dissipation may be as low as ~10^{-6} zJ/nm of travel for each ~nanometer-scale charge carrying device (Section 3.4.3).

6.4.3.2 Electromagnetic Tethers

Optical energy may be piped from one place to another by allowing light to enter a narrow solid fiber of clear plastic or fused silica. Light undergoes total internal reflection at the glass-air boundary and follows the contours of the light pipe, with losses due to scattering and absorption in the material as each photon undergoes up to ~10^5 reflections/meter during transit. The scattering minimum in commercial ultrapure silica fiberoptic cable occurs at ~1500 nm, or ~2 x 10^{14} Hz, in the near infrared. These losses are roughly equivalent to transmission in clear air, negligible over distances of relevance in nanomedicine: measurable amounts of energy may be transmitted through single fibers ~100 km long.

At the lowest frequencies, the cutoff frequency for electromagnetic waveguides of diameter d_{guide} filled with material of dielectric constant κ_e, below which frequency the waveguide cannot transmit photons (velocity c = 3 x 10^8 m/sec in vacuo, and slightly lower in various dielectric materials at various frequencies), is ν_{cutoff} = c / 2 κ_e d_{guide} ~ 7.5 x 10^{13} Hz (λ = 1000 nm) in the near infrared—close to the scattering minimum at 1500 nm—for d_{guide} = 2 microns and κ_e ~ 1. This cutoff applies only to waveguides; coax (shielded single wire) or triax (shielded twisted pair) lines can conduct frequencies all the

This "maximum" may be quite conservative: "A single crystal metal wire surrounded by a strongly bonded, lattice-matched sheath should be stable at far greater current densities than a conventional wire of the same material".[10]

way down to DC and all the way up to near-infrared (Section 7.2.5.1.)

More specifically, if a nonmagnetic weak dielectric (~air) fills the space between two coaxial cylindrical conductors, with inside wire of radius r_{in}, outer jacket of radius r_{out} and line current I_{line}, then the average transmitted power[727] is given by:

$$P_E = 30\, I_{line}^2 \ln\left(\frac{r_{out}}{r_{in}}\right) \quad \text{(watts)} \qquad \text{\{Eqn. 6.43\}}$$

In coax theory,[727] r_{out}/r_{in} = 1.65 allows maximum power to be carried at a given breakdown voltage gradient across the dielectric (most appropriate for power transmission), whereas r_{out}/r_{in} = 3.6 gives the lowest attenuation due to conductor losses for a given outer diameter (most appropriate for communications applications). Thus for a 1-micron power coax, r_{out} = 0.5 micron implies r_{in} ~ 0.3 micron; assuming I_{line} ~ 10^8 amps/m^2 on the inside wire, P_E ~ 10^4 pW at ~1 millivolt and the line has a characteristic impedance of 30 ohms.

For the highest frequencies, optical fibers may be as small as ~0.5-1 micron in diameter, roughly the photon wavelength—a dielectric rod can serve as a waveguide crudely analogous to the hollow metal pipes used at rf frequencies. Blue photons (~400 nm) carry ~500 zJ of energy, almost enough to break C-C bonds (~550 zJ). Ultraviolet (UV) wavelengths shorter than ~300 nm are greatly attenuated for fiber lengths >1 meter due to heavy absorption, and intense prolonged UV irradiation of silica creates defects (color centers) in the material that lead to further absorption of the laser light in the fiber.

In biomedical applications, silica fibers are used to conduct photons from excimer lasers, the brightest known sources of UV radiation.[3539,3540] Typical maximum continuous power intensities are ~30,000 watts/m^2 for corneal sculpting, ~10^5 watts/m^2 for bile duct cholangiocarcinoma tumor surgery, and ~10^6 watts/m^2 for arterial debulking, laser dental machining and laser lithotripsy for kidney stones,[645,646] so ~0.01-1 microwatts may be delivered to medical nanodevices using a single ~1 micron^2 optical tether transmitting UV photons. The maximum transmittable power intensity is approximated by Eqn. 6.40; taking e_r = 0.80 for silica, $A_w^{1/2}$ = 1 mm diameter fiber, L = 1 meter and T_{max} - T_0 = 20 K at room temperature for a handheld surgical instrument, then P_{Aw} ~ 4 x 10^5 watts/m^2, in line with the above figures for excimer lasers assuming a ~40% duty cycle. For a nanomedical optical power cable with $A_w^{1/2}$ = 1 micron diameter fiber, L = 1 meter, T_0 = 310 K and T_{max} ≤ 373 K, then P_{Aw} ~ 10^9 watts/m^2 and a maximum of P ~ 1 milliwatts may be delivered down the fiber. However, at this high fluence there is tremendous risk of localized tissue incineration, should the fiber detach in vivo and the photon flow is not immediately halted—a good argument for limiting optical power tether intensities to <10^5 watts/m^2 or less. A thin adjacent backchannel fiber could serve as a fuse, rupturing simultaneously with the main fiber and cutting off the feedback control signal.

6.4.3.3 Hydraulic and Acoustic Tethers

Power is easily conveyed to medical nanodevices through tethers by simple hydraulic means. For example, a virtually leakproof thick-walled fullerene nanotube measuring $2r_{tube}$ = 1 micron in diameter and l_{tube} = 1 meter long could safely transport pressurized fluid of absolute viscosity η = 6.9 x 10^{-4} kg/m-sec (310 K water) at a fluid pressure p_{tube} = 5 atm to drive a mechanical turbine or valved reciprocating piston system, establishing an energy density of 0.5 pJ/micron^3 and delivering $P_n = \pi\, r_{tube}^4\, p_{tube}^2 / 8\, \eta\, l_{tube}$ ~ 10 pW to a V_n = 1 micron^3 nanorobot power plant at a fluid flow velocity of $v_{fluid} = r_{tube}^2\, p_{tube} / 8\, \eta\, l_{tube}$ ~ 20 microns/sec and producing a power density of ~10^7 watts/m^3, assuming Poiseuille flow.

Acoustic waves could be delivered by tether, but slightly larger tubes are required. Consider a water-filled pipe with dimensions as defined in the previous paragraph which is excited at one end by a vibrating piston operating at a frequency $\nu_p << v_{sound}/r_{tube}$ (~1 GHz for $2r_{tube}$ = 1 micron). For such small tubes, the inertia and kinetic reaction of the fluid may be neglected in favor of the frictional force (e.g., Poiseuille flow; Eqn. 9.25), since the compressions and rarefactions of the fluid are practically isothermal on account of the almost perfect heat conduction, and the power transmission is given by:

$$P_n = P_0\, e^{(-2\, \alpha_{tube}\, l_{tube})} \quad \text{(watts)} \qquad \text{\{Eqn. 6.44\}}$$

with the attenuation coefficient given by Rayleigh's classical formulation:[649,650]

$$\alpha_{tube} = \left(\frac{8\, \pi\, \gamma\, \eta\, \nu_p}{\rho\, v_{sound}^2\, r_{tube}^2}\right)^{1/2} \qquad \text{\{Eqn. 6.45\}}$$

where γ is the ratio of specific heats (1.004 for water, 1.009 for seawater), v_{sound} = 1500 m/sec and ρ = 993.4 kg/m^3 for water at 310 K. Maximum energy transfer (like a rigid bar) occurs at integral multiples of half-wavelengths of the incident sonic waves, in other words, at ν_p = n v_{sound} / 2 l_{tube}, where n = 1 is the fundamental frequency or first harmonic, n = 2 is the first overtone or second harmonic, and so forth. Minimum attenuation occurs at n = 1, the first harmonic.

A periodic source pulse of an intensity low enough to avoid cavitation in pure water (~10^4 watts/m^2; Section 6.4.1) applied as input power P_0 across a tube area of $\pi\, r_{tube}^2$ produces a 10 pW output power for l_{tube} ≤ 300 microns at ν_p = 2.5 MHz and r_{tube} = 0.5 microns with P_0 = 8000 pW and α_{tube} ~11,000 m^{-1}. To get l_{tube} = 1 meter length requires r_{tube} = 15 microns and ν_p = 750 Hz to deliver 10 pW at the output. (A three-phase "alternating current" acoustical power transmission system using 100 Hz waves traversing three water-filled pipes was patented by M. Constantinesco in 1920.)[650]

Diamond rods can also make nearly lossless acoustic power transmission lines (Section 7.2.5.3).

6.4.3.4 Gear Trains and Mechanical Tethers

Lengthy nanoscale gear trains may transmit power over great distances because mechanical efficiency for steric nanogear pairs may be ~99.997% (Section 6.3.2). Thus the initial mechanical input power only falls to 94% after passing through a sequential gear train of 2000 units, a 10-micron long train assuming each gear is ~5 nm in diameter.

Torque power may also be transmitted via a long rotating cable inside a fixed tubular sheath, somewhat resembling an automobile speedometer cable or a dentist's drill (~10-100 Hz). (Reciprocating cables are briefly treated in Section 7.2.5.4.) Two modes of power transmission are readily distinguished—first, a twist-and-release or "AC" strategy, resulting in the propagation of a torsion wave which looks locally like a shear wave, and second, a constant-twist or "DC" strategy, in which a driver end turns the cable at a constant rate (up to the bursting velocity) and the cable is maintained at constant torque (up to the shear strength limit). In the following analysis, we consider a cylindrical transmission cable of radius r_{cable}, length L_{cable}, and density ρ, with shear modulus G and working stress σ_w. The author thanks J. Soreff for helpful clarifications.

The AC case may be thought of as the propagation of a shear sound wave with maximum shear σ_w and maximum strain $s_{max} = \sigma_w/G$, traveling at $v_{shear} \sim (G/\rho)^{1/2}$, the transverse wave velocity in the cable medium. The maximum power passing through the cable is $P_{AC} = \pi\, r_{cable}^2\, D_E\, v_{shear}$, where energy density $D_E \sim G\, s_{max}^2 = \sigma_w^2 / G$, hence:

$$P_{AC} \sim \frac{\pi\, r_{cable}^2\, \sigma_w^2}{\rho^{1/2}\, G^{1/2}} \quad \text{(watts)} \qquad \{\text{Eqn. 6.46}\}$$

limiting maximum cable operating frequency to $\sim v_{shear}/L_{cable}$ or:

$$\nu_{AC_m} \lesssim \frac{G^{1/2}}{\rho^{1/2}\, L_{cable}} \quad \text{(Hz)} \qquad \{\text{Eqn. 6.47}\}$$

In the DC case, the maximum surface speed of a spinning cable is the flywheel bursting speed $v_{burst} \sim (\sigma_w / \rho)^{1/2}$ and the maximum shear stress is $\sim\sigma_w$. Ignoring the minor complication that a real cable cannot withstand maximum static shear and maximum tangential velocity simultaneously, the maximum power passing through the cable is approximated by $P_{DC} \sim \pi\, r_{cable}^2\, \sigma_w\, v_{burst}$, so:

$$P_{DC} \sim \frac{\pi\, r_{cable}^2\, \sigma_w^{3/2}}{\rho^{1/2}} \quad \text{(watts)} \qquad \{\text{Eqn. 6.48}\}$$

limiting maximum cable operating frequency to $\sim v_{burst} / 2\,\pi\, r_{cable}$ or:

$$\nu_{DC_m} \lesssim \left(\frac{\sigma_w}{2\, p^2\, \rho\, r_{cable}^2} \right)^{1/2} \quad \text{(Hz)} \qquad \{\text{Eqn. 6.49}\}$$

Hence $P_{DC}/P_{AC} \sim (G / \sigma_w)^{1/2} \sim 7$, taking $G = 5 \times 10^{11}$ N/m^2 and $\sigma_w \sim 10^{10}$ N/m^2 for a diamondoid cable, so the initial conclusion is that the DC strategy allows transmission of ~1 order of magnitude higher mechanical power than the AC strategy, for a given cable size and material. A cable, secured at one end and twisted through a maximum angle θ_{max} at the other end, acquires at maximum stress an energy $E_{cable} = (1/2)\, k_{torsion}\, \theta_{max}^2$ where $k_{torsion} = \pi\, G\, r_{cable}^4 / 2\, L_{cable}$; setting $E_{cable} = \pi\, r_{cable}^2\, L_{cable}\, D_E$ gives $\theta_{max} = 2\, L_{cable}\, \sigma_w / r_{cable}\, G \sim 4$ radians for an L_{cable} = 1 micron and r_{cable} = 10 nm diamondoid cable.

The AC cable may suffer transmission losses due to shear wave radiation from an oscillating torque.[10] However, this radiation can be suppressed by imposing the torque between the cable and a coaxial sheath, or by imposing opposite torques on a pair of cables, both going from the same transmitter to the same receiver. In either case, no net torque need be imposed on the surrounding medium; even startup transients may be cancelled in the latter case. Thermally induced transient irregularities may still interact with the moving cable to radiate some power, but this remains a minor effect. A rotating cable suffers small additional transmission losses due to frictional interactions with the jacket in which it is encased, but drag power losses are much less than shear wave radiation losses in most nanoscale applications,[10] so transmission efficiency is very nearly 100%. In some cases, there may be an additional strain limit imposed by supercoiling. Interestingly, double-stranded free DNA in vivo behaves much like a cable under torsional stress, with one negative superhelical turn per 100-200 base pairs (34-68 nm of "cable"); torsional stress is relieved by unwinding the double helix.[997]

However, thermal safety of in vivo mechanical power tethers is also of paramount concern. Under severe braking, loading or jamming of a cable, significant heat may be released. For a cable in vivo, a temperature rise of 63 K at the outer jacket surface (e.g., in contact with body fluids) boils water. Even a $\Delta T > 10$ K may constitute an unacceptable risk in a conservative nanomedical design, as this is more than enough to trigger biological responses, for example by heat-shock proteins (HSPs). (Activation of HSPs in some cases may be beneficial to human health, but conservative nanomedical design requires minimizing all such unplanned side-effects.)

In the most optimistic scenario, power is immediately shut off the instant a fault is detected, instantly converting a DC cable into a half-cycle AC cable under relaxation. To prevent stored energy from causing damage in the event of a heat pulse, a DC cable should never be operated faster than the fastest physically equivalent AC cable, e.g., $\nu_{DC} \lesssim \nu_{AC_m}$.

In the most pessimistic scenario, the cable jams at a single pointlike defect and then radiates the entire power flux from a sphere of radius $\sim r_{cable}$; the practical effect is to preclude power cables altogether, because total cable power could not be allowed to exceed the heat flux from a droplet of water of radius $\sim r_{cable}$ whose temperature had been raised by ΔT.

An intermediate, yet conservative, scenario allows that the entire power flux (not just the energy already stored in the cable) must be dissipated, but that the whole length of the cable may be employed as the radiator during a dissipative event—as, for example, if power continues to be transmitted after the fault but the cable jacket retains physical integrity. In this scenario, a cable carrying power flux I_{power} (W/m^2) through a medium of heat capacity C_V and thermal conductivity K_t overheats the immediate environment in a time $t_{overheat} \sim L_{cable}\, C_V\, \Delta T / I_{power}$, but thermal equilibration time $t_{EQ} \sim X_{bio}^2\, C_V / K_t$ where X_{bio} is a characteristic thermal conduction path length (e.g., minimum-size biological elements of size $X_{bio} \sim 1$ micron). Requiring for safety that $t_{overheat} > t_{EQ}$, then $I_{power} < (K_t\, L_{cable}\, \Delta T / X_{bio}^2)$, which defines considerably more restrictive operating frequency limits for cables.

For an AC cable in the intermediate thermal scenario, the energy density per cycle is $\sim(1/2)\, D_E$, giving at maximum frequency ν_{AC_t} a power flux of $I_{AC} = \nu_{AC_t}\, L_{cable}\, \sigma_w^2 / 2\, G$, hence:

$$\nu_{AC_t} \lesssim \frac{2\, G\, K_t\, \Delta T}{\sigma_w^2\, X_{bio}^2} \quad \text{(Hz)} \qquad \{\text{Eqn. 6.50}\}$$

For a DC cable in the intermediate thermal scenario, power flux is $I_{DC} = \sigma_w\, v_{burst} = 2\,\pi\, \nu_{DC_t}\, r_{cable}\, \sigma_w$, hence:

$$\nu_{DC_t} \lesssim \frac{L_{cable}\, K_t\, \Delta T}{2\,\pi\, r_{cable}\, \sigma_w\, X_{bio}^2} \quad \text{(Hz)} \qquad \{\text{Eqn. 6.51}\}$$

Adopting the intermediate scenario, the general conclusion is that very small cables tend to be thermally limited, while very large cables are both thermally and mechanically limited. In the following configurations, we assume a diamondoid cable with $\Delta T = 10$ K, $\rho = 3510$ kg/m^3 for diamond, $K_t = 0.623$ W/m-K for water at 310 K, and X_{bio} = 1 micron.

An AC cable carrying a power throughput of $\pi\, r_{cable}^2\, I_{AC}$ = 1000 pW (near-peak nanorobot requirement) with r_{cable} = 5 nm and L_{cable} = 2 microns is thermally limited to an operating frequency of $\nu_{AC_t} \lesssim 60$ KHz ($\ll \nu_{AC_m} \sim 6$ GHz), giving a power density of $I_{AC} / L_{cable} = 6 \times 10^{12}$ W/m^3. The same cable in DC mode is thermally limited to an operating frequency of $\nu_{DC_t} \lesssim 40$ KHz ($\ll \nu_{DC_m} \sim 70$ GHz) with the same power density. If thermal limits were ignored, the cable could carry 0.2 milliwatts in AC mode and 1 milliwatt in DC mode.

Similarly, an AC cable carrying a power throughput of $\pi\, r_{cable}^2\, I_{AC}$ = 100 watts (human basal requirement) with r_{cable} = 4 microns and L_{cable} = 0.4 meter is mechanically limited to an operating frequency of $\nu_{AC_m} \lesssim$ 30 KHz (< ν_{AC_t} ~ 60 KHz), again giving a power density of I_{AC} / L_{cable} = 6 x 10^{12} W/m^3. The same cable in DC mode is thermally limited to an operating frequency of $\nu_{DC_t} \lesssim$ 10 MHz (< ν_{DC_m} ~ 100 MHz) with the same power density. If thermal limits were ignored, the cable would still carry only 100 watts in AC mode but could carry up to 700 watts in DC mode.

The refractive index profile of a sufficiently wide (Section 6.4.3.2) rotating diamond cable could be engineered, and might possibly be made sufficiently transparent, to also act as a photonic channel simultaneously conveying optical power or communications signals.

6.4.3.5 Chemical Tethers

Chemical energy may also be delivered by tether at power densities > 10^{10} watts/m^3. Single tethers could bring ATP, glucose, or synthetic energy storage molecules (Section 6.2.3) directly to nanodevices in vivo. Double-tether cables could carry two hypergolic fuels, or a separate fuel and oxidizer, in a paired cable under pressure with the components mixed on site to release their stored energy. At 1000-10,000 atm pressures, most organic substances should undergo a hypergolic (spontaneous) reaction with oxygen piped in at equivalent pressure; safety would be a primary concern with this approach. Chemical tethers may also be used to resupply macroscopic energy organs (Section 6.4.4), or to exchange chemicals with an artificial nanoliver or other chemical modulating, processing, or synthesizing implanted nano-organs.

6.4.3.6 Power Tether Configurations In Vivo

If an application requires only a very small number of nanodevices operating in a very limited tissue volume for a brief period of time, then direct tethered power supply might be preferred. Tethered devices may employ simpler onboard energy conversion systems, hence may be appropriate for devices of more primitive design such as may exist in the early years of nanomedical technology development. Tethered power systems could be useful when working inside a tissue volume that has been drained of indigenous useful chemical energy resources and which has no bloodflow or active homeostatic processes, such as amputated limbs, massively ischemic organs, or cryogenically preserved tissues or bodies. Tethered power might also be acceptable for operations inside tissues with incomplete, non-existent, or low-density vascularization, such as the epidermis, or inside tissues with incompetent or compromised immune systems, such as an embryo or fetus. In cyto slaved nanodevices may transmit/receive power or data to/from an extracellular master nanorobot via transmembrane tethers (Section 9.4.5.6).

The two principal drawbacks to tethered supplies are physical vulnerability and tissue irritation (see also Section 7.3.3). Tethers may kink, break, or become tangled; failures in rotating cable tethers may include "drilling" and "weed-whacker" modes, chemical tethers can detach and leak, and so forth. If billions or trillions of medical nanodevices are deployed, these vulnerabilities are enhanced. In addition, tether volume may equal or exceed nanorobot volume, increasing intrusiveness and reducing nanorobot mobility. For instance, a 10 cm long tether measuring 20 nm in diameter that might be used to power a ~1 micron^3 device has a volume of ~30 micron^3—a clear case of the tail wagging the dog. Limb/organ macromotions and tissue micromovements may produce a microscale sawing action of tether fibers against tissues, causing irritation, inflammation (including leukokine release with macrophage and fibroblast mobilization), and possibly a granulomatous reaction unless tethers can be made with variable compliance to match the stiffness of the tissues through which they pass, adding greatly to design complexity. Mobile tethers deployed inside cells can mechanically excite cytoskeletal elements, eventually triggering unwanted gene expression cascades in the nucleus. Tethers deployed through blood vessel walls or cell membranes may face similar challenges regardless of the chemical biocompatibility of their exterior or sheathing surfaces.

The simplest tethered configuration for powering large numbers of nanorobots is to transmit external power into an energy organ (Section 6.4.4) using a single tether connection. A complete analysis of networks and configurations of more complex tethered nanorobot power supplies is beyond the scope of this book. However, several simple configurations include Cartesian, fractal, and hub systems. A Cartesian system is laid out along a regular gridwork using a rectangular, cylindrical, spherical, helical, or other coordinate system as appropriate to the biotopology. A fractal system resembles a branching vascular-like "power tree" inside the body, with tendrils following blood or lymph vessels and natural tissue graining. A hub system (aka "mother ship") employs an array of isolated distribution nodes, with numerous individual nanorobots directly connected to one or another node.

Tethers must be directed entirely through tissue; placement in the active bloodflow may precipitate prompt thrombosis from microturbulence shear forces or netting action with formed elements. Macrophagic responses characteristic of wound repair (Chapter 24) would likely be stimulated within hours of tissue entry as cellular shear force sensors activate cytokine signaling mechanisms in response to mechanical stresses. To avoid massive granulomatous reaction, tethers cannot be abandoned after use and probably must be spooled out during deployment and respooled during retraction, adding additional potential failure modes and increasing the time required for deployment or retraction, a major drawback in emergency situations.

It might be possible to carefully install a biocompatible electrical or fiberoptic power network throughout a patient's body (Section 7.3.1) as a permanent augmentation without causing irreparable damage. The presence of great numbers of isolated current-carrying wires creates numerous stray electrical fields that could affect cellular processes and possibly stimulate a macrophagic response; however, electric fields are minimal outside a well-shielded 1-micron-diameter coax or twisted-pair triax cable. If ~1 micron stray-field-free cables or optical fibers are used, a total network volume of ~10 cm^3 of fiber (~0.01% of human body volume) has ~13,000 kilometers of length; assuming ~1-meter strands and a simple Cartesian distribution, fibers have a mean lateral separation of ~80 microns between nearest neighbors (~4 cell widths).

6.4.4 Dedicated Energy Organs

Delivery of energy to in vivo nanorobots via tethers necessarily involves a hierarchical distribution network of some kind, ranging from maximum span (e.g., maximally horizontal hierarchy: all units directly connected to the external source) to minimum span (e.g., maximally vertical hierarchy: all units connected in series). Many intermediate network topologies are readily imaginable. Networks typically are most efficient at some optimum mix of spans and levels. To support this optimum mix, dedicated energy storage organs positioned at network nodes can add stability and longevity to the system and provide load buffering. Energy organs may act as distribution or routing devices, simply passing power down the line, or they may act as output nodes which are periodically encountered or revisited by in vivo nanorobots to recharge or refuel depleted onboard energy stores.

For example, we may envision a permanent macroscopic implanted device with a transdermal connector port. Through this port, the user recharges the internal energy organ by plugging in a source of compressed gas, by connecting through the port to a battery or a household electrical wall outlet, or by attaching an antenna system to facilitate the receipt of acoustic, mechanical, inductive, rf, infrared, or optical power signals. Chemical tethers could also resupply these energy organs: Assuming Poiseuille flow (Eqn. 9.25), ~40 mm^3/sec of stoichiometric oxyglucose fuel supply at 1000 atm pressure differential flowing (separately) through a double-tether ~1 meter in length and ~60 microns in diameter supplies the entire 100-watt human basal power requirement assuming 50% chemical energy conversion efficiency at the receiving end, with the glucose supplied in a saturated 70% aqueous solution at 310 K. Chemical tether power density ~ 4×10^{10} watts/m^3.

Inside the body, components of the implant may protrude into tissues or the bloodstream to supply power to internal nanorobots. These protrusions could act in broadcast mode, emitting acoustic or electrical power intracorporeally. Circumaortic current-carrying loops could energize bloodborne nanorobots as they passed through the vascular solenoid, although energy transfer efficiency may be low (Section 6.4.2) and possible biological effects of these electric fields on cellular systems should be studied further. Energy organ protrusions could release manufactured artificial energy-rich molecules (Section 6.2.3) or microscale fuel tankers containing energetic compounds directly into the bloodstream. Protrusions might act as "energy teats" to which nanorobots could dock and refuel or recharge, although this will require navigational beacons, docking mechanisms, transfer conduits, etc., thus increasing system complexity. Energy organ protrusions could also serve as catalytic or conversion nodes, transducing one form of energy into another, or as manufacturing nodes, converting less energetic chemicals into more energetic chemicals through the application of externally supplied energy. In all these cases, biocompatibility is a critical issue that must be fully addressed[3234] (Chapter 15).

Dedicated energy organs may range in size from hundreds of microns up to several centimeters, depending on the position in the distribution hierarchy and the task to be performed, and may themselves be recharged from other larger energy organs positioned higher up in the hierarchy, or directly from external sources. Given the maximum conventional energy storage density of ~10^{11} joules/m^3 (Section 6.2), the human basal energy requirement of ~2000 Kcal for one day could be stored in a (>4.4 cm)^3 cube. A special case is the nuclear powered energy organ containing a similar volume of Gd^{148} radionuclide, which could provide the same basal requirement for ~centuries (Section 6.3.7.1). Although a nuclear-powered organ is unlikely to be implemented in this manner, from Eqn. 6.27 a sphere of Gd^{148} emitting ~100 watts with a 75-year half-life and measuring 3.41 cm in diameter with a 5-micron Pt shield glows at 1326 K (e_r for Pt at 1326 K is 0.156; Gd melting point ~1585 K, Pt melting point ~2042 K); this is approximately the decomposition temperature of diamond (into graphite) and well above the combustion point for diamond in air (Section 6.5.3), so Pt-coated sapphire (sapphire melting point ~2310 K[1602]) may provide a more stable first wall for the radionuclide energy organ. Carnot thermal efficiency for a heat engine using this source could reach, at most, ~76%.

6.5 Design Energetics Assessment

6.5.1 Power in Biological Cells

Table 6.8 summarizes the total power outputs and power densities of various cells in the human body, adapted from numerous experimental studies on tissue metabolism using assumed cell volumes as listed. Relatively inactive red cells produce only ~0.01 pW, while thermogenic fat cells may release 8 million times more energy during shivering. Muscle cells and platelets have very low basal rates, but are capable of brief bursts of high power density. The typical human tissue cell operates at ~30 pW and at this power level has ~2000 sec of free glucose energy available solely from internal stores without requiring external resupply, assuming ~50% energy conversion efficiency. Biological power densities range from 10^2-10^6 watts/m^3, with the typical tissue cell operating at about 3800 watts/m^3. The active flight muscle of the honeybee has the highest known power density in biology (3.4 million watts/m^3).

6.5.2 Thermogenic Limits In Vivo

Consider nanorobots at work inside a single biological cell of size L_{cell}, volume $V_{cell} = L_{cell}^3$, and thermal conductivity $K_t = 0.623$ watts/m-K (water) immersed in a large isothermal heat sink. The maximum temperature differential ΔT_n between core and periphery caused by the intracellular release of P_{cell} (watts) due to nanorobot activity is:

$$\Delta T_{cell} = \frac{P_{cell}}{6\, L_{cell}\, K_t} = \frac{D_{cell}\, L_{cell}^2}{6\, K_t} \quad \text{(kelvins)} \qquad \text{\{Eqn. 6.52\}}$$

where D_{cell} is total cellular energy density (watts/m^3). A typical ~20 micron diameter human tissue cell produces 30-480 pW, giving ΔT_{cell} = 0.3-6.0 microkelvins. The data in Table 6.8 indicates that individual cells appear to safely tolerate internal energy releases up to D_{cell} ~ 10^6 watts/m^3, which leads to the following proposed thermogenic limit for in cyto operations:

$$P_{cell} \lesssim 10^6\, V_{cell} \quad \text{(watts)} \qquad \text{\{Eqn. 6.53\}}$$

Thus, for example, using the proposed limit an isolated 20-micron tissue cell can safely host in its interior a set of active nanorobotic machinery that in total generates P_{cell} ~ 8000 pW and raises cell temperature by ΔT_{cell} ~ 100 microkelvins, which seems extremely conservative.

If many cells in a given block of tissue contain active nanomachinery, as will often be the case, then the assumption of an isothermal heat sink no longer holds because the nanorobots will collectively warm up their operating environment. In the limit of an entire human body, a 100-watt total nanorobot power expenditure giving a whole-body 1000 watt/m^3 incremental power density (Table 6.8) seems quite conservative since 50,000-100,000 watts/m^3 is considered the safe therapeutic range for medical diathermy.[819] A temperature rise in the tissues triggers an increase in blood flow, which in turn produces a cooling effect. The maximum thermal load that an adult can dissipate under room temperature conditions without an increase in body temperature is a whole-body exposure of 100 watts/m^2,[822] or ~2000 watts/m^3. Thus a 100-watt whole-body nanorobot power budget normally will produce no measurable increase in body temperature.

Table 6.8 Estimated Power Output and Measured Power Density of Biological Cells and Human Tissues

Organelle, Cell or Object	Estimated Power Output (picowatts)	Assumed Volume (micron^3)	Measured Power Density (watts/m^3)	Compiled, Computed or Estimated from: (References)
Myosin muscle motor	0.000001	5×10^{-7}	2.0×10^6	578
Bacterial flagellar motor	0.0001	5×10^{-5}	2.0×10^6	581
S. faecalis bacterium (basal)	0.00035	0.2	1.8×10^3	798
Platelet (resting)	0.003-0.09	3	$0.1\text{-}3.0 \times 10^4$	791,792,796
Red blood cell	0.008	94	8.5×10^1	789
E. coli bacterium (basal)	0.05	2	2.5×10^2	797
Mitochondrion organelle	0.1-1.1	1	$0.1\text{-}1.1 \times 10^6$	781,786
S. faecalis bacterium (maximum growth)	0.23	0.2	1.2×10^6	798
Chondrocyte	0.3	670	4.0×10^2	744
Platelet (activated)	0.7-7.0	3	$0.2\text{-}2.3 \times 10^6$	790
Skin cell	1-3	1000	$1.0\text{-}3.1 \times 10^3$	744,783,794,818
Skeletal muscle cell (resting)	1-10	2000	$0.5\text{-}4.9 \times 10^3$	526.744.818
Neutrophil leukocyte	2-9	450	$0.4\text{-}2.0 \times 10^4$	753,792,796
Osteocyte (bone)	2-38	30,000	$0.08\text{-}1.3 \times 10^3$	744,818
Pancreatic cell	9	1000	8.9×10^3	745
Relaxed resting cardiac muscle cell	16	8000	2.0×10^3	788
Diaphragm muscle cell	20	2000	1.0×10^4	744
Liver cell (hepatocyte)	45-115	6400	$0.7\text{-}1.8 \times 10^4$	744,745,782,783,818
Typical Tissue Cell (basal)	***30***	***8000***	$\boldsymbol{3.8 \times 10^3}$	***744,745,782***
T-Cell lymphocyte (basal)	40	200	2.0×10^5	470,777
Bone marrow cell	45	8000	5.6×10^3	745
Intestine/Stomach cell	46-52	8000	$5.7\text{-}6.5 \times 10^3$	745
Testicular cell	46-149	8000	$0.6\text{-}1.9 \times 10^4$	745
Lung cell	56-78	8000	$7.1\text{-}9.7 \times 10^3$	744,745,782
Brown fat cell (resting)	60	200,000	3.0×10^2	745,818
Spleen cell	60-80	8000	$7.5\text{-}9.9 \times 10^3$	745
Neuron cell (basal)	70-110	14,000	$5.0\text{-}7.9 \times 10^3$	744,745,747,779,782
Thymus cell	74	8000	9.3×10^3	745
Heart muscle cell (typical)	87-290	8000	$1.1\text{-}3.6 \times 10^4$	744,782,783,795,818
Skeletal muscle cell (max., voluntary)	113	2000	5.7×10^4	818
Thyroid cell	130	8000	1.6×10^4	745
T-Cell lymphocyte (antigen response)	130	200	6.5×10^5	470,777
Adrenal cell	150	8000	1.9×10^4	745
Kidney cell	155-346	8000	$1.9\text{-}4.3 \times 10^4$	744,745,782,818
Neuron cell (maximum)	255-330	14,000	$1.8\text{-}2.4 \times 10^4$	746,779
Typical Tissue Cell (maximum)	***480***	***8000***	$\boldsymbol{6.0 \times 10^4}$	***745,780,782***
Skeletal muscle cell (max., tetanic)	2300	2000	1.2×10^6	526
Honeybee flight muscle cell	3400	1000	3.4×10^6	---
Heart muscle cell (maximum)	3500-5000	8000	$4.4\text{-}6.3 \times 10^5$	783,787
Pancreatic islet (multi-cell)	50,000-90,000	8,000,000	$0.6\text{-}1.1 \times 10^4$	793
Brown fat cell (thermogenic)	64,000	200,000	3.2×10^5	786
Human brain	15-25 watts	1.4×10^{-3} m^3	$1.1\text{-}1.8 \times 10^4$	746,747,784,785
Human body (basal)	100 watts	0.1 m^3	1.0×10^3	780
Human body (maximum)	1600 watts	0.1 m^3	1.6×10^4	780
Gasoline-powered automobile	200,000 watts	10 m^3	2.0×10^4	Author's 1969 Oldsmobile
The Sun	3.92×10^{26} watts	1.41×10^{27} m^3	0.28	1662

Operated at its peak output of 1600 watts,[780,865] the human body's core temperature rises ~3.5 K.[821] Even assuming a simple linear relation, a whole-body 100-watt nanorobot power budget would correspond to an increase in core body temperature of at most ~0.2 K, far smaller than the mean normal diurnal variation of ~1 K (Section 6.3.1) and less than the ~0.2-0.5 K load error in the human thermoregulatory control system.[865] Since glucose-powered nanorobots may compete with tissues for fuel, a 100-watt total withdrawal also represents ~2000 Kcal/day, near the limit of what can be conveniently replaced dietetically on a long-term basis.

A proper comprehensive analysis of energy flows[818] requires a detailed model of body geometry, incident radiation, skin emissivity, convection currents, heat exchange by conduction, evaporative cooling, respiratory heat losses, physiological and behavioral thermoregulatory responses, work done by the patient, and the precise distribution, clumping patterns and activities of in vivo nanorobots, all of which is very complex and quite beyond the scope of this book. However, a simple log-linear interpolative relation with correct endpoints ($D_{tiss} = 10^6$ watts/m^3 at $L_{tiss} = 20$ microns and $D_{tiss} = 10^3$ watts/m^3 at $L_{tiss} = 0.5$ meters) suggests the following proposed crude maximum thermogenic limits for nanorobot operations in human soft tissue:

$$P_{tiss} \lesssim V_{tiss} D_{tiss} \quad \text{(watts)} \qquad \text{\{Eqn. 6.54\}}$$

$$D_{tiss} \sim 10^{[2.77 - 0.687 \log_{10}(L_{tiss})]} \quad \text{(watts/m}^3\text{)} \qquad \text{\{Eqn. 6.55\}}$$

$$\Delta T_{tiss} \sim \frac{P_{tiss}}{1800\, L_{tiss}^{\pi/2}} \quad \text{(kelvins)} \qquad \text{\{Eqn. 6.56\}}$$

where $V_{tiss} = L_{tiss}^3$ for the total volume of soft tissue in which all deployed nanorobots are active. (Eqns. 6.52 through 6.56 are summarized in Figs. 6.14 and 6.15). Thus, for example, medical nanorobots deployed solely in the thyroid gland ($L_{tiss} \sim 2.6$ cm; Table 8.9) should be restricted to a maximum total power budget $P_{tiss} \sim 0.1$ watt which elevates thyroid temperature by $\Delta T_{tiss} \sim 0.02$ K. Higher in vivo power densities may sometimes be justified in hospital or emergency medical situations (Chapter 24), and a few other special circumstances (e.g., Chapter 21).

6.5.3 Nanorobot Power Scaling

As an initial, crude order-of-magnitude estimate of nanorobot power consumption, allometric scaling of metabolism in biology for whole organisms follows a 3/4 power law.[698,3242] Normalizing to P = 100 watts for an m = 70 kg human body mass and assuming ~water density for nanorobots, then $P = (4.13)\, m^{3/4} = 23$ pW for a 1 micron^3 nanorobot, a power density of $D_n \sim 2 \times 10^7$ watts/m^3.

Surface power intensity considerations drive maximum nanorobot onboard power density. For instance, the maximum safe intensity for ultrasound is 100-1000 watts/m^2 (pain threshold for human hearing ~100 watts/m^2) (Section 6.4.1) and the conservative maximum safe electromagnetic intensity is also ~100 watts/m^2 (Section 6.4.2). Additionally, a surface at 373 K (boiling water) relative to a 310 K environment radiates 100-1000 watts/m^2 at emissivities $e_r = 0.1$-1 (Eqn. 6-19). Conservatively taking 100 watts/m^2 as the maximum safe energy flux across the surface of a spherical nanorobot of radius r_n, then the maximum nanorobot power density is

$$D_n = \frac{300}{r_n} \sim 10^9 \quad \text{(watts/m}^3\text{)} \qquad \text{\{Eqn. 6.57\}}$$

for a device ~1 micron in diameter—the largest safe whole-device power density that should be developed in vivo. A 10^9 watt/m^3 maximum implies a ~1000 pW limit for 1 micron^3 nanorobots. Interestingly, the energy dissipation rate required to disrupt the plasma membrane of ~95% of all animal cells transported in forced turbulent capillary flows is on the order of ~10^8-10^9 watts/m^3.[1185]

For chemically powered foraging nanorobots, another fundamental constraint on power density is imposed by diffusion limits on fuel molecules. From Eqn. 3.4, the maximum diffusion current of glucose molecules of energy content $E_{fuel} = E_{glu}$ (4765 zJ; Eqn. 6.16), burned at efficiency e% ~ 0.50 (50%) in oxygen, to the surface of a spherical nanorobot of radius r_n will support a maximum onboard power density of:

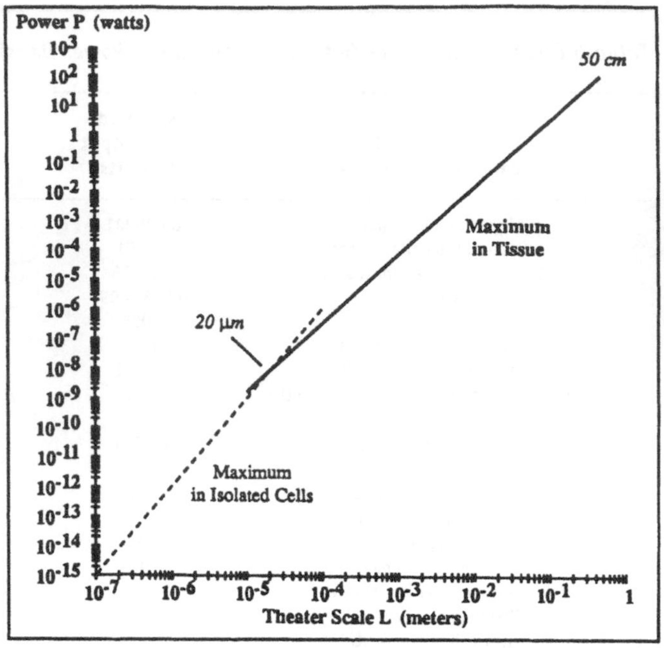

Fig. 6.14. Recommended maximum total nanomachinery power consumption in isolated cells and in human tissue.

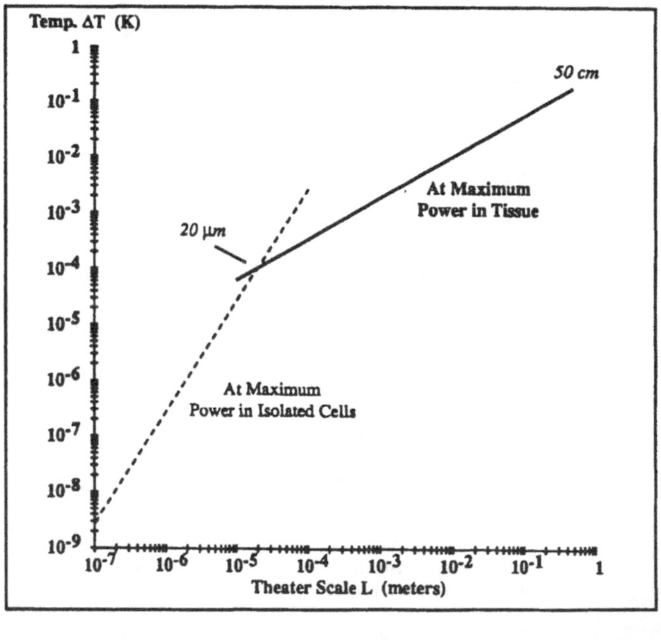

Fig. 6.15. Maximum temperature change produced by nanorobot power released in isolated cells and in human tissue.

$$D_{diff} = \frac{3\, e\%\, E_{fuel}\, D\, C}{r_n^2} \quad \text{(watts/m}^3\text{)} \qquad \text{\{Eqn. 6.58\}}$$

For $D = 7.1 \times 10^{-10}$ m^2/sec for glucose in water at 310 K (Table 3.3), $C = (0.67)\ 3.5 \times 10^{24}$ molecules/m^3 in (newborn and) adult

Since oxyglucose foraging nanorobots are not seriously glucose-limited, there is little to be gained by enabling energy organs or cooperative nanorobot populations to secrete insulin/glucagon hormones (mimicking the pancreas), cortisol hormones, etc. to artificially manipulate serum glucose levels. Available oxygen also may be artificially manipulated using nanorobotic compressed gas dispensers[1400] or by other means (Chapter 22).

***Note that as nanodevices get smaller, their surface/volume ratio expands. Thus the Square/Cube law predicts that smaller nanodevices can admit more energy (e.g., chemical, acoustic, electromagnetic) through their surfaces per unit enclosed volume of working nanomachinery, hence can have higher power densities, as illustrated by Eqn. 6.58.*

human blood plasma (Appendix B), and $r_n \sim 0.5$ micron, D_{diff} = 1-7 x 10^{10} watts/m^3. However, because oxygen dissolves only slightly in blood plasma and interstitial fluid, the oxyglucose engine is more severely diffusion-limited by its oxygen requirements than by its glucose requirements.* Applying Eqn. 6.58 and using (for oxygen) D = 2.0 x 10^{-9} m^2/sec (Table 3.3), C = 7.3 x 10^{22} molecules/m^3 in arterial blood plasma (Appendix B), $E_{fuel} \sim E_{glu}/6$, and $r_n \sim 0.5$ micron, D_{diff} = 7 x 10^8 watts/m^3. Once again, ~10^9 watts/m^3 appears to be a correct upper limit for whole nanorobots.**

The disposition of combustion byproducts, particularly CO_2, may provide another weak constraint on chemical systems. For example, a 10-pW glucose-burning nanorobot generates ~10^7 molecules/sec of CO_2. Pressurized to 1000 atm, this production rate fills ~0.001 $micron^3$/sec of onboard storage space, assuming no venting. If CO_2 is vented from a population of 10^{12} 10-pW nanorobots uniformly distributed throughout a ~0.1 m^3 human body volume, then local CO_2 concentration rises by ~2 x 10^{-7} M/sec, reaching 0.0003 M after 1 hour of continuous operation assuming no physiological removal—still well below the normal ~0.001M blood plasma CO_2 concentration.

By implication, these limits also drive the maximum number density of nanodevices deployable in human tissue. For example, at 10^9 watts/m^3 the hottest 1-micron nanorobot develops 1000 pW; assuming a ~0.1 watt power budget when restricted to the thyroid gland (Section 6.5.2), 100 million nanodevices may be deployed in the gland giving a maximum number density of ~10^{13} nanorobots/m^3. Nanorobot power consumption may range from ~0.1 pW for simple respirocytes[1400] (Chapter 22) up to ~10,000 pW or more for the largest and most sophisticated repair and defensive in vivo devices (Chapter 21), but the typical simple micron-scale nanorobot may develop ~10 pW (roughly in line with biologically-derived allometric scaling laws giving $D_n \sim 10^7$ watts/m^3) and thus could safely achieve a number density of ~10^{15} nanorobots/m^3 (~10 micron mean interdevice separation). Recall that the maximum diffusion-limited total power draw for a population of oxygen-unrestricted glucose-energized foraging nanorobots in cyto is ~70,000-300,000 pW (Section 6.3.4.1).

Minimum powerplant size varies with requirements. Assuming $\gtrsim 10^{12}$ watts/m^3 energy conversion for chemical (Section 6.3.4) or electrical (Section 6.4.1) power transducers, then a 100 pW power supply subsystem inside a working nanorobot may be as small as (~50 nm)^3 in size.

Macroscale masses of working nanodevices may grow extremely hot, placing major scaling limits on artificial nano-organs and other large-scale nanomachinery aggregates (Chapter 14). As a somewhat fanciful example, consider a macroscopic ball of radius R consisting of N tightly-packed nanodevices each of mass density ρ and whole-nanorobot power density $D_p \sim 10^9$ watts/m^3, of which nanodevices some fraction f_n are active, all suspended in mid-air. The ball grows hotter as R (~$N^{1/3}$) rises, until at some "critical combustible mass" $M_{crit} = (4/3)\,\pi\,\rho\,R_{crit}^3$ the surface temperature exceeds the maximum combustion point for diamond in air (T_{burn} = 1070 K)[691] and the solid ball of nanorobots bursts into flame. (Sapphire devices cannot burn, but have a $T_{melt} \sim 2310$ K;[1602] as a practical matter, nanomachinery may fail at temperatures significantly below T_{burn}.)

From simple geometry and neglecting ~2% air conduction losses, the maximum noncombustible aggregate radius R_{crit} is:

$$R_{crit} \sim \frac{3\,\sigma\,e_r\left(T_{burn}^4 - T_{environ}^4\right)}{f_n\,D_p} \qquad \text{\{Eqn. 6.59\}}$$

For e_r = 0.97 (e.g., carbon black) to maximize heat emission at the lowest possible temperature and $T_{environ}$ = 300 K, then R_{crit} = 0.22 mm for f_n = 100%. Assuming a full cold start, critical time to incineration is $t_{crit} = C_V\,(T_{burn} - T_{environ})\,/\,f_n\,D_p$ = 1.4 sec for f_n = 100% if nanorobot heat capacity C_V = 1.8 x 10^6 joules/m^3-K (~diamondoid). Decreasing D_p to a more reasonable 10^7 watts/m^3 or simply switching off 99% of the nanorobots (f_n = 1%) increases R_{crit} to ~22 cm.

6.5.4 Selection of Principal Power Source

In selecting the ultimate source of power for a given application, the appropriate energy acquisition strategy must first be decided. Two overall strategies are readily distinguished: (1) nonrefuelable and (2) refuelable.

A nonrefuelable strategy implies that all nanorobot power is drawn from internal energy storage. Such a nanorobot simply stops when its internal energy stores are depleted. The relevant parameter is onboard energy storage density, which should be maximized. From Section 6.2, chemical energy storage produces the highest energy density, up to ~10^{11} joules/m^3. (Nuclear storage has a much higher theoretical energy density, but in medically "safe" fissile systems the rate of energy withdrawal from the store cannot be precisely regulated using known technology, thus limiting the effective energy density of this potential source.) A 1 $micron^3$ store of chemical energy at a conservative 10^{10} joules/m^3 powers a 10 pW nanorobot for ~10^3 sec, which may be sufficient in some applications.

A refuelable strategy implies that onboard energy stores serve mainly as buffers, which are refilled periodically or continuously from external chemical, sonic, electrical, or tethered sources. A relevant parameter is now the rate of energy transfer, or environmental power density, which should be maximized consistent with safety. Again, at least two strategies can be distinguished: (2A) in vivo sources and (2B) ex vivo sources. In vivo power sources may include free-flowing chemical fuels (e.g., bloodstream glucose circulating once every 60 seconds represents ~2 x 10^5 watts/m^3), encapsulated chemical fuels, or implanted dedicated energy organs. Ex vivo power sources may include acoustic ($\lesssim$2 x 10^4 watts/m^3), electromagnetic ($\lesssim$2 x 10^3 watts/m^3), or tethered sources. For tethered sources, a safe properly configured 1-meter tether 1 micron in diameter transfers hydraulic energy at ~10^5 watts/m^3 (at 1000 atm), fiberoptic photonic energy at ~10^6 watts/m^3, electrical energy at ~10^7 watts/m^3 (silver wire, ~10^7 amp/m^2 at ~1 volt), chemical energy at ~10^8 watts/m^3 (at 1000 atm), or mechanical energy up to ~10^{10} watts/m^3.

However, this is only the first step of the analysis because the initial energy, once received, must be transduced into other useful forms which may be used to drive onboard systems. Most nanorobot designs will involve energy transduction chains of various lengths, so the efficiency of the entire chain is also a relevant parameter driving the choice of initial power source. Consider, for example, a nanorobot requiring electrical power for some internal function. While the maximum available electrical power density in the environment may be comparatively low, the advantage of a much higher available chemical power density may be offset by a relatively low direct chemoelectric transduction efficiency (Section 6.3.4.5). On the other hand, the relative efficiency of the chemoelectrical pathway may be improved by using a glucose engine to generate mechanical motions, which motions may then be converted to electrical energy via highly efficient mechanoelectrical transduction (Section 6.3.2).

6.5.5 Electrical vs. Mechanical Systems

Because of the ubiquity of electrochemical processes in biological systems, it is natural to assume that electrical power would be the energy of choice to drive nanomedical systems. However, it is clear that mechanically powered nanorobots are competitive because mechanical energy may be transmitted at very high efficiency over nanoscale distances. Fully mechanical motors, pumps, actuators, manipulators, and even computers have been designed.[10]

The principal disadvantages of electrically-powered nanorobots include:

A. *Bioelectric Interactions* — Electrical systems can create stray fields which may activate bioelectric-based molecular recognition systems in biology. While electrical systems allow ready coupling with electrochemical systems in the body, stray fields also may provoke unintended electrokinetic interactions. For example, all galvanic sources have been found to provoke a significant host reaction, including formation of layers of necrotic debris, free neutrophils, granulation tissue and complete fibrous connective tissue encapsulation of long-term implants.[590,3512] Microelectrophoretic interactions with possible natural rf oscillations of cells[683] could present additional complications. Stray high-frequency vibrations from purely mechanical systems may be less provocative.

B. *Electrical Interference* — Electrical nanorobots are susceptible to electrical interference from external sources such as rf or electric fields, EMP pulses, and stray fields from other in vivo electrical devices. (Digital cellular telephones have been reported interfering with implanted cardiac pacemakers, causing the pacemakers to speed up, slow down, or even turn off.[3495-3498]) Cosmic rays can provoke arc discharges in systems operated at high electrical potential.

C. *Thick Insulators* — Very thick insulation is required to prevent electron leakage, especially serious at the smallest sizes where significant quantum mechanical tunneling can occur. Without careful design, the high conductivity of the in vivo medium* can cause sudden power loss, e.g., by "shorting out."

D. *Thick Wires* — Relatively thick wires are needed to conduct significant power levels without overheating, although future room-temperature superconductors might reduce this disadvantage.

The principal advantages of electrically-powered nanorobots include:

E. *Speed of Operation* — Electronic field configurations have a velocity near the speed of light ($c \sim 3 \times 10^8$ m/sec), much faster than mechanical logic rods which may move as slow as 1 m/sec. Even the classical electron drift speed v_d in a bulk metallic conductor at high current density I_d may be faster than mechanical rod motions: $v_d = I_d / n_e e$, where $n_e = 8.4 \times 10^{28}$ electrons/m^3 for copper and $e = 1.6 \times 10^{-19}$ coul/electron, giving $v_d \sim 100$ m/sec at $I_d \sim 10^{10}$ amps/m^2, near the maximum current density. (A more typical $I_d \sim 10^6$ amps/m^2 gives $v_d \sim 1$ cm/sec.) And the mobility of an electron confined to a one-dimensional wire or patterned diamondoid channel can be much higher than in the bulk material, up to $\sim 10^6$ m/sec or ~0.3%c.[1097,1098] Thus applications demanding the greatest speeds may require electrical systems.

F. *Electromagnetic Coupling* — Detection of photons and electric/magnetic fields is more easily mediated by an electrical transmission device than a mechanical device. For instance, a photocell or rhodopsin antenna absorbs photons to directly create moving charges. This is probably more efficient than using a piezoelectric transducer backwards as a detector, but involves handling higher-energy packets of energy which is inherently riskier.

G. *Transmission Attenuation* — Electrical signals at sub-MHz frequencies are only modestly attenuated during passage through human tissue.

6.5.6 Power Analysis in Design

An important part of any nanodevice design exercise is a detailed assessment of power requirements and heat dissipation. Such an assessment might typically include the following elements:

A. *Molecular Transport* — Sorting rotors, internal transport mechanisms, sieving or nanocentrifugation, and receptor-based transport have specific power requirements (Chapter 3). Sorting rotors operating at full speed ($\sim 10^5$ rev/sec) dissipate $\sim 10^{10}$ watts/m^3. However, it should be possible to boost efficiency in some continuous molecular exchange systems by recovering most of the sorting energy by compressing (or concentrating) one species using energy derived largely from the decompression (or deconcentration) of the other via differential gearing.

B. *Chemical Transformations* — Drexler[10] estimates that the energy dissipation caused by chemical transformations involving carbon-rich materials is ~1000 zJ/atom or $\sim 10^8$ joules/kg of final product using readily-envisioned irreversible methods in systems where low energy dissipation is not a design objective, but may in theory be as low as ~1 zJ/atom or $\sim 10^5$ joules/kg "if one assumes the development of a set of mechanochemical processes capable of transforming feedstock molecules into complex product structures using only reliable, nearly reversible steps." However, R. Merkle notes that essentially all current proposals are quite dissipative. Most interactions with biological molecules may also have relatively low energy densities because common cut-and-repair operations can involve only a small number of covalent bonds on a single macromolecule. For example, forging just one new 1000-zJ covalent bond on a single 500-residue protein molecule containing ~10,000 atoms has a net molecular transformation cost of only ~0.1 zJ/atom. Transformations involving noncovalent bonds can have even lower per-atom energy costs.

C. *Mechanical Operations* — As a crude rule, physically active nanocomponents such as rotating roller bearings generate $\sim 10^5$ watts/m^3 of waste heat; inactive parts produce no waste heat. Larger mechanical assemblages such as nanomanipulator arms dissipate $\sim 10^9$ watts/m^3 in normal continuous operation,[10] or ~1 megawatt/kg for active diamondoid nanomachinery. Energy required for locomotion, actuation and manipulation is described in Chapter 9; energy requirements for shape-changing or other metamorphic activities must also be assessed (Chapter 5).

---

*The purest water (e.g., distilled and deionized) has a specific resistance of 2.5×10^5 ohm-m.[390] It is normally difficult to obtain and store water with resistivity exceeding $\sim 10^4$ ohm-m because of the absorption of CO_2 and other air gases, and of alkali and other electrolytes leached from glassware; ordinary distilled water in equilibrium with air has resistivity ~1000 ohm-m.[390] These values may be compared to 1.59×10^{-8} ohm-m for silver at 293 K,[763] 3.5×10^{-5} ohm-m for amorphous carbon at 293 K,[1662] 0.0893 ohm-m for 1M KCl in water at 298 K and 68.1 ohm-m for 0.001M KCl solution[390] (human blood is ~0.15M NaCl), 10^7-10^8 ohm-m for synthesized diamond (depending on the growth process used), and $>10^{18}$ ohm-m dark resistivities in natural diamond.[537]

D. *Communication and Navigation* — There must be a design assessment of the energy required, if any, for internal navigation (Chapter 8) and for all communication tasks (Chapter 7) including intradevice and interdevice signaling, inmessaging and outmessaging, plus allocation of systemic overhead for communications and navigational networks.

E. *Computation* — Mechanical nanocomputers using rod logic in the design described by Drexler[10] dissipate ~10^{12} watts/m^3 at ~GHz clock rates, yielding ~10^{10} MIPS/watt or ~10^4 instructions/sec per pW (~10^{28} instructions/sec-m^3). R. Merkle suggests that the use of nearly reversible computational operations[713] may reduce energy requirements per instruction by at least two orders of magnitude, at the cost of a slower clock cycle. With standard logic, dissipative irreversible operations can approach a minimum energy dissipation of ln(2) kT ~ 3 zJ per operation at 310 K, and in principle with reversible logic a computer can dissipate arbitrarily less energy per logic operation (Section 10.2.4.1). Nevertheless, total nanorobotic power demand will often be dominated by computational energy requirements (Section 10.2).

F. *Component Assembly* — Fabricating nanoscale diamondoid parts using hydrogen-rich organic feedstock molecules and oxygen generates energy, because the process involves a controlled, but highly-exoergic, combustion reaction. In a well-known example given by Drexler,[10] "burning" hydrocarbon to make diamondoid liberates 17 MJ/kg of gross energy, less 1.7 MJ/kg of local entropy decrease in the reactants, giving ~15 MJ/kg of free energy; assuming 3 MJ/kg dissipated in the mills, rotors, and computers needed to drive the manufacturing process, a net output of 12 MJ/kg of surplus energy is produced. However, subsequent higher-order assembly processes using this diamondoid material are endoergic. In the worst case, assembly of larger diamondoid structures from 1-nm cubes may cost ~9 MJ/kg, although with proper technique most of this energy can be recovered as mechanical work, reducing the cost of block assembly of larger structures to as low as ~0.5-1.0 MJ/kg.[10] Leaving aside the initial exoergic energy production, then depending upon computation, materials handling, and other requirements in a particular implementation, assembling prefabricated diamondoid part-like or module-like components into larger structures will probably cost ~1-3 MJ/kg of energy[10](Chapter 19).

6.5.7 Global Hypsithermal Limit

Finally, it is possible to derive a limit to the total planetary active nanorobot mass by considering the global energy balance. Total solar insolation received at the Earth's surface is ~1.75×10^{17} watts (I_{Earth} ~ 1370 W/m^2 ± 0.4% at normal incidence[887,1945]). Global energy consumption by mankind reached an estimated 1.2×10^{13} watts (~0.02 W/m^2) in 1998. This latter figure may also be regarded as the total heat dissipation of all human technological civilization worldwide, as distinct from the ~10^{12} watt metabolic output of the global human biomass. The evidence for global warming remains controversial,[887] but it is clear that as the waste heat from human-built machinery continues to grow, the climate will begin to change. Technological heat plumes from asphalt-covered major cities already have demonstrable impact on local weather and thermal patterns.

Leaving aside all considerations of changing concentrations of various atmospheric components (e.g., CO_2, H_2O, O_3), one might ask at what point anthropogenic energy releases could begin to seriously affect the global energy balance. (Climatologists sometimes call this the "hypsithermal limit.") Global warming data remain inconclusive but certainly suggest that the present ~10^{13} watts may lie within an order of magnitude of an important threshold. The power dissipation of all terrestrial vegetation is ~10^{14} watts,* and it is well-known that such vegetation plays a major role in the planetary energy equation. Climatologists have speculated that an anthropogenic release of ~2×10^{15} watts (~1% solar insolation) might cause the polar icecaps to melt. A high upper limit is provided by Venus, which receives ~3.3×10^{17} watts at its cloudtops, producing a surface temperature of ~700 K and a hellish ~100 atm sulfurous atmosphere—despite its close geological and size similarity to Earth. As a fairly liberal estimate,[3100,3101] the maximum hypsithermal limit for Earth is taken to be ~10^{15} watts.

The hypsithermal ecological limit in turn imposes a maximum power limit on the entire future global mass of active nanomachinery or "active nanomass." Assuming the typical power density of active nanorobots is ~10^7 W/m^3, the hypsithermal limit implies a natural worldwide population limit of ~10^8 m^3 of active functioning nanorobots, or ~10^{11} kg at normal densities. Assuming the worldwide human population stabilizes near ~10^{10} people in the 21st century and assuming a uniform distribution of nanotechnology, the above population limit would correspond to a per capita allocation of ~10 kg of active continuously-functioning nanorobotry, or ~10^{16} active nanorobots per person (assuming 1 micron^3 nanorobots developing ~10 pW each, and ignoring non-active devices held in inventory).** Whether a ~10-liter per capita allocation (~100 KW/person) is sufficient for all medical, manufacturing, transportation and other speculative purposes is a matter of debate.

The hypsithermal active nanorobot population limit cannot be defeated by heroic artifices of planetary engineering such as giant Earth-orbiting sunscreens or planetary-scale heat pumps, which would devastate global photosynthetic activity or climate while not significantly reducing thermal energy density at the Earth's surface. Likewise, significantly reducing the atmospheric concentration of the most important natural greenhouse gases, especially CO_2 and H_2O, on a worldwide basis is not possible if the present ecology is to remain essentially undisturbed, but even the complete elimination of such gases would raise the hypsithermal limit by at most a factor of 10-20. Specifically, if Earth had no atmosphere at all, then to maintain the global mean surface temperature at its current value of T_{Earth} ~ 288 K,[3097] an additional nanorobogenic power of $P_{noatm} \sim \pi R_{Earth}^2 (4 \sigma T_{Earth}^4 - I_{Earth}) \sim 2 \times 10^{16}$ watts could be released at the Earth's surface, where $R_{Earth} = 6.37 \times 10^6$ m (radius of Earth) and $\sigma = 5.67 \times 10^{-8}$ W/m^2-K^4 (Stefan-Boltzmann constant). Still more unrealistically, if Earth's surface were an atmosphere-free black body surrounded by a perfect mirror (e.g., albedo = 1.00, vs. ~0.31 for natural Earth), an additional nanorobogenic power release (underneath the mirrored barrier) of $P_{mirror} \lesssim 4 \pi R_{Earth}^2 (\sigma T_{Earth}^4 - I_{geol}) \sim 2 \times 10^{17}$ watts would allow maintenance of the current mean global surface temperature T_{Earth}; $I_{geol} = 0.05$ W/m^2,[3123] the mean geological heat flow at Earth's surface due to radioactive decay (e.g., U^{238}, K^{40}) in the crust. Reductions in nanorobot waste heat made possible by low-dissipative molecular manufacturing and reversible computing may be offset by popular

**Global photosynthetic fixation of CO_2 by plants is ~3.85×10^{14} kg CO_2/yr, ~46% by ocean flora;[1720] CO_2 fixation requires ~794 zJ/molecule (Eqn. 6.16) or ~1.1×10^7 J/kg CO_2, giving a global vegetative total of ~1.4×10^{14} watts.*

***Note that a global population limit of ~10^{26} 10-pW nanorobots represents only ~100 moles of active devices; for 1000-pW devices (~10^9 W/m^3 power density), the upper population limit is only ~1 mole of 1-micron^3 active nanorobots worldwide. Facile talk of controlling localized "mole quantities" of nanodevices is thus highly misleading.*

insistence on adherence to a more conservative global limit, perhaps ~10^{13} watts (today's level), to better preserve the terrestrial habitat. Consistent with long-term ecological maintenance the hypsithermal limit ultimately can only be avoided by continuing human technological progress in space, which seems an excellent idea in any case.

CHAPTER 7

Communication

7.1 Nanorobot Communications Requirements

Communication is an important fundamental capability of medical nanorobots. At the most basic level, nanomachines must pass sensory and control data among internal subsystems to ensure stable and correct device operation. They must also exchange messages with biological cells, communicating with the human body at the molecular level. Nanodevices must be able to communicate with each other in order to:

1. coordinate complex, large-scale cooperative activities,
2. pass along relevant sensory, messaging, navigational, and other operational data, and
3. monitor collective task progress.

Finally, nanorobots must be able to receive messages from, and transmit messages to, both the human patient and external entities including antennas and telecommunications links, laboratory or bedside computers, and attending medical personnel.

It is instructive first to examine the gross information flows likely to be required in typical nanomedical situations. Nanorobot onboard computers are likely to generate from $\dot{I} \sim 10^4$ bits/sec for the simplest systems to $\sim 10^9$ bits/sec for the most complex systems and tasks (Chapter 12), which sets broad limits on internal communications requirements. Assuming onboard data storage of 10^5-10^9 bits, rewriting an entire nanorobot memory in ~1 second demands information flows of 10^5-10^9 bits/sec. Communications with human cells may take place at many levels, ranging from 10-1000 bits/sec for individual neuronal impulses (Section 4.8.6) up to brief bursts at $\sim 10^6$ bits/sec (~MHz frequencies) for intracellular processes involving enzyme action or molecular gating. Inter-nanorobot communications are unlikely to require data transfer rates exceeding 10^3-10^6 bits/sec; explicit exchanges between nanodevices and the human user are restricted by the maximum data processing rate of the conscious mind, variously estimated as 1-1000 bits/sec (Chapter 25), although dermal and retinal displays may transfer visual information to the patient at up to $\sim 10^7$ bits/sec (Section 7.4.6). Communications with external entities may include monitoring or data transfer operations. For example, the ~525 x 390 = 204,750 pixel/frame of standard halftone black-and-white broadcast television transmitted at 30 frames/sec with ~1 bit/pixel mandates a $\sim 6.1 \times 10^6$ bit/sec (6.1 MHz) digital transfer rate (~6.1 MHz transmission bandwidth)*; downloading an entire uncompressed human genome during cytogenetic repair operations (Chapter 20) in ~1000 sec requires a $\sim 10^7$ bits/sec transfer rate.

According to classical information theory for channel capacity on a dissipative transmission line with additive equilibrium thermal noise,[699] the minimum erasure energy required per transmitted bit is

$$E_{bit} \geq kT \ln(2) = 3 \text{ zJ/bit} \qquad \{\text{Eqn. 7.1}\}$$

where k = 0.01381 zJ/K (Boltzmann constant), T = 310 K, and 1 zeptojoule (zJ) = 10^{-21} joule. Thus the maximum $\dot{I}_{max} \sim 10^9$ bits/sec bandwidth requirement noted earlier must draw $\gtrsim 3$ picowatts (pW), well within the anticipated 1-1000 pW power budget of typical in vivo medical nanodevices (Section 6.5.3). Slower bit rates can draw even less power. The design challenge is to closely approach this minimum theoretical limit.**

In this Chapter, an analysis of the most common nanorobotic communication modalities (Section 7.2) and communication network architectures (Section 7.3) is followed by a brief discussion of the many specific communication tasks to be performed (Section 7.4).

7.2 Communication Modalities

As a general principle, any method by which materials or power can be transferred into, around, or out of the human body also may be employed as a mode of communication by imposing a time-varying modulation on the flow. For in vivo communications, the leading candidates are free-tissue chemical, acoustic, and electromagnetic broadcast, nanomechanical and cable systems, and dedicated communicytes. An extensive treatment of data protocol systems,[1652] such as TCP/IP or any layered communication protocol, as they might apply to medical nanorobotic systems, would be interesting but is beyond the scope of this Volume.

7.2.1 Chemical Broadcast Communication

Chemical broadcast communication is widely used in the human body, as for example, in cellular communications using cytokines and other mechanisms (Section 7.4.5), hormones, neuropeptides, immune system components and pheromones. Consider the simple case of in vivo nanorobots attempting to communicate with each

** Although treated as approximately equal for simplicity in this book, the digital transfer rate is distinct from the transmission bandwidth. The bandwidth needed to handle a specific transfer rate is related to the actual coding and modulation technique selected. The simplest modulation techniques can indeed approach ~1 bit/sec per Hz of bandwidth, but much more efficient techniques are available. For instance, a typical 1998-vintage PC modem used complex coding and modulation schemes to transmit 33 KB/sec over a voice-grade transmission line that was only 4 KHz wide, thus achieving a transfer rate of ~8 bits/sec per Hz of bandwidth; ~100:1 data compression algorithms are currently available for voice transmissions.*

*** Landauer[700] points out that in theory there is no minimum energy required to transfer a bit; but see also Levitin[2318] and the discussion of reversible computing in Section 10.2.4.1.*

other exclusively by chemical means. In this model, the sender releases a coded messenger molecule of some type into the cytosol, interstitial fluid, or bloodstream, and this molecule travels via diffusion and convective transport to its intended recipient, whereupon the messenger molecule is recognized, absorbed and decoded.

7.2.1.1 Ideal Messenger Molecule

The ideal chemical messenger molecule will have several important characteristics. First, its structure will contain a distinctive "head" or "flag" that permits easy recognition and binding by nanorobot molecular receptor systems such as molecular pumps or sorting rotors (Section 3.4), so that the entire message need not be read in order to identify the intended recipient. Second, it will be relatively bioinactive, thus not readily broken down by natural processes before the message is likely to be received. Third, it should be easily eliminated from the body, thus preventing potentially toxic accumulations; however, the molecule and any likely breakdown products should also be inherently nontoxic in anticipated maximum concentrations.* Finally, the molecule should be capable of easy extension to larger sizes, permitting significant entire messages to be written on the molecule, as the statistical nature of the transport process implies a relatively long time between assured detections of the messenger molecule.

One possible candidate messenger is the partially fluorinated polyethylene molecule originally suggested by Drexler [10] for nanocomputer tape bulk memory systems, although others have been investigated.[1200] Such molecules can store one bit per carbon atom using an H atom to represent a "0" and an F atom to represent a "1" on one side of the carbon-chain backbone, with all H atoms occupying the other side of the backbone to facilitate easy reading. The message may be a single linear chain or may include branching structures representing conditionals or prioritizations embedded in the message. Assuming molecules (averaging 50%/50% H/F atoms on the read side) are of the form $CH_3(CHX)_nCH_3$ (with X = H or F atoms) and can store 1 bit per unit (with n units/molecule), then message molecule density $r_{message} \sim 1000$ kg/m^3 and message molecule volume $V_{message} \sim (3.82 \times 10^{-29})n$ (meter^3), giving an information density of $D_{message} \sim 26$ bits/nm^3 (~3 bits/nm of linear message molecule length). (By comparison, linear DNA achieves ~1 bit/nm^3.) Message molecule molecular weight $MW_{message} \sim n\,MW_{unit}$ (kg/mole) for n >> 1, where $MW_{unit} = 0.023$ kg/mole for (CHX), ignoring the end caps and again assuming 50%/50% H/F atoms.

Hydrofluorocarbon message molecules with n > 20 may be strategically crosslinked in a standardized pattern across the all-H backbone and folded into a maximally compact spheroidal configuration in preparation for transmission. Alternatively, the polymer could be wound up onto a bobbin or reel, allowing more convenient reading and a high packing density.[10] The read-write mechanism may require ~10^4 nm^3 of nanomachinery, providing a readout rate of $\dot{I}_{read} \sim 10^9$ bits/sec by scanning the message molecule at a ~30 cm/sec read rate,[10] although the complete tape-handling mechanism may require up to 10^5 nm^3 of nanomachinery. Two-dimensional information-bearing fluorinated hydrocarbon molecules have also been considered.[2182]

Are hydrofluorocarbon molecules biocompatible? Fluorinated hydrocarbon perfusants with n < 20 such as Fluosol-DA or the commercial solvent polyfluoro-octobromide (Perflubron) are FDA-approved and have been used as reversible oxygen carriers in artificial blood formulations for years.[704,705] Such fluorocarbons are characterized by high chemical and biochemical inertness, absence of metabolism, and rapid excretion.[704] The rate of excretion has been shown to decrease exponentially with increasing molecular weight, with the exception of fluorocarbons containing a lipophilic substituent such as Br (e.g., Perflubron) or a hydrogenated fragment in their molecular structure.[704] These water-insoluble compounds usually consist of 8-10 carbon atoms with molecular weights of ~450-500 daltons; clinical administrations typically reach maximum bloodstream concentrations of 70-400 gm/liter.[705] (cf. LD50 ~ 700 gm/liter estimated from acute single-dose toxicity studies[707]), many orders of magnitude in excess of the levels anticipated for nanodevice chemical communication applications. Interestingly, mice survive immersion in fluorocarbon through which oxygen is bubbled,[2183] and rats breathing 95% oxygen have survived total blood replacement with fluorocarbon fluid.[2184] The boiling point of perfluoropentane (C_5F_{12}) is 29.2°C, but is >37°C for n>5—e.g., 56.6°C for perfluorohexane (C_6F_{14}).

Fluorocarbons and fluorocarbon moieties have very strong intramolecular bonds and very weak intermolecular interactions,[2940] hence should display low particle aggregation. Fluorinated surfactants are less hemolytic and less detergent than their hydrocarbon counterparts,[2940] and fluorosurfactants appear unable to extract membrane proteins.[2940] The stability and permeability of fluorinated liposomes has been widely studied.[2941-2944] For example, anionic double chain glycophospholipids with either two hydrocarbon or two perfluorocarbon chains, or a mixed double chain (one fluorinated, one hydrogenated), readily give vesicles 30-70 nm in diameter when dispersed in water, with maximum tolerated IV doses up to 0.5 gm/kg body weight in mice (~5 gm/liter blood volume); hemolytic activity sharply decreases with increasing degree of fluorination.[2943] Many fluorinated surfaces such as Teflon are simultaneously hydrophobic and lipophobic.[2940]

Fluorocarbons are typically administered in the form of emulsions of 0.1-0.2 micron droplets dispersed in a physiologic solution, similar to fat emulsions routinely used for parenteral nutrition. A compact folded messenger molecule of spherical radius $r_{message}$ can store approximately

$$I_{message} = \frac{4}{3}\,\pi\, r_{message}^3 D_{message} \quad \text{(bits)} \qquad \text{\{Eqn 7.2\}}$$

and may display $I_{surface} \sim (3\,\pi^{1/2}\, I_{message}/4)^{2/3} \sim 1.2\, I_{message}^{2/3}$ (bits) on a compact spherical packet surface. For $r_{message} = 0.2$ micron, $I_{message} \sim 10^9$ bits/molecule (e.g., "genome packets") with $I_{surface} \sim 10^6$ bits. Of this number, at most ~1000 bits may be required for recipient identification, time stamping, "destroy by" dating, or other message packet flagging or header information. For the $(CHX)_n$ core fragment, $I_{message} = n$ (bits).

Hydrofluorocarbon messenger molecules will not be readily metabolized. The smaller molecules are cleared rapidly from the circulation with brief retention in the mononuclear phagocyte system,[706] mainly in the liver, spleen and bone marrow. They are then reintroduced into the circulation by lipid carriers in the blood at a rate that appears to depend on the fluorocarbon's solubility in fat, with some concentration in adipose tissues. Eventually, they are excreted through the lungs with the expired air[709] as a vapor (for short message segments of low molecular weight), with an intravascular persistence of 4-12 hours for present oxygen-carrying emulsions.[704] (Linear mixed

** M. Krummenacker notes that if a common standard format is established for design economy, then any stray messenger molecules that are released intact into the environment could trigger unwanted action in other bodies, and at inappropriate times, if inhaled or ingested by someone other than the original patient. Such "information toxicity" can be reduced by judicious degradation and deflagging of all messenger molecules prior to final excretion, by recycling, and by employing validity-checking security protocols (Chapter 12) before permitting any action to be stimulated or influenced by received messenger molecules.*

fluorocarbon-hydrocarbon amphiphiles have demonstrated at least some bloodstream persistence in vivo of up to 4 months.[712]) Massive single doses or repeated administration can cause saturation and transient blockade of the reticuloendothelial system (RES), temporarily depressing this component of the host-defense system.[710] Message-carrying fluorocarbons should be extremely inert, although there is some evidence that macrophages which have ingested perfluorocompounds show loss of phagocytic function and possible release of cytokines and other immune mediators.[708] Fluosol has been found to elicit anaphylactoid-type reactions is a small percentage of patients at blood concentrations as low as ~0.1 gm/liter.[711] Irregular Teflon $(CF_2)_n$ granules measuring 4-100 microns (equivalent to $n = 10^{12}$-10^{16}) employed clinically in periurethral injection [944] have produced granulomatous reaction, embolization, and migration to the lungs.[945-946] This implies a maximum size limit on large naked messenger molecules and a possible requirement for encapsulation in a biocompatible shell prior to release. R. Bradbury suggests that such a shell might include a lipid membrane with "docking tags" similar to viral attachment proteins. These tags should be engineered to be incapable of binding by antibodies, to have minimal affinity for common cell receptors, and to be indigestible by the regular cellular protein breakdown and recycling machinery (and thus be incapable of generating long-term immunity).

A hydrofluorocarbon messenger molecule with a lengthy stretch of exposed hydrogens might display increased toxicity, as some short-chain linear paraffin hydrocarbons (C_nH_{2n+2}) are considered "poisonous"[2945] with an official NFPA Health Hazard Rating of 1 or "slightly toxic" (scale 0-4).[2947] Animal toxicity of pure propane (C_3H_8) occurs with inhalation exposures to concentrations >10% and includes mild respiratory tract irritation and irregular respiration, cardiac sensitization to catecholamine-induced arrhythmias, analgesia and hypotension,[2947,2948] although the principal risk is simple asphyxia and cold burn during bulk exposures. Typical OSHA workplace air exposure concentration limits for propane and butane are 0.06%-0.1%.[2946,2947] Inhalation toxicity to pentafluoroethane (C_2F_5H) in rats is 70.9% (4-hour ALC), with no significant toxicological effects under <5% concentration.[2948] Toxicity mechanisms may differ for short-chain and long-chain hydrocarbon molecules.

This entire area deserves an in-depth toxicology study. If long-term toxicity is found to be unacceptable, the solution may be to engineer "digestible" but non-immunogenic packages, reducing bit density but increasing the available molecular pool of raw materials for building messenger molecules in vivo. As a possible alternative to hydrofluorocarbons, R. Bradbury suggests using unusual protein or polysaccharide chains (which can compactly encode large quantities of data; Section 8.5.2.2)[3122] that are easily read by nanorobots but also are easily digestible by cells as "food." If patient immunotype is known, then protein sequences can be designed which cannot be bound by MHC molecules (Section 8.5.2.1), preventing the patient from developing an immunity to them, and which look like self-shapes or are nonbinding to antibodies.

7.2.1.2 Diffusion-Limited Broadcast Rate

Given $I_{message} \sim 10^9$ bits for $r_{message} = 0.2$ micron from Eqn. 7.2, it is clear that onboard stores of messenger molecules will be quickly exhausted at the highest broadcast bit rates unless the communication system architecture makes substantial use of messenger molecule recycling. Without recycling, emission of hydrofluorocarbon message molecules is fluorine-limited, because carbon and hydrogen atoms are readily available from glucose and water molecules. The bloodstream concentration of fluoride is $\sim 4.5 \times 10^{-7}$ gm/cm^3 (Appendix B) or $\sim 1.4 \times 10^{22}$ F atoms/m^3. From Eqn. 3.4, the maximum diffusion current to the entire surface of a spherical nanodevice of radius R = 1micron and diffusion constant $D \sim 2 \times 10^{-9}$ m^2/sec (est. from Table 3.3) is $J = 3.6 \times 10^8$ F atoms/sec or 1.1×10^{-17} kg/sec, enough fluorine to manufacture 2.7×10^{-17} kg/sec representing a continuous long-term maximum broadcast rate of $\dot{I} \sim 7.2 \times 10^8$ bits/sec of $(CHX)_n$ 1-bit/unit hydrofluorocarbon messenger molecules.

Even in the unlikely event that all 8.3×10^{22} atoms of fluorine present in the human body (Table 3.1) were somehow converted to hydrofluorocarbon messenger molecules and released into the bloodstream simultaneously, the bloodstream concentration would reach ~1.2 gm/liter, well below the ~700 gm/liter LD50, though admittedly exceeding the ~0.1 gm/liter limit that occasionally triggers anaphylactoid-type reactions.

In 1963, Bossert and Wilson[703] completed the first systematic analysis of chemical communication in the context of animal olfactory communication in air, later extended by Bossert[725] in an analysis of maximum possible bit rates. In the following discussion, their results are adapted to the problem of in vivo chemical communication among medical nanodevices.

7.2.1.3 Instantaneous Stationary Source in Stationary Medium

Consider a chemomessaging nanorobot that releases $Q_{message}$ messenger molecules (each carrying $I_{message}$ bits/molecule) in a single puff as a point source at time t = 0. This is the ideal design for an alarm-type message or for messages requiring rapid fade-out. For simplicity, the human body is taken to be a continuous, isotropic, unbounded, stationary aqueous medium; a more detailed treatment is beyond the scope of this book. The spatial density of message molecules as a function of time t and distance r from the point source is

$$U_{message} = \frac{Q_{message}}{(4\pi D t)^{3/2}}\, e^{-\frac{r^2}{4Dt}} \quad (\text{molecules/m}^3) \quad \{\text{Eqn. 7.3}\}$$

where D = the translational diffusion coefficient for message molecules, which are assumed to be roughly spherically packed, estimated from Eqns. 3.5 and 7.2 as

$$D = \left(\frac{kT}{\eta}\right)\left(\frac{D_{message}}{162\,\pi^2\, I_{message}}\right) \quad \{\text{Eqn. 7.4}\}$$

For $I_{message} = 100$ bits, $D = 2.2 \times 10^{-11}$ m^2/sec; for $I_{message} = 10^9$ bits, $D \sim 1.0 \times 10^{-13}$ m^2/sec. Because the detection of molecules by receptor-based chemical sensors requires a concentration-dependent minimum sensor cycle time t_{EQ} approximated by Eqn. 4.3, then there exists some minimum threshold concentration (c_{min}) of message molecules that can be detected by a chemical sensor in some minimum waiting time $t_{sensor} = t_{EQ}$, given by

$$c_{min} = \left(\frac{N_{encounters}}{r_{message}^2\, t_{sensor}}\right)\left(\frac{I_{message}\, MW_{unit}}{4\pi kT N_A}\right)^{1/2} \quad \{\text{Eqn. 7.5}\}$$

For $N_{encounters} \sim 100$,[10] $N_A = 6.023 \times 10^{23}$ molecules/mole (Avogadro's number), $r_{message}$ from Eqn. 7.2 and taking $t_{sensor} = 1$ sec, then $c_{min} \sim 1 \times 10^{-9}$ molecules/nm^3 for $I_{message} = 100$ bits and $c_{min} \sim 9 \times 10^{-11}$ molecules/nm^3 for $I_{message} = 10^9$ bits. The concentration of message molecules exceeds c_{min} within an expanding diffusive sphere. In a time $t_{rec} = (0.0293 / D)\,(Q_{message} / c_{min})^{2/3}$ this expanding sphere reaches a maximum size $R_{max} = (0.419) (Q_{message} / c_{min})^{1/3}$, after which it begins to contract as the puff dissipates;[703] the concentration eventually falls below c_{min} everywhere at $t_{fadeout} = e\ t_{rec}$, where e = 2.718...

10^{12} nanorobots uniformly distributed throughout a 0.1 m^3 human body have a mean interdevice separation of ~50 microns. For simple messages ($I_{message}$ = 100 bits) and R_{max} = 50 microns, then $Q_{message} \sim 2 \times 10^6$ message molecules emitted, $t_{rec} \sim 20$ sec ($\dot{I} \sim 5$ bits/sec), and $t_{fadeout} \sim 50$ sec. If R_{max} = 1 mm, then $Q_{message} = 2 \times 10^{10}$ molecules and $t_{rec} \sim 8000$ sec to receive the signal ($\dot{I} \sim 0.01$ bits/sec). For complex messages ($I_{message} = 10^9$ bits), $Q_{message} \sim 1 \times 10^5$ molecules but $t_{rec} \sim 4000$ sec (~1 hour) for the message to be transported R_{max} = 50 microns ($\dot{I} \sim 3 \times 10^5$ bits/sec).

A simple alarm signal ($I_{message}$ = 100 bits) released within an individual tissue cell is received everywhere throughout the cytosol—an assumed ~(20 micron)^3 cell volume—in $t_{rec} \sim 0.8$ sec ($\dot{I} \sim 100$ bits/sec) with $t_{fadeout} \sim 2$ sec, using a single alarm puff of $Q_{message} \sim$ 17,000 message molecules (computed with $R_{max} \sim 10$ microns) which molecules may be stored in a (40 nm)^3 volume per puff. As a practical matter, the cytosol is quite crowded with macromolecules and cytoskeletal components (Section 8.5.3); exclusion effects will increase diffusion times by as yet unknown amounts, to be determined experimentally.

7.2.1.4 Instantaneous Stationary Source in Flooded Tube

For a source at the end of a long water-filled tube with non-absorbent walls, cross-sectional area A_{tube}, and length $X_{max} = (0.484)\ Q_{message} / A_{tube}\ c_{min}$, then $t_{rec} = (0.117 / D) (Q_{message} / A_{tube}\ c_{min})^2$ and $t_{fadeout} = e\ t_{rec}$,[703] using c_{min} from Eqn. 7.5. Hence a simple message ($I_{message}$ = 100 bits) passing through a tube of area A_{tube} = 1 micron^2 and length X_{max} = 50 microns requires $Q_{message}$ = 130 message molecules and is received in $t_{rec} \sim 60$ sec ($\dot{I} \sim 2$ bits/sec).

7.2.1.5 Continuous Stationary Source in Stationary Medium

Consider a source of message molecules emitting continuously at the constant rate $\dot{Q}_{message}$ (message molecules/sec) into the idealized stationary medium described in Section 7.2.1.3. Such a source might be useful for status telemetry, navigational beacons, or periodic sampling monitors. If the source continues for a long time then the detectable threshold concentration sphere[703] of message molecules around the point source asymptotically approaches a maximum radius $R_{max} = \dot{Q}_{message} / (4\ \pi\ D\ c_{min})$. The time for the expanding detectable concentration sphere to reach a radius $R = f_R\ R_{max}$ (where $0 \leq f_R \leq 1$ is the fractional radial expansion of the message sphere), the exact solution for which involves the complementary error function, is approximated reasonably well by $t_{rec} \sim (1.1\ f_R\ \dot{Q}_{message} / 8\ \pi\ c_{min}\ (1\text{-}f_R)\ D^{3/2})^2$ for $0.1 < f_R \leq 1$, using D from Eqn. 7.4 and c_{min} from Eqn. 7.5. Thus for simple messages ($I_{message}$ = 100 bits) with R_{max} = 100 microns and R = 50 microns (f_R = 0.5), then $\dot{Q}_{message} \sim 4 \times 10^4$ message molecules emitted per second and $t_{rec} \sim 140$ sec ($\dot{I} \sim 1$ bit/sec). For complex messages ($I_{message} = 10^9$ bits), $\dot{Q}_{message} \sim 10$ message molecules emitted per second and $t_{rec} \sim 8.4$ hours ($\dot{I} \sim 3 \times 10^4$ bits/sec).

7.2.1.6 Continuous Mobile Source in Stationary Medium

Consider a mobile nanorobot traveling through a stationary aqueous medium at velocity v_n (m/sec), emitting message molecules continuously at the rate of $\dot{Q}_{message}$ (molecules/sec). The cigar-shaped molecular trail envelope has a maximum length $X_{fadeout} = \dot{Q}_{message} / 4\ \pi\ D\ c_{min}$, and at a distance $X_{max} = X_{fadeout} / e$ behind the moving source the message molecules diffuse outward to a maximum detectable radius $R_{max} = (0.342) (\dot{Q}_{message} / v_n\ c_{min})^{1/2}$ as measured from the motion axis; for distances $>X_{max}$ the radius of the detectable message molecule envelope declines to zero at $X_{fadeout}$, with $t_{fadeout} = X_{fadeout} / v_n$. Thus, a nanorobot velocity v_n = 10 microns/sec and an $X_{fadeout}$ = 1000 microns requires $\dot{Q}_{message} = 4 \times 10^5$ molecules/sec for simple message molecules ($I_{message}$ = 100 bits) giving $R_{max} \sim 60$ microns at X_{max} = 370 microns and $t_{fadeout}$ = 100 sec.

These equations[703] also apply to a continuous stationary source in a nonstationary medium, where the medium moves past the source with a slow, constant velocity with perfect laminar nonturbulent flow in the absence of nearby boundary surfaces, an idealized instance of the case described in Section 7.2.1.7.

7.2.1.7 Continuous Stationary Source in Nonstationary Medium

A nonstationary transporting medium does more than just move message molecules in the direction of flow—it also may create turbulence in the medium, adding a component of turbulent diffusivity that overwhelms simple Brownian diffusion, giving a total diffusivity that is more a property of the flow structure of the medium and the boundary surfaces than of the substance of the medium, a complex analytical problem. Consider a continuous point source emitting a constant $\dot{Q}_{message}$ (molecules/sec) from a fixed position near the luminal surface of a blood vessel of radius R_{vasc}. From the relations given in[703] and as a crude approximation assuming plume width << boundary wall separation, $\dot{Q}_{message} \sim (0.0396)\ v_{vasc}\ c_{min} X_{fadeout}^{7/4}$ to create an ellipsoidal message molecule plume of maximum detectable length $X_{fadeout}$ in a medium flowing along the x-axis with fluid velocity v_{vasc}. The widest part of the plume occurs at $X_{max} \sim (3.57)\ F^{4/7}$, $Y_{max} \sim (0.686)\ F^{1/2}$, and $Z_{max} \sim (0.341)\ F^{1/2}$, where $F = \dot{Q}_{message} / v_{vasc}\ c_{min}$. Message receipt time $t_{rec} \sim X_{fadeout} / v_{vasc}$.

Thus a simple message ($I_{message}$ = 100 bits, $c_{min} \sim 10^{-9}$ molecules/nm^3 for t_{sensor} = 1 sec) broadcast from the luminal surface of the common carotid artery ($v_{vasc} \sim 0.2$ m/sec, $R_{vasc} \sim 3$ mm; Table 8.2) with a desired plume length $X_{fadeout}$ = 100 microns requires at least $\dot{Q}_{message} \sim 10^9$ molecules/sec, producing a very narrow plume with $Y_{max} \sim 40$ microns, $Z_{max} \sim 20$ microns (the radial direction), and $t_{rec} \sim 0.5$ millisec ($\dot{I} \sim 100$ bits/sec, limited by t_{sensor} = 1 sec). For a complex message ($I_{message} = 10^9$ bits, $c_{min} \sim 9 \times 10^{-11}$ molecules/nm^3 for t_{sensor} = 1 sec), $\dot{Q}_{message} \sim 7 \times 10^7$ molecules/sec at $t_{rec} \sim 0.5$ millisec ($\dot{I} \sim 10^9$ bits/sec, limited by t_{sensor} = 1 sec).

7.2.1.8 Assessment of Chemical Broadcast Messaging

Chemical broadcast messaging in theory permits information transfers up to 10^9 bits/sec but appears to be extremely energy-inefficient. The assembly of $(CHX)_n$ messenger molecule units may require 1-1000 zJ/bit (Section 6.5.6 (B)). For instance, replacing C-H (642 zJ) with C-F (876 zJ) costs ~234 zJ, but recycling CH_3F molecules into C-CH_2F chains actually produces 97 zJ of energy. A feedstock of CH_3F and CH_4 will release energy when the tape is first assembled, but will cost energy to tear apart into its fundamental subunits. R. Bradbury believes that the net cost of tape production and recycling can be reduced to 10-50 zJ/bit, given sufficient space to store lots of tape subunits: "If the assembly process is efficient at harvesting the energy produced, and the molecules don't get lost to cellular recycling machinery, then you could produce a system with very high overall efficiency, though you will have to worry about distribution of harvested energy and feedstock."

However, since ~10^6 molecules must be released to ensure receipt of at least one message molecule by an intended recipient ~50 microns away (e.g., Section 7.2.1.3), the energy cost per received bit rises sharply to ~10^6-10^9 zJ/bit, which is >> 3 zJ/bit, the theoretical minimum (Eqn. 7.1). Thus a 1-pW communications power budget limits steady-state bandwidth to ~1 bit/sec across ~50-micron transmission ranges. Additional disadvantages of chemical communications are slowness of transmission (except in nonstationary media or across short distances) and the ability to be delayed or blocked by semipermeable or impermeable barriers, or by absorptive nanorobotic agents active in the environment. Noise on chemical channels may almost be eliminated by using artificial messenger molecules, reducing the natural background nearly to zero, though noise may still be present due to the presence of old signals, interference or cross-talk from other man-made devices, or even from intentional medical or military jamming. The encoding mechanism of "genome packets" would act less like email, and more like FTP, because the amount of information transferred per messenger molecule is so large.[1652] Finally, used messenger molecules must be degraded by nanomachines (or other means) after the "destroy by" date has been passed; the number of messenger molecules to be captured and degraded or recycled by the messaging nanorobot population must approximate the number of messenger molecules released.

Nanorobot-to-nanorobot chemical broadcasts may be useful in the case of nanorobots working in close quarters where low emission rates will suffice, as in bacterial quorum sensing.[3236] For example, achieving the minimum detectable concentration $c_{min} \sim 10^{-9}$ molecules/nm^3 for 100-bit message molecules inside a (20 micron)^3 human tissue cell requires emission of only ~10^4 molecules (Section 7.2.1.3), costing ~1 pJ to manufacture and representing just 10^{-7} % of tissue cell volume. Chemical communications may also be useful in various special applications such as "silent alarms" using premanufactured messenger molecules vented from onboard storage tanks, thus moving the manufacturing energy cost ex vivo. Assuming 0.1 micron^3 tankage per nanorobot, each device may store ~10^8 100-bit message molecules available for ready release, enough to signal ~10^4 in cyto alarm events. Each such alarm signal may permeate the entire cytosol in ~1 sec.

Chemical broadcast messaging may be most useful when the high energy cost of creating the message molecules is borne by some external or macroscale agency, thereby requiring individual nanorobots only to receive the chemical signal but not to send it. For example, messenger molecules manufactured in the laboratory, treatment clinic, or implanted dedicated communication organ (Section 7.3.4) may be injected into the bloodstream in sufficient concentration to ensure receipt. Given $c_{min} \sim 1 \times 10^{-9}$ molecules/nm^3 ($I_{message}$ = 100 bits/molecule) or $c_{min} \sim 9 \times 10^{-11}$ molecules/nm^3 ($I_{message} = 10^9$ bits/molecule), the minimum number of messenger molecules needed to promptly raise the entire bloodstream concentration to c_{min} (assuming no absorption by the body) is >7×10^{15} 100-bit messenger molecules (a ~0.006 mm^3 injection) or >5×10^{14} 10^9-bit messenger molecules (a 4 cm^3 injection producing ~0.9 gm/liter concentration, somewhat exceeding the ~0.1 gm/liter threshold that occasionally produces anaphylactoid-type reactions). By comparison, a single nanorobot with a 1 pW power budget can only manufacture ~10^4-10^7 100-bit message molecules/sec.

In 1998, chemical messaging was only starting to be applied in robotics. For example, in one experiment simple pheromone-guided macroscale mobile robots could follow a scent plume using silkworm moth antennae wired into an electronic neural network.[2163]

7.2.2 Acoustic Broadcast Communication

Communication by acoustic waves is a highly useful channel for information transfer in nanomedicine. Previous Chapters have described the reception of acoustic energy in sensing (Sections 4.5, 4.8.2 and 4.9.1) and in the transfer of power (Sections 6.3.3, 6.4.1 and 6.4.3.3). Issues remaining to be addressed here include the generation of ultrasonic radiation by nanorobots (Section 7.2.2.1) and free-tissue acoustic channel bandwidths available in the human body (Section 7.2.2.2). Acoustic cables and transmission lines are treated in Section 7.2.5.3.

7.2.2.1 Acoustic Radiators

The acoustic power generated by any vibrating source is $P_{out} = U^2 R_A$ (RMS watts), where U is the rate of oscillatory volume displacement of the fluid, measured in RMS m^3/sec, and R_A is the acoustic radiation resistance seen by the source, measured in MKS acoustic ohms.[889] Two basic generators are the vibrating piston and the pulsating sphere, both of radius r. From Stokes Law (Eqn. 9.73) the input power required to propel a circular piston through water at velocity v is $P_{in} \sim 6 \pi r \eta v^2$, or $P_{in} \sim 24 \pi r \eta v^2$ for a radially oscillating sphere. Hence $U = \pi r^2 v = (\pi r^3 P_{in} / 6 \eta)^{1/2}$ for a vibrating piston to which P_{in} watts of mechanical input power are delivered, and $U = (2 \pi r^3 P_{in} / 3 \eta)^{1/2}$ for the pulsating sphere.

The radiation resistance $R_A = \pi \rho \nu^2 / k_r v_{sound}$, where k_r = 2 (piston) or 4 (sphere) and ν is acoustic frequency (Hz). This equation is valid only when $r/\lambda << 1$ (e.g., radiator size is very small in comparison to acoustic wavelength $\lambda = v_{sound} / \nu$); for r = 1 micron and ν = 1 MHz, then $r/\lambda \sim 0.001$ in water. Sound energy generated from a source with dimensions small compared with the wavelength of the vibration in the medium produces an intensity uniform in all angular directions; such a generator is considered to be a point source. Formulas for radiators having $r/\lambda >> 1$ are also provided by Massa.[889]

Combining these results with Eqn. 4.53, transmitted acoustic pressure (A_p), output power (P_{out}), and power intensity (I_p) at the radiator surface are given by

$$A_p = \left(\frac{\pi \rho^2 \nu^2 r P_{in}}{3 k_r \eta} \right)^{1/2} \quad (\text{N/m}^2) \qquad \{\text{Eqn. 7.6}\}$$

$$P_{out} = \frac{k_r \pi^2 \rho \nu^2 r^3 P_{in}}{24 \eta v_{sound}} \quad (\text{watts}) \qquad \{\text{Eqn. 7.7}\}$$

$$I_p = \frac{4 P_{out}}{k_r^2 \pi r^2} \quad (\text{watts/m}^2) \qquad \{\text{Eqn. 7.8}\}$$

For example, a vibrating piston radiator of radius r = 1 micron and input power P_{in} = 10 pW operating at ν = 1 MHz in vivo produces A_p = 0.0007 atm radiation pressure, P_{out} = 0.005 pW (giving e% = P_{out} / P_{in} = 0.0005 (0.05%) and an acoustic intensity of I_p = 0.002 watts/m^2 at the surface of the radiator, assuming ρ = 993.4 kg/m^3, $\eta = 1.1 \times 10^{-3}$ kg/m-sec and $v_{sound} \sim 1500$ m/sec for human interstitial fluid at 310 K. Figure 7.1 summarizes Eqn. 7.6 for various parameter choices.

7.2.2.2 Free-Tissue Acoustic Channel Capacity

Figure 7.1 (with blood pressure variations compared; Section 4.9.1.2) and Eqn. 7.7 illustrate the well-known result in acoustics that for a given driving amplitude, micropistons and microspheres are more powerful sound radiators at higher frequencies. That is, input power (driving the radiator) is more efficiently transduced into output power (waves in the medium) both at higher frequencies and at larger radiator sizes. Thus to achieve the highest acoustic channel capacity per unit of input power, the highest practical frequency and the largest possible radiator should be used for nanorobot-to-nanorobot acoustic communications. Of course, at higher frequencies, attenuation becomes more severe and eventually limits the value of ever higher frequencies.

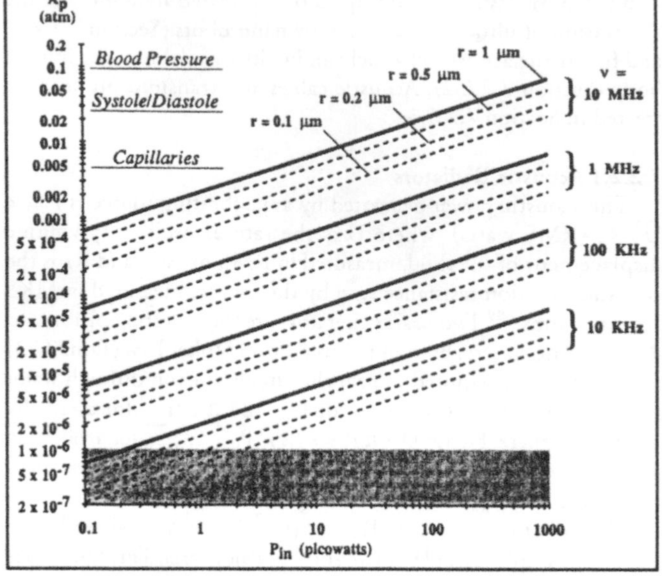

Fig. 7.1. Acoustic pressure (A_p) at the surface of a cylindrical vibrating piston acoustic radiator of radius r and input power P_{in} for ΔP_{min} ~10^{-6} atm in water at 310 K (from Eqn. 7.6).

An acoustic sensor of radius r located a distance X_{path} from a transmitter of like size must receive at least kT e^{SNR} ~ 30 zJ within a ν^{-1} (sec) integration time in order to receive information at frequency ν (bits/sec) for SNR = 2 (Section 4.5.1). If acoustic energy conversion efficiency e% = P_{out}/P_{in} (Eqn. 7.7), receiver duty cycle is f_{duty}, and acoustic attenuation in the medium is given by Eqns. 4.52 and 4.53 with α_{tiss} = 8.3 x 10^{-6} sec/m for soft tissue (Table 4.2), then to satisfy the above criterion requires that

$$P_{in} = \left(\frac{\nu f_{duty}}{e\%}\right)\left(kT\, e^{SNR}\right)\left(\frac{X_{path}^2}{r^2}\right) e^{2\,\alpha_{tiss}\,\nu X_{path}} \quad \text{(watts)} \qquad \text{\{Eqn. 7.9\}}$$

For f_{duty} = 10%, r = 1 micron, X_{path} = 100 microns, taking ν = 10 MHz gives e% ~ 0.05 (5%), P_{in} ~ 6000 pW continuous, and $\dot{I}$ ~ 10^6 bits/sec. Increasing ν to 100 MHz improves e% to at least ~50% and $\dot{I} = f_{duty}\,\nu$ ~ 10^7 bits/sec without increasing P_{in}, giving a maximum safe acoustic power intensity of ~e% $P_{in} / \pi r^2$ ~ 1000 watts/m^2 (Section 6.4.1) at the transmitter surface. Further increases in ν cause $\dot{I}$ to decline, because e% cannot improve beyond a maximum of 100%.

These results imply that nanorobot-to-nanorobot acoustic communications will generally take place at ~10-100 MHz frequencies over 10-100 micron path lengths in vivo. Acoustic messaging over longer path lengths require mobile signal amplifiers such as communicytes (Section 7.2.6), dedicated fixed-position communication organs with repeater protocols, or packet routing networks analogous to the Internet (Section 7.3).

7.2.3 Electromagnetic Broadcast Communication

The receipt of externally-generated radiofrequency (rf) power signals up to ~MHz frequencies by nanorobot antennas has already been considered in Section 6.4.2. Such signals are readily adapted to communication and may carry ~MHz signals into the human body, allowing information transfers to in vivo nanorobots of up to ~10^6 bits/sec from an external signal intensity of $\gtrsim$0.1 watts/m^2. Eqn. 6.32 suggests that rf signals pass through soft tissue with negligible absorption, leaving most of the signal energy available for detection by nanorobot receivers. (See also Section 4.7.1.)

While externally-generated rf signals may be detectable by nanorobots, onboard submicron-scale broadcast antennas probably cannot generate rf signals of sufficient power for meaningful device-to-device communications. For example, low-frequency electromagnetic waves of wavelength λ_{rf} and frequency ν_{rf} customarily are generated using a simple electric dipole of length $d_E << \lambda_{rf} / 2\pi$, or using a magnetic dipole loop antenna of diameter $d_M << \lambda_{rf} / 2\pi$. If the current carried by either antenna is I_{dipole}, then the average transmitted power for each radiator is given by[727]:

$$P_E = \frac{1}{3}\pi \mu_0 c \left(\frac{d_E}{\lambda_{rf}}\right)^2 I_{dipole}^2 \quad \text{(watts)} \qquad \text{\{Eqn. 7.10\}}$$

$$P_M = \frac{1}{12}\pi^5 \mu_0 c \left(\frac{d_M}{\lambda_{rf}}\right)^4 I_{dipole}^2 \quad \text{(watts)} \qquad \text{\{Eqn. 7.11\}}$$

$$\frac{P_E}{P_M} = \frac{4\lambda_{rf}^2 d_E^2}{\pi^4 d_M^4} \qquad \text{\{Eqn. 7.12\}}$$

where μ_0 = 1.26 x 10^{-6} henry/m (permeability constant), and c = 3 x 10^8 m/sec (speed of light). For ν_{rf} = 1 KHz and $d_E = d_M$ = 1 micron, P_E / P_M ~ 10^9 and the electric dipole is strongly preferred over the magnetic dipole radiator; at high frequencies, the relative power emission of the electric dipole is even greater.

An electric dipole antenna of length 1 micron and cross-section 1 micron^2 carrying a fairly aggressive current density of ~10^8 amp/m^2 consumes ~200 pW to produce an rf output power of only P_E ~ 10^{-11} pW. Not only is this extremely energy-inefficient, but the signal is too weak for detection by neighboring nanorobots. The 430-nm electret pendulum antenna described by Eqn. 6.34 has a theoretical minimum incident power detection limit of ~0.01 pW at 0.7 MHz; a limit of kT e^{SNR} = 30 zJ/cycle for a 10^{-11} pW signal implies a maximum operating frequency of ~0.0003 Hz, too low to convey any meaningful information. (Here, signal-to-noise ratio SNR = 2 (20 dB); error-corrected digital signals can provide virtually perfect communications even below 10 dB.) Furthermore, simple scaling predicts nanoelectric antennas will have nondirectional radiation patterns, since antenna gain G ~ A / λ; for A = 1 micron^2 antenna surface, then $\lambda \gtrsim$ 1 micron (3 x 10^{14} Hz) to achieve G $\gtrsim$ 1.

The reciprocity theorem in electromagnetic field theory predicts that the radiation pattern of an antenna will have the same shape as the response of that antenna when used as a receiver. W. Ware points out that a group of antennas tuned to a given resonant frequency, if illuminated by an external source at that frequency, will reradiate at that frequency, essentially echoing the signal. Thus a ~1 watt external source may induce 10^9 micron-scale antennas (one antenna per nanorobot, with a billion nanorobots reporting) to reradiate a total of ~0.01 pW at the same frequency, in theory detectable by a single nanorobot rf receiver and certainly detectable by macroscale instruments situated external to the body. (For comparison, television signals entering home TV antennas typically provide ~10-10,000 pW to the receiver). Near-coherence of the echo is virtually assured because the external rf interrogation signal passes through 30 cm of tissue in ~10^{-9} sec, so ~MHz antennas located anywhere in the body will lie at worst ~0.1% from perfect coherence. Interrogation pulses at many different rf frequencies may simultaneously poll echoing nanorobots programmed to monitor various internal phenomena of interest (and to adjust their antenna resonances accordingly prior to interrogation) in order to establish spatial distributions of those phenomena—which may include temperature, pressure, biochemical concentrations, bloodflow velocities, detection of specific cell types or metabolic processes. In 1999, the 250-micron microtransponders under development by PharmaSeq[3432] were expected to be interrogated at a throughput rate of $\gtrsim$1000/sec.

Aside from the environmental sources of electrical noise already described in Section 4.7.1, two additional potential sources deserve brief mention. First, radio, television, radar and other broadcast sources in developed countries produce a frequency-dependent broadband background (e.g., a carrier-frequency spike for each source) across a 0.01-1000 MHz spectrum up to ~10^{-11} watts/m^2-Hz which at $\lesssim$MHz frequencies passes through the human body largely unattenuated (Section 6.4.2). However, a ~1 micron^2 antenna employing a ~1 MHz channel receives at most ~10^{-5} pW of this rf broadcast energy, only ~0.002 kT/cycle which is almost certainly undetectable. In other words, micron-scale nanorobots probably cannot directly receive commercial TV, radio, or satellite broadcasts or GPS signals unless mediated by a macroscale communication organ (Section 7.3.4) or assemblage. Hence such broadcasts should generate no detectable noise at these frequencies.

Second, electrical discharges associated with muscular and neural action throughout the body cause electrical potentials to appear at the skin[3508] which are typically detected in a medical context during electrocardiographs (ECG or EKG, ~10^{-3} volt), electroencephalographs (EEG, ~10^{-4} volt), and biofeedback monitoring with frequencies ranging from 1-40 Hz. These surface waves also may reach ~10^{-11} watts/m^2-Hz, producing an undetectable 10^{-9} pW signal in a ~1 micron^2 antenna using a 100-Hz channel—although an electric field strength of >10^{-2} volts/m is in principle detectable by living cells (Section 4.7.1). Thus, micron-scale nanorobots can sense individual neural discharges nearby but probably cannot directly monitor global brainwave, ECG, gastroelectric or intestinal electrical wave patterns (which require a macroscale electrosensory organ or, possibly, cellular eavesdropping).

Electromagnetic modulations ν_{rf} >> 10-100 MHz (which must be imposed upon microwave, infrared, or optical carrier waves) may be difficult to generate, control and detect using submicron nanorobot components if those components are limited to mechanical ~GHz motions (Section 10.1.2.2); electronic components may cycle faster. Such carrier waves are 99% absorbed by soft tissue for path lengths ranging from ~10 cm for 100 MHz waves, to ~1 mm for infrared, or ~40 microns for optical photons. Energetic carriers also face a sharply declining count rate at the receiver due to the increasingly particle-like nature of the nondirectional transmission carrier at higher frequencies. For example, while micron-scale solid-state lasers are available, from simple geometry, an omnidirectional 1-micron^2 optical photon (~10^{14} Hz) emitter with a 1-pW power budget producing 10^7 photons/sec transmits only ~10^3 photons/sec to a 1-micron^2 receiver located 100 microns away (~maximum mean free path in tissue; Section 4.9.4). This limits information transfer to ~10^3 bits/sec at an energy cost of ~10^6 zJ/bit. Short bursts at much higher bit rates also satisfy the stated power budget; using this strategy, photon intensity must still be held below ~100 watts/m^2 (Section 6.4.2) at the source, so for a 1 micron^2 transmitter the maximum transfer rate is ~10^5 bits/sec in a ~0.01 second burst, with bursts repeatable only once per second.

Relatively slow modulations impressed on high-frequency electromagnetic waves might provide another useful communications channel. For example, nanorobots may detect each other's heat signatures, so modulations of those signatures can be used to transmit messages. Consider a nanorobot immersed in a medium of thermal conductivity K_t and heat capacity C_V, producing P_n watts of thermal power at a distance R_{detect} from a second nanorobot equipped with a thermal sensor of temperature sensitivity ΔT_{min}. The maximum detection range is

$$R_{detect} = \frac{P_n}{4 \pi K_t \Delta T_{min}} \qquad \text{\{Eqn 7.13\}}$$

For K_t = 0.623 watts/m-K for water at 310 K, ΔT_{min} = 10^{-6} K (Section 4.6), and P_n = 10-1000 pW, then R_{detect} ~ 1-100 microns. If P_n is pulsed on and off to send a message, the thermal time constant $\tau_{thermal} = 4 \pi R_{detect} C_V / K_t$ = 0.0001-1 sec for $C_V = 4.19 \times 10^6$ watts/m^3-K in water at 310 K. Assuming single-channel bandwidth ~ $1 / \tau_{thermal}$, then detectable signals range from ~10 KHz (~10^4 bits/sec) at a distance R_{detect} = 1 micron from a 10-pW modulated heat signature down to 1 Hz (~1 bit/sec) at a distance R_{detect} = 100 microns from a 1000-pW modulated heat signature.

7.2.4 Nanomechanical Communication

Internal communications (or interdevice communications through hard junctions between linked devices; Section 5.4.2) are readily achieved via sliding or rotating mechanical rods and couplings. A thin diamondoid rod producing 1-nm displacements and oscillating longitudinally at ~1 m/sec may transfer information at ~GHz frequencies. Similarly, a diamondoid transmission line carries acoustic compression pulses at ~17,300 m/sec, providing a >10 GHz bandwidth channel sufficient to support the ~GHz clocking speeds typical of sensors and nanomechanical computers (Section 10.1).

A simple communication mode between unlinked nanorobots operating in close quarters is simple physical tapping. During a 1 microsecond contact event, transfer of 1000 bits is allowed at a 1 GHz line frequency assuming single-threaded transmission; arrays of isolated transmission lines can transmit much more information. Cleavage energies for diamond range from E_{cleave} = 10.6 J/m^2 for the {111} crystal plane up to 18.4 J/m^2 for the {100} plane.[536] Adopting the more conservative number to estimate the minimum hammer/anvil cleavage velocity v_{cleave}, and as a crude approximation, a rodlike diamondoid signal hammer 100 nm in length moving at velocity v_{hammer} with tip area A_{tip} = 100 nm^2 and mass m_{hammer} ~ 3.5×10^{-20} kg impacting a diamondoid anvil at speeds of:

$$V_{hammer} < V_{cleave} = \left(\frac{2 E_{cleave} A_{tip}}{m_{hammer}} \right)^{1/2} = 246 \text{ m/sec} \qquad \text{\{Eqn. 7.14\}}$$

cannot cause cleavage in an unfractured anvil structure. The smallest detectable impact for this hammer has energy $kT e^{SNR} = (1/2) m_{hammer} v_{hammer}^2$, giving minimum detectable v_{hammer} ~ 1.3 m/sec for SNR = 2 (Section 4.3.1) at T = 310 K. At this speed, and neglecting anvil mass, a hammer cycled at ν_{hammer} = 1 GHz (~10^9 bits/sec) against a spring-loaded receiver anvil has a displacement stroke of:

$$\Delta x = \left(\frac{kT e^{SNR}}{2 m_{hammer} v_{hammer}^2} \right)^{1/2} = 670 \text{ pm} \qquad \text{\{Eqn. 7.15\}}$$

well above the minimum detectable displacement of 10 pm (Section 4.3.1), giving a maximum power cost of $kT e^{SNR} \nu_{hammer}$ ~ 32 pW (~32 zJ/bit).

Mechanical communication can also be achieved by more passive means, as for example the posting of Braille-like tactile-readable information mechanically on the nanorobot surface which may be scanned by neighboring nanorobots using compliant read tips at the distal ends of flexible manipulator arms (Section 5.3.2.5).

7.2.5 Cable Communication

Signals may be imposed upon any tethered power transmission (Section 6.4.3), allowing the transfer of information as well as energy. This Section examines the ability of various cable carriers to transmit information. The drawbacks of tethered power transmission systems enumerated in Section 6.4.3.6 also apply to in vivo communication cables.

7.2.5.1 Electrical Cables

Uninsulated wires risk electrical leakage and unnecessary heat transfer; unshielded wires produce stray fields that may attract unwanted attention from mobile elements of the immune system, e.g., electrosensitive leukotaxis (Section 4.9.3.1). Thus coaxial cable or "coax" is the proper transmission line for in vivo electrical cable communications. Unlike waveguides, coaxial cable is not a resonant device, hence the traveling wave frequencies it carries may be varied continuously down to DC. The electric fields within a coax line have axial symmetry. However, serious design complications may arise if the transmitted wavelength (λ) is less than the circumference of the annular dielectric space between the conductors, because a second (nonaxial) mode of rf propagation with diametral symmetry can then be excited simultaneously. To avoid this complication, a 1-micron diameter coax should be held to a practical upper frequency limit of $c / \pi d_{coax} < 1 \times 10^{14}$ Hz for cable lengths >> λ.

Intracoaxial scattering and absorption are negligible, so for single-channel bandwidth the maximum coaxial bit rate $\dot{I}_{max}$ consistent with a nanorobot onboard communication power budget P_{comm} using rf or microwave photons ($h\, \nu_{coax} / kT \ln(2) << 1$) occurs at the full-power transmission frequency

$$\nu_{coax}(\sim \dot{I}_{max}) = \frac{P_{comm}}{kT \ln(2)} \quad \text{(Hz)} \qquad \text{\{Eqn. 7.16\}}$$

Thus the maximum coaxial transmission frequency is 0.1 GHz (10^8 bits/sec) for P_{comm} = 0.3 pW, 1 GHz at 3 pW, and 100 GHz (10^{11} bits/sec) for P_{comm} = 300 pW (>3 zJ/bit).

7.2.5.2 Infrared and Optical Cables

Photon energy equals thermal noise ($h\, \nu_{equal} / kT \ln(2) = 1$) in the far infrared, specifically, at $\nu_{equal} = 6 \times 10^{12}$ Hz for T = 310 K. At still higher frequencies, the cost per bit becomes the energy per photon, or $h\, \nu_{optical}$, hence the maximum transmission frequency becomes

$$\nu_{optical} = \left(\frac{P_{comm}}{h}\right)^{1/2} \quad \text{(Hz)} \qquad \text{\{Eqn. 7.17\}}$$

Silica optical fibers are damaged by near-UV photons at frequencies exceeding ~10^{15} Hz (λ ~ 300 nm), giving an upper limit on optical information transfer rates. Transmitting 10^{15} UV photons per second requires a power budget of P_{comm} = 1 milliwatt; holding intensity to <10^5 watts/m^2 for safety reasons (Section 6.4.3.2) mandates a fiber >100 microns in diameter. Cables this large are suitable primarily for relatively short internodal trunk lines (Section 7.3.1). At ~10^5 watts/m^2 a 1 micron^2 fiber can safely continuously transmit ~10^5 pW, enough to generate 10^{13} photons/sec at 10 THz (~10^{13} bits/sec), or ~10 zJ/bit. Note that below ν_{equal}, the energy cost per bit is constant; above ν_{equal}, the energy cost per bit rises linearly with frequency. Regenerative systems could in theory recover and reuse some of this energy.

7.2.5.3 Acoustic Cables and Transmission Lines

Consider an acoustic compression signal of frequency ν_{acoust} traveling down a fluid-filled transmission cable of length l_{cable} and radius r_{cable}. In order to be detected at a signal/noise ratio SNR = 2, each pulse cycle must transfer a minimum energy $kT\, e^{SNR}$ to a receiver of volume L^3 at the cable terminus; hence from Eqn. 4.29, the maximum detectable pulse frequency $\nu_{acoust} = I_{rec} L^2 / kT\, e^{SNR}$ (Hz), where I_{rec} is the acoustic power intensity at the receiver. To obtain this intensity at the receiver, the input signal power at the other end of the cable must be $P_0 \geq \pi\, r_{cable}^2\, I_{trans}$ (watts) where I_{trans} is the power intensity of the signal transmitter. Combining these relations with Eqn. 6.44 for acoustic attenuation in cables gives

$$\nu_{acoust} \leq \left(\frac{L^2}{kT\, e^{SNR}}\right) I_{trans}\, e^{-2\, \alpha_{tube}\, l_{cable}} \quad \text{(Hz)} \qquad \text{\{Eqn. 7.18\}}$$

where α_{tube} is given by Eqn. 6.45 with a ~$\nu_{acoust}^{1/2}$ dependency. To avoid cavitation in pure water (Section 6.4.3.3) and to ensure safety in the unlikely event of cable detachment in vivo, maximum I_{trans} = 10^4 watts/m^2 of acoustic energy (Fig. 6.8). For a cable of diameter 1 micron terminating on a receiver of volume (680 nm)^3 sensitive to 10^{-6} atm displacements (Section 4.5.1), then ν_{acoust} ~ 1 GHz (10^9 bits/sec) for a cable of length l_{cable} = 14 microns (~8000 zJ/bit). A 1000-micron long cable can transmit up to ~1 MHz; ν_{acoust} ~ 1 KHz at l_{cable} ~ 5 cm; and ν_{acoust} ~ 1 Hz at l_{cable} ~ 2 meters. For intradevice communications, ν_{acoust} ~ 1 GHz for L = 300 nm, l_{cable} = 1 micron, and r_{tube} = 50 nm, though pure diamond fiber may be more efficient in this case.

A solid diamond acoustic transmission line transfers signals over great distances at GHz frequencies with almost no power losses, in part because of the extreme stiffness of diamond. Consider a rod of volume V_{rod} at temperature T_{rod}, made of a material with a thermal coefficient of volume expansion β and heat capacity C_V, to which a pressure pulse ΔP is applied at one end that travels at velocity v_{sound} (~17,300 m/sec for diamond) to the other end. In the worst-case thermodynamic cycle, Drexler [10] gives the total energy dissipation per pulse W_{max} as

$$W_{max} = \frac{T_{rod}\, V_{rod}\, \beta^2\, \Delta P^2}{C_V} \quad \text{(joule/cycle)} \qquad \text{\{Eqn. 7.19\}}$$

For diamond at T_{rod} = 310 K, $\beta = 3.5 \times 10^{-6}$ /K and $C_V = 1.8 \times 10^6$ joule/m^3-K.[460,567] Thus a 1-atm pulse that is applied to a transmission line consisting of a diamond rod 1 micron in length and (10 nm)^2 in cross sectional area ($V_{rod} = 10^{-22}$ m^3) requires a pulse input energy of ~10,000 zJ, but suffers an energy loss during transmission of at most $W_{max} = 2 \times 10^{-6}$ zJ. Under smooth mechanical cycling, nanomechanical systems may approach the isothermal limit and significantly reduce dissipation still further,[10] to ~1% W_{max} at ~1 GHz and ~0.001% W_{max} at ~1 MHz. Thus even at ν_{rod} ~ 1 GHz the losses using 1-atm pulses amount to only ~20 zJ and the transmission of energy is still ~99.8% efficient.

7.2.5.4 Mechanical Cables

Information may be transferred mechanically by modulating the turning frequency of a rotating cable. In this case the mechanical load is applied by the receiver at the cable terminus as it measures frequency changes in the received signal (e.g., FM modulation). Section 6.4.3.4 discusses cable operating modes, frequencies, dimensions, and power requirements. For example, a rotating cable 2 nm in diameter and ~50 nm long (suitable for internal data transmissions) operated in AC mode can convey 6×10^4 bits/sec at a power cost of 1 pW (~16,000 zJ/bit).

Power and control signals can also be transmitted through a stiff reciprocating member, operating in the manner of a bicycle brake or derailleur cable. Molecular control cables using polyyne rods encased in single-walled carbon nanotube (Section 2.3.2) sheaths is one simple example.[2281] Polyyne is a chain of carbon atoms with alternating single (0.1377 nm) and triple (0.1192 nm) bonds, hence the polyyne cable has ~7.8 carbon atoms and a mass of $\sim 1.5 \times 10^{-25}$ kg per nanometer of length. The stretching stiffness of the single bond is ~824 N/m, the triple bond ~1560 N/m, and the length of a bond pair is 0.2569 nm, giving the compliance for a cable of length L of (7.2×10^6) L (m/N), or the stiffness as $k_s = (1.4 \times 10^{-7}) / L$ (N/m). Thus an L = 1 micron polyyne cable stretches by ~1 nm when a tensile force of 140 pN is applied. Thermal noise produces an uncertainty in the position of the end of the polyyne cable, which varies approximately[10] as $\Delta x \sim (kT / k_s)^{1/2} \sim 0.18$ nm in the previous example, at 310 K.

7.2.5.5 Chemomessenger Cables

Unlike the chemical messaging described in Section 7.2.1, which was dominated by diffusive effects, information transfer using chemical messenger molecules that are confined within sealed pipes is controlled by the laminar bulk flow rate of the rapidly-moving carrier fluid.

Consider a chemomessenger cable of length l_{cable} and radius r_{cable} carrying a fluid of viscosity η at a volumetric flow rate of $\dot{V}$ maintained by a pressure differential of p_{cable} between the two ends of the cable. Assuming the fluid is a 10% suspension of messenger molecules of information density $D_{message} \sim 26$ bits/nm^3 (Section 7.2.1.1) with viscosity similar to human plasma, then net fluid information density $D_{fluid} \sim 2.6 \times 10^{27}$ bits/m^3; from the Hagen-Poiseuille law (Section 9.2.5) the maximum information transfer rate is

$$\dot{I}_{chemo} = \frac{\pi\, r_{cable}^4\, p_{cable}\, D_{cable}}{8\, \eta\, l_{cable}} \quad \text{(bits/ sec)} \qquad \text{\{Eqn. 7.20\}}$$

Assuming a safe, ultraconservative p_{cable} = 1 atm and taking r_{cable} = 0.5 micron and $\eta = 1.1 \times 10^{-3}$ kg/m-sec, then $\dot{I}_{chemo} = 10^{14}$ bits/sec through a cable of length l_{cable} = 50 microns, with power consumption $P_{chemo} = \pi\, r_{tube}^4\, p_{cable}^2 / 8\, \eta\, l_{cable}$ = 4500 pW (~0.04 zJ/bit). For a cable 0.5 meter in length, $\dot{I}_{chemo} = 10^{10}$ bits/sec and P_{chemo} = 0.4 pW (~0.04 zJ/bit). If p_{cable} is more liberally raised to 1000 atm, a cable 0.5 meter in length can transfer $\dot{I}_{chemo} = 10^{13}$ bits/sec requiring P_{chemo} = 450 nanowatts (~40 zJ/bit). While these are phenomenal information transport rates compared to other methods, two important caveats are in order.

First, such high transfer rates are purchased at the price of significantly increased receiver complexity and message processing time, since the message molecules must be captured, oriented, unspooled, fed past a read head at relatively slow speed, then stored, recycled, or disposed of properly. Data carrier fluid must be returned to the transmitter using a second cable; a double-cable pair establishes a complete fluidic circuit. The additional transmitter complexity and extra power required for chemical modifications of message carriers may be confined to external facilities and hence do not significantly constrain in vivo operations.

Second, the message travel speed from one end of the cable to the other is limited to the fluid flow velocity $v_{fluid} = r_{tube}^2\, p_{cable} / 8\, \eta\, l_{cable}$. Thus a given message requires a travel time $t_{message} = l_{cable} / v_{fluid} = 8\, \eta\, l_{cable}^2 / r_{cable}^2\, p_{cable} \sim 0.001$ sec to pass through a 50-micron-long 1-micron-diameter cable; a 10^9 bit message molecule measuring ~0.4 micron in diameter (Eqn. 7.2) travels at ~5 cm/sec and therefore only transfers the message information at $\sim 10^{12}$ bits/sec, or ~5 zJ/bit, near the theoretical minimum. Similarly, $t_{message}$ ~ 4 days through a 1-meter-long micron-wide cable at 1 atm driving pressure (~6 minutes if driving pressure is raised to 1000 atm).

R. Merkle points out that these two restrictions may be ameliorated by employing a cable transporting monomeric units that can adopt one of two or more distinct physical conformations. In particular, if the monomeric units are flat (e.g., small bits of graphite), are held together by short sections of polyyne (carbyne rods), and if the cable is formed in a flat housing, then one bit of information can be transmitted by rotating each monomeric unit into one of two positions which are separated by 180°. Minimal energy should be required to rotate a monomer entering the cable input, or subsequently to read the rotational state of a transported monomer exiting the cable output. A monomer transport speed of v = 1 m/sec and a 1-nm separation between successively arriving bit-carrying monomeric units allows a v_{cable} ~ GHz data transfer rate. From Eqn. 3.19, $P_{drag} \sim 10^{-16}$ watts per monomeric unit giving a total cable power dissipation of $P_{cable} = P_{drag}\, l_{cable}\, v_{cable} / v \sim 10^5$ pW (10^5 zJ/bit) taking l_{cable} = 1 meter, v_{cable} = 1 GHz and v = 1 m/sec.

7.2.6 Communicytes

A useful supplemental means of information transport throughout the body is a mobile mass-storage memory device called a communicyte. Communicytes may serve an analogous function to postal carriers—messages are delivered to them, passed among them, and eventually delivered by them to the intended recipients. Mass mailings to selected recipient subpopulations are also possible. Classes of communicyte mass memory may include rapidly spooled hydrofluorocarbon memory tape (Section 7.2.1.1), dense banks of diamondoid register rods forming a random access memory (RAM) (Fig. 10.2), or other means (Section 10.2).

In the first case, a 1 micron^3 storage block could contain a 10^{10} bit, 0.4-micron^3, 3-meter length of memory tape, with the remaining 0.6-micron^3 volume occupied by read/write heads, spool drivers, housing and the like. With a read speed[10] of ~30 cm/sec ($\sim 10^9$ bits/sec) the entire data cache may be offloaded in ~10 sec. The energy cost to rewrite the tape is 1-1000 zJ/bit (Sections 6.5.6 (B) and 7.2.1.8), hence the entire tape may be erased and overwritten in 1-1000 sec assuming a 10 pW tape-handling power budget, giving a write speed of 10^7-10^{10} bits/sec.

In the second case, register rods of cross-section ~1 nm^2 (described in Drexler[10]) require ~4 nm of length to accommodate a single input/output rod pair and can store at least ~1 bit/40 nm^3. Thus a 0.4 micron^3 block of tightly-packed register-rod RAM may hold 10^7 bits, with the remaining 0.6 micron^3 of the 1 micron^3 storage block reserved for springs, latches, and other essential mechanisms (including address-decoding logic) to access the stored data, and housings. Read and write speeds are $\sim 10^{10}$ bits/sec; full-cycle energy losses are ~5 zJ/bit assuming 1 bit/register,[10] a ~50 pW power draw during the ~1 millisec required to read or write the entire onboard data cache.

Communicytes may also incorporate mechanisms allowing data transfers among themselves or between themselves and living or artificial entities (Section 7.4). Communicytes will normally be deployed as components of a communication network of such devices, as described in Section 7.3.2, although they may also serve as mobile data repositories or software libraries.

7.3 Communication Networks

To maintain a continuous information flow for sensor data sharing, mission monitoring and wide-area control, it is convenient to establish a communication network in vivo that facilitates point-to-point and broadcast messaging. Two distinct physical network architectures are readily discerned—fiber networks (Section 7.3.1) and mobile networks (Section 7.3.2).

7.3.1 Fiber Networks

Fiber networks may employ fixed-topology data-conducting cables (Section 7.2.5) of virtually any description, including electrical, optical, acoustical, mechanical, or chemical. A complete design analysis of each of these network classes is beyond the scope of this book. The following discussion focuses on high-frequency electrical and optical cables, which most clearly exemplify the salient characteristics of fiber networks.

Suppose that a simple three-dimensional hierarchical Cartesian grid of electromagnetic communication fibers of radius r_{fiber} is embedded in a block of tissue of volume V_{tiss} (m^3) with a mean separation between adjacent parallel fibers of x_{fiber1} in the rectangular grid. This defines a total of $V_{tiss} / x_{fiber1}{}^3 = N_{node1}$ intersection nodes and an equal number of cubic voxels, each of volume $x_{fiber1}{}^3$ (m^3) and bounded by $N_{seg1} = 3\ N_{node1}$ fiber segments each of length x_{fiber1}.* Total fiber volume is $V_{fiber1} = 3\ \pi\ r_{fiber}{}^2\ V_{tiss} / x_{fiber}{}^2$ and total fiber length $L_{fiber1} = 3\ V_{tiss} / x_{fiber1}{}^2$. Allowing a maximum power budget of P_{net1} (watts) for the network, then each internodal fiber segment may dissipate up to $P_{seg1} = P_{net1}\ x_{fiber1}{}^3 / 3\ V_{tiss}$. A cable energy dissipation of E_{bit1} (joules/bit) implies a maximum data traffic of $\dot{I} = P_{seg1} / E_{bit1}$ on each segment between nodes.

For whole-body installation in a human being, $V_{tiss} \sim 0.1\ m^3$. For the first subnetwork, x_{fiber1} = 100 microns, r_{fiber} = 0.5 microns, and P_{net1} = 1 watt, giving total fiber length $L_{fiber1} = 3 \times 10^7$ meters, fiber volume V_{fiber1} = 24 cm^3, and $N_{seg1} = 3 \times 10^{11}$ internodal fiber segments defining $N_{node1} = 10^{11}$ communications voxels. This network may be emplaced by $\sim 10^{11}$ installer nanorobots (Chapter 19) of size ~1000 $micron^3$ that travel through tissue at 1-100 microns/sec (Section 9.4.4). Each installer unspools ~300 microns of internally stored fiber (~240 $micron^3$) in 3-300 sec while consuming <<1 pW of motive power (Section 9.4.4.2), then briefly conjugates (Section 9.4.4.4) with other installers to make the nodal connections. Using GHz nanocoax (diameter ~1 micron) with E_{bit1} ~ 3 zJ/bit, internodal traffic has a capacity of $\dot{I}_1 \sim 10^9$ bits/sec (~1 GHz). Cable power density is ~40,000 W/m^3; power intensity is ~4 W/m^2.

Three additional subnetworks are interleaved with the first, each passing messages to the others through appropriate nodal junctions:

In subnetwork #2, x_{fiber2} = 1 mm, giving total fiber length $L_{fiber2} = 3 \times 10^5$ meters and 10^8 communications voxels. For P_{net2} = 1 watt and using a single IR line or a bundle of ten 100 GHz lines (diameter ~3.6 microns) with E_{bit2} ~ 3 zJ/bit, $\dot{I}_2 \sim 10^{12}$ bits/sec.

In subnetwork #3, x_{fiber3} = 1 cm, giving total fiber length $L_{fiber3} = 3 \times 10^3$ meters and 10^5 communications voxels. For P_{net3} = 1 watt and using a bundle of ten 10-THz optical cables (Section 7.2.5.2; bundle diameter ~3.6 microns) with E_{bit3} ~ 10 zJ/bit, $\dot{I}_3 \sim 10^{15}$ bits/sec.

In subnetwork #4, x_{fiber4} = 10 cm, giving total fiber length L_{fiber4} = 30 meters and 100 communications voxels. For P_{net4} = 1 watt and using a bundle of 100,000 10-THz optical cables (bundle diameter ~360 microns) with E_{bit4} ~ 10 zJ/bit, $\dot{I}_4 \sim 10^{18}$ bits/sec, and power intensity $\sim 10^5\ W/m^2$, the maximum deemed safe for in vivo applications (Section 6.4.3.2).

Assuming 5 zJ/bit switching losses at each node, total power dissipation of all nodes in each subnetwork is ~0.5 watts, or ~2 watts for nodes at all four levels. Combining the four subnetworks into a single well-linked network gives the ability to transfer 10^9 billion-bit (e.g., "genome packet") messages per second across the entire installation volume—providing $\sim 10^{18}$ bits/sec along the optical backbone with a 6-watt power budget. By comparison, in 1997 the Internet backbone (admittedly much larger in physical extent) could transfer only $\sim 10^{10}$ bits/sec, average global communications traffic was $\sim 10^{12}$ bits/sec, total worldwide Ethernet capacity was $\sim 10^{13}$ bits/sec, and worldwide data storage in all movies, recordings, corporate and government databases, and personal files was informally estimated by Michael Dertouzos,[983] Philip Morrison,[1649] and Michael Lesk[3130] as $\sim 10^{19}$ bits.

Messages are transmitted acoustically from in vivo nanorobots present within a (100 micron)^3 communications voxel to the nearest local network node. These nonoptical links are the principal bottleneck in the system. In the worst case, a nanorobot lies at most L_n / 2 = ($3^{1/2}$ / 2) x_{fiber1} from the nearest local node (Section 5.2.1 (F)). From Eqn. 7.9, taking ν = 100 MHz, f_{duty} = 1%, r = 1 micron and X_{path} = 87 microns, then P_{in} = 550 pW per voxel. Each communications voxel contains up to ~100 (20 micron)^3 tissue cells, so one nanorobot per cell communicating continuously on a 10^4 bit/sec channel produces 10^6 bits/sec of message traffic, just 0.1% of rated capacity of each local node. At this maximum bit rate, local acoustic power dissipation totals ~55 watts, giving a total of ~60 watts for the network. If nanorobots can physically dock at a node, the need for acoustic links is eliminated; bit rate per channel rises to $\sim 10^7$ bits/sec and network power draw falls to ~6 watts.

Assigning one nanorobot in each tissue cell ($\sim 10^{13}$ nanorobots) a unique address requires each message packet to contain a $\log_2$ (10^{13}) = 44-bit sender identifier plus a 44-bit recipient identifier, mandating a ~100-bit header allowing 12 check bits, the absolute minimum message packet size for a comprehensive cell-addressible network. At a 1 MHz acoustic nodal access rate, a simple 200-bit message takes ~0.2 millisec to upload or download, plus ~2 meters / ~c = $\sim 10^{-8}$ sec to pass through the network at ~0.67c, where c = 3 x 10^8 m/sec (speed of light). Nodal read/write functions should operate at 10-10,000 MHz (Section 7.2.6) and optical switching may be even faster, so signal passage through at least the local nodes should impose no significant additional delays. Hence simple messages may be passed between any two specific nanorobots in ~0.4 millisec; a complex 10^9-bit message requires ~1000 sec. By comparison, simple adjacent internodal Internet "pinging" takes ~10 millisec. (Again, node-docked nanorobots with no acoustic intermediaries can exchange messages several orders of magnitude faster.)

Communication with bloodborne nanorobots is most convenient during capillary passage (once every ~60 sec), when nanorobots should remain within the operating range of local nodes during the entire transit owing to the narrow width of such vessels (4-15 microns). Capillaries are typically ~1 mm long with flow rates of 0.2-1.5 mm/sec, so the passing nanorobot has 0.7-5 sec to upload or download

---

** This network design, with each node having 6 connecting fibers, may be unduly redundant, resulting in excess fiber usage. Single nodes may need no more than 4 connecting fibers, forming a tetrahedral grid.*

messages. Given the ~0.2 millisec echo time, a nanorobot entering a capillary can announce its position and begin receiving its email before it has traveled more than ~0.2 micron through the narrowest vessels; messages of up to ~5 x 10^6 bits may be sent or received during each capillary transit.

Communication from the arterioles (average ~100 microns diameter) requires contacting the nearest local node which may be 150 microns away, boosting required nanorobot acoustic transmitter power to ~1600 pW at 100 MHz. Energy costs become prohibitive in the arteries and larger veins and other special locations such as the cardiac chambers, the bursae, and the bladder. Simple 200-bit messages might possibly be transacted by nanorobots immediately adjacent to the 25,000-micron diameter aortal wall; maximum flow velocity of ~1 m/sec carries an unanchored nanorobot beyond the 100-micron operational radius of a medial local node in just ~10^{-4} sec. Under conditions of bradycardia or cardiostasis, communications improve significantly in the vascular regions because bloodborne nanorobots remain longer in the vicinity of nearby embedded nodes.

Subdermal networks may be useful in some specialized applications, but the skin area (~2 m^2) is relatively small in comparison with various internal surfaces such as the vascular network (~300 m^2).

Fiber nodes may store considerable quantities of useful data. For instance, in the above example there are 10^{11} local network nodes. If each node stores just ~2600 bits on hydrofluorocarbon memory tape at 26 bits/nm^3 (Section 7.2.1.1) accessible in <10^{-5} sec (Section 7.2.6), this cache occupies a volume of ~100 nm^3 per node and the entire local nodal network storage capacity is ~3 x 10^{14} bits, or ~one Library of Congress.

7.3.2 Mobile Networks

In a fiberless network, mobile communicytes may be deployed in tissue and blood, and serve as communications nodes. Devices enter a tissue and station themselves for optimum data transfer. All nodal and internodal traffic is acoustic. With a spacing of 100 microns between nodes, continuous internodal message transmission at 100 MHz with f_{duty} = 1% using an r = 1 micron radiator requires ~600 pW (Eqn. 7.9). From relations given in Section 7.3.1, a whole-body installation with V_{tiss} ~ 0.1 m^3 requires ~10^{11} communicytes uniformly distributed throughout the tissues, a maximum network dissipation of ~60 watts plus another 0.5 watts for node switching losses. Since broadcasts are necessarily omnidirectional for transmitters smaller than ~v_{sound} / ν = 15 microns at 100 MHz, the network is entirely uniform with no backbone and total long-distance message capacity is ~10^6 bits/sec in broadcast mode. Limits on broadcast power can minimize bandwidth overlap and crosstalk between nonadjacent nodes. At 100 MHz and f_{duty} = 10%, a whole-body network capacity of 10^7 bits/sec generates an uncomfortable ~600 watts of waste heat; if these communicytes are installed in only <17% of the body volume, then local 10^7 bit/sec networks may be made available at <100 watts. There may be many conceptual similarities to telephonic cellular networks,[1650,1651] including frequency re-use, handoff algorithms, and the likelihood of large numbers of point-to-point ~10^6 bit/sec communication sessions through different modes without straining the system. Such design details, while interesting, are beyond the scope of this book.

Non-communicyte mobile nanorobots access the network via acoustic channels as in the fiber network. The ν f_{duty} = 1 MHz/node limit implies that long-distance communications will be sharply curtailed within the tissues. However, local-area communications may have quite satisfactory bit rates. For example, each of 100 nanorobots present in one (100 micron)^3 communications voxel can send continuous ~100 bit/sec messages (using only ~100 Hz of available bandwidth) simultaneously to each of 100 nanorobots located in an adjacent voxel. Thus total mononodal traffic over all 10^{11} nodes can approach the ~10^{18} bits/sec of the optical fiber backbone throughout the entire installation volume. At a 0.01 MHz/channel nodal access rate for each of 100 nearby nanorobots, a simple 200-bit message takes 20 millisec to upload or download, plus ~200 microns / v_{sound} ~10^{-7} sec to pass between adjacent communications voxels at the speed of sound (v_{sound} ~ 1500 m/sec in soft tissues and whole blood; Table 6.7). Hence simple messages may be passed between any two specific nanorobots in nearby cells in ~40 millisec, though a complex 10^9-bit message requires an impractical ~10^5 sec.

Bloodborne communicytes provide a supplementary long-distance messaging capability. Deployment of ~10^{10} 5-micron^3 communicytes in a 5.4-liter blood volume (<0.001% concentration by volume) gives a mean interdevice separation of ~80 microns. Communicytes passing through a 1 mm capillary (averaging 10 embedded nodes along its length) in ~ 1 sec can upload or download ~10^5 bits at each node. Each bloodborne communicyte has a patrol volume of (80 microns)^3 = 500,000 micron^3, about ten times the volume of the average capillary, so a fresh communicyte enters each capillary about once every 10 seconds and can receive messages totalling 10^6 bits during each transit. The fixed patrol volume per bloodborne communicyte implies that these devices will not remain in continuous contact with their bloodborne neighbors while in transit through vessels much smaller than ~80 microns in diameter (e.g., terminal arterioles, metarterioles, capillaries, and the postcapillary and collecting venules; Section 8.2.1). For example, in a 40 micron-diameter terminal arteriole the mean interdevice spacing grows from ~80 microns to ~400 microns, resulting in a temporary communications blackout between bloodborne neighbors during transit through the microvasculature. The blackout may normally last 5-10 seconds (Section 8.2.1.1).

Once received by a bloodborne communicyte, simple long-distance messages are quickly rebroadcast (post-blackout) throughout the bloodstream communicyte fleet (which draws ~6 watts continuous), the signal propagating at near the speed of sound, finally reaching the one communicyte situated nearest to the intended recipient node in at most ~2 meters / v_{sound} ~ 10^{-3} sec. Assuming a 10 microsec delay between rebroadcasts due to reading a 10-bit routing header at 1 MHz implies an additional rebroadcast delay of at most ~0.2 sec through a chain of ~20,000 communicytes over a ~2 meter path length. Allowing up to ~10 sec to enter and traverse the entire length of the relevant capillary, then long-distance point-to-point messaging requires at most ~11 sec and allows transfer rates of ~10^5 bits/sec or better systemwide. Total long-distance capacity is limited to acoustic bandwidth and the maximum transfer rate of each communicyte, say, at f_{duty} = 1%, or ~10^6 bits/sec (Section 7.2.6) equivalent to ~0.01% of the entire Internet backbone in 1997. Bloodborne communicytes also provide a useful messaging facility for bloodborne non-communicyte nanorobots.

Besides serving as mobile message repeater stations, bloodborne communicytes may further boost total system capacity by acting as physical message carriers. For example, a single communicyte bearing messages totalling 10^{10} bits (Section 7.2.6) circumnavigates the entire vascular circuit once every ~60 seconds. Thus, in theory, point-to-point messages may be carried throughout the entire operational volume at an effective ~10^8 bits/sec rate in this manner, most useful for nanorobots in peripheral tissues attempting to send messages to devices (or postal depots) located in the heart or lungs (organs which the entire blood volume reliably transits once every circuit). (Acoustic downloading at the destination is limited to

10^6 bits/sec at f_{duty} = 1%, but modest locomotion skills and maneuverability would permit physical docking with nodes allowing up to ~10^{10} bit/sec mechanical downloading rates; purely statistical collision-mediated data transfer is not efficient at these low bloodstream concentrations.) A total of 10^{20} (message-carrier) bits may be in transit at any one time in the blood. Except for this message-carrier function and the "blackout" effect in the microvasculature, communicyte network performance is not significantly affected by conditions of bradycardia or cardiostasis.

As in the fiber network, communicyte nodes may store considerable quantities of data. Assuming up to ~10^{10} bits for each of 10^{11} nodal devices, either network has a maximum total storage capacity of ~10^{21} bits. A single dedicated (4 mm)^3 library nodule (Section 7.3.4) implanted anywhere in the body can also contain ~10^{21} bits.

7.3.3 Networks Assessment

Fiber networks excel at high-capacity long-distance communication, with additional capacity readily added to the design by multiplying the number density or bundle density of fibers. Acoustic mobile relay networks have relatively low and fundamentally limited bandwidth. An additional advantage of the fiber network is speed—point-to-point fiber messaging takes ~10^{-4} sec vs. up to ~10 sec for the mobile network. Both of these advantages may be important in transdermal communication and whole-body diagnostic monitoring applications.

However, fiber and mobile networks may provide roughly equivalent local transmission speed and capacity if both must employ acoustic nodal access, as this provides the highest endogenously transmitted bit rate per unit power consumption for mobile nanorobots that are arbitrarily positioned network users. Thus in applications requiring predominantly local information transfers, the choice of basic network architecture may be driven by factors other than system total capacity and speed.

Fiber networks also have many significant disadvantages. Both fibers and mobile nanodevices can be made immunochemically biocompatible, but fibers are physically vulnerable and can cause serious physical tissue and cellular irritation (Section 6.4.3.6). It is well-known in dermatology that subdermally-placed, but incompletely absorbed, "dissolvable" stitches can work their way back to the surface of the skin; fiber network elements could be similarly ejected from the body. Some of these mechanical difficulties possibly may be overcome using a helical coil or a fiber which is coupled to a biocompatible sheathing using compliant internal springs; large-diameter fibers could be installed within bones where they would experience minimal flexing and immune system exposure, although transmissions across joints or tissues with high flexure or vascularization might still be required to be acoustic.

Networks with mobile components are easier and quicker to install, to reconfigure, to upgrade while in vivo, or to remove in the event of malfunction or change in medical objectives, than fiber networks with immobile components. On the other hand, communication protocols may need to be substantially more complicated to provide the necessary reliability with drifting nodes.

The fixed physical positions of fiber network nodes is also a major disadvantage because tissue movement is ubiquitous inside the human body, causing progressive fiber misalignment. Examples of such movement include untreated metastasizing tumors or benign growing tumors, angiogenesis in injured or heavily exercised tissue, enlargement and shrinkage of tissue channels or prelymphatics after wounding or edema, adipocyte deposition, and the breakdown or buildup of muscle tissue; cell loss and tissue modifications in the brain, sclerotic livers, radiation-damaged bone marrows, chancres and blisters, hematomas, and the uterus and related tissues during pregnancy; normal periodic movements in muscle-laden tissues such as the biceps, cardiac tissue, arterial walls, and the thoracoabdominal diaphragm; and other nonpathological but irregular movements such as tissues which may rapidly inflate with fluid, including the sex organs and related tissues, the bladder, and to a lesser extent the lungs. With such movement, nodal positional assignments quickly become obsolete and nodes may be carried out of acoustic range. Fiber spatial distributions may develop undesirable clumping and rarefactions. Fiber-embedded tissues which slough off in the normal course of events (e.g., epidermal, endometrial, placental, gastrointestinal) may carry fibers out into the uterine or intestinal canals, or expose them to air in the case of the epidermis.

The paradoxical conclusion is that overall fiber network reliability may be improved by adding nodal mobility. One crude biological analog is the filopodia of embryonic axons which can drag their fibrous neural cargo through embryonic tissue at ~0.1 micron/sec.[3296] While adult tissue may in theory have a more solidified extracellular matrix (ECM) and greater intercellular connectivity, making dragging more difficult, leukocyte and fibroblast mobility through ECM is typically 0.05-0.70 microns/sec (Section 9.4.4.2).

7.3.4 Dedicated Communication Organs

By analogy to implanted energy organs (Section 6.4.4), dedicated macroscopic organs may be installed in the human body to facilitate internal communications. Such organs could serve as high-capacity data storage, computation, and retransmission nodes in internal networks; as storage bays or reprogramming facilities for communicytes; as transdermal links to the outside world to permit rapid inmessaging and outmessaging, offloading of major data processing tasks to ex vivo computational resources or to dedicated computational organs (Section 10.2.5), or integration with external sensory, communications, and navigational facilities; as rf, TV, or satellite broadcast receivers, for example to receive Global Positioning System (GPS) signals or personal email; as radio signal transmitters for outmessaging; as convenient foci for multisystem or autogenous control, coordination, or data distribution; or as library nodules or personal medical history information storage devices.

7.4 Communications Tasks

Nanomedical messaging tasks fall into three broad categories:

1. nanorobots communicating with externalities including physicians, laboratory machines, external computers, or even the conscious perception of the patient himself;
2. nanorobots communicating with other nanorobots; and
3. nanorobots communicating with human organs, tissues, or cellular systems.

Communications data flowing into a nanorobot from some extrarobotic source is called inmessaging; outward-bound data transfers are called outmessaging. A comprehensive examination of all these possibilities is beyond the scope of this book. The present discussion is limited to a brief overview of the following elementary situations: inmessaging from external sources (Section 7.4.1), inmessaging from patient or user (Section 7.4.2), intradevice messaging (Section 7.4.3), interdevice messaging (Section 7.4.4), biocellular messaging (Section 7.4.5), outmessaging to the user (Section 7.4.6), outmessaging to an external receiver (Section 7.4.7), and transvenue outmessaging (Section 7.4.8). Some of the examples presented may appear whimsical from a 20th century perspective, but they illustrate the incredible variety and power inherent in the technology. A discussion of user interfaces is largely deferred to Chapter 12.

7.4.1 Inmessaging from External Sources

Inmessaging occurs when information is conveyed from a source external to the human body, or external to working nanodevices, to a nanorobotic receiver located inside the human body. Security protocols (Chapter 12) are a strong necessity here. The receiver may be associated with medical nanodevices, either individually or collectively, or with specialized communications organs.

Methods of modulating power sources to achieve data transmission have already been examined at length in Section 7.2. To summarize a few of the many possibilities—commands, data, software, processed results of extensive computations, and messages from medical personnel may be conveyed into the human body by:

A. *Chemical Inmessaging*— communicytes or messenger molecules encased in pills or suspended in ingestible liquids, injectable or IV fluids, mouthwashes, earwashes, eyedrops, inhalants, nasal sprays, dermal patches, suppositories or enemas; or artificially vascularized data secretion glands transdermally linked to external control mechanisms.

B. *Acoustic Inmessaging* — dermal ultrasound transducers including handheld units, cuffs or bracelets, or transmission through water baths; vibrating treatment tables, beds or chairs; ingestible sonosondes; osteoimplanted acoustic radiators or implanted dental vibrators with rf or direct cable external links; or implanted circumvascular acoustic radiators.

C. *Electromagnetic Inmessaging* — broadcasts from external rf and microwave sources including epidermally-placed electrodes (Section 4.7.1); optical laser arrays pressed against the skin; ingestible radiosondes[638] and radio telemetry pills;[3333] whole-body electrical current flows including transosteal intercellular transmissions; transdermal multi-tesla oscillating magnetic fields; electromagnetic emanations from implanted rf or microwave emitter organs under external control; or direct linkages to internal networks via permanent transdermal access ports.

D. *Cable Inmessaging and Message Depots*— information may be transported directly into the body through chemical, acoustic, electrical, optical, or mechanical cables or tethers feeding implanted communications organs, message depots, data distribution centers or bulletin boards; such depots may have biocompatible termini in the bloodstream, brain, or intercellular regions to facilitate message exchanges with mobile nanorobots.

E. *Eavesdropping*— continuous nanorobot monitoring of normal physiological sensory traffic (imported by human sensory organs) with specific sensitivity to defined control or keyed patterns that might have been inserted into the natural data stream, such as modulated visual, auditory, or tactile cues, periodic dermal pain or temperature sensations, or oscillating taste and scent signals.

F. *Macrosensing* — external modulation of physiological or environmental parameters which can be directly sensed by in vivo nanorobots but controlled by external agencies, including pharmacologically-modulated heartbeat or respiration rate, mental alertness or stage of sleep, atmospheric humidity or pressure, chemical composition of the air, gravity or centrifugal acceleration, particulate radiation flux, or geographical position and altitude (see Section 4.9).

7.4.2 Inmessaging from Patient or User

Autogenous command and control (Chapter 12) gives a patient or user the ability to issue instructions directly to nanodevices present in his or her body. Patient or user inmessaging is an important enabling technology for autogenous control, wherein a human being manipulates a consciously controlled variable, which manipulation is then detectable by in vivo nanodevices. Once the message is received by even a single nanorobot, the information may be rapidly multiplied and passed along to other nanorobots using an internal communications network.

7.4.2.1 Mechanical Inmessaging

Perhaps the simplest example of user inmessaging is finger-drumming on a hard surface such as a tabletop, a method which we will now examine in some detail. A ~15 gm finger may be drummed at a maximum of ~5 Hz[920,921] over a 2 cm path length at a maximum velocity of ~0.2 m/sec; if the impacting finger is brought to a halt within 1 mm of the ~1 cm^2 fingertip and ~50% of the kinetic energy is converted into acoustic energy, the phalangeal impact produces a maximum compression wave of ~0.3 atm (~300 watts/m^2). The lightest audible tapping produces a pressure wave of ~0.01 atm (~0.3 watts/m^2). Either pulse is easily detectable by ~10^{-6} atm-sensitive nanorobot acoustic sensors (Section 4.5.1) located in the patient's hand or arm.

Consider five sensor-equipped nanorobots each positioned ~2 mm below the epidermis in the soft tissue just beyond the distal phalanx of five different fingers, and each with access to a local communications network (Section 7.3) spanning the hand. An impact pulse applied to a given finger reaches the sensor stationed in that finger in ~1 microsec by conduction through soft tissue at ~1540 m/sec. The acoustic pulse then travels down the phalanges and metacarpals, crosses the distal row of carpals, then travels back up through the metacarpals and phalanges of the other fingers mostly via bone conduction at ~3550 m/sec (Table 6.7), reaching the adjacent sensors 90-110 microsec after the initial impact. The pulse does not travel exclusively in bone as it must pass through 8-11

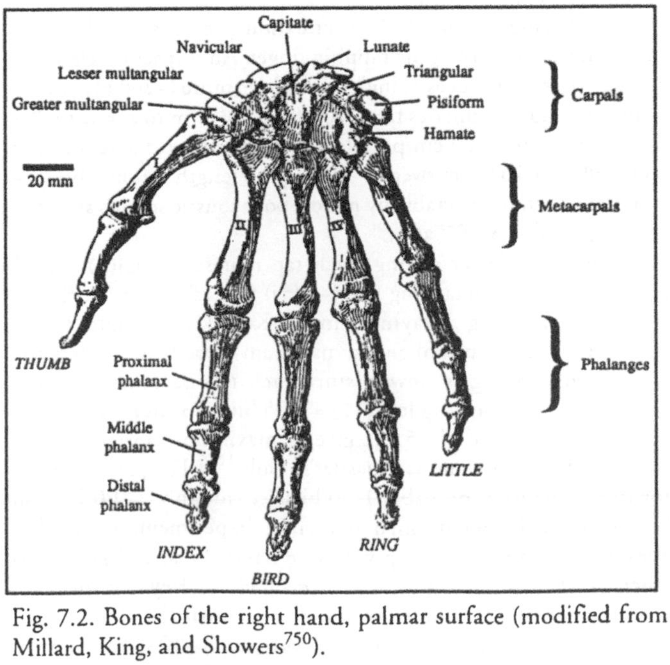

Fig. 7.2. Bones of the right hand, palmar surface (modified from Millard, King, and Showers[750]).

Table 7.1. Temporal Signature of a Detectable Mechanical Pulse Conducted Mostly through Bone, which is Applied to One Finger and Received by Nanorobot Sensors Distally Located in Each of the Five Fingers of the Hand

	Mechanical pulse is applied to finger (tapping finger):									
	Finger #1 (Thumb)		Finger #2 (Index)		Finger #3 (Bird)		Finger #4 (Ring)		Finger #5 (Little)	
Pulse is detected by sensor on finger #:	X_{path} (cm)	Arrival Time (μsec)	X_{path} (cm)	Arrival Time (μsec)	X_{path} (cm)	Arrival Time (μsec)	X_{path} (cm)	Arrival Time (μsec)	X_{path} (cm)	Arrival Time (μsec)
1	0.2	1	34.3	97	37.5	106	39.5	111	38.7	109
2	34.3	97	0.2	1	34.8	98	36.5	103	36.8	104
3	37.5	106	34.8	98	0.2	1	34.3	97	35.3	99
4	39.5	111	36.5	103	34.3	97	0.2	1	32.3	91
5	38.7	109	36.8	104	35.3	99	32.3	91	0.2	1

diarthrodial articulations (see Figs. 7.2, 8.25). Approximating each as a bone/soft-tissue interface with R = 66% reflection loss across each interface (Section 6.4.1), the 0.01-0.3 atm pressure pulse is reduced by at most 10^{-4}, still detectable even at the lightest tapping pressure.

Assuming nanorobots may possess synchronized internal clocks with at least 1-10 microsec accuracy (Section 10.1), then data sharing of pulse arrival times among the five nanorobots via the network allows the reconstruction of five unique temporal signatures of an impact event at any particular finger (Table 7.1). Conduction also occurs through soft tissue pathways which may be ~15 cm shorter than the typical osteal path length (X_{path}) used in Table 7.1, and may also produce much less signal attenuation. These soft-tissue pulses arrive ~120-160 microsec post-impact because of the slower conduction speed and thus should not be confused with the osteal signal. Still other pathways with widely varying conduction velocities will increase noise levels, but a brief training session should produce acceptable signal/noise ratios for event recognition especially since maximum pulse extinction time (~200 microsec) << pulse repetition time at ~5 Hz (~0.2 sec).

Interphalangeal amplitude attenuation provides an additional check on the identity of the tapping finger. An impact deceleration in ~5×10^{-3} sec produces a single ~5 millisec pulse (~200 Hz) which from Eqn. 4.52 attenuates from $10{,}000 \times 10^{-6}$ atm to at most 9997×10^{-6} atm over a ~20 cm path length through soft tissue, or to at most ~9900×10^{-6} atm over a ~35 cm path length through bone—either of which is detectable by nanorobot acoustic sensors sensitive to changes of ~1×10^{-6} atm.

With single-finger coding, each tap represents $\log_2(5)$ = 2.32 bits/tap; a maximum tapping rate (~5 Hz) for each of the five fingers simultaneously (e.g., playing Rimsky-Korsakov's "Flight of the Bumblebee" on the piano) gives a maximum capacity of ~58 bits/sec. Multifinger coding is slower, since each tap becomes a 5-digit binary word representing $\log_2(31)$ = 4.95 bits/tap, and a maximum multifinger tap rate of ~5 Hz gives a maximum capacity of ~25 bits/sec, about the same as Quastler's result.[1265] The practical limit for this modality is probably 1-50 bits/sec, roughly 2-100 English words/min or 10-500 decimal digits/min. Experiments by the MIT Wearable Computers Group with one-handed chorded keyboards (such as The Twiddler, manufactured by HandyKey[1595]) suggest a requirement of ~5 minutes of training to learn the alphabet, ~1 hour to learn to touch type, and ~3 days to reach ~10 words/minute.

Many conceptually similar methods of mechanical inmessaging may be employed by a patient whose in vivo nanorobots have been appropriately programmed and positioned, including clapping/slapping of hands/feet (~3 bits/sec), mandibular clicking (~2 bits/sec), tongue-tapping on palate (~2 bits/sec), eyelid or eyebrow flapping (~2 bits/sec), dental/dermal drumming using a rigid object (~1 bit/sec), epiglottal pulsing (~1 bit/sec), thoracoabdominal diaphragmatic contractions (~1 bit/sec), or toe tapping (~0.5 bit/sec).

Other mechanical stimuli at the skin—including pressure, touch, vibration, and tickle (see Schmidt[1633])—may also be eavesdropped by medical nanorobots. Interestingly, the frequency response of these receptors may range as high as 800 Hz for Pacinian corpuscles (sensory organs located at the skeletal joints, tendons, and in the muscles;[1634] Table 7.3). Thus an eavesdropping subdermal nanorobot could receive ≳100 Hz modulated signals through this channel that would only be perceived as "flat stimulus" by the conscious human patient.

7.4.2.2 Kinesthetic Inmessaging

With the support of an internal communications and navigational network, proprioceptive nanosensors resident in selected human tissues permit the direct detection of gross limb positions, limb velocities, and body orientation in space with t_{meas} ~ 10^{-3} sec or better (Sections 4.9.2 and 8.3.3). Thus, for example, data may be rapidly inmessaged using a highly literal manual sign language[3297] designed for minimum ambiguity and maximum precision, with a minimum number of discrete symbols to memorize. (Native American sign language has ~400 root signs and other gestural languages have ~2000 signs,[731] though a manual alphabet is also used.) Fingers and limbs can be comfortably moved at 0.1-1 m/sec; if ~1-cm positional increments can be adequately controlled by a patient and thus can be employed to convey one bit of information, then the maximum channel capacity of signing is 10-100 bits/sec per finger or 100-1000 bits/sec for all ten fingers. This estimate compares favorably with the ~100 bits/sec achieved by hearing-impaired signers translating speech at a conversational rate of ~150 words/min, and also with the record manual typing speed of 216 words/minute (~173 bits/sec) achieved on an IBM Selectric typewriter.[739] Nanorobots may also eavesdrop on proprioceptive information detected by Pacinian proprioceptors.

Properly monitored voluntary large body motions such as break-dancing or karate programs, or lesser displacements such as head rolling or shrugging movements, leg jiggling or calisthenic exercises, rapid periodic lung inflations, anal sphincter contractions, blinking or eyeball rotations can similarly transfer useful information into the body at ~1 bit/sec. In combination with real-time retinal displays (Section 7.4.6.5), eyeball movement nanosensors can allow patients to use their eyes as an "ocular mouse" to point to an icon or array of alphanumeric characters superimposed on the visual field. This will allow them to initiate a programmed function or to spell out words or numbers. In 1997, an analogous system, known as the Ocular Vergence and Accommodation Sensor (OVAS) manufactured by Applied Modern Technologies Corp. of Garden Grove, California, used 12.5 W/m^2 IR laser beams reflected from each eye's retina to provide information about eye movement and other biometric data. The OVAS design included a 12-component optics system and a Pentium processor with algorithms for processing data on the accommodative state, movements, and vergence of the eyes, as well as 10 other ocular functions.[1295] In 1998, Canon EOS cameras used eye-control focus sensors to detect where in the frame the photographer was looking, and autofocus there, instead of defaulting to the center of the frame. Superimposing retinal displays over normal vision need not prove confusing to the patient. Experiments with head-mounted displays show identical ergonomic efficiency and accuracy for pointing tasks when control characters are projected either on a dark background screen or on a translucent background through which moderately distracting objects and moving traffic are visible.[1307]

7.4.2.3 Acoustic Inmessaging

A wide variety of sounds may be generated voluntarily by the patient and be detected by in vivo nanorobots, such as coughing, grunting, humming, various other mechanical body noises (Section 4.9.1.4) and even vocalizations including direct voice commands spoken aloud by the user (Section 4.9.1.5); 1-100 bit/sec inmessaging rates appear feasible by these methods. Intracochlear nanodevices can also be used for high-capacity inmessaging (Section 7.4.6.3).

Soundless subvocalizations may also be detected using kinesthetic techniques (Section 7.4.2.2) to measure ~0.5 mm movements in tongue position and the muscles of the larynx that produce adjacent distinguishable tones in the vocal cords. The triangular waveform harmonics emitted by the larynx are modified during passage through sub- and supraglottal cavities, the shape of which may be voluntarily altered by submillimeter muscular movements — again, well within the range that nanorobots can detect (Section 4.9.2.1). Data sharing by multiple nanorobots using a communication network should permit reconstruction and estimation of the intended vocalization with sufficient reliability to transfer useful noncritical data or commands into the network. In 1998, radar microchips operating at ~2 GHz were already used for soundless speech recognition—the system recognized and interpreted motions of the human glottis, lips, tongue, jaw, and velum in real time.[1648]

The field of voice recognition is active, and no systematic review will be attempted here.[1654-1658,1710] In 1998, IBM's speech recognition technology, including the VoiceType Dictation and Personal Dictation systems (IPDS), was well-known and commercially available,[1659,1660] as was Kurzweil's VoiceCommands and VoicePro[3131] and NaturallySpeaking from Dragon Systems.[3132]

7.4.2.4 Chemical Inmessaging

Ingestion or inhalation of chemical messenger molecules is another way the patient can control the flow of information and commands into his body. The patient could provide the desired data or commands to a desktop manufacturing appliance, which appliance then encodes the information onto billions of copies of a hydrofluorocarbon messenger molecule suspended in a carrier fluid or solid pill, which the patient subsequently inhales or ingests. Messages up to ~10^9 bits may be distributed throughout the body in ~one circulation time (~60 sec), a data transfer rate up to ~10^7 bits/sec. Patients without access to personal manufacturing appliances could be given fluid ampules, standardized pill sets or inhalers whose contents are designed to trigger specific predetermined nanorobot behaviors. Such sets must contain personal security codes to prevent their unauthorized use on other patients (see Chapter 12).

A related technique for chemical inmessaging is to allow naturally inhaled or ingested molecules (e.g., gustation or olfaction) to trigger specific nanorobot actions. For example, if continuously circulating detoxification nanorobots are programmed to begin removing alcohol from the bloodstream whenever the presence of garlic compounds is detected, then the patient can voluntarily trigger the detox response by sniffing or chewing a clove of garlic. (A population of 10^{12} bloodborne nanodevices with aggregate storage volume ~6 cm^3 can reduce serum alcohol from 0.2% to 0.005% in ~1 second by prompt onboard sequestration, followed by metabolization of the entire inventory in ~10 minutes within a systemic caloric budget of ~200 watts, although outflows from ethanol-soaked body tissues into the bloodstream and other factors complicate the process; see Chapters 19 and 25.) Similarly, nanorobots with selected chemical sensors stationed in the vomeronasal organ,[1971] vallate papillae or olfactory epithelium could directly detect and respond to specific flavors, perfumes, pheromones[1972] or other chemical substances—even molecules which humans are normally incapable of tasting or smelling, including artificial or engineered substances.

Binary message sequences employing the five basic gustatory stimuli (Section 7.4.6.4) must use one of the stimuli as a positional spacer to avoid confusion. For example, a patient sipping the 8-taste sequence "sweet (1), salty (/), sweet (1), salty (/), sour (0), salty (/), sweet (1), salty (/)" has just transferred the binary sequence "1101" into his body. ("Salty" is used as the spacer because salt sensitivity is most widely distributed over the surface of the tongue. "Sour" is used because saltiness partially suppresses perception of bitterness, and because sweet and bitter taste messages are transmitted by the same transducer protein, called α-gustducin.) This inmessaging modality is probably limited to ~0.1 bit/sec but may be boosted considerably by employing complex artificial gustatory stimuli (akin to messenger molecules) which only lingually-embedded nanorobot sensors can detect.

Human olfactory receptors can probably detect ~1000 different smells (Section 7.4.6.4); exposure to a new olfactory stimulus every 1-10 seconds, with each smell worth $\log_2(1000)$ = 10 bits/symbol, allows information transfer up to ~1-10 bits/sec. Individual chemical assay nanorobots that can detect ~10^7 different molecules (Section 4.2.4) allow greater diversity and specificity of signal carriers, but at most only ~double the bit rate because $\log_2(10^7)$ = 23 bits/symbol. However, the bit rate using long-chain digitally coded artificial messenger molecules is vastly higher, and probably only thermogenically (heat of manufacture and access; Sections 7.2.1.8 and 7.2.6) and biocompatibility (Chapter 15) limited.

7.4.2.5 Electromagnetic and Thermal Inmessaging

The human body does not emit voluntary electrical or electromagnetic radiation except for modest dermal potentials associated with ECGs and EEGs which probably cannot be directly detected by individual in vivo nanorobots (Section 7.2.3). Simple voluntary actions that might allow electromagnetic inmessaging to subdermally-implanted nanorobots include placing a hand near a heated stove, then pulling it away; or blinking a flashlight beam on and off while the flashlight is pressed against the skin, for nanorobots positioned at most 1-2 cm below the epidermis (Section 4.9.4); or moving a bar magnet across a patch of skin (Section 4.7.2)—all allowing ~0.1-1 bit/sec transfer rates. A thermographic system might also detect the slightly elevated dermal temperature caused by touching a hand to the face or thigh, much like a simple demarcation strategy (Section 8.4.1).

7.4.2.6 Neural Inmessaging

The most comprehensive inmessaging capability may be afforded by eavesdropping on selected neural sensory traffic (Section 4.9.5). Noninvasive monitoring of neuroelectric impulses (Section 4.8.6) by nanorobots stationed near afferent neurons can detect and interpret any sensory stimulus that can be consciously perceived by the patient. Virtually every inmessaging stimulus described elsewhere in Section 7.4.2—including finger-drumming, hand-signing, vocalized or olfactory signals, dermal heat sensations, scalp/eyebrow myopotentials, and the like—may be indirectly detected by suitably positioned and configured neural monitors. For instance, finger-tapping generates electrical activity in a specific ~1 cm^2 patch of neurons in the primary motor cortex[1090]—although nanorobots suitably positioned in the brachial plexus, or lower in the tree near critical junctions of the median nerve (above the digital, thumb, and palmar cutaneous branches) and the ulnar nerve (above the muscular, dorsal cutaneous, superficial palmar and deep palmar branches), may achieve more rapid and reliable monitoring of motor impulses. Neurons may fire at >100 Hz, so, ignoring significant electrical spike redundancy, inmessaging rates up to ~100 bits/sec per monitored neuron can in theory be achieved with this approach.

Nonsensory volitional neural inmessaging channels are also available to nanorobot monitors stationed in the brain. For example, by consciously recalling a specific series of numbers, letters, names, words, concepts, images, or events, a well-defined constellation of neural impulses of certain frequencies may be caused to pass repeatably through the same, say, (~200 micron)^3 blocks of brain tissue for each recalled item. Brain tissue contains numerous "dominance columns" on approximately this scale which appear to represent functionally associated fiber bundles.[1036,1039] For example, 300-500 micron wide columns have been described in the striate and inferotemporal cortex of the macaque monkey;[742,1037] organized patterns of action potential waves have been observed via calcium imaging in rodents, measuring 100-300 microns wide in the retina and ~50 microns wide in the cortex.[771] An experiment using a context-recall memory task in monkeys suggested that an ensemble of as few as 16 motor cortical cells could perfectly classify (i.e., 100% accuracy) all the items in a sequence of five stimuli ;[3184] nanorobotic monitors stationed at those 16 cells could in theory discriminate all five-stimulus sequences.

Thus, without being able to understand any of the higher-order meanings of these signals (e.g., to "read human thoughts"), nanorobots detecting such reproducibly neurographically-localized impulse trains may pool their readings and interpret specific combinations of such localized trains as data or as command strings (a ~0.1-1 bit/sec channel) and then take appropriate action. Biofeedback monitors,[1661] volitional scalp EEG multiband user interfaces, PET scanners and functional magnetic resonance imaging (fMRI) operate on a crudely analogous principle, but without the benefit of precise impulse localization that is made possible by molecular nanotechnology. In 1998, a glass cone electrode filled with neurotrophic factors (which encouraged neural ingrowth) was implanted in a patient's motor cortex; the patient learned to mentally operate the output signal as a binary switch.[3074] Another system using cortical potentials achieved transfer rates of ~2 characters/min.[3121]

7.4.2.7 Macroscale Inmessaging Transducers

Inmessaging signals from patient to nanorobot may also be mediated using macroscale communications interfaces. These interfaces may be fixed or mobile, and may be either stable or reconfigurable. A crude example of a fixed, stable inmessaging transducer would be a ~1 cm dermally- or cranially-mounted coaxial cable connector which allows data to flow into an implanted dedicated communication organ for subsequent distribution to in vivo nanodevices via an internal communications network. Data passes into the patient through a simple rf or microwave coax cable which is plugged directly into the patient's socket, readily achieving ~10^{10} bit/sec transfer rates (Section 7.2.5.1) directed from a computer operated by the patient or physician. Up to ~10^{13} bit/sec transfers are available using fiberoptic (Section 7.2.5.2) or chemocable (Section 7.2.5.5) ports. Other fixed transducers may incorporate photoelectric or olfactory sensors, microphones, neural taps, or manipulable tactile elements such as buttons or switches.

At the other extreme of maximum inmessaging versatility, a dermal transducer may be configured upon request and presented to the patient on any part of his body. For example, a tattoo-like ~30 cm^2 dermal control panel comprised of ~3 billion communication-linked kinesthetically-sensitive chromomorphic nanorobots spaced ~5 microns apart could be assembled under a clear flat patch of epidermis such as the back of the hand. This panel could take the shape of a touch-sensitive alphanumeric keypad resembling a laptop computer keyboard or a touch-tone telephone or home-security keypad, complete with a touch-sensitive grid of visually-readable inscribed characters. (See details in Section 7.4.6.7.) Similarly, a wristwatch-shaped device could accept accept and interpret verbal commands, then translate them into modulated electromagnetic signals displayed on a 2-D array of photodiodes or microlasers on the back of the watch; the signals could then be received by a nanorobot dermal transducer panel (Section 7.4.6.7) and passed along to the rest of the in vivo network.

7.4.3 Intradevice Messaging

Intradevice messaging has already been briefly described in the context of metamorphic control (Section 5.3.3), lengthy gear trains (Section 6.3.2), sliding and rotating control rods (Section 7.2.4), acoustic transmission lines (Section 7.2.5.3), and mechanical cables (Section 7.2.5.4), and does not appear to present any major fundamental or conceptual difficulties.

To summarize, internal communications within an individual nanorobot may be achieved by impressing modulated low-pressure acoustical spikes on the hydraulic working fluid of the power distribution system, or by mechanically actuating simple networks of rods and couplings, easily achieving transfer rates of >10^9 bits/sec.[10] Single-channel mechanical, hydraulic or acoustic cables ~10 nm in diameter can be bundled together into a flexible 100-nm diameter 100-channel data bus suitable for controlling flexible manipulators or for maintaining control during metamorphic shape shifts; nested doped buckytube fibers could provide a similar multiplicity of electrical conduction channels. Internal fluid chambers can distribute pressure actuation signals in the manner of the latching ratchet/pawl and vernier ratchet threshold-active pressure actuator mechanisms proposed by Drexler.[10]

7.4.4 Interdevice Messaging

Physically-linked nanomachines may communicate with each other through their tethers or network connections. Messaging between physically separated in vivo nanodevices will normally take place via acoustic or chemical, and occasionally mechanical or optical, modalities.

Interdevice communications has been extensively discussed in both free-tissue (broadcast) and cable contexts for chemical messaging (Sections 7.2.1 and 7.2.5.5), acoustic messaging (Sections 7.2.2 and 7.2.5.3), electromagnetic messaging (Sections 7.2.3 and 7.2.5.1-2), mechanical tapping and cable messaging (Sections 7.2.4 and 7.2.5.4), metamorphic surface reconfigurations (Section 5.3.2.5) and network configurations (Section 7.3). The general conclusion is that untethered free nanorobots will typically have maximum interdevice communication ranges on the order of ~100-200 microns; interdevice messaging much beyond that distance probably must be handled by a local or wide-area communications network.

7.4.5 Biocellular Messaging

Nanodevices can also directly communicate with cells by intercepting, modulating, or initiating the flow of natural chemical messenger molecules. Because cells are the fundamental unit of biological organization, it is useful first to examine the various modalities of cellular chemical communication in general terms (Section 7.4.5.1). Properly designed and positioned nanodevices can receive chemical messages from cells (Section 7.4.5.2), send chemical messages into cells (Section 7.4.5.3), modulate natural cellular message traffic (Section 7.4.5.4), or communicate directly with neurons (Sections 7.4.5.5 and 7.4.5.6). Information can also be transferred mechanically into the cell via links between the extracellular matrix (ECM) and the cytoskeleton in ways that have yet to be fully elucidated.[942]

7.4.5.1 Natural Cellular Communications

Cells communicate chemically with each other in two ways—contact signaling and secretory signaling. In the first category, chemical messages may be passed between cells in direct contact through gap junctions that directly join the cytoplasms of the interacting cells (Section 5.4.2). As in the case of foreign or self-antigen presentation (Sections 5.3.6 and 8.5.2.1), cells may also display plasma-membrane-bound molecules on their surfaces which may be "read" by other cells that come into physical contact with them. Signals may also be transduced into cells directly from the ECM.[942,984-986]

In the second category—the principal focus of this Section—there are four basic classes of secretory signaling molecules in the human body, as described briefly below and incompletely listed in Table 7.2. Normal human bloodstream concentrations of some of these molecules are given in Appendix B. At least several hundred different chemical messengers are known to be used in the human body, and many thousands may exist. Biologist Dennis Bray of Cambridge University believes that up to ~50% of the human genome may code for proteins involved in cell signaling,[776] but 10%-20% for "classical" communication pathways is probably more reasonable. For example, the now-sequenced 97-megabase genome of the nematode *Caenorhabditis elegans* has ~19,099 protein-coding genes,[3138] of which ~11% are involved in signal transduction and another ~11% in transport and secretion .[3139]

The first class of secretory signaling molecules is comprised of the endocrine hormones, which are usually secreted by exocytosis and travel through the bloodstream to distant target cells (e.g., "volume transmission") where they act as direct effectors on cell activity. For example, a steroid hormone, upon entering a target cell, binds to a complementary receptor protein. Binding induces conformational changes in the receptor and activates it, increasing the receptor's affinity for DNA and allowing it in turn to bind to specific genes in the nucleus, thus directly regulating their transcription.[3140] This process is extremely wasteful because many activated receptors bind to DNA at sites where their presence has no effect;[531] Lewin[997] notes that activated receptors have a tenfold increased affinity for nonspecific DNA.

The second class consists of local chemical mediators or paracrines, which travel only a short distance (up to ~1 mm) to neighboring cellular targets. This group also includes the autocrines which act upon a cell's own receptors, such as the prostaglandins which are made by cells in all tissues. The single largest group in this class is the cytokines. Cytokines are soluble proteins or glycoproteins, produced by leukocytes and other cell types, which act as chemical communicators between cells but not as effector molecules in their own right.[767] Cytokines include secretory peptides formerly classified as lymphokines, monokines, interferons, colony-stimulating factors, chemotactic factors and growth factors; over 150 different cytokines had been cloned by 1998.

The third class of chemical signaling molecules is the neurotransmitters, including the 60+ known neuropeptides (typically up to 30-40 residues long), which mediate communications between nerve cells and other cells. Interestingly, a single neurotransmitter signaling molecule may have different effects on different target cells. For instance, acetylcholine stimulates the contraction of skeletal muscle cells but decreases the contraction rate and force in heart muscle cells.[531] The immune and neuroendocrine systems produce and respond to similar signal molecules (e.g., neuropeptides and cytokines). Neuropeptides have been shown to effect immune responses through their influence on cytokine production and action, and cytokines are known to induce or influence the production of peptidergic messenger substances.[768]

The fourth class is the intracellular messengers, also known as intracellular mediators or second messenger substances. While small hydrophobic signaling molecules like the steroids and thyroid hormones pass through the cell membrane and activate receptor proteins inside the cell, hydrophilic signaling molecules such as neurotransmitters, most hormones and local chemical mediators activate receptor proteins on the surface of the target cell. (Cell surface receptors for these signaling molecules may be either diffusely distributed or localized to specific regions of the membrane, and their number can vary from 500 to more than 100,000 per cell for a specific ligand.) Because cell surface receptors cannot regulate gene expression directly, they must emit a second messenger molecule into the cytosol which can then trigger the desired regulatory action. Cyclic AMP (cAMP), an intracellular messenger that tells certain types of cells to break down their glycogen stores in response to receipt of epinephrine at the cell surface, is perhaps the best-known example (Section 7.4.5.4). Another example is the voltage-gated Ca^{++} ion channel (Sections 3.3.3 and 7.4.5.3), which participates in nerve pulse events but also in signal transduction via the inositol-phospholipid pathway for more than 25 different types of cell surface receptors of hormonal signals.[531] For instance, excitation-contraction coupling in skeletal muscle cells requires the release of Ca^{++} ions through ryanodine receptor channels in the SR (sarcoplasmic reticulum; Section 8.5.3.5), each of which opens to provide 4-8 picoamp Ca^{++} ion currents in 1-2 millisec bursts, through the SR membrane.[1965]

7.4.5.2 Inmessaging from Cells

Nanodevices can receive the natural chemical messages transmitted from and between cells simply by eavesdropping on the natural molecular message traffic. (Of course, mechanical (e.g., cytoskeletal) and electrical (e.g., ionic) cellular emanations may also be detectable by nanodevices.)

For instance, consider a ~0.1 micromole puff of epinephrine (aka adrenalin, $C_9H_{13}NO_3$, MW = 183 daltons) released into the human bloodstream from cells in the adrenal medulla located above the kidneys. Epinephrine is an emergency hormone emitted in response to stressful conditions which acts to increase heart rate, decrease the blood flow to the gut, increase blood flow to skeletal muscles, increase circulation of oxygen and nutrients to other organs, and mobilize the production of metabolic fuels such as fatty acids and glucose (by causing liver and muscle cells to break down glycogen)—establishing the primitive mammalian "fight or flight" response.

As bloodstream concentrations rise over 1-10 sec to a peak of $c_{ligand} \sim 10^{-8}$ molecules/nm^3 (Appendix B), then from Eqn. 4.3 a bloodborne nanorobot with a single epinephrine chemical sensor having just ~0.4 nm^2 of active surface area can detect the peak concentration in $t_{EQ} \sim 0.3$ sec. A patch of 260 such receptors measuring ~500 nm^2 in total physical surface area can detect the peak concentration within ~1 millisec of its occurrence, or can detect 10% of peak concentration within 10 millisec from the start of the ramp-up. Epinephrine and most other signaling molecules cannot be directly measured by nanorobots stationed within the cytosol because the molecule is hydrophilic and cannot pass through the cellular membrane (unlike the steroids). For the most rapid possible response to changing hormone levels, chemosensor-equipped nanorobots should be positioned on or inside the cells and organs which produce specific signals of interest, with the results of positive detections of increased activity quickly passed along through the in vivo communications network (Section 7.3).

For the rarest cytokines or steroid hormones present at $c_{ligand} \sim 10^{-12}$ molecules/nm^3 in the bloodstream or cytosol (equivalent to ~8 molecules inside one (20 micron)^3 tissue cell or ~1 molecule inside a single leukocyte), a ~5000 nm^2 sensor patch containing ~100 individual receptors (each having ~6 nm^2 of active area) can register a detection in ~10 sec for a single cytosol-based nanorobot. However, cellular signaling molecules are more commonly present in the cytosol at ~10^{-8} molecule/nm^3 levels,[531] enabling ~1 millisec detections using this sensor configuration. By comparison, the typical target tissue cell has ~10,000 steroid receptors (each binding one steroid molecule) floating in the cytosol.

Nanodevices may also eavesdrop on morphogenic signals. For example, simple changes in the extracellular protease/antiprotease concentration ratio (which causes endothelial cells to detach from their parent vessel and invade their underlying stroma during angiogenesis) are readily detected using chemical nanosensors. Continuous monitoring of the relevant natural cytokine traffic can help nanorobots maintain a complete picture of current cellular activities and states. Indeed, the principal design challenge is likely to be sensory traffic data management rather than sensor speed or specificity. Living cells are awash in a sea of messages from hormones, cytokines, growth factors, and a host of other message-carrying molecules, all of which must be transmitted through complex chemical networks of intermediates and multiple signal pathways into the cell's interior.

7.4.5.3 Outmessaging to Cells

Individual micron-scale nanorobots have insufficient chemical release volume or manufacturing capacity to transmit endocrine-like chemical signals throughout the entire bloodstream (Section 7.2.1.8), although simultaneous coordinated chemical releases may be made from large numbers of in vivo nanomachines for special purposes. Nanodevice outmessaging to cells thus will normally be limited to localized paracrine-like, neurotransmitter, or intracellular messaging, and of course nucleic molecules which may have a direct control function. Indeed, the most efficient outmessaging to cells may involve the assembly of customized RNA molecules or their antisense variants (using locally available raw materials such as RNA bases and amino acids) to up- or down-regulate specific gene activities (Chapter 12) thus taking advantage of the cell's inherent amplification by the ribosomes.

As a simple example, Ca^{++} serves as an intracellular mediator in a wide variety of cell responses including secretion, cell proliferation, neurotransmission, cellular metabolism (when complexed to calmodulin), and signal cascade events that are regulated by calcium-calmodulin-dependent protein kinases and adenylate cyclases. The concentration of free Ca^{++} in the extracellular fluid or in the cell's internal calcium sequestering compartment (which is loaded with a binding protein called calsequestrin) is ~10^{-3} ions/nm.^{3} However, in the cytosol, free Ca^{++} concentration varies from 6 x 10^{-8} ions/nm^3 for a resting cell up to 3 x 10^{-6} ions/nm^3 when the cell is activated by an extracellular signal; cytosolic levels > 10^{-5} ions/nm^3 may be toxic,[531] e.g., via apoptosis (Sections 10.4.1.1 and 10.4.2.1).

To transmit an artificial Ca^{++} activation signal to a typical tissue cell in ~1 millisec, a single nanorobot stationed in the cytoplasm must promptly raise the cytosolic ion count from 480,000 Ca^{++} ions to 24 million Ca^{++} ions, a transfer rate of ~2.4 x 10^{10} ions/sec which may be accomplished using ~24,000 molecular sorting rotors (Section 3.4.2) operated in reverse, requiring a total nanorobot emission surface area of ~2.4 micron^2. Or, more compactly, pressurized venting or an ion nozzle may be employed (Section 9.2.7). Onboard storage volume of ~0.1 micron^3 can hold ~2 billion calcium atoms, enough to transmit ~100 artificial Ca^{++} signals into the cell after ionization (2877 zJ/ion double-ionization energy)[763] even assuming no recycling.

In addition to the amplitude modulation (AM) of Ca^{++} signals noted above, De Koninck and Schulman[1121] have discovered a mechanism (CaM kinase II) that transduces frequency-modulated (FM) Ca^{++} intracellular signals in the range of 0.1-10 Hz. Fine tuning of the kinase's activity by both AM and FM signals (either of which is readily detected or generated by in cyto nanorobots) may occur as the molecule participates in the control of diverse cellular activities.

Nanorobots may also mechanically outmessage to cells. The cytoskeleton of living cells and nuclei are hard-wired such that a mechanical tug on cell surface receptors can immediately change the organization of molecular structures inside the nucleus and the cytoplasm[942] and can dramatically alter cellular electrical conductivity.[1100] The intermediate fiber network (Section 8.5.3.11) alone is sufficient to transmit mechanical stress to the nucleus.[942] The minimum force required to initiate signal transduction may be as low as ~10 pN (Section 9.4.3.2.1), well within the ~100 nanonewton capacity of the nanomanipulator arm described in Section 9.3.1.4.

7.4.5.4 Cell Message Modification

Properly configured in cyto nanorobots can modify natural intracellular message traffic according to preprogrammed rules or by following external commands issued by the attending physician. In the case of steroids and thyroid hormones, this may involve the direct manipulation of the signaling molecules themselves (after they

Table 7.2. The Four Major Classes of Human Cell Secretory Signaling Molecules[531,755,767,769]

I. Endocrine Hormones

STEROIDS

Aldosterone
Catecholestrogens
Cholecalciferol (vitamin D_3)
Cortisol (hydrocortisone)
Dehydroepiandrosterone (DHEA)
11-Deoxycorticosterone
Dihydrotestosterone
Estradiol & Estriol
Estrone
Progesterone
Testosterone

AMINO ACID DERIVATIVES

Epinephrine (adrenalin)
Thyroid Hormone (thyroxine)

PEPTIDES AND PROTEINS

Adrenocorticotropic hormone (ACTH)
Antimullerian hormone
Arg-Vasopressin (AVP)
Arg-Vasotocin
Atrial natriuretic factor (ANF)
Autoimmune antiinsulin
Cacitonin (CT)
Enteroglucagon (GLI)
Follicle-Stimulating hormone (FSH)
Gastric Inhibitory Polypeptide (GIP)
Gastrin
GH Releasing Factor (GRF)
Growth Hormone (GH, somatotropin)
Glicentin
Human Chorionic Gonadotropin (hCG)
Human Placental Lactogen (hPL)
Inhibin
Insulin
Leptin
Lipotropin (LPH)
Long-Acting Thyroid Stimulator (LATS)
Luteinizing Hormone (LH)
Melanocyte-Stimulating Hormone (MSH)
Motilin
Osteoclast-Activating Factor (OAF)
Ovarian Growth Factor
Pancreatic Glucagon
Pancreatic Polypeptide (PP)
Parathyroid Hormone (PTH)
Platelet Growth Factor
Proinsulin
Prolactin-Releasing Factor (PRH)
Relaxin
Secretin
Somatomedins
Thymic Humoral Factor (THF)
Thyroid-Stimulating Hormone (TSH)
Thyrotropic-Releasing Hormone (TRH)

II. Local Chemical Mediators

FATTY ACID DERIVATIVES

Leukotriene A_4(LTA_4)
Leukotriene A_5 (LTA_5)
Leukotriene B (LTB)
Leukotriene C (LTC)
Leukotriene C_5 (LTC_5)
Prostacyclin (PGI_2)
Prostaglandin A_2 (PGA_2)
Prostaglandin E_1 (PGE_1)
Prostaglandin E_2 (PGE_2)
Prostaglandin $F_{1\alpha}$ ($PGF_{1\alpha}$)
Prostaglandin $F_{2\alpha}$ ($PGF_{2\alpha}$)
Thromboxane A_2 (TXA_2)
Thromboxane B_2 (TXB_2)

AMINO ACID DERIVATIVES

Histamine

CYTOKINE FAMILIES (Peptides & Proteins)

<u>Hematopoietin Family</u>: Erythropoietin, IL-2 (Interleukin), IL-3, IL-4, IL-5, IL-6, IL-7, IL-9, IL-10, IL-13, G-CSF, GM-CSF (Granulocyte-Macrophage Colony Stimulating Factor), M-CSF, CNTF, OSM, LIF (Leukemia Inhibitory Factor), IFNα (Interferon), IFNβ, IFNγ

<u>EGF Family</u>: Epidermal Growth Factor (EGF, or urogastrone), TGFα (Transforming Growth Factor)

<u>β-Trefoil Family</u>: FGFα (Fibroblast Growth Factor), FGFβ, IL-1α, IL-1β, IL-1Rα

<u>TNF Family</u>: TNFα (Tumor Necrosis Factor), TNFβ, LTβ

<u>Cysteine Knot Family</u>: NGF (Nerve Growth Factor), TGFβ1, TGFβ2, TGFβ3, PDGF (Platelet Derived Growth Factor), VEGF (Vascular Endothelial Growth Factor)

<u>Cheomkine Family</u>: IL-8, MIP-1α (Macrophage Inflammatory Protein), MIP-1β, MIP-2, PF-4, PBP, I-309/TCA-3, MCP-1, MCP-2, MCP-3, γIP-10

<u>Other Cytokines</u>: Angiopoietin, Eosinophil Chemotactic Factor, Eosinophil Stimulator Promoter, Fibrinopeptide B, Insulinlike Growth Factors (IGF), Kallikrein, Leukocyte Inhibitory Factor, Lymphocyte Stimulating Factor, Macrophage Activating Factor (MAF), Macrophage Growth Factor (MGF), Macrophage Stimulatory Protein (MSP), Neutrophil Chemotactic Factor, Platelet Activating Factor, Proliferation Inhibitory Factor, Thrombopoietin (TPO), Thymopoietin

III. Neurotransmitters

NEUROTRANSMITTERS

Acetylcholine
Acetylserotonin
γ-Aminobutyric acid (GABA)
Dopamine
Glutamic acid
Glycine
Histamine
Melatonin
Nitric Oxide
Norepinephrine (noradrenaline) (NEP)
Octopamine
Serotonin

NEUROPEPTIDES

ACTH
Angiotensin II
Bombesin
Bradykinin
Cacitonin
Carnosine
Cholecystokinin (CCK, pancreozymin)
Corticotropin Releasing Factor (CRF)
Dynorphin
β-Endorphin
Enkephalin
Galanin
Gastrin & Gastrin Releasing Peptide
GH Releasing Hormone (GHRH)
Glucagon & Insulin
Kyotorphin
LH Releasing Hormone (LHRH)
Lipotropin
Motilin
Neurokinin A & B
Neuropeptide Y & P
Neurotensin
Oxytocin
Proctolin
Prolactin (PRL)
Secretin
Somatostatin
Substance P
Tachykinins
Vasoactive Intestinal Peptide (VIP)
Vasopressin

IV. Intracellular Messengers

Arachidonic acid
Ca^{++} (w/ or w/o calmodulin)
Cyclic AMP
Cyclic GMP
Diacylglycerol
Diadenosinetetraphosphate
GTPase-Activating Proteins (GAPs)
Guanine Nucleotide Exchange Factors (GEFs)
Inositol triphosphate

have passed through the cell membrane) or their bound receptor complexes. However, most signaling molecules are absorbed at the cell surface, initiating a signal cascade which must be modulated by manipulating the second-messenger molecules or other components of the signal cascade. A complete analysis of the modifications that nanorobots may impose upon normal intracellular message traffic is beyond the scope of this book. However, a few basic examples of modifying action may be illustrated using the familiar cyclic AMP (cAMP; $C_{10}H_{11}N_5O_6P$, MW = 328 daltons) messaging system.

A. *Amplification* — A single epinephrine molecule received by a β adrenergic receptor at a cell surface transduces the activation of dozens of G-protein α subunits, each of which in turn activates a single adenylate cyclase enzyme which cyclizes hundreds of ATP molecules into cAMP molecules. The intracellular population of cAMP (in muscle or liver target cells) is normally $\lesssim 10^{-6}$ M or ~5 million molecules for a typical (20 micron)^3 tissue cell. Stimulation by epinephrine raises the cAMP population to ~25 million molecules in a few seconds. Upon detecting this rising tide of cAMP in a few millisec, a single in cyto nanorobot could amplify this existing chemical signal by instantly releasing 20 million cAMP molecules (occupying ~0.01 micron^3) from onboard inventories—decreasing cellular response time by several orders of magnitude.*

B. *Suppression* — Similarly, upon detection of rising cAMP levels in target cells, resident nanorobots could use molecular rotors to rapidly remove cAMP from the cytosol as quickly as it is formed, even under maximum adrenal stimulation. From Eqn. 3.4 the diffusion-limited intake current at the basal concentration (~6 x 10^{-7} molecules/nm^3) for a cAMP-absorbing spherical nanodevice 1 micron in radius is ~4 million molecules/sec, so a single such device could probably keep up with natural cAMP production rates and thus completely extinguish the response by preserving a flat basal concentration. (As a practical matter, it may be more efficient to simply control epinephrine generation at its glandular source unless it is desired to interface with just a single tissue type.) Simultaneously, the cAMP-absorbing nanorobot may hydrolyze the stored cAMP (hydrolysis energy is ~11.1 Kcal/mole or ~77.1 zJ/molecule)[3298] in the manner of the cAMP phosphodiesterases (c.f. nanofactories, Chapter 19), then excrete these deactivated AMP messenger molecules back into the cytosol. Similar methods might be useful in ligand-gated ion channel desensitization or in disease symptom suppression (Chapter 24)—as for example, in suppressing the prolonged elevation of cAMP in intestinal epithelial cells associated with the cholera toxin, that produces severe diarrhea by causing a large influx of water into the gut.

C. *Replacement* — Combining suppression and amplification, an existing chemical signal may be eliminated and replaced by a different—even an opposite—message pathway using nanorobot mediators. Alternative pathways may be natural or wholly synthetic. Novel responses to existing signals may be established within the cell to enhance functionality or to improve stability or controllability. For example, detection of one species of cytokine by a nanorobot could trigger rapid specific absorption of that cytokine and a simultaneous fast release of another (different) species of cytokine in its place. Such procedures must take into account the redundant signaling pathways and backup systems (e.g., developmental signals, immune system, blood clotting). Medical nanorobotics will allow the replacement of many redundant pathways with more refined and specific responses.

D. *Linkage* — Previously unlinked signal cascades may be artificially linked using in cyto nanodevices. As a fanciful example, the receipt of epinephrine by nanorobots located in the capillaries of the brain could trigger these devices to suppress the adrenalin response while simultaneously releasing chemical messengers producing message cascades that stimulate production of enkephalins or other opioids, thus encouraging a state of psychological relaxation rather than the "fight or flight" response to certain stressful conditions.

7.4.5.5 Inmessaging from Neurons

Inmessaging from neurons to nanodevices has already been considered in Sections 4.8.6, 4.9.5 and 7.4.2.6. In these discussions, it was concluded that at least half a dozen different methods should permit nanorobot sensors to noninvasively detect, measure, and count the passage of nerve impulses. Neurographics, neuroinformatics,[1298] connectivity mapping and individual neural targeting are described in Chapter 25.

7.4.5.6 Outmessaging to Neurons

In vivo nanorobots can outmessage to neurons as well. The most direct method is synaptic stimulation. In excitory cholinergic synapses, perhaps the most common type, the arrival of a presynaptic nerve impulse stimulates the release of up to ~10^5 molecules of acetylcholine ($C_7H_{16}NO_2$, MW = 146 daltons) from synaptic vesicles into the synaptic cleft in ~1 millisec, producing a local concentration of ~3 x 10^{-4} molecules/nm^3 (~0.0005 M).[531] The acetylcholine molecules diffuse across the cleft to the postsynaptic membrane (Section 4.8.6.4), where they bind to specific receptor proteins (Section 3.3.3), opening ion channels within 0.1 millisec[313] and partially depolarizing the cell, increasing local Na^+ permeability. When depolarization reaches ~15% of full voltage range (e.g., from -60 mV down to about -40 mV), voltage-activated sodium channels open, making the membrane highly permeable to Na^+ ions. These ions rapidly flow into the cell and initiate the ~100 nanoamp[799] action potential spike. These channels close spontaneously after a short interval to reduce permeability, thus allowing the membrane voltage to be restored to its normal resting potential (Section 3.3.3).

A sorting-rotor-tipped manipulator (Section 3.4.2) or pressurized nanoinjector (Section 9.2.7.1) placed in the vicinity of the synaptic cleft can emit a puff of ~10^5 acetylcholine molecules (~20,000 nm^3), producing partial depolarization and initiating nerve impulses at will. (This is preferable to the use of unnatural depolarizing agents such as veratridine.) A 1-micron^3 storage volume contains ~5 billion molecules, sufficient to induce ~50,000 discharges or ~1 hour of continuous firing at 15 Hz. The initiating mechanism must provoke a discharge in ~1 millisec, a throughput rate of 10^8 molecules/sec requiring, say, ~100 sorting rotors with total manipulator tool tip area ~10^4 nm^2. At 15 Hz continuous firing, ~10^6 molecules/sec are

* *From a practical standpoint, R. Bradbury notes that designers should have knowledge of the biochemical pathways that are most critical in the response to a signal, hence nanorobots may be able to skip the intermediate steps required in the biological system. In the present example, the cascade is typically intended to increase the glucose available for muscles, so it might make more sense to skip the cAMP step and simply commence disassembly of glycogen (in the liver and muscles) and accelerate the pumping of glucose into the bloodstream (from the liver).*

** *Under controlled mechanochemical conditions (Chapter 19) where the effective heat of protonation of the buffering system can be ignored, the net enthalpy of hydrolysis at 298 K and pH 7 may fall as low as ~1.95 zJ/molecule, or ~0.28 Kcal/mole.*[3142]

consumed. Sorting rotors placed near the cleft can also absorb the two breakdown products (acetate and choline) of acetylcholinesterase activity (~150 microsec turnover time [3143]) and recycle them into new molecules of acetylcholine. Taking the enthalpy of hydrolysis under physiological conditions** as ~70 zJ/molecule (~10 Kcal/mole) for the acetylcholinesterase-mediated hydrolysis reaction,[3142] the power requirement for continuously recycling 10^6 molecules/sec is ~0.07 pW. A similar rotor transport mechanism may also be used to rapidly extract acetylcholine molecules from the synaptic cleft, thus extinguishing a passing nerve impulse. Note that to exert control over nerve impulses, neurotransmitter injectors must be placed very close to the post-synaptic surface because the effective diffusion radius of acetylcholine is only a few microns, due to the high efficiency of local acetylcholinesterase.[803]

Many compounds other than acetylcholine may serve as neurotransmitters (Table 7.2), including nitric oxide and possibly carbon monoxide.[1125,1129] Catecholamines such as dopamine, norepinephrine and epinephrine, synthesized in the adrenal gland and elsewhere, act as neurotransmitters at adrenergic synapses which are found at the junctions between nerves and smooth muscles in internal organs such as the intestine and in nerve-nerve junctions in the brain. There are also histaminergic neurons found exclusively in the hippocampus.[1123] Most tissues in the human body are innervated by several different types of nerve cells, each using a different neurotransmitter, allowing a great diversity of signals and responses. But synaptic-resident nanorobots should be able to monitor, stimulate, or extinguish all of these signals, even given the confusing geometries entailed by synaptic clusters.

While some synapses use excitory neurotransmitters that elicit an electrical signal, others use different neurotransmitters such as GABA, glycine, or the enkephalins that deliver an inhibitory signal, suppressing electrical response. Some molecules work both ways. For example, acetylcholine is excitory at neuromuscular junctions but may be excitory or inhibitory in the central and peripheral nervous system. A nerve cell may receive thousands of these excitory and inhibitory chemical inputs, and their relative number determines the probability of axonal firing. Again, selections from the complete known library of neurotransmitters of all types may be made available for storage, synthesis, absorption or release by properly configured nanorobots.

Neuropeptides, which can act as highly specific triggers for complex patterns of activity in the nervous system (including memory, learning, perception, mood, and behavior) and allow long-term chemical modulation of synaptic sensitivity, add yet another complication to neural outmessaging by nanorobots. Neuropeptides are manufactured by ribosomes on rough endoplasmic reticulum within the neuron cell body and must be transported to axon terminals for release by "fast axonal transport"—a journey that may take a day or more for a long axon. They are stored in intracellular vesicles from which they are released to the extracellular space of peptidergic neurons. Neuropeptides released into the synaptic cleft serve as neuromodulators (to inhibit the action of excitory neurotransmitters) or neuromediators (to prolong the action of neurotransmitters), both functions easily duplicated by nanorobots. However, neuropeptides released into the bloodstream act as long-range neurohormones, and neuropeptides released into the extracellular space act as paracrines and enter both pharmacodynamic and pharmacokinetic cascades.[770] Nanorobot management of these more diffusely distributed tissue neuropeptide concentrations (e.g., by mimicking the action of natural peptidases of broad substrate specificity) is a more difficult, though not intractable, task.

There are many other methods by which in vivo nanorobots can outmessage to neurons:

1. Periodic manipulation of electric (Section 4.8.6.1) and magnetic (Section 4.8.6.2) fields may trigger neural impulses.[3328]

2. An excess population of Na^+ ions outside the myelinated nerve fiber establishes an intra-axonal resting potential of -60 mV. The net movement of Na^+ associated with a single neural impulse is ~0.3 ion/micron^2 in ~0.5 millisec,[526] so the direct injection of a few electric charges should produce local depolarization, initiating a neural impulse. Note that the voltage balance is maintained by differing concentrations of several ions, not just Na^+, although the inrush of Na^+ is the primary cause of membrane voltage change during the discharge spike.

3. Membrane ionic currents may be pharmacologically manipulated by nanodevices permanently stationed within the cytosol. For example, sodium pumps are completely inhibited by the injection of 10-100 nM of cardioactive steroids such as ouabain and strophanthidin.[805] Injection of ~300 nM tetrodotoxin inhibits sodium currents while leaving potassium currents unchanged; inserting tetraethylammonium blocks only the potassium currents, while leaving sodium currents unchanged.[804]

4. Establishing a localized ~100 mV circumaxonal (external) superexcess of positive charge may present an electrical barrier steep enough to quench a depolarization wave, thus extinguishing a passing nerve impulse. Techniques of electronic anesthesia, such as transcutaneous electronic nerve stimulation (TENS) and cell demodulated electronic anesthesia (CEDETA), involve crude applications of similar principles.[3299,3300]

5. Long-term electrical stimulation of neurons using electrodes to apply 0.1-Hz pulses for ~10^5 sec reduced the expression of neural cell adhesion molecule L1 (NCAM) by a factor of ~13.[1063]

6. Direct ultrasonic stimulation of neurons.[3535]

7.4.6 Outmessaging to Patient or User

In many applications, in vivo medical nanodevices may need to communicate information directly to the user or patient. This capability is crucial in providing feedback to establish stable and reliable autogenous command and control systems (Chapter 12). Outmessaging from nanorobot to the patient or user requires the nanodevice to manipulate a sensory channel that is consciously available to human perception, which manipulation can then be properly interpreted by the patient as a message.

Sensory channels available for such communication include sight, audition, gustation and olfaction, kinesthesia, and somesthetic sensory channels such as pressure, pain, and temperature. Nanodevice-originated data may be superimposed upon the natural sensory traffic by:

1. generating an artificial sensory stimulus,

2. direct stimulation of the receptor in the absence of actual sensory stimulus, or

3. triggering artificial action potentials in the afferent nerves that carry information from the sensor to the CNS.

7.4.6.1 Somesthetic Outmessaging

Human skin contains about 700,000 pressure or touch receptors, mostly concentrated on the fingers (~17,000 receptors on all fingertips) and on the face—especially the lips and the tip of the tongue.

In addition to information about the presence of tactile stimuli, touch receptors can also discriminate both intensity and spatial direction of the stimulus (Table 7.3). Meissner's corpuscle, located in the papillae of the corium just beneath the epidermis, is a receptor for light touch. The Pacinian corpuscle is a deep touch or pressure receptor located in the deep parts of the dermis, in the connective tissue around muscles, tendons, and joints, and in the mesenteries supporting the visceral organs.

A networked population of outmessaging nanorobots, with each nanorobot positioned near a Meissner's or Pacinian corpuscle and capable of triggering artificial nerve impulses (Section 7.4.5.6), could create coordinated spatial and temporal patterns of pressure sensations that could be interpreted by the patient as specific messages. For example, nanorobots neurally emulating the sensation of pressure in the fingers in the sequence Thumb-Thumb-Ring-Index-Thumb are communicating the message "11421" to the user at a transfer rate of 1-10 bits/sec. Similarly, stimulating the arrector muscles artificially triggers the nerve plexus surrounding epidermal hair follicles (which register hair motion), creating well-defined and potentially communicative patterns of "gooseflesh" on the skin.

Mild stimulation of pain receptors (nociceptors), consisting of unmyelinated free sensory nerve endings with pain sensation mediated by the peptide nociceptin, could also produce interpretable messages. For instance, some C fibers when sufficiently stimulated produce burning pain, while small D fibers signal a prickling pain. (There are ~228 pain receptors/cm^2 in the neck region, ~188/cm^2 on the back of the hand, ~95/cm^2 on the radial surface of the middle finger, and ~44/cm^2 on the tip of the nose).[869] Heat receptors (brushes of Ruffini) and cold receptors (end bulbs of Krause) also may be employed for outmessaging. Cold spots outnumber warm spots by a factor of 4-10, with temperature receptors concentrated on the face and hands and specific regions showing marked differences in the mix of sensor types (e.g., the forehead contains 0.6 warm receptors/cm^2 but 8.0 cold receptors/cm^2). Nanorobots could employ these neural channels to communicate temporally- and spatially-ordered sensations of burning pain, prickly pain, or heat and cold. The maximum serial transfer rate of each of these outmessaging channels to the conscious human mind may be only ~1 bit/sec, although complex spatial and temporal patterns using multiple parallel channels involving significantly higher data flows may be employed in creating full-immersion virtual reality simulations and in related applications (Chapter 25).

The Optacon (Optical-to-Tactile Converter), originally developed by NASA, scanned normal inkprint and converted the characters into a tactile format on a 24 x 6 vibrating-pin array, enabling the blind to feel-read without Braille. Average users achieved ~30 words/min, or up to ~100 words/min in exceptional cases. The Optacon was first sold in 1970 by Telesensory Inc. but is no longer manufactured. Blazie Engineering, Inc., which acquired all rights to the Optacon in 1998, also sells Power Braille, an 81-character 8-dot refreshable Braille display for desktop computer applications.

7.4.6.2 Kinesthetic Outmessaging

Direct stimulation of kinesthetic sensory neural channels for outmessaging may prove disorienting, disturbing, confusing, or even nauseogenic to the user, as for example a periodic manipulation of the vestibular ganglion (creating synthetic vertigo), muscular stretch receptors (creating "phantom limb" effects), or reflex arcs (e.g., sneezing, knee jerks, lactation, pupillary dilation, or orgasm). Patients might be slightly more comfortable if nanorobots generate a genuine sensory stimulus which can then be detected as a true sensory reading. Examples might include the creation of patterned nervous tics by triggering small-muscle spasms in the face or limbs (twitches), temporally-structured subvocal hiccups by stimulating and inhibiting the phrenic nerve causing tiny spasms in the diaphragm muscle, or periodic blepharospasms (winking) by stimulating the orbicularis palpebrarum muscle (ring muscle) of the eye.

Selective activation of motor neurons controlling the ~400 skeletal muscles in the human body can produce involuntary macroscopic limb motion. To take a familiar example, properly positioned neurostimulatory nanorobots may trigger in sequence the extensor indicis and the flexor indicis muscles, causing the second and third phalanges of the index finger first to extend, then to retract; or trigger

Table 7.3. Tactile Receptors in the Human Skin[854,869,1633-1637]

Skin Receptor Type	Receptor Class	Skin Type	Probable Sensory Correlation	Receptive Field, Range (and Median)	Frequency Range (and Most Sensitive)	# of Fingertip Receptors (and on Palm)
Pacinian corpuscles	PC	G, H	Vibration, tickle	10-1000 mm^2 (100 mm^2)	40-800 Hz (200-300 Hz)	21/cm^2 (9/cm^2)
Meissner's corpuscles	RA	G	Touch, tickle, motion, vibration	1-100 mm^2 (13 mm^2)	10-200 Hz (20-40 Hz)	140/cm^2 (25/cm^2)
Hair follicle nerve	RA	H	Touch, vibration	~ 0.01 mm^2	10-100 Hz (?)	10/cm^2 200/cm^2 (scalp)
Ruffini ending	SA II	G, H	Stretch, shear, tension (?)	10-500 mm^2 (60 mm^2)	7 Hz	49/cm^2 (16/cm^2)
Merkel's cells	SA I	G	Pressure, edge (?)	2-100 mm^2 (11 mm^2)	0.4-100 Hz (7 Hz)	70/cm^2 (8/cm^2)
Tactile disks	SA I	H	Pressure, edge (?)	3-50 mm^2	1-100 Hz (?) (10 Hz) (?)	70/cm^2 (?) (8/cm^2) (?)

PC = Pacinian afferents; RA = rapidly-adapting afferents; SA II = slowly-adapting, large receptive field afferents; SA I = slowly-adapting, small receptive field mechanoreceptive afferents; G = glabrous (hairless) skin; H = hairy skin.

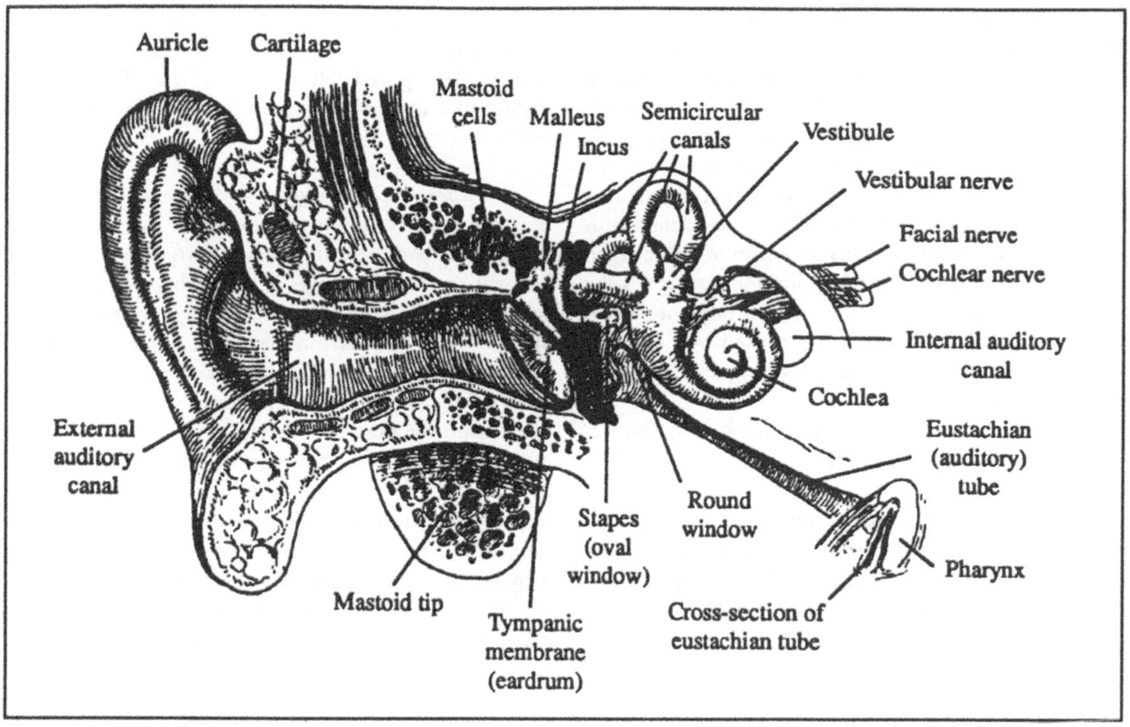

Fig. 7.3. Cross-section of the human ear (redrawn from Davis and Silverman[868]).

the extensor minimi digiti and the flexor brevis minimi digiti muscles, causing the second and third phalanges of the little finger to extend, then the first phalanx of the little finger to flex; or trigger the extensor pollicis brevis and the flexor pollicis brevis muscles, causing the base of the first phalanx of the thumb to extend, then retract. These artificially induced finger movements may be directly interpreted as messages by a trained user at a 1-10 bit/sec transfer rate, or else the patient may grasp a handheld device that translates the controlled sequence of forced gripping motions into a correct alphanumeric or voiced message.

7.4.6.3 Auditory Outmessaging

The human ear consists of an air-filled external auditory canal terminating on the ~1 cm^2 tympanic membrane (~100 microns thick), whose vibrations are transmitted through the bony ossicles of the ~2 cm^3 middle ear to the membranous oval window of the inner ear (Fig. 7.3). From there, sound energy enters the cochlea as compressional waves in the perilymph, an incompressible watery fluid that fills most of the ~100 mm^3 spiral cochlear tube. This ~35-mm long tube resembles a snail shell, coiled two and a half times around the modiolus, itself the center axis along which pass the cochlear nerves and blood vessels. About 24,000 hair cells (multifiber stereocilia) on the basilar membrane under the tectorial membrane (Fig. 7.4) inside the cochlea resonate in response to different acoustic frequencies. These cells make complex synaptic contacts with neurons of the spiral ganglion, which passes this aural information into the auditory (8th cranial) nerve and thence to the brain for decoding.

A large nanodevice (~20-50 microns) stationed in the perilymph of the cochlea can "speak" directly into the human ear, loud enough to be heard. Total acoustic power delivered to the tympanic membrane during normal audition is ~10^{-4} pW (0 dB) at the threshold of hearing, ~0.1 pW for whispering (30 dB), and ~100 pW for normal conversation (60 dB). At the low frequencies (30-10,000 Hz) common to human speech, micron-scale acoustic radiators are very inefficient (Section 7.2.2.1) although there are virtually no attenuation losses (Eqn. 4.52). Even so, from Eqn. 7.7 a cochlear nanodevice able to apply an input power of 2000 pW to an acoustic omnidirectional piston radiator 20 microns in diameter can generate 10 KHz sound waves at an output power ~ 0.1 pW, approximately the intensity level of whispering. At a more comfortable 3 KHz (the peak sensitivity of human hearing), P_{in} must rise to ~22,000 pW or piston diameter must increase to 45 microns to maintain P_{out} ~ 0.1 pW, or a duty cycle substantially less than 100% must be employed. If linked to a communication network, the cochlear nanodevice can receive information to be audibilized from the network. This device can also be used for acoustic inmessaging by allowing it to intercept sound waves before they reach the basilar membrane, then passing this information immediately to the network (which thus receives the signal sooner than the brain). Perilymph contains glucose for power at roughly serum concentrations; alternatively, the cochlear device can absorb and store the natural ambient acoustic energy present in the auditory canal (Section 7.4.8).

Similarly, a nanorobot located in the endolymph-filled scala media, the innermost of the three parallel chambers of the cochlea, can attach itself to the reticular lamina of the organ of Corti and physically manipulate the stereocilia to produce the desired audible stimulus. Stereocilia are spaced over the organ of Corti at a linear density of ~1 cell/micron along the 30 mm length of the cochlear spiral tube.[585] Continuously stimulating all ~100 cells within reach of a 20-micron diameter nanorobot with bidirectional 40-micron long extensible manipulators should produce a narrow-frequency tone up to ~0.4% of maximum pressure amplitude, close to normal conversational levels. Hair cells have a membrane time constant of ~0.5 millisec,[772] in theory permitting a transfer rate of up to ~2000 bits/sec if all stereocilia are manipulated coherently as a single channel. Careful design should prevent unwanted stimulation of tinnitus.

Direct neural stimulation of some of the ~31,000 spiral ganglion cells allows transduction of information into the human auditory system. Each ganglial cell carries temporal and amplitude information on a narrow band of acoustic frequencies received by the ear, essentially a crude Fourier transform of the original audio signal. Properly positioned nanorobots can superimpose artificial signals on this natural traffic which may be perceived by the patient as a frequency-reconstructed voice of limited tonal range speaking words or numbers. Nanorobots stationed at the saccule, an otolithic organ in the vestibule of the inner ear, can stimulate direct ultrasonic hearing in humans up to ~108 KHz.[1372] In 1998, cochlear implant devices were in wide use, with audible sounds transmitted by FM radio waves to an electrode array in the inner ear, providing direct electrical stimulation of the auditory nerves.[1891-1893]

A review of current technology in artificial speech synthesis[1653,1654] is beyond the scope of this text.

7.4.6.4 Gustatory and Olfactory Outmessaging

In theory it would be possible to insert artificial flavors onto the lingual surface, or to release artificial scents into the nasal epithelium. However, human taste buds have a lifetime of ~10 days, requiring constant repositioning of resident chemical emission devices. Human olfactory receptors are located at the back of the nose (Fig. 8.11), covered by a sheet of mucus, adding signal time delays and dispersion (due to finite and differential molecular diffusion rates) to high-frequency olfactory messages. Additionally, frequent large-volume chemical emissions from individual nanorobots is not feasible due to scaling factors (Section 7.2.1.8).

In this case it appears more efficient to stimulate the gustatory and olfactory nerves directly. This minimizes power consumption, reduces the required volume of chemical releases by many orders of magnitude, and permits rapid multiplexing of numerous distinct synthetic sensory signals.

A. *Gustatory Outmessaging* — There are ~12,000 taste buds innervated by nerve fibers that lose their myelin sheaths as they pass through the basement membrane. Large fibers end on two or more bud cells, with the endings of small fibers invaginating the receptor cell membrane. The large taste fibers from the anterior two-thirds of the tongue branch from the lingual nerve to form a slender nerve, the chorda tympani, which traverses the eardrum as part of the facial (7th cranial) nerve en route to the medulla. The afferent fibers from the posterior third of the tongue collect in the lingual branch of the glossopharyngeal (9th cranial) nerve, through the petrosal ganglia and into the medulla. Since taste buds have a response repertoire of only five known distinct sensations (sweet, sour, bitter, salt, and umami*), nanorobots seeking to artificially provoke these sensations may proceed to the chorda tympani or petrosal ganglia with the objective of triggering a higher-level confluent signal on each of a handful of distinct ganglial positions corresponding to the five primary stimuli plus a small set of mixed-sensitivity combinations. Proper identification of the nerve bundles carrying information on each of the five primary stimuli may require a brief training session or prior connectivity mapping (Chapter 25). Note also that natural taste response time is diffusion-limited to ~1 sec (~1 Hz, ~1 bit/sec), and it is not yet known whether the natural

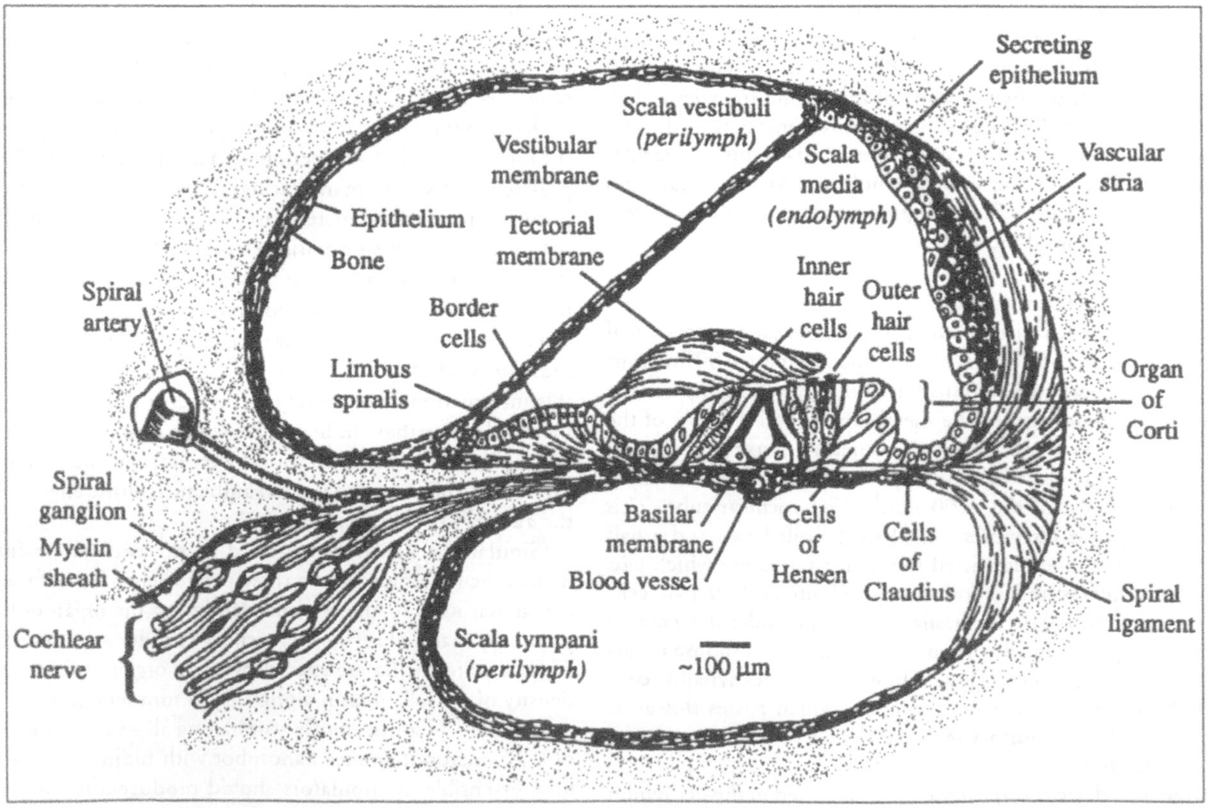

Fig. 7.4. Cross-section of the cochlear duct (redrawn from Wilson[526]).

*Umami, a complex "meaty" or "savory" tastiness factor, was first identified by a Japanese scientist, Professor Ikeda, at the University of Tokyo.[3030-3034] Umami is specifically associated with monosodium glutamate (MSG)[3035], sodium inosinate, and sodium guanylate. Specific taste bud receptors (e.g., mGluR4) for umami have been discovered.[3033,3034]

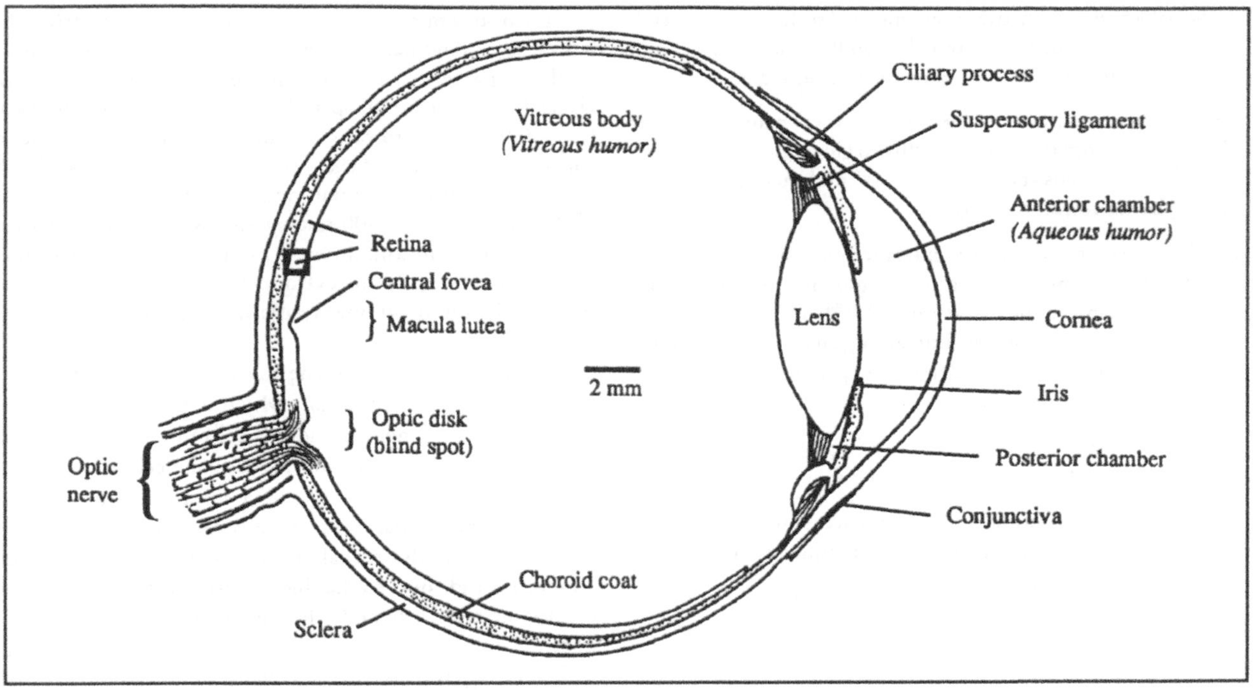

Fig. 7.5. The human eyeball (redrawn from Leukel[869]).

conscious brain can be educated to process multiplexed high-frequency (up to 10-100 Hz, or ~10-100 bits/sec) artificially-stimulated taste signals.

B. *Olfactory Outmessaging* — Humans have up to 50 million olfactory sensors spaced an average ~3 microns apart in the olfactory epithelium (~2.5 cm^2/nostril) located in the upper part of the nasal cavities on the surface of the superior conchae and upper part of the septum (see Figure 8.11). Each sensor protrudes a long and extremely thin olfactory nerve fiber. These fibers are grouped into ~20 filaments in each nasal cavity, and the filaments pass through the cribriform plate of the ethmoid bone into the olfactory bulb (the terminus of the olfactory (1st cranial) nerve) in the forebrain in the cranial cavity. The nasal epithelium also contains a few bare nerve endings from fibers of the trigeminal (5th cranial) nerve. The responses of olfactory receptor neurons are rarely specific to only one odor; the majority of cells respond to a broad range of substances.[3433]

The olfactory nerve fibers enter the olfactory bulb to end in a series of intricate basketlike synaptic terminations or antenna-shaped dendritic clusters called glomeruli. Each olfactory glomerulus receives impulses from about 26,000 receptors and sends them on through 24 mitral cells and 68 tufted cells, thus showing a high degree of neural convergence.

The number of such glomeruli (~1000) may approximate the number of nonmultiplexed distinct olfactory sensations available to man. Humans can identify over 10,000 structurally distinct odorant ligands[807]—some have claimed as many as 400,000 discernible odors[3134,3135]—but this does not imply an equally large repertoire of odorant receptors, because structurally related odorants may bind to the same receptor molecules.[1120] Indeed, individual neurons respond strongly to closely related groups of odorants and weakly or not at all to many others.[807] Sensory neurons with similar ligand specificities project to common glomeruli. The family of 7TD membrane proteins, which is localized to the olfactory cilia and shares homology with the superfamily of neurotransmitters and neuropeptide 7TD receptors,[808] constitutes an extremely large multigene family likely to encode odorant receptors that transduce intracellular signals by interacting with cellular transmembrane G proteins which then activate second messenger systems inside the cell. This family of putative odorant receptors could constitute one of the largest gene families in the genome, with perhaps as many as 500-1000 genes,[809] approximately one receptor type for each glomerulus.

If each glomerulus may be treated as the locus for a single unique olfactory sensation, this may provide an essentially clear output channel for a neurostimulatory nanodevice. Such a device could trigger action potentials in a single glomerulus producing a perception of a rapidly pulsing (possibly up to ~10-100 Hz, or ~10-100 bits/sec) rare scent. Such signals would no longer be diffusion limited (to ~1 Hz, ~1 bit/sec) as is the case with natural olfaction, and rapid adaptation caused by receptor saturation would also be eliminated for these signals since the signals are inserted at the glomeruli and don't pass through the sensory receptors at all. A thousand coordinated nanorobots positioned one at each glomerulus could provide complete olfactory sensation control and the potential for massive multiplexing. As with taste messaging, it is unknown whether the natural conscious brain can be trained to process such multiplexed high-frequency smell signals. In 1998, studies of the human olfactory (combinatorial) code were in progress.[3207]

7.4.6.5 Ocular Outmessaging

Nanorobots may send messages to the patient by emitting photons directly into the eye (Fig. 7.5), generating an artificial visual stimulus. Retinal displays could be broadcast by photoemissive nanodevices located:

1. in the palpebral conjunctiva (inner mucosal surface) of the eyelid, where access to nutrients from the capillary bloodflow is still available in muscular tissue below the fibrous plates;
2. on the exterior surface of the cornea, when nanorobots may obtain power from transcorneal-diffused glucose and other sugars in the lacrimal fluids at $c_{ligand} \sim 2.9 \times 10^{-4}$ molecules/nm^3 (~10% blood plasma concentration);[585]
3. on the interior corneal or exterior lens surface (c_{ligand} = 1.6-3.7 x 10^{-3} molecules/nm^3 for glucose in the aqueous humor, ~plasma concentration),[585,3284] or in the anterior chamber in front of the lens (implanting an artificial lens in the anterior chamber was considered an experimental vision correction procedure in 1998);
4. inside the lens which is 68% water (c_{ligand} = 0.8-2.0 x 10^{-3} molecules/nm^3 for glucose,[585] ~50% plasma concentration);
5. the interior lens or retinal surface with access to glucose in the vitreous humor (~same concentration as aqueous humor); or
6. within the individual rod (dim light, monochromatic) and cone (bright light, color-sensitive) cells — retinal glucose is stored in glial Muller cells and is supplied upon demand.[3260]

Oxygen is available at ~5% of normal plasma concentration via solvation in the lacrimal fluids and diffusion into the aqueous humor; CO_2 and lactate exit by the same route. Formation of potentially signal-blocking scar tissue is avoided by using mobile nanorobots with active, biocompatible exterior surfaces[3234] (Chapter 15).

We shall now consider four different methods for ocular outmessaging:

A. *Extraretinal Projection* — Photoemissive nanodevices must generate a photon flux intensity sufficient to equal or exceed ambient background illumination levels. With the eyelid lightly closed, normal indoor illumination transmitted through this thin muscular fibrous tissue produces a background retinal flux of at least $I_{min} \sim 10^{-2}$ watts/m^2. With eyes open in a normally lighted room, the background flux may be ~1 watt/m^2 or even higher (Section 4.9.4).

Normally the lens of the eye can accommodate viewing distances no closer than $X_{min} \sim 10$ cm (measured from posterior lens surface) in adults. Photons emitted from nanodevices located in the eyelid ($X_{object} \sim 8.6$ mm), exterior corneal surface ($X_{object} \sim 7.3$ mm), interior corneal surface ($X_{object} \sim 6.2$ mm), or exterior lens surface ($X_{object} \sim 3.8$ mm) cannot be brought to focus inside the eye unless they are tightly collimated. A cylindrical emitter of length h_e = 25 microns and radius r_e = 0.5 micron can produce a collimated beam with an axial divergence angle $\varphi_e = 0.5 \tan^{-1} (2 r_e / h_e) \sim 1°$ (2° full-width divergence), which is geometrically equivalent to rays passing through a pupil aperture d_{pupil} = 5-6 mm after emanating from an object located at a distance $X_{object} = d_{pupil} / 2 \tan (\varphi_e)$ = 12-15 cm which is $\gtrsim X_{min}$, hence is focusable. One major difficulty with eyelid projection is that tight flexing of the corrugator supercilii muscle (which draws the eyebrow downward and inward) causes the eyelid tissue to ripple and fold, potentially producing significant optical distortions. A large projector suspended in the anterior chamber might offer greater spatial stability. These devices are probably small enough to avoid stimulating lid edema or blepharitis.

Present-day micron-scale LEDs emit up to ~1 watt/m^2 (Section 5.3.7), so extraretinal displays from such emitters are comfortably read by patients. If the emitters overwrite 10% of the visual field, then total optical power input through the lens is $P_{out} \sim$ 0.03-3.0 microwatts. Assuming a very conservative energy conversion efficiency of e% ~ 0.01(1%) for LEDs (Section 5.3.7), the emitters consume a total input power (and radiate waste heat) of $P_{in} = P_{out}$ / e% = 3-300 microwatts, well below the conservative 2000 microwatt maximum for 0.1 cm^3 of eyelid tissue (Eqn. 6.54). Emitter power density ranges from ~0.4 megawatts/m^3 at 10^{-2} watts/m^2 intensity up to ~40 megawatts/m^3 at 1 watt/m^2 intensity.

B. *Foveal Projection* — The fovea is a small pit in the macula lutea, opposite the visual axis, which is the spot of most distinct vision (Fig. 7.5). There are no rod cells in the fovea and relatively few in the near-foveal region. Foveal cone cells have diameters of 1-5 microns[585] (average $d_{fov} \sim 3$ microns) with a minimum center-to-center separation of ~2.6 microns (average $x_{sep} \sim 5.2$ microns) across the foveal surface of the retina. The retina is arranged "inside out" so that light must pass through nine layers of connecting nerve cells and other tissue to reach the receptors which lie at the deepest level (Fig. 7.6, enlargement of box in Figure 7.5). This covering tissue is $x_{tiss} \sim 130$ microns deep across the fovea (the ganglion and bipolar layers are pushed aside, directly above the fovea) and $x_{tiss} \sim 300$ microns thick elsewhere on the retina. The foveal and near-foveal region extends ~2° (~0.55 mm^2) around the visual axis, comprising ~20,000 cone cells and providing a resolvable visual angle of 0.5-2.3 minutes of arc (sufficient for reading printed text) and creating a 140 x 140 pixel writeable billboard.

Consider a cylindrical emitter of diameter ~1 micron affixed to the retinal surface over the fovea. This emitter produces a collimated beam with an axial divergence angle $\varphi_e \sim 1°$, which diverges to a width $w_{beam} = x_{tiss} \tan (2 \varphi_e) \sim 5.2$ microns after traveling a distance x_{tiss} = 130 microns into the fovea. Each cylindrical emitter can target one foveal cone cell with no overlap, so ~20,000 photoemissive nanorobots are required for complete control of all foveal cone receptors. A population of 20,000 photoemissive nanodevices ~1 micron in diameter attached to the inner retinal membrane above the foveal surface blocks only ~3% of photons entering the fovea via the lens, an unnoticable diminution of the natural incident intensity that is visible to the patient.*

Given that $d_{fov} < w_{beam}$ and $\pi r_e^2 < 1$ micron^2, achieving 0.01-1 watts/m^2 intensity at the receptor cells to overcome the natural illumination background requires an emitter photonic intensity of 0.04-4 watts/m^2, already within state-of-the-art in 1998. At a very conservative e% = 0.01(1%) ergophotonic efficiency, P_{in} ~ 3-300 pW per nanodevice or 0.06-6 microwatts for the entire population, well below the ~0.1 watt recommended thermogenic limit for the eyeball from Eqn. 6.54. If the nanorobot employs an oxyglucose power supply, continuous foveal control consumes ~10^{10}-10^{12} glucose molecules/sec which would exhaust the ~10^{19} glucose molecules present in the vitreous humor in ~0.3-30 years but would more quickly exhaust the oxygen supply (Section 6.5.3) in ~0.5-50 days even if there were no diffusive resupply from the surrounding tissues; fortunately, such resupply appears highly likely.

If the photoemissive foveal nanorobot population is extended to cover the rest of the retinal surface (with most devices not emitting photons most of the time), then real-time ocular and cranial positional

* *J. Logajan points out that if the cylindrical emitter has a photodetector on the end facing the lens, then even the 3% loss could be largely retrieved by amplification; the emitters could also serve as dark-area amplifiers, providing improved night vision or infrared-to-visible light conversion (Chapter 30).*

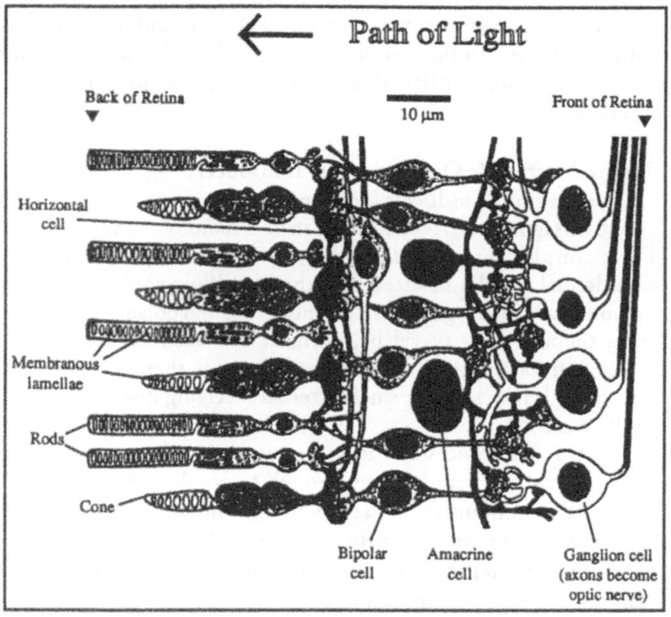

Fig. 7.6. Above, the human retina (redrawn from Vander et al[866] and Feynman et al[538]).

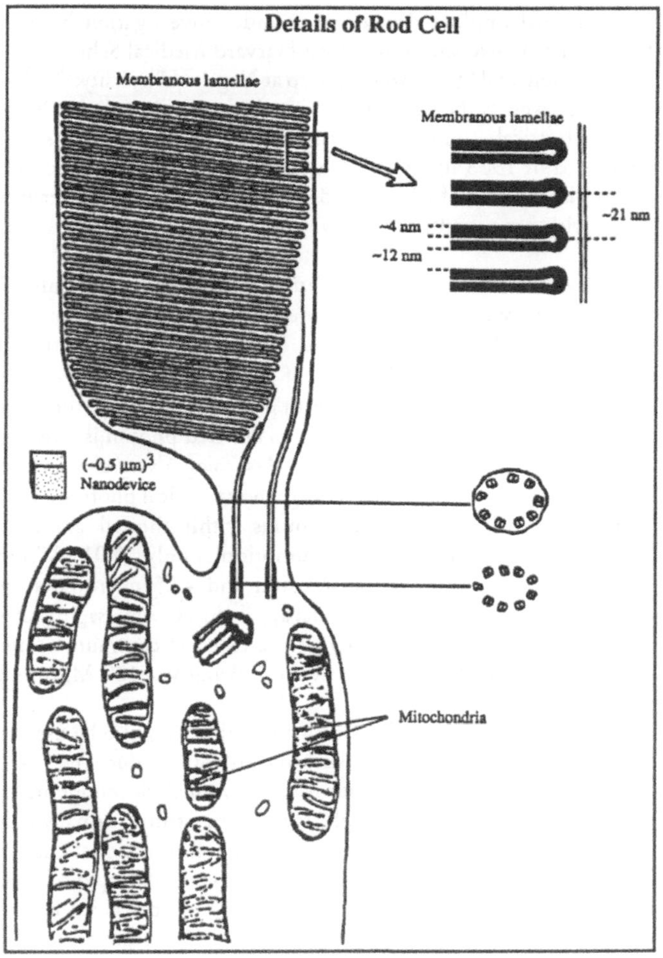

information provided by kinesthetic macrosensors (Section 4.9.2.1) via the communication network can be used to shift displayed images in synchrony with eye and head movements, allowing displays to appear fixed in the field of view as in normal viewing of external objects. (Information gleaned from the oculomotor, trochlear, trigeminal, abducens, and spinal accessory nerves may assist in this control process.) Accommodation sensors (Section 7.4.2.2) assist in maintaining proper focus. Foveal nanorobots should be designed to avoid stimulation of uveitis or retinitis.

C. *Ganglionic Stimulation* — Because of the inverted structure of the retina, neurostimulatory nanorobots attached to the inner retinal membrane can trigger artificial action potentials directly in the axons of afferent ganglia carrying information from rods and cones to the optic (2nd cranial) nerve. It is useful to briefly review the basic structure of the human retina (Fig. 7.6).

Starting with the outermost layer and moving inward toward the vitreous humor that fills the eyeball, the choroid layer (Fig. 7.5) is covered with a very sensitive optically absorbing pigmented epithelium which bleeds and detaches easily from the retina if physically disturbed by overpressures of ~10 mmHg. Above and covering the pigment layer lie about 250 million rod cells and 6 million cone cells. Rod and cone cells communicate by electronic conduction, not by action potentials. Rod and cone receptor cells converge in a complex synaptic network on bipolar and horizontal cells. Bipolar cells are depolarizing (inhibited by rod/cone neurotransmitters) or hyperpolarizing (excited by rod/cone neurotransmitters), allowing the transmission of positive and negative signals to amacrine and ganglion cells. Horizontal cells laterally connect rods and cones to bipolar cells, allowing lateral inhibition in the retina. Amacrine cells connect bipolar cells to ganglion cells. Numerous types of ganglion cells react to contrast borders, intensity changes and color contrasts. Preprocessed visual information flows into ~1 million ganglion cells whose fibers collect into a giant bundle and exit the eyeball under the ~1.5 mm-diameter optic disk or "blind spot", forming the optic nerve. Convergence is maximal at the periphery of the retina—rods outnumber cones by more than 10:1 in the periphery, and up to 10^3-10^4 rods may report to a single ganglion cell. Convergence is minimal in the fovea, where one cone cell may synapse with a single ganglion cell through a single bipolar cell.

Low-level signal processing aided by amacrine and horizontal cells in the bipolar layer thus reduces the optic data traffic from 256 million to only 1 million channels at the ganglionic axons which lie closest to the nanorobots attached to the inner retinal membrane. The ganglia are spaced from ~3 microns apart bordering the fovea to ~100 microns apart at the farthest periphery of the retina, averaging ~30 microns. For simplicity, if we regard each ganglion as carrying the equivalent of a single pixel of data in a 1000 x 1000 pixel visual field, then a comprehensive retinal ganglionic management system comprising ~10^6 neurostimulatory devices installed within each eyeball allows complete control of the entire human visual field with a refresh rate close to the flicker frequency for rods of ~15 Hz,[585] with ocular data transfer near ~10^7 bits/sec which is near the practical upper limit for in vivo mobile communication networks (Section 7.3.2). Assuming up to P_{in} ~ 30 pW for each neurostimulatory nanorobot (Section 7.4.5.6) a continuously operated retinal ganglionic control system consumes at most ~30 microwatts, comparable to ocular projection systems described in (A) and (B), so energy supply and heat generation are not significant design limitations.

As of 1998, prototype retinal implant components had been installed and tested in rabbits. These test devices delivered ~10 microamps per electrode directly to ganglion cells and produced measurable activity in the visual cortex of the animals' brains.[1044]

Other retinal implant devices were under investigation by Rolf Eckmiller at Universitat Bonn, by a Harvard Medical School/MIT collaboration, and by a Japanese group at Nagoya University;[1887-1890] Eckmiller expects the first implant in a human volunteer by 2001. Direct electrical stimulation of the human visual cortex was first attempted in 1968 using 100 Hz pulses applied in 200 microsec bursts via an array of 81 electrodes implanted in a blind person's brain, with poor results.[1713]

D. *Direct Photoreceptor Stimulation* — A single photoemissive nanorobot may be carefully stationed in each of the 256 million rod and cone cells of the human eye. If the nanorobot is positioned in the pigment-rich apical region of the cell,* (e.g., the ~9-nm thick double-membranous lamellae, or planar structures, of the outer segment of the rod cell; Figure 7.6) its emitted photon is likely to be detected even without collimation. Assuming a very conservative 1% energy conversion efficiency to generate optical photons, 10% absorption efficiency of optical photons within the cell, and a 25 Hz image refresh rate, power consumption is only ~0.01 pW per nanorobot for continuous transmission and ~2.5 microwatts for complete control of the human visual apparatus. Outmessaging rates are limited by the peak capacity of the external communications link, ~10^7 bits/sec for a mobile network using ν ~ 100 MHz and f_{duty} = 10% (Section 7.3.2).

Chemical or mechanochemical stimulation may also be used in place of photons. For example, such means could induce the 11-*cis* to 11-*trans* torsional isomerization of the retinal chromophore in rhodopsin, the first step in photoreceptor stimulation, which occurs naturally in ~0.2 picosec.[1692] This conformational change opens a calcium channel in the rod cell membrane; the rapid calcium ion influx triggers a nerve impulse, and light is perceived by the brain.[996] (Each rod rises1-2 microkelvins in temperature during the heat burst following a light flash causing 180-1800 rhodopsin photoisomerizations per rod.[3470])Direct nanorobot modulation of intracellular concentrations of α-transducin, the G-protein that transduces the light signal in retinal cells, or directly opening an artificial transmembrane Ca^{++} channel allowing a Ca^{++} influx (mediated by a membrane-spanning nanorobot) may be even more efficient.

7.4.6.6 Artificial Symptoms

The triggering of artificial symptoms in the human body offers at best a primitive, noisy, misinterpretable, and low bit rate outmessaging channel. Outmessaging protocols may allow a population of in vivo nanorobots to communicate systemwide status (e.g., "low serum oxygen," "low serum glucose," "immune system under attack,") or specific conditions (e.g., "cancer tumor detected in breast," "breach of intestinal wall detected") directly with the patient by inducing recognizable physiological cues (e.g., fever, nausea, shivering, tingling, gasping, tinnitus, hypothalamic "reward" center stimulation). But message noise level is high because these signals are readily confused with natural symptoms that may normally communicate the presence of entirely unrelated conditions. One suggestion to improve the signal/noise ratio is to insert artificial genes that code for enzymes producing a harmless but chromatic signaling compound that colors the urine when excreted, or which adds an unusual color to hair or fingernails as a diagnostic telltale.[2991] Nanodevices also could "manually" trigger such a gene, or manufacture the colorant themselves. Alternatively, coordinated nanorobot-induced neural firings might produce externally-measurable changes in the cranial radiative electric field.[3472] All these sorts of information transfer are very energy inefficient and are about as informative as "Indian smoke signals."[731] Artificial symptoms have only limited utility as a primitive channel for nanodevice outmessaging.

7.4.6.7 Macroscale Outmessaging Transducers

Inmessaging transducers (Section 7.4.2.7) may also be employed as outmessaging interfaces between in vivo nanorobots and patients. For example, a simple transduction organ (e.g., macroscale transdermal needle) inserted into the bloodflow could chemically or acoustically interrogate passing nanodevices and obtain information from them as they travel by, without the need for nanodevice removal or locomotion. This information may then be transferred out through the skin to a small external receiving device accessible to the patient.

In vivo nanodevices can also join together to form coordinated aggregates which may be large enough to emulate the action of a macroscale communications device. In some instances, this approach will produce only energy-inefficient marginally-feasible results. For example, consider the concept of the subdermal nanospeaker or "talking tattoo." The minimum acoustic power output that can be heard as a whisper is ~0.1 microwatts (Section 4.9.1.5). From Eqn. 7.7, a 1-micron acoustic radiator driven by 1000 pW of input power at 3000 Hz produces ~4 x 10^{-18} watts/radiator. The sound waves then lose 99.9% of their power passing through the skin-air interface (Section 4.9.1.6), so ~22 trillion devices are required to generate the required ~0.1 microwatt (by coherent emission) in order to be heard. But this many 1000-pW devices operated simultaneously produce 22,000 watts, well in excess of the suggested 100-watt whole-body thermogenic maximum. However, if the radiators position themselves near the skull to employ bone conduction into the tympanum, most of the skin-air interface loss is avoided reducing the required radiator count to 22 billion and total power to 22 watts, which might be acceptable. Such radiator nanorobots occupying 10% of local tissue volume make a patch ~350 microns deep covering the area of a postage stamp (~1 $inch^2$). (Skin-air interface losses may also be avoided by acoustic nanoradiators positioned exclusively supraepidermally.) The "talking wristwatch" approach (Section 7.4.2.7) is another possibility.

A more efficient nanorobot-aggregate user interface is the programmable dermal display. Pigment tattoos,[96] port-wine stains, strawberry marks (common hemangiomas), and other birthmarks constitute an existence proof that small biocompatible particles can be permanently implanted in the dermis and do not migrate on timescales of decades or longer. This suggests that dermal displays can be positionally stable over very lengthy periods of time.

Consider a population of ~3 billion display nanorobots embedded 200-300 microns below the surface of the epidermis covering a 6 cm x 5 cm rectangle on the flat part of the back of the hand or on the smooth medial surface of the forearm. The nanorobots are ~1 $micron^3$ in volume and occupy only 1% of the 300 mm^3 local tissue deployment volume. Each device consumes ~10 pW when generating visible photons of desired colors at a comfortable visible intensity of ~1 pW/$micron^2$ or ~1 watt/m^2 (Section 5.3.7), assuming an improved 10% ergooptical conversion efficiency. Visible photons are completely scattered in 10-100 microns but almost none are absorbed, producing a diffuse glow as ~50% of the scattered photons eventually exit the surface of the skin. For installation and stationkeeping, display nanodevices require at least limited mobility, and a few additional nanodevices may be required to assist with computation,

* *The tips of rod cells are renewed at the end of each night, the tips of cone cells at the end of each day, as regulated by the diurnal circadian clock (Section 10.1.1).[1664] Resident nanorobots should avoid being sloughed off during this process.*

data storage and external communications, and other housekeeping chores.

If powered by continuously available chemical fuels, the display would only be operable for 0.1-10 sec before exhausting the entire oxyglucose supply present in the limited tissue deployment volume. Consequently, it is necessary to include a large energy storage buffer constituting 40% of device volume (assuming 10^{10} joule/m^3 stored energy density; Section 6.2.3) which allows ~1000 sec of operation if only 20% of all pixels are radiating at any given time. This power can be reabsorbed from local oxyglucose supplies in ~1 day, giving a long-term ~1% duty cycle for the display (~14 min/day) although the buffer can operate the display for up to ~21 minutes before being exhausted. This power restriction may be entirely avoided by adding supplemental power from, say, a wristwatch-sized extradermal acoustic source (Section 6.4.1), a dedicated transvascular energy organ (Section 6.4.4), photoelectric collectors (~30 pW/micron^2 in cloudless noontime sunlight, ~1 pW/micron^2 in a well-lighted room; Sections 4.9.4 and 6.3.6), or by employing a passive (reflective) display which might be satisfactory for some purposes.

The array of 3 billion nanorobots may be programmed to adopt any of many thousands of different displays. Each display configuration is capable of

1. presenting output data received from the larger in vivo nanorobot population scattered throughout the body (via a communication network), and
2. accepting input data from the patient to be conveyed (through the communication network) to appropriate internal nanorobot subpopulations.

Full-motion animation or video may also be projected, up to the 10^7 bit/sec maximum limit of the mobile communication network; fiber networks may allow up to ~10^9 bit/sec data transfer rates (Section 7.3.1). Figure 7.7A shows a small sample of alternative displays (at actual size) from among the many thousands that are conceivable. Acquisition of the information displayed requires a population of

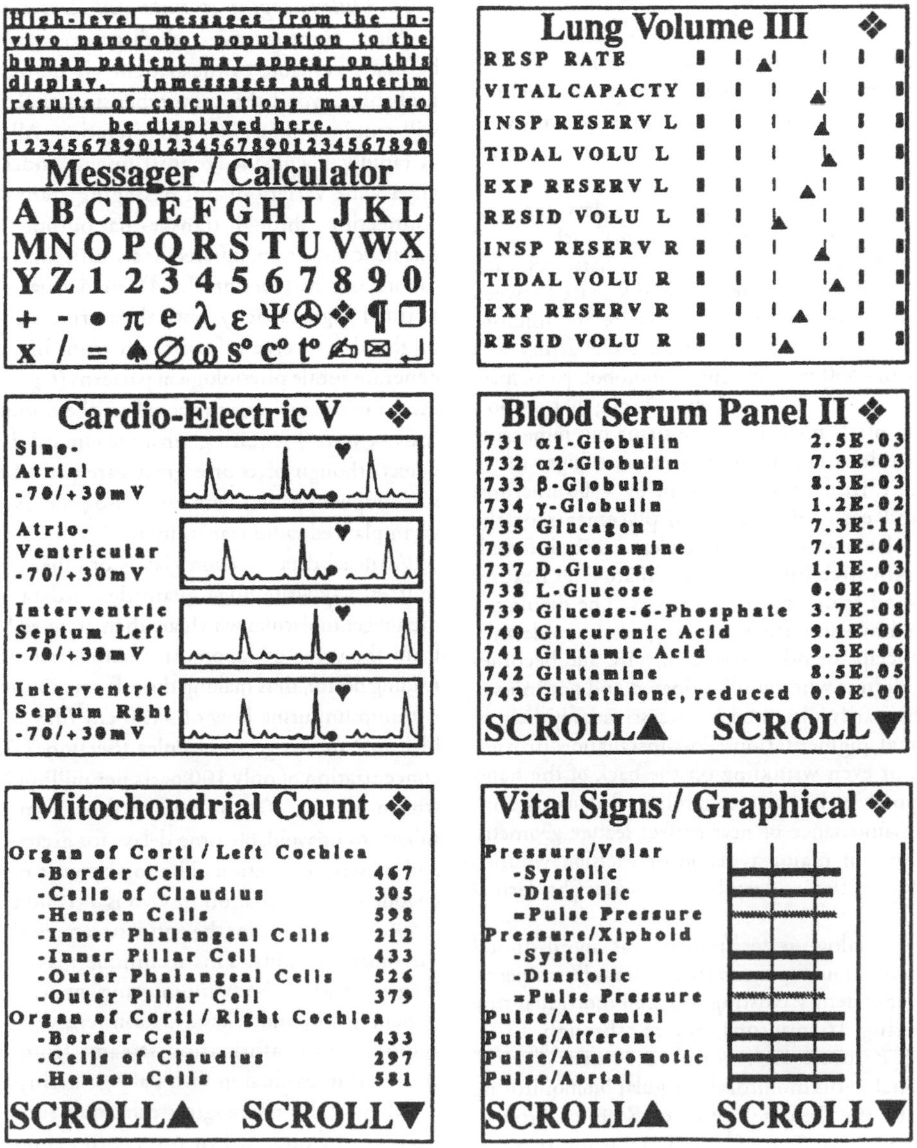

Fig. 7.7A. A selection of possible dermal display screens.

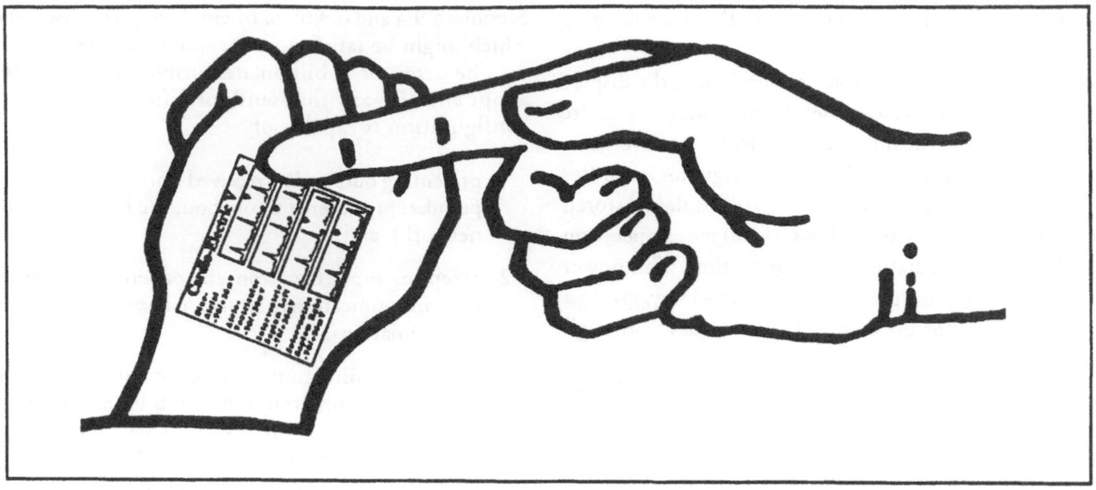

Fig. 7.7B. A dermal display screen in use.

sensory nanodevices distributed throughout the body and linked by a communications network. For instance, the "Vital Signs" panel requires at least one telemetering nanorobot stationed in each of the several hundred arteries of the human body (or possibly behind each vein valve cusp (Fig. 8.3) throughout the venous system), with each device reporting local blood pressure conditions on a periodic basis.

As for the display itself, in the first example ("Messager/Calculator") there are 60 input keys measuring $(0.5\ cm)^2$ each and a 2 cm x 6 cm output panel that can print 7 rows of 30 characters, each character measuring $(2\ mm)^2$ with 1 mm of blank space between each line. Line segments used to write characters are 500 microns wide, more than ten times the limit of human visual acuity at a reading distance of 30 cm; ~500 million active nanorobots participate in drawing the images of the 60 input keys. Display nanorobots have a mean separation of ~5 microns in the tissue but remeasure their relative positions at least ten times per second; a finger-touch on an input key (Fig. 7.7B) depresses the skin by ~500 microns, producing massive and easily detectable displacements of the underlying nanodevices from which the chosen key may be inferred. Non-message related skin stretchings and proximate limb flexures are readily distinguished from input fingerings. The display is activated or deactivated by using finger tapping on the epidermis, temporally coded handclaps or other similar means, and becomes invisible under the epidermis when unilluminated and not in use.

The display may be partly obscured by excessive body hair or particularly dark dermal pigmentation. Post-installation bruises, scabs, incisions, scars, or even wrinkling on the back of the hand may slightly or temporarily impair readability. But nanorobot stationkeeping allows maintenance of near-perfect feature geometry during any trauma short of major avulsion or excision wounds involving significant loss of tissue, deep burns, or outright dermal excoriation or flaying.

In 1998 the closest analogous technology was an all-digital chip-mounted ~1 cm^2 projection display, created by Texas Instruments, which operated by independently twisting 307,200 individual tiny mirrors, each measuring 16 microns square, through ±10°, reflecting pulses of colored light onto a screen.[1062,1974] Wristwatch-sized personal status monitors for regular biomonitoring were being developed by the Defense Advanced Research Projects Agency (DARPA) in the United States,[3301] and in the private sector for sports medicine.[3323]

7.4.7 Outmessaging to External Receivers

Much of the extensive self-diagnostic data that could theoretically be made available to the patient via dermal displays (Fig. 7.7) is probably beyond the comprehension of the typical user and thus will require professional interpretation. All such information may be rapidly downloaded to instruments under the physician's control via a wide variety of outmessaging transducers including cable connections through transdermal output ports (Section 7.4.2.7), magnetic induction, infrared or acoustic links with internal communications organs (Section 7.3.4), or dermal displays configured for optimal high-capacity optical external data transfers. Physicians might also receive information from in vivo nanorobots which generate subtle physiological patterns (e.g., an artificial electrical or mechanical signal superimposed on the normal cardiac or respiratory "carrier wave") requiring sensitive clinical diagnostic equipment to detect, though of course great care must be taken to ensure that such imposed patterns are non-nosogenic. Nanorobots could operate an implanted radio transmitter.

Artificial data secretion glands or other distributed data secretion sources may write huge quantities of data onto nonmetabolizable messenger molecules which are then excreted by the patient, recovered from the urine by laboratory nanodevices, then passed through a reading device, thus making the information available to the physician. A minimum urine flow of ~120 cm^3/day containing $D_{message}$ ~ 26 bits/nm^3 messenger molecules (Section 7.2.1.1) at an innocuous concentration of only 100 parts per million by volume allows a data stream of ~4 x 10^{15} bits/sec to flow from patient to physician—subject to unavoidable time delays for excretion, materials processing and message extraction. The total power requirement to originally encode this information in vivo is 1-1000 zJ/bit (Section 7.2.6) or 4-4000 microwatts for the entire stream, well within safe whole-body thermogenic limits. This technique may be especially valuable in long-term whole-body monitoring, neural recording and archiving (Chapter 25), and related data-intensive applications that require acquisition of information streams from millions or billions of scattered individual in vivo data-gathering sources.

Many of the inmessaging techniques summarized in Section 7.4.1 may also be operated in reverse to achieve outmessaging to the physician from in vivo nanodevices.

7.4.8 Transvenue Outmessaging

Can nanorobots stationed inside one patient communicate with nanorobots stationed inside another patient? Other than simple linkages of previously described standard inmessaging and outmessaging modalities, remote communication between two fully physically disjoint sets of intracorporeal nanorobots can probably be ruled out. However, in vivo and epidermal nanorobots can in theory be programmed to take advantage of serendipitous opportunities using mobile communicytes. Such opportunities for extracorporeal contacts may include patient-to-patient communicyte exchange by direct physical contact (e.g., handshaking or sexual activity), by indiscriminate broadcast transfers (e.g., sneezing, bleeding, desquamation, or sharing tools or utensils), by serendipitous anonymous contacts (e.g., doorknobs, public toilet seats, library books), or by deliberate airborne nanorobot migrations (Section 9.5.3). Security protocols (Chapter 12) are especially important in these applications.

Data is also readily transferred purposely between patients, as for example via matching dermal communications patches embedded in the palms of each patient's hands which are briefly pressed together while shaking hands. In 1998, IBM's Personal Area Network (PAN) used near-field oscillating galvanic potentials with a low carrier frequency (~330 KHz), inducing ~50 picoamp currents from a ~1.5 milliwatt power source, to exchange a few hundred bytes of personal data between users during a handshake.[2700]

Communication among large numbers of airborne exodermal nanorobots (Section 9.5.3) is a particularly interesting and useful application (e.g., Chapter 21). Such communication may be accomplished by chemical means (Section 8.6.2), but here we will review only optical and acoustic methods.

Consider a cloud of aerial nanorobots with number density n_{bot} (nanorobots/m^3) and mean separation $X_{path} = n_{bot}^{-1/3}$ (meters) that is stationkeeping around a human user (Section 9.5.3). Each nanorobot has a communications energy budget of P_{comm} (watts) and broadcasts photons (or sound waves) of frequency ν from a circular transmitter of radius $r_{antenna}$ to a receiver of similar size located a mean distance X_{path} away.

In the case of optical communication, the information transfer rate $\dot{I}$ may be regarded as the number of photons received per second from a neighboring device, or

$$\dot{I} \sim \frac{e\% \, P_{comm} \, r_{antenna}^2}{4 \, h \, \nu \, X_{path}^2} \quad \text{(bits/sec)} \qquad \text{\{Eqn. 7.21\}}$$

where e% is the ergophotonic efficiency of photon generation and $h = 6.63 \times 10^{-34}$ joule-sec (Planck's constant). Conservatively taking e% = 0.01(1%), P_{comm} = 10 pW, $r_{antenna}$ = 1 micron, and assuming red photons with $\nu = 4.3 \times 10^{14}$ Hz (λ = 700 nm, ~280 zJ/photon), then inter-nanorobot $\dot{I}$ ~ 10 bits/sec for X_{path} = 100 microns, or $n_{bot} = 10^{12}$ nanorobots/m^3. A nanorobot cloud of this density should appear visually dense, possibly nearly opaque, since 10^{12} nanorobots each of cross-sectional area ~$\pi \, r_{antenna}^2$ ~ 3 micron^2 may occult >1 m^2 looking through a 1 m^3 cubic cloud having a face area of 1 m^2. The maximum broadcast optical intensity of a ~1 meter column uniformly distributed at this number density is ~0.1 watts/m^2, which is safe for the human eye. Nanorobot cloud waste heat at this number density, due to communications activities, is ~10 watts/m^3.

In the case of acoustic communication, the efficiency of ergoacoustic transmission efficiency e% = P_{out} / P_{in}, as defined by Eqn. 7.7, and the input power budget for communication $P_{comm} = P_{in}$ from Eqn. 7.9, except that in air the exponential attenuation must be replaced with $e^{2 \alpha_{air} \nu^2 X_{path}}$ as described in Section 4.9.1.3 for pure fluids. Using variables as previously defined, then $\dot{I} \sim \nu \, f_{duty}$ and

$$P_{comm} = f_{duty} \left(\frac{24 \, \eta \, \nu_{sound} \, X_{path}^2 \, kT \, e^{SNR}}{\pi^2 \, k_r \, \rho \, \nu \, r_{antenna}^5} \right) e^{2 \alpha_{air} \nu^2 X_{path}} \quad \text{(watts)} \qquad \text{\{Eqn. 7.22\}}$$

which is valid in pure fluids if $r_{antenna}/\lambda << 1$. We assume $\eta = 0.018 \times 10^{-3}$ kg/m-sec and ν_{sound} ~ 343 m/sec for air at 20°C,[763] kT ~ 4.3 zJ, SNR = 2, k_r = 2 for a piston radiator, ρ = 1.3 kg/m^3, $r_{antenna}$ = 1 micron, and $\alpha_{air} = 1.4 \times 10^{-10}$ sec^2/m (Table 4.2). For any given X_{path}, there is an optimum transmission frequency ν that minimizes P_{comm}.* Taking X_{path} = 100 microns ($n_{bot} = 10^{12}$ nanorobots/m^3), internanorobot $\dot{I}$ ~ 40 bits/sec at an optimum frequency of 4.2 MHz and f_{duty} = 0.001% duty cycle (P_{comm} ~ 7 pW). Note that Eqn. 7.22 is extremely sensitive to antenna size. At $r_{antenna}$ = 2 microns, $\dot{I}$ ~ 2000 bits/sec at 4.2 MHz for X_{path} = 100 microns.

What is the maximum acoustic intensity at the ear? Measuring from the outermost boundary of the nanorobot cloud and moving inward, ultrasound power extinguishes rapidly, falling to an intensity e^{-1} (~37%) in a distance $\lambda_x = (2 \, \alpha_{air} \, \nu^2)^{-1}$ ~ 200 microns at ν = 4.2 MHz. If the nearest boundary of the cloud is maintained a distance X_{ear} from the tympanic membrane of the human ear, then the acoustic intensity reaching the eardrum surface is approximately:

$$I_{cloud} \sim P_{comm} \, \eta_{bot} \, \lambda_x \, e^{-X_{ear}/\lambda_x} \quad \text{(watts/m}^2\text{)} \qquad \text{\{Eqn. 7.23\}}$$

If the cloud fills the auditory canal, then X_{ear} = 0 and I_{cloud} ~ 10^{-3} watts/m^2 (~93 dB, "shouting"), which is probably safe enough for the human ear and is inaudible at 4.2 MHz. At X_{ear} = 3 mm, I_{cloud} ~ 10^{-9} watts/m^2 (~30 dB, "whispering"); if the cloud remains entirely outside the auditory canal, then X_{ear} ~ 2 cm and I_{cloud} ~ 10^{-46} watts/m^2.

Photonic or acoustic modalities may serve as the basis for ex vivo mobile communication networks (Section 7.3.2). Since bit rates are significantly enhanced by proximity (e.g., smaller X_{path}), it may be useful to assign circumcorporeal aerial nanorobots to condensed geometric or traffic patterns, and to allow opportunistic conferencing among them as required, which might appear to the user as irregular or stellate aggregations, diaphanous tendrils, ordered rows or clump arrays at Cartesian grid vertices, evanescent toroidal cloudlets, or other floating geometries conducive to rapid and effective data sharing. In the earlier examples given above, reducing X_{path} to 10 microns raises the optical transfer rate to 900 bits/sec and the acoustic transfer rate to 50,000 bits/sec at 13.4 MHz, for $r_{antenna}$ = 1 micron.

These modalities could also be used by a circumcorporeal nanorobot cloud to communicate visual and auditory messages directly to the user.

**Airborne nanorobots traveling at a $\Delta v \sim 1$ m/sec relative velocity will incur a Doppler shift in the received frequency of $\nu \, (1 + (\Delta v / v_{sound})) \sim (1.003) \, \nu$, defining a ± 3 KHz per MHz band bracketing the intended frequency.*

CHAPTER 8

Navigation

8.1 Navigating the Human Body

It is difficult to imagine any significant application of medical nanodevices which does not involve navigation, however crude. Devices intended to monitor somatic states, assemble artificial internal structures, remove tumors or foreign matter, combat infections, or perform repairs, must normally be extremely tissue- or cell-specific. Navigation is also required to execute many control protocols (Chapter 12), to locate dedicated energy, communication, or navigational helper organs, or to stationkeep and coordinate with other nanodevices. Even bloodborne nanorobots intended to operate solely at the systemic level—such as nanobiotics or immunocytes (Chapter 19) and respirocytes (artificial red cells;[1400] Chapter 22)—must know if they have been prematurely ejected from the vasculature so that they may cease functioning or at least modify their activities.

Perhaps the most important challenge of in vivo navigation is to determine how physicians may best direct nanorobots to specific target sites needing treatment within the human body. Two alternative strategies appear most likely to produce the best clinical results (both of which will be considered in this Chapter).

The first strategy is positional navigation, in which the nanorobot knows its position inside the human body to ~micron accuracy at all times in some clinic-centered or body-centered coordinate grid system. The nanodevice relies upon dead reckoning, cartotaxis, microtransponder network alignment, or triangulation on external beacon signals to establish its position continuously. This method requires some onboard computation, at least a basic set of sensors (e.g., acoustic), and probably also a good clock (Section 10.1). However, it is hardly foolproof—if the target coordinates are poorly specified or the beacon signals are misaligned or poorly calibrated, the nanorobots may go to the wrong place.

The second strategy is functional navigation, in which nanodevices seek to detect subtle variations in their environment, comparing diverse sensor readings with the profile of the target tissue or cell and congregating wherever this very precisely defined set of preconditions exists. These preconditions may be thermal, acoustic or barostatic, cytochemical or immunochemical, mechanical or topological, or even genetic. The crudest forms of functional navigation may be called demarcation, wherein the doctor manually creates detectable artificial conditions at or near the target site such as dermal hot spots, injected chemical plumes, or focused ultrasonic beam spots of appropriate magnitudes and frequencies. Demarcation strategies can be implemented using extremely simple onboard sensors and control devices, possibly not even requiring a nanorobot computer, thus may prove useful early in nanomedical technology development.

More sophisticated forms of functional navigation can be extraordinarily flexible because targets may be specified without the physician having to know their exact physical location in the body—e.g., nascent cancer tumors, T cells reactive to specific antigens, infected deep-thoracic lymph nodes, bacteria of a particular species, broken capillary vessels, or virus particles having a specified protein coat chemistry. The physician need not know the exact number of targets, nor even if any targets are present at all. These forms of functional navigation require onboard computation, a resident database of relevant parameters and operational details, and a wider assortment of sensors and control protocols. But they also offer the greatest benefit at lowest risk for the patient and thus must be regarded as the preferred approach once the technology is available.

This Chapter opens with a survey of human somatography (Section 8.2), followed by general discussions of positional (Section 8.3) and functional (Section 8.4) navigation, cytonavigation (Section 8.5), and finally ex vivo navigation (Section 8.6).

8.2 Human Somatography

Somatography is, quite simply, the "geography" or map of the anatomical spaces, as seen from the viewpoint of a microscopic traveler in those realms. The human body is a complex and fascinating place to visit. The nanomedical theater of operations in adult patients may range in size from an extremely small ~0.005 m^3 (Lucia Zarate, 5.9 kg, in January 1883 at age 20) to an extremely large ~0.5 m^3 (Robert Earl Hughes, 485 kg, in February 1958 at age 32),[739] but averages ~0.06 m^3 of navigable volume for the standard 70 kg adult male having 15% body fat, medium build and good health.[817] (The more typical tall but overweight late 20th-century American male (6-ft, 220 lbs, 25% body fat) measures ~0.1 m^3 in size.) Thus the volume normally available for nanorobot navigation in a single patient is ~10^{17} $microns^3$.

The first fully digitized comprehensive three-dimensional map of the human body was compiled in the early 1990s as part of the National Library of Medicine's Visible Human Project.[1304] During this effort, a male and female cadaver were frozen in blocks of gel, sectioned into thousands of thin slices and digitally scanned in MRI (magnetic resonance imaging), CT (computerized x-ray tomography) and anatomical modes (optical photography), slice by slice.

The male data set, released in 1994, consists of axial MRI images of the head and neck taken at 4 mm intervals and longitudinal sections of the rest of the body also at 4 mm intervals; each MRI image is 256 x 256 pixels with a 12-bit grey scale per pixel. The CT data consists of 512 x 512 pixel axial CT scans of the entire body taken at 1 mm intervals, also with a 12-bit grey scale per pixel. The axial anatomical images are 2048 x 1216 pixels with a 24-bit color scale per pixel, representing ~60 megabits per image. The anatomical cross-sections are also at 1 mm intervals and coincide with the CT axial images. There are 1871 cross-sections for each mode (CT and anatomy) obtained from the male cadaver, a ~0.112 terabit data set for the anatomical images (~111 million $micron^3$ per voxel).

The female data set, released in 1995, has the same characteristics as the male set except that the axial anatomical images were obtained at 0.33 mm intervals instead of 1.0 mm intervals, resulting in more than 5,000 anatomical images and a data set of ~0.336 terabits. Even though this map has a resolution of only 37 million micron^3 per voxel, this is still sufficient to resolve all terminal veins and terminal arterial branches in the body and all major gross anatomical features, and thus provides a good start toward a human somatographic atlas.

A complete human somatographic static map to cellular resolution in theory requires ~20 micron increments, a ~100 terabit data set using 8-bit 8000 micron^3 voxels assuming a fixed scanning geometry and ignoring the indexing tables. Recording all major structural details in the capillary terminal bed demands ~4 micron resolution, a ~10,000 terabit data set assuming 8-bit voxels. A 10,000 terabit data set may be stored on a ~26 bit/nm^3 hydrofluorocarbon memory tape (Section 7.2.1.1) in a cubic volume of ~(72 micron)^3 within an in vivo ~(100 micron)^3 library nodule. Divided into ~10^6 independent spools, a datum located anywhere on the 3300-kilometer total tape length could be accessed in ~10 seconds assuming a read speed of ~30 cm/sec (Section 7.2.6). A smaller 100 terabit library nodule requires only ~(16 micron)^3 of tape, with ~1000 spools and similar access times as in the previous example. Topological or functional mapping may permit data compression by a factor of 10-100 (e.g., Sections 8.2.1.2 and 8.3.2) without increasing access time or seriously reducing map utility.

A 1 micron^3 storage block that could conveniently be carried aboard an individual medical nanorobot can hold ~0.01 terabits (Section 7.2.6), enough memory to contain a three-dimensional map of the entire human body to ~430 micron resolution or a map of a 1-kg organ to ~100 micron resolution, using 8-bit voxels. The required resolution for a given application is very mission-dependent. Additionally, two types of map are likely to be of value. The first is a precise static map of some generic reference cadaver, as described above, that may provide general navigational guidance. The second is a detailed map of the individual patient, assembled by exploratory or "surveyor" nanorobots (Chapter 19) prior to the deployment of therapeutic nanorobots which would be given this information to allow very specific navigational guidance. Map stability is an important issue (Section 8.2.1.2; Chapter 19).

The remainder of this Section offers a quick guided tour of the larger navigable volumes inside the human body, along with some useful quantitative details. The different regions of the body appear to have enough structural and chemical dissimilarity to allow a nanorobot traversing these volumes to determine its position to at least ~mm accuracy, based solely on simple landmark recognition, chemonavigational cues, and bifurcation and topological information, even without resorting to the precision positional systems described in Section 8.3.

8.2.1 Navigational Vasculography

Medical nanorobots may access the interior of the human body principally via the blood-carrying vasculature, representing ~5.4 liters or ~9% of total body volume. The blood vessels are of three types, each characterized by functional and structural differences. First, there is the high-pressure distributing system, made up of the arteries and smaller branches called arterioles, which convey oxygenated blood from the heart to all regions of the body (Section 8.2.1.1). Second, there is a network of minute vessels, called capillaries, through which biologically important materials are exchanged between blood and tissues (Section 8.2.1.2). Third, there is a low-pressure collecting system made up of veins and smaller branches called venules, which return the blood to the heart (Section 8.2.1.1). The lymphatic system, an additional 3.3 liters of very low-pressure vasculature (Section 8.2.1.3), returns cell-filtered plasma to the main circulatory system.

8.2.1.1 Arteriovenous Macrocirculation

Topologically, the arteriovenous circulatory system resembles a "figure-eight" with a four-chambered heart positioned at the central junction. In the top half of the "figure-eight," oxygen-depleted blood is pumped from the heart to the lungs via the pulmonary artery. Oxygen-rich blood leaves the lungs and returns to the heart via the left and right pulmonary veins. In the bottom half of the "figure-eight," oxygen-rich blood received from the lungs is pumped into the aorta for distribution to the tissues, as shown in Figure 8.1. Oxygen-depleted blood is collected by the venous network (Fig. 8.2) and returns to the heart via the vena cava. (In both Figures, superficial vessels are drawn as solid lines and deep vessels as broken lines.) Most veins 1 mm in diameter or larger are fitted with a series of one-way valves to prevent backflow (Fig. 8.3). Such valves are most numerous in the lower extremities: the vena cava and the mesenteric, pulmonary and portal veins. Arteries have no valves. The smaller arteries are heavily anastomosed except across the midline of the body.

Table 8.1 provides a summary of the ~19,000 kilometers of human arteriovenous vasculature (mostly capillaries); additional data for a few selected major vessels is in Table 8.2. Singhal et al[828] have carefully surveyed the complete branching structure of the pulmonary arterial network, spanning the entire range from principal artery to final capillary (Table 8.3). These data may provide a useful model for estimating capillary branching systems in other tissues, bearing in mind that pulmonary capillaries are generally wider and shorter than capillaries found elsewhere in the body, and that capillary bed geometries are unique to each organ (Section 8.2.1.2). The measured thickness of the glycocalyx of the endothelium of the systemic

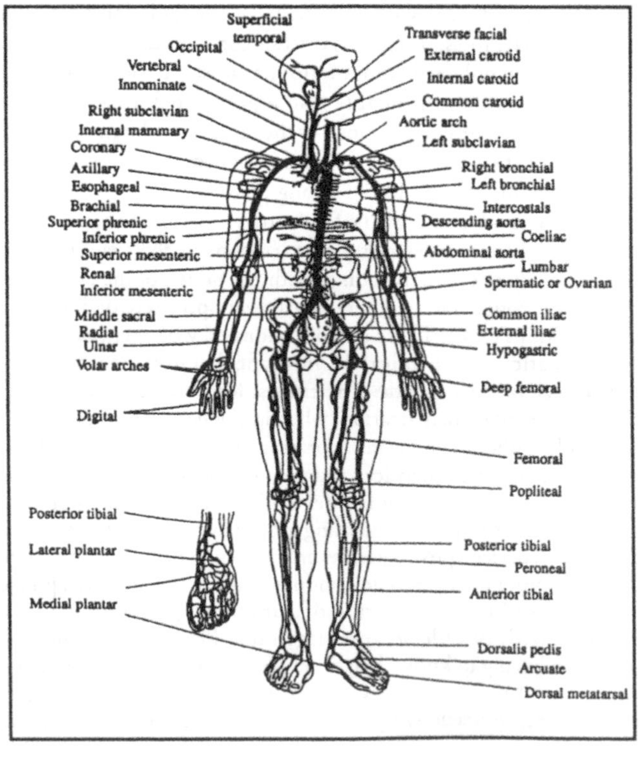

Fig. 8.1. Human arterial system.

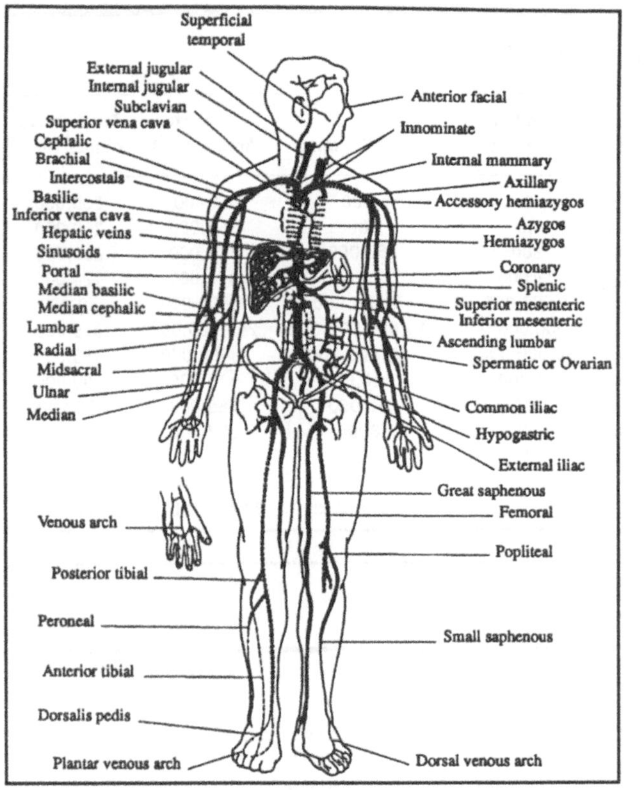

Fig. 8.2. Human venous system.

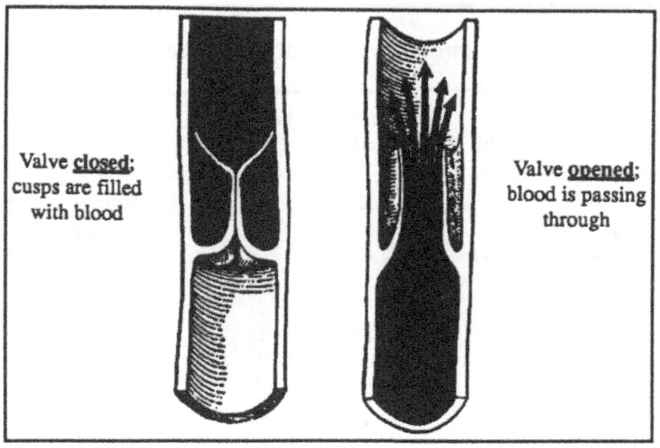

Fig. 8.3. Vein valve architecture.

arteries and vena cava may also be utilized for navigational purposes. For example, the thickness of rabbit glycocalyx ranged from 45 ± 1 nm in the coronary artery to 81 ± 2 nm in the carotid; the glycocalyx was 20 ± 1.5 nm thicker on the downstream side of intercostal ostia than on the upstream side.[3164]

How much time does a nanorobot flowing with the blood take to transit individual organs and the entire vascular circuit? It is generally accepted that the round-trip circulation time through the entire "figure-eight" averages ~60 seconds under resting conditions,[398] a time that appears constant for nearly all mammals.[362] During heavy exercise, the minimum circulation time may fall to 11-15 sec along most pathways primarily due to vasodilation.

Tissue transit times have been widely studied.[839] For example, bloodborne particles in the lung normally take only 1-2 seconds to pass the alveolar sheet but 5-10 seconds to transit the entire pulmonary vasculature.[361,780] Lung transit time is not significantly reduced if heart rate is simply increased;[829] however, during strenuous exercise the alveolar transit time falls to 0.3 sec and the maximum lung transit time falls from 10 sec to 2 sec due to vasodilation. Organ transit times are dominated by capillary flow speeds which range from 0.20-1.50 mm/sec (Table 8.2). Given that capillaries average ~1 mm in length, minimum organ transit times are 0.7-5.0 seconds.

8.2.1.2 Arteriovenous Microcirculation

In most cases, the true capillaries do not directly join arterioles to venules. Rather, oxygenated blood passes out of the terminal branches of the arterioles (terminal arterioles are ~10-50 microns in diameter) into metarterioles (10-20 microns), "preference channels" whose walls contain smooth muscle fibers in declining numbers from proximal to distal, which eventually merge with the non-contractile postcapillary (8-30 micron) and collecting (10-50 micron) venules (Fig. 8.4). Capillaries branch off directly from the metarterioles through precapillary sphincters constructed of single muscle fibers; other than these, there are no contractile elements in the capillaries. The state of contraction of the sphincters controls the rate of fluid flow through the capillaries. In skeletal muscle, with its widely varying oxygen requirements, there are 8-10 capillaries per metarteriole; in the mesenteric circulation, a stable metabolism requires only 2-3 capillaries per metarteriole; in the nail bed, the ratio is 1:1.[832] The topology of the arterioles that supply the capillaries, and of the venules that drain them, is usually special for each tissue. Some beds are structured as trees, while others are organized into arcades, sinuses, or portal systems. Thus the vasculature of each organ is unique—useful navigational information for medical nanorobots.

The wall of a capillary vessel is a tube consisting of a single layer of rolled-up endothelial cells. Endothelial cells may be less than 1 micron thick with a flat surface area of 300-1200 micron^2, so the entire ~313 meter^2 vascular surface may be comprised of up to 0.25-1 trillion endothelial cells. Endothelial cells are laterally apposed to each other with a 10-20 nm gap between neighboring cell membranes. These junctions are also somewhat organ-unique. There are three major types.

1. First, there is the continuous type with cells joined tightly together. Striated muscles may have flat thin cells, while in postcapillary venules the cells are cuboidal, forming a thick layer.
2. Second, there is the fenestrated type, with cells so thin that internal vesicles form small pores 25 nm thick and 100 nm in diameter (typically ~1000 pores/micron^2, compared to ~190 pores/micron^2 in arteriole endothelium and ~645 pores/micron^2 in postcapillary venule endothelium).[838] This type is found in the renal medulla, endocrine glands, and in structures engaged in the production or absorption of fluids such as the renal glomerulus, choroid plexus of the brain, and the intestinal villus.
3. Third, there is the discontinuous type with distinct intercellular gaps and a broken basement membrane, commonly found in sinusoid vessels and in organs such as the liver, spleen, and bone marrow whose functions include injection or extraction of whole cells, large molecules and extraneous particles from the blood.

Capillaries average 8 microns in diameter, but what is the minimum human capillary diameter? This question is important because it sets an upper limit on the size of bloodborne nanorobots. For example, in one experiment 97% of all 15-micron radiolabelled

Table 8.1. Approximate Quantification of the Human Arteriovenous System[830-833,835,836,838,1616]

Human Blood Vessel	Diameter (mm)	Length (mm)	Wall Thickness	Internal Pressure	Number of Vessels	Total Length (mm)	Total Surface Area (mm^2)	Total Blood Volume (mm^3)
Aorta	25.0	400	1500 µm	100 mmHg	1	400	31,400	200,000
Large arteries	6.5	200	1000 µm	100 mmHg	40	8000	163,000	260,000
Main artery branches	2.4	100	800 µm	95 mmHg	500	50,000	377,000	220,000
Terminal artery branches	1.2	10	125 µm	90 mmHg	11,000	110,000	415,000	120,000
Arterioles	0.1	2	20 µm	60 mmHg	4,500,000	9,000,000	2,800,000	70,000
Capillaries	0.008	1	1 µm	30 mmHg	19,000,000,000	19,000,000,000	298,000,000	375,000
Venules	0.15	2	2 µm	20 mmHg	10,000,000	20,000,000	9,400,000	355,000
Terminal veins	1.5	10	40 µm	15 mmHg	11,000	110,000	518,000	190,000
Main venous branches	5.0	100	500 µm	15 mmHg	500	50,000	785,000	1,590,000
Large veins	14.0	200	800 µm	10 mmHg	40	8000	352,000	1,290,000
Vena cava	30.0	400	1200 µm	5 mmHg	1	400	37,700	280,000
Heart chambers	--	--	--	120 mmHg	--	--	--	450,000
TOTALS						**~19,000 km**	**312,900,000**	**5,400,000**

hypothetical male, age 30, weight 70 kg, blood volume 5.4 liters

Table 8.2. Additional Data on Selected Blood Vessels[386,834]

Blood Vessel or Element	Diameter (mm)	Mean Flow Rate (mm^3/sec)	Mean Flow Velocity (mm/sec)	Velocity Range (mm/sec)	Mean Tube Reynolds Number
Ascending aorta	23.0-43.5	364,000	630	245-876	3210-6075
Inferior vena cava	20.0	34,000-50,000	135	107-160	323-482
Descending aorta	16.0-20.0	54,000-85,000	270	--	1200-1500
Common carotid	5.9	5100	187	99-388	332
Carotid sinus	5.2	3300	156	85-325	244
Femoral artery	5.0	3700	188	-350 to 1175	283
External carotid	3.8	1800	157	83-327	180
Large veins	5-10	4000-12,000	150-200	--	210-570
Large arteries	2-6	1600-5700	200-500	--	110-850
Small arteries	0.3	3.5	50	--	2.3
Arterioles	0.025-0.10	0.025	5	--	0.038
Capillaries	0.004-0.015	0.000075 to 0.00057	0.2-1.5		0.00036 to 0.0027

microspheres reaching the eye were trapped during the first pass.[842] Standard anatomy and physiology textbooks variously report that the minimum capillary lumen measures 5-7 microns,[834,839] 4-9 microns,[836] 4-8 microns,[517] or 4-6 microns[841,843] in diameter. There are also references to capillaries as narrow as 3 microns for laboratory rodents and other mammals.[834,840]

Theoretical calculations[841,844] suggest that a cylindrical vessel must be at least 2.7 microns in diameter to allow maximally deforming human red cells normally averaging 7.82 microns in diameter [362] to pass. This theoretical minimum assumes a mean cell (surface) area (MCA) of ~135 micron^2 and a mean cell volume (MCV) of ~94 micron^3 for human erythrocytes, and allows for a maximum surface stretch of 10 micron^2 to a total of MCA ~ 145 micron^2.* From simple geometry for a red cell compressed into a hemisphere-capped cylinder during tube passage, the minimum tube diameter D_{tube} is given by

$$MCV = \left(\frac{MCA}{4}\right) D_{tube} - \left(\frac{\pi}{12}\right) D_{tube}^3 \quad (m^3) \qquad \text{\{Eqn. 8.1\}}$$

Experiments using polycarbonate sieves and micropipettes confirm that a tube diameter of at least 2.3 microns is necessary to avoid plugging.[374]

However, the above theoretical computation assumes mean erythrocyte geometry and ignores the considerable dispersion in volume and surface area of individual physiological red cells around the mean value. Specifically, the largest 1% of human red cells have diameter d_{RBC} ~ 9.65 microns, MCA ~ 182 micron^2 and MCV ~ 132 micron^3, [362]

** Different species have red cells differing slightly in diameter, thickness, surface area and volume.[840] For example, dogs have 7.2-micron red cells with MCA ~ 123 micron^2 and MCV ~ 69 micron^3, giving (assuming surface elasticity characteristics similar to the human erythrocyte) a theoretical minimum passable tube diameter of 2.4 microns. Cats have 5.6-micron red cells with MCA ~ 83 micron^2 and MCV ~ 43 micron^3, giving D_{tube} ~ 2.2 microns, a full 0.5 micron less than for human red cells.*

Table 8.3. Branching Structure of the Pulmonary Arterial Network Entering the Lungs[828]

Pulmonary Branching Order	Number of Branches of Each Order	Number of End Branches of Each Order	Length of Pulmonary Vessel (mm)	Diameter of Pulmonary Vessel (mm)
1	1	300,000,000	90.5	30.0
2	3	100,000,000	32.0	14.83
3	8	30,210,000	10.9	8.06
4	20	13,760,000	20.7	5.82
5	66	3,983,000	17.9	3.65
6	203	1,159,000	10.5	2.09
7	675	347,000	6.6	1.33
8	2290	89,160	4.69	0.85
9	5861	48,050	3.16	0.525
10	17,560	16,040	2.10	0.351
11	52,550	5358	1.38	0.224
12	157,400	1787	0.91	0.138
13	471,300	598	0.65	0.086
14	1,411,000	200	0.44	0.054
15	4,226,000	67	0.29	0.034
16	12,660,000	24	0.20	0.021
17	300,000,000 (*alveolar*)	1	0.13	0.013

giving a theoretical minimum passable tube diameter D_{tube} ~ 3.1 microns for these cells. The largest cell in a population of 10^8 cells (there are a total of ~300,000 of these largest cells in circulation at any given time, a not inconsiderable number) has d_{RBC} ~ 16 microns, MCA ~ 500 micron^2, MCV ~ 450 micron^3,[362] giving D_{tube} ~ 3.7 microns. Thus if human capillaries were as small as 2.3-3.7 microns, a significant number of red cells would be unable to navigate passage and would quickly plug the tubes, resulting in angionecrosis. Experiments have also shown plugging by human leukocytes at tube apertures much below ~5 microns.[845,846] Thus the minimum viable human capillary diameter appears to be ~4 microns.

The average density of capillaries in human tissue is ~600/mm^3,[832] which implies a mean separation of ~40 microns between adjacent capillaries averaging ~1 mm in length. Most living tissue cells lie within ~1-3 cell widths of a capillary. To reach a particular cell, bloodborne nanorobots may normally travel most of the distance through the vascular network, then exit the capillary and cross at most one or two cells to reach the desired target cell. Capillary density varies considerably in the vascular beds of different organs. For instance, microvascular density is 2500-3000/mm^3 in the brain, kidneys, liver, and myocardium; 300-400/mm^3 in phasic units of the skeletal musculature; and <100/mm^3 in bone, fat, connective tissue, and in tonic units of the skeletal musculature.[832] Blood flow rate per gram of tissue (Table 8.4) is very roughly proportional to the relative microvascular density in each organ or tissue. More than 70% of the water of the blood is exchanged with extravascular water every minute—the walls of smaller capillaries are veritable sieves with respect to water.[2229]

What is the size (in bits) of the minimum topological map needed to reliably navigate the entire ~19,000 kilometers of human blood vasculature? Map size is driven by the number of bifurcations (decision junctions; see Section 8.3.4) and capillaries. Taking the pulmonary arterial tree (Table 8.3) as representative, traveling from the heart to a final capillary requires passage through approximately 17 forks with an average of 3.2 branches per fork. In a simple bifurcation map with 17 forks and at most 4 branches per fork, each capillary can be assigned a unique topological address using 17 digits with each digit having $\log_2(4) = 2$ bits, a 34-bit address vector. This specification is very compact because the minimum number of bits required to name each of 19 billion capillaries in the body is also $\log_2$(19 billion vessels) ~ 34 bits. Using run-length coding, we can have 4^{17} addresses of length 34 bits, 4^{16} addresses of length 32 bits, and so forth, giving a whole-body minimum of: 34 bits (4^{17}) + 32 bits (4^{16}) + ... + 2 bits (4^1) = 763,549,741,512 bits for a single comprehensive bifurcation map.

Assuming some data redundancy (e.g., parity check bits) and an allowance for special cases (e.g., arterial anastomoses, shunts, or arteriovenous fistulas which are direct connections between a small artery and a small vein), a complete map of the human vasculature

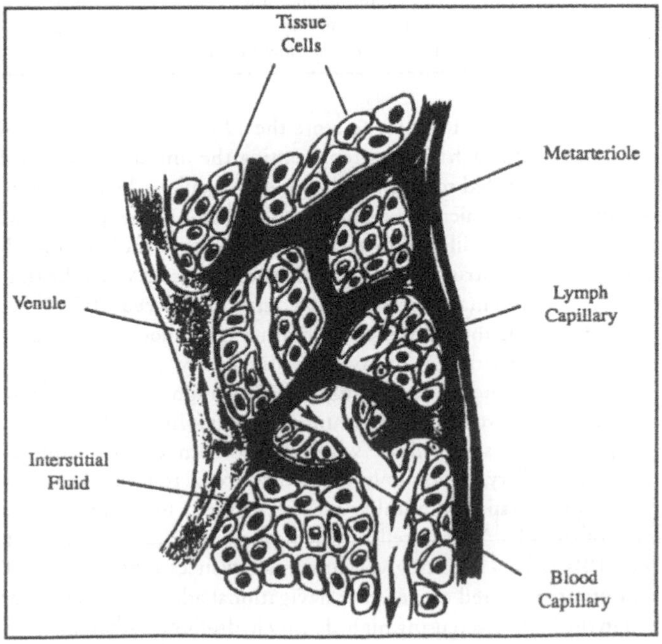

Fig. 8.4. Metarterioles, venules, and lymph capillaries (redrawn from Tortora[853]).

Table 8.4. Typical Blood Perfusion Rates for Various Tissues and Organs[818,837]

Tissue Type	Anatomical Location or Organ	Specific Blood Flow Rate (mm^3/sec-gm)
Adipose tissue	Abdomen, 10-29 mm thick	0.507
	Abdomen, 30-49 mm thick	0.358
	Abdomen, >40 mm thick	0.307
	Thigh, 11 mm thick	0.93
	Thigh, 20 mm thick	0.33
	Thigh, 43 mm thick	0.15
Bone	Humerus, marrow flow only	0.055
Connective tissue	Typical, basal (max)	0.50 (2.5)
Joint	Knee, avg. @ 303 K skin temp.	0.222
	Knee, avg. @ 308 K skin temp.	0.487
Muscle	Calf, anterior, resting flow (max)	0.46 (9.15)
	Forearm, resting flow (max)	0.53 (8.38)
	Thigh, anterior, resting flow (max)	0.43 (6.00)
	Typical, basal (max)	0.50 (10.0)
Organ	Brain, basal (max)	9.0-9.2 (18.3)
	Gastrointestinal tract, basal (max)	6.7 (26.7)
	Heart, basal (max)	13.3-14.0 (64.0)
	Kidney, basal (max)	67-70 (100)
	Liver, basal (max)	9.6-14.2 (54.5)
	Lung, basal (max)	90 (490)
Skin	Abdomen, resting flow	1.44
	Arms, resting flow	1.40
	Calf, resting flow	1.77
	Face, resting flow	11.7
	Foot, dorsal surface, resting flow	2.38
	Forearm, sunburned (max)	9.22 (46.7)
	Hands, resting flow	3.35
	Head, resting flow	7.15
	Thigh, resting flow	1.6
	Thorax, resting flow	6.45
	Typical, resting flow (max)	1.7 (25.0)

probably requires ~1 terabit to store the addresses of all 19 billion capillaries, with each address representing the unique navigational instructions needed to reach each vessel. This allows localization to within a ~50,000 micron^3 volume or ~(40 micron),^{3} the approximate volume of each capillary. However, map stability at the lowest levels of the branching structure becomes a serious concern when the time interval between map compilation and map use exceeds 10^5-10^6 sec (1-12 days), due to angiogenesis and other continuous natural tissue remodeling activities, or in cases of tissue injury.

An arteriovenous vasculographic map might also provide an excellent framework for determining cytographic location in the body, since all tissue cells lie within a few diameters of a capillary and each capillary services only ≲500 tissue cells. To make a complete cytographic map, the number of bits required to uniquely name each of the ~10^{13} tissue cells in the human body (Section 8.5.1) is $\log_2(10^{13}$ cells) ~ 43 bits; given similar allowances as before, ≲1000 terabits are required to store the navigational address of every fixed cell in the body. Even using high-density hydrofluorocarbon memory tape it does not appear feasible for individual bloodborne nanorobots to carry a whole-body vasculographic or cytographic map onboard (the latter of which might require ~40,000 micron^3 of data storage volume). However, a modest 0.1-micron^3 10^9-bit map will allow a bloodborne nanorobot to retain the addresses (with complete navigational instructions) of up to 30 million individual capillaries (~50 cm^3 of typical tissue) or ~20 million individual cells (~0.2 cm^3 of cell-dense tissue) for the duration of its mission. Note that sequential passage through ~10 million different named capillaries of average length ~1 mm at a swimming speed of ~1 cm/sec (Section 9.4.2.6) requires ~12 days, a not unreasonable mission duration.

8.2.1.3 Lymphatic System

The lymphatic system consists of a branching series of closed endothelium-lined vessels. These vessels slowly drain lymph (composition discussed below) from the extracellular spaces and convey it back to the arteriovenous circulation, a sluggish current easily navigated by lymphborne medical nanodevices. The lymphatic vessels have a total capacity of ~2 liters of lymph,[852] vs. ~3.7 liters of fluid capacity for all the veins. No detailed quantitative summation of the lymphatic system is readily available in the literature, so Table 8.5 must be regarded as an estimate consistent with data gleaned from a variety of sources[363,838,848,850,853-860,874] but possibly still containing significant errors.

Lymphatic vessels resemble veins in structure but are greater in number. Compared to veins, lymphatics of similar size have thinner walls, more valves, much greater variation in their caliber but a less sinuous course through the tissue. They also contain lymph nodes at various intervals along their length. Lymph vessels are frequently connected with one another by short anastomotic branches.[857] Lymphatics of the skin travel in loose subcutaneous tissue and generally follow veins and venules. Lymphatics of the viscera generally follow arterioles, forming plexuses (extensive two-dimensional meshworks) around them.

However, the lymph drainage system actually begins with the prelymphatics. The prelymphatics are a randomly interconnected network of non-endothelialized tissue channels 0.1-0.2 microns in diameter penetrating the cell masses of the body, although in certain regions where lymphatic capillaries are absent (e.g., the brain, eye, and bone), the prelymphatics take over the role of the capillaries and eventually discharge into them, outside the regions in question.[861] In the viscera, these interstitial channels will normally be very short since there are frequent arteriovenous and lymphatic capillaries—for example, ~30 microns long in the capsules of knee joints (~0.02-0.05 channels/micron^3). In the muscles, the prelymphatics are longer since the lymphatic capillaries extend only into the larger regions of connective tissue. In the brain the channels may be 10-30 cm long since they must reach (in the case of the brain) from the depths of the cortex to the outside of the skull.[861] Following injury, tissue channel volume may enlarge as much as ~400 times in a week, in response to a simple incision wound.[1339]

Drainage of the prelymphatics is done by the lymphatic capillaries, thin-walled irregularly-contoured valveless endothelial tubes varying in diameter from 15-75 microns. The lymphatic capillaries are blind sacs (Fig. 8.4) with an inferred mean separation of ~86 microns or ~4 tissue cell widths. Their walls are more porous than those of blood capillaries, so that larger molecules and particles may pass (Fig. 8.5). The resting gap of the open junction of adjoining lymphatic endothelial cells usually ranges from ~0.1 micron to several microns.[361] However, Allen[851] injected intraperitoneally a variety of particles of various sizes up to 22.5 microns in diameter, and all sizes later appeared in the diaphragmatic lymph. This suggests that the peritoneal mesothelium and the lymphatic endothelium on either side of the fenestrations of the basement membrane can open

Table 8.5. Approximate Quantification of the Human Lymphatic System

Human Lymphatic Vessel or Lymphatic Component	Diameter (mm)	Length (mm)	Wall Thickness	Lymph Flow Rate (mm^3/sec)	Number of Vessels, Tissues or Objects	Total Length (mm)	Total Lymph Volume (mm^3)	Flow Velocity (µm/sec)
Cervical portals:								
Thoracic duct	4.0	450	500 µm	21.4	1	450	5700	1700
Right lymphatic duct	3.0	14	500 µm	1.7	1	14	100	250
Main lymphatic trunks:								
Subclavian (left & right)	2.5	50	~300 µm	0.7	2	100	500	100
Jugular (left & right)	2.3	40	~300 µm	0.7	2	80	330	200
Intestinal	2.3	85	~300 µm	14.0	1	85	350	3400
Bronchomediastinal (left & right)	2.2	125	~300 µm	2.0	2	250	950	500
Lumbar (right & left)	1.9	100	~300 µm	0.3	2	100	570	100
Cisterna chyli (thoracic)	8-13	50-75	~500 µm	14.0	1	60	1700	500
Minor lymphatic trunks:	1.0	10	~100 µm	0.2	100	1000	800	300
Post-Lymphonodal collecting ducts	0.5	~3	15-50 µm	0.01	1700	5100	1000	70
Pre-Lymphonodal collecting ducts	0.5	~3	15-50 µm	4×10^{-5}	617,000	1,850,000	363,000	0.2
Precollecting ducts	0.15	~1	~5 µm	3×10^{-7}	68,000,000	68,000,000	1,200,000	0.02
Lymphatic capillaries	0.02	0.5	1 µm	3×10^{-7}	6,800,000,000	3,400,000,000	425,000*	0.03
Lymphatics, subtotal				23.1		~3500 km	2,000,000	~10 (avg)
Pre-lymphatic channels	0.1-0.2 µm	30 µm- 30 cm	--	3×10^{-14}	8×10^{14}	24×10^{12}	(370,000)	0.002
Lymphocytes	~10 µm	--	--	--	7×10^{11}	--	(350,000)	--
Lymph nodes	4.0	--	--	0.05	450	--	(15,000)	10
Spleen	66	--	--	--	1	--	(75,000)	--
Thymus	22	--	--	--	1	--	(10,000)	--
Lymphatic vessel walls	--	--	--	--	--	--	(460,000)	--
Total Lymphatic System							**~3,300,000**	

estimated for hypothetical adult male, weight 70 kg, consistent with references cited in text; * final volume after an assumed 90% fluid reabsorption

at least this wide, so micron-sized nanorobots should find easy passage into the lymphatic system through these pores.

Lymph capillaries originate throughout the body, though not in avascular tissue, the central nervous system, splenic pulp or bone marrow. They may occur singly or in plexuses, especially in regions where the connective tissue is lobulated (e.g., glands) or arranged in cylinders (e.g., muscles). Each lymphatic capillary plexus is typically 320-640 microns wide, encompassing 2-6 blood capillary loops. The terminal lymphatic network has different geometric patterns in different tissues. In the mesentery, it conforms to the modular configuration of the blood capillary network. In the skeletal muscle, lymphatics are found in the immediate neighborhood of the arterioles; in the dermis, near the venules. In the lung, the terminal lymphatics lie at the junctions of interalveolar septa.[363] Simple observation of the local lymphocapillary topology (Section 8.3.4) might enable nanorobots to identify which tissue they are passing through.

The precollecting ducts are short vascular segments with valves (like all subsequent lymphatics) at intervals of 0.4-1.5 mm that connect the capillary plexuses to the larger collecting ducts. The lymphatic collecting ducts are denoted either prenodal or postnodal, though there are no morphological or structural differences between the two. Collecting ducts display many swellings and strictures along their course which alter their profile, due to the presence of valves. (Valve-counting may offer useful navigational information.) There is an inner and an outer muscular layer. The collecting ducts empty

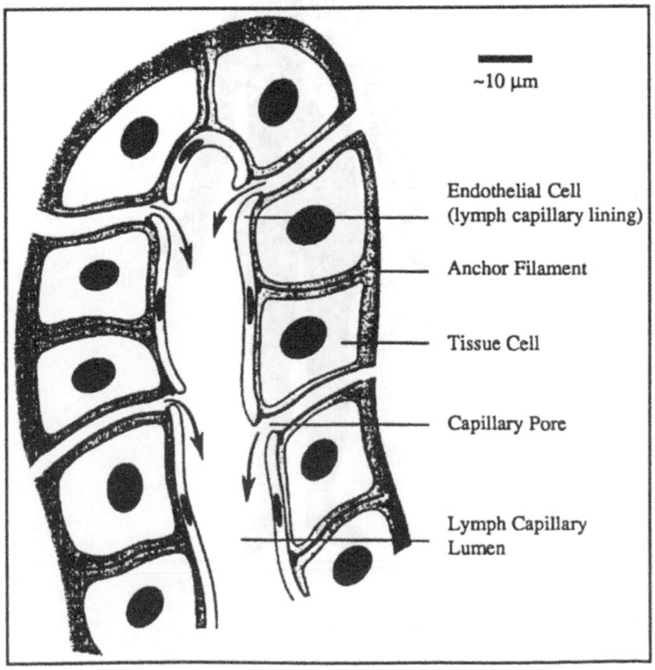

Fig. 8.5. Details of a lymph capillary (redrawn from Tortora[853]).

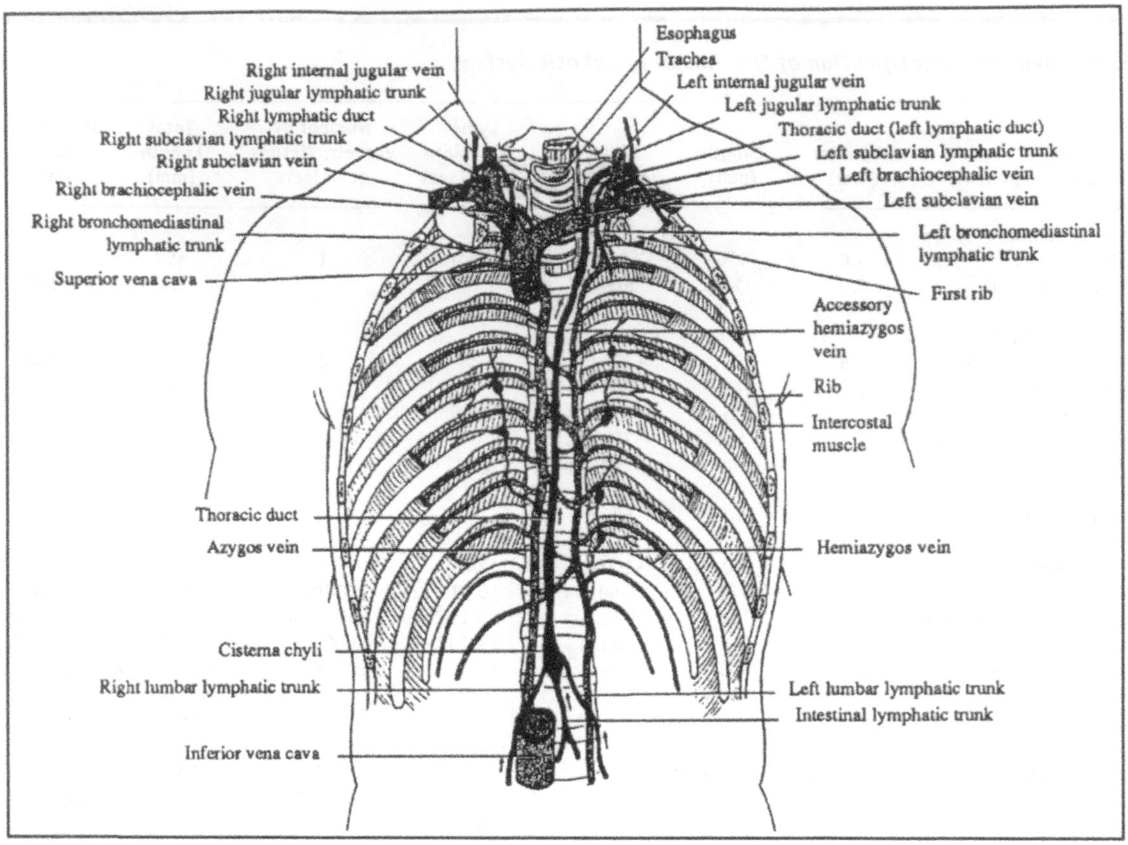

Fig. 8.6. Main trunks of the human lymphatic system (redrawn from Tortora[853]).

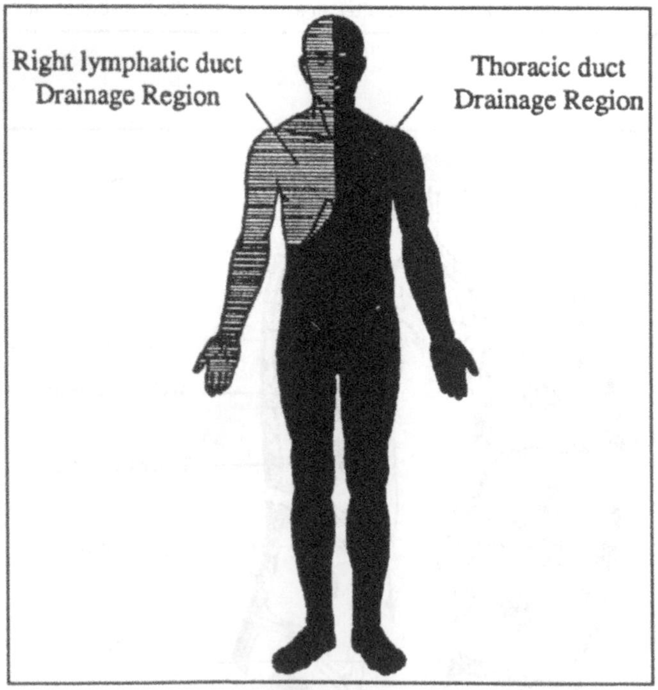

Fig. 8.7. Lymphatic drainage regions.

into the lymphatic trunks, larger and thicker-walled vessels which receive the lymph drained from entire regions of the body.

By their confluence, the lymphatics form progressively larger vessels, which ultimately converge at two cervical portals (Fig. 8.6). The first is the right lymphatic duct, which is relatively short and typically opens into the right brachiocephalic vein at the junction of the right internal jugular and right subclavian veins. It carries lymph drainage from the right upper portion of the body (Fig. 8.7). The second is the thoracic duct, which arises in the abdomen and courses upward along the anterior aspect of the vertebral column (with valves every ~3 cm along its length),[857] through the thorax into the base of the neck, where it typically joins the venous system at the junction of the left jugular and subclavian veins. At its termination, a bicuspid valve faces into the vein to prevent or reduce reflux of blood, although after death blood regurgitates freely into the thoracic duct, which then looks like a vein.

The thoracic duct is ~5 mm in diameter at its abdominal commencement, but becomes narrower at mid-thoracic levels, then in ~50% of patients grows slightly wider again before its termination.[854] There is a tremendous variation in structure from one patient to another. The duct may divide in its mid-course into two unequal vessels which soon re-unite, or into several small branches which form a plexus before combining again to form one short wide trunk. Higher in the body, the duct occasionally bifurcates, the left branch ending as usual, the right branch diverging to join one of the right lymph trunks or even the right lymphatic duct, with the combined vessel opening into the right subclavian vein. After performing 529 human dissections, Kinnaert[856] found that the thoracic duct terminated on the internal jugular vein in 36% of the cases, the subclavian vein

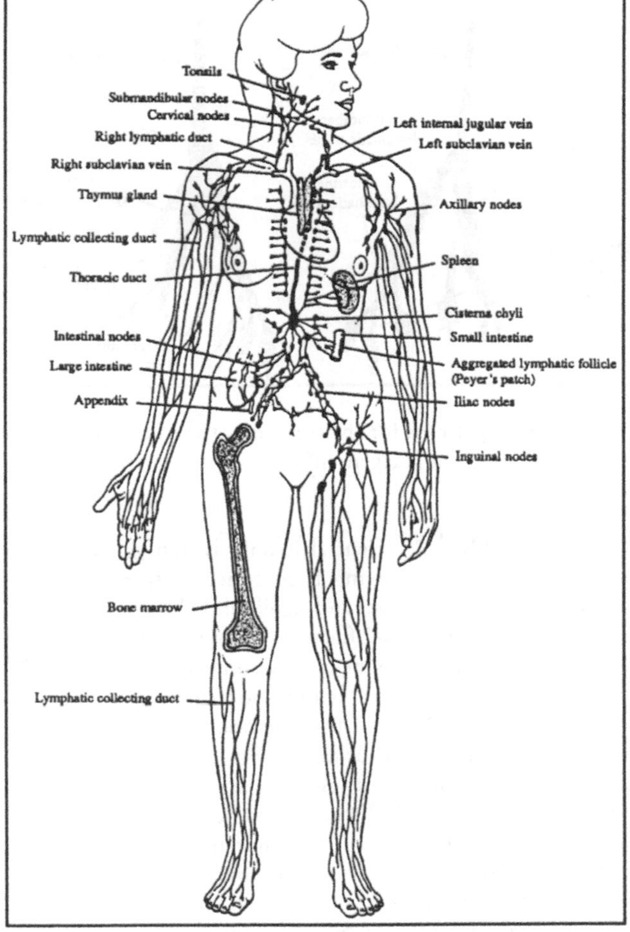

Fig. 8.8. Main organs of the human lymphatic system (redrawn from Tortora[853]).

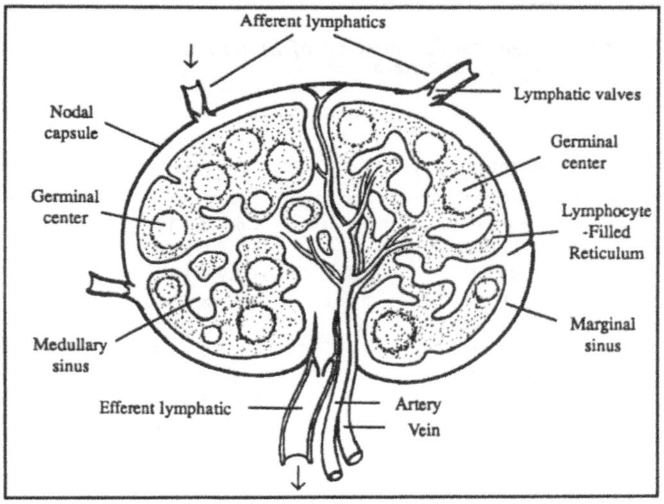

Fig. 8.9. Details of a lymph node (redrawn from Haagensen[857]).

in 17% of the cases, the jugulo-subclavian junction in 34% of the cases, both veins 8% of the time, and the transverse cervical vein in 2% of the cases where the thoracic duct terminated on the left. In 21% of the cases, the terminal openings were multiple; in the rest of the cases, the single thoracic duct terminus diameter ranged from 2-5 mm.[856]

Various lymphatic organs are located along the length of the lymphatic system (Fig. 8.8). A major function of these organs is the production of lymphocytes which are added to the lymph passing through the vessels. Lymphatic tissue is a loose-structured material consisting of a spongelike stroma and free cells in the meshes of the stroma, and is part of the reticuloendothelial system (RES). Phagocytic cells in the sinuses serve as filters that scavenge particles from the lymph and destroy them. Such particles include red blood cells, pathogenic bacteria, and larger dust particles imported by the respiratory tract and collected by macrophage cells of the bronchial nodes. Lymphborne nanorobots can avoid these traps (Chapter 15); the Reynolds number of lymph flow[3303] is typically only ~0.0025.

The most numerous of the lymphatic organs is the lymph node, designed as a bacterial/particulate filter with channels, sinuses, valves, and fluid entering via 6-10 afferent lymph vessels (Fig. 8.9). Lymph nodes vary enormously in their size and structure, probably averaging ~4 mm in diameter but occasionally reaching 30-40 mm.[857] A normal young adult body contains ~450 lymph nodes distributed as follows: ~30 nodes in the arm and superficial thoraco-abdominal wall down to the umbilicus; ~20 nodes in the legs and superficial buttocks, infraumbilical abdominal wall and perineum; 60-70 nodes in the head and neck; ~100 nodes in the thorax, including deep walls and contents; and ~230 nodes in the abdomen and pelvis, including deep walls and contents.[854]

There is also the 10 cm^3 of lymphoid tissue in the bilobate thymus gland, and additional lymphoid tissue in the 80-300 cm^3 spleen.[854] (The spleen slowly enlarges during alimentary digestion and varies in size with the content of blood and state of nutrition, being large in well-fed patients and small in starved patients.) About 10% of the population has accessory spleens; these ~1 cm^3 spleniculi may be numerous and widely scattered in the abdomen.[854] Other lymphoid tissues include the lymph nodules or the lymph follicles in the intestines (Section 8.2.3), the subepithelial lymphoid aggregates including the palatine, lingual, and nasopharyngeal (e.g., adenoids, tonsils), and the lymphoid tissue in the submucosa of the appendix and in the bone marrow.

What, exactly, is lymph? Lymph is essentially an alkaline ultrafiltrate of the blood plasma formed by continual seepage of fluid constituents of the blood across the capillary walls and into the surrounding interstitial spaces. The lymph fluid has much the same composition as the interstitial fluid. Like blood, lymph consists of a plasmatic part and a corpuscular part (Table 8.6). Lymph contains almost no platelets but has about one-third the fibrinogen and five times the prothrombin as in blood serum, hence will thrombose spontaneously forming a yellowish clot. Lymph has 0.02-0.10% as many red cells as arterial blood, but most have passed near cells and become thoroughly deoxygenated, especially given the ~1 day transit time through the lymphatic system for cells. There is still some dissolved oxygen in the lymph water, however, roughly the same concentration as in blood plasma (see Appendix B). Glucose may be present in lymph at slightly higher concentration than in blood serum, so lymphoresident nanorobots have access to plenty of chemical fuel energy (Section 6.3.4). Lymph is slightly less viscous[3304] than blood plasma, with specific gravity 0.016-1.023.[2223]

In a fasting patient, the lymph coming from the intestine is a clear, transparent fluid. After a meal containing fat has been ingested, the intestinal lymph becomes white or milky. This is termed chyle—chyle is just lymph containing a surge (5-15% by volume) of emulsified fat which is transported in the form of chylomicrons measuring 0.5-0.75 microns in diameter.[749] In ~65% of all patients, the intestinal trunk (which drains lymph from the stomach, intestines,

Table 8.6. Chemical Compostion of Human Thoracic Lymph[585,847,848]

Component of Lymph	Concentration (gm/cm^3)
Albumin	$1.6\text{-}4.2 \times 10^{-2}$
Bilirubin	$5.0\text{-}8.0 \times 10^{-6}$
Calcium	7.7×10^{-5}
Chloride	3.4×10^{-3}
Cholesterol	7.5×10^{-4}
Creatinine	$0.8\text{-}3.0 \times 10^{-5}$
Fibrinogen	$0.16\text{-}1.1 \times 10^{-3}$
Globulin	$1.2\text{-}2.6 \times 10^{-2}$
Glucose	$0.95\text{-}1.4 \times 10^{-3}$
Iron	9.4×10^{-7}
Nitrogen, non-protein	2.3×10^{-4}
Phosphorus, inorganic	3.9×10^{-5}
Potassium	1.8×10^{-4}
Protein, total	$2.8\text{-}5.1 \times 10^{-2}$
Prothrombin	5.1×10^{-4}
Sodium	2.9×10^{-3}
Uric acid	$3.3\text{-}5.0 \times 10^{-5}$
Water	8.6×10^{-1}
Component of Lymph	**Concentration ($cells/cm^3$)**
Erythrocytes (red cells)	
-Normal, mean	$1\text{-}5 \times 10^{6}$
-Normal, max	7×10^{7}
-Leukemic	1.5×10^{9}
Lymphocytes	$0.19\text{-}2.0 \times 10^{7}$
Neutrophilic granulocytes	$0.2\text{-}4.0 \times 10^{5}$
Platelets	~ 0

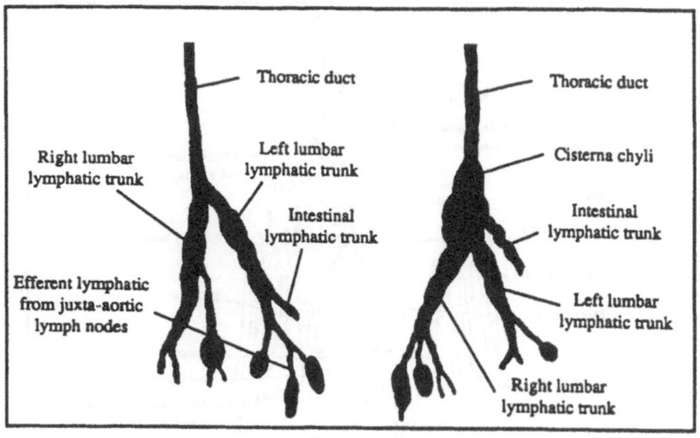

Fig. 8.10. Two patterns for the junction of the lumbar lymphatic trunks (redrawn from Haagensen[857]).

pancreas, spleen, and visceral surface of the liver) empties separately into the thoracic duct immediately above the junction of the two lumbar trunks, and so the thoracic duct widens to a diameter of 8-13 mm, forming a cisterna chyli.[857,874] In the other ~35% of cases, the intestinal trunk joins the left lumbar trunk and there is no cisterna chyli (Fig. 8.10), a navigationally distinctive characteristic.

The chemical composition of lymph plasma varies significantly at different locations in the lymphatic system, reflecting changes in source of drainage and variations in capillary permeabilities. This provides another ready source of useful navigational information for lymphborne medical nanorobots (Section 8.4.3). For example, thoracic lymph is rich in histaminase originating in the kidneys and gut, while cervical duct lymph contains only very low concentrations of histaminase, as in blood plasma.[848] In humans, fibrinogen is 4.1 mg/cm^3 in blood plasma, 1.1 mg/cm^3 in thoracic duct lymph; in dogs, prothrombin concentration expressed as a percentage of serum concentration was measured experimentally as 93.2% in hepatic lymph, 51.2% in thoracic lymph, and 7.6% in leg lymph.[848] The enzyme tributyrinase has high concentration in the intestinal lymph and significantly lower concentrations elsewhere.[847] Insulin is more plentiful in pancreatic lymph.[847]

Cervical, leg, renal, and right duct lymph has 33%-50% of the protein concentration of blood plasma, while intestinal and thoracic duct lymph contains ~67% as much protein as the blood plasma.[860] Protein is generally lowest in the capillary lymph, increasing in several steps with travel upstream toward the main trunks. Hepatic lymph has the highest protein content (about equal to blood plasma), as would be expected in view of the high permeability of the capillaries of the liver sinusoids.[847,860] Central (trunk) lymph generally differs from blood plasma in having high concentrations of sodium, cholesterol, and tributyrinase, and significantly lower concentrations of total protein, albumen α-2 fraction, potassium, nitrogen, aldolase, pyruvic transaminases, choline esterase, amylase, and diastase.[847]

The cellular composition of lymph also changes dramatically with lymphatic location. Most of the prenodal duct lymph contains ~1×10^6 $cells/cm^3$, except for hepatic lymph which has $4\text{-}6 \times 10^6$ $cells/cm^3$. The majority of these cells are red cells, but a small proportion, perhaps 10-20%, are nucleated cells. Such cells include ~85% lymphocytes, ~13% monocytes and macrophages, and ~2% neutrophilic granulocytes. The postnodal duct lymph has ~12 times more nucleated cells than the peripheral lymph, perhaps ~3×10^6 nucleated $cells/cm^3$. The central lymph has $8\text{-}11 \times 10^6$ nucleated $cells/cm^3$.[847]

How fast does lymph move? Of the 20 liters/day of plasma water that leaves the blood circulation through ultrafiltration, 18 liters/day are reabsorbed[862] by passing back out of the lymphatic capillaries and into the venous capillary loops; the remaining 2 liters/day returns to the circulation as lymph that passes through the entire lymphatic system. In other words, relatively little lymph reaches the collecting ducts compared with the total amount entering the lymphatic capillaries;[850] much more lymph is formed in the periphery than ever reaches the main lymph ducts.[849] Basal lymph flow rates are ~2 liters/day,[847,848] rising to a 6-12 liter/day rate during heavy exercise.[848] Summing the vessel crossing times (~length/velocity from Table 8.5), it takes ~24 hours for a node-inert particle entering a lymphatic capillary to drift to the final terminus of the thoracic duct and rejoin the venous flow.

What moves the lymph? Valves are essential to the function of the lymph vascular system, which has no pump comparable to the heart. In the collecting ducts, one-way valves are spaced roughly 2-3 mm apart[857] and can oppose retrograde pressures of up to 20 mmHg.[855] Lymph flow in the extremities depends largely on the massaging effect of movement of the surrounding tissues that results from muscle contraction. Such movements can be produced indirectly by the motion of nearby arterioles, or by the contraction of the skeletal muscles, or by movement of the organs (e.g., motion of the arms or legs, peristalsis of the intestine, or breathing of the lung). Arterial pulsations contribute 1.5-2.2 mmHg pressure variation to the lymphatic ducts between systole and diastole.[848] Larger collecting lymphatics are innervated, so movement can also be induced by contractions of smooth muscles in the lymphatic vessel wall.[848] The contractile activity seems to depend on the volume of lymph produced. If this is small, the vessel walls are quiescent, but slight distension initiates rhythmic contractions at ~0.1-0.2 Hz[838,848,863] and can raise the lymphatic pressure by up to ~5 mmHg.[855] By comparison, the mean interstitial hydrostatic pressure is ~1.4 mmHg and the mean intralymphatic pressure is ~0.9 mmHg.[526,847,860]

The minimum topological map required to reliably navigate the entire ~3500 kilometers of human lymphatic vasculature should be roughly comparable to that required for a comprehensive blood capillary map, or ~1 terabit (Section 8.2.1.2).

8.2.2 Navigational Bronchography

Medical nanorobots may access the human body via the respiratory system. The airway begins at the mouth and nose, extends through the pharynx, larynx, the trachea and bronchial branchings, and ends at the alveoli. The conducting zone from the top of the trachea to the beginning of the respiratory bronchioles contains no alveoli, so gas exchange with the blood does not occur there. Gas exchange occurs only in the respiratory zone, which extends from the respiratory bronchioles down to the alveolar sacs.

Weibel[864] provided the first quantitative measurements of the length, diameter, and area of successive segments of the human airway. Each branch gives rise to two narrower daughter branches which may vary considerably in length. However, the summary in Table 8.7 assumes mean values of length and diameter. Generations 0-16 are the conducting airways, while generations 17-23 constitute the respiratory airways which have alveoli on their walls. Generation 23 terminates in alveoli.

The respiratory airflow begins in the mouth and nose. In the nose are two nasal cavities (totalling ~160 cm^2 in area,)[863] one of which is illustrated in Figure 8.11. The nasal cavities are divided by a partition called the nasal septum, from which diverge three winglike projections called the conchae. The endings of the olfactory nerve lie in the mucosa in the cilia-free region near the ~1 cm^2 olfactory bulb above the superior concha. The nasal passages are flanked by four sinuses which may swell up during infection or inflammation, closing off the air passages and necessitating breathing through the mouth. Lacrimal ducts drain tears and other secretions from the eyes into the nose via the nasolacrimal duct, requiring noseblowing after crying. The ≤1 mm human vomeronasal organ, located near the base of the nasal septum in adults,[1971] transduces pheromonal signals,[1972] although apparently this organ is not present, is inactive, or is very insensitive in some people.

Air passing through the nasal cavities is warmed to within 1 K of body temperature by an extensive capillary vasculature, and is humidified by nasal mucous glands (e.g., goblet cells which secrete mucoid fluid) to within ~1% of full saturation, before the air enters the pharynx. Coarse particles are removed from incoming air by nose hairs. Smaller particles are removed by turbulent precipitation, wherein obstacles in the nasal passages force the airflow to execute many sharp turns which the particles are too heavy to negotiate. The particles hit the nasal mucous membrane and become embedded in the mucus. The nasal turbulence mechanism is so effective that

Table 8.7. Approximate Quantification of the Human Bronchial System[864]

Pulmonary Branch	Generation	Number	Branch Diameter (mm)	Branch Length (mm)	Cumul. Length (mm)	X-Section Area (cm^2)	Volume (cm^3)	Cumul. Volume (cm^3)	Air Speed (cm/sec)	Reynolds Number
Trachea	0	1	18	120.0	120	2.6	31	31	393	4350
Main bronchus	1	2	12.2	47.6	167	2.3	11	42	427	3210
Lobar bronchus	2	4	8.3	19.0	186	2.2	4	46	462	2390
	3	8	5.6	7.6	194	2.0	2	47	507	1720
Segmental bronchus	4	16	4.5	12.7	206	2.6	3	51	392	1110
	5	32	3.5	10.7	217	3.1	3	54	325	690
Bronchi w/cartilage	6	64	2.8	9.0	226	4.0	4	57	254	434
in wall	7	128	2.3	7.6	234	5.1	4	61	188	277
	8	256	1.86	6.4	240	7.0	4	66	144	164
	9	512	1.54	5.4	246	9.6	5	71	105	99
	10	1020	1.30	4.6	250	13	6	77	73.6	60
Terminal bronchus	11	2050	1.09	3.9	254	19	7	85	52.3	34
	12	4100	0.95	3.3	257	29	10	95	34.4	20
Bronchioles w/muscle	13	8190	0.82	2.7	260	44	12	106	23.1	11
in wall	14	16,400	0.74	2.3	262	70	16	123	14.1	6.5
	15	32,800	0.66	2.0	264	113	22	145	8.92	3.6
Terminal bronchiole	16	65,500	0.60	1.65	266	180	30	175	5.40	2.0
Respiratory bronchiole	17	131×10^3	0.54	1.41	267	300	42	217	3.33	1.1
Respiratory bronchiole	18	262×10^3	0.50	1.17	269	534	61	278	1.94	0.57
Respiratory bronchiole	19	524×10^3	0.47	0.99	270	944	93	370	1.10	0.31
Alveolar duct	20	1.05×10^6	0.45	0.83	271	1600	139	510	0.60	0.17
Alveolar duct	21	2.10×10^6	0.43	0.70	271	3200	224	734	0.32	0.08
Alveolar duct	22	4.19×10^6	0.41	0.59	272	5900	350	1085	0.18	0.04
Alveolar sac	23	8.39×10^6	0.41	0.50	273	12,000	591	1675	0.09	--
Alveoli, 21 per duct	--	300×10^6	0.28	0.23	273	--	3200	4800	--	--

average of five normal human lungs; includes both lungs; air speed and Reynolds number at 1 liter/sec flow.

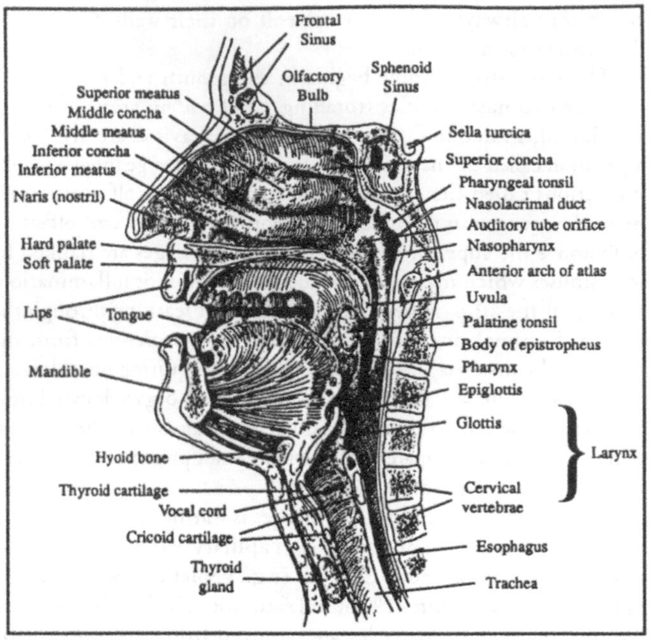

Fig. 8.11. Sagittal section through mouth, nasal cavity, pharynx and larynx (redrawn from Millard, King, and Showers[750]).

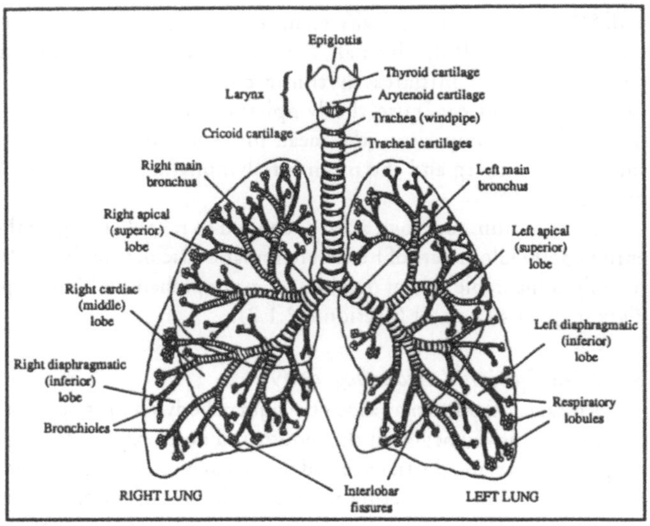

Fig. 8.12. Lung lobes and the bronchial tree (crude schematic, redrawn from Guyton[863]).

almost no nasally-inhaled particles larger than 2-5 microns reach the lower airway.

Most of the surfaces of the nasal airway are covered by a layer of ciliated, pseudostratified columnar epithelium cells. Each epithelial surface cell has 25-100 cilia that beat forcefully and continually toward the pharynx at ~10 Hz.[3556,3557] Respiratory cilia are ~0.2 microns in diameter and ~2-5 microns long (having a ~31 nm apical glycocalyx),[3587] with a mean separation between cilia of ~2-5 microns. The film of particle-carrying nasal mucus ≳200 microns thick [3167] is moved toward the pharynx by the cilia at a speed of ~1-3 cm/min,[863,3167] where it is then swallowed down the esophagus. Mucus velocity increases with luminal depth. In unciliated areas such as the front of the nose, where temperatures fall below levels the cilia can tolerate, the mucous layer creeps along the surface solely through traction from neighboring ciliated areas. Swallowed mucus volume totals ~0.1 cm^3/min. The absolute viscosity of normal mucus is typically ~1 kg/m-sec, rising as high as ~500 kg/m-sec in the thick sputum of cystic fibrosis patients.[1081] Mucus rheology and mucociliary clearance mechanisms of the respiratory tract have been widely studied,[3168] along with the energy dissipation per cilium in the periciliary fluid.[3170] Airflow contributes little to mucus transport during normal breathing ,[3168] except in patients with bronchial hypersecretions,[3167] although high-frequency ventilation and coughing may make significant contributions.[3167-3169]

During inspiration, air passes through the nose or mouth into the pharynx (throat). The posterior wall of the pharynx rests against the cervical vertebrae; the lateral wall has openings communicating with the middle ear (auditory or eustachian tube). The pharynx branches into two tubes—the esophagus (through which food passes to the stomach; Section 8.2.3) and the larynx (part of the airways). The larynx houses the vocal cords, two strong bands of elastic tissue (covered by stratified scalelike epithelium) stretched horizontally across its lumen. The flow of air past the vocal cords causes them to vibrate, producing sounds. The ventricular folds or false vocal cords (in mid-glottis) point downward. When closed by the action of sphincter muscles, the folds form an exit valve that permits the building up of abdominal pressure as in straining at stool or in expulsion of the fetus. Coughing involves releasing the air explosively through the folds.

After passing the larynx, air enters the trachea, a cylindrical tube with 16-20 circumferential cartilaginous rings shaped like horseshoes and embedded in an external fibroelastic membrane (Fig. 8.12). The trachea branches into two main bronchi, one of which enters each lung. The right bronchus is shorter, wider, and more nearly vertical in direction than the left bronchus; both (and subsequent branchings) are supported by complete rings of cartilage to prevent collapse under high levels of suction. There are more than 20 generations of branchings in the lungs, each resulting in narrower, shorter, and more numerous tubes (Table 8.7). When the bronchi become smaller than ~1 mm in diameter, they lose their cartilage, and become bronchioles.

The lungs themselves are cone-shaped organs which lie in the pleural cavities of the thorax. The base of each lung contacts with the upper surface of the diaphragm, extending to the level of the 7th rib anteriorly and the 11th rib posteriorly. The right and left pleural cavities are formed by two serous sacs into which the lungs are invaginated. Two layers of pleura are separated by a thin layer of fluid from ~20-80 microns thick. Pleural fluid is formed on the parietal pleural surface at a rate of 7-11 cm^3/hr, with up to 20-25 cm^3 normally present in the pleural space;[2180,3305] glucose is present at serum levels (Appendix B) and there are topographic differences in pleural pressure.[3402] The right lung, larger in size than the left, is divided into three lobes; the left lung has only two lobes (Fig. 8.12), presumably to make room for the heart. The interlobar surfaces are covered with visceral pleura where the lobes contact one another and are lubricated with the same thin mucoid pleural fluid that lubricates the outer surface of the lungs. The lobes slide against each other in the same way that the entire lungs slide within the thoracic cavity. The diaphragm is the principle respiratory muscle. Contraction of the diaphragm elongates the lungs, forcing them to inflate. Other muscles elevate the anterior thoracic wall or compress the abdomen, raising the ribs from an inferiorly slanting position to a horizontal position that increases the anteroposterior diameter of the chest.

Returning to the airflow, bronchiole walls are composed of smooth muscle and connective tissue. This smooth muscle normally

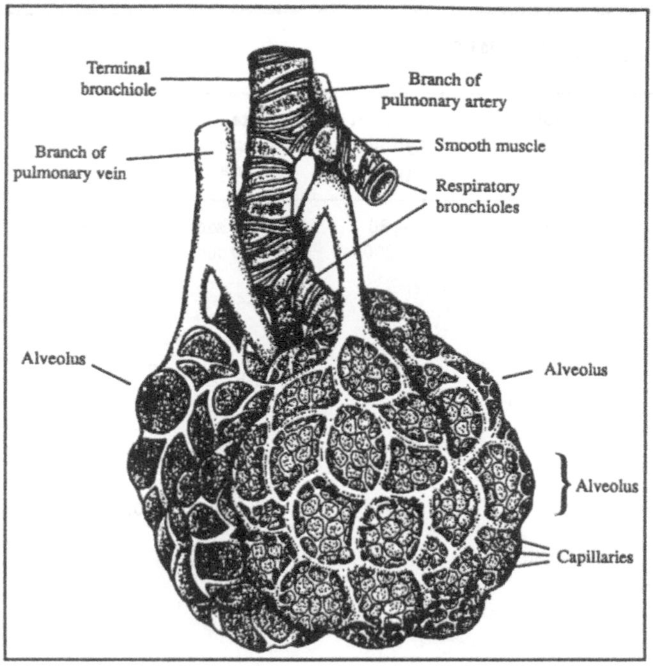

Fig. 8.13. Expanded view of the respiratory lobules (redrawn from Vander, Sherman, and Luciano[866]).

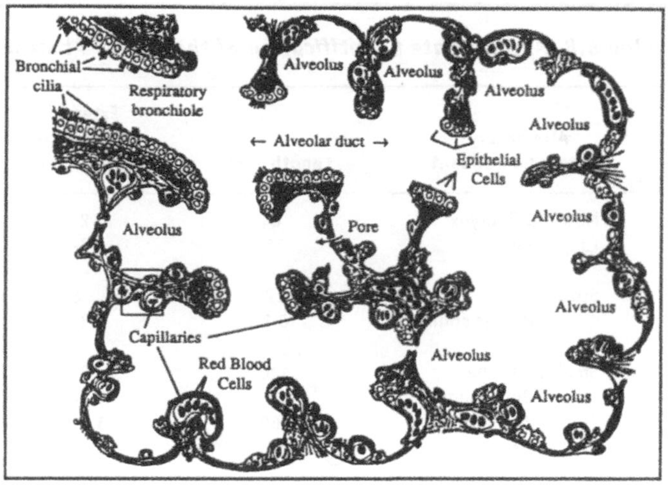

Fig. 8.14. Expanded view of the alveolus (redrawn from Greep and Weiss[867]).

remains relaxed so that the bronchioles stay open, although particles of irritating substances entering these passageways can cause bronchiolar spasms (as in patients with asthma). The bronchioles branch several times. The last bronchiolar branch that still has a complete muscular coat is the terminal bronchiole. This too branches into several respiratory bronchioles with sparse smooth muscle. These bronchioles are the entryways into the respiratory lobules, the final air spaces of the lungs (Fig. 8.13). The walls of all parts of the respiratory lobules form the respiratory membrane which totals ~70 m^2 in total surface area in both lungs combined.[361,863] The membrane is so thin (≤1 micron) that oxygen and carbon dioxide can diffuse freely between the air inside the lobule and the blood in the capillary surrounding the lobule.

As in the nasal passages, the bronchial tree from the lower pharynx down to the end of the respiratory bronchioles is lined with ciliated columnar epithelial cells. These cilia also wave constantly toward the pharynx, moving secreted mucus at ~1.4 cm/min which replaces the entire mucoid coating once every ~20 minutes. A second protective mechanism is provided by mobile phagocytes present in the airways and in the alveoli, that engulf inhaled particles and bacteria (≤100/cm^2 in a healthy person[360]) and thus prevent this foreign matter from gaining access to other lung cells or from entering the blood by conveying this matter into the lymph system. Ciliary activity may be inhibited for several hours by smoking a single cigarette. Phagocytes are also injured by cigarette smoke, air pollution, and other noxious agents. Below the respiratory bronchioles, the ciliated columnar epithelium gives way to a nonciliated cuboidal epithelium.

Alveoli first begin to appear in the respiratory bronchioles, attached to the walls, and their frequency increases in the alveolar ducts until the airways end in grapelike clusters of alveoli (Fig. 8.13). The alveoli are tiny hollow sacs 100-300 microns in diameter that open onto the lumina of the airways (Fig. 8.14). Typically the air in two alveoli is separated by a single wall. The moist air-facing surfaces of the alveolar wall are lined by a continuous layer, one cell thick, of squamous type I epithelial cells (Fig. 8.15, enlargement of box in Figure 8.14). The alveolar surface contains smaller numbers of thicker specialized type II epithelial cells that secrete a detergent-like substance, or surfactant (a complex of protein with dipalmityl lecithin) in a fluid layer ~70 nm thick, which physically stabilizes alveoli of different sizes during inflation and deflation. (See also Section 9.2.3.)

The alveolar walls also contain capillaries, the endothelial linings of which are separated from the alveolar epithelial lining only by a basement membrane and a very thin interstitial space containing interstitial fluid and a loose meshwork of connective tissue (Fig. 8.15). In places, the interstitium is absent and the alveolar epithelium fuses with the capillary endothelium, with total thickness ≤1 micron. In some of the alveolar walls there are pores that permit the flow of air between alveoli, an important route when the airway leading to an alveolus is occluded by disease.

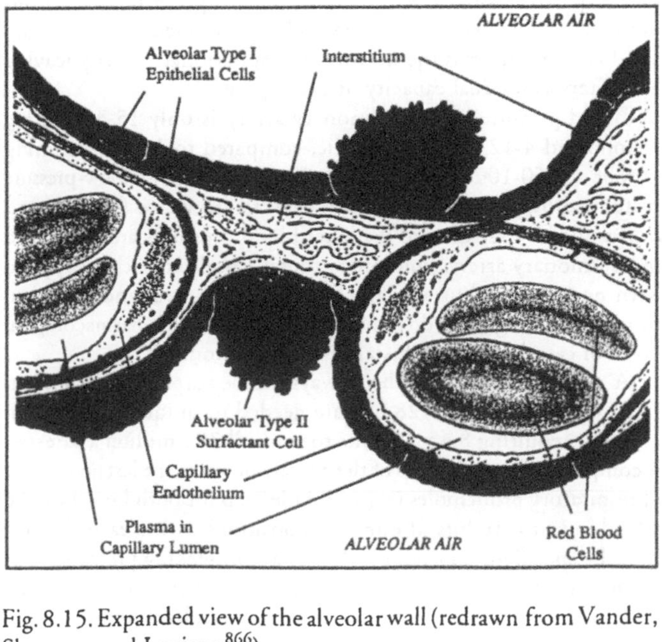

Fig. 8.15. Expanded view of the alveolar wall (redrawn from Vander, Sherman, and Luciano[866]).

Table 8.8. Approximate Quantification of the Human Alimentary System[750,853,863,870,874,2122]

Alimentary System Component	Length (cm)	External Diameter or Width (cm)	Internal Volume (cm^3)	Luminal Cylinder (cm^2)	Contents Passage Time	Velocity of Contents (cm/sec)
Mouth & Pharynx	8	2-5	~ 50	~ 80	1-10 sec	1-8
Esophagus	25	1.3-2.5	~ 100	~ 200	5-20 sec	3-5
Stomach	12	8	230-1000	~ 600	2-6 hrs	~ 0.001
Pyloric sphincter	0.3	1.3-2.0				
Small Intestine	400	3-6	1100	~ 3500	3-5 hrs	0.03
Duodenum	25	3.8-6.0				
Jejunum	160	3.2-3.8				
Ileum	215	2.5-3.2				
Large Intestine	~ 150	5.0-7.5	300	~ 2000	10-20 hrs	0.004-0.008
Cecum	6	7.5				
Appendix	8-9	~ 0.8	0.07-0.60			
Ascending colon	13-20	~ 7				
Transverse colon	50	~ 6.5				
Descending colon	23-30	~ 6				
Sigmoid colon	41	~ 5				
Rectum	16-20	2.5-3.8	40	~ 100	~ 1 hr	0.006
Rectal canal	13-16	3.8				
Anal canal	3-4	2.5				
Total, Average, or Range:	**~ 600**	**~ 3.5**	**1800-2600**	**~ 6500**	**16-32 hrs**	**~ 0.01**

estimated for 70 kg adult male.

At rest, ~4 liters/min of air enter and leave the alveoli, while 5.4 liters/min of blood, the entire cardiac output, flows through pulmonary capillaries which total ~2400 kilometers in length and ~150 cm^3 in volume. During heavy exercise, the air flow to the alveoli can increase to 120-160 liters/min and the blood flow to 25-30 liters/min.[866] The volume of air taken in with each breath (resting tidal volume) is ~0.4 liter/breath at a respiration rate of 18/min (12-15/min during sleep). Volume flow may rise to ~3.2 liters/breath at a respiration rate of up to 62/min during the most strenuous exercise.[780] The two human lungs hold a combined ~6 liters of gas, of which ~3.7 liters is the maximum inspirational capacity leaving ~2.3 liters as residual capacity or dead space.

Blood pressure in the pulmonary artery is only 15-30 mmHg systolic and 4-12 mmHg diastolic, compared to 100-150 mmHg systolic and 60-100 mmHg diastolic in the aorta.[361] This low-pressure system allows pulmonary capillaries to be quite flexible and thin-walled—they distend if higher blood pressures are applied to the pulmonary artery. Pulmonary blood vessels are richly supplied with nerve fibers but are largely free from neural and chemical control—although they do respond to hypoxia and to pharmacological doses of catecholamines, histamine and serotonin.[361]

A navigational map of the airways can be surprisingly compact. Only $\log_2(300 \times 10^6) \sim 28$ bits are needed to uniquely name each alveolus, requiring 8.4×10^9 bits to store all 300 million addresses. A complete bifurcation map of the airways down to the last generation of respiratory bronchioles (e.g., a lobule map for both lungs) can be stored in just ~10^7 bits. If numerous positions within each alveolus must be specified, for example during a scan seeking pre-cancerous epithelial cells, the required map could be much larger. However, C. Phoenix notes that if nanorobots are given individual instructions to scan a certain set of cells for cancer, a contiguous (nonrandom) tissue volume could be searched, specified by a small number of partial addresses. For instance, if 10^7 nanorobots were tasked to scan 30 (unnamed) alveoli each, within the contiguous volume, then each nanorobot must store one ~23 bit hardcoded kernel address plus one ~5 bit alveolus extension address (total 28 bits/alveolus) and one 30-bit cell address for each cancerous cell discovered, a modest memory requirement. On the other hand, general surveyor nanorobots lacking individualized instructions can keep track of the forks they pass and the branches they take as they enter the lungs, assembling the final address (of any cancer cell they ultimately discover) as they go. Upon reaching the terminus of the bronchial system and encountering another nanorobot already at work, the newcomer moves on to another location, keeping track of its current address (~28 bits). Once a cancer is detected, treatment nanorobots can follow the surveyor's address to return to the specific cancer cell without requiring a comprehensive map of the rest of the lung. Thus a treatment protocol can be executed without any overall map of the lung, although the assignment of individual search territories may prove more efficient, and multiple connectivities within the bifurcation tree may demand storage of additional bits or require post-survey data compression.

8.2.3 Navigational Alimentography

Medical nanorobots may also access the human body via the alimentary canal—a ~6 meter long musculomembranous digestive tube which begins at the mouth and ends at the anus. With its accessory glands and organs, the alimentary system controls the intake, mastication, digestion, absorption and elimination of foods.

An approximate quantification of the gastrointestinal system is given in Table 8.8. (Passage times are for normal digestion and exclude pathological conditions such as constipation or diarrhea.) The general

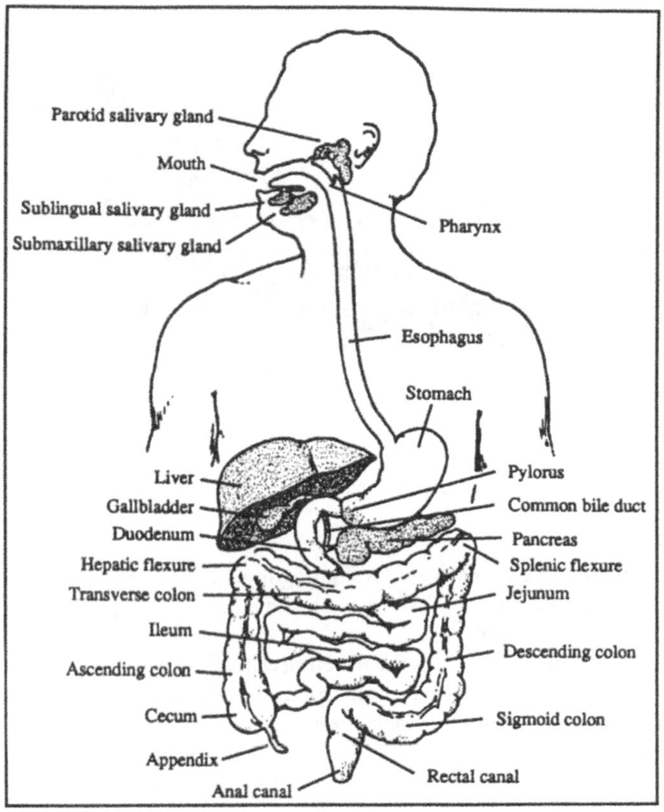

Fig. 8.16. Overview of the alimentary system from mouth to rectum (redrawn from Janowitz[871]).

plan as shown in Figure 8.16 is topologically very simple. The alimentary canal is formed by the mouth, pharynx, esophagus, stomach, small intestine, large intestine, and rectum. Associated with the canal are accessory structures and glands including the salivary glands, liver, gallbladder and pancreas. The tube itself has four layers in radial aspect. Starting at the luminal surface these include the mucosal (superficial epithelium and cells secreting mucus and digestive juices), submucosal (connective tissue with blood and lymphatic vessels), muscular (smooth muscle in circular and longitudinal layers) and serous (parietal and visceral peritoneum) layers. The entire tract, glands, and muscle are innervated from the involuntary or autonomic system and are also influenced by hormones, some from the tract itself and some secreted by glands elsewhere in the body.

It is instructive to imagine the "view" from a medical nanorobot as the nanodevice navigates the entire length of the alimentary system. The journey begins in the mouth (the sphincter oris) where food (typical viscosity 0.01-100 kg/m-sec[3309-3313]) is chewed and mixed with saliva secreted by one of the three pairs of major salivary glands (Fig. 8.17). (There are also the minor salivaries consisting of the labial, buccal, molar, lingual, and palatine glands).[935] After consulting its map, the nanorobot first explores a duct (~1 mm wide, ~25 mm long) in the anteroinferior dental arch leading into the walnut-sized submaxillary salivary gland situated mostly under the lower jawbone. The gland is organized as several thousand separate small secretory units called acini. Each acinus with its microduct forms a single parenchymal unit called a salivon.[935] The lumens of salivons flow together to form progressively larger ducts (all surrounded by contractile myoepithelial cells and a basal lamina), finally reaching the main salivary duct that empties into the mouth. Passing under

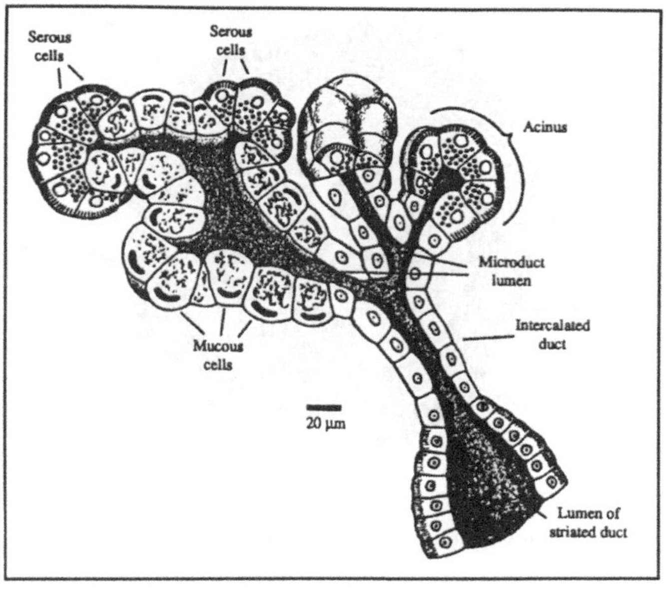

Fig. 8.17. Midplane section of a terminal portion of the submaxillary salivary gland (myoepithelium omitted; redrawn from Guyton[863]).

the tongue, our mobile nanodevice traverses multiple ducts (~0.5 mm wide, ~5 mm long) leading from the sublingual, the smallest gland located in the floor of the mouth. After climbing up to the soft palate in the roof of the mouth, the nanorobot reaches a pair of ducts (~1 mm wide, 15-20 mm long) leading from the parotid glands—the largest of the three glands, lying anteroinferior to each ear.

The six major salivary glands together typically produce 500-1500 cm^3/day of saliva in response to mechanical, thermal, and chemical stimuli applied to the mucous membrane of the mouth, or as the result of psychological or olfactory stimuli.[749,751,1975] Unstimulated flow is 10-50 cm^3/hr during waking hours and 1-2 cm^3/hr during sleep,[749,873] but may rise as high as 290 cm^3/hr during eating.[585] Salivary fluid specific gravity is 1.01-1.02, mean viscosity is ~ 4×10^{-3} kg/m-sec but up to 7.4×10^{-3} kg/m-sec in bulimic patients,[3306] and pH averages 6.8 (range 5.6-7.6).[585,751] Plenty of chemical energy (Section 6.3.4) is available to power a nanorobot exploring these ducts—including 1.96 (1.13-2.81) x 10^{-4} gm/cm^3 of glucose, 7.5 (2.5-9.0) x 10^{-5} gm/cm^3 of cholesterol, and 2-4 x 10^{-3} gm/cm^3 of protein for stimulated secretions,[585,749] or 1 x 10^{-3} gm/cm^3 of glucose and 8 x 10^{-3} gm/cm^3 of cholesterol for unstimulated secretions.[943] Saliva is 99.4% (99.1%-99.6%) water,[585] but duct secretions vary enough in composition along the length of each duct and between glands to be useful in crude chemonavigation (Section 8.4.3). For example, the submaxillary glands secrete 2.7 (0.8-6.0) x 10^{-3} gm/cm^3 of mucopolysaccharide (mucin) derived from mucous cells within the glands, plus a small amount of the important digestive enzyme ptyalin (salivary amylase) from serous cells. By comparison, the parotid glands are purely serous glands that secrete no mucin, while the sublingual glands secrete mostly mucus.[585,863] The salivary microbial population is ~ $10^6/cm^3$.[360]

After food has been chewed, moistened, and reduced to a semi-liquid state, the tongue rolls it into a 1-10 cm^3 bolus[3312] and pushes it backward into the pharynx (Fig. 8.11). During the act of deglutition (swallowing), the uvula is pushed backward against the posterior pharyngeal wall, closing the nasal passages; the larynx elevates and the epiglottis folds back, forming a protective ledge

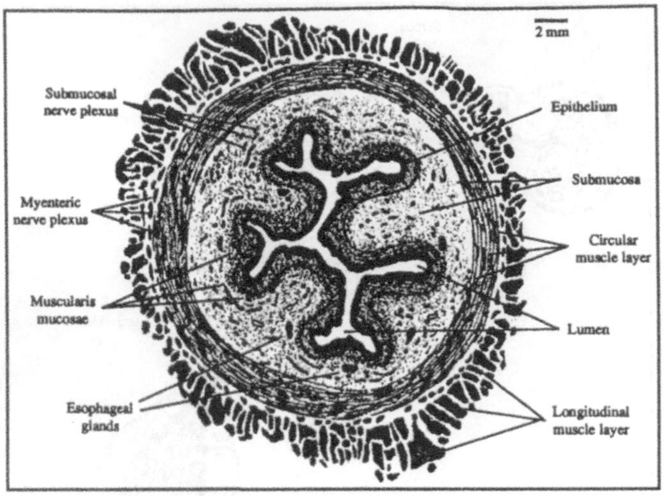

Fig. 8.18. Cross-section of the esophagus (redrawn from Guyton[863]).

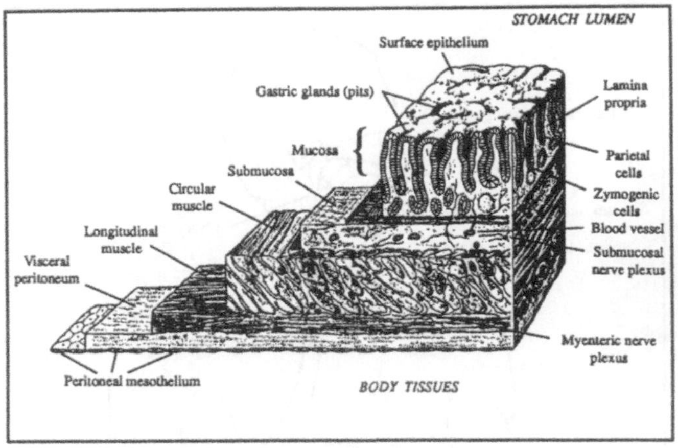

Fig. 8.19. Layers of the stomach lining (redrawn from Guyton[863]).

that covers the windpipe. The esophagus opens to receive the food, and contracting muscular waves convey the bolus to the stomach. These waves are strong enough to oppose at least several g's of negative vertical acceleration; esophageal manometry shows normal contractions of up to ~190 mmHg in the distal esophagus.[2122] With each swallow, 2-5 cm^3 of air are ingested.[2180]

Like the mouth and pharynx, the esophagus is lined with mucus-coated stratified squamous epithelium which is part of the mucous membrane. Figure 8.18 illustrates a cross-section of the esophagus, showing a number of longitudinal pleats to allow radial stretching. Note that when no food is present, the tube is almost completely squeezed shut. The tube readily distends to a width of 1-2 cm to permit the passage of a bolus of food or drink. The movement of food from the bottom of the esophagus into the stomach is controlled by the opening and closing of a muscular ring called the lower esophageal or cardiac sphincter. At the approach of the bolus, the cardiac sphincter relaxes, the opening widens, and the food is shot into the stomach. Normal sphincter pressure is 10-50 mmHg.[2122,2180]

The stomach is an irregularly pear-shaped bag located at the level of the lowermost ribs with its upper end just below the heart. It has a central portion (the body), a balloonlike portion to the left (the fundus), and a constricted portion to the lower right (the pylorus, or lower quarter of the organ). The upper part of the stomach is usually puffed out a bit with gas, even when the stomach is empty, so it protrudes slightly above the cardiac sphincter. However, when the stomach is filled with food in a man standing erect, the organ assumes an almost vertical position with a tubular shape.

When greatly stretched, the stomach of a normal male can store as much as 1000 cm^3 of food and fluid, up to 1500 cm^3 for very large people but as little as ~60 cm^3 in newborns;[863,870] however, 500 cm^3 usually gives a person a sense of fullness.[863] The inner wall of the empty stomach has longitudinal expansion pleats called rugae. As the stomach fills with food, the rugae flatten out and disappear, leaving a ~600 cm^2 smooth mucous membrane surface when the organ is full.

The uppermost epithelial layer of the stomach lining is the mucosa, several millimeters thick (Fig. 8.19). Almost all of the epithelial cells that line the surface are simple columnar mucous cells that secrete mucus. The gastric mucus is especially viscous, ~50-100 microns thick,[3165] and is highly resistant to both the digestive juices and the acid secreted by the stomach itself. Absorption through the almost impermeable stomach wall is slight, although the stomach does absorb small amounts of water, electrolytes, certain drugs such as aspirin, and alcohol.

The mucosa contains the secreting cells of the stomach, arranged in small tubular units to form the gastric glands. Within these glands, the chief or zymogenic cells are simple columnar cells forming a continuous lining for the tubule, and secrete important protein-digesting enzymes such as pepsin and rennin (chymosin), and lipid-digesting enzymes such as lipase. The parietal cells are scattered along the tubule and secrete ~0.5% hydrochloric acid solution.[749] Both the movements of the stomach and the flow of gastric juice may be stimulated by the nerve plexuses and by hormones such as gastrin and histamine.[751]

Each day ~35 million gastric glands secrete 1000-3000 cm^3 of gastric juice;[1975] a residuum of 50 cm^3 is always present in the stomach, even after lengthy fasting.[749] Secretion rates in young adults average 77 cm^3/hr (male) and 70 cm^3/hr (female) while fasting, 54 cm^3/hr (male) and 38 cm^3/hr (female) while sleeping, and 114 cm^3/hr (male) and 99 cm^3/hr (female) after eating.[585] (The gender distinction is at least partly due to differences in mean body size.) Gastric juice is 99% water with specific gravity ~1.006 (1.004-1.010) and pH ~2.0.[585,751] Glucose content of gastric juice is 0.33-1.19 x 10^{-3} gm/cm^3.[585]

If the stomach has been empty for some time, it contracts and produces uncomfortable sensations (hunger pangs). Soon after food is taken, the pangs cease and gastric peristalsis begins as a ring of constriction around the middle of the stomach. This ring progresses toward the pylorus, growing measurably deeper as it moves. These mixing waves recur at ~3/minute, each taking ~1 minute to travel from its origin to the pylorus, so there are usually 3-4 moving waves of contraction simultaneously present on the human stomach. This kneading of the food can produce a gurgling sound because of the gas that is usually trapped in the stomach.

The well-churned food mixture, now called chyme, is ejected through the pyloric valve into the duodenum of the small intestine. Nervous and hormonal signals (e.g., enterogastrone) arising mainly from the duodenum, but also partly from the stomach, control the degree of contraction of the pyloric sphincter and thereby control the rate at which the chyme is emptied from the stomach into the duodenum of the small intestine.

About 8-10 cm downstream from the pyloric sphincter, the cruising nanorobot pauses to investigate a small elevation called the duodenal papilla. The orifice at the summit of the papilla is surrounded by muscle fibers which form the sphincter of Oddi, beyond which lies the 6-mm-wide ampulla of Vater and the common bile duct, a tube ~3 mm wide and ~60 mm in length that carries various glandular secretions directly into the duodenum. About 10 mm up the ampulla of Vater the pancreatic duct (duct of Wirsung) veers to the left side of the body and runs ~15 mm to the pancreas, where it continues on for the length of the organ, another ~90 mm. In some patients, the narrower accessory pancreatic duct (duct of Santorini, draining the head of the pancreas) runs ~15 mm from the pancreas and empties into the duodenum ~25 mm upstream from the duodenal papilla. Through the ~2 mm wide pancreatic duct passes ~1000-1500 cm^3/day of pancreatic juice.[853,1975] This juice contains pancreatin, a mixture of the three digestive enzymes trypsin (which digests protein), lipase (which digests fat), and amylase (which digests starch). The specific gravity of the fluid is 1.008, mean viscosity is 1.61×10^{-3} kg/m-sec (up to 5.8×10^{-3} kg/m-sec in patients with chronic pancreatitis[3315]), the pH is 7-8, and the glucose content is $0.85\text{-}1.8 \times 10^{-4}$ gm/cm^3.[585] Juice flows on signal from the hormone secretin, manufactured by the mucous membrane of the duodenum which sends its message as soon as partially digested food enters from the stomach.

Moving ~55 mm up the common bile duct from the ampulla of Vater, the nanorobot passes through the sphincter of Boyden and next encounters the cystic duct, a ~2 mm wide tube ~35 mm in length branching to the right that leads through the spiral valve directly to the gallbladder. The branch to the left (of the body) continues as the ~25 mm long common hepatic duct, which then bifurcates to form the left and right hepatic ducts (~2 mm wide) leading directly to the liver (Section 8.2.5), each duct up to ~50 mm in length. Some patients also have a few direct connections between the liver and the cystic duct, called the ducts of Luschka.[935]

The gallbladder is a 7-10 cm long pear-shaped bag composed of muscle and membrane lodged in a hollow on the underside of the right lobe of the liver behind the lower ribs, that serves as the reservoir for bile that is secreted continuously by the liver. The cystic duct carries bile both to and from the gallbladder, depending upon whether the sphincter of Oddi is open or closed. The liver secretes 800-1000 cm^3 of bile each day,[853] but the bile duct delivers only ~500 cm^3/day of bile to the duodenum.[870] The excess is shunted to the gallbladder, which holds up to ~50 cm^3 of tenfold bile concentrate (more than 90% of the water and salts are reabsorbed from the excess flow). The gallbladder empties by contraction of the smooth muscle contained in its walls, when stimulated by the hormone cholecystokinin, which serves as the signal that bile is needed. This signal in turn is triggered by the passage of chyme over the duodenal papilla in the small intestine. Only about 10% of the bile is permanently lost in the feces; 90% is reabsorbed and returned to the liver.

Bile is a bitter yellowish fluid that helps to emulsify and digest fats to hasten their absorption from the intestines, to activate the pancreatic enzyme lipase, to stimulate intestinal movements, and to inhibit fermentation of the bowel contents. The specific gravity of bile is 0.998-1.062; absolute viscosity ranges from $0.843\text{-}2.342 \times 10^{-3}$ kg/m-sec; and pH averages 7.5 (6.2-8.5) for hepatic bile, 6.0 (5.6-8.0) for gallbladder bile.[585] Hepatic bile contains $1.7\text{-}5.2 \times 10^{-4}$ gm/cm^3 sugars and 1.2 (0.8-1.7) $\times 10^{-3}$ gm/cm^3 cholesterol, while gallbladder bile contains 8×10^{-4} gm/cm^3 sugars and 6.3 (3.5-9.3) $\times 10^{-3}$ gm/cm^3 cholesterol,[585] plus 0.3-3% lipids.[749] Thus the various biles are chemonavigationally distinguishable.

The nanorobot resumes its journey down the small intestine. The small bowel extends from the pylorus of the stomach all the way to the large intestine and occupies the greater portion of the abdominal cavity. About 90% of all digestion and absorption takes place in the small intestine, including up to 6 liters/day of the 8-10 liters/day of water that flows into it from swallowed saliva, ingested water, the acid fluid secreted by the stomach, bile and pancreatic juice, as well as fluid secreted by the upper small bowel itself. Food is passed along by muscular contractions in waves known collectively as peristalsis, with waves progressing arhythmically for distances varying from 10-100 cm in length, and occasionally over the entire length of the small intestine. Food is also broken up by rhythmic segmentation contractions within the irregular peristaltic motions, which are ringlike contractions of the circular muscle ranging in frequency from 10-30/minute, with higher rates at the upstream end of the bowel.

The small intestine is a continuous tube with three well-defined sections—the duodenum, jejunum, and ileum (Table 8.8). The total length is commonly reported as ~7 meters, but this measurement is for tissues taken from cadavers which have lost all muscle tone. In the living body, the small intestine is only 3-5 meters in length.[863] In the duodenum and jejunum the submucosa elevates into a series of permanent transverse pleats called circular folds, plicae circulares, or Kerkring's folds (Fig. 8.20). These ridges do not disappear when the wall is distended by the passage of food, and may stand up to ~10 mm high in the mucosa. Some folds wrap all the way around the intestine, while others extend only partly around. Starting a short distance past the pylorus, the circular folds are numerous and high in the distal portion of the duodenum and in the proximal portion of the jejunum, after which they gradually become less numerous and smaller; by mid-ileum, they fade out completely. Thus the number and depth of the folds may be used as crude navigational surface markers of range from the pylorus. The folds increase the local absorptive area by about threefold and further enhance absorption by causing the chyme to spiral as it passes downstream,[853] crudely analogous to a spinning bullet passing down a rifled bore. A nanorobot traversing the folded intestinal surface must travel at least ~3 times farther than another nanorobot pursuing a more linear axial course through the luminal (chymous) contents of the tube.

The duodenum is the first short part of the small intestine, arranged in a horseshoe shape enclosing the head of the pancreas. The acidic chyme is neutralized following exposure to the alkaline pancreatic juices and bile fluid. Hence the pH of the chyme

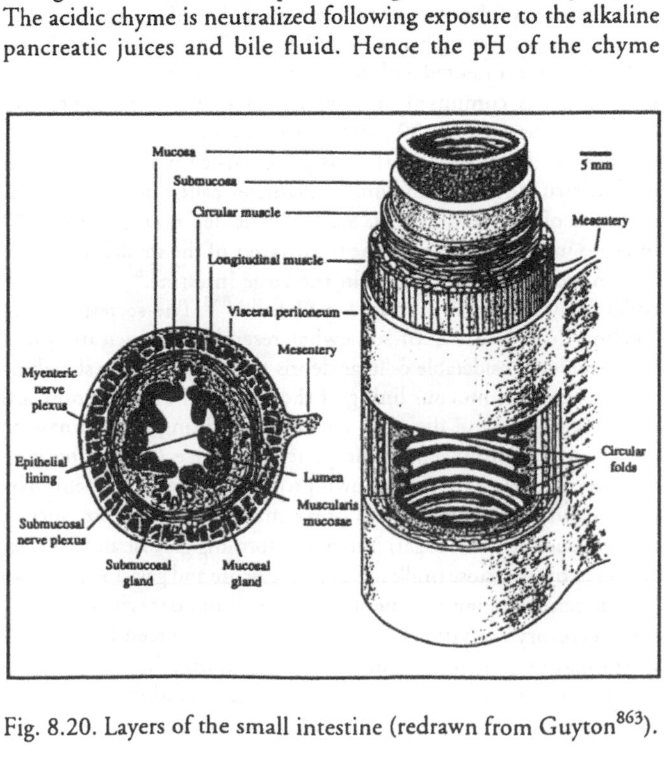

Fig. 8.20. Layers of the small intestine (redrawn from Guyton[863]).

increases along the length of the duodenum, a fact which may be useful for chemonavigation (Section 8.4.3). The duodenal glands (Brunner's glands) are found only in the duodenum. They are tortuous and branching; their mucus-containing secretion has a pH of 5.8-7.6, a specific gravity of 1.01, and a highly variable cholesterol concentration of 3.61 (0-31.5) x 10^{-4} gm/cm^3.[585] Total unstimulated secretory volume is ~30 cm^3/hr, rising to 181 cm^3/hr (male) and 126 cm^3/hr (female) with secretin stimulation.[585]

In the jejunum, fats, starches, and proteins are broken down to their smallest components (or small peptides) and are absorbed by the lining cells of the bowel. Of particular interest, absorption of sugars takes place chiefly in the upstream portion of the small intestine, specifically in the duodenum and upper jejunum. Hence the concentration of glucose in the chyme peaks and then sharply declines in the jejunum because starches of all molecular sizes are enzymatically reduced to the simplest sugars there, prior to absorption, although the disaccharides are not as readily absorbed. Cholesterol is also absorbed mainly in the jejunum.

In the ileum, water is absorbed (~0.07-0.40 cm^3/sec) along with calcium, other minerals, and vitamins (especially vitamin B_{12}). Bile is recaptured and returned to the liver via the hepatic portal vein and the lymphatic thoracic duct systems. Fat is also absorbed more rapidly in the ileum than in the duodenum or jejunum. These spatially differential absorptive properties of the small intestine produce numerous luminal chemical gradients that may be useful for both axial and radial chemonavigation by nanorobots traveling with the chyme flow.

Four additional somatographic features will be encountered by nanorobots crawling across the surface of the small intestine. First, lymphoid tissue is present in the form of nodules or follicles throughout the luminal wall. These may appear as solitary nodules that may extend into the submucosa all over the intestine, averaging 0.4-2 mm in diameter, up to 3-5 nodules/cm^2 of mucous membrane, ~2400-4500 per patient.[848] The nodules become larger and more numerous as the nanorobot travels downstream. Aggregated nodules are found chiefly in the lower ileum, penetrating the mucosa, always located on the side of the intestinal wall opposite to the line of attachment of the mesentery. These oval-shaped aggregates, called Peyer's patches, are slightly elevated areas 12-38 mm in length and 8-25 mm wide, oriented with the long axis pointing downstream.[874] Each patch is composed of 8-60 nodules in varying degrees of fusion.[874] There are 20-30 patches per patient.[874]

Second, the mucosal surface is pockmarked with ~100 million pit-like structures ~50 microns in diameter called intestinal glands or crypts of Lieberkuhn (Fig. 8.21). Their depth ranges from 100 microns in the mucosa near the headwaters of the small intestine to 700 microns far downstream in the large intestine.[872] The glands collectively secrete 2-3 liters/day of fluid.[853] The secretion is an alkaline fluid (pH ~ 7.6) somewhat resembling pancreatic juice, but includes considerable cellular debris resulting from the sloughing of cells from the mucous lining of the intestine. The secretion also contains mucus and digestive enzymes including enterokinase to activate the trypsinogen of the pancreatic juice (converting it to trypsin), peptidases to break down protein fragments left behind by pepsin and trypsin, maltase to break maltose into glucose, sucrase to break sucrose (table sugar) into halves forming glucose and fructose, lactase to break lactose (milk sugar) into glucose and galactose, and two nucleic acid digesting enzymes (ribonuclease and deoxyribonuclease). The secretory activity of the intestine is influenced by nervous, hormonal (e.g., enterocrinin), and mechanical stimuli, and again provides many navigationally-useful chemical gradients.

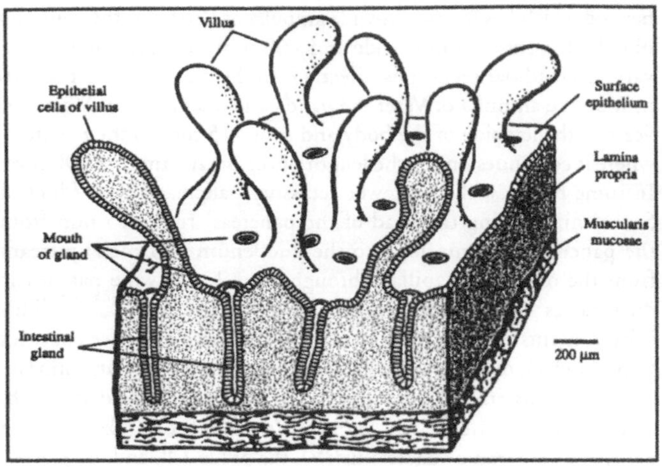

Fig. 8.21. Expanded view of the surface of the small intestine (redrawn from Mitchell and Arey[872]).

Third, there are ~5 million villi studding the entire mucosa of the small intestine (Fig. 8.21). Each villus is a fingerlike outgrowth of the mucous membrane averaging ~200 microns wide and ~1000 (range 500-1500) microns in length. (For comparison, a micron-scale nanorobot is about the size of one of the stipple dots in Figure 8.21.) Villi are taller and more numerous in the duodenum and jejunum (~20-40/mm^2) than in the ileum (~15-30/mm^2),[848] and collectively increase the effective absorptive surface of the small intestine to ~10 m^2. They are leaf-shaped in the proximal duodenum, change to tongue-shaped by the upper jejunum, and finally become slender and finger-shaped in the ileum[936]—probably all morphologically distinguishable for navigational purposes using a high-resolution navigational network (Section 8.3.3). Villi have a skin of simple columnar epithelial cells adapted for nutrient absorption and contain a capillary loop, a central lymphatic (lacteal) and connective tissue. Each villus is also provided with a small lengthwise strip of smooth muscle. During fasting, the villi lie flat on the mucosal surface and are inactive; when exposed to the intestinal contents during digestion, they become erect and perform a lashing movement driven by rhythmical shortenings and lengthenings. These movements accelerate the flow of blood and lymph, and mechanically assist absorption by stirring the liquids of the gut in the immediate neighborhood.

Fourth, the surface area covered by the absorptive mucosal cells of the villi is also increased many times, estimated to be 14- to 39-fold, by the striated or brush border which consists of minute processes or microvilli projecting vertically into the lumen (not shown in Figure 8.21). These microvilli are extremely regular in size and evenly spaced: ~1 micron long, ~0.1 micron in diameter,[848] and numbering ~1000 microvilli/cell.[938]

Our touring nanorobot now leaves the ileum and enters the headwaters of the large intestine (the colon) through the ileocecal valve (valvula Bauhini), moving into the cecum. The ileocecal sphincter normally remains mildly contracted to slow the passage of chyme into the cecum. Immediately after a meal, a gastroileal reflex forces any chyme that remains in the ileum out into the cecum, and intensifies ileal peristalsis; the stomach hormone gastrin also relaxes the valve.[853] Thus ileocecal-resident nanorobots can usually infer the taking of a meal, even though the ileocecal sphincter contracts more tightly if the cecum becomes distended. In many animals, the bulbous cecum is a storehouse where fermentation can take place. In humans, the cecum is of no particular use. At the bottom of the cecum (~20-30 mm from the ileocecal valve) a small appendage is attached, the vermiform appendix, a twisted and coiled vestigial tube that also serves no useful purpose but often becomes clogged and infected, causing acute appendicitis (see also Section 1.2.2).

There is almost no digestion in the large intestine. The task of the colon is to absorb most of the remaining fluid and electrolytes from the chyme. Each day ~2000 cm^3 of loose watery material is dehydrated and compacted in the ascending colon, and temporarily stored in the transverse colon. All but ~100 cm^3 of the 500-1500 cm^3 of the water that enters the colon daily is absorbed, mostly in the cecum and ascending colon.[853,2180]

Structurally, the colonic tube is shirred into sacculations known as haustra, ~16 mm long segments running along the tube axis. Each haustrum is defined internally by opposing semilunar folds (corresponding to the creases on the outer surface) that act as mechanical baffles to hold the feces steady against lateral accelerations. There are mixing movements comprised of haustral contractions of the recesses of the colon, somewhat resembling the segmenting contractions of the small bowel. Three or four times a day mass peristalsis occurs, long-wave contractions that begin at the middle of the transverse colon and drive the more solid contents of the transverse colon into the descending colon and sigmoidal colon. Food in the stomach triggers this reflex action. The large intestine is generally quiet between meals except for mild peristalsis at 3-12 contractions/minute.[855]

The mucous epithelium of the colon has a single layer of columnar cells, some of which have become specialized as unicellular slime glands (goblet cells); the colon coats feces with a thin layer of mucus to ensure smooth movement. (Amoeba move readily through the colonic mucus layer,[3316] which has an experimentally-measured mean thickness increasing from 107 microns in the ascending colon to 155 microns in the rectum.[3317]) The large intestine has no villi and no circular folds,[750] although absorptive cells on the colonic surface have a thin striated border (microvilli).[935] Intestinal glands are present, but they secrete mostly mucus. Lymphoid tissue is present as scattered solitary nodules but there are no aggregated nodules.

The bacterial population[2198] is also of navigational significance. From the esophagus to the ileocecal valve, the upper tract is relatively sterile with few live bacteria. That's because gastric acids whose main purpose is to break down food more rapidly also act as a disinfectant to prevent the growth of microbes. The human colon, however, contains at least 400 species of bacteria,[360,3050] with ~15 types of these accounting for the majority of the intestinal microflora. These bacteria ferment any remaining carbohydrates and produce surplus vitamins (e.g., vitamins K and B_{12}) and useful amino acids which are absorbed in the colon, so the relationship is quite symbiotic. About one-third of the material in the colon is microbial mass, and up to half of the stool consists of bacteria.

Having passed through the sigmoidal colon, the traveling nanorobot finally enters the rectum. The muscular wall of the rectum is stronger than that of the colon, and that of the anal canal is thicker still. The rectum has 3-4 crescent-shaped folds (Houston's valves) that support the weight of the fecal matter and prevent its movement toward the anus, where its presence excites a sensation demanding discharge. The anus is guarded by two sphincters, internal and external. The internal (involuntary) sphincter is smooth muscle tissue formed by a thickening of the circular fibers of the muscular coat. The external (voluntary) sphincter is striated muscle tissue formed by a separate muscle encircling the lower end of the rectum. The act of defecation is preceded by a voluntary effort consisting of relaxation of the external anal sphincter and usually compression of the abdominal contents by means of straining efforts. Peristaltic waves then appear in the colon. The entire distal colon, from the splenic flexure to the anus, may be emptied at one time. The normal frequency of bowel movements is 3-12 per week among the general population.[2180]

The 100-200 grams of feces excreted daily are 65-75% water, 5-10% fatty material, and 20%-50% bacterial bodies, with a normal pH of 7.0-7.5.[585,749,2180] Even while fasting, 7-8 grams of feces are excreted daily. (Further details are in Chapter 26.) The dark brown color of the normal stool is due chiefly to stercobilin and urobilin, the reduction products of the action of bacteria on the bile pigment bilirubin; the high-molecular-mass fraction most responsible for fecal viscosity is bacterial peptidoglycan.[3308]

Defecation is also accompanied or preceded by the escape of intestinal gases, or flatus. Normal volume is 500-1500 cm^3/day, with normal frequency 6-20 per day.[2180] Up to ~500 cm^3 of flatus is nitrogen and some oxygen from swallowed air—it takes ~10 minutes for swallowed air to descend to the colon.[873] Flatus contains other gases such as carbon dioxide, inflammable hydrogen and methane. The unpleasant fecal odor is due mainly to skatole and indole, produced by bacterial action in breaking down amino acids, but hydrogen sulfide and methyl mercaptan (more pronounced on a high-protein diet) also contribute. All of these chemical substances may be quantitatively measured in real time (Section 4.2) by medical nanorobots traversing the alimentary canal.

A simple map of the ~0.65 m^2 cylindrical luminal surface of the gut (Table 8.8) to ~(200 micron)^2 villiary resolution requires just ~16 million pixels or ~130 million bits assuming 8-bit pixels. This data store can be compactly encoded on ~0.005 micron^3 of hydrofluorocarbon memory tape (Section 7.2.1.1) and may be carried aboard a micron-scale nanorobot in a storage device only ~0.01 micron^3 or ~(0.2 micron)^3 in volume. A complete map of the ~10 m^2 absorptive surface to ~(20 micron)^2 cellular resolution (excluding the brush border) requires ~25 billion pixels or ~0.2 terabits assuming 8-bit pixels.

8.2.4 Navigational Osteography

The skeleton is the single largest organ system, representing ~14% of total mass and ~11% of the navigable volume of the human body. The bony skeleton supports and protects the vital organs—the skull protects the brain; the spinal column shields the spinal cord and maintains erect posture; the ribs shelter the heart, lungs, and liver; pelvic bones protect the kidneys and internal sexual organs.

The total number of bones varies at different ages. At birth, the human body contains ~270 bones. This number declines slightly during infancy as a few separate segments join to form single bones. From young childhood through puberty, the bone count increases as wrist and ankle bones develop. Post-adolescence, the bone count steadily declines again with the gradual union of independent bones.

The adult skeleton (Fig. 8.22) consists of 206 bones: 28 skull bones (8 cranial, 14 facial, and 6 ear ossicles); the horseshoe-shaped hyoid bone of the neck (which breaks during hanging, choking the victim to death; see Figure 8.11); 26 vertebrae (7 cervical or neck, 12 thorax, 5 lumbar or loins, the sacrum which is five fused vertebrae, and the coccyx, our vestigial tail, which is four fused vertebrae); 24 ribs plus the sternum or breastbone; the shoulder girdle (2 clavicles, the most frequently fractured bone in the body, and 2 scapulae); the pelvic girdle (2 fused bones); and 30 bones in each of the four extremities (a total of 120). The paired bones include the 12 ribs on either side, 8 wrist bones, 5 hand bones, 14 finger bones, 7 ankle bones, 5 foot bones, 14 toe bones, 3 auditory ossicles, and the parietal, temporal, palatine, lacrimal, nasal, upper jaw, cheek, lower nasal concha, collarbone, shoulder blade, hip, arm, outer and inner

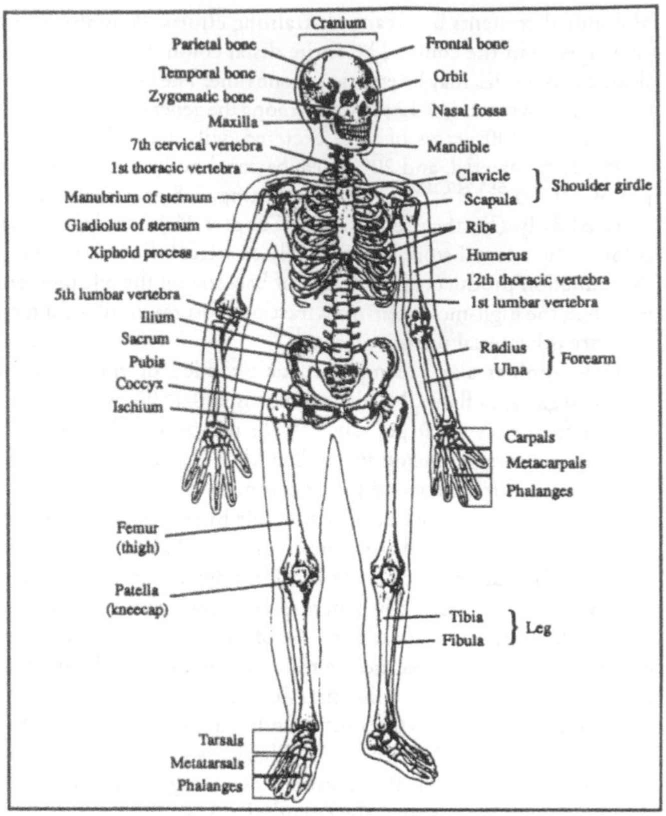

Fig. 8.22. Anterior view of the human skeleton (redrawn from Guyton[863]).

forearm, thigh, kneecap, calf, and shin bones. There are also a variable number of sesamoid bones, ranging from 8-18 in number, which are small rounded masses embedded in certain tendons and usually related to joints.

The total mass of the skeleton is ~10,000 gm; skeletal density averages ~1.45 gm/cm^3, so total volume is ~6875 cm^3 (Table 8.9). The total exterior surface area of the bones is ~1 m^2, which may be mapped to ~(20 micron)^2 cellular resolution using 2.5 billion pixels, requiring ~0.02 terabits of onboard nanorobot memory assuming 8-bit pixels.

More interesting are the interior spaces of bones in which medical nanodevices may travel. Bone is composed mainly of ~50 nm long crystals of very dense calcium salts having the hardness of marble (mostly hydroxyapatite, ~45% of bone mass) held together by bone matrix containing large numbers of extremely strong ~200 nm-wide collagenous fibers arranged in a dense mat together with a mucopolysaccharide cement sometimes called "ground substance." In living bone, ~25% of bone weight is water and another ~30% is organic material.[870]

Embedded in this mineral structure are bone cells of three types.[863] Osteoblasts, which secrete the substances that make up the bone matrix, line the outer surfaces of bone and also line many of the surfaces inside the internal cavities of the bone. Osteocytes, the most numerous bone cell type, originate from osteoblasts when those cells become trapped within small irregular matrix cavities called lacunae. After the trapped cells transform into osteocytes, they stop forming new bone but continue to support normal bone metabolism. Finally the osteoclasts (large multinucleated cells lining ~3% of internal bone cavity surfaces) remove old bone when it needs repair. Osteoclasts may be stimulated by parathyroid (endocrine) hormone to cause bone absorption when extra calcium ions are needed in the extracellular fluid. Bone is continually being resorbed and rebuilt to maintain its structural integrity.

Most of the compact bone is laid down in concentric layers, or lamellae, both on the outer surfaces of the bone and around the internal blood vessels that supply nutrition.[863] Figure 8.23 illustrates this lamellar structure of bone, showing that the lacunae (irregular spaces) containing the osteocytes lie between the successive lamellae and are interconnected from one layer to another and between lacuna by small fluid-filled canaliculi averaging ~0.3 microns (range 0.1-1.0 micron) wide.[935-936] The largest (Haversian) canal lies at the center of each system of concentric lamellae. Haversian canals are ~20 microns wide and carry blood vessels, lymph vessels, nerves, and also connect with the lacunae via the canaliculi. All osteocytes lie within ~200 microns of a blood capillary.[936] The entire Haversian system allows nutrient and calcium flow through the bone interior volume and provides convenient navigable channels which medical nanorobots may utilize to gain direct access to bone cells and matrix materials.

Compact bone (providing the principal structural bearing strength of the body) is formed on the exterior of all bones. Deeper inside, the bone becomes a more open latticework with large spaces, called spongy or cancellous bone, whose solid parts nevertheless have an internal structure similar to compact bone. In the long bones of the extremities, the epiphyses (end knobs) are composed of spongy bone covered by a thin layer of compact bone. The diaphysis (central shaft) is made up almost entirely of compact bone surrounding a cavity containing marrow. Covering the entire bone is the periosteum, a nutrient-carrying fibrous membrane investing the surfaces of bones, except at the points of attachment of tendons and ligaments (where cartilage is substituted). The periosteum has an outer fibrous layer composed of dense fibrous tissue with blood vessels and an inner osteogenic layer containing many fibroblasts.[750] Blood vessels

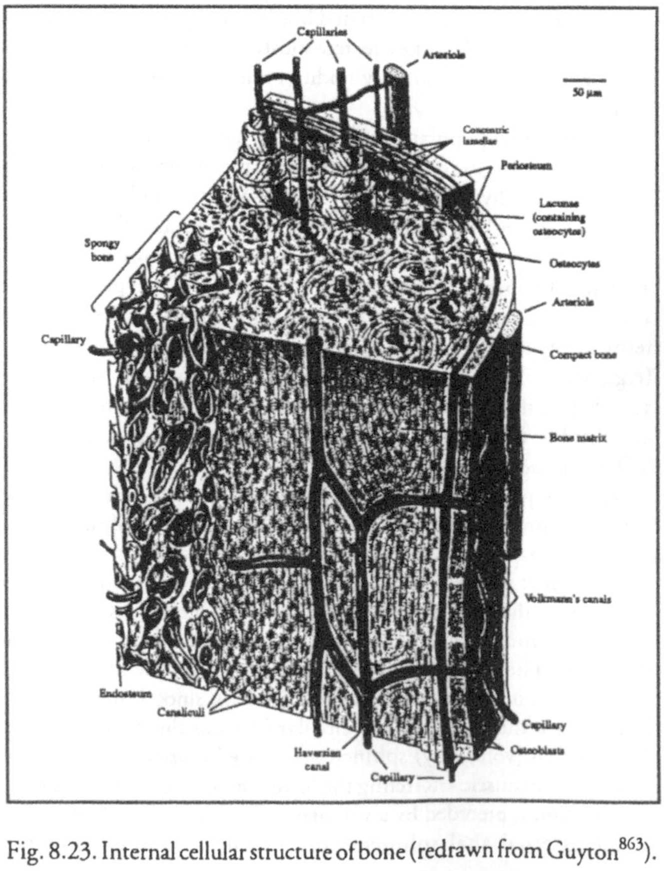

Fig. 8.23. Internal cellular structure of bone (redrawn from Guyton[863]).

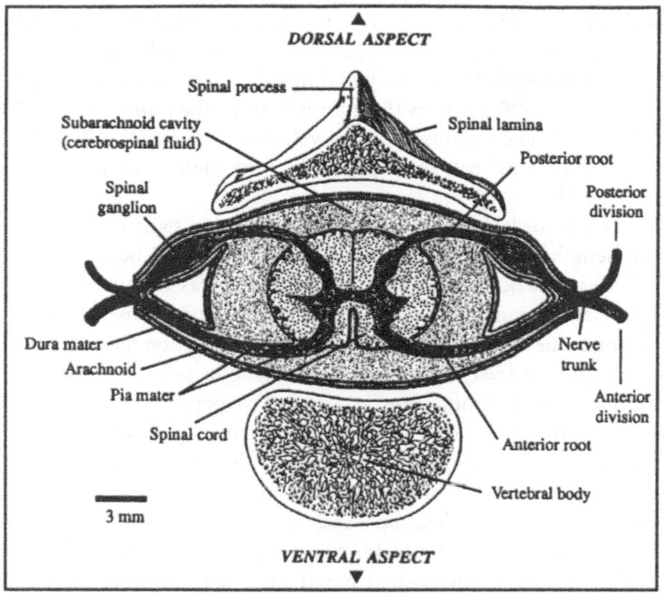

8.24. Cross-section of spinal cord (redrawn from Millard, King, and Showers[750]).

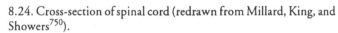

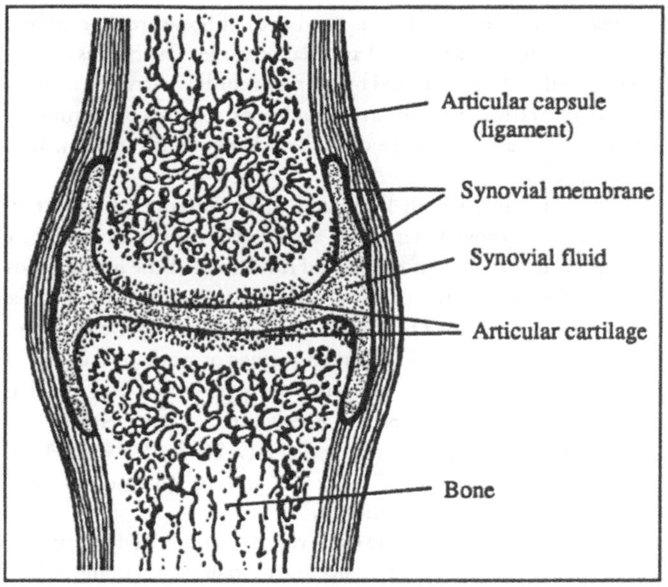

Fig. 8.25. Diagram of diarthrodial joint (redrawn from Millard, King, and Showers[750]).

traversing the periosteum enter the bone and pass through channels called Volkmann's canals to enter and leave the Haversian canals. In humans, there are few true voids in the bones.

Bone marrow fills the spaces of spongy bone and the medullary (marrow) cavity of long bones. It is composed of a supporting framework of reticular tissue in which there are blood vessels and blood cells in various stages of development. A thin membrane called the endosteum, more delicate than the periosteum but resembling it in structure, lines the medullary cavity. In the adult, there is red and yellow marrow.[750] Red cells and some white cells are formed in the red marrow; in the newborn all marrow is red, but in the adult the red marrow is found in the spongy bone such as the proximal epiphyses of long bones and in the sternum, ribs, vertebrae and diploe of the cranial bones. Yellow marrow contains many fat cells and is found in the medullary cavity of long bones, producing macrophages and granulated white cells. There is ~3 kg of marrow in the adult body,[817] occupying a volume of ~2400 cm^3.

Even the relatively low capillary density of <100/mm^2 in bone[832] implies a total investiture of ~3×10^8 skeletal capillaries and a total luminal surface area of ~8 m^2 for the entire vasculature, which would require a ~0.16 terabit vascular map at cellular resolution. A full cellular map identifying each individual osteocyte in the entire skeletal system requires ~1 terabit.

An interesting navigable volume within the skeletal system is the human spine, which averages 71 cm in length in men and 60 cm in women with remarkably little variation.[870] The body of each vertebra has a ring-shaped neural arch, through which passes the spinal cord. The spinal cord, measuring ~46 cm long and ~1 cm in diameter, descends from the brain and medulla oblongata through the foramen magnum and passes through the hollows of the spinal column, giving off 31 pairs of spinal nerves until it reaches the level of the disc between the first and second lumbar vertebrae, where the lower end tapers off to a point called the conus medullaris. The cord itself (Fig. 8.24) is composed of H-shaped gray matter in the center, extending forward as the anterior nerve roots (motor control) and backward as the posterior nerve roots (sensory), with solid white tracts of nerve fibers descending from the brain or ascending to it.

Cerebrospinal fluid (CSF) fills the ventricles of the brain and the subarachnoid cavity surrounding the spinal cord. The fluid is formed mainly by the choroid plexuses (large, reddish tufted organs) in the four ventricles of the brain. The plexuses are rich in blood vessels and separated from the cavity of the ventricles by only a single layer of secretory cells, thus affording ready access to the fluid by medical nanorobots (Chapter 16). The fluid, once formed in the brain, is later mostly reabsorbed by the arachnoid villi in the brain, but a small amount drifts slowly downstream along the spinal cord and is absorbed by the arachnoid villi through the spinal regions. Among other things, CSF is regarded as "the drainage system of the brain," crudely analogous to urine, and the entire fluid volume is replaced once every ~30,000 sec.

The human body contains 90-150 cm^3 of cerebrospinal fluid, normally maintained at an average pressure of 11 mmHg (range 5-13 mmHg[1712]). The fluid is clear and watery, normally containing 1-10 white cells/mm^3 (all mononucleocytes) and similar chemical constituents as blood plasma, but with only 0.4% as much protein as the plasma; to first approximation, it may be regarded as an almost protein-free filtrate of the blood. The specific gravity of cerebrospinal fluid is 1.007 (1.0062-1.0082); viscosity at 310 K typically ranges from $0.7\text{-}1 \times 10^{-3}$ kg/m-sec;[3325] and pH averages 7.4 (7.35-7.70), with ~1% (0.85-1.7%) total solids, 6×10^{-4} gm/cm^3 glucose, $2.4\text{-}5.0 \times 10^{-6}$ gm/cm^3 cholesterol, and no acetylcholine or fibrinogen.[585] Protein content increases from 1.0×10^{-4} gm/cm^3 in the ventricles of the brain, to 1.5×10^{-4} gm/cm^3 in the cisterna of the upper spinal column, to a high of 2.5 (2.0-4.0) $\times 10^{-4}$ gm/cm^3 in the lumbar vertebrae[585]—a potentially useful chemonavigational gradient.

Most of the ~150 bone joints in the human body are freely movable diarthroses (Fig. 8.25). There are ball and socket joints, saddle joints, ~40 hinge joints,[870] and pivot joints. In the diarthrodial joint, two or more bones are united by an encircling band of fibrous tissue called the articular or fibrous capsule. The articular capsule is lined with synovial membrane, and the apposed ends of bone are covered by a layer of hyaline cartilage, called articular cartilage. The fibrous capsule is reinforced and strengthened by ligament cords woven into it. Joint cavities sometimes extend into pouches or recesses or communicating bursae, and the shape of the sac changes with motion, as in the knee joint.

Synovial fluid, which lubricates and nourishes the joint, is exuded by the synovial membrane and fills the capsule cavity. There may be a total of ~30 cm^3 of synovial fluid in all of the human body joints. Synovial fluid is a colorless, viscid mucin-containing material resembling egg white. The human knee contains ~1.1 cm^3 (range 0.13-3.5 cm^3) of synovial fluid at an average osmotic pressure of 11 mmHg (9-13 mmHg). The specific gravity of the fluid is 1.008-1.015; absolute viscosity is highly variable but averages ~160 (4-800) x 10^{-3} kg/m-sec; pH is 7.39 (7.29-7.45); with 3.4% (1.2%-4.8%) total solids, 0.7-1.0 x 10^{-3} gm/cm^3 glucose, 8.5 x 10^{-3} gm/cm^3 mucin, and no fibrinogen.[585]

There are also ~140 bursae (synovial sacs) in the body, located in fibrous tissue wherever friction occurs, probably containing at least ~20 cm^3 of additional synovial fluid. The best-known include the subdeltoid bursa, which lies beneath the shoulder muscle; the prepatellar bursa, located in front of the kneecap; and the Achilles bursa, which lies between the heel bone and the Achilles tendon at the back of the heel.

8.2.5 Organography and Histonavigation

Measured by volumes, the typical ~0.06 m^3 adult male body contains ~38% hydrated protein, ~15% fat, ~14% expandable volumes and ~13% fluids. More importantly, ~60% of the volume of the human body is comprised of well-defined and highly specialized organs (Table 8.9) if skin and blood are included, as is commonplace.

Earlier Sections have described numerous physical routes through which all the organs can be accessed by a traveling medical nanorobot. Simple maps describing each of these routes can be made available to the nanodevice within a modest onboard data storage budget.

In addition to map-reading and precision positional navigation to ~3 micron accuracy (Section 8.3.3), with the help of a navigational network a nanorobot might verify that it had arrived at its intended organ by detecting various asymmetries that exist throughout the human body. As trivial examples, the heart lies mostly on the left side of the chest while the liver lies mostly on the right.* The larger right lung has 3 lobes with 10 secondary bronchi segments, while the left lung has only 2 lobes and 9 secondary bronchi segments. The left ventricle of the heart has a muscular wall twice as thick as the right ventricle. The right lobe of the liver is much larger than the left lobe, and has a completely different shape. The right ear statistically is slightly more sensitive than the left ear,[827] undoubtedly involving small-scale anatomical asymmetries. The left and right halves of the face have distinct physiognomies.

Aside from such gross anatomical measurements, there are many other (and more convenient) ways for a nanorobot to determine its histological location in the body. For example, in the kidney, the tissue pressure (easily measurable by nanosensors) is lower than the pressure under the tight renal capsule, and tissue pressure is lower in the brain than in the surrounding cerebrospinal fluid.[363] (See also Section 8.4.2.) The speed of sound varies markedly from tissue to tissue (Table 6.7). For instance, a grid of nanorobots equipped with acoustic radiators and ~nanosecond clocks (Section 10.1) could measure and distinguish the speed of sound in the brain (1550 m/sec), the kidney (1575 m/sec), and muscle (1600 m/sec) over a grid distance of ~100 microns (Section 8.3.3). In the human eye, at 20 MHz, the highest acoustic sound velocities are found in the sclera (1597 ± 20.3 m/sec); the lens exhibits the highest attenuation in the eye.[483]

Each tissue has a unique spectral transmission signature at optical wavelengths. For example, liver looks distinct from bowel because of differences both in absorbance and in the way the tissue scatters light (see Section 4.9.4), making feasible automated discrimination among tissue types.[738] Both scattering and absorption measurements will require at least ~100 micron path lengths (~5 cell widths) for reliable tissue discrimination, requiring a cooperative activity among several nanorobots using timed test pulses. A ~1 pW radiator power budget producing up to ~10^7 optical photons/sec omnidirectionally using a ~1 $micron^2$ emitter transmits up to ~10^3 photons/sec to a ~1 $micron^2$ receiver located ~100 microns away (Section 7.2.3), which should be adequate for tissue-type discrimination. Tissues might also be distinguished based on cell membrane electrical conductivity (Section 4.8.7).

Each organ has a unique macroscale chemical signature. For instance, the anterior lobe of the pituitary gland (the adenohypophysis) is particularly rich in endocrine hormones including somatotropin (growth hormone), thyroid-stimulating hormone (TSH), adrenocorticotropic hormone (ACTH), follicle-stimulating hormone (FSH) and luteinizing hormone (LH). By contrast, the posterior lobe of the pituitary gland (the neurohypophysis) is rich in neuropeptides such as oxytocin and vasopressin.[750] Grey matter, white matter, and myelin in human brain tissues have distinctive lipid compositions.[1014]

In some cases, the local distribution of vitamin concentrations alone might be probative. Table 8.10 gives vitamin concentrations for various tissues,[585] which may reflect chemical variations present in the intracellular fluids, the constituent cells, or both. Thiamine (B_1) occurs both free and phosphorylated,[749] with elevated concentrations in the heart, liver, and kidneys, and low amounts in the stomach and skin; larger stores of riboflavin (B_2) exist in the kidney and liver than elsewhere; niacin (B_3) is more prominent in the liver and skeletal muscle; inositol is concentrated most heavily in the brain, kidney, and spleen. Cobalamin (B_{12}) is stored primarily in liver, kidney, lungs, and spleen.[752] Vitamin A (retinol) is fat-soluble and is stored principally in ester form in the liver but also in the lungs and kidneys.[749] Water-soluble vitamin C (ascorbic acid) is present in highest concentration in tissues of high metabolic activity, most notably the adrenal and pituitary glands and in the intestinal wall.[749] Vitamin D (cholecalciferol) is most concentrated in the skin,[752] while vitamin E is stored mainly in the heart, lungs, muscles, and fatty tissues,[749] and vitamin K is absorbed through the colon and stored in the liver;[752] all three are fat-soluble. With enough chemical markers to choose from, a nanorobot equipped with suitable chemosensors can make high-probability locational inferences.

Tissues also have unique extracellular matrices (ECM) that can be sampled and identified by traveling nanorobots (Section 9.4.4.2). For example, 19 different forms of collagen have been identified in various tissues, including 5 fibrillar types, 1 network-forming type, 4 fibril-binding types, 2 short-chain types and 1 long-chain anchoring type.[971,1497,1498] Types III and VIII are found only in cardiovascular tissue, Type VII is found only in the skin, and so forth.[521]

** Normally the major lobe of the liver is on the right side of the abdomen and the spleen is on the left side, but about one in 10,000 patients is born with situs inversus—a reversal of the left-right positions of these organs.[1127]*

Glycosaminoglycans (a component of the glycocalyx and ECM, usually complexed with proteins to form mucoproteins) are also tissue specific. For instance, chondroitin sulfates are found in cartilage, bone, and cornea. Keratin sulfate I is found in the cornea, keratin sulfate II in loose connective tissue, heparin in mast cells, heparan sulfate in skin fibroblasts and the aortic wall, and hyaluronic acid in synovial fluid, vitreous humor, and loose connective tissue.[996] It appears that ECMs contain embedded structures and glycoproteins (e.g., osteonectin, tenascin) unique to each tissue type that should be recognizable to nanorobots even in the complete absence of cells. Intermediate filaments comprising the cytoskeleton inside the cell are also tissue-specific (Section 8.5.3.11).

Finally, organs may be identified by examining the surface antigens of their constituent cells. This is the most powerful technique. For

Table 8.9. Mass, Volume, and Scale Size of the Organs of the Human Body[749,817,854,881,1973]

Fluid, Tissue, Organ, or Organ System	Total Mass (gm)	Total Volume ($L^3 \sim cm^3$)	Size Scale per Organ ($L \sim cm$)
Avg. Adult Male Body	70,000	60,000	~ 40
Muscle	30,000	23,000	--
Fat	10,500	12,000	--
Integument (total:)	6,100	5,500	--
Skin	2,000	1,800	--
Subcutaneous tissue	4,100	3,700	--
Skeleton (total:)	10,000	6,875	--
Cortical bone	4,000	2,235	--
Red marrow	1,500	1,200	--
Yellow marrow	1,500	1,200	--
Cartilage	1,100	845	--
Trabecular bone	1,000	670	--
Periarticular tissue	900	725	--
Lymph	~ 2,000	~ 2,000	--
Lymphoid tissue	1,400	1,350	--
Gastrointestinal tract	2,000	1,800	--
Contents (chyme/feces)	~ 2,000	~ 2,000	--
Blood vessels	1,800	1,700	--
Contents (blood)	5,600	5,400	--
Liver	1,650	1,470	11.7
Brain	1,400	1,350	11.1
Nerve trunks	340	330	--
Cerebrospinal fluid	90-150	90-150	--
Spinal cord	38	36	--
Lungs (2)	825	775	9.8
Contents (air)	~ 7.7	~ 6,000	--
Heart	330	300	6.7
Chamber volume	--	450	--
Kidneys (2)	300	270	5.2
Spleen	155	145	6.6
Urinary bladder	150	140	~12
Contents (urine)	~ 500	~ 500	--
Digestive fluids	~ 150	~ 150	--
Pancreas	110	100	4 x 15
Salivary glands (6)	50	48	2.0
Synovial fluid	~ 50	~ 50	--
Teeth (32)	42	14	0.8
Thyroid gland	40	36	3.3
Testes (2) male	40	37	2.6
Uterus (virgin/post-preg.)	35/110	30/100	~5
Eyes (2)	30	27	2.4
Hair (avg. haircut)	21	16	--
Prostate gland	20	18	2.6
Adrenal gland (2)	20	18	2.1
Thymus gland	16	14	2.4
Ovaries (2) (female)	8	7.2	1.5
Gallbladder	7	7	3 x 8
Contents (bile)	~ 50	~ 50	--
Fingernails & toenails (20)	1.1	0.9	0.3
Pituitary gland	0.61	0.57	0.8
Pineal gland	0.2	0.18	0.5
Parathyroid glands (4)	0.15	0.14	0.3

estimated for 70 kg adult male.

Table 8.10. Vitamin Concentration in Various Human Organs[585]

Human Tissue	Thiamine (gm/cm^3)	Riboflavin (gm/cm^3)	Niacin (gm/cm^3)	Biotin (gm/cm^3)	Inositol (gm/cm^3)	Pantothenic acid (gm/cm^3)
Serum	0.01-0.09 x 10^{-6}	0.03-0.04 x 10^{-6}	0.02-0.15 x 10^{-5}	0.09-0.16 x 10^{-7}	0.03-0.07 x 10^{-4}	0.06-0.35 x 10^{-6}
Whole blood	0.03-0.10 x 10^{-6}	0.15-0.60 x 10^{-6}	0.5-0.8 x 10^{-5}	0.07-0.17 x 10^{-7}	--	0.15-0.45 x 10^{-6}
Mammary gland	0.43 x 10^{-6}	2.4 x 10^{-6}	1.0 x 10^{-5}	0.4 x 10^{-7}	2.7 x 10^{-4}	3.9 x 10^{-6}
Skin	0.52 x 10^{-6}	1.2 x 10^{-6}	0.86 x 10^{-5}	0.22 x 10^{-7}	2.0 x 10^{-4}	3.1 x 10^{-6}
Ileum	0.55 x 10^{-6}	4.2 x 10^{-6}	1.9 x 10^{-5}	0.6 x 10^{-7}	7.5 x 10^{-4}	5.3 x 10^{-6}
Stomach	0.56 x 10^{-6}	5.2 x 10^{-6}	1.9 x 10^{-5}	1.9 x 10^{-7}	7.6 x 10^{-4}	6.1 x 10^{-6}
Ovary	0.61 x 10^{-6}	4.3 x 10^{-6}	1.8 x 10^{-5}	0.25 x 10^{-7}	5.8 x 10^{-4}	3.9 x 10^{-6}
Seminal duct	0.69 x 10^{-6}	1.0 x 10^{-6}	0.92 x 10^{-5}	0.15 x 10^{-7}	<1.0 x 10^{-4}	2.0 x 10^{-6}
Testicle	0.80 x 10^{-6}	2.0 x 10^{-6}	1.6 x 10^{-5}	0.9 x 10^{-7}	16.0 x 10^{-4}	5.0 x 10^{-6}
Colon	1.0 x 10^{-6}	2.1 x 10^{-6}	1.3 x 10^{-5}	0.9 x 10^{-7}	7.8 x 10^{-4}	5.0 x 10^{-6}
Spleen	1.1 x 10^{-6}	3.6 x 10^{-6}	2.3 x 10^{-5}	0.6 x 10^{-7}	10.3 x 10^{-4}	5.4 x 10^{-6}
Skeletal muscle	1.2 x 10^{-6}	2.0 x 10^{-6}	4.7 x 10^{-5}	0.35 x 10^{-7}	4.5 x 10^{-4}	12.0 x 10^{-6}
Smooth muscle	1.2 x 10^{-6}	2.3 x 10^{-6}	3.1 x 10^{-5}	0.6 x 10^{-7}	5.8 x 10^{-4}	6.2 x 10^{-6}
Lung	1.5 x 10^{-6}	1.9 x 10^{-6}	1.8 x 10^{-5}	1.9 x 10^{-7}	4.0 x 10^{-4}	5.0 x 10^{-6}
Adrenal gland	1.6 x 10^{-6}	8.2 x 10^{-6}	2.4 x 10^{-5}	3.5 x 10^{-7}	6.9 x 10^{-4}	8.0 x 10^{-6}
Brain	1.6 x 10^{-6}	2.5 x 10^{-6}	2.0 x 10^{-5}	5.8 x 10^{-7}	15.1 x 10^{-4}	15.0 x 10^{-6}
Liver	2.2 x 10^{-6}	16.0 x 10^{-6}	5.8 x 10^{-5}	7.4 x 10^{-7}	6.6 x 10^{-4}	43.0 x 10^{-6}
Kidney	2.8 x 10^{-6}	20.0 x 10^{-6}	3.7 x 10^{-5}	6.7 x 10^{-7}	12.4 x 10^{-4}	19.0 x 10^{-6}
Heart	3.6 x 10^{-6}	8.3 x 10^{-6}	4.1 x 10^{-5}	1.7 x 10^{-7}	5.0 x 10^{-4}	16.0 x 10^{-6}

instance, T cell receptors may be organ-specific: those comprised of γ 2 subchains are found in the spleen, γ 3 in the skin, γ 4 in the female reproductive organs and the tongue, and γ 5 in the lining of the intestinal tract.[882] Protein components of the matrix, such as laminin and fibronectin, bind to specific integrin molecules on cell surfaces; through these 20+ integrins, the ECM transduces signals that regulate intracellular tissue-specific gene activity.[971] The plasma membrane class B scavenger receptor for high-density lipoproteins, known as SR-BI, is expressed primarily by liver, ovarian, and adrenal cells.[1038] Cell type identification is a major topic that is addressed at length in Section 8.5.2.2.

Must a bloodborne nanorobot exit the bloodstream and enter the tissues in order to determine its proximity to the target organ? Most endothelial cells that coat the blood vessels servicing an organ or tissue system are likely to display organ-specific antigens on their luminal surfaces (Section 8.5.2.2). In these cases, organ homing can be accomplished without exiting the blood vessels, simply by sampling the antigenic signature of the vessel luminal walls. However, in some cases it may be necessary for a nanorobot to penetrate the endothelial layer and directly examine the surfaces of the underlying tissue cells or the underlying ECM to determine proximity to the target organ.

Once a nanorobot verifies that it has arrived at the intended organ, the next major challenge is intraorgan navigation. This may be accomplished by following standardized maps which may be customized to the individual patient by prior somatographic surveys (e.g., Section 8.4.1.4) and supplemented with direct positional and chemonavigational techniques. A complete somatographic description of all the organs in the body is beyond the scope of this book, especially since relevant material is readily available in the well-known *Handbook of Physiology* series published by the American Physiological Society, and in anatomy,[853,854,863,866] histology[867,935,936] and cytology[531,938,939] textbooks generally. However, it is instructive here to convey a sense of place and scale by briefly reviewing the internal structure of the largest gland in the human body, the liver (see position in Figure 8.16).

The liver is a soft, plastic organ whose surface is pushed in by the surrounding organs. Thus the smaller left lobe bears concave impressions of the esophagus and stomach, while the larger right lobe bears concave impressions of the duodenum, the transverse colon, and the kidney.

Histologically, the liver is comprised of ~250 billion hepatic cells averaging ~18 microns in size. The human liver contains ~6 different cell types, but hepatocytes constitute ~80% of the cell population of the liver.[935] The hepatocyte has 1-3 spherical nuclei (depending

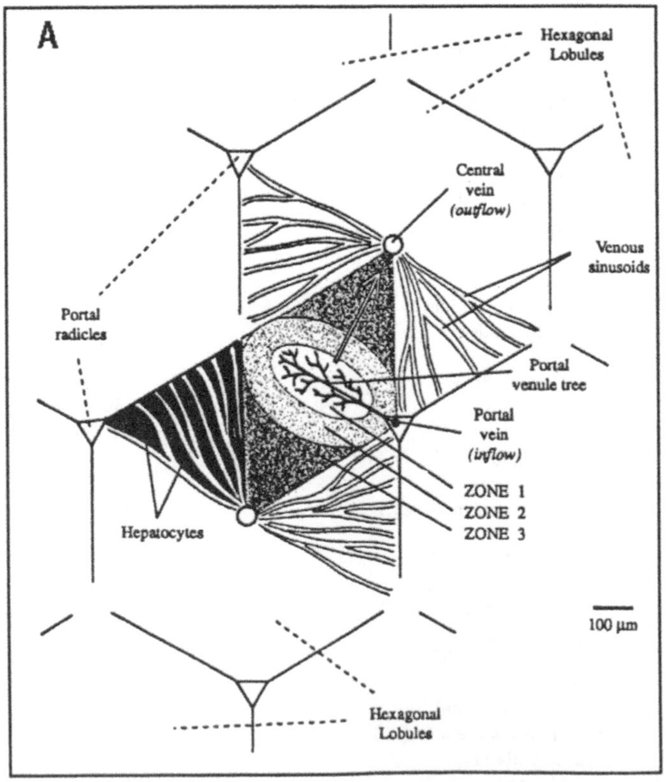

Fig. 8.26A. Geometric arrangement of hexagonal lobules in the liver (redrawn from Cormack[936]).

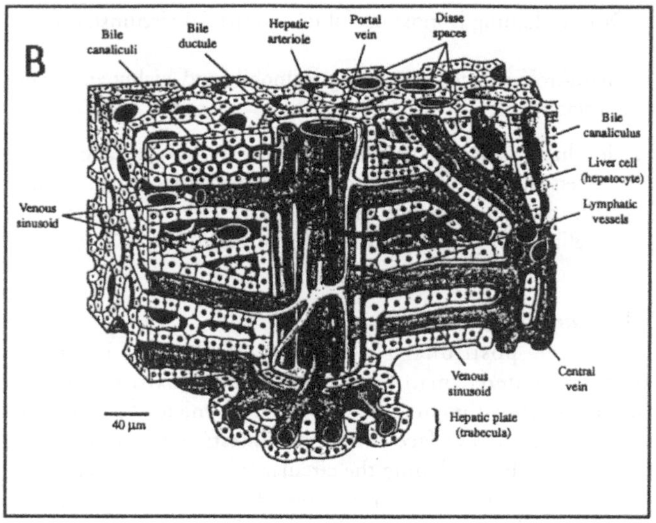

Fig. 8.26B. Plate structure of a liver lobule (redrawn from Guyton[863]).

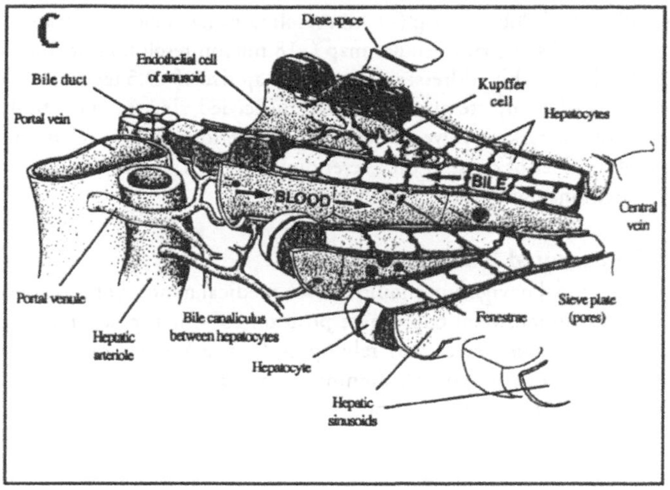

Fig. 8.26C. Schematic of flow geometry across a liver lobule (modified from Cormack[936]).

upon cell volume and position in the structure), each containing a nucleolus. These cells are bathed in flowing blood and arranged into ~1 million roughly hexagonal functional units ~1 mm wide called hepatic lobules (Fig. 8.26A). There are no interlobular septa (membranes separating the lobules) in the human liver.[936]

Around each hepatic lobule, liver cells form single-cell thick trabecular or hepatic plates (Fig. 8.26B). Portal blood from the gastrointestinal tract enters the portal vein through the hepatic plate, carrying absorbed nutrients into the portal venules. Each portal venule opens directly into large numbers of venous sinusoids (open cavities) formed by liver cells. The hepatic sinusoids form rich vascular networks with extensive but irregular anastomoses, making a three-dimensional spongework. Blood filters through the sinusoids and exits via the central vein (Fig. 8.26C), from which it flows into the hepatic venous system and from there into the inferior vena cava. Hepatic arterioles diverging from the hepatic artery supply an additional ~25% of the blood flow through the lobule, enriching the venous blood with freshly oxygenated red cells.

Bile canaliculi 1-2 microns wide[936] lie between adjacent liver cells, forming networks of polygonal meshes each surrounding an individual hepatic cell. The canaliculi empty into a bile ductule at the periphery of the lobule. The ductules, in turn, join other ductules, producing vessels of increasing diameter, leading eventually to the wide hepatic duct and the common bile duct beyond.

The lymphatic system of the liver begins in the spaces of Disse, which lie between the surfaces of the hepatic plates and the endothelial walls of the venous sinusoids (Fig. 8.27). This perisinusoidal space contains blood plasma but no red cells or platelets, and is lined with vast numbers of microvilli projecting from the sinusoidal surface of the hepatocytes bordering the space.[936] The spaces of Disse empty into small lymphatic vessels that run alongside the portal venules.

The sinusoid endothelial cells are flat and thin, with only their nuclei protruding slightly into the sinusoid lumen. Their walls are perforated with large fenestrae (~1 micron openings) numbering ~0.1/micron^2. The fenestrations are dynamic structures that undergo changes in size and number in response to hormones and cytoskeletal fiber inhibitors.[884,885] There are also numerous smaller pores measuring ~0.1 microns in diameter, mostly organized into groups of 10-15 pores called sieve plates (Fig. 8.27). Sieve plates are ~0.7 microns wide and number ~0.3 plates/micron^2.[936] These openings admit particulate material into the Disse space, for disposal by Kupffer cells.

Kupffer cells are ~15-20 micron stellate macrophagic cells, mechanically attached to the sinusoid endothelial cells. They partially occlude the sinusoid lumen but have no functional attachments to the endothelial cells or the hepatocytes. Kupffer cells are motile and have the ability to phagocytize (engulf and digest) particles of dirt, inert nanodevices (engulf and transport; Chapter 16), worn-out blood cells, and bacteria. Their customary positioning, predominantly at the periportal end of the sinusoids, confirms that they monitor arriving blood, looking for particles to remove from the flow. There are ~25 billion Kupffer cells in the liver,[884,886] with a lifepsan of many months.

With ~10^6 hepatic lobules each containing ~250,000 liver cells, a connectivity map listing every hepatocyte requires a 20-bit lobular address plus an 18-bit cellular address (within the lobule). Thus a

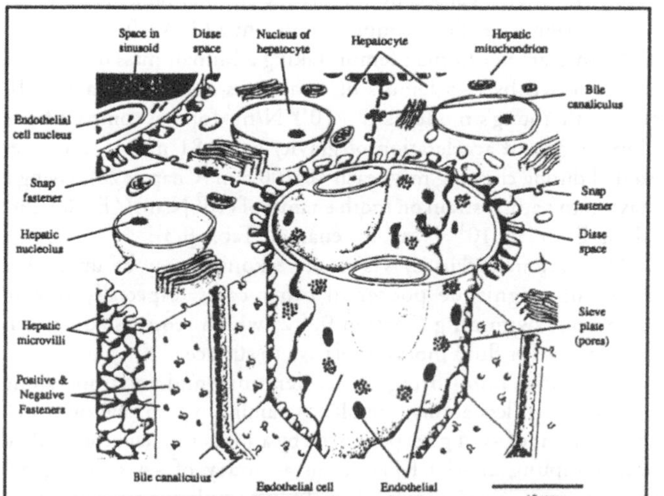

Fig. 8.27. Expanded view of hepatocyte neighborhood (Kupffer cells omitted; modified from Elias[883]).

simple hepatic lobular map (~1 mm resolution) takes just 20 megabits but a complete hepatic cellular map (~18 micron resolution) requires 250 billion 38-bit addresses, for a total map size of ~9.5 terabits. Of course, such complete maps may rarely be needed, since most medical nanorobotic tasks involve operations to be performed on a relatively small number of cells, or on a serendipitous basis, or can be guided by chemonavigation (Section 8.4.3).

8.3 Positional Navigation

Positional navigation should allow a medical nanorobot to know its three-dimensional coordinate position to ~micron accuracy at all times. A nanodevice may rely upon dead reckoning, cartotaxis, microtransponder network alignment, or triangulation on external beacon signals, as described below.

8.3.1 Dead Reckoning

Perhaps the simplest but least accurate method of positional navigation is dead reckoning—the determination of position by keeping an account of the distance and direction traveled, without reference to any exogenous sources of information other than the beginning point. For example, starting from a well-defined initial location, a legged nanorobot counts the exact number of footfalls taken in all directions; the measured length of each footfall gives the distance traveled. However, anchor points on biological membranes are positionally unstable (Section 9.4.3.1), so a micron-sized bipedal walker with a 100-nm leg stride that achieves even a very optimistic 1% footpad positional stability (~1 nm) during each leg placement cycle will find that the accumulated error in its computed position has reached one body length (~1 micron) after just 1000 strides, or ~100 microns (~100 body-lengths) of locomotion. This level of accuracy is equivalent to ~one cell-width of error per ~2 mm (~20,000 strides) of travel.

Accuracy may be at most 2 orders of magnitude better when negotiating hard or very firm surfaces such as tooth enamel or bone. The classical positional variance of a telescoping nanomanipulator capable of 100 nm of horizontal travel is at best 0.01 nm (Section 9.3.1.4); a device stiffness of ~10 nN/nm gives a limb deflection of ~0.1 nm if ~nN forces are applied, resulting in a measurement error of 0.01%-0.1% at each footfall. Additional measurement errors due to varying strains caused by fluctuating normal bone loads are of similar magnitude. For example, strain ~ m g / E A ~ 0.01% for the ~2.5-cm diameter human femur, taking a human mass of m ~ 10^2 kg supported by two femurs of total cross-sectional area A ~ 10 cm^2, with Young's modulus E ~ 10^{10} N/m^2 for wet compact bone (Table 9.3) and acceleration of gravity g = 9.81 m/sec^2. Pressures exerted during chewing may reach 10-100 atm (Chapter 28), giving a maximum natural strain on tooth enamel of (10^7 N/m^2) / E ~ 0.01%, taking E = 7.5 x 10^{10} N/m^2 for enamel (Table 9.3).

Navigational accuracy via dead reckoning may be up to 1-2 orders of magnitude poorer in other cases, especially during nanorobot swimming (Section 9.4.2) which requires additional corrections for fluid motions relative to surfaces.

Sequential monitoring of accelerations and rotations alone produces even less accurate results. Assuming typical environmental accelerations of ~0.4 g's experienced by a 1-micron nanorobot, then data sampling at ~10 KHz to an accuracy of ~4 x 10^{-5} g per measurement (Section 4.3.3.2) yields a cumulative error of ~0.4 g after ~10^4 measurements, a mere 1 second of travel. Pendular orientation sensors accurate to ~2 milliradian (Section 4.3.4.2) produce ~1 radian of accumulated error after a non-recalibrated chain of just 500 measurements.

Dead reckoning is most useful in two special circumstances:

1. hard-frozen tissues presenting immobile and highly anchorable surfaces; and
2. localized navigation requiring only very short distances to be traversed, such as locomotion between organelles in cyto or where abundant functional or positional cues allow frequent recalibration of the estimated current location.

8.3.2 Cartotaxis

Another positional navigation technique is simple landmark-centered map-following, or cartotaxis. Consider a nanorobot that wishes to crawl to a specific 1 $micron^2$ patch on the subvilliary mucosal surface of the small intestine. Ignoring the villi and microvilli but including the circular folds, the mucosal surface of the small intestine is ~1 m^2 (Section 8.2.3), at worst requiring a map of ~8 terabits to achieve 1 $micron^2$ resolution using 8-bit pixels.

A more compact map might include only the positions, sizes and shapes each of the ~100 million 50-micron-wide intestinal glands dotting the surface of the small intestine at least ~100 microns apart. These dots form a pattern unique to each person that changes slowly over time. After defining a two-dimensional intestinocentric coordinate system, two coordinates of $\log_2 (10^6)$ ~ 20 bits each can specify a location to 1-micron accuracy on a 1 m^2 surface. Using 20 bits each for the two surface coordinates, 20 bits each for the major and minor elliptical axes framing the gland aperture, and another 920 bits to record unique topographic features of each hole, a complete small intestinal gland map requires at most ~1000 bits/gland or ~0.1 terabits.

This data storage requirement may be significantly further reduced by recognizing that on its way to its destination, an efficient ~10 $micron^3$ surface-walking nanorobot need pass over at most 0.002% of the 1 m^2 of small intestinal surface recorded on the map described in the previous paragraph, even assuming a maximum-length 4-meter whole-intestine traverse, passing at most a total of 4 m / 100 microns = 40,000 identified glands each requiring ~1000 bits to describe. Hence the minimum intestinoglandular map required for this longest traverse could in theory contain as few as ~40 megabits of data for a perfectly navigating nanorobot using a perfectly compiled and absolutely stable map. As a practical matter, to ensure reliability the onboard map conservatively should contain complete intermediate annular ring segment recalibration maplets at least ~500 microns in length along the tube axis and spaced ~2 cm apart, to be sequentially encountered axially while traveling down the tube. Nanorobots use dead reckoning to navigate between these guide rings until the ring closest to the destination is reached, analogous to the mid-course correction areas employed by cruise missiles. Having arrived at this nearest ring, the nanorobot follows a final map swath ~500 microns wide leading directly to the three glands lying closest to the destination patch; the final 1 $micron^2$ target patch is reached by interpolation and dead reckoning between these last three glands. Reliability and efficiency are enhanced by using large numbers of intercommunicating nanorobots simultaneously (Sections 7.3.2 and 8.3.3). This ~1 gigabit "practical map" contains complete descriptions of ~1 million individual intestinal glands and may be stored in a ~0.1 $micron^3$ onboard data spool using hydrofluorocarbon memory tape (Section 7.2.1.1).

The above scenario describes the ideal case. In actual living systems, biological surfaces are constantly in motion, are coated with slime, and are frequently being remodeled. Some mucosal surfaces may replace their entire luminal cell population every ~10^5 sec (~1 day).* Thus the precise shapes and features of individual intestinal glands are constantly changing, although their larger structures and the pore pattern may remain intact for considerably longer periods of time. Intestinal glands are easily located by moving in the direction of rising concentration of enzyme-loaded intestinal juice, a basic chemonavigational technique (Section 8.4.3), and villiary trunks are available to provide additional cartographic guidance. But cartotaxic nanorobots will achieve the best results by using only the most recently prepared maps.

8.3.3 Microtransponder Networks

The archetypal high-resolution (~3-micron) internal navigational network may be described as a set of ~10^{11} mobile acoustic transponder nanodevices, or navicytes, uniformly deployed throughout a ~0.1 m^3 human body volume with an average 100-micron spacing. (Power consumption rises sharply for much larger spacings.) Total navicyte fleet volume is a relatively unobtrusive ~1 cm^3. Navicytes emitting omnidirectional ~100 MHz acoustic signal packets using r = 1 micron radiators are ~50% energy efficient (Section 7.2.2). Navigational signal packets are ~1 microsec in duration (conveying ~100 bits/packet) and repeat at ~1 millisec intervals (~1 KHz), giving a duty cycle of f_{duty} ~ 0.1% which leaves plenty of clear air time for positional information inquiries from non-navigational nanorobots, communications and sensor traffic, local acoustic microscopy and the like, and also to allow staggered time slots to avoid noise and crosstalk.

How is a 100 MHz packet signal detected in a 1 nanosec signal processing time? At SNR = 2 (Section 4.5.1), a navicyte acoustic sensor must receive at least kT e^{SNR} ~ 30 zJ within a 1 nanosec integration, an energy influx rate of ~30 pW at the receiver. To produce 30 pW at a 1-micron receiver located 100 microns away, a transmitter of equal area must radiate ~300,000 pW of acoustic output (see Section 4.9.1.5) or ~10^5 watts/m^2 for ~1 nanosec. Thus, each navigational signal packet is prefaced by a triangular pulse ~1 nanosec in duration. This triangle pulse is used for ranging. Because the transmitter is ~50% efficient, each triangle pulse requires ~600,000 zJ of input energy to the transmitter in order to produce an acoustic output energy of 300,000 zJ/pulse at the transmitter surface. Broadcasting ~1000 pulses/sec brings the required transmitter input power to ~600 million zJ/sec or ~0.6 pW continuous. Transmitting the non-pulse portions of all packets costs ~60 pW (Section 7.2.2.2). Note that the 1 nanosec triangular ranging pulse has the highest frequency that can be used without significant absorption. Given a pulse which deposits a small fixed multiple of kT at the receiver, then using the highest frequency produces the least uncertainty in distance. Very roughly, a pulse which is just barely detectable can have its timing localized to ~1 pulse width.

The triangle pulses make ~9 atm acoustic spikes in water, probably low enough to avoid transient cavitation at this frequency and too brief for shock wave formation or stable cavitation (Section 6.4.1)—though it might be a good precaution to vary the time intervals between packets to preclude any possibility of unexpected resonances. Acoustic torque and related effects (Section 6.4.1) cannot yet be ruled out in this application and should be investigated further. Each triangular pulse represents an energy discharge event requiring a momentary power density of ~10^{12} watts/m^3 inside a ~(0.8 micron)^3 powerplant, comparable to power densities available in mechanical (Section 6.3.2), chemical (Section 6.3.4.5), and electrical (Section 6.3.5) systems. At ~100 pW/navicyte, total navicyte network system power consumption is ~10 watts, well within proposed in vivo thermogenic limits (Section 6.5.2).

How is the navigational network established? For convenience, a navigational Prime Centrum is established on the ventral surface of the 10th thoracic vertebra (T-10) at the midsagittal plane of the vertebral body (see Figures 8.22 and 8.24), defining a permanent origin for a body-centered coordinate system. This origin is centrally located, lying directly posterior to the xiphoid process (Fig. 8.22) and the liver, directly inferior to the heart and between the two lungs. The site is easily accessible by bloodborne nanorobots, well-supplied with oxygen and glucose for power, securely anchorable due to the dense bone, and reasonably well-protected from injury; also, movements in the thoracic vertebrae are the most restricted because the ribs and costal cartilages resist distortion.

The Prime Centrum is comprised of four "monument" type bloodborne navicytes which are injected, or migrate stochastically using cytoidentification (Section 8.5.2), or are directed to the site by demarcation or other means. These nanorobots congregate around the chosen navigational origin approximately at the vertices of a square. Each monument navicyte attaches one end of a retractable fullerene cable rule to each of its three brethren and crawls backward on an approximately radial course, paying out the slippery cable and adjusting mutual positions until the two diagonals measure exactly 141.42 microns center-to-center and the four normals measure exactly 100.00 microns center-to-center, guaranteeing a perfect 100-micron square with exact 90.00° corners. The four navicytes then secure themselves to the bone beneath the periosteum using biocompatible permanent anchors, becoming fully sessile, and retract the cable rules. If vertebral curvature radius R ~ 2 cm and diagonal navicyte separation S = 141.42 microns, then maximum anteroposterior geometric deviation due to off-sagittal positioning is R(1-sin((π/2)-(S/R))) = 0.5 micron. The square may not be precisely aligned with the conventional anatomical coordinate axes. At least 10 independent navicyte monument quartets should be established as alternate or backup sites on T-10 to satisfy customary redundancy requirements (Chapter 13). Additionally, ~10^4 regional monuments are established at ~cm intervals at fixed positions on all major skeletal surfaces of the body. Relative positions of regional monuments vary only within well-defined envelopes depending upon macroscopic joint rotations and limb flexures, or almost not at all on inflexible surfaces such as the diaphysis of the long bones.

Mobile navicytes deployed throughout the remaining body volume receive message packets emitted by neighboring devices, which in turn have received packets from their neighbors, ultimately stretching back in an unbroken chain to a regional monument or to the Prime Centrum. Assuming a simple cubical array, each stationary navicyte has two neighbors per directional axis—a total of six neighbors within acoustic communication range (100 microns). Navicyte positional stability is enhanced by stationkeeping activities to avoid drift (~1 micron/sec for a 1-micron nanorobot due to Brownian motion; Section 3.2.1), and anchorage to nonsignalling elements of the omnipresent extracellular matrix.

Each navicyte possesses an onboard clock capable of continuous Δτ ~ 1 nanosec temporal accuracy between recalibrations or over mission times of ≳10^3 sec (Section 10.1). Message packets received

* *In the fundus, the cell turnover cycle is ~5 days, while in the body of the stomach the whole cycle takes ~1 day. The time required for complete renewal of intestinal epithelium is ~2.3 days for the duodenum and ~2.8 days for the ileum.[359] At the other extreme is the lens of the eye—one of the few structures containing cells that is preserved without turnover.[531]*

periodically from each neighbor include data describing the exact universal time of packet transmission. Since each recipient has a synchronized clock (Section 10.1.3), the triangle pulse travel time between navicytes (τ ~ 65 nanosec) is known to an accuracy of ~1 nanosec. The speed of sound v_{sound} ~ 1540 in soft tissue (Table 6.7), so the ~1 nanosec temporal uncertainty adds ($v_{sound}\,\Delta\tau$) ~ 1.5 microns of uncertainty to the range estimate.

The speed of sound varies between 1400-1600 m/sec for most nonosseous tissues. This speed is reasonably uniform within specific tissues (Table 6.7) over time, and is essentially frequency-independent over the nanomedically-relevant range. Knowledge of its own approximate histological location (based on chemical sampling, etc.) allows a navicyte to consult an onboard data table or a previously-compiled low-resolution map (see Chapter 19) to estimate local sound velocity to within ~25 m/sec. Also, two navicytes (at least one of which is mobile) can directly measure the local speed of sound by briefly conjugating (Section 9.4.4.4), extending a cable rule of known length between them, then transmitting and timing a test pulse traveling through the medium. A 100-micron rule length allows local sound velocity to be measured to an average Δv_{sound} ~ 25 m/sec accuracy using a 1-nanosec clock. A measurement uncertainty of ~25 m/sec in the local speed of sound adds another ($\Delta v_{sound}\,\tau$) ~ 1.6 micron of positional uncertainty, giving a total of ΔX_{min} ~ 3 microns uncertainty in each range estimate. Additional small uncertainties in sound velocity and in acoustic reflection and refraction power losses may occur when capillaries or other microvessels cross the line of sight between two navicytes.

Only four of the six neighbors are absolutely required for positional triangulation. The data packet received by a navicyte from its first neighbor (containing that neighbor's correct three-dimensional coordinates) narrows the navicyte's possible position to a spherical surface of radius equal to the computed range, centered on the first neighbor. The data packet received from the second neighbor defines a second geometric sphere, further narrowing the navicyte's possible position to a circle formed by the intersection of the first and second spheres. The data packet from the third neighbor adds a third sphere, reducing the possibilities to two points on the intersection circle, and the signal packet from the fourth neighbor selects one of these two points as the navicyte's true position. Additional minor corrections may be made for the bending of sound waves crossing known thermal, pressure, or salinity gradients (Section 6.4.1).

What positional accuracy can this system achieve? Consider the simplest case with many parallel coplanar rows of N navicytes lying ~X_{row_i} apart, each row of total length L_{row} ~ ΣX_{row_i} emanating from a common tangential surface and extending deep into the tissues. The terminal navicyte of each row estimates its cumulative length as L_{row} which also contains an unknown range error ε_{row}. The series of randomly distributed errors in the positions of each navicyte in the row, individually of magnitude $\pm\Delta X_{min}$, do not cancel to zero but instead constitute a random walk with maximum error excursion from the mean of ε_{row} ~ $2\,N^{1/2}\,\Delta X_{min}$. The longest rows will occur in the viscera, farthest from any bony surface. Taking L_{row} = 15 cm, ΔX_{min} = 3 microns and X_{row} = 100 microns, then N = L_{row}/X_{row} = 1500 navicytes per row and ε_{row} ~230 microns. Hence in this simple case, the minimum accuracy at the terminus of each row is 15 cm ± 230 microns, or ~0.2%. Shorter rows accumulate less error at the terminus—the cumulative error at ~2 mm from the common surface is at worst ~27 microns (~1 cell width). The average error per navicyte in a 15-cm row is only ε_{row} / N ~ 0.2 microns. Even for L_{row} = 2 meters (~longest possible transverse path length in the human body), N = 20,000 and ε_{row} = 800 microns. Note that an additional small systematic error in position may accrue if there is a systematic change in local sound velocity between recalibrations and if the subject viscera have a free surface unbounded by bone. For example, bruised tissue in which foreign fluids are accumulating will produce a slightly warped coordinate system; sound velocity differentials between, say, blood and interstitial fluid may be as large as 70 m/sec (Table 6.7).

Accuracy within each row may be significantly improved by introducing active error checking and continuous recalibration. Consider the terminal navicytes of two parallel rows A and B. As before, the rows lie ~X_{row} apart in their common plane. Each terminal navicyte computes that its total length is precisely L_{row}, but in fact navicyte B is in error by a distance ε_B along the row. Given the minimum range error ΔX_{min}, terminal navicyte B can only detect that an error exists when its range measurement to neighboring terminal navicyte A increases from X_{row} to $X_{row} + \Delta X_{min}$, whereupon from simple geometry:

$$\varepsilon_B = \left[(X_{row} + \Delta X_{min})^2 - X_{row}^2\right]^{1/2} \qquad \text{\{Eqn. 8.2\}}$$

For X_{row} = 100 microns and ΔX_{min} = 3 microns, then ε_B ~25 microns or ~1 cell width. This range error is relatively insensitive to X_{row}; for instance, if X_{row} increases to 110 microns then ε_B only rises to ~26 microns.

However, row terminus errors (measured in integral units of ε_B) are likely to be normally distributed between $\pm\varepsilon_{row}$ ~ 230 microns in the earlier simplest-case example. The error correction procedure involves nearest neighbors collectively polling the nearest n_{row} ~ 6000 rows (a bundle with termini covering ~0.6 cm^2 when X_{row} = 100 microns) for their measured ε_B's and then computing the mean of the distribution, which has an uncertainty of ε_{row} / $n_{row}^{1/2}$ ~ 3 microns = ΔX_{min}, matching the uncertainty of a single range measurement, the smallest possible error. The estimated mean is used to produce a correction factor which is applied to the erroneous estimated value of L_{row}, yielding a corrected L_{row} accurate to ~ ΔX_{min} or ~3 microns. This corrective process is repeated:

a. for each row,

b. for planar cross-sections at ~2 mm increments along the entire row length (to eliminate error compression or rarefaction waves), not just along the terminal plane, and

c. at regular time intervals (~3 sec) to ensure continuous recalibration to ~3 microns at all points in each row.

Note that parts of the human body frequently may deform up to ~30% during normal activities, so X_{row} is not constant but may vary between 85-115 microns in as little as 0.1-1 sec in working situations.

Detailed specification of a complete recalibration protocol [1624] is beyond the scope of this book. One procedure to further improve row-length measurement accuracy is to use the navicyte grid as a phonon gain medium by configuring each navicyte as a repeater station during the calibration cycle, effectively allowing the propagation of row-long pulses thus permitting independent row-length measurements. Multiple measurements can reduce independent row-length measurement error to arbitrarily low levels. Alternatively, J. Soreff suggests treating the entire calibration bundle as a coherent amplifier using lower acoustic frequencies to increase range. This enables phase detection to within ~1 nanosec if phase-locked detection is used and if a few kT of energy are present in the time resolution window, allowing navicytes to hear a propagating plane wave averaged across an entire bundle. An analysis of soliton-like systemic effects analogous to intrinsic local modes in lattices [3036] is beyond the scope of this text.

The ability to make the corrections described above assumes that navicytes can distinguish $-\varepsilon_B$ from $+\varepsilon_B$, an angular spread of $\pm$ 14° for ε_B ~ 25 microns and X = 100 microns. Since sound crosses the width of a micron-sized nanorobot in ~1 nanosec, the relative angular location of a distant acoustic source can be directly measured by placing two sensors on either side of the nanodevice at precisely calibrated separations. For angles of acoustic wave incidence $\lesssim\theta$, measured from the axis joining the two sensors which are separated by a width x_{sensor} on either side of the nanorobot, the wave arrival times will differ by more than $\Delta\tau$ ~ 1 nanosec and thus will be received as two distinct pulses, rather than one. For incidence angles $>\theta$, the wave arrival times at either side cannot be distinguished. θ thus defines a permissive angular detection cone of size

$$\theta = \frac{\pi}{2} - \sin^{-1}\left(\frac{\Delta\tau\, v_{sound}}{x_{sensor}}\right) \qquad \{\text{Eqn. 8.3}\}$$

For $\Delta\tau$ = 1 nanosec and v_{sound} = 1540 m/sec, a sensor separation of x_{sensor} = 1.59 microns allows up to θ = 0.25 radian = 14° to be distinguished. The uncertainty in v_{sound} of ~25 m/sec imposes a minimum measurement uncertainty of $\Delta\theta$ ~ 3°. The permissive detection cone shrinks to θ = 0° at x_{sensor} = 1.54 microns.

Relative navicyte angle can also be computed from the coordinates of neighbors by simple geometry. Using the coordinates of a nearest neighbor with range $X_{range} = X_{row}$ ~ 100 microns and lateral positional uncertainty $X_{error} = \Delta X_{min}$ ~ 3 microns, then relative navicyte angle can only be computed to an accuracy of $\Delta\theta \sim \sin^{-1}(X_{error} / X_{range})$ ~ 1.7° (~30 milliradians). However, relative angle uncertainty is reduced if the coordinates of more distant neighbors are available to the navicyte. For example, using a neighbor located 15 rows away ($X_{range} = 15\, X_{row}$) and again taking the minimum X_{error}, then $\Delta\theta$ ~ 0.1° (~2 milliradians). Coordinates from a distant-neighbor navicyte with $X_{range} = L_{row}$ ~ 15 cm with an uncorrected lateral positional uncertainty $X_{error} = \varepsilon_{row}$ ~ 230 microns would give $\Delta\theta$ ~ 0.09° (~2 milliradians); taking $X_{error} = \Delta X_{min}$ = 3 microns in the ideal case, $\Delta\theta$ ~ 0.001° of arc (~0.02 milliradian). By comparison, from Eqn. 3.2 Brownian tumbling of a micron-scale nanorobot amounts to ~$10^{-6°}$ (~0.02 microradian) in ~1 nanosec, or ~1° (~20 milliradians) between ~1 millisec signal packet repeat intervals.

Each navicyte obtains its own orientation relative to gravity using onboard gravity sensors, which are accurate to within ~2 milliradians of verticality, with new measurements available every ~0.1 millisec (Section 4.9.2.2) or up to the limits of the communication network capacity (e.g., recalibration protocols). Regional monuments monitor and disseminate the local grid's angular orientation relative to the gravity field at ~1 millisec intervals, thus fixing each navicyte's orientation to the local grid on a virtually continuous basis. Absolute spatial orientation relative to a fixed onboard standard such as a nanogyroscope (Section 4.3.4.1) may be determined to 1-100 microradian accuracy during nonrecalibrated deployment lifetimes of 10^3-10^7 sec. Direct gyrostabilization may be possible in some applications (Section 9.4.2.2).

8.3.4 Vascular Bifurcation Detection

The ~5 billion navicytes circulating in the 5400 cm^3 blood volume can be used to form a dynamic transluminal geometric "virtual lattice" (with constantly changing membership) that remains positionally stationary near the bifurcation of each blood vessel whose diameter exceeds X_{row} ~ 100 microns. A spatial progression of such rows allows the bifurcation break point to be registered at most ~100 microns past the junction and in at most ~20 millisec after leaving the larger-diameter vessel, for nanorobots drifting with the blood flow in arterioles. In the high velocity aorta (Table 8.2), minimum bifurcation detection range increases to ~630 microns in a detection time of ~1 millisec. Transmission of local navicyte coordinates allows traveling nanorobots to determine which branch of the bifurcation they are about to enter, or have already entered. (Major organs, lymphatic topology, and other important landmarks can be accurately located by similar methods.)

Bifurcations involving capillaries and other vessels with diameters less than X_{row} may be readily detected by direct acoustic reflection echolocation from vessel walls (Section 4.8.2). Echoes from red blood cells are relatively weak (though still measurable)[3044] in comparison with those from the solid tissues within the body because the characteristic impedance of red blood cells is very similar to that of the plasma in which the cells are suspended.[570]

8.3.5 Macrotransponder Networks

It has been proposed [888] that a macroscopic acoustic signal source could be used by individual medical nanorobots to determine their location within the body, much as handheld radio receivers can use satellite transmissions (e.g., the 24-satellite Global Positioning System or GPS)[1310] to determine their position on Earth's surface. Such a system might involve externally generated signals from beacons placed at fixed positions outside the skin, or could employ dedicated internally-installed emitter organs. As described in the microtransponder example (Section 8.3.3), at least four beacon signals must be detectable simultaneously to allow a fix to be determined in three-dimensional space. Macrotransponder networks may be useful in some applications, but also have several important drawbacks as described below.

Since in a macrotransponder system the nanorobots determine their positions by direct detection of beacon range signals rather than by polling their neighbors, accuracy may be solely a function of the total range measurement uncertainty ΔX_{min}. As before (Section 8.3.3), given a typical signal path length X_{path} ~ 15 cm and a mean v_{sound} ~ 1540 m/sec, signal travel time (τ ~ 97,400 nanosec) is known to an accuracy of $\Delta\tau$ ~ 1 nanosec if beacon clocks and nanorobot clocks are stable and synchronized, adding ($v_{sound}\, \Delta\tau$) ~ 1.5 microns of range uncertainty.

However, by far the greatest source of uncertainty in a macrotransponder system is the variation in the speed of sound along the randomly chosen linear paths through the human body which the beacon signals must follow. The speed of sound is reasonably uniform within specific tissues or local regions, but an arbitrary 15-cm path through the body may plausibly involve sound velocities ranging from 630 m/sec for a path entirely through the lungs up to ~4090 m/sec for a path entirely through the densest skull bone (Table 6.7). This implies a velocity uncertainty range of Δv_{sound} ~ 3460 m/sec and thus a maximum range uncertainty of $\Delta v_{sound}\, \tau$ ~ 33.7 cm—approximately the anteroposterior thickness of the human body. There is also some variation in v_{sound} as a function of temperature (Section 10.5.5) and other factors.

While local (~100 micron range) sound speed may be measured on site by one or a small number of nanorobots (Section 8.3.3), the net sound speed along an arbitrary ~15 cm path cannot be similarly assessed without a comprehensive survey effort. Pathwise uncertainty in sound velocity is somewhat reduced by completing a whole-body survey of v_{sound} as a function of position, then loading this map into each nanorobot using the navigational system.* In some cases, standardized maps with modest customization will suffice. A whole-body v_{sound} map to ~(100 micron)^3 resolution, giving Δv_{sound} ~ 25 m/sec,

** This suggests some interesting open problems requiring further computer science research. For instance, how might individual nanorobots know which section of the map is relevant for them, before they are able to determine their position?*

would require ~1 terabit of onboard storage, a minimum 38 micron^3 memory tape volume inside a (~4 micron)^3 memory mechanism. Assuming a more reasonable ~1 micron^3 tape volume allows a ~0.026 terabit velocity map to be stored onboard, providing ~(340 micron)^3 resolution and giving Δv_{sound} ~ 84 m/sec. Unfortunately, a measurement uncertainty of ~84 m/sec in the local speed of sound still adds (Δv_{sound} τ) ~ 8 mm of positional uncertainty to each ~15 cm range measurement, a ~5% error. Shortening the average beacon-nanorobot distance to X_{path} ~ 1 cm (e.g., by installing ~60,000 internal emitter organs, which may be unduly intrusive) reduces positional uncertainty to ~500 microns, possibly sufficient in some applications.

Adequately stable surfaces on the skin or even inside the body may be difficult to find for large macroscopic transmitters, causing significant source movement and degrading the positional accuracy of the beacons as system monuments. This problem is partially overcome by using acceleration compensators (e.g., gimbals and gyros to "float" transmitters), thus neutralizing the effects of minor body motions. However, because of the minimum ~8 mm range uncertainty noted above, it will be difficult for beacons to mutually recalibrate their own positions to high accuracy, so there will be unavoidable unmonitorable monument movements especially during rapid joint rotations and limb flexures. And macroscopic transmitters are physically more responsive to the small random centrifugal and gravitational forces normally experienced by the body than are microtransmitters, adding to their moment-by-moment positional uncertainty.

By now, the alert reader will be wondering if measurements of just the angular positions of at least three externally located macroscopic acoustic beacons, taken without regard to range measurements, can suffice for accurate navigation. The answer is that an angles-only system is quite possible, but unfortunately offers little improvement. (GPS uses 4 satellites so that inexpensive handheld receivers don't need accurate clocks and thus can avoid ranging errors. Orbiting satellites do have atomic clocks and transit time codes, but the ground-based receiver need only compare time differences between received signals.)

Consider an acoustic sensor pair with x_{sensor} = 1.54 micron, giving the minimum possible angular measurement error $\Delta\theta$ ~ 3° (Section 8.3.3). The positional uncertainty Δx of the nanorobot is then

$$\Delta x \sim \frac{X_{path}\,\sin(\Delta\theta)}{\sin\left(\frac{\pi}{2} - \Delta\theta\right)\left(\frac{1}{3}N_{beacon}\right)^{1/2}} \qquad \text{\{Eqn. 8.4\}}$$

where X_{path} is the average distance between beacon and nanorobot and N_{beacon} is the number of noncollinear beacons sampled during each measurement cycle. Assuming an epidermal beacon network with X_{path} = 15 cm, Δx ~ 8 mm for N = 3 beacons; Δx ~ 400 microns for N = 1000 beacons.

Beacon signals will also travel many adjacent pathways with sound speeds that differ only very slightly, producing a multiplicity of received pulses and a smearing effect, further degrading signal quality. Signals suffer refraction over such lengthy courses, causing the beam to bend significantly from its original path in unknown amounts. By contrast, the acoustic energy received from a pulse traversing a ~100 micron path lies close to the sensor detection limit; these signals are rapidly attenuated by the medium beyond this limit, and thus produce no confusing detectable signal at the next navicyte station located ~200 microns from the transmitter. Another problem with macrobeacons is that they must use lower frequencies (~100 KHz; Section 6.4.1) due to the long path lengths their signals must traverse unamplified, hence maximum data flow rate may be up to ~1000 times slower than for the microtransponder system. Finally, macrobeacons permit only a one-way flow of navigational information, a major limitation.

8.3.6 Dedicated Navigational Organs

By direct analogy to communication organs (Section 7.3.4), dedicated macroscopic organs may be implanted in the human body to facilitate navigation. One important function of such organs would be to act as central clearinghouses for systemic information that is normally available only regionally or to individual navicytes. This information might include updated positions of all regional monuments, orientations of various grid sectors relative to gravity, or information on macroscopic rotation rates (e.g., compasses, gyros) to allow centrifugal and gravitational forces to be distinguished. Highly accurate chronometers could also be maintained in these organs (Section 10.1.4) to allow periodic systemwide resynchronization.

Dedicated navigation organs could serve as the "map rooms" of the body, collating and organizing new information as it comes in, maintaining accurate navicyte grid maps, organ maps, vascular maps, functional maps (Section 8.4), and so forth, possibly in coordination with dedicated computational organs (Section 10.2.5). A 1 mm^3 navigational library node can contain up to ~10 million terabits of map data, which may be downloaded to nanorobots berthed at docking ports at rates of up to 0.01 terabit/sec drawing ~50 pW per docking port during the transfer (Section 7.2.6).

Dedicated navigation organs may be employed as direct interfaces between internal navigational systems and related macroscopic external modalities including operating theaters, clinical equipment, various environmental entities, satellite uplinks, radio antennae, transportation vehicles, and the like. They could also serve as emitter organs in GPS-like acoustic navigational systems (Section 8.3.5).

8.4 Functional Navigation

Functional navigation allows a medical nanorobot to detect and respond to subtle variations in tissue characteristics, often in the absence of precise positional knowledge. Such tissue characteristics may include thermal, acoustic or barostatic, cytochemical or immunochemical, electrical (Section 4.9.3.3) or magnetic,[1256] mechanical or topological variations. A few of the many possibilities are described below.

8.4.1 Thermographic Navigation

8.4.1.1 Thermography of the Human Body

The human body presents a complex and temporally varying spatial temperature field. The external parts of the body have a lower mean temperature than the internal parts, with temperature decreasing along the longitudinal axis of the extremities, producing both axial and radial temperature gradients. The differing heat production of individual organs, geometric irregularities, changes in insulation and evaporation, convective heat transport via the blood, and the diurnal and other periodic variations[3327] add further complexities to the thermal map.[890]

The homeothermic core of the body is distinguishable from the shell, which most readily responds to environmental fluctuations. The core generally consists of the interior of the thorax and abdomen, the brain, and part of the skeletal muscles. With moderate changes in ambient temperature, the shell normally comprises the outermost 20%-35% of the human body.[894,895] However, during extreme chilling, the shell may enlarge to ~50% of total body volume, equivalent to a mean layer thickness of 2.5 cm.[890] Figure 8.28 shows the overall distribution of tissue temperatures as a series of isotherms.

Skin temperatures display the greatest thermographic variability in response to external factors. For example, nude humans standing for 3 hours in a cold room (5°C, 50% relative humidity, 0.1-0.2 m/sec wind speed) experience skin temperature differentials up to 15°C (= 13°C to 28°C), with the lowest temperatures in fingers and toes, the highest in trunk and forehead, and average core/surface gradient ~15°C;[896] heat loss is ~10% lower for females due to their thicker layer of subcutaneous fat, making their cold-room skin temperature slightly lower than for males.[898] After 3 hours in a hot room (50°C), skin temperature differentials amounted to only 2.5°C (= 35°C to 37.5°C), with an average core/surface gradient of ~1°C.[896] With normal clothing in a room at 15-20°C, mean skin temperature is 32-35°C.

Skin thermography of the human head was first reported by Edwards and Burton;[897] skin vs. rectal temperatures at various ambient temperatures are well-studied.[893,898] Skin temperature patterns in neonates reflect near uniform heat conduction through the tissues.[917] In childhood, specific patterns develop into a stable, permanent adult pattern.[916] The dermothermal patterns differ in lean and obese patients, and exhibit a continual state of small rhythmic change. These changes —probably a result of active vasodilation due to sympathetic innervation over most of the human skin area[919]—are observed over the arms, hands, trunk and head, but are not all in phase with each other, nor even of the same amplitude.[918,919,3334-3338] Skin thermology, including infrared thermography, is now an important branch of medical diagnostic imaging.[899,912] Subcutaneous (shell) temperatures generally increase with depth.

Human core (rectal) temperature averages 37.0°C,[894] but this simple number hides considerable natural variation (Table 8.11). The temperatures of inner organs vary by 0.2-1.2°C under normal room conditions, and by up to 0.9°C within individual organs.[890] Temperature gradients within the brain amount to 1.4°C; the cortex is cooler than the basal regions, with incoming blood cooler than the central brain tissue.[900] Brain temperature also decreases during sleep

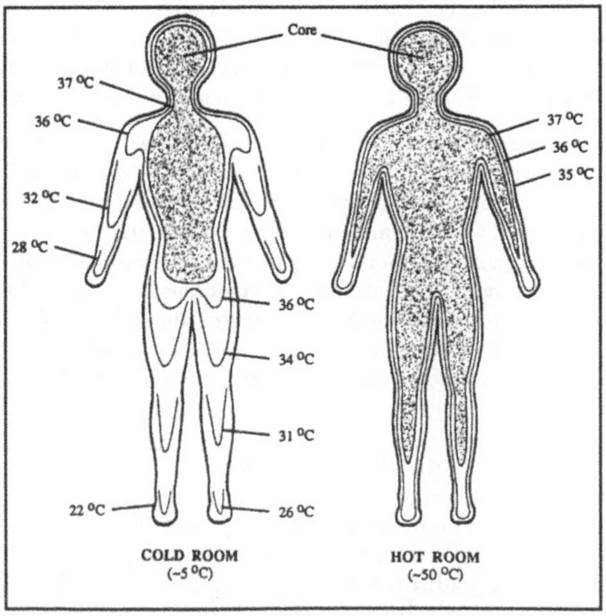

Fig. 8.28. Distribution of isotherms in a human body placed in cold or hot environment (modified from Wenger and Hardy,[865] and from Aschoff and Wever[891]).

Table 8.11. Core Temperatures of Organs and Blood Vessels in the Human Body[890,894,904,907]

Blood Vessel, Organ or Tissue	Normal Temperature
Skin	32-35°C
Scrotum	34.0°C
Sternum	34.5°C
Subclavian vein	36.4°C
Liver	36.4-36.8°C
Oral cavity	36.5-36.6°C
Transverse facial artery	36.5-36.8°C
Superior vena cava	36.65°C
Urine	36.75°C
Esophagus	36.75°C
Aorta	36.75°C
Inferior vena cava	36.75°C
Pulmonary artery	36.75°C
Lungs	36.75°C
Pulmonary vein	36.75°C
Heart, right ventricle	36.75°C
Femoral artery	36.75°C
Common carotid	36.8°C
Kidney	36.85°C
Spinal cord	36.95°C
External jugular vein	37.0°C
Hepatic vein	37.0°C
Stomach	37.0°C
Rectum, mean	**37.0°C**
Rectum, range	36.2-37.8°C
Hypothalamus	37.3°C
Brain	37.3°C
Uterus	37.3°C

and rises during periods of emotional arousal.[901] Cooling or warming the skin of the head causes temperature changes in the tympanic membrane (Fig. 7.3) of up to 0.4°C due to the returning venous blood.[909] Oral temperature can have wide variation, depending for example on the thermal character of recently ingested food and drink, and thus has little direct correlation with swings in rectal temperature.[910] Liver temperatures lie 0.2-0.6°C subrectal,[902] possibly due to heat loss via the respiratory tract through the diaphragm. The temperature of the testes in the scrotum is ~3°C lower than that of the abdominal cavity.[890] The temperature of the hypothalamus, the seat of human thermoregulation, might be the most logical choice as a reference value.[890]

Human blood temperature also displays considerable variation. Outflowing blood is warmer than inflowing blood in organs with high metabolic rates, so the blood has a cooling effect in these organs, the opposite of the skin. Venous blood temperature in the extremities may be ~3°C lower than the arterial supply, but even the arterial blood can sink to 22°C in human extremities at cold room temperatures .[903] Blood in the common carotid artery remains within 0.2°C of oral temperature, but falls 0.2-0.5°C as it cools the face and possibly also due to cooling from the internal jugular vein.[905] However, inhalation of cold air has little effect on pulmonary blood temperature; even for patients in rooms cooled to -18°C, blood in the pulmonary vein and artery differ at most by 0.03°C.[906]

There are also periodic variations in body temperature. The diurnal fluctuation is the best known. This cycle is absent in neonates, but develops during the first weeks of life.[913] Children have higher daytime temperatures than adults and a daily range of 1.7°C,[890] with the daily range peaking near the age of 1 year.[894] Precisely standardized tests on young adults found that rectal core temperature fluctuated between 36.83-38.32°C in males (range 1.49°C) and 37.16-38.36°C (range 1.20°C) in females,[908] with temperatures normally reaching their lows near 6 AM local time and their highs near 6 PM.[915] (The timing is keyed to environmental influences such as light/dark cycles, not personal activity.) The menstrual cycle also involves a complex long period fluctuation. During this monthly cycle, morning core temperature falls from 37.0°C to 36.7°C just before and during menstruation, after which there is an abrupt dip to ~36°C at midperiod near ovulation, followed by a return to normal levels for the remaining ~2 weeks. Menstrual-related skin temperature pattern variations are also observed.[3329]

Finally, there are various irregular influences on body temperature. Rectal temperature may rise up to 3.5°C during the most extreme exercise,[821] or may fall 2°C after ~1 hour immersion in water at 23°C. Ingesting food elevates skin temperature, and to a lesser extent the rectal temperature, for 1-2 hours. Alcohol ingestion raises skin temperature but lowers core temperature, while nicotine ingestion (e.g., smoking) lowers skin temperature in the extremities by 2-7°C. In persons with fever, the temperature may rise from 37.0°C up to 41.5°C,[916] with daily fluctuations of 2.8-5.0°C, usually peaking in late afternoon. Transient elevations to 44-45°C have been recorded but are very rare.

In view of this measurable spatial and temporal variability, maintaining a high-resolution whole-body thermal map in real-time is impractical using in vivo nanodevices. Given the availability of ~microkelvin sensors with ~microsecond measurement cycles (Section 4.6.1), sensor technology is not the limiting factor. Map stability is the main concern. A volumetric map with only ~1 mm^3 resolution, comparable to the best thermographic images, requires 10^8 voxels and 17 bits/voxel for 0.001°C accuracy. A hand placed on a stove produces thermal gradients >10°C/sec in the shell, but periodic temporal variations are 0.1-40 microkelvins/sec in the core and 0.005-1°C/sec in the shell during changes in physical exercise levels (~3°C in 10-100 sec), movement between hot and cold environments (~10°C in 10-100 sec), and fevers (~5°C in ~1000 sec). Thus to maintain a map that reports all changes of $\gtrsim$1 millikelvin requires the entire field to be resampled every 0.001°C / (1°C/sec) = 1 millisec, generating ~2 terabits/sec. This dataflow possibly could be accommodated by a dedicated high-capacity fiber network (Section 7.3.1) but would rapidly overwhelm both a mobile acoustic network and the data storage capacity of individual bloodborne nanorobots. Maintaining a hematothermographic map employing capillary-volume resolution to millikelvin accuracy generates an even more intractible $>10^{15}$ bits/sec.

8.4.1.2 Thermal Demarcation

Thermographic navigation to a target site is possible without the use of any maps. Simple thermal demarcation is a good example of this. In a controlled room-temperature clinical setting, the relatively narrow homeostatically-maintained temperature band of 36-38°C allows easy demarcation of selected target regions by applying thermal stimuli lying just outside the normal band. Examples might include hot (T > 38°C) or cold (T < 36°C) packs applied to the skin; diathermic tissue heating using different frequencies to achieve selective heating at various tissue depths (Section 6.4.2); adaptive phased array (APA) heating of small target volumes deep inside the body;[1518] thermally active catheter probe tips inserted transdermally or otherwise, directed to specified internal targets; or multiple intersecting focused infrared, visible photon, or ultrasound beams directed to specific convergence volumes for maximum heating effect. Depending upon the technique employed and the target tissue, volumes as small as ~1 mm^3 may be demarcated in this manner. Nanorobots of relatively simple design may be injected near the target or allowed to circulate in the bloodstream, and will detect the outlier temperature data and gather in the vicinity of the target at a statistically determined accumulation rate and number density.

Outside of controlled environments or during prolonged treatment periods, simple demarcation becomes less reliable for several reasons:

1. Error in the physical placement of the instrument of demarcation will produce erroneous nanorobot localization, which may increase the likelihood of treatment error. Such iatrogenic mistakes are especially likely during time-critical or emergency crises, or in situations where the diagnosis is unclear, or in cases of self-administered medical care.

2. Even when initially correctly placed, the artificial hot or cold region will diffuse outward from the original spot, enlarging the radius of action in imprecisely known directions (due to nonisotropic tissue conductance), again increasing the risk of iatrogenic effects.

3. Load error in the human thermoregulatory control system is ~0.2-0.5°C.[865] Any thermal deviation of this magnitude or larger from local temperatures will provoke a natural counteractive response to restore the local temperature, including capillary sphincter action (both vasodilator and vasoconstrictor activity), increased sweat gland secretions, accelerated counter-current exchanges, more rapid heart rate, or local thermogenesis.

4. Increased susceptibility to spoofing, as when a patient enters a hot shower or bath[3331], lies down on snow or on a cold concrete surface, washes his hands and face with hot water, drinks a hot or cold beverage, basks in the sun, and so forth. Temperatures hot or cold enough to definitively prevent spoofing might damage tissues if maintained for very long. This problem can be avoided by employing an oscillating artificial thermal gradient instead of a time-invariant source (especially across layers of highly insulating subcutaneous fat), but at the cost of increased required overall nanorobot sophistication to detect the oscillating demarcation. For energy delivered to a target L ~ 1 mm from the source in a medium of heat capacity C_V and thermal conductivity K_t, the maximum frequency that may be resolved is $\nu_{thermal} \sim K_t / C_V L^2 \sim 0.15$ Hz for aqueous tissue at 37°C.

General positional information is also available to nanorobots equipped with thermal sensors in the absence of any maps. For instance, assuming the temperature of the external environment has been measured and disseminated via the communication network (Section 7.3), a nanorobot traveling within a microvolume of blood can crudely infer its distance from the epidermis based on the local blood temperature, especially when passing through the thermal shell of the body surrounding the core. Other cues including velocity measurements or histonavigational data may allow further refinement of the estimate.

8.4.1.3 Low-Resolution Thermographics

Even simple thermographic maps may have great utility. If the deviation from mean temperature to 3 significant figures (~0.01°C accuracy requiring ~10 bits/measurement) is resampled at ~10 Hz, then 0.1°C/sec gradients may be detected in each of ~10^5 voxels (volume ~1 cm^3/voxel) using ~10^5 resident thermographicytes, producing a 10^7 bit/sec dataflow. A dermal thermographic network divided into 1 cm^2 squares requires ~20,000 resident nanorobots and produces a ~2 x 10^6 bit/sec whole-network dataflow at

0.01°C accuracy (vs. 0.5-1.0°C accuracy for traditional thermograms).[899] In either case, each thermographicyte in the network (Section 7.3) maintains in its ~10^{10}-bit memory (Section 7.2.6) the entire continuously updated network map and can store ~1 hour of historical data (~7 x 10^9 bits) for the whole-body thermographic map or ~1 year of historical data (~3 x 10^9 bits) taken at its own position.

Measured skin temperature can be used for macrosensing (Section 4.9). As a simple example, knowledge of average skin temperature allows estimation of the environmental wind chill (air temperature and velocity) and relative wind direction using the theoretical equation given by Lampietro[890] or the experimental data compiled by Mitchell et al[893] over the range of 10-50°C and wind velocities of 1-5 m/sec, although the presence of clothing may be a complicating factor.

Thermal patterns appearing on centimeter-resolution volume or surface maps may be useful either for macrosensing or for the determination of various medically relevant states. Some examples of measurable patterns include:

1. bimodal thermal variations on the soles of the feet, while the patient is standing on a cold concrete floor or a hot asphalt pavement;
2. cooling of the back and seat after settling into a chair whose surface is initially at room temperature (chair material may be inferred from the subsequent temperature warm-up profile);[3330]
3. warm pattern of a hand placed on the chest while patient hears the national anthem at a sports event;
4. cool vertical lines caused by tears running down cheeks;
5. asymmetric temperature profile caused by lying on one side or the other, in bed or at the beach;
6. warmth or coolness on palm and thumb of one hand while carrying a hot or cold plate of food, or grasping a cold can of beer;
7. cool knee spots while kneeling on a cold floor;
8. comparison of facial and scalp temperatures permitting inference of hair length and coiffure;
9. patterns of muscle warmth indicating physical activity involving specific tendons, limbs or appendages;
10. approximate arrangement and density of clothing;[3332]
11. increased warmth of the sexual organs, during excitation or tumescence, or of the skin, stomach, and liver, following a meal;
12. dangerous thermal gradients (e.g., hand placed on stove) detected in 0.1 sec, faster than the usual ~0.2 sec human response time; and
13. specific thermographic dermal patterns that signal the presence of a wide variety of medical conditions such as ischemic limbs, Raynaud's Syndrome, cerebral apoplexy, reflex sympathetic dystrophy, muscular injuries, abnormal joints, ankylosing spondylitis (Pott's disease), spinal root syndrome, osteoarthritis, tennis elbow, osteoid osteomas, headaches, breast cancers, or melanomas.[899]

Assuming exogenous positional information is available to fixed thermographicytes, a population of these devices can constitute a permanent monitoring network that can issue alerts and detect:

1. temperature profiles of internal or external lesions located anywhere in the body;
2. thermal anomalies reflecting the presence of interior hematomas, lipomas, myomas, edemas and hydromas, new fibrous deposits or air pockets, or dental caries;
3. slowly growing tumors (e.g., by searching for localized, shallow, but monotonic thermal gradients in the ~microkelvin/sec range in the historical data);
4. unusual skin patterns due to defects in nervous control of the peripheral circulation;
5. intestinal surface patterns reflecting identifiable thermal characteristics of materials passing through the bowels, or alterations in cell metabolism resulting from food toxins or inflammatory reactions; or
6. alterations in the thermal behavior of individual organs at specific times of day, under varying workloads, or over long timespans, possibly indicating a change in functionality or general health (measurable by taking advantage of the different thermal characteristics of body tissues; Table 8.12).

Mobile nanorobots passing near any thermographicyte can interrogate the device's thermographic data library and thus may examine all or part of the current whole-body coarse thermal map. Similarly, historical and current data can be transmitted to medical personnel who interrogate the network.

8.4.1.4 High-Resolution Thermographics

High-resolution maps can be assembled in designated tissue monitoring volumes, using a network of fixed thermographicytes whose physical positions are accurately known (Section 8.3.3). If L_{therm} = 100 microns is the mean spacing between devices, then for a maximum transorgan temperature differential ΔT ~ 1°C for an organ with scale size d_{organ} ~ 10 cm (Table 8.9) the largest endogenously generated temperature differential between neighboring thermographicytes is $\Delta T\ L_{therm}\ /\ d_{organ}$ ~ 10,000 microkelvins; the smallest detectable thermal variation of ~1 microkelvin (Section 4.6.1) corresponds to a fluctuation of ~60 watts/m^3 in power density within the 0.001 mm^3 monitoring volume (the equivalent power output of ~100 mitochondria). Recording a single temperature measurement to microkelvin accuracy requires at most ~24 bits.

Many useful configurations of such a network are readily conceived. As a simple example, consider a monitoring unit consisting of 100 thermographicytes reporting at ~1 KHz to one centrally located data processing nodule. The thermographicytes transmit a total of 2.4 megabits/sec to the nodule from within their 0.1 mm^3 patrol volume. A nodule with ~8 $micron^3$ of storage tape can retain up to ~1 day's worth of historical data generated within its monitoring unit. Nodule nanocomputers can scan the data for a wide range of specified anomalies and thresholds, emitting an appropriate alert message (containing all relevant details) when one is found. In principle, an expanding (warm) tumor could be detected* after

---

** Tumors which are metabolically less active are harder to detect by this means. Also, measuring heat from tumors located in organs having high metabolic activity (e.g., liver, kidney) is even more difficult, especially given the large caloric variations after consuming food or drink, or during normal hormonal responses, and given the relatively high normal rate of cell division in some organs (e.g., liver, gut) that must be distinguished from abnormal tumor growth.*

Table 8.12. Thermophysical Characteristics of Various Body Tissues, Organs, and Other Materials[460,567,817-819,1865,2153]

Material, Organ or Tissue	Thermal Conductivity K_t (watts/m-K)	Heat Capacity C_V (MJ/m^3-K)	Approx. Density (kg/m^3)
Skin			
Very warm	2.80	3.77	1000
Normal hand	0.960	3.77	1000
Cool	0.545	3.77	1000
Upper 2 mm	0.376	3.77	1000
Cold hand	0.335	3.77	1000
Subcutaneous fat			
High values	0.450	--	901
Pure fat	0.190	1.96	850
Muscle			
Living muscle	0.642	3.94	1050
Excised, fresh	0.545	3.64	1050
Skeletal muscle, living	0.372	--	1070
Bone			
Mineral	--	--	2982
Cortical	2.28	2.70	1790
Average	1.16	2.39	1500
Cancellous	0.582	2.07	1250
Blood			
Water at 310 K	0.623	4.19	993.4
Plasma (Hct = 0%) at 310K	0.599	4.05	1025
Whole blood (Hct = 40%)	0.549	3.82	1050
Organs			
Heart (excised, near fresh)	0.586	3.94	1060
Liver (excised, near fresh)	0.565	3.78	1050
Kidney (excised, near fresh)	0.544	4.08	1050
Abdomen core	0.544	3.89	1050
Brain (excised, near fresh)	0.528	3.86	1050
Brain (living)	0.805	--	--
Lung (excised, bovine)	0.282	2.24	603
Whole body (average)	--	4.12	1156
Air	0.009246	0.00119	1.18
Cotton fabric at 310 K	0.0796	0.0267	160
C_{60}/C_{70} bulk compacts/crystals	0.1-0.4	2.3-2.5	1540-1676
Rubber	0.156	2.41	1200
Ethanol at 310 K	0.163	1.96	789
Teflon	0.399	2.20	2180
Concrete	0.934	1.93	2310
Glass, plate	1.09	1.94	2520
Ice at 249 K (-42°C)	2.21	1.76	913
Sapphire (normal to c axis) at 310 K	2-20	2.89	3970
Stainless steel	13.8	3.68	7910
Aluminum	204	2.45	2710
Silver	405	2.59	10,500
Diamond, natural	2000	1.82	3510

growing to a volume of at most L_{therm}^3, a maximum pathological cell count of ~100. Each monitoring unit consumes at most ~20,000 pW, including 100 pW/thermographicyte and 10,000 pW in the nodule for a ~1 micron^3 computational facility drawing ~1000 watts/m^3-Hz (Section 6.5.6 (E)) and operating internally at a ~10 MHz clock speed. For continuous surveillance of an entire organ to microkelvin accuracy, up to ~16 million monitoring units are required, dissipating at most ~0.3 watts, which must also be taken into account. (The liver, for example, generates ~10 watts metabolically.)

Patients may also receive thermographicytes installed in a mobile configuration, with the nanodevices constantly traversing the tissues looking for anomalies, outmessaging only when such anomalies are detected, and accurately fixing their location to within ~3 microns at all times by interrogating a separate microtransponder positional navigation network (Section 8.3.3). At the extreme limits of accuracy, nanorobot waste heat may contribute significant error to thermal measurements. A nanorobot generating waste heat P_{heat} = 100 pW produces a ΔT = 10 microkelvin temperature differential over an $X = P_{heat} / K_t \Delta T$ = 16-micron aqueous path; this nanorobot heat is dissipated by thermal conduction to below measurable levels in ~$C_V X^2 / K_t$ ~ 2 milliseconds, approximating the ~1 KHz sampling time.

8.4.2 Barographic Navigation

The internal pressure field of the human body (already briefly summarized in Sections 4.9.1, 6.3.3, and 8.2) is as complex as the temperature field. (Section 9.4.1 discusses the rheology of the circulation.)[361] In general, fluid pressures range from 60-150 mmHg in the heart, arteries and arterioles; ~30 mmHg in the capillaries and 5-20 mmHg in the veins; 4-30 mmHg in the pulmonary artery; 9-13 mmHg in the cerebrospinal and synovial fluids; ~1.4 mmHg in the interstitial fluid between cells; and ~0.9 mmHg mean pressure in the lymphatics, with arterial pulsations contributing 1.5-2.2 mmHg oscillations with a maximum of ~5 mmHg in the lymphatics. (Systolic pressure may reach a maximum of ~230 mmHg during the heaviest exercise.)

As in thermographics, simple barographic demarcation provides a ready means for directing medical nanorobots to a desired treatment location within the body. Simply pressing down on the surface of the skin creates an anomalous region of elevated tissue pressure; tapping, slapping, or palpitating the body's surface is also detectable by in vivo nanorobots (e.g., Section 7.4.2.1). Acoustically active catheters inserted transdermally can place a sonic beacon signal near almost any target location. Highly focused but relatively low power (to reduce reflection echo detection) ultrasonic columnar or planar beams of, say, three different frequencies can be directed into the body on various trajectories and from various sources. The tiny spot where all three frequencies are audible at precisely equal intensity marks the target, providing $\lesssim 1$ mm^3 localization accuracy at frequencies $\gtrsim 1.5$ MHz. Focused ultrasound surgery (FUS) and high-intensity focused ultrasound (HIFU) may use ~2-second bursts of 1.7-MHz, 150-mm-deep focused beams at 5×10^7 watts/m^2 to occlude blood flow or destroy tumors by creating a spot of intense heat so small that there is a boundary of only ~6 cells between destroyed tissues and completely unharmed tissues, a ~100 micron spatial resolution.[1647]

As in the case of temperature fields, low-resolution and high-resolution barographic maps can be compiled and stored by barographicytes, then used to diagnose a wide variety of medically relevant states in organs and throughout the body including tumors, edemas, excess cranial pressure, general hypertension or hypotension, swollen lymph glands, muscle spasms and the like. Such maps are also useful in macrosensing, as for instance to help determine if the patient is sitting,[3330] standing, prone, inverted, falling, or floating (Section 4.9.2). Blood pressure increases in patients who are exercising, eating a meal, or emotive (e.g., angry), and decreases in patients who are relaxing or sleeping. The typical daily readings in a hypertensive 35-year-old male might be 150-220 mmHg systolic and 90-140 mmHg diastolic.

However, the amplitude and timing of pressure waves in the blood vessels permit somewhat clearer positional inferences than is possible with thermographics, in part because the heart is such a strong, reliable, and stably-positioned acoustic pulse generator.* Functional hemobaric mapping thus may provide useful positional information regarding vascular range estimates.

For example, Figure 8.29 shows the change in shape and amplitude of the pressure wave with increasing distance downstream from the aortic valve (where the left ventricle of the heart initially discharges into the descending aorta). There are three features of interest. First, each successive profile shifts to the right, suggesting wave propagation. Second, the sharp dicrotic notch in the pressure record (marking the closure of the aortic valve) is gradually lost in successive profiles, a clear navigational marker of aortic range.

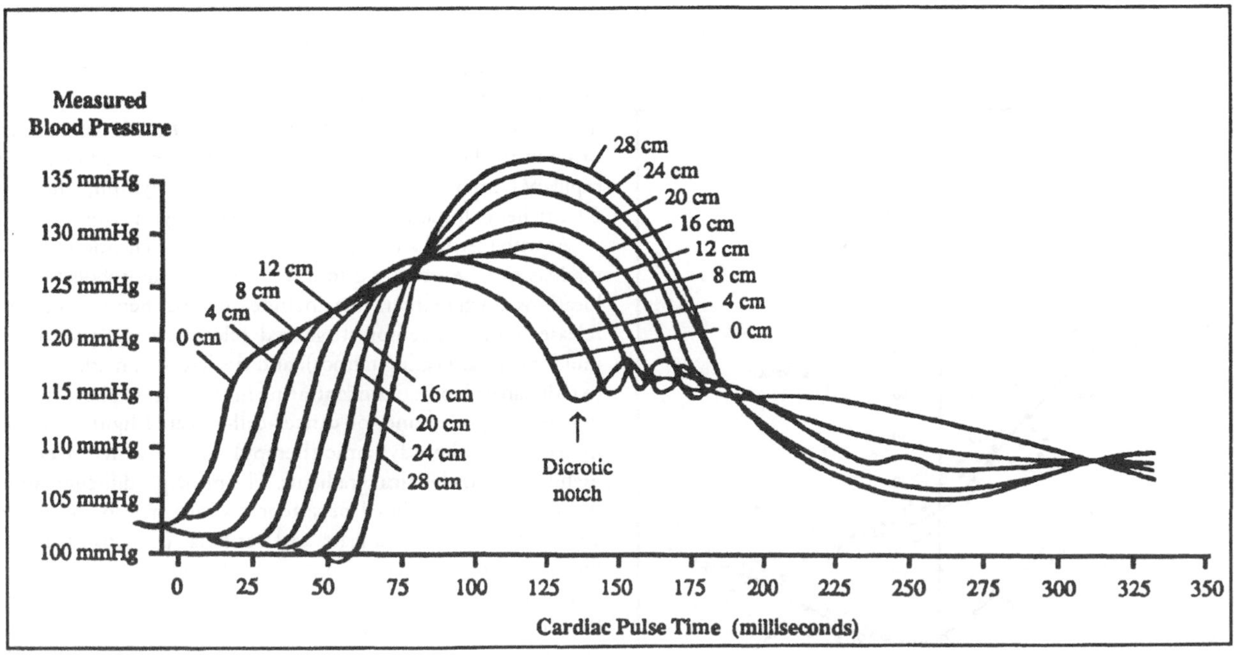

Fig. 8.29. Blood pressure profiles recorded at various distances along the aorta (data from dog aorta; distances measured from beginning of descending aorta; modified from Olson[923]).

* *In 1998, heart sounds originating from multiple sites within the four chambers of the heart, its valves and the great vessels remained difficult to analyze. Despite the close coincidence of valve closure and high frequency components in the first heart sound (echocardiographic corroboration), the exact mechanism of sound production was poorly understood.[1302] Phonocardiograms (PCGs) are distorted during transmission through the chest wall; cardiac auscultation, traditionally used to detect a wide variety of normal and pathological heart conditions, was still more art than science.[3339-3342]*

Third, there is a steepening and increasing of amplitude in successive profiles, indicating a rise in peak systolic pressure with distance from the heart. This counterintuitive increase is a dynamic phenomenon of an elastic branching system with tapered tubes—with steady flow in a rigid tube of similar diameter and taper, pressure always decreases in the direction of flow unless there is deceleration.[361] Note that the mean pressure averaged over a full heartbeat still decreases with increasing distance from the aortic valve—by ~4 mmHg over the full length of the aorta—while the amplitude of the systolic/diastolic pressure oscillation nearly doubles.[361] Measurements in dogs show that this peak pressure pulse amplification process continues until about the third generation of arterial branchings, after which both the oscillation and the mean pressure decrease gradually downstream along the arterial tree.[361] These pulse profiles can probably be resolved with sufficient accuracy to allow a medical nanorobot equipped with appropriate pressure sensors to fix its position along all the main trunks of the arterial tree to within at least ~1 cm, and perhaps better.

Pressure and velocity waveforms change in different ways along the branches of the tree,[924] in part due to reflection at bifurcations, which may allow bloodborne nanorobots to distinguish the organ in which they currently reside. For instance, the waveforms found in the renal and iliac arteries are quite distinct.[924]

Approximate position in the venous tree is readily inferred as well. For example, mean pressure in the venules is ~18 mmHg with fluctuations of amplitude ~3 mmHg; by the time bloodborne nanorobots reach the upper vena cava, near the right atrium of the heart, the mean pressure has fallen to ~2.2 mmHg with pressure fluctuations of amplitude ~5 mmHg.[361]

Microvascular position can also be estimated from various local pressure measurements.[929] For instance, Figure 8.30 shows a typical pressure-velocity distribution in arteriovenous microvessels 8-60 microns in diameter in the cat mesentery. Knowledge of mean local pressure and flow velocity identifies vessel diameter to within ± 5 microns. Additionally, these pressure distribution profiles differ

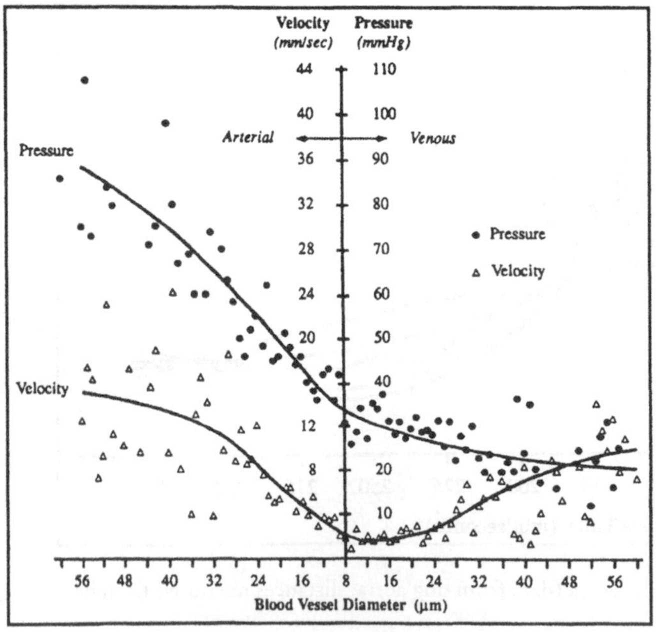

Fig. 8.30. Pressure-velocity distribution in microvasculature (data from cat mesentery; each point represents the average value of 3-5 measurements; modified from Zweifach and Lipowsky[925]).

markedly from one tissue to another (Fig. 8.31). Comparison of the measured profile against a library of such profiles will at least narrow the possibilities, if not produce a unique tissue identification.

Local hematocrit (the volume fraction of red cells in whole blood, or Hct) varies as a function of microvessel diameter (Fig. 8.32). Simple omnidirectional echolocation (Section 4.8.2) measures the average distance to the nearest red blood cell over many samples—e.g., the mean center-to-center distance between red cells is ~9.8 microns at Hct 10%, ~6.8 microns at Hct 30%. An acoustic test pulse travels ~1.5 microns in 1 nanosec, hence Hct 10% and Hct 12.7% are distinguishable using one round-trip measurement, allowing a medical nanorobot to estimate the local microvessel diameter to within approximately ± 10 microns. Given the scatter in the data, multiple measurements should improve the accuracy of the estimate.

Maps of mechanical properties such as strain fields in tissues can also provide useful navigational information but will be more difficult for individual nanorobots to employ directly. Magnetic resonance elastography (MRE) has already been used experimentally to map the shear modulus field of a porcine kidney using shear wave excitation at 200-400 Hz.[928] Shear waves with displacements under 100 nm were readily observed, and it is believed the technique may be useful in mapping other viscoelastic parameters such as attenuation and dispersion, allowing more detailed tissue characterization. Elastographic parameters are highly variable in time as well as space. For example, the viscoelasticity of cervical mucus secretions swings widely over the course of the menstrual cycle, with a major feature occurring at mid-period near ovulation time,[922] mirroring the temperature changes (Section 8.4.1.1)

8.4.3 Chemographic Navigation

The human body is a cauldron of chemical complexity. Of particular interest to us here are those extracellularly occurring chemical species reliably associated with specific locations, functions, or processes that might be useful in navigation. As trivial examples, high concentrations of hormones or neuropeptides are found in the endocrine glands or in the nerve tissues; lactic acid is produced in muscles driven anaerobically; uric acid is heavily concentrated in urine in the bladder (although high blood levels may indicate gout); capillary lymph is more watery than thoracic lymph, which in turn is far richer in histaminase than cervical duct lymph (Section 8.2.1.3).

As with thermal and pressure markers, crude chemical demarcation markers may be employed to direct medical nanorobots to particular locations. Such markers may include injected chemical plumes, time release implants, remote-triggered releasers (e.g., pressure-release multi-chemical-bearing tattoos), and tissue-coded markers (analogous to radiolabeled iodine concentrating in the thyroid gland, alkali metal ions seeking out bone, or cancer-cell-targeted light-sensitive drug molecules in photodynamic therapy)—all of which may establish useful localized chemical gradients. The principle difficulty for natural signal molecules is signal persistence, which may be relatively brief unless continuous broadcast and artificial (nonabsorbable) signal molecules are employed. Continuous broadcast creates a detection sphere of maximum radius R_{max} around the broadcast emission point (Section 7.2.1.5). Use of artificial non-biodegradable molecules maximizes the signal/noise ratio. Diffusion causes small molecules to drift ~1 cell width in ~1 second, or ~1 mm in ~1000 seconds (Section 3.2 and Table 3.4); bulk flow microconvection and increased effective diffusivity due to natural stirring (Section 3.2.2) further limit positional precision.

Use of chemical beacons for chemonavigational triangulation is not efficient over large distances, since the required volume of signal

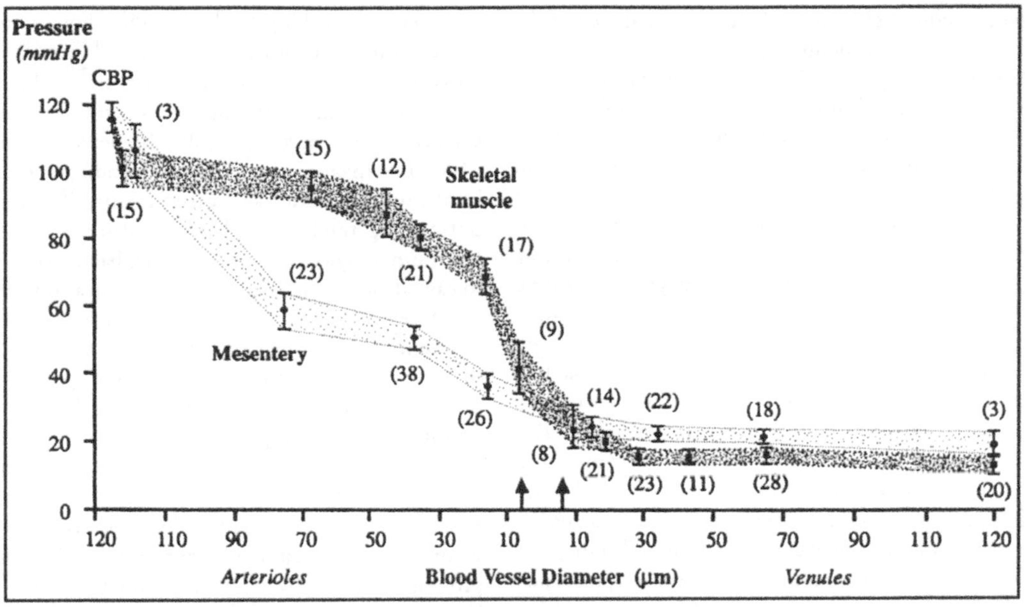

Fig. 8.31. Micropressure distribution profile while passing through two different tissues (data from mesentery and skeletal muscle of the cat; number of measurements in parentheses; central blood pressure (CBP) is average central arterial pressure from all experiments; modified from Fronek and Zweifach[926]).

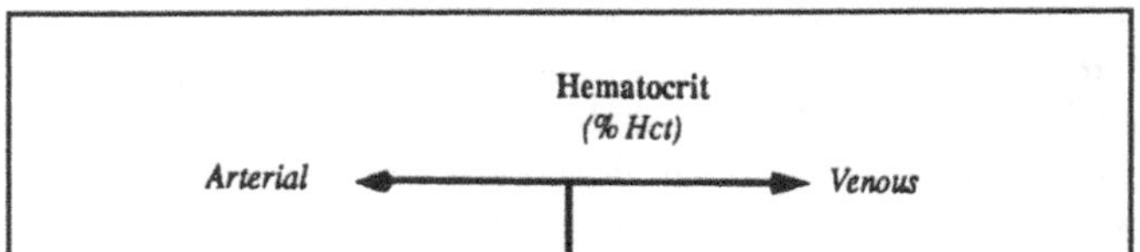

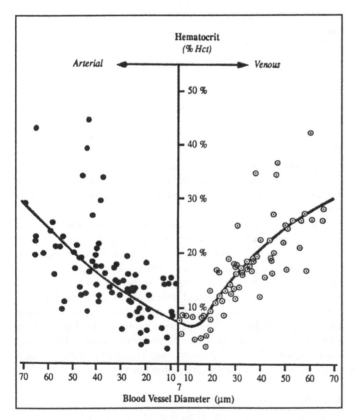

Fig. 8.32. Hematocrit distribution profile in microvasculature as a function of vessel diameter (data from cat mesentery; modified from Lipowsky, Usami, and Chien[927]).

chemical rises as the cube of the range. However, chemical localization may be moderately useful in close quarters. For instance, a micron-size nanorobot equipped with two antipodal chemical sensors can angularly resolve two periodic sources of dissimilar signal molecules to the limit of nanodevice rotation during a Brownian motion-limited measurement time (Section 3.2.1). A pair of 10-probe sensors taking measurements every ~1 millisec (concentration differential $\Delta c / c \sim 20\%$ over the full nanomedically-relevant range of $K_d = 10^{-4}$ to 10^{-13} molecules/nm^3; Section 4.2.1) can resolve $\Delta\alpha \sim 3°$ of arc (Eqn. 3.2), or two chemical point-emitters separated by $X_{path} \sin(\Delta\alpha) \sim 1$ micron at a range of $X_{path} \sim 20$ microns (~1 cell width) from the nanorobot.

Chemonavigation can also provide useful positional information. For example, glucose absorption in the jejunum establishes chemical gradients both in the radial and axial directions in the lumen and also across the surface of the small intestine (Section 8.2.3). If chyme leaving the duodenum starts with 1% glucose concentration and exits the upper jejunum at 0.01% concentration ~50 cm downstream, then the same 10-probe chemical sensor as above can measure 25 distinguishable glucose levels as a function of distance from the pylorus. This allows jejunal position to be estimated to within ~2 cm using glucose concentration alone.

Chemical navigation in the gut may incur significant positional uncertainties due to the large chemical variation of ingested foodstuffs, the generation and transport of gases, the volume and character of liquids consumed with the food, the state of mind (and bowel peristalsis) of the patient, the presence of biochemistry-altering disorders, and other factors. On the other hand, the results of measurements of nutrient levels in the stomach and duodenum may be broadcast downstream to jejunal nanorobots, allowing real-time assessment of the efficiency of digestive processes and thus reducing positional uncertainties. Similar gradients allow positional chemonavigation in gland ducts such as the salivary and pancreatic ducts.

Sulfate groups are more numerous on the surfaces of the rabbit aortic arch and carotid than on the surfaces of the rest of the systemic arteries, and post-staining fluorescence intensity (measuring abundance of sialyl groups in the endothelial glycocalyx) is 1.65 times higher in the carotid than in the aorta.[3164] In cyto chemonavigation is possible as well. For example, intracellular diffusion gradients of O_2 and ATP that appear under some conditions[3068] could be useful for detecting the distribution and clustering of mitochondria.

Detailed chemomapping of individual patients may allow customization of standardized human chemographic profiles, e.g., to identify problem areas. Chemographicytes may assist in the mapping process at up to ~KHz sampling frequencies (Section 8.5.2.1; see also Chapter 19). For instance, regions of hypoxia develop in all solid tumors where rapidly dividing cells are supplied by inadequate or poorly developed vasculature. A continuously updated tissue oxygenation map allows recognition of growing hypoxic regions, permitting prompt detection of nascent tumors, myocardial and cerebral ischemia, cardiorespiratory failure, and rheumatoid arthritis (e.g., loss of fluids that provide joint oxygenation). Similarly, a whole-body map of the concentration of intracellularly sampled telomerase (or associated proteins such as TRF1/TRF2,[3051,3052] Ku, and tankyrase,[3053] or even telomerase mRNA levels) may provide a good first-cut toward a whole-body late-stage cancer map,* since 85%-90% of all primary tumors display this biochemical marker.[3058] Cancer cells also display above-normal concentrations of β_1 integrins, survivin, sialidase-sensitive cancer mucins and leptin receptors such as galectin-3, and below-normal concentrations of β_4 integrins. Other examples include GM2 ganglioside, a glycolipid present on the surface of ~95% of melanoma cells, with the carbohydrate portion of the molecule conveniently jutting out on the extracellular side of the melanoma cell membrane.[1403] GM2 and another ganglioside, GD2, are expressed in several types of cancer cells including small-cell lung, colon, and gastric cancer, sarcoma, lymphoma, and neuroblastoma.[1403] Numerous specific markers of disease (an emerging field known as molecular epidemiology)[1112] are available for detection and mapping by nanorobots.

Another example is the chemographic mapping of organs. In the liver, hepatocytes located close to the portal vein (acinal Zone 1; Figure 8.26A) are bathed in blood that is comparatively rich in oxygen and nutrients, with only minimum exposure to metabolic waste products. In Zone 2, the blood is less fresh and wastes are more plentiful. In Zone 3, which extends to the central vein, the blood has little oxygen or nutrients but the highest concentration of metabolites.[936] Metabolic and exocrine secretory activity creates distinct chemical and thermal gradients, clearly defining each lobule. This allows medical nanorobots to navigate between lobules by simply counting the number of lobules traversed, and to navigate within a chosen lobule by gradient averaging. Changes in measured gradients may evidence a recent ingestion of alcohol or other toxins, or may record the progression of hypoxia or cirrhosis which invariably begins in Zone 3.[936]

Chemical localization to specific organs or tissues appears practical (Sections 8.2.5 and 8.5.2.2), as does chemical macrosensing of systemic states. For instance, a rise in serum adrenalin accompanied by surges in lactic acid production or oxygen consumption in the lower extremities might raise the reasonable inference that the patient is panicky and possibly fleeing from something that may be chasing him. Measurement of the concentration of thiocyanate in salivary secretions can distinguish smokers (~9×10^{-3} gm/cm^3) from non-smokers (~2×10^{-3} gm/cm^3).[943] Measurement of leptin concentrations (a hormone secreted by fat cells) in the blood allows nanorobots to estimate the total amount of fat currently stored in the body, relative to the normal baseline of a given person.[3265]

Chemical tracking is also feasible. For example, a "bacterium moves through the water (or the liquid interior of your body) in a greasy cloud of its own waste products,"[2973] due to the excretion of metabolic byproducts through transmembrane pores. Such microbial exhaust plumes might plausibly be detectable for distances up to ~100-1000 microns downstream, depending upon bacterial emissions, local fluid flow rates and other factors (Section 7.2.1), possibly permitting tracking and interception by medical nanorobots. Interestingly, quorum sensing among bacteria enables some microbes to eavesdrop on the chemical communications of other species.[3236]

Developing embryos demonstrate a sophisticated "biological positioning system" by which each cell determines its location relative to other cells to eventually produce the appropriate tissue, organ, or nerve. For example, members of the "Wnt" and "Hedgehog" families of signaling proteins help cells (in developing limbs and organs) to distinguish up from down. As another example, neuron migrations within the developing embryo are thought to be guided by chemical signposts such as the proteins reelin (released near the destinations of migrating neurons), mDab1 (which may be a docking protein activated by reelin),[949] and the homeodomain proteins DLX-1 and DLX-2.[950] Neuroblast cells that divide in the subventricular zone of the lateral ventricle in the brain of adult mice migrate a distance of ~3-5 mm to the olfactory bulb; these migrating neuroblasts remain organized in chains until they reach the core of the olfactory bulb, after which they separate and migrate radially as individual cells to more peripheral layers, then halt and differentiate into neurons.[947] During this process, the neural precursors are not guided by radial glial or axonal fibers, suggesting chemonavigational guidance here too. Similarly, developing neurons shoot out axons whose tips are steered to their destinations by an array of guidance molecules that are fixed on cell surfaces, or are located within the extracellular matrix, or are secreted by the axon's targets—such as the netrins (a chemoattractant group of proteins) and the semiphorins such as collapsin (a chemorepellant protein).[951,1055] There is also a chemical "area code" [1495] that is used for cell localization during extravasation of leukocytes from blood vessels (Section 9.4.4.1). Medical nanorobots can be programmed to follow and to interpret any such positional chemical signposts normally used by motile cells.

Chemonavigation may also be aided by the detection of isozymes—physically distinct forms displaying the same catalytic activity that may be present in different tissues of the same organism, in different cell types, or in different subcellular compartments in a human being. Isozymes are common in the sera and tissues of all vertebrates, insects, plants, and unicellular organisms. They are commonly used in clinical diagnosis, as, for instance, to distinguish normal serum and serum from patients with a myocardial infarct or with liver disease, using a lactate dehydrogenase (LDH) electropherogram,[996,3343-3348] although more recently the utility of isoenzymes in some clinical applications has been questioned.[3349,3350]

8.4.4 Microbiotagraphics

While high-speed nanomedical prophylactic measures against pathogens will be readily available (e.g., Section 10.4 and Chapter 19), in some cases the physician may wish to obtain an infection map before beginning treatment. It may also be useful to prepare maps of particular symbiotic, commensal, or parasitic bacterial species,

* *Telomerase is a ribonucleoprotein enzyme found principally in the cell nucleus. Telomerase is present in ciliated protozoa in concentrations of ~0.004-1 enzyme molecule per telomere;[3054,3055] with 92 chromosome-tip telomeres, telomerase-active human cell nuclei may contain only 1-100 copies of the enzyme. About 10% of human cancer cells maintain their telomeres without telomerase.[3056] Additionally, while telomerase is not expressed in most human somatic tissues,[3057,3058] certain normal human stem cells and germline populations are telomerase positive[3058-3062] and telomerase has been reported in normal human white blood cells and in some noncancerous liver diseases;[3063-3065] stem cells have low but detectable telomerase activity but continue to exhibit telomere shortening throughout life,[3060] hence telomerase expression per se is not oncogenic.[3066]*

or native mobile cellular elements, in the human body, whether for scientific or for diagnostic purposes.

For example, leukocytes and macrophages are readily recognized (Section 8.5.2.2) and could be statistically sampled to produce a crude whole-body leukographic map. A fleet of 2 trillion mapping nanorobots evenly distributed throughout a 0.1 m^3 body volume gives each nanorobot a patrol volume of 50,000 $micron^3$ (~1 capillary volume). At 310 K, a 1-micron nanorobot of normal density has an average thermal velocity of ~500 microns/sec (Eqn. 3.3). Assuming a cross-sectional area of ~1 $micron^2$, in 1 second a motile device traveling at this speed may trace out a nonrepeating zigzag path ~500 microns in length, or ~1% of its patrol volume, even while diffusing an additional radial distance of only ΔX ~ 1 micron (Eqn. 3.1). During its zigzag course, the device may collide at least once with ~1% of the motile body cells or microbiota present within the patrol volume. If ~10 collisions are required to ensure a positive identification of a cellular coat, then ~0.1% of the entire target cell population present in the patient's body may be physically sampled, positively identified, affirmatively counted, and directly associated with a specific map voxel in ~1 sec—a sufficient statistical sample for most purposes, even given the likelihood of substantial double-counting. A whole-body white-cell-count map to ~1 cm^3 voxel resolution requires ~10^6 bits to describe and may be retrieved by the physician in $\lesssim$1 sec using an in vivo mobile acoustic communication network; a ~1 mm^3 resolution map (~10^9 bits) fine enough to discover even the smallest macroscale infection site requires ~100-1000 seconds to outmessage in this manner. A sequence of readouts at regular intervals provides a clear strategic overview of the developing infection—some bacterial infections cause a selective increase in neutrophils, while infections with some protozoa and other parasites cause a selective increase in eosinophils.[531]

Whole-body vascular (e.g., bloodstream only) surveys of red cells, white cells, platelets or pathogens will proceed ~10 times faster using a nanorobot fleet of similar number density, owing to the reduced search volume, though at the cost of slightly increased onboard computational complexity needed to compensate for the moving reference frame.

Discussion of possible protein coat marker modifications that bacteria or other pathogens might evolve in a nanomedical technology-rich treatment environment as a defensive tactic is deferred to Chapter 17.

8.5 Cytonavigation

Cytonavigation is the study of navigation in and around the individual cell. The topic is large and the present work can only scratch the surface. After a brief cytometric overview (Section 8.5.1), the discussion here addresses four important issues—distinguishing whether an encountered cell is self or nonself (Section 8.5.2.1), determining the exact cell type of an encountered cell (Section 8.5.2.2), the significant features and landmarks inside living cells, called cytography (Section 8.5.3), and special considerations involved in navigating the cellular nucleus, called nucleography (Section 8.5.4). Issues relating to membrane penetration and cell entry by medical nanorobots are largely deferred to Section 9.4.5.

8.5.1 Cytometrics

How many cells are there in the human body? Serious estimates vary from a low of 10 trillion[312,931,2185] up to 50 trillion,[870] 75 trillion,[71,863] and even 100 trillion.[836,932,938,2022] The numbers show considerable spread because some authors refer only to tissue cells while others may refer to all cells physically present, both native and foreign.

The single most common native cell in the human body is the red blood cell (RBC), or erythrocyte. The average adult male carries ~5.2 x 10^9 RBCs/cm^3 (Appendix B) in his ~5400 cm^3 blood volume (Table 8.1), giving ~28.1 trillion RBCs. The spleen has an additional ~70 cm^3 of noncirculating RBC storage volume, giving another 0.4 trillion RBCs for a total of ~28.5 trillion RBCs in the body. Also confined to the bloodstream are a median ~2.5 x 10^8 platelets/cm^3, ~7.0 x 10^6/cm^3 leukocytes including neutrophils, eosinophils, basophils, lymphocytes and monocytes (Appendix B), plus another ~0.7 trillion platelets sequestered in a circulation-accessible pool in the spleen,[2122] giving ~2.1 trillion platelet cells in the human body and a white cell count of 0.4 trillion in the blood. There are also ~0.7 trillion lymphocytes in the lymphatic system (Table 8.5) and ~0.2 trillion macrophages and other reticuloendothelial (mononuclear phagocyte) cells throughout the human tissues.[743] Thus there are ~31.5 trillion native nontissue cells in the human body. There are also ~40 trillion foreign single-celled bacteria inhabiting the human colon, assuming ~35% of the ~340 cm^3 colorectal contents are bacteria each averaging ~1.8 microns in diameter.

As for tissue cells, a 70 kg adult male reference body includes ~28.8 kg of body cell mass (BCM), defined as the amount of body tissue calculated to contain potassium at a concentration of 120 mEq (millimole)/kg.[817] This figure is favored over the LBM (lean body mass) because BCM defines the component of body composition that contains the oxygen-containing, potassium-rich, glucose-oxidizing, work-performing tissue and contains all cellular elements concerned with respiration, physical and chemical work, and mitotic activity.

Most human cells fall within a size range of 2-120 microns.[866] Platelets are ~2 microns, red cells ~3 microns x ~8 microns, neutrophils ~8-10 microns, lymphocytes ~6-12 microns in size, exocrine cells ~10 microns, fibroblasts 10-15 microns, osteocytes ~10-20 microns including processes, chondrocytes and liver cells ~20 microns, goblet and ciliated cells ~50 microns long and 5-10 microns wide, macrophages at ~20-80 microns, hematopoietic stem cells ~30-40 microns, and adipocytes filled with stored lipid are typically 70-120 microns in diameter (but may be up to five times larger in very obese people).[935-936] Neurons vary enormously in size and shape, their bodies ranging from 4-120 microns in diameter with axonal processes varying between ~0.1-20 microns in diameter and ranging in length from a few microns up to ~1 meter;[799] muscle cells (~30% of all tissue cells) also vary from 10-100 microns in diameter and may run up to ~50 cm in length. However, the "average" tissue cell, if such a thing may be said to exist, is probably ~20 microns in diameter,[313] weighing ~10 nanograms.

Since the reference human has a mean density of 1064 kg/m^3 excluding bone minerals,[817] a BCM of 28.8 kg makes ~0.027 m^3 of cells; taking 8000 $micron^3$ per cell gives a total of ~3.4 trillion tissue cells. Thus the human body contains ~35 trillion native cells, of which only ~10% are tissue cells, plus ~40 trillion foreign (mostly bacterial) cells in the colon for a grand total of 75 trillion cells. The number of tissue cells comprising each organ listed in Table 8.9 may be crudely estimated by multiplying tissue volume by the mean tissue cellular number density, or ~125 million cells/cm^3.

8.5.2 Cytoidentification

Before entering and navigating a cell, a medical nanorobot must first determine whether the cell belongs to the patient or is a foreign cell (Section 8.5.2.1). The nanorobot must also determine which type of cell it has encountered, either to verify its location in a desired target organ or tissue, or to ensure that a targeted cell type has been found (Section 8.5.2.2). Fortunately, the plasma membrane (the cell's outermost coat; Section 8.5.3.2) is an open book for nanodevices equipped to read it.

8.5.2.1 Identification of Self

The cytochemical distinction between self and nonself is mediated by the histocompatibility molecules.[939,953-955,997] These antigens are genetically coded in the major histocompatibility complex (MHC), a cluster of ~28 genes located on chromosome 6 and comprising ~0.1% of the entire human genome. There are three broad classes (I, II, and III) of MHC genes that encode self antigens. The major function of the MHC-I and MHC-II molecules[439] is the presentation of antigenic peptide fragments, derived from internal (MHC-I) or external (MHC-II) foreign proteins, to the immune system. It is the combination of an MHC molecule plus a foreign peptide fragment that appears antigenic to the immune system. (See Chapter 15.)

Most important are the MHC Class I molecules—glycoproteins encoded by several separate genetic loci which comprise the HLA (histocompatibility locus antigens, formerly "human leukocyte antigens") complex. The three classical loci within the HLA complex are called HLA-A, HLA-B, and HLA-C. Essentially all adult nucleated cells in the human body (including white cells but excluding cells in the nervous system and cells of some tumors) display the classical MHC molecules of the A, B, and C regions on their surfaces in varying amounts.* Class I glycoproteins account for up to 1% of the total protein of the plasma membrane.[939] Figure 8.33 shows the structure and orientation of a Class I MHC glycoprotein. Each MHC Class I molecule has two parts. The first part is a long folded glycosylated polypeptide chain of molecular weight ~45,000 daltons (~340 residues). This chain has a short (~30 residue) hydrophilic tail inside the cell and a ~40 residue hydrophobic transmembrane segment. The extracellular portion has three ~90-residue segments designated α_1, α_2, and α_3 with intrasegment disulfide bridges. Alloantigenic sites (carrying determinants specific to each individual) are located primarily in the α_1 domain and to a lesser extent in the α_2 domain, and there is a carbohydrate unit attached to the α_2 domain. The α_3 domain is relatively invariant. The second part of the MHC Class I molecule is a nonglycosylated 96-residue peptide called β_2-microglobulin, of molecular weight ~12,000 daltons, which is noncovalently bound to the α_3 domain of the longer glycosylated chain nearest the outer surface of the cell membrane. β_2-microglobulin is not part of the active antigenic site of the HLA molecule but is essential for the expression of specificity.

MHC Class II molecules are also glycosylated integral membrane proteins (Fig. 8.34). These proteins are coded by at least six expressed genes located in the D region of the MHC cluster, each of which encodes either a ~34,000-dalton α chain or a ~28,000-dalton β chain. Each MHC Class II polypeptide consists of two external 90-residue domains, a 30-residue transmembrane domain, and a cytoplasmic domain with 10-15 amino acids. There are four serologically-determined Class II subtypes: HLA-DR and HLA-D (one α and several β chains), HLA-DQ (one α and one β chain), and HLA-DP (at least one α and one β chain). Each Class II glycoprotein molecule consists of at least two of these transmembrane polypeptide chains bound together noncovalently. Only the shorter β chains contain the alloantigenic sites, and both chains have carbohydrate units.[955] MHC Class II molecules are less widely distributed than those of Class I, being found primarily on dendritic cells, glial cells in the brain, some epithelial and endothelial cells (e.g., Langerhans cells in the epidermis), monocytes, macrophages (including tissue macrophages such as the Kupffer cells of the liver), melanoma cells, activated (but not resting) T cells, and most B lymphocytes.[953,955] Other cells may be induced to express MHC Class II proteins when exposed to γ interferon.[956] Most parenchymal cells do not express MHC Class II molecules.[953]

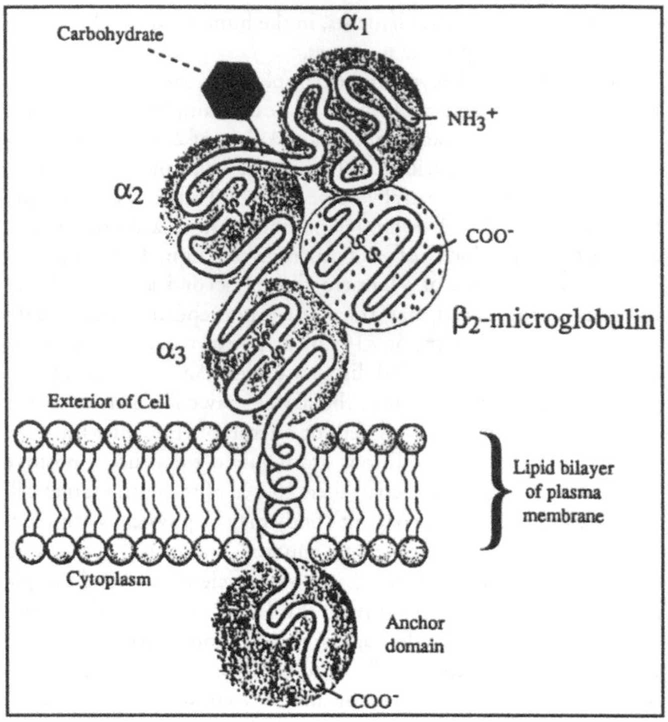

Fig. 8.33. Stucture and orientation of an MHC Class I glycoprotein molecule (modified from Becker and Deamer[939]).

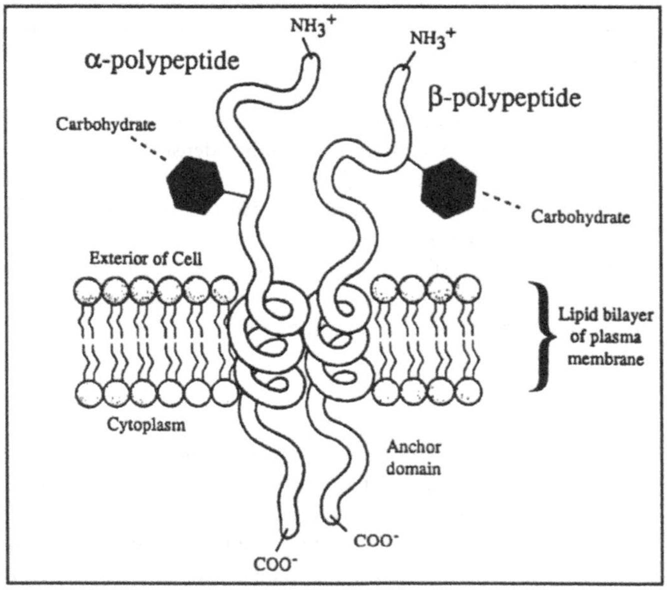

Fig. 8.34. Structure and orientation of an MHC Class II glycoprotein molecule (modified from Becker and Deamer[939]).

* *Classical HLA tissue typing relied solely upon observations of cytotoxic reactions of human alloantisera with live lymphocytes. By 1998 it was apparent that this approach fails to distinguish all HLA alleles, and typing based on nucleotide sequences had begun to replace serological methods.*[1028]

Table 8.13. Recognized HLA Specificities

A. Specificities Based on Classical Serological Alloantisera Typing[956]

Class I Proteins							**Class II Proteins**						
HLA-A		**HLA-B**				**HLA-C**	**HLA-D**		**HLA-DR**		**HLA-DQ**	**HLA-DP**	
A1	A28	B5	B38	B5102	B65	Cw1	Dw1	Dw14	DR1	DR12	DQ1	DPw1	
A2	A29	B7	B39	B5103	B67	Cw2	Dw2	Dw15	DR103	DR13	DQ2	DPw2	
A203	A30	B703	B3901	B52	B70	Cw3	Dw3	Dw16	DR2	DR14	DQ3	DPw3	
A210	A31	B8	B3902	B53	B71	Cw4	Dw4	Dw17	DR3	DR1403	DQ4	DPw4	
A3	A32	B12	B40	B54	B72	Cw5	Dw5	Dw18	DR4	DR1404	DQ5	DPw5	
A9	A33	B13	B41	B55	B73	Cw6	Dw6	Dw19	DR5	DR15	DQ6	DPw6	
A10	A34	B14	B42	B56	B75	Cw7	Dw7	Dw20	DR6	DR16	DQ7		
A11	A36	B15	B44	B57	B76	Cw8	Dw8	Dw21	DR7	DR17	DQ8		
A19	A43	B16	B45	B58	B77	Cw9	Dw9	Dw22	DR8	DR18	DQ9		
A23	A66	B17	B46	B59	B7801	Cw10	Dw10	Dw23	DR9	DR51			
A24	A68	B18	B47	B60			Dw11	Dw24	DR10	DR52			
A25	A69	B22	B48	B61	Bw4		Dw12	Dw25	DR11	DR53			
A26	A74	B27	B49	B62	Bw6		Dw13	Dw26					
		B35	B50	B63									
		B37	B51	B64									

Total Number of Protein Types = 26 + 57 + 10 + 26 + 24 + 9 + 6 = 158 types
Total Number of Combinations = 26 x 57 x 10 x 26 x 24 x 9 x 6 = 499,374,720 combinations

B. Specificities Based on Modern Nucleotide Sequence Typing[1028]

HLA Class I Alleles				**HLA Class II Alleles**			
Locus	**Number of of Alleles**	**Locus**	**Number of of Alleles**	**Locus**	**Number of of Alleles**	**Locus**	**Number of of Alleles**
HLA-A	67	HLA-F	1	HLA-DRA	2	HLA-DPA	8
HLA-B	149	HLA-G	6	HLA-DRB	179	HLA-DPB	69
HLA-C	39			HLA-DQA	18	HLA-DMA	4
HLA-E	5			HLA-DQB	29	HLA-DMB	5
		Total:	**266**			**Total:**	**314**

Number of Class I sets = 11,680,110 six-allele sets
Number of Class II sets = 2,063,111,040 eight-allele sets
Total Number of Combinations = 2.41 x 10^{16} fourteen-allele combinations

MHC Class III genes encode the ~20 proteins that comprise the complement system, including Bf, C2, C4A and C4B. These are functionally related in that they are each involved in the activation of the C3 component (Chapter 15). They allow human cell membranes to be distinguished from nonhuman (e.g., bacterial) membranes, a crude form of self identification, but are nonspecific and thus play no role in distinguishing the cells of one patient from those of another.

The >3.8 megabase gene locus of the MHC is the most polymorphic (having alternative types) in the human genome; the number of observed MHC (HLA) types appears to be near the optimum number based on evolutionary simulation experiments using a cellular automaton model of antigen-lymphocyte interactions.[958] Table 8.13 summarizes classical serological and modern nucleotide-based HLA specificities that were recognized as of 1998. (Not shown are several "public antigens" such as HLA-DRw52 and DRw53 which, like MHC Class III proteins, are essentially nonspecific.) The HLA-uniqueness of an individual patient can only be estimated because the specificities do not occur with equal probability. For example, 16% of the human population has HLA-A1 but only 10% have HLA-B8.[955] As an additional complication, the specificities are not strictly independent—given the above probabilities, the combination A1B8 should occur with a frequency of 1.6%, but the actual observed frequency is 8.8%.[955] Members of the same geneological family are also far more likely to have matching MHC Class II proteins than randomly selected unrelated individuals. Subject to these provisos, the existence of ~500 million distinct classical HLA combinations originally seemed to imply that only ~10 people in a worldwide population of 5 billion people shared exactly the same self-molecules, making each person literally "one in a billion." However, based on nucleotide sequencing, as of 1998 there were estimated to be >10^{16} known combinations, making each person quite histocompatibility-unique.

MHC Class I and Class II self-molecules are manufactured in the rough endoplasmic reticulum (Section 8.5.3.5) and are then delivered to the plasma membrane (Section 8.5.3.2) for presentation to the extracellular environment. A typical cell may have 15,000-30,000 Class I molecules (~10-20/micron^2) at its surface; a cell expressing Class II proteins may display 50,000-500,000 Class II molecules (~40-400/micron^2) at its surface.[439,3453] A nanorobot chemotactic sensor pad (with appropriate reversible binding sites; Section 4.2.8) measuring 50-300 nm in diameter pressed against a cell surface will overlay at least one of each class of self-molecule. Vesicle-transported proteins (like MHC proteins) have an estimated lateral diffusion coefficient in the cell plasma membrane of ~2 x 10^{-14} m^2/sec,[531] so an MHC molecule (assumed diameter ~10 nm) experiences an effective absolute viscosity of $\eta_{antigen}$ ~ 2.3 kg/m-sec (Eqn. 3.5) and thus migrates across the plasma membrane surface under the sensor pad from center to periphery of the sensor pad in 20-600 millisec (vs. 0.01-0.5 millisec for phospholipid molecules in the membrane; Eqn. 3.1), allowing a single binding event and hence a detection in much less than a second.

Consider a chemotactic sensor pad of area A_{pad} overlaying $N_{antigen}$ antigen molecules, comprising an array of N_{sensor} chemosensors each of area A_{sensor}. If a single detection event requires $\tau = 3 \pi \eta_{antigen} R_{antigen} \Delta X^2 / kT$ seconds (Eqn. 3.1) where ΔX is the mean antigen migration distance in the cell membrane, then the time needed to measure N_{spec} specificities assuming a minimum of $N_{encounter}$ contact events to ensure a binding event is $t_{meas} = \tau (N_{spec} N_{encounter} / N_{sensor})$. Since $N_{sensor} = A_{pad} / A_{sensor}$ and $\Delta X^2 = A_{sensor} N_{spec} / N_{antigen}$, then:

$$t_{meas} = \frac{3 \pi \eta_{antigen} R_{antigen} N_{encounter} N_{spec}^2 A_{sensor}^2}{A_{pad} N_{antigen} kT} \quad \text{(sec)}$$

{Eqn. 8.5}

Taking $R_{antigen}$ = 5 nm, $N_{encounter}$ = 10, A_{sensor} = 100 nm^2, A_{pad} = 90,000 nm^2, $N_{antigen}$ = 1, and T = 310 K, then t_{meas} ~ (3 x 10^{-5}) N_{spec}^2. A nanorobot searching for a particular set of 7 HLA proteins (N_{spec} = 7) thus requires t_{meas} ~ 0.001 sec to make the self/nonself determination for a particular cell membrane it has encountered. A nanorobot seeking to determine the HLA type of the membrane (e.g., in mapping mode) must in the worst case search all (266 + 314 =) 580 HLA protein types (N_{spec} = 580), requiring at most t_{meas} ~ 10 sec.

The principal exceptions to the MHC system are the red blood cells, the most numerous native cells in the human body (Section 8.5.1). Red cells do not express HLA proteins. Rather, the erythrocyte surface expresses a complex set of at least 22 blood group systems and 7 antigen collections, as listed in Table 8.14, plus 47 additional high-prevalence (public) and low-prevalence (private) antigens not associated with known systems or collections, also grouped into numbered series (not shown in the table).[957] Some of these antigen systems are carbohydrates, like the familiar ABO system, which is coded by genes located on chromosome 9; others are nonglycosylated proteins, glycoproteins or glycosphingolipids. Each system or collection is expressed on every erythrocyte surface, so an exhaustive assay of all 30+ antigen systems allows at least ~10^{19} different combinations to be distinguished. Most combinations are extremely rare, so the practical net specificity of the entire blood group set is considerably less in the human population, though probably still much higher than the HLA system.

ABO is the best-known blood group system. Erythrocytes are typed as A, B, AB, or O, the latter indicating a lack of expression of either A or B. The H antigen is the precursor of A and B (Fig. 8.35) and is found on all red cell surfaces (up to ~1.7 x 10^6 antigens/RBC, or ~18,000/micron^2) except those of patients with the rare O_h Bombay or H-null phenotype. Because H is a precursor of A and B, type O erythrocytes have more H antigen than A or B erythrocytes, which in turn have more H antigen than AB erythrocytes (which express both A and B antigens). The number of A and B antigens on the red cell surface ranges from 1-2 x 10^6 (~10,000-20,000/micron^2); in 75% of Type A individuals, "double-length" A antigens are also present (~500/micron^2). MNSs factor antigens range from ~2700-5400/micron^2, Rh factor antigens ~100-300/micron^2, Lewis factor antigens ~30/micron^2, and so forth. Again assuming a ~(300 nm)^2 chemotactic sensor pad, from Eqn. 8.5 a nanorobot searching for a particular set of ~30 blood group antigens (N_{spec} = 30) requires t_{meas} ~ 0.03 sec to make the self/nonself determination for a particular red cell membrane it has encountered. A nanorobot seeking to determine the complete blood group type of the membrane (e.g., in mapping mode) must in the worst case search all 254 known blood antigen types (N_{spec} = 254), requiring at most t_{meas} ~ 2 sec.

Direct detection of blood group antigens, or of antibodies to blood group antigens in body fluids, permits at least partial self-recognition by bloodborne nanorobots without the need for any direct cell contact, which may be useful in establishing theater protocols (Chapter 12). ABH, Lewis, I and P blood group antigens are found in blood plasma, and serum IgM-class antibodies associated with the carbohydrate antigens of the ABO, Lewis, and P blood group systems are almost universal. Anti-M and anti-N are common, anti-Sd^a is found in 1-2% of normal people, and anti-V^w or anti-Wr^a is found in ~1% of patients.[960] In persons who previously have been

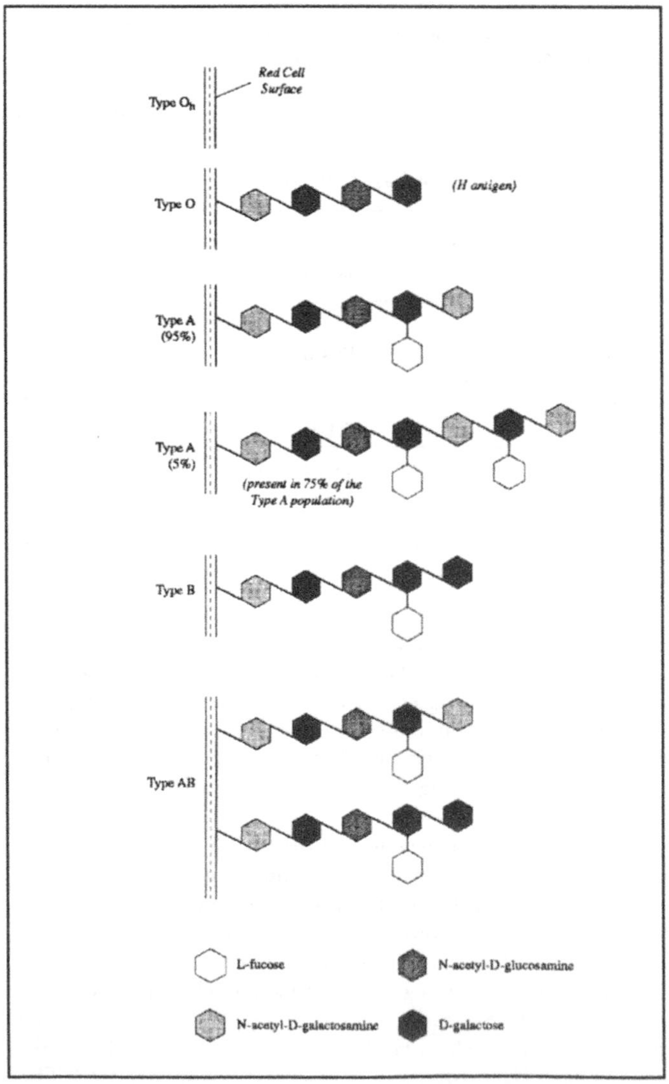

Fig. 8.35. Structure of ABO blood system red cell surface carbohydrate antigens (modified from Cunningham[959]).

Table 8.14. Blood Group Systems and Antigen Collections Recognized in 1997[957]

Conventional Name	Total # of Antigens	Common Antigens	Common Phenotypes	% Frequency	# of Antigen Sites/RBC
Blood group systems:					
ABO	4	A	A	40%	ABO: 1-2 x 10^6
		B	B	11%	H: 1.7 x 10^6
			AB	4%	
		H	O	45%	
Rh	47	D	R_1 DCe	42%	D: 1 x 10^3
		C,c,C^W	r dce	37%	R_2R_2: 15-33 x 10^3
		E,e	R_2 DcE	14%	R_1R_1: 14-19 x 10^3
		f(ce)	R_0 Dce	4%	R_0r: 12-20 x 10^3
		V(ce^S)	r′dCe	2%	R_1r: 9-14 x 10^3
			r″ dcE	1%	cc: 70-85 x 10^3
			R_z DCE	rare	Cc: 37-53 x 10^3
			r^ydCE	rare	ee: 18-24 x 10^3
					Ee: 13-14 x 10^3
MNSs	37	M	M+N-	28%	MN: 5 x 10^5
		N	M+N+	50%	Ss: 2.5 x 10^5
		S	M-N+	22%	
		s	S+s-	11%	
		U	S+s+	44%	
			S-s+	45%	
			S-s-U-	<1%	
P	1	P_1	P^k+P+P_1+(P_1)	79%	
		P	P^k+P+P_1-(P_2)	21%	
		P^k	P^k-P-P_1-(p)	rare	
			P^k+P-P_1+($P_L{}^k$)	more rare	
			P^k+P-P_1-($P_2{}^k$)	most rare	
Lewis	3	Le^a	Le(a+b-)	22%	Le^a: 3 x 10^3
		Le^b	Le(a-b+)	72%	
			Le(a-b-)	6%	
			Le(a+b+)	rare	
Kell	21	K	K-k+	91%	2-6 x 10^3
		k	K+k+	8.8%	
		Kp^a	K+k-	0.2%	
		Kp^b	Kp(a-b+)	97.7%	
		Js^a	Kp(a+b+)	2.3%	
		Js^b	Kp(a+b-)	rare	
			Js(a-b+)	100%	
			Js(a+b+)	rare	
			Js(a+b-)	very rare	
Duffy	6	Fy^a	Fy(a+b-)Fy3+	17%	Fy^a: 7-13 x 10^3
		Fy^b	Fy(a+b+)Fy3+	49%	
		Fy^3	Fy(a-b+)Fy3+	34%	
		Fy^4	Fy(a-b-)Fy3-4+	rare	
			Fy(a-b-)Fy3-4-	very rare	
Kidd	3	Jk^a	Jk(a+b-)Jk3+	28%	Jk^aJk^a: 14 x 10^3
		Jk^b	Jk(a+b+)Jk3+	49%	
		Jk^3	Jk(a-b+)Jk3+	23%	
			Jk(a-b-)Jk3-	very rare	
Lutheran	18	Lu^a	Lu(a-b-)Lu3+	0.15%	Lu^b: 0.8-4 x 10^3
		Lu^b	Lu(a+b+)Lu3+	7.5%	
		Lu^3	Lu(a+b-)Lu3+	92.3%	
			Lu(a-b-)Lu3-	very rare	
Diego	2				
Cartwright	2				
Xg	1				
Scianna	3				
Dombrock	5				
Coulton	3				
LW	3				
Chido/Rogers	9				
H	1				
Kx	1				
Gerbich	7				
Cromer	10				
Knops	5				

Table 8.14. Blood Group Systems and Antigen Collections Recognized in 1997[957] (cont'd)

Conventional Name	Total # of Antigens	Common Antigens	Common Phenotypes	% Frequency	# of Antigen Sites/RBC
Antigen collections:					
Indian	2				
Cost	2				
Ii	2	I	I adult(+I-i)	common	I adult: 1-5 x 10^3
		i	I_{int}(+I-i)	rare	
			i cord (-I+i)	common	
			i adult(-I+i)	<0.01%	
Er	2				
(P,P_k,LKE)	3				
(Lewis-like: Le^c, Le^d)	2				
Wright	2				
Low-prevalence (private)	36				
High prevalence (public)	11				

Total Number of Antigens = 254
Total Number of Combinations > 1.84 x 10^{19}

pregnant or transfused, 0.16-0.56% have anti-D (Rh group) and 0.14-0.60% have anti-E and anti-C (Rh system), anti-K and anti-Fy^a, and several other antibodies in serum.[960] Body secretions contain ABH, I and Lewis antigen but no P system antigens; Sd^a antigen is found in most body secretions, with the greatest concentration in the urine.[960]

Other partial exceptions to the MHC system are the keratinocytes, smooth muscle cells, and fibroblasts, which do not constitutively express HLA Class II molecules.[967] As a result, foreign fibroblasts cannot induce the generation of required helper T cells and thus stimulate no rejection response when transplanted between hosts.

8.5.2.2 Identification of Cell Type

How many different cell types are there in an adult human body? The usual estimate based on histological studies is that there are ~200 distinct kinds of cells that show alternate structures and functions.[312,531,866] These represent discrete categories of cell types of markedly different character, not arbitrary subdivisions along a morphological continuum. Traditional classification is based on microscopic shape and structure, and on crude chemical nature (e.g., affinity for various stains), but newer immunological techniques have revealed, for instance, that there are more than 10 distinct types of lymphocytes. Pharmacological and physiological tests have revealed many different varieties of smooth muscle cells—for example, uterine wall smooth muscle cells are highly sensitive to estrogen and (in late pregnancy) oxytocin, while gut wall smooth muscle cells are not. Appendix C presents a catalog of the cells of the human body, slightly modified from an original compilation by Alberts et al.[531] The catalog is organized by cellular function and omits subdivisions of smooth muscle cells, neuron classes in the CNS, various related connective tissue and fibroblast types, and intermediate stages of maturing cells such as keratinocytes (only the stem cell and differentiated cell types are given). Otherwise, the catalog is said to represent an exhaustive listing of the ~219 cell varieties found in the adult human phenotype. (Complexity theory and phylogenetic comparisons suggest that the maximum number of cell types $N_{cell} \sim N_{gene}^{1/2}$ = 370 cell types for humans with $N_{gene} \sim 10^5$ genes).[1266,766]

Medical nanorobots can probably distinguish all of these cell types by surface chemical assay using chemosensor pads (Section 4.2.8). Antigenic specificities exist for species (xenotype), organ, tissue or cell type for almost all cells—possibly involving as many as ~10^4 distinct antigens. A comprehensive analysis of the cytoimmunography of all cell types is beyond the scope of this book, but a few examples of cell type-specific antigenic markers can be given to illustrate the tremendous power of this approach.

In the case of red blood cells, antigens in the Rh, Kell, Duffy, and Kidd blood group systems are found exclusively on the plasma membranes of erythrocytes and have not been detected on platelets, lymphocytes, granulocytes, in plasma, or in other body secretions such as saliva, milk, or amniotic fluid.[960] Thus detection of any member of this four-antigen set establishes a unique marker for red cell identification. MNSs and Lutheran antigens are also limited to erythrocytes with two exceptions: GPA glycoprotein (MN activity) also found on renal capillary endothelium,[961] and Lu^b-like glycoprotein which appears on kidney endothelial cells and liver hepatocytes.[962] In contrast, ABH antigens are found on many non-RBC tissue cells such as kidney and salivary glands.[955] In young embryos ABH can be found on all endothelial and epithelial cells except those of the central nervous system.[963] ABH, Lewis, I and P blood group antigens are found on platelets and lymphocytes, at least in part due to adsorption from the plasma onto the cell membrane. Granulocytes have I antigen but no ABH.[960]

Platelets also express platelet-specific alloantigens on their plasma membranes, in addition to the HLA antigens they already share with body tissue cells. Currently there are five recognized human platelet alloantigen (HPA) systems that have been defined at the molecular level (Table 8.15). The phenotype frequencies given are for the Caucasian population; frequencies in African and Asian populations may vary substantially. For instance, HPA-1b is expressed on the platelets of 28% of Caucasians but only 4% of the Japanese population.[964] A medical nanorobot that detects a

Table 8.15. Complete Listing of Recognized Human Platelet Alloantigen (HPA) Systems[956]

Alloantigen System	Allelic Forms	Former Names	Phenotype Frequency
HPA-1	HPA-1a	$P1^{A1}$ or Zw^a	a/a = 72%
			a/b = 26%
	HPA-1b	$P1^{A2}$ or Zw^b	b/b = 2%
HPA-2	HPA-2a	Ko^b	a/a = 85%
			a/b = 14%
	HPA-2b	Ko^a	b/b = 1%
HPA-3	HPA-3a	Bak^a or Lek^a	a/a = 37%
			a/b = 48%
	HPA-3b	Bak^b or Lek^b	b/b = 15%
HPA-4	HPA-4a	Pen^a or Yuk^b	a/a = 99%
			a/b < 0.1%
	HPA-4b	Pen^b or Yuk^a	b/b < 0.1%
HPA-5	HPA-5a	Br^b or Zav^b	a/a = 80%
			a/b = 19%
	HPA-5b	Br^a, Zav^a, or Hc^a	b/b = 1%

representative antigen from any of these five HPA antigen groups on an encountered surface can be certain that it has found a platelet.

Lymphocytes with a particular functional activity can be distinguished by various differentiation markers displayed on their cell surfaces. For example, all mature T cells express a set of polypeptide chains called the CD3 complex. Helper T cells also express the CD4 glycoprotein, whereas cytotoxic and suppressor T cells express a marker called CD8.[939] Thus a nanorobot that detects the phenotype $CD3^+CD4^+CD8^-$ has positively identified a helper T cell, whereas the detection of $CD3^+CD4^-CD8^+$ uniquely identifies a cytotoxic or suppressor T cell. All B lymphocytes express immunoglobulins (their antigen receptors, or Ig) on their surface and can be distinguished from T cells on that basis, e.g., as Ig^+ MHC Class II^+.[939]

Lymphocyte surfaces also display distinct markers representing specific gene products that are expressed only at characteristic stages of cell differentiation. For example, Stage I Progenitor B cells display $CD34^+PhiL^-CD19^-$; Stage II, $CD34^+PhiL^+CD19^-$; Stage III, $CD34^+PhiL^+CD19^+$; and finally $CD34^-PhiL^+CD19^+$ at the Precursor B stage.[965]

There are neutrophil-specific antigens and various receptor-specific immunoglobulin binding specificities for leukocytes. For instance, monocyte FcRI receptors display the measured binding specificity $IgG1^{+++}IgG2^-IgG3^{+++}IgG4^+$, monocyte FcRIII receptors have $IgG1^{++}IgG2^-IgG3^{++}IgG4^-$, and FcRII receptors on neutrophils and eosinophils show $IgG1^{+++}IgG2^+IgG3^{+++}IgG4^+$.[955] Neutrophils also have β-glucan receptors on their surfaces.[1403]

Tissue cells display specific sets of distinguishing markers on their surfaces as well. Thyroid microsomal-microvillous antigen is unique to the thyroid gland.[955] Glial fibrillary acidic protein (GFAP) is an immunocytochemical marker of astrocytes,[947] and syntaxin 1A and 1B are phosphoproteins found only in the plasma membrane of neuronal cells.[1079] Alpha-fodrin is an organ-specific autoantigenic marker of salivary gland cells.[968] Fertilin, a member of the ADAM family, is found on the plasma membrane of mammalian sperm cells.[2143] Hepatocytes display the phenotypic markers $ALB^{+++}GGT^-CK19^-$ along with connexin 32, transferrin, and major urinary protein (MUP), while biliary cells display the markers $AFP^-GGT^{+++}CK19^{+++}$ plus BD.1 antigen, alkaline phosphatase, and DPP4.[966] A family of 100-kilodalton plasma membrane guanosine triphosphatases implicated in clathrin-coated vesicle (Section 8.5.3.7) transport include dynamin I (expressed exclusively in neurons), dynamin II (found in all tissues), and dynamin III (restricted to the testes, brain, and lungs), each with at least four distinct isoforms; dynamin II also exhibits intracellular localization in the trans-Golgi network.[1193] Table 8.16 lists numerous unique (to one or the other cell type) and shared antigenic markers of hepatopoietic (e.g., hepatoblast) and hemopoietic (e.g., erythroid progenitor) cells. There are many tumor-specific antigens, a fact exploited in conventional peptide-guided chemotherapy.[1143]

Bacterial membranes are also quite distinctive, including such obvious markers as the family of outer-membrane trimeric channel proteins called porins in Gram-negative bacteria like *E. coli*[1045,1053] and other surface proteins such as *Staphylococcal* protein A [1046] or endotoxin (lipopolysaccharide or LPS), a variable-size carbohydrate chain that is the major antigen of the outer membrane of Gram-negative bacteria. Mycobacteria contain mycolic acid in their cell walls.[2134] In addition, only bacteria employ right-handed amino acids in their cellular coats, which helps them resist attack by digestive enzymes in the stomach and other organisms. Peptidoglycans, the main structural component of bacterial walls, are cross-linked with peptide bridges that contain several unusual nonprotein amino acids and D-enantiomeric forms of Ala, Glu, and Asp.[1718] D-alanine is the most abundant D-amino acid found in most peptidoglycans and the only one that is universally incorporated.[1719]

At least four major families of cell-specific cell adhesion molecules had been identified by 1998—the immunoglobulin (Ig) superfamily (including N-CAM and ICAM-1), the integrin superfamily, the cadherin family and the selectin family (see below).

Integrins are ~200 kilodalton cell surface adhesion receptors expressed on a wide variety of cells, with most cells expressing several integrins. Most integrins, which mediate cellular connection to the extracellular matrix, are involved in attachments to the cytoskeletal substratum. Cell-type-specific examples include platelet-specific integrin ($\alpha_{IIb}\beta_3$), leukocyte-specific β_2 integrins, late-activation ($\alpha_L\beta_2$) lymphocyte antigens, retinal ganglion axon integrin ($\alpha_6\beta_1$) and keratinocyte integrin ($\alpha_5\beta_1$).[975] At least 20 different heterodimer integrin receptors were known in 1998.

Table 8.16. Unique and Shared Antigenic Surface Markers of Hepatopoietic and Hemopoietic Human Cells[966]

	Hepatopoietic Cells (e.g., Hepatoblasts)	Hemopoietic Cells (e.g., Erythroid Progenitors)
UNIQUE Antigenic Markers:	α-fetoprotein, albumin, stem cell factor, hepatic heparan sulfate-PGs (syndecans/perlecans), IGF I, IGF II, TGF-α, TGF-α receptor, α_1 integrin, α_5 integrin, connexin 26 and connexin 32	OX43 (MCA 276), OX44 (MCA 371, CD 37), OX42 (MCA 275, CD118), c-Kit, stem cell factor receptor, hemopoietic heparan sulfate-PG (serglycin), GM-CSF, CSF, α_4 integrin, and red blood cell antigen
SHARED Antigenic Markers:	all known oval cell antigens, tranferrins, γ glutamyl transpeptidase (GGT), glucuronyl transferases (some isoforms), glutathione-S-transferases, ligandins, cEBP isoforms, IL-1 receptor, IL-6 receptor, interferon receptor, HGF receptor, insulin receptor, MDR1 and MDR2 (multidrug resistance genes), and connexin 43	

The cadherin molecular family of 723-748-residue transmembrane proteins provides yet another avenue of cell-cell adhesion that is cell-specific.[977] Cadherins are linked to the cytoskeleton. The classical cadherins include E- (epithelial), N- (neural or A-CAM), and P- (placental) cadherin, but in 1998 at least 12 different members of the family were known.[980] They are concentrated (though not exclusively found) at cell-cell junctions on the cell surface and appear to be crucial for maintaining multicellular architecture. Cells adhere preferentially to other cells that express the identical cadherin type. Liver hepatocytes express only E-; mesenchymal lung cells, optic axons and neuroepithelial cells express only N-; epithelial lung cells express both E- and P-cadherins. Members of the cadherin family also are distributed in different spatiotemporal patterns in embryos, with the expression of cadherin types changing dynamically as the cells differentiate.[977]

Carbohydrates are crucial in cell recognition. All cells have a thin sugar coating (the glycocalyx; Section 8.5.3.2) consisting of glycoproteins and glycolipids, of which ~3000 different motifs had been identified by 1998. The repertoire of carbohydrate cell surface structures changes characteristically as the cell develops, differentiates, or sickens. For example[415]:

1. The array of carbohydrates on cancer cells is strikingly different from that on normal cells.
2. A unique trisaccharide (SSEA-1 or Le^x) appears on the surfaces of cells of the developing embryo exactly at the 8- to 16-cell stage when the embryo compacts from a group of loose cells into a smooth ball.
3. Bacterial pathogens often use cell-specific sugars[981] to guide them to their preferred targets—*E. coli* are abundant in tissues surrounding the ureters leading from kidneys to bladder but are rarely found in the upper respiratory tract; group A *streptococci*, which colonize only the upper respiratory tract and skin, rarely cause urinary tract infections; the gonorrhea organism *Neisseria gonorrhoeae* adheres only to cells of the genital and oral epithelia but not to cells of other organs.[415] These bacterial carbohydrate specificities (e.g., carbohydrate-specific bacterial adhesins, lectins, and glycoconjugates) have been at least partially catalogued.[981,3356-3370] and molecular dynamics studies have begun.[3353-3355]

Carbohydrate motifs are in theory more combinatorically diverse than nucleotide- or protein-based structures. While nucleotides and amino acids can interconnect in only one way, the monosaccharide units in oligosaccharides and polysaccharides can attach at multiple points. Thus two amino acids can make only two distinct dipeptides, but two identical monosaccharides can bond to form 11 different disaccharides because each monosaccharide has 6 carbons, giving each unit 6 different attachment points for a total of 6 + 5 = 11 possible combinations. Four different nucleotides can make only 24 distinct tetranucleotides, but four different monosaccharides can make 35,560 unique tetrasaccharides, including many with branching structures.[415] A single hexasaccharide can make ~10^{12} distinct structures, vs. only 6.4 x 10^7 structures for a hexapeptide; a 9-mer carbohydrate has a mole of isomers.[3122]

The coded sugar coating of red cells has already been described (Fig. 8.35). As another example, the CD44 family of transmembrane glycoproteins are 80-95 kilodalton cell adhesion receptors that mediate ECM binding, cell migration and lymphocyte homing. CD44 antigen shows a wide variety of cell-specific and tissue-specific glycosylation patterns, with each cell type decorating the CD44 core protein with its own unique array of carbohydrate structures.[972,973] Distinct CD44 cell surface molecules have been found in lymphocytes, macrophages, fibroblasts, epithelial cells, and keratinocytes. CD44 expression in the nervous system is restricted to the white matter (including astrocytes and glial cells) in healthy young people, but appears in gray matter accompanying age or disease.[972] A few tissues are CD44 negative, including liver hepatocytes, kidney tubular epithelium, cardiac muscle, the testes, and portions of the skin.[972]

The selectin family of ~50 kilodalton cell adhesion receptor glycoprotein molecules[976,978] can recognize diverse cell-surface antigen carbohydrates and help localize leukocytes to regions of inflammation (leukocyte trafficking). Selectins are not attached to the cytoskeleton.[980] Leukocytes display L-selectin, platelets display P-selectin, and endothelial cells display E-selectin (as well as L and P) receptors. Cell-specific molecules recognized by selectins include tumor mucin oligosaccharides (recognized by L, P, and E), brain glycolipids (P and L), neutrophil glycoproteins (E and P), leukocyte sialoglycoproteins (E and P), and endothelial proteoglycans (P and L).[976] The related MEL-14 glycoprotein homing receptor family allows lymphocyte homing to specific lymphatic tissues coded with "vascular addressin"—cell-specific surface antigens found on cells in the intestinal Peyer's patches, the mesenteric lymph nodes, lung-associated lymph nodes, synovial cells and lactating breast endothelium. Homing receptors also allow some lymphocytes to distinguish between colon and jejunum.[937,974] Selectin-related interactions, along with chemoattractant receptors and with integrin-Ig, regulate leukocyte extravasation (Section 9.4.4.1) in series, establishing a three-digit "area code" for cell localization in the body.[1495]

Viral capsid proteins are readily recognized, permitting identification of many virus species.[3371-3375] Enveloped viruses, which have acquired a lipid membrane coating borrowed from the host cell upon release,[1969,3375] will be more difficult to detect by simple surface marker sensing. A lipid-penetrating sensor or a host-cell "decoy" sensor (activating membrane fusion protein release (Section 9.4.5.4) by the virus, thus revealing its true identity) may be more useful.

Finally, cells may be typed according to their indigenous transmembrane cytoskeleton-related proteins. For example, erythrocyte membranes contain glycophorin C (~25 kilodaltons, ~3000 molecules/micron^2) and band 3 ion exchanger (90-100 kilodaltons, ~10,000 molecules/micron^2);[980,3655] platelet membranes incorporate the GP Ib-IX glycoprotein complex (186 kilodaltons); cell membrane extensions in neutrophils require the transmembrane protein ponticulin (17 kilodaltons); and striated muscle cell membranes contain a specific laminin-binding glycoprotein (156 kilodaltons) at the outermost part of the transmembrane dystrophin-glycoprotein complex.[980] There are also a variety of carbohydrate-binding proteins (lectins) that appear frequently on cell surfaces, and can distinguish different monosaccharides and oligosaccharides.[415] Cell-specific lectins include the galactose (asialoglycoprotein)-binding and fucose-binding lectins of hepatocytes, the mannosyl-6-phosphate (M6P) lectin of fibroblasts, the mannosyl-N-acetylglucosamine-binding lectin of alveolar macrophages, the galabiose-binding lectins of uroepithelial cells, and several galactose-binding lectins in heart, brain and lung.[415,970,981,3361]

Each cell expresses a different set of genes from the genome, and each gene normally represents a different protein (although in some cases alternate splicing can generate several proteins from the same gene; Chapter 20). Thus it seems plausible to conclude that each different cell type uses a unique constellation of proteins in its construction which can be detected as a set by nanorobot chemosensors, thus unambiguously identifying the cell type.

(Of course, possibly up to ~50-70% of the proteins in different cells may be the same, serving common "housekeeping" functions.) If there are ~400 cell types (including all varieties of smooth muscle cells, neuron cells, and other cytochemically distinct cell subcategories not fully enumerated in Appendix C), then every cell type in the catalog may be uniquely identified using as few as $\sim\log_2(400) \sim 9$ binary antigenic markers. Given that Nature has employed ~580 markers among the HLA specificities and ~254 markers in the blood group systems to distinguish self from nonself, it is clear that biological systems may employ considerable multifunctionality and redundancy. By 1998 a complete catalog of all cell-specific antigens had not yet been compiled. However, the completion of sequencing of ~90% of the human genome by the spring of 2000[3186] (with the complete version finished by 2002-2003[3186,3187]), and foreseeable advances in DNA chip technology (used to sample gene expression patterns), should allow the rapid determination of unique sets of cell-specific antigens by circa 2002-2005.

In the worst case, 9 unique antigenic markers would be required for each of at most ~400 cell types, giving a maximum of 3600 antigenic markers needed to positively identify all cell types. From Eqn. 8.5, a $\sim(300\ \text{nm})^2$ chemotactic pad with $N_{spec} = 3600$ implies a maximum cell typing measurement time $t_{meas} \sim 400$ sec in mapping mode. If a more plausible working set of ~300 key antigenic markers will suffice, then $t_{meas} \sim 3$ sec in mapping mode. On the other hand, a nanorobot searching for a particular set of $N_{spec} = 9$ binary antigenic markers (e.g., seeking only liver cells, rejecting all nonliver cells) requires just $t_{meas} \sim 0.002$ sec to make the cell-type determination.

8.5.3 Cytography

Cytography is concerned with the "geography" of the cell and directing navigation through the intracellular spaces. Discussion of the nucleus, the largest and most important cellular organelle, is deferred to Section 8.5.4. Methods of cell entry are described in Section 9.4.5.

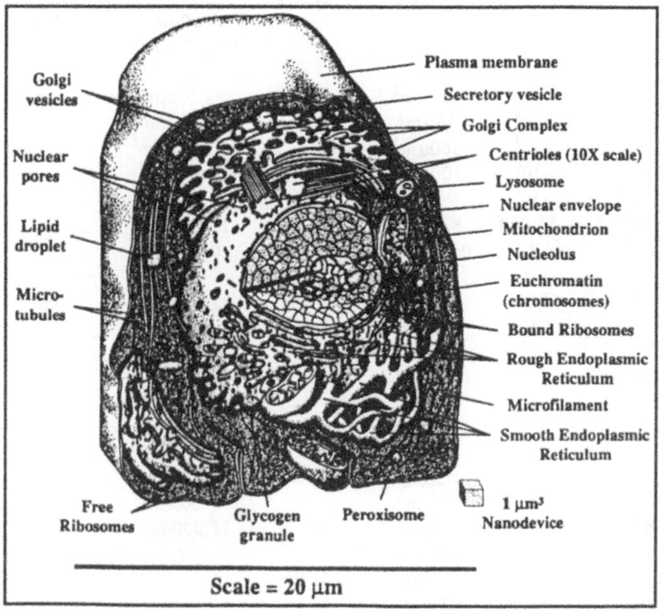

Fig. 8.36. Schematic cutaway view of a typical human cell (redrawn from Guyton[863]).

8.5.3.1 Overall Cellular Structure

As recently as the late 1970s, the cell was often incorrectly described as a water-filled membranous sac enclosing a loosely structured population of discrete organelles. In reality, the interior of a cell is extremely compact, only a few times more open than a hydrated protein crystal.[941] The cell interior is crisscrossed by many tens of thousands of cytoskeletal filaments of various gauges, attaching organelles to the nucleus, the plasma membrane, the ECM, and to each other.[942]

Cells also have various shapes. Most cells are surrounded by and are anchored to neighboring cells. Such immobilized cells usually assume a polyhedral shape. Specialized cells adopt shapes related to the specific functions they perform. A dramatic example is the nerve cell, which has one or more cylindrical processes extending from the cell like the branches of a tree, which processes allow the cell to receive and to transmit electrical signals.

From the nanomedical perspective, the cell (Fig. 8.36) may be regarded as a large machine constructed of many smaller machines.[182] These smaller machines are the organelles. Organelles are typically 0.5-3 microns in diameter, roughly the same size as the largest bloodborne medical nanorobots. Table 8.17 is a very approximate quantification of the known classes of cellular organelles and other major cellular components. Cytoskeletal number densities are crude but self-consistent estimates. Actual data may differ widely from the values given in the table depending upon:

1. size, age, and type of cell;
2. global and local respiration, nutrition and energy demand;
3. tissue and organ location;
4. environmental factors such as temperature, pressure, salinity, ECM activity, and extracytosolic toxicology; and
5. cellular secretory and mitotic status.

Organelles represent the principal metabolic and structural machinery of the cell. Each organelle type or cellular component is engineered to carry out specific functions while maintaining a specific structure, as described briefly below.

The small size of most organelles makes intra-organelle locomotion by whole nanorobots difficult or impossible, with the possible exception of the nucleus (Sections 8.5.4 and 9.4.6). This does not

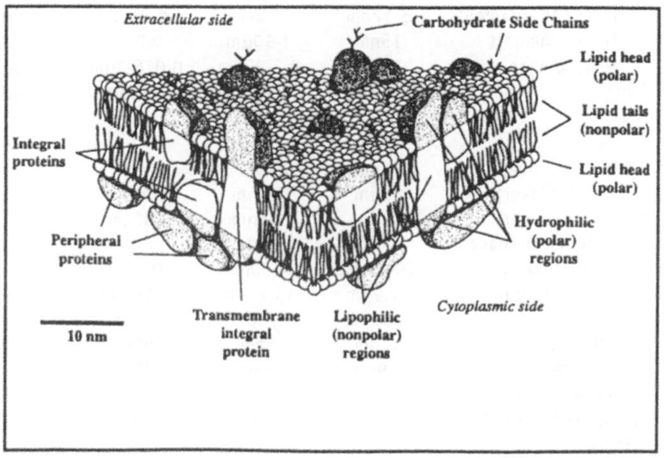

Fig. 8.37. Fluid mosaic model of the lipid bilayer membrane, with embedded proteins (redrawn from Murray et al[996]).

Table 8.17. Approximate Quantification of the Components of a Typical 20-μm Human Tissue Cell[531,997]

Cellular Component or Organelle	Typical Diameter	Typical Length or Thickness	Typical Surface Area	Typical Volume	Typical Number per Cell	Total Item Volume in Cell	Total Item Volume as a %	Total Item Surface Area in Cell	Total Item Surface Area as a %
Glycocalyx (external to cell)	~20μm	10-50nm	2400μm^2	12-120μm^3	1	12-120μm^3		2400μm^2	0.5%
Plasma membrane *(~900 kg/m^3)*	20μm	6-10nm	2400μm^2	14-24μm^3	1	~20μm^3	0.3%	2400μm^2	0.5%
Ribosomes	25nm	15-30nm	0.002μm^2	8000nm^3	~10^7	80μm^3	1.0%	20,000μm^2	4.3%
Rough endoplasmic reticulum	~μm	--	--	1120μm^3	1	1120μm^3	14.0%	--	
Cisternae	--	--	--	720μm^3	--	720μm^3		--	
Membrane	--	5-6nm	70,000μm^2	400μm^3	--	400μm^3		70,000μm^2	14.9%
Smooth endoplasmic reticulum	~μm	--	--	420μm^3	1	420μm^3	5.3%	--	
Cisternae	--	--	--	240μm^3	--	240μm^3		--	
Membrane	--	5-6nm	32,000μm^2	180μm^3	--	180μm^3		32,000μm^2	6.8%
Golgi complex *(~1090 kg/m^3)*	~μm	--	--	410-510μm^3	1-300 stks	450μm^3	5.6%	--	
Cisternae	--	--	--	300-400μm^3	--	350μm^3		--	
Membrane	--	avg. 8nm	14,000μm^2	110μm^3	--	110μm^3		14,000μm^2	3.0%
Golgi vesicles *(~1120 kg/m^3)*	30-80nm	--	0.008μm^2	65,000nm^3	~200,000	13μm^3	0.2%	1400μm^2	0.3%
Secretory vesicles *(~1120 kg/m^3)*	0.1-1μm	--	0.13μm^2	0.004μm^3	~50,000	210μm^3	2.6%	6000μm^2	1.3%
Glycogen granules *(1560 kg/m^3)*	10-40nm	--	0.002μm^2	10,000nm^3	~100,000	1μm^3	0.01%	200μm^2	0.04%
Lipid droplets *(850 kg/m^3)*	0.2-5μm	--	~1μm^2	0.1μm^3	~100?	10μm^3	0.1%	100μm^2	0.02%
Vaults	55nm	30nm	0.003μm^2	50,000nm^3	~3000	0.16μm^3	0.002%	10μm^2	0.002%
Lysosomes *(1120 kg/m^3)*	0.5-1μm	--	--	0.31μm^3	~300	~90μm^3	1.1%	--	
Body	--	--	--	0.30μm^3	--	~90μm^3		--	
Membrane	--	5-6nm	2.2μm^2	0.01μm^3	--	0.017μm^3		600μm^2	0.1%
Proteasomes	~11nm	~36nm	0.002μm^2	3400nm^3	~10^7	~20μm^3	0.2%	8000μm^2	1.7%
Peroxisomes *(1250 kg/m^3)*	0.5-1μm	--	--	0.31μm^3	~300	~90μm^3	1.1%	--	
Body	--	--	--	0.30μm^3	--	~90μm^3		--	
Membrane	--	5-6nm	2.2μm^2	0.01μm^3	--	0.017μm^3		600μm^2	0.1%
Mitochondria *(1190 kg/m^3)*	0.5-1μm	2-3μm	6.3μm^2	~1μm^3	300-3000	1000μm^3	12.5%	--	
Outer membrane		5-6nm	6.3μm^2	0.035μm^3	--	--		6000μm^2	1.3%
Inner membrane		5-6nm	30μm^2	0.17μm^3	--	--		(30,000μm^2)	
Cytoskeleton, total	--	--	--	--	1	875μm^3	10.9%	280,000μm^2	59.2%
Superfine filaments	2-4nm	10-100nm	400nm^2	450nm^3	~10^8	45μm^3		40,000μm^2	
Microfilaments	5-7nm	~μm	0.02μm^2	36,000nm^3	~10^7	360μm^3		200,000μm^2	
Intermed. filaments	8-12nm	~μm	0.03μm^2	100,000nm^3	~10^6	100μm^3		30,000μm^2	
Thick filaments	15nm	1-10μm	0.2μm^2	900,000nm^3	<10^4	--		--	
Microtubules	25nm	0.2-25μm	0.016-2μm^2	0.0001-0.02μm^3	~50,000	370μm^3		10,000μm^2	
Centrioles	150nm	300-500nm	0.22μm^2	0.007μm^3	2	0.014μm^3	0.0002%	0.44μm^2	
Nucleus, total	8μm	--	--	268μm^3	1	268μm^3	3.4%	27,500μm^2	5.9%
Nuclear envelope	8μm	--	--	--	1	--		400μm^2	
(Outer layer)	~8μm	7-8nm	200μm^2	1.5μm^3	--	1.5μm^3		200μm^2	
(Inner layer)	~8μm	7-8nm	200μm^2	1.5μm^3	--	1.5μm^3		200μm^2	
Perinuclear space	--	20-40nm	--	6μm^3	1	6μm^3		--	
Nuclear pores	70-90nm	~100nm	~40,000nm^2	0.0005μm^3	2000-4000	1.5μm^3		120μm^2	
Nuclear cortex	~7.9μm	30-40nm	196μm^2	6.9μm^3	1	6.9μm^3		196μm^2	
Nucleolus	<5μm	--	<78μm^2	25-65μm^3	1	45μm^3		--	
Nucleosomes	10nm	6nm	350nm^2	400nm^3	2.5 x 10^6	10μm^3		8750μm^2	
Chromatin	1.9nm	65mm	390μm^2	0.18μm^3	46	8.3μm^3		18,000μm^2	
Nucleoplasm	--	--	--	~206μm^3	1	~206μm^3		--	
Cytosol *(~1020 kg/m^3)*	--	--	--	~3348μm^3	1	~3348μm^3	41.9%	--	
Cytoplasm	--	--	--	~7712μm^3	1	~7712μm^3	96.4%	--	
Cell, total *(~1064 kg/m^3)*	~20μm	~20μm	2400μm^2	8000μm^3	1	8000μm^3	100%	469,000μm^2	100%

preclude insertion of specialized sensory tools or small manipulatory devices into organelle interiors.

8.5.3.2 Cell Membrane

The cell and most organelles are individually surrounded by their own thin envelope. The envelope surrounding the entire cell is called the plasma membrane.[1968] According to the fluid mosaic model,[1189] all membranes are composed of a double layer of lipid molecules, called the lipid bilayer, in which proteins are embedded (Fig. 8.37). The lipid bilayer acts as a barrier to the diffusion of polar solutes, whereas the embedded proteins provide the pathways for

1. the selective transfer of certain molecular substances through the lipid barrier, and
2. the mechanical transfer of information from the ECM into the interior of the cell.

The plasma membrane actually represents only a tiny fraction of the total membrane surface in the cell. For example, the combined membrane surface area of the endoplasmic reticulum (Section 8.5.3.5) is 44 times larger than the plasma membrane surface area for a typical human cell (Table 8.17).

Lipid bilayer plasma membranes are 6-10 nm thick. The major membrane lipids are phospholipids, fatty acid chains in the range of 16-18 carbons long; chains with fewer than 12 carbons cannot form a stable bilayer.[939] Phospholipid chains are amphipathic molecules—one end, the head, has a negatively-charged (polar) region, while the remainder of the molecule, the tail, consists of two (nonpolar) long fatty acid chains. The phospholipids in cell membranes self-organize into a bimolecular layer, with the nonpolar fatty acid chains in the middle. The polar regions are oriented toward the membrane surfaces due to their attraction to the polar water molecules in the extracellular and cytosolic fluids (Fig. 8.37).

The plasma membrane also contains other lipids (Table 8.18). For example, cholesterol, a steroid lipid, acts as a "mortar" that fills in small gaps in the phospholipid structure, thus improving membrane impermeability to small water-soluble molecules like glucose by a factor of ten. Cholesterol also acts as a membrane antifreeze agent, decreasing bilayer fluidity at higher temperatures (e.g., raising lipid bilayer "melting point") and preventing hydrocarbon chains of phospholipids from aggregating at lower temperatures (e.g., lowering membrane "freezing point"). Plasma membranes may contain up to ~1 cholesterol molecule for each phospholipid molecule. The precise lipid composition of plasma membranes varies from one cell type to another, and also varies among the membranes of organelles within each cell type (Table 8.18). Medical nanorobots equipped with suitable chemosensors may access this information, both for cell type identification during extracellular navigation and for organelle type identification during intracellular navigation.

There are ~5 x 10^6 lipid molecules in a 1 micron^2 area of lipid bilayer[531] or ~2.5 bilayer lipid pairs/nm^2 of cell membrane surface. Thus the plasma membrane of a typical 20-micron human tissue cell contains ~10 billion lipid molecules. Phospholipids are not covalently bound to each other, so each lipid molecule is free to move independently, resulting in considerable random lateral movement parallel to the bilayer surfaces. The long fatty acid chains each include one unsaturated bond, producing a kink in the otherwise straight chain that prevents close packing (and solidification). The chains also wiggle back and forth, so the lipid bilayer has fluidlike characteristics much like a layer of oil on a water surface. Movement of hydrophilic head groups through the hydrophobic interior of the membrane is thermodynamically unfavorable. Such flip-flopping, or transverse diffusion, does occur in membrane lipids but is relatively slow. For instance, a typical phospholipid molecule undergoes transverse diffusion (one flip flop between monolayers) once every several hours in a lipid bilayer. By contrast, lateral diffusion of phospholipids (movement within each monolayer) is so rapid that a lipid molecule can move 10 microns (the equivalent of ~12% of cell circumference) in a few seconds.[939] (But see Section 9.4.3.3 regarding the membrane-skeleton fence model.)

Membrane proteins are embedded in the lipid bilayer plasma membrane. Indeed, it has been said that the lipid bilayer serves as a "solvent" for membrane proteins.[531] The plasma membrane contains roughly equal masses of lipid and protein (Table 8.18). However, the mass of an individual protein molecule is much larger than the mass of any lipid molecule, so there are 10-100 times more lipid molecules than protein molecules.[997] The plasma membrane of a typical 20-micron human tissue cell contains ~0.1 billion protein molecules.

There are two classes of membrane proteins: Integral (intrinsic) membrane proteins and peripheral (extrinsic) membrane proteins.

Integral membrane proteins are closely associated with membrane lipids and cannot be extracted from the membrane without disrupting

Table 8.18. Mass % Biochemical Composition of Cell and Organelle Membranes[531,939,996,997]

Type of Membrane Molecule	Liver Cell Plasma Membrane	Red Cell Plasma Membrane	Myelin Sheath	Mitochondrion Inner/Outer Membranes	Endoplasmic Reticulum Membrane	*E.coli* (Bacterial Membrane)
Lipid	--	40%	~81%	~24%/~48%	--	--
Protein	~50%	52%	~19%	~76%/~52%	~50%	~50%
Carbohydrate	--	8%	--	--	--	--
Lipid Class:						
Cholesterol	17%	23%	22%	3%	6%	0%
Phospholipids						
Phosphatidylethanolamine	7%	18%	15%	35%	17%	70%
Phosphatidylserine	4%	7%	9%	2%	5%	trace
Phosphatidylcholine	24%	17%	10%	39%	40%	0%
Sphingomyelin	19%	18%	8%	0%	5%	0%
Glycolipids	7%	3%	28%	trace	trace	0%
Other lipids	22%	13%	8%	21%	27%	30%

the lipid bilayer. Like phospholipids, integral proteins are amphipathic. Polar amino acid side chains lie in one region of the molecule and nonpolar side chains are in a separate region. Thus integral proteins vertically align with the amphipathic lipids in the plasma membrane—protein polar regions position themselves at the surfaces in association with polar water molecules, while the protein nonpolar regions are attracted to the interior in association with the nonpolar fatty acid chains at the center of the lipid bilayer membrane (Fig. 8.37; see also Figures 8.33 and 8.34). Many integral proteins can move laterally in the membrane; others are immobilized by links to a network of peripheral proteins located near the cytoplasmic surface of the membrane. How fast do embedded proteins laterally diffuse? If a single hybrid cell is created by fusing two cells having radiochemically-tagged membrane protein molecules, ~1 hour is needed for the two populations of transmembrane protein molecules to become thoroughly randomly intermixed.[939]

Most integral proteins are transmembrane proteins with polar regions at each end and a nonpolar region in the middle, spanning the entire membrane. These polar regions may extend up to 10-20 nm beyond the surface of the lipid bilayer, forming channels through which water, ions, or chemical signals can pass into the cell (Section 3.3.3). A few integral proteins do not cross the entire membrane and are found only in the outer or inner layer, performing functions localized to only one membrane surface. These proteins are also amphipathic and oriented parallel to the lipid molecules. Some are anchored to the membrane by covalent bonds with phospholipids. For example, in the red blood cell membrane, glycophorin spans the entire membrane, all glycolipids and most of the phosphatidylcholine are in the outer monolayer, and the majority of the phosphatidylethanolamine and phosphatidylserine molecules are in the inner monolayer where most of the proteins reside. (Cholesterol is distributed about equally between the two layers.) The number of different integral proteins in a membrane ranges from 6-8 in the sarcoplasmic reticulum to over 100 in the plasma membrane (including enzymes, transport and structural proteins, antigens and receptors), many of which are present in only a few copies per cell, although the 135 $micron^2$ red cell surface has ~1 x 10^6 copies of the glycophorin A molecule and ~1 x 10^5 copies of glycophorin B.[1091]

Peripheral membrane proteins are bound to the hydrophilic regions of integral membrane proteins or to the hydrophilic heads of membrane lipids by weak electrostatic forces.[939] Most peripheral proteins are located near the cytoplasmic surface of the plasma membrane rather than on the extracellular surface and mediate such properties as cell shape and motility. Peripheral proteins are not amphipathic and do not associate with the hydrophobic regions of the lipids in the membrane interior.

Both lipid and protein components of the plasma membrane are continually removed and replaced. Turnover allows the cell to continuously change out damaged components. This is a highly selective process, since the rate of turnover varies for different proteins and lipids. For instance, the half-life of some phospholipids in membranes is ~10,000 sec;[939] the "off-rate" (half-life) for cholesterol from a lipid bilayer (e.g., the red cell surface) into the cytoplasm is ~7200 sec at 310 K.[1113] Protein turnover half-lives may range from several minutes to several years, but the "typical" protein has a turnover half-life of ~200,000 sec[531,939] or ~2 days. Protein replacement is carried out by protease enzymes located in the cytoplasm and in lysosomes. Replacement rates also depend upon cell type. For example, the plasma membrane surface of the macrophage has an unusually fast mean turnover time, ~1800 sec, vs. ~5400 sec for fibroblasts.[996]

The plasma membrane also contains small amounts of carbohydrate. This carbohydrate is covalently linked to some of the membrane lipids and proteins. Carbohydrate portions of the membrane glycoproteins (e.g., Section 8.5.2) are always located at the extracellular surface, forming the glycocalyx (together with collagen proteins and glycosaminoglycans, aka "mucopolysaccharides"). The red cell membrane, for instance, contains 52% protein, 40% lipid, and 8% carbohydrate by weight.[939] A small proportion of membrane carbohydrate is glycolipids, but most is in the form of glycoproteins. The sugar units are usually short oligosaccharide chains attached to serine, threonine, or asparagine side chains.

The glycocalyx, or fuzzy coat, lies exterior to the plasma membrane. In most cell types, the glycocalyx is 10-100 nm thick consisting of tangled strands of up to ~10,000-atom glycoproteins each measuring 5-8 nm thick and up to 100-200 nm in length.[531,998] The experimentally-measured thickness of the glycocalyx of various cells ranges from ~6 nm for human blood-group A erythrocytes,[3163] to 13 nm in *Eimeria* microgametes,[3588] 20-30 nm for chick fibroblasts,[3589] 30-60 nm for human bladder cells,[3590] 40-70 nm for human lymphocytes,[3591] ~50 nm for human myocardial cells,[3592] 56 nm for frog mesenteric microvessels,[3593] >70 nm for rat vasculature,[3594] ~81 nm for rabbit endothelial cells of the systemic arteries (e.g. carotid),[3164] and 90 nm for human cochlear hair cells.[3595] The most prominent glycocali are found in intestinal epithelial cells, where the fuzzy coat may reach 150 nm in thickness and consists primarily of oligosaccharide chains 1.2-2.5 nm in diameter.[939] (There is one report of rat venule endothelial cells with glycocali up to 870 nm thick,[3594] and a few macroscopic parasites such as the fork-tailed cercariae of the blood fluke *Schistosoma mansomi* have glycocali 500-2000 nm thick.[3596])

The glycoproteins of the glycocalyx provide a set of highly specific biological markers that are readily recognizable by suitably equipped medical nanorobots. These markers assist normal cellular interactions by allowing blood group recognition, bacterial and toxin binding sites, egg recognition by sperm, immune responses, guidance of embryonic development, and cellular lifespan determination (e.g. the red cell coat thins with age which may serve as an RBC removal signal for phagocytes and in the liver).[940]

The cell's surface is also strewn with numerous pits and indentations. For example, one class of these is the "coated pits" whose inner surfaces are covered by a dense layer of the protein clathrin, important in receptor-mediated endocytosis wherein proteins and other large molecules are imported into the cytoplasm (Section 8.5.3.7). Another class of membrane indentation is the ~50 nm caveolae ("tiny caves") that serve to draw substances such as vitamins and signal transduction molecules into the cell's interior.[1137,3376-3379] Caveolae are coated with a unique membrane marker protein called caveolin, making them easy for nanorobots to identify.

8.5.3.3 Cytosol

In traditional cell biology, the "cytoplasm" is the filling substance in the large space enclosed by the plasma membrane and surrounding the cell nucleus. It includes all non-nuclear cell organelles plus all fluid surrounding these organelles. Every point inside the cell, except the nucleus, is considered part of the cytoplasm. The "cytosol" is the liquid that fills all of the cytoplasmic region, except for fluids filling the interior of the cell organelles. Finally, the term "intracellular fluid" refers to all of the fluid inside a cell—the cytosol plus the fluid inside each organelle, including the nucleus. Internal hydrostatic pressure in the cytosol ranges from ~23 N/m^2 in the human erythrocyte cell[1452] up to ~1.6 x 10^5 N/m^2 in *Amoeba proteus*.[1453]

Fulton[941] points out that in an average protein crystal ~40% of crystal mass is solvent water—half strongly absorbed by the protein in the hydration shell and half resembling bulk water in its properties. Protein crystals may range from 20-90% solvent, or 10-80% protein, by weight. Muscle cells are ~23% protein, red cells ~35%, and actively growing cells contain 17-26% protein by weight.[938] Thus the cytosolic environment more closely resembles proteinaceous crystals than dilute solutions (e.g., <0.1% proteins).

Hydration water is not immobile water like ice, but it does have reduced mobility, different solvating characteristics, a higher heat capacity, and is generally more ordered than bulk water.[1936] Water of hydration coats the macromolecular cell components such as carbohydrates, nucleic acids, and the proteins of membranes, and is required for enzyme activity. Mammalian cells can maintain glycolysis and normal respiration down to 60% dehydration, which suggests that in a typical cell the cytosol may consist of ~60% bulk water and ~40% water of hydration. Distribution of ordered water in the cell is a heterogeneous and dynamic process, possibly cytonavigationally useful. For instance, ~55% of the water of the vegetal pole region of the frog oocyte is bound water, with only ~25% bound near the animal pole cytoplasm and ~10% bound in the nucleus.[1937]

Minton[1010] showed that the volume occupied by proteins affects the activity of the other proteins in solution by "crowding" them into a smaller volume where they have less freedom of movement, forcing them into compact configurations that would occur far less frequently in dilute solutions. These effects can produce 50-100-fold excesses in protein activity over the values predicted from dilute solutions. Crowding also reduces diffusion mobility—60%-70% of glycolytic enzymes are freely diffusing (30%-40% are immobilized on the matrix) in squid axoplasm that contains 2% protein by weight, but only 20% of cytoplasmic proteins are freely diffusing in oocyte cytoplasm that contains 30%-40% protein by weight.[941] Crowding effects could be nonspecific and due simply to protein number density, or they could be specific and maintained by selection. McConkey[1011] estimates that about half of the polypeptides in the cell may participate in specific associational structures. For instance, many enzymes exist in complexes that may involve a dozen or more proteins, potentially complicating required nanorobotic actions; according to the substrate channelling hypothesis, these complexes can help speed up reactions.

Even without these crowding effects, cells display localized biochemical gradients that are cytonavigationally significant. Specific molecules, organelles and physiological processes may be localized to defined zones within the cell. This regional cytoplasmic differentiation is regulated in part by cytosolic Ca^{++} ion and by H^+ ion (pH) spatial gradients.[1076,1077] As another example, the cytosol immediately surrounding the Golgi apparatus is compositionally distinct from the cytosol that closely encircles the cell nucleus.[531] Active chemical processing taking place within most cellular organelles produces persistent concentration gradients that may be used by in cyto nanorobots to establish proximity to specific organelles. Microsecond-cycle chemical nanosensors (Section 4.2.1) can sample the local environment far faster than the typical time required for a molecule to diffuse a distance of ~1 micron, the mean separation between adjacent major organelles inside human cells. Taking cytoplasm absolute viscosity $\eta \sim 6 \times 10^{-3}$ kg/m-sec,[362] then from Eqn. 3.1 the 1-micron diffusion time $\tau_{diffuse} >> t_{meas}$ (~1 microsec) for small molecules like amino acids or glucose ($\tau_{diffuse} \sim 5000$ microsec) or for 100,000-dalton macromolecules measuring ~10 nm in diameter ($\tau_{diffuse} \sim 130{,}000$ microsec).

Control proteins such as the transcription factors that regulate gene expression are typically present in only ~300-3000 copies of each type per cell. More common cytosolic proteins may be present in numbers up to 10^6-10^7 copies of each type per cell.

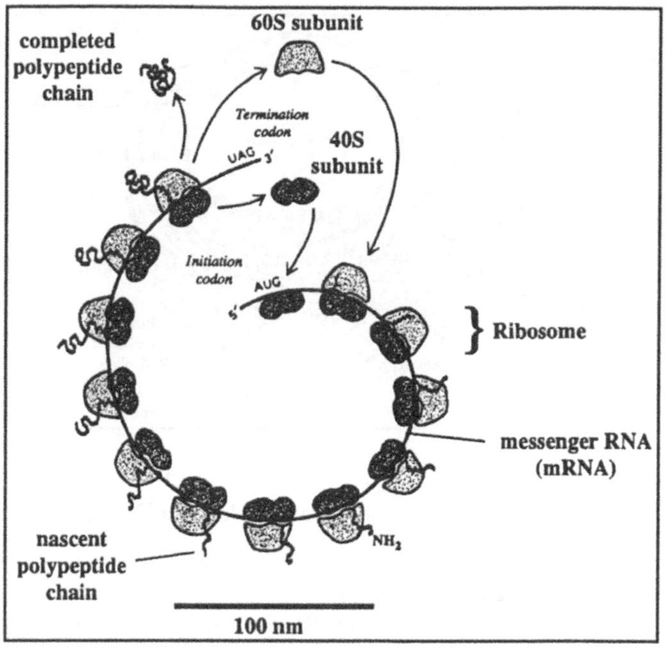

Fig. 8.38. Schematic of polyribosome (redrawn from Alberts et al[531]).

8.5.3.4 Ribosomes

Ribosomes are the smallest and most numerous "organelle" (macromolecular assembly) in the human cell. A typical liver cell contains 10^7 ribosomes constituting ~5% of the total dry mass of the cell. Cells less actively involved in protein synthesis have correspondingly fewer ribosomes. Some ribosomes float freely in the cytosol, making proteins for intracellular use. Others are attached to membranes or to the cytoskeleton, synthesizing proteins destined for membranes or for export from the cell.

Ribosomes are ~25 nm in diameter. Each of the several types of ribosome (containing rRNA) is constructed of two subunits that fit snugly together. A typical ribosome might have a mass of 4.2 million daltons, comprised of 2.8 million daltons for the large ribonucleoprotein 60S subunit (~23 nm diameter) and 1.4 million daltons for the small ribonucleoprotein 40S subunit (~9 nm diameter).[938,996] There is no intrinsic difference between free cytosolic ribosomes (50% or more of the total) and membrane-bound ribosomes—it is the "signal" sequence on the end of the protein being synthesized that directs a free ribosome to become a bound ribosome.

The ribosome is an ATP-powered protein-assembling machine (Fig. 2.2). Amino acids drawn from the cytosol are presented to the ribosome, which incorporates them one by one into polypeptides at ~20 Hz.[531] The complete synthesis of an average-sized protein takes 20-60 seconds. Even during this short period, multiple initiations take place, with a new ribosome hopping onto the 5' starting end of an mRNA (messenger) molecule almost as soon as the preceding ribosome has translated enough of the amino acid sequence to get out of the way, thus allowing the assembly of many copies of the same protein to proceed almost in parallel.[531] Thus, under physiological conditions, actively translated mRNA is found in polyribosomes, or polysomes, formed by gangs of multiple ribosomes spaced as close as 80 nucleotides apart along a single messenger molecule (Fig. 8.38). Further discussion of ribosomes may be found in Volume II.

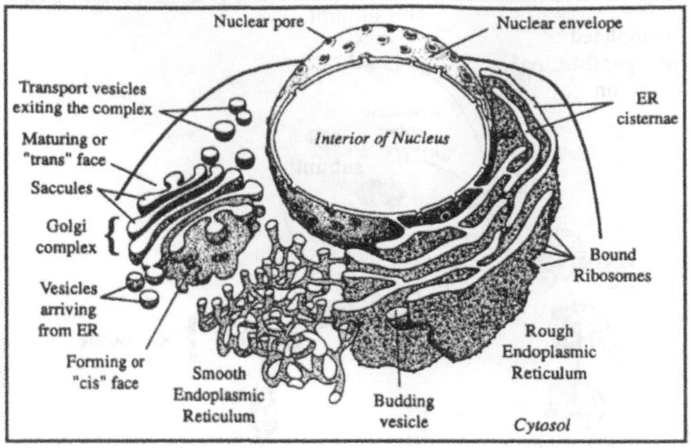

Fig. 8.39. Schematic of rough and smooth endoplasmic reticulum, and the Golgi complex (redrawn from Becker and Deamer[939]).

8.5.3.5 Endoplasmic Reticulum

The endoplasmic reticulum (ER), the principal protein manufacturing facility of the cell (aside from free ribosomes), is the most spatially extensive cytoplasmic organelle (Fig. 8.39). The ER is an interconnecting membranous network of fluid-filled vesicles, branching tubules, and flattened sacs or cavities called cisternae, possessed by almost all eukaryotic cells. The 5-6 nm thick membrane of the endoplasmic reticulum typically constitutes more than half of the total membrane surface area present in a cell. The membranes enclose a space that is continuous throughout the network and connects with the perinuclear space between the two membranes of the nuclear envelope (Section 8.5.4.1), allowing transport of manufactured substances throughout the cell. The fluid occupying the luminal or cisternal space of the ER, which is typically 20-40 nm wide but ranges from 10-70 nm, is called the reticuloplasm. There are ER-specific luminal proteins called reticuloplasmins found only in the reticuloplasm[999]—if these proteins are detected, a nanorobot has localized its position uniquely to this space. For example, molecular chaperones that assist in protein folding and are unique to the ER lumen include immunoglobin heavy-chain binding protein (BiP) and calnexin.[1080] BiP bears the "KDEL" amino acid sequence (Lys-Asp-Glu-Leu) at its C-terminus, a tagging sequence specifying that a protein is intended for attachment to the luminal surface of the ER cisterna.[996] There is evidence that specific compartments or subdomains within the ER may perform specialized functions and may also bear unique chemical markers,[1138] thus allowing nanorobots to distinguish different regions of the ER.

There are two varieties of endoplasmic reticulum—rough or "granular" ER, and smooth or "agranular" ER, both present in the same cell. One variety or the other may predominate in a given cell type depending on the specific functions performed by the cell, and the mix may change within the same cell during different periods of cell activity. Both are anchored to and mobilized by cytoskeletal motor proteins.

Rough ER is an extensive membranous network of flattened sheets with a flattened sac appearance and a continuous cisternal space that communicates directly with the perinuclear space. Ribosomes are bound to the ER membrane only on the cytosolic surface, loosely attached by short cylindrical conduits comprised of the Sec61 trimeric protein complex[1024] spanning the ER membrane and produced exclusively in the granular ER. Ribosome-produced proteins enter the cisternal space through these conduits, called translocons,[1018] in the ER membrane. Found in all nucleated cells except sperm, rough ER synthesizes proteins and packages proteins destined to be secreted by cells. The rough ER is also the site of the initial steps in the addition of sugar groups to glycoproteins by dolichol, a hydrophobic lipid that resides in the ER membrane with its active group facing the ER lumen.[997] Rough ER is especially abundant in cells that are specialized for protein secretion such as the pancreatic acinar cells and antibody-secreting plasma cells, or that are specialized for extensive membrane synthesis such as the immature egg cell or the retinal rod cell. In such cases, almost half of the total ribosomes present in the cell may be bound to the granular ER. Glycoproteins produced in the rough ER become encapsulated by bits of ER membrane, which bud off and migrate along cytoskeletal elements to the Golgi complex for further processing.

Smooth ER has a branched, tubular structure with no ribosomes on its surface, though its interior is continuous with the granular ER. Agranular ER has enzymes in the cisternal side of its membrane that allow it to synthesize carbohydrates, lipids (including neutral fats, phospholipids and steroids), and lipoproteins (in liver cells), and that allow it to assist in drug detoxification in the liver and kidney.[940] Muscle cells have a specialized, elaborate smooth ER called the sarcoplasmic reticulum that sequesters Ca^{++} (which controls muscle contraction) from the cytosol. Cells in the testes that synthesize steroid hormones from cholesterol have an expanded smooth ER compartment to accommodate enzymes needed to synthesize cholesterol and then to modify it to make steroid hormones.

8.5.3.6 Golgi Complex

The Golgi complex (GC) is a multicisternal membranous structure crudely similar to the rough ER (minus the ribosomes). Substances synthesized by the ER usually pass via vesicles traversing the cytoplasm on microtubule tracks to the Golgi complex, where they are further processed, concentrated, sorted, containerized in appropriate self-identifying new vesicles, and then shipped out to various destinations. Some oligosaccharides are synthesized in the ER, while extensive portions of the same structures are degraded in the Golgi—competing sets of reactions that are crucial in fixing the "address" of the intracellular compartment to which a newly synthesized macromolecule will be sent. Thus the GC serves as a production editor, allowing several successive sorting steps to take place while reducing the overall cytomanufacturing error rate. The Golgi acts as a "countercurrent" fractionation system to separate proteins destined for the plasma membrane from those to be retained in the ER.[1116]

Morphologically, the Golgi complex consists of a series of flattened, membranous saccules, forming disk-shaped cisternae that are stacked together to form a cup-shaped structure. Cisternal boundaries are morphologically distinct and are only rarely, if at all, connected.[3439,3440] A series of 5-8 saccules comprises a single Golgi stack or dictyosome, typically measuring ~1 micron in diameter and ~250 nm thick. As with the ER, the size and number of Golgi complexes vary according to cell type and metabolic activity. All eukaryotic cells have a GC. Some cells have just one stack; others, particularly those especially active in secretion, may have hundreds.[531] One enzyme, thiamine pyrophosphatase, occurs only in Golgi membranes,[939] and galactosyl transferase is found only in the GC.[996] These may be used by nanorobots as unique cytochemical markers of the Golgi complex.

The Golgi complex is a dynamic structure. The saccules of the GC form by the fusion of vesicles budded off from the ER. As these vesicles reach the GC and fuse, they give rise to new saccules on the forming ("cis") face of the organelle. Existing saccules move forward (outward) in the stack. Meanwhile, on the maturing ("trans") face of the GC, vesicles bud off the tips of the saccules continuously and exit the complex, transported on cytoskeletal elements through an interaction with motor proteins. This is known as the "cisternal maturation model."[2347,3443-3445] Within the Golgi, net membrane flow can be quite rapid. In certain mucus-secreting cells of the intestinal mucosa, it takes only ~2000 sec for membrane components to move from the forming face of a Golgi stack to the maturing face.[939] Vesicles exhibiting COPI (coat protein I) apparently transport some proteins backwards, both within the Golgi stack and also from the Golgi to the ER.[2347] One study counted ~400 individual vesicles in transit within ~0.2 microns of a ~4 micron^3 region containing 2 stacks of 7 cisternae.[3440]

The two faces of a Golgi stack are biochemically distinct. Specific enzymes and receptor proteins are concentrated in the cisterna on the "cis" face of the stack (the "receiving" end), while other proteins are localized mainly in the cisterna on the "trans" face (the "shipping" end). For example, the receptor protein for the carbohydrate mannose-6-phosphate (M6P) is present only in the forming cisterna of the Golgi stack, thus allowing the stack to recognize these proteins and target them to the lysosomes.[939] A 28,000-dalton protein called GS28 acts as one of the targeting receptors involved in the recognition of ER-derived vesicles that are destined for fusion with the cis-Golgi membrane.[1033] By 1998, more than two dozen different members of the small G protein superfamily (including the Rab and Arf protein families) had been implicated in the regulation of intracellular vesicular trafficking and membrane recognition. The Golgi complex also contains substantial amounts of cholesterol and sphingolipids, making a rising gradient from cis to trans.[1117] Various Golgi compartments are defined by the presence of particular enzymes (e.g., glycosidases, glycosyltransferases, and others involved in protein modification or sphingolipid synthesis) that are localized to one or more compartments, often in a graded manner.[1118,1119] While all cisternae are fenestrated and display coated buds, the trans-most cisterna produces exclusively clathrin-coated buds, whereas the others display only nonclathrin coated buds.[3440] Such distinctions will allow in cyto medical nanorobots with suitable transmembrane chemical sensor tools to readily establish Golgi stack configuration, polarity, and physical extent.

The Golgi stack has other easily detectable asymmetries. Since the GC mediates the flow of secretory proteins from the ER to the cell exterior, the GC displays spatially variant protein and lipid compositional gradients along the Golgi polarity axis. Specifically, the saccule membranes at the forming face resemble those of the ER in morphology and composition—~5-6 nm thick membranes defining a relatively narrow ~30-80 nm cisternal space, with ~20% phosphatidylcholine in the membrane. At the maturing pole, the saccule membranes more closely resemble the plasma membrane, ~10 nm thick, with a much wider cisternal space (>100 nm) and with ~10% phosphatidylcholine in the membrane. (Variable membrane thickness is part of the control mechanism for spatially anisotropic budding).[1113] Another asymmetry: Swarms of ~50 nm diameter membrane-bound vesicles always cluster on the side of the Golgi stack abutting the ER and along the circumference of a stack near the dilated rims of each cisterna.

8.5.3.7 Vesicles, Granules, and Vaults

For most membranes, such as those of the Golgi complex and lysosomes, the transfer of manufactured lipid and protein from the rough ER occurs by means of 30-80 nm transport vesicles that pinch off from the rough ER and fuse with the target membranes. Some of these vesicles are coated with a bristlelike polyhedral lattice of clathrin subunits.[3450,3451] Clathrin, a 180,000-dalton protein, is a distinctive feature of vesicles involved in a variety of intracellular transport processes. Besides bringing secretory proteins from the ER to the GC, clathrin-coated vesicles also transport membrane proteins from the GC to lysosomes (Section 8.5.3.8), to the plasma membrane (Section 8.5.3.2), and to other cellular destinations. In each case the clathrin coat forms a basket or cage around the vesicle, and transport involves cytoskeletal elements. Clathrins are cell specific—for example, neuron clathrins have 12 pentagons and 20 hexagons, liver clathrins have 30 hexagons, and fibroblast clathrins have 60 hexagons and thus may be distinguished by medical nanorobots. In cultured cells, assembly of a free clathrin-coated vesicle takes ~1 minute, and >300-1000/min can be formed.[3448,3449]

Cellular products are concentrated and packaged before being discharged to the outside of the cell, a process known as exocytosis. Concentration occurs as structures called condensing vacuoles located on the periphery of the Golgi complex fill with concentrated protein, then fuse with one another to form larger secretory granules and vesicles. Outbound vesicles are given unique membrane compositions, including high-specificity targeting molecules that can bind only to receptor molecules located on the appropriate surface of the target acceptor compartments. A well-known example is the synaptic vesicle targeting protein synaptobrevin (VAMP 1 and 2) which binds only to the neuron-specific plasma membrane proteins syntaxin 1A and 1B, thus ensuring proper vesicle docking and fusion at the neuron cell plasma membrane.[1079] In general, the fusion of two distinct lipid bilayers is energetically unfavorable in the absence of these specialized targeting proteins.

In some cells, the complementary process of endocytosis is also important.[3452] In endocytosis, the cell ingests extracellular materials by invaginating the plasma membrane, then budding off vesicles, vacuoles (phagocytic, pinocytotic, etc.), or "endosomes" to the interior of the cell from these sites. Endocytosis and exocytosis produce opposite membrane flows, the former reducing plasma membrane mass and the latter increasing it via fusion. The net membrane flow can be rather large in cells that carry out both processes actively. For instance, in cultured macrophages an amount of membrane equivalent to the entire surface area of the cell is replaced in ~1800 sec, and macrophages may ingest ~25% of their volume per hour.[996]

Storage granules are also important in the cell. For example, glycogen is the storage polysaccharide of the animal body, also known as animal starch. It is a polymer of glucose. In many cells, large individual molecules of polymerized glucose measuring 10-40 nm in diameter appear as granules. The enzymes needed to carry out the synthesis and degradation of glycogen (including the synthetic enzyme glycogen synthase and the degradative enzyme glycogen phosphorylase) are bound to the surface of these glycogen granules in a ~5 nm-thick shell. These granules constitute up to 4-6% by weight of liver cells (~5 million granules), up to 0.7-1% of muscle cells, with lesser amounts in other cells (typically <10^5 granules) and only very small amounts in the brain, and are absent in some cells.

Another storage vesicle found floating in the cytoplasm is the lipid droplet containing triglyceride, the main storage form of fatty acids in cells. In many cells, these insoluble triglycerides coalesce in the cytosol to form large, anhydrous droplets from 0.2-5 microns in diameter. In adipocytes, the cells specialized for fat storage, these droplets can be as large as 80 microns, occupying virtually the entire cytosol and constituting up to ~99% of the cell's organic matter.[938]

Other intracellular storage vessels include melanin pigment granules found in certain cells of the skin and hairs; zymogen (enzyme-containing) granules synthesized in pancreatic cells, then transported into the small intestine; inflammatory toxins stored as intracellular granules in eosinophil leukocytes; ferritin molecules containing cellular iron stores (each ~610-690 kilodalton molecule is comprised of 24 subunits of 18,500 daltons each, which surround in an 8-nm-diameter-cavity micellar form some 3000-4500 ferric atoms);[996,3380] and water vacuoles, mucus vesicles, and crystals of various types. The smallest observed effective hydrodynamic radius of sonicated phospholipid vesicles is ~10.25 nm independent of hydrocarbon chain length for synthetic even-numbered 12-18 carbon-chain phosphatidylcholines, and ~10.7 nm for egg-yolk phosphatidylcholine vesicles.[2949]

Finally, a related cell component is the vault, numbering in the thousands in human cells.[3381] Vaults are barrel-shaped particles measuring ~55 nm x 30 nm, assembled from 96 copies of MVP (major vault protein) plus some integral RNA. Vaults look like pairs of unfolding flowers, each half having 8 petals attached to a central ring with a small hook. Vaults were first discovered in the mid-1980s and their exact function was not yet known in 1998. However, their structure suggested an ability to open and close as a natural part of their function in the cell,[1410] and their size and shape would be an almost perfect match to dock at the nuclear pore complex[3382] (Section 8.5.4.2), which suggested to some investigators that vaults might serve to ferry mRNA around the cell.[1001,3381]

In 1998, the chemical content of individual vesicles was analyzed regularly using a combination of optical trapping, capillary electrophoresis separation, and laser-induced fluorescence detection.[1263]

8.5.3.8 Lysosomes and Proteasomes

Lysosomes are Golgi-budded organelles that contain ~40 digestive enzymes[531] capable of degrading all major classes of biological macromolecules — including at least 5 phosphatases, 4 proteases, 2 nucleases, 6 lipases, 12 glycosidases, and an arylsulfatase.[939] These enzymes are needed both to degrade materials brought into the cell from the outside and to degrade internal cellular structures that are damaged or are no longer needed. Lysosomal enzymes are acid hydrolases stored inside the lysosome as small granules 5-8 nm in diameter—protein aggregates of the hydrolytic enzymes with a pH optimum around 5, representing over 60% of organelle mass.[531] The lysosomes can release these enzymes after fusion with endosomes containing foreign matter, or to digest dead portions of the cell or malfunctioning organelles, or to destroy abnormal substances such as bacteria that enter the cell. An unusual oligosaccharide containing mannose-6-phosphate (M6P) serves as a recognition marker or address that targets all such enzymatic proteins to the lysosomes, and sorting nexins are proteins containing lysosomal targeting codes using either tyrosine- or di-leucine-based motifs.[1032] These membrane markers are readily detectable by nanorobots suitably equipped with transmembrane sensory tools, although it is important not to destroy the membrane integrity or to allow leaks (Section 9.4.5.5) which may alter fluid pH, during any probing. Since intralysosomal pH is different from the rest of the cell, chemosensors intended to probe the lysosomal interior may require a different design (or different detection parameters) than cytosolic chemosensors. In general, nanorobots can exploit the same biochemical markers that the cell normally uses to transport organelles to specific locations within the cell. Organelle surface chemosensing is most valuable for navigation and identification, while chemosensing of the organelle interior is also important for diagnosis and treatment (Chapter 21).

Lysosomes are spherical or nearly spherical organelles, typically 0.5-1 microns (range 50 nm—3 microns) in diameter. They vary greatly in appearance and content according to cell type and also in relation to the physiological state of a particular cell. The lysosome has a unique 5-6 nm three-layered membrane[938] with a special transmembrane transport protein that uses ATP to pump H^+ into the organelle lumen, thereby maintaining the internal pH at 5. The lysosomal membrane also has special docking marker acceptor proteins that mark a lysosome as a target for fusion with specific transport vesicles in the cell. Soluble products of digestion can cross the membrane, exit the organelle, and enter the cytosol for recycling into the cellular metabolism. Indigestible material slowly accumulates in the cytoplasm as lipofuscin pigment granules and other residual bodies. Lysosomes are present in most cells except red cells.

Although it is normally quite stable, the lysosome membrane can become more fragile when the cell is injured or deprived of oxygen or when excessive amounts of vitamin A are present. Lysosomes were once called "suicide sacs" because lysosomal rupture can result in self-digestion of the cell, a process known as autolysis. However, it is now known that lysosomes are part of the normal cellular digestion apparatus relating the process of endocytosis to the processes of intracellular synthesis, storage, and transport,[938] and structural deterioration of lysosomes does not occur rapidly in ischemic or post-mortem cells.[2019,2020] Most of the digestive enzymes require the low pH of the lysosomal or peroxisomal vesicles for activation (just as some proteases require the low pH of the stomach).

In addition to the lysosomal degradation system, there is also a large number of small cytosolic proteasomes (each having a 700,000-dalton 20S core complex ~11 nm in diameter). This serves as an extra-lysosomal ATP-driven system for selectively degrading endogenous ubiquitinated proteins in virtually all human cells[1087,1088,3383] (Chapter 13). Indeed, the ~2 megadalton 26S proteasome complex (containing 30-40 different proteins) appears to be the major protease of the nuclear and cytoplasmic compartments of the eukaryotic cell—proteasomal degradation controls the lifetime of most cellular proteins, including many regulatory proteins, and generates peptide antigens for presentation by MHC Class I molecules to $CD8^+$ cytotoxic T cells.[2915] Proteasomes are ubiquitous and very abundant, comprising up to 1% of total cellular protein.[1087,2916,2917] The entire 26S complex is 30-44 nm in length.

8.5.3.9 Peroxisomes

Peroxisomes (also called microbodies)[1000] are rough ER-budded organelles typically 0.1-1 microns in diameter.[531] Peroxisomes occur in most cells, but are most prominent in liver and kidney cells which are active in detoxification. The organelle destroys cytotoxic chemicals such as hydrogen peroxide, methanol, ethanol, formate, formaldehyde, nitrites and phenols, as well as D-amino acids which are not found in proteins and are not recognized by enzymes involved in the degradation of the more common L-amino acids. Peroxisomes also catalyze 25-50% of all fatty acid breakdown in cells (the remainder occurs in the mitochondria). The organelle is a concentrated source of three oxidative enzymes found in liver cells—D-amino acid oxidase, urate oxidase (usually present in a distinctive crystalline core), and catalase (which is up to 40% of total peroxisomal protein and most of the catalase present in a cell).

Peroxisomes may also protect cells from toxic oxygen levels,[3069-3072] since peroxisomal O_2 consumption is directly proportional to cellular oxygen concentration,[939] unlike mitochondrial respiration. In case of excessive O_2 levels, peroxisomal respiration is greatly stimulated, reducing the intracellular oxygen tension.

8.5.3.10 Mitochondria

Mitochondria are the principal chemical energy transducers of the eukaryotic cell under aerobic conditions.[3384] Except for the 10 reactions of the glycolytic pathway, all of the ATP-generating capacity of eukaryotes lies within the mitochondria. Mitochondria are scattered throughout the cytoplasm in virtually all aerobic cells, with numbers ranging from ~300/cell for relatively inactive cells like lymphocytes up to 2000-3000/cell for very active cells such as liver, kidney tubule and cardiac muscle cells (where mitochondria may occupy up to 20% of total cell volume).[531] Mitochondria are often clustered within the cell in regions of intense metabolic (hence ATP) demand. For instance, in muscle cells the mitochondria are organized in rows between adjacent contractive myofibrils in order to minimize the required diffusion distance for ATP molecules that are powering the activity. Similar localization appears in sperm tail flagella, in cilia, and at the base of kidney tubule cells where exchange with the blood is most rapid. Except for plant chloroplasts, mitochondria are unique among organelles in having their own DNA genomes, ribosomes and tRNAs that are quite different from those found in the cytoplasm.

After the nucleus, the mitochondrion is the largest organelle in most animal cells. The typical time-averaged dimensions are roughly cylindrical, with a 0.5-1.0 micron diameter and a ~3 micron length (and rarely, up to 10 microns)[939]—about the size of a bacterium or modest-sized medical nanodevice. Mitochondria are usually depicted as tiny kidney-bean- or sausage-shaped organelles, but in living cells they squirm, flex, elongate, and change shape almost continuously (Fig. 8.40) in part due to cytoskeletal interactions. Mitochondria may be shuttled around a cell at up to ~10 microns/sec via dynein motors[453] riding on microtubules (Section 8.5.3.11), bulging the plasma membrane as they travel.[1249]

Mitochondria have four functional compartments: outer membrane, intermembrane space, inner membrane, and the matrix. The outer surface is a smooth, featureless, 5-6 nm thick membrane[938] embedded with many copies of a transport protein that forms large aqueous channels through the lipid bilayer, so the membrane is permeable to all molecules of mass <10,000 daltons (which includes all metabolites pertinent to mitochondrial function). Since mitochondria do not grow by fusion with vesicles synthesized elsewhere in the cell, transfer of phospholipids from the endoplasmic reticulum to the mitochondrion requires special phospholipid transfer proteins in the outer membrane (e.g., glycerolphosphate acyltransferase and monoacyl glycerolphosphate acyltransferase) that can recognize a specific kind of phospholipid, remove it from a vesicle membrane and add it to the mitochondrial membrane. Special enzymes such as monoamine oxidase, acyl-CoA synthetase, and phospholipase A_2 are also present.[996] The first 32 N-terminal amino acids of cytochrome c1 constitute a fixed "leader sequence" that is recognized as a matrix targeting signal and allows the tagged molecule admission through the outer membrane.[997] Thus, as with other organelles, the outer coat of the mitochondrion should be immediately and uniquely recognizable by in cyto nanorobots equipped with suitable chemosensors (Section 4.2).

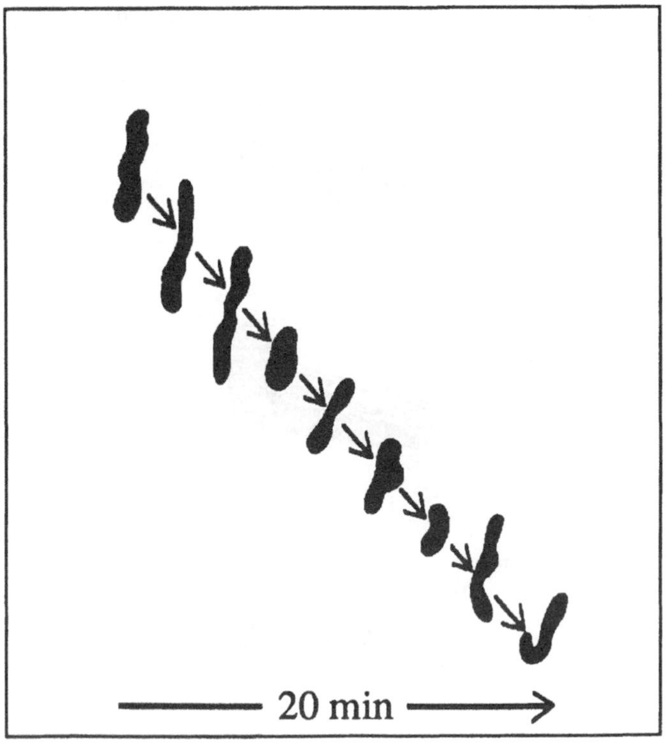

Fig. 8.40. Mitochondrial shape changes in living cells (redrawn from Alberts et al[531]).

The intermembrane space also contains numerous unique proteins, as for example the essential multispanning carrier (chaperone) proteins Tim10p and Tim12p.[1142]

The 5-6 nm thick inner membrane is highly convoluted, forming a series of ~30 infoldings (each fold ~100 nm wide) known as cristae, which extend into the inner compartment or matrix, roughly quintupling the active surface area of the outer membrane (Fig. 8.41). The inner membrane is rich in cardiolipin, a phospholipid that accounts for 10% of the membrane lipid content and renders it unusually impermeable to most solutes. The inner membrane also contains a variety of special transport proteins that make it selectively permeable to those particular small molecules that are metabolized by mitochondrial enzymes concentrated in the matrix space,[531] such as the integral membrane proteins Tim17, Tim 23, and Tim22p.[1142] All of these membrane-specific proteins are readily detectable by nanorobots that are extending manipulators tipped with appropriately configured chemical sensors through the intermembrane space (Section 9.4.5).

The inner membrane is the locale of electron transport and ATP synthesis. A single mitochondrion has ~10,000 large protein F_1 (ATP synthase) complexes embedded in its inner membrane, randomly distributed and typically measuring ~10-20 nm in diameter.[939] These integral proteins freely diffuse laterally within the inner membrane. Mobility is high—protein complexes collected at one end of a membrane by externally imposed electrophoretic forces return to a random distribution in just a few seconds.[939]

The prominence of cristae is correlated with the relative metabolic activity of the cell or tissue. Heart, kidney, and muscle cells have high respiratory activity levels, and their mitochondria have correspondingly large numbers of prominent cristae.[531] The number of cristae is three times greater in the mitochondria of cardiac muscle cells than in hepatic mitochondria, reflecting the greater demand for ATP in heart tissue. The cristae of mitochondria in different cell types are not only different in number and deepness, but also in basic morphology (Fig. 8.42).[531,3385-3388]

The interior of the mitochondrion is filled with a semifluid gel-like matrix that contains a concentrated mixture of hundreds of different enzymes related to aerobic cellular respiration and oxidation, plus several identical copies of the mitochondrial DNA genome, special mitochondrial ribosomes, tRNAs, and various enzymes required to express the mitochondrial genes. The mitochondrial genome[3073] consists of a circular DNA molecule of ~11 million daltons, coding for about a dozen polypeptides. It has 16,569 base pairs and a contour length of ~5 microns. Mitochondria are self-replicating organelles (with the help of cell-supplied proteins and lipids). When cellular requirements for ATP increase, mitochondria pinch in half (a process called fission) to increase their number, then both halves regrow to the former full size.[940]

Mitochondria also are sometimes found as extended reticular networks[3177-3179] which are extremely dynamic in growing cells (such as mammalian fibroblasts), with tubular sections dividing in half, branching, and fusing to create a fluid tubular web.[3179,3180]

8.5.3.11 Cytoskeleton

In addition to the membrane-enclosed organelles described above, the cytoplasm of most cells is packed with filaments of various sizes collectively called the cytoskeleton. Much as the bony skeleton occupies ~11% of the human body volume (Section 8.2.4), the cytoskeleton likewise occupies ~11% of cell volume (Table 8.17). This elaborate three-dimensional webbing of filaments and tubules forms a highly structured yet dynamic matrix that extends throughout the cytoplasm, stretching from the nuclear envelope to the plasma membrane. The cytoskeleton helps to establish and maintain shape and plays important roles in cell movement, cell division, metabolism and growth,[1426-1429] and even gene expression by accepting mechanical signals (e.g., through membrane proteins such as the integrins) originating in the extracellular matrix and transducing them into the nucleus.[942] Cellular shape appears to be maintained by an architecture known as tensional integrity or "tensegrity"—a system that achieves mechanical stability because of the way compressive and tensional forces are distributed and balanced within the cell.[1020,1021] Forcing cells to adopt different shapes causes the cells to switch between different active genetic programs.[718,1425]

The cytoskeleton also serves as a framework for positioning, anchoring, and actively moving organelles and vesicles within the cytoplasm, for muscle contraction and the beating of cilia (Section 9.3.1.1) and flagella (Section 6.3.4.2), and for chromosomal movements. It has been estimated that up to 80% of unbound cytoplasmic proteins are not freely diffusible but are associated in some way with the cytoskeleton, and up to 20-40% of cytoplasmic water may be bound to the filaments and tubules of the cytoskeleton.[939] The most radical example of cytoskeletal dynamics may be the complete remodeling of the cellular microtubular array during replication—from a network radiating throughout the cell in interphase to the compact bipolar mitotic spindle during mitosis.

There are five recognized classes of filaments, grouped according to their diameter and by the types of protein they contain. In order of size, starting with the thinnest, they are

1. superfine filaments,
2. microfilaments,
3. intermediate filaments,
4. muscle thick filaments, and
5. microtubules.

Microfilaments and microtubules can be rapidly assembled and disassembled, allowing a cell to modify its cytoskeletal framework according to changing requirements. The other filament types, once assembled, are less readily disassembled.

A. *Superfine Filaments* — Superfine filaments are short segments measuring 2-4 nm in diameter and up to 100 nm in length. Superfine filaments such as plectin[1194,3389] serve to interconnect other filaments and microtubules, stabilize the nucleus,[3391] regulate actin dynamics,[3392] and also provide the means by which the membranes of organelles may be attached to stable or moving elements of the cytoskeleton.[938,3389,3390]

B. *Microfilaments* — Microfilaments are the smallest of the major cytoskeletal components, measuring 5-7 nm in diameter and up to several microns in length. They are F-actin polymers of the contractile monomer protein G-actin, a single polypeptide consisting

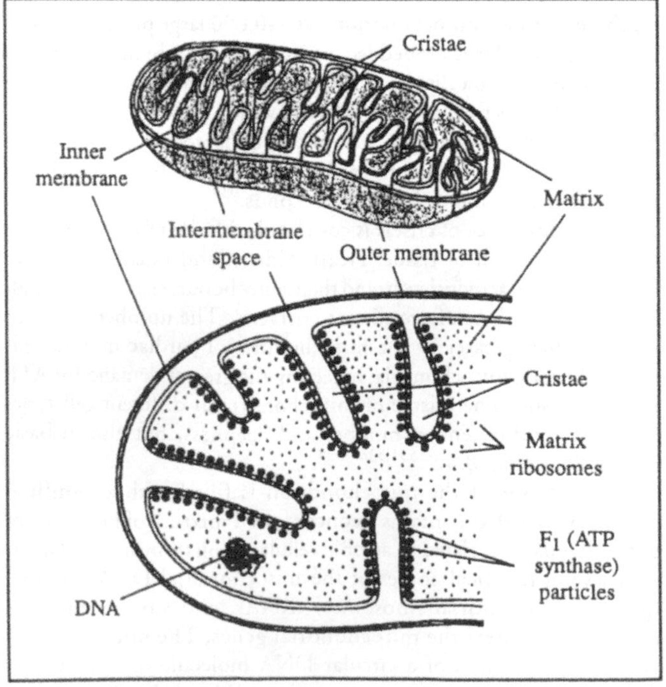

Fig. 8.41. Mitochondrial structure (redrawn from Vander, Sherman, and Luciano,[866] and from Becker and Deamer[939]).

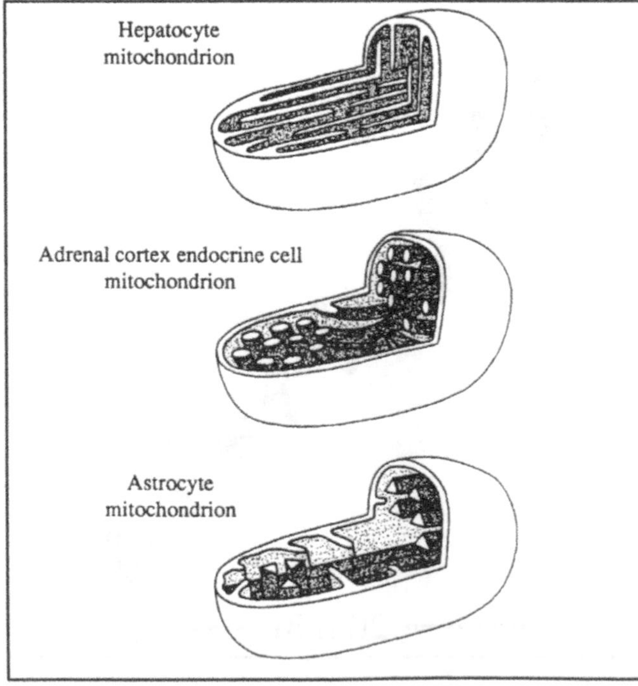

Fig. 8.42. Morphologically distinct mitochondrial cristae (from rat tissues; redrawn from Alberts et al[531]).

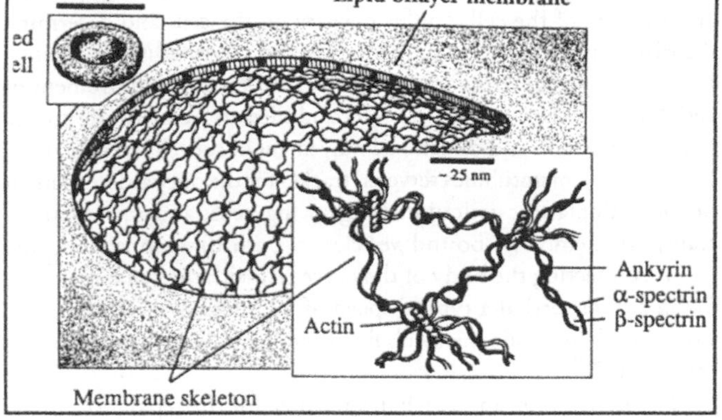

Figs. 8.43. Above, a schematic of microfilaments in the erythrocyte cell cortex, below, schematic of microfilaments in the erythrocyte cell cortex (redrawn from Schmidt et al[1126] and Becker and Deamer[939]).

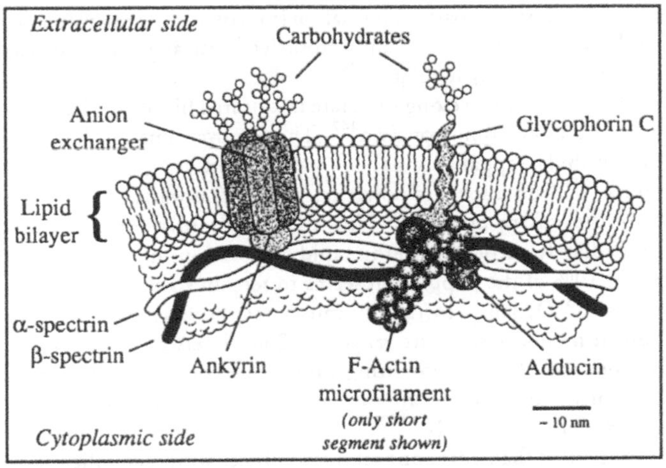

of 375 amino acid residues with a molecular weight of ~42,000. Actin is the most abundant protein in most cells, usually comprising more than 5% of the total cellular protein.[939] Polymerization at the "plus" end and depolymerization at the "minus" end occur spontaneously, driven by local G-actin concentration. This produces a treadmilling action, wherein a given actin monomer is incorporated at the "plus" end, transfers slowly along the microfilament from one end to the other, and finally is lost by depolymerization at the "minus" end.[939] Assembly speed for microfilaments of the actin cytoskeleton is 0.1-1 micron/sec.[942] Tensile failure strength of a single strand is ~108 pN,[362] while the compressive load force or "stall force" applied during polymerization by a single actin fiber is typically ~10 pN.[1203]

Microfilaments make up a major portion of all cell cytoskeletons and are best known for their role in the contractile fibrils of muscle cells. They can form connections with the plasma membrane and thereby influence locomotion, amoeboid movement, and cytoplasmic streaming. They produce the cleavage furrows that divide the cytoplasm of cells after chromosomes have been separated by the spindle fibers during mitosis. Microfilaments also help develop and maintain cell shape by acting as tensile elements in the cellular tensegrity structure, pulling the plasma membrane and all of the cell's internal constituents toward the nucleus at the core.[1021] Microfilaments also conduct mechanical signals throughout the cell at propagation speeds of 100-1200 m/sec, allowing 0.01-2 Hz signals to cross a cell in 2-20 nanosec.[1202]

Most cells have a dense network of subsurface microfilaments called the cell cortex, which includes actin-binding peripheral proteins such as spectrin (in erythrocytes) or filamin and vinculin (in fibroblasts) just below the plasma membrane. In the case of the red cell, the membrane skeleton (Fig. 8.43) is a highly organized two-dimensional triangulated network of actin oligomers tethered to spectrin tetramer filaments interconnecting ~70,000 nodes[1136] or microfilament junctional complexes comprising an equal number of triangular ~50 nm-wide meshes[1126] (mean mesh size 3000-4800 nm^2).[3612]

The cell cortex confers structural rigidity on the cell surface and facilitates shape changes and bulk movement. In some cells, microfilaments are ordered into long parallel bundles called stress fibers, which may span the entire length of the cell. Stress fibers also comprise the core of microvilli. Each cell has its own arrangement of microfilaments, thus no two cells are exactly alike.[940] Indeed, the microfilament network itself may form a complete tensegrity substructure within the larger cytoskeletal network.[1021]

C. *Intermediate Filaments* — Tough, insoluble intermediate filaments (IFs) have a diameter of 8-12 nm with a mean intertubule spacing of perhaps ~50-100 nm. They are the most stable of the cytoskeletal elements, not being subject to constant de-/re-polymerization, with a tensile failure strength of ~100 pN per fiber (Table 9.3). With their high tensile strength and comparative positional stability, IFs act as internal guy wires to resist mechanical stress on the cell[940] and thus are regarded as a scaffold supporting the entire cytoskeletal framework, with polysomal ribosomes located at IF junction control nodes (Fig. 8.44). IFs also have a tension-bearing role in some cells, as intermediate filaments are most extensively developed in those regions of cells most subject to mechanical stress. Another specific function of IFs is to maintain the position of the nucleus within the cell. Intermediate filaments form a ring around the nucleus with branches extending outward through the cytoplasm, and possibly extending downward into the pores of the nuclear envelope (Section 8.5.4.2) to connect with the nuclear cortex (Section 8.5.4.3). Intermediate filaments constitute ~1% of total protein, although in some cells (e.g., epidermal keratinocytes, neurons) IFs may represent up to 85% of the total protein of fully differentiated cells.[1543]

In contrast to microtubules and microfilaments, intermediate filaments differ in their composition from one tissue to another.

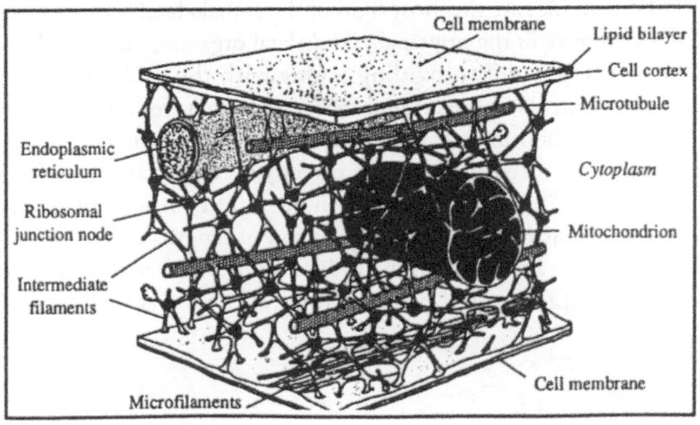

Fig. 8.44. Cytoskeletal network in the cell (redrawn from Loewy et al[938] and Marieb[940]).

The known classes of IF protein (based on biochemical and immunological criteria) include the keratins of which there are at least 15 different varieties in each of the acidic and basic/neutral subclasses (in the tonofilaments of epithelial cells); vimentin, which is found in fibroblasts, connective tissue and other cells of mesenchymal origin; desmin, in muscle cells; glial fibrillary acidic (GFA) protein, in glial cells; neurofilament (NF) protein, present in the neurofilaments of nerve cells; and nuclear lamins A, B and C, which are found in the nuclear cortex of all cells.[939] Most cells contain at least two different types of IF proteins: the three lamins in the nucleus, plus the cytoplasmic IF protein appropriate to the specific cell type. Because of this tissue specificity, cells from different tissues can be distinguished almost solely on the basis of the IF proteins present[3393]—intermediate filament typing via immunofluorescence microscopy is a useful diagnostic tool in detecting cancer and prenatal birth defects.[3394-3397] In cyto nanorobots can use this same information to continuously verify the cell type in which they are resident.

D. *Muscle Thick Filaments* — Muscle thick filaments, ~15 nm in diameter and composed of the very large contractile protein myosin, are found mainly in striated muscle cells and occasionally in the cortex of nonmuscle cells.[3398-3400] Myosin molecules not in filament form are also present in many, if not most, other cells where they interact with microfilaments to produce local forces and movements.

E. *Microtubules* — Microtubules are straight hollow cylinders with an outer diameter of 25 nm and an inner diameter of 15 nm. They vary greatly in length. Some are less than 200 nm long, while others, particularly in nerve cells (where they provide the framework that maintains the cell's cylindrical shape), can be as long as 25 microns. Mean intertubule spacing is at least 200-300 nm, with a minimum radius of curvature of ~0.2 microns.[1437] Each microtubule is composed of a helical arrangement of the αβ-tubulin heterodimer protein, with 13 tubulin subunits in each rotation of the tight helix.[1092] The uniform orientation of the tubulin molecules confers an inherent polarity on the microtubule. Placed in a tubulin-rich environment, the "plus" end of the tubulin polymer (β-tubulin) will elongate much more rapidly than the "minus" end (α-tubulin).[1124] In the living cell, the ends of the microtubules farthest away from the center of the cell are always the "plus" ends. Microtubules radiate out as lacelike threads toward the periphery of the cell from a microtubule-organizing center (MTOC) near the nucleus.[939] The best-known MTOC is the centrosome, which consists of granular material surrounding two centrioles (Fig. 8.36). Other examples of MTOCs include the kinetochore and the poles of the mitotic spindle.

Microtubules are the most rigid of the cytoskeletal filaments and thus often serve as the principal cytoskeletal organizers and backbone elements (Fig. 8.44), providing (along with the ECM) the compressive elements of the cellular tensegrity structure. Tensile failure strength is ~1000 pN per fiber (Table 9.3). The flexural rigidity of individual microtubules has been directly measured as $\kappa_{rigid} = 3.4 \times 10^{-23}$ N-m^2,[1468] which is higher than the rigidity of actin filaments. What does this mean? For an elastic rod of length L attached to a wall by a pivot about which the rod is completely free to rotate, the magnitude of the critical buckling force of the rod is:[642,1468]

$$F_{buckle} \sim \frac{\pi^2 \kappa_{rigid}}{L^2} \qquad \text{\{Eqn. 8.6\}}$$

Hence a 1-micron long microtubule will not begin to buckle until an axial load of $F_{buckle} \gtrsim 340$ pN is applied.

Microtubules define and maintain the overall shape and architecture of the cell, confer polarity on the cell, and determine the distribution of the microfilaments and intermediate filaments. By providing a radiating system of fibers to guide the movement of vesicles and other organelles, microtubules also contribute to the spatial disposition and directional movement of subcellular structures. For example, microtubules serve as "tracks" for the outward movement of the endoplasmic reticulum in growing cells, and microtubules transport membrane-bound vesicles in both directions along the axons connecting the body of the nerve cell with the synaptic knobs (axonal transport) at a typical speed of ~2 microns/sec.[939] Particles easily switch from one microtubule to another intersecting one during transport.[1448]

The structure immediately responsible for the separation of the chromosomes, the spindle fibers, is composed of microtubules, as are the organelles (the centrioles) that generate the spindle fibers at the time of cell division. (Each cell has two centrioles, solid structures composed of microtubules. Prior to cell division, the centrioles replicate and then produce the intracellular architectural skeleton called the mitotic apparatus that guides the cell through mitosis.) Spontaneous spatial pattern formation from oscillating microtubules has been observed,[1071,1073] and cytoskeletal rearrangements appear to be biochemically regulated.[1083]

The microtubule elongation rate in cultured fibroblasts has been measured as ~0.06 microns/sec.[1423] The turnover time for the entire microtubular apparatus has been estimated as ~900 sec (0.25 hour),[1423] with a specific power output of ~0.6 watts/m^3 averaged over the entire array.[1424] Not all cytoplasmic microtubules immediately participate in this rapid turnover during interphase—about 10% of the population seems to remain stable for at least 2 hours.[1423] Dynamic instability causes microtubule shortening in human monocytes, in the range of ~260 dimers/sec[1446] or ~0.15 microns/sec.[1447] Depolymerizing microtubules can drive kinetochore movements towards the minus end at ~0.5 microns/sec, exerting forces of up to ~100 pN.[1593]

Superfine filaments connect microtubules with each other, with intermediate filaments, and with adjacent organelles.[1439,1440] The filaments extend from the microtubular surface and prevent direct contact with other cellular structures.[1441] This forms a narrow exclusion zone around microtubules that is devoid of other structures, and often appears as a clear halo[1442] with a radius from ~10 nm in insect cells[1443] up to ~50 nm in neurons.[1444] High molecular weight microtubule-associated proteins (MAPs) define zones of exclusion around microtubules and may help maintain the observed spacing between microtubules and cell organelles.[1445]

8.5.3.12 Cytonavigational Issues

Cytonavigational requirements are strongly mission-driven. A nonexhaustive list of mission classes might include:

1. examination or modification of the plasma membrane or cell cortex, including chemical testing for toxins or poisons in cell receptors and transport channels;
2. cytosolic chemical or pathogenic assay, chemical injection or extraction, or other selective cytosolic modification;
3. biocellular messaging or eavesdropping using chemical, mechanical, or other means;
4. organelle counting, dimensional measuring, and general cytocartography;
5. circumorganelle chemical assay;

6. organelle-specific surface membrane analysis or intraplasmic chemical assay;
7. dynamic functional or structural testing of cellular components;
8. sampling, diagnosis, chemoinjection, replacement or repair operations to be performed upon an individual organelle or cytocomponent located at a specific cellular physical address;
9. cytoassembly or structural editing;
10. establishment of direct functional control over some or all of normal cellular functions, including metabolism, secretion, and mitotic cycling;
11. comprehensive cellular reconstruction;
12. long-term cytoplasmic materials or equipment storage;
13. sentinel or cytodefensive functions; or
14. activities involving the nucleus (Section 8.5.4). Each of these mission classes has very specific, and often quite different, navigational requirements.

Medical nanorobots can certainly undertake many useful tasks without physically entering the cell, relying solely upon diffusion, transport via cellular pumps, endocytosis and pinocytosis, or even nanoinjectors or manipulator appendages inserted through the plasma membrane (Section 9.4.5) while the nanorobot remains securely anchored outside the cell. However, it is well-known that motile entities are capable of entering and navigating the interiors of living cells for long periods of time without ill effect. For example, one description[848] from early microscopic investigations included the following observation: "...lymphocytes entered the cells and circulated inside them for hours at a time. This odd relationship of lymphocytes to other cells, sometimes moving around them, sometimes entering them, they termed 'emperipolesis'." (Emperipolesis[3286-3293] is a rarely observed and still poorly understood phenomenon that may only occur in pathological conditions.) Micron-scale bacterial pathogens that invade nonphagocytic cells, once free in the cytoplasm, are propelled "harmlessly" through the cytosol via continuous cytoskeleton-linked actin polymerization[1012] (Section 9.4.6). While delivery of treatment "packages" to extracellular spaces may be an early use of medical nanorobotics, subsequent development will allow nanorobots to enter and operate inside the cell. Ultimate applications would permit delicate sensing and repair of DNA or organelles (Chapter 21).

The interior of a cell is a unique and intuitively unfamiliar environment. Figure 8.36, drawn primarily for conceptual clarity, erroneously makes the cell appear spacious and relatively empty. In reality, cellular components are fairly closely packed. Even though cells may consist of up to 70% water, only some of this is bulk water and the cytosol more closely resembles a proteinaceous crystal (Section 8.5.3.3). The mean separation of adjacent organelles (of all types) is <1 micron, roughly the size of the nanorobot itself. Forward travel is further impeded by the presence of a dense cytoskeletal network. This includes sheetlike ~30 nm meshes of microfilaments intertwined and bonded with peripheral proteins comprising the cell cortex, plus additional three-dimensional networks of intermediate filaments (~100 nm mesh) and microtubules (~300 nm mesh) throughout the body of the cell (Fig. 8.44). There may be only a few multi-micron-scale "freely swimmable" spaces for nanorobots within the cell.

A medical nanorobot bears about the same size relationship to a cell as a human body bears to a swimming pool. Consider this fanciful analogy to a common macroscale experience, imagining a "nanorobot" of roughly human size: The subsurface robot does not find itself traversing a large swimming pool of water, encountering an occasional submerged obstacle. Rather, it finds itself crawling through a swimming pool mostly filled with thick-skinned water balloons separated by its own width, or slightly less, of fluid. The water balloons are of many different sizes and shapes but average an equivalent volume as the nanorobot itself, with almost all of the balloons embedded in and loosely tethered to a dense three-dimensional multilevel webbing of threads, strings, cords, and 1-cm gauge ropes arranged in a progressive semirandom 1-10 cm mesh. To employ a slightly different and even more imprecise metaphor, navigating the interior of a cell may more closely resemble hacking through a dense jungle than strolling in an open garden.

Given the tight spacing of the multilevel cytoskeletal webbing, it will be almost impossible for a micron-scale medical nanorobot to enter cells and freely navigate therein without disrupting the cytoskeletal framework that lies across its path. Some disruption cannot be avoided even if useful nanodevices or their extensible appendages can be metamorphically compressed as narrow as ~100 nm in width (Section 5.3.1.2). However, cytoskeletal disruption can be minimized by employing active and continuous breach-sealing polymerization protocols during passage (Section 9.4.6). The nanorobot must also avoid applying excessive forces to the cytoskeleton, as these forces could transmit mechanically-mediated signal cascades into the nucleus and activate unwanted stress responses via regulated genetic circuits.[1956] Some details regarding cytopenetration (Section 9.4.5), in cyto locomotion (Section 9.4.6), and biocompatible nanorobot surfaces[3234] (Chapter 15) are presented elsewhere.

How can a nanorobot determine its intracellular position? If a high-resolution microtransponder network (Section 8.3.3) has been installed in the surrounding tissue, in vivo nanorobots can acoustically fix their cytographic position to within ~3 microns, although a gigahertz acoustic chirp system may allow localized accuracies as close as ~100 nm in some cases (Section 8.5.4.7). A 3-micron grid size divides a 20-micron cell volume into ~300 distinguishable voxels with each voxel encompassing an average of ~10 individual major organelles.

Because of the close spacing of cellular organelles, a micron-scale nanorobot typically may be in direct physical contact with at least one organelle at all times. The nanorobot can uniquely identify any organelle type based on membrane composition, intraplasmic biochemistry, or physical structure, and can also estimate which additional organelles may be in the neighborhood based on peri-organelle chemogradients. In the case of the nucleus or the ER, where there may be only one organelle of that type per cell, organelle detection provides relative positional localization in the radial dimension (although the ER has multiple layers). In the angular dimensions, and in the case of multiple organelles, cytoskeletal network topology provides additional positional and orientational cues. The circumnuclear ring of intermediate filaments and the microtubule-organizing centers (MTOCs) have already been mentioned. Center-to-periphery orientation is readily established by comparing the net polarity of the local microtubule array with a previously assembled gross map of cellular microtubular topology.

Dead reckoning (Section 8.3.1) may also be used to estimate transit positions and to create internal maps accurate to ~100 nm, the typical internodal separation of the junctions of the intermediate fibers (the most persistent component of the cytoskeletal network). The mean separation of cytoplasmic free ribosomes is also ~100 nm. However, even positional localization as crude as ~1 micron resolution will uniquely locate all individual major organelles within the cytoplasm. This may be sufficient for most purposes, since random hydrodynamic flows induced by thermal fluctuations inside a cell have velocities of ~10 microns/sec in a time range of ~10 millisec with a characteristic length of ~1 micron.[1069]

A volumetric cytographic map using $(100\ nm)^3$ voxels requires 8 million 8-bit voxels or ~64 megabits of memory. A 1 $micron^3$ nanorobot moving at ~1 micron/sec would require ~8000 sec to volumetrically survey the entire interior of a 20-micron cell using an efficient nonoverlapping scanning pattern, or ~300 sec to scan a region having the same volume as the nucleus. A volumetric map would allow computation of the shortest path to the plasma membrane in order to exit the cell quickly and with minimum disruption. Such maps might help the nanorobot to identify the axodendritic polarity of a neuron, locate the nucleus or a specific part of a membrane—for instance, a part of the membrane that is connected via intercellular junctions to adjacent cells, or which is adjacent to bone or digestive juices. Volumetric maps could also allow the nanorobot to return to the exact site of unwanted natural deposits (e.g., lipofuscin) or to sites where foreign objects are lodged, although long-term map stability is problemmatical.

The cytoplasmic membranes present inside a 20-micron tissue cell have a total surface area of ~180,000 $micron^2$, plus another ~280,000 $micron^2$ of cytoskeletal fiber surfaces (Table 8.17). Assuming 8-bit pixels, the totality of internal cellular surfaces could be instantaneously described using 1 $micron^2$ pixels with a 4 megabit map, or with $(100\ nm)^2$ pixels using a 400 megabit map (requiring ~0.02 $micron^3$ of hydrofluorocarbon memory tape). However, high-resolution cytographic surface survey maps are not as useful because of their short half-lives. Membrane lipids and transmembrane protein molecules have lateral diffusion speeds (Section 8.5.3.2) averaging ~3 microns/sec and ~0.02 micron/sec, respectively; giving a 0.3-50 sec half-life for a 1 $micron^2$ resolution surface map. Surface folds and other gross morphological features on the nuclear envelope, the endoplasmic reticulum and the Golgi complex may have half lives of $\sim 10^3$-10^5 sec, so maps of these features may have modest operational utility but still will have minimal archival utility. In any case, many malfunctions in these three organelles may require biochemical rather than mechanical interventions (Chapter 21).

For multiple-copy organelles, statistical sampling to acquire census data may provide the most useful information. Semipermanent structures such as mitochondria may be examined one by one to measure size and number density, to verify biochemical composition, and to test functionality. If a population of N cellular objects is independently and randomly sampled one by one by a population of N_{nano} in cyto nanorobots, taking a time t_{exam} for each examination, then the probability that any one object has not yet been examined after n selections is $p_x = (1 - N^{-1})^{(n\ N_{nano})}$, the total examination time $T = n\ t_{exam} / N_{nano}$, and the average number of times the same object is examined $n_{po} = n\ N_{nano} / N$. For a cell containing N = 1000 mitochondria, mean travel distance between these organelles is $X_{travel} \sim 2$ microns in a 20-micron cell, or $t_{travel} \sim 2$ sec travel time at a travel speed of ~1 micron/sec. Conservatively taking $t_{exam} \sim 10$ sec, then reducing the probability of nonexamination of any mitochondrion to $p_x = N^{-1} = 0.1\%$ requires n ~ 7,000 examinations or an average of $n_{po} = 7$ examinations per mitochondrion, and requires T = 70,000 sec ~ 19 hours to complete all the examinations using a single in cyto nanorobot ($N_{nano} = 1$). A census sampling that reaches only $p_x = 50\%$ completeness requires just n ~ 700 examinations, $n_{po} = 0.7$ examinations per mitochondrion and T = 7000 sec ~ 2 hours using one nanorobot. An $n_{po} \sim 1\%$ sampling of a population of 10^6 cytoplasmic free ribosomes requires n = 10,000 examinations and T ~ 10,000 sec ~ 3 hours assuming $t_{exam} \sim 1$ sec ($t_{travel} \sim 0.2$ sec) for a single in cyto nanorobot. These times compare well even against the rapid multiplication rate of proliferating tissue cells (e.g., human embryonal cells, ~24 hours). Post-examination individual target object tagging (e.g., using anchored messenger molecules) without physical sequestration reduces t_{exam} only slightly but does not reduce t_{travel}, hence has no significant impact on T. Note that successive mitochondrial samplings will generally be independent if X_{travel} (~2 microns) >> $\Delta X_{diffuse}$; from Eqn. 3.1, mitochondrial diffusion displacement is of order $\Delta X_{diffuse} \sim 20$ nm, taking $\tau = t_{exam} \sim 10$ sec, R ~ 1 micron, and $\eta \sim 10$ kg/m-sec (in cyto, at 310 K; Table 9.4), hence the independence condition is usually satisfied.

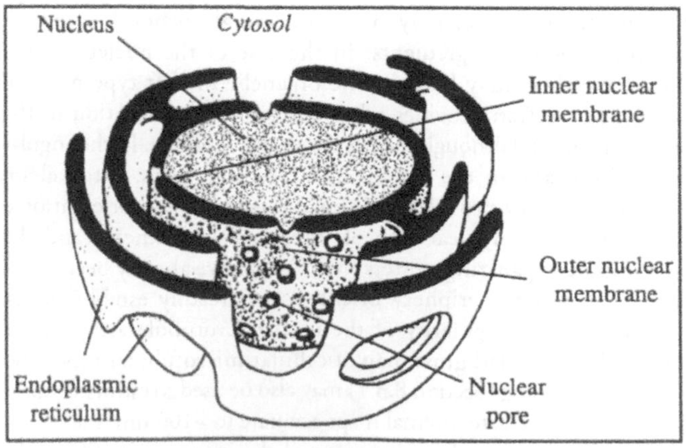

Fig. 8.45. Endoplasmic reticulum surrounds the nucleus (redrawn from Alberts et al[531]).

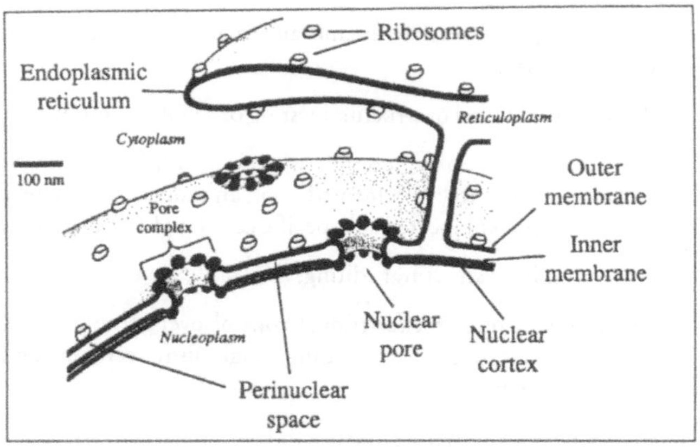

Fig. 8.46. Nuclear pores and the perinuclear space (redrawn from Becker and Deamer[939]).

8.5.4 Nucleography

Nucleography is the "geography" of the cell nucleus. The nucleus, 5-8 microns in diameter for a 20 micron tissue cell and up to 10 microns for a fibroblast cell, is the largest cellular organelle and the only one that is voluminous enough, in theory, to admit a micron-scale medical nanorobot into its interior. The nucleus is usually a large spherical or ovoid structure surrounded by its own nuclear membrane, although its shape generally conforms to the shape of the cell. For example, if a cell is elongated, the nucleus may be extended as well.[940]

Almost all cells contain a single nucleus, whose primary function is the storage and expression of genetic information. However, a few cell types have multiple nuclei of similar size, such as skeletal muscle cells, osteoclasts, megakaryocytes, and some hepatocytes.[935] A few cell types have no nucleus, such as red blood cells, platelets, keratinized squamous epidermal cells, and lens fibers.

In 1998 the finer details of nuclear structure were just beginning to be understood.[1529] Thus the following discussion of nucleography must be regarded as a very tentative work in progress.

8.5.4.1 Nuclear Envelope

The nuclear envelope enclosing the nucleus is a lipid bilayer similar in structure to the cell membrane, except that it is a double-layered membrane which is topologically more convenient for dissolution during mitosis and subsequent reassembly from vesicles. Each of the two lipid bilayer membranes is 7-8 nm thick. The outer nuclear membrane is occasionally continuous with the rough endoplasmic reticulum and is almost entirely surrounded by it (Fig. 8.45). Like the rough ER, the outer membrane is often studded on its outer surface with ribosomes involved in protein synthesis.[939] Intermediate filaments extend outward from the outer membrane into the cytoplasm, anchored on the other end to the plasma membrane or other organelles, thus positioning the nucleus firmly within the cell and increasing its mechanical stiffness almost tenfold.[942]

The perinuclear space (or perinuclear cisterna) between the two membranes ranges in width from 10-70 nm but is usually a gap of 20-40 nm. This fluid-filled compartment is continuous with the cisternae of the rough ER (Fig. 8.46), thus providing one possible avenue for transporting substances between the nucleus and different parts of the cytoplasmic compartment.

The nuclear envelope disassembles at the onset of mitosis and is reassembled at the end of mitosis.[1140]

8.5.4.2 Nuclear Pore Complexes

The most distinctive feature of the nuclear envelope is the presence of numerous nuclear pores (Fig. 8.46), small cylindrical channels with eightfold symmetry that extend through both membranes and provide direct contact between cytoplasm and nucleoplasm.[1003,3403-3405] Each pore complex marks a point of fusion between the inner and outer membranes. Elements of the cytoskeleton appear to be attached to many pores, possibly allowing direct mechanical regulation of pore activity.[3406,3407]

Each nuclear pore complex is a huge multimolecular assemblage measuring 70-90 nm in diameter, with a mass of 125 million daltons, ~34 times the size of a ribosome. Up to 100 different nucleoporin protein molecules make up the structure.[1004] Early experiments with passive gold particles showed that cytoplasmic particles with diameters of 5-6 nm passed into the nucleus in ~200 sec, those with diameters of 9-10 nm took ~10^4 sec, but particles larger than 15 nm didn't seem to enter at all.[939] Closer examination has revealed that the pores are actually large enough to allow the passage of substrates as large as 23-26 nm,[1003,1004] but this is still much too narrow for nanorobots or their flexible processes to pass through without damaging the mechanism. The nuclear localization sequence (NLS), a molecular tag consisting of 1-2 short sequences of amino acids, marks cytoplasmic proteins for active transport through the nuclear pores. Small (~40 nm) arm-like import receptors (cytoplasmic filaments) ringing the mouth of the pore bind to a protein cargo tagged with an NLS, then flex toward the pore to shove the cargo into the mouth.[1264,3408,3409]

The density of pores across the surface of the nuclear envelope varies greatly, depending mainly on cell type and the amount of RNA being exported to the cytoplasm. Values range from 3-4 pores/micron^2 in some white cells up to 50 pores/micron^2 in oocytes and a theoretical maximum density of 60 pores/micron^2.[939] A typical ~20 micron human cell has 2000-4000 pores embedded in its nuclear surface,[1004] a mean density of 10-20 pores/micron^2. Pore structures may protrude at most ~100 nm into the nucleoplasmic space.

8.5.4.3 Nuclear Cortex

The nuclear cortex is an electron-dense layer of intermediate filaments (composed of the nuclear lamins common to most cell types) on the nucleoplasmic side of the inner nuclear membrane.[1004] The cortex, also called the nuclear lamina or karyoskeleton, is up to 30-40 nm thick in some cells but is difficult to detect in others.[939] Its proteinaceous fibers are arranged in whorls that may serve to funnel materials to the nuclear pores for export to the cytoplasm. These fibers may also be involved in pore formation. The nuclear cortex helps to determine nuclear shape, and also binds to specific sites on chromatin, thereby guiding the interactions of chromatin (Fig. 8.47) with the nuclear envelope.[531] Chromatin binding sites on the nuclear cortex avoid the immediate vicinity of nuclear pores to ensure unobstructed passage of materials through the pores.[531]

8.5.4.4 Nucleoplasm and Chromatin

The nucleoplasm is the semifluid matrix in the interior of the nucleus. It contains some condensed but mostly extended chromatin (called heterochromatin and euchromatin, respectively), as well as a structural nuclear matrix of nonchromatin (mostly protein) material (Section 8.5.4.6). The chromatin represents chromosomes as they exist between cell divisions. Chromosomes assume a highly condensed (compact) state as the cell prepares to divide, but after mitosis most of the chromosomes relax into a highly extended state. The nucleus of the human cell contains 46 chromosomes of varying lengths, in 23 pairs. Each of these in turn are composed principally of a single deoxyribonucleic acid (DNA) molecule. The DNA contains the genes of the cell, and all ~100,000 genes are represented, though not expressed, in each nucleated cell. The nucleosol, or fluid com-

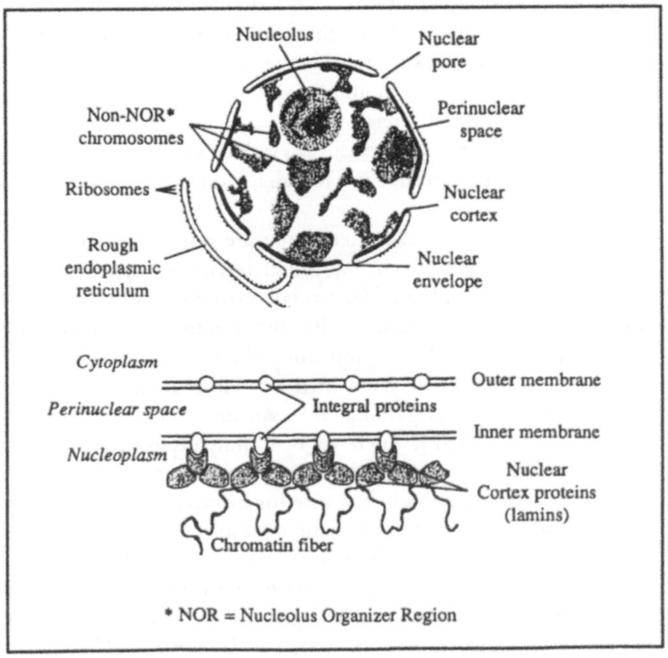

Fig. 8.47. Schematic of chromatin distribution in the nucleus (redrawn from Alberts et al[531]).

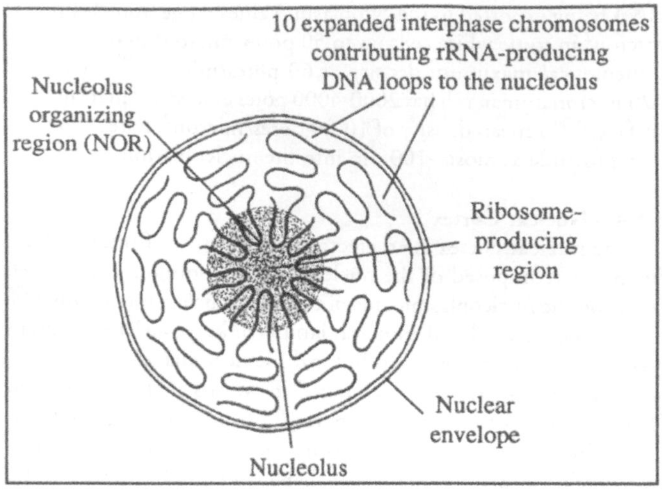

Fig. 8.48. Schematic of human nucleolus structure (redrawn from Alberts et al[531]).

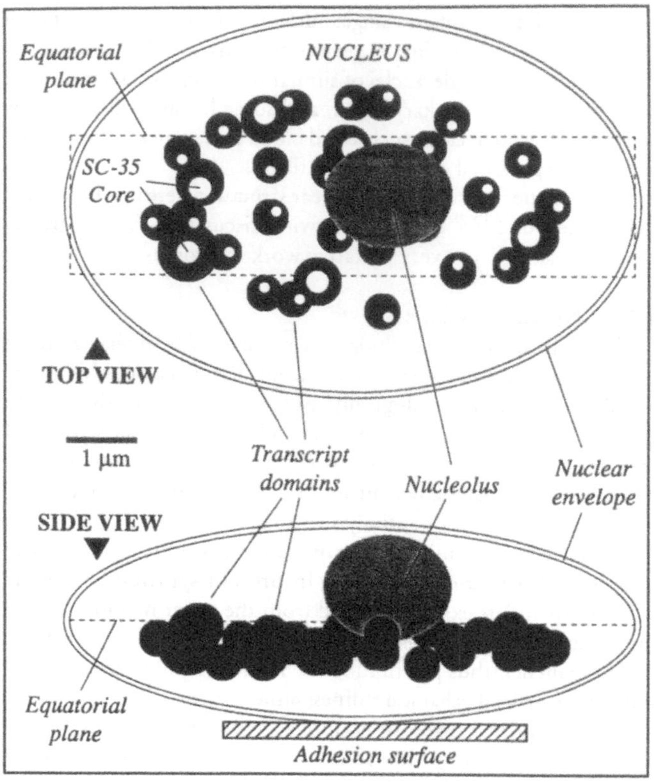

Fig. 8.49. Schematic topology of nuclear transcript domains (after Carter et al[1135]).

ponent of the nucleoplasm, contains salts, nutrients, and other needed biochemicals. A number of different granules are also present.[938]

During interphase (e.g., between cell divisions), individual chromosomes occupy compact, discrete territories within the nucleus that may range up to 4 microns in diameter (Fig. 8.47).[2464-2467,3410-3417] The structure and location of these territories is specific for both cell type and mitotic stage,[3412,3413] and may be arranged in the same spatial order as is found in the wheel-shaped ring aggregate known as the chromosome rosette at the time of mitotic prometaphase.[1060] It has been proposed that active genes are preferentially localized to the periphery of the chromosome territories; RNA templates would be preferentially produced at the surfaces of these territories and then shed into interchromosomal domain channels for further processing and transport.[1529] Others have argued against this.[3414] But knowledge of any such spatial orderings, which was woefully incomplete in 1998, might permit intranuclear nanorobots to approximate their position inside the nucleus once the locations of three or more specific chomosomes have been definitively established. The diameter of a territory $D_{territory} \sim D_{nucleus} (c_{chromosome} / c_{genome})^{1/3} \sim 3$ microns, where $c_{chromosome}$ is chromosome size and c_{genome} is genome size, both measured in base pairs, and $D_{nucleus}$ is the diameter of the nucleus.[2464]

Note, however, that these territories are not rigid. Changes in the relative positions of chromosomal territories often occur at ~0.3-0.4 nm/sec, and intraterritorial movement and flexing of subchromosomal foci measuring 400-800 nm in diameter have also been observed.[1529,3415] Both cytoplasm and nucleoplasm may contain numerous as yet undiscovered intricate substructures that could provide many new navigational aids. An important task for early nanomedicine-oriented research will be to fully explore and elucidate this fine structure, and to determine whether or not it is stable enough to be relied upon in any way for intracellular navigation.

In its most relaxed state, chromatin resembles a network of bumpy threads weaving their way through the nucleoplasm. Chromatin is composed of roughly equal amounts of negatively charged DNA (comprising the chromosomes) and globular histone proteins (basic proteins which carry a positive charge at the normal pH found in the cell).[938] Nucleosomes, the fundamental units of chromatin, are spherical clusters of eight histone proteins, connected like beads on a string by a DNA molecule that winds around each of them. The average cell nucleus contains 25 million nucleosomes, also called histone octamers. Each nucleosome is encircled by 146 base pairs of DNA. Nucleosomes have a mass of 206,000 daltons. About half of nucleosome mass is protein and half is DNA. Each human chromosome contains DNA with an average contour length of ~75 mm. (See Chapter 20 for more details.)

8.5.4.5 Nucleolus

The largest and most prominent "nuclear organelle" is the nucleolus, a highly coiled structure associated with numerous particles but not surrounded by a membrane.[1141] The nucleolus is a ribosome-manufacturing machine. Assembly of precursor ribosomal subunits within the nucleolus requires ~1800 sec, while the complete assembly of a large ribosomal subunit (needing only protein to make a completed ribosome) takes ~3600 sec.[531]

The nucleolus is composed of DNA, RNA, and proteins. It also has a granular component (each granule ~150 nm thick) and a fibrillar component, and a variable internal structure.[1141] The granular component consists of ~15-nm particles that are ribosomal subunits in the process of maturation. The fibrillar component consists of rRNA molecules that have already become associated with proteins to form fibrils with a thickness of ~5 nm. The size of the nucleolus correlates with its level of activity. In cells characterized by a high rate of protein synthesis and hence by the need for many ribosomes, the nucleolus can occupy 20-25% of nuclear volume (3-5 micron diameter in a 20-micron cell), mostly comprised of the granular component. In less active cells, the nucleolus is much smaller—as small as 0.5 micron in a mature lymphocyte.[1141] Nucleoli are frequently located at or near the nuclear envelope, adhering directly to the

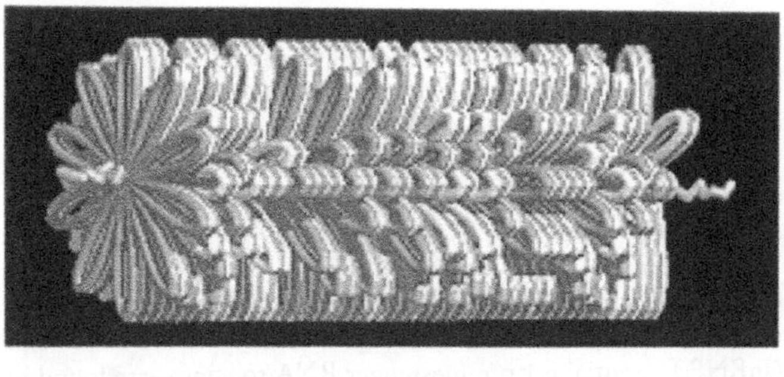

Fig. 8.50. MLS model of human chromosome 15 in its condensed state during mitosis (courtesy of Tobias A. Knoch, Division of Biophysics of Macromolecules, German Cancer Research Centre, Heidelberg, Germany ©1999).[2465]

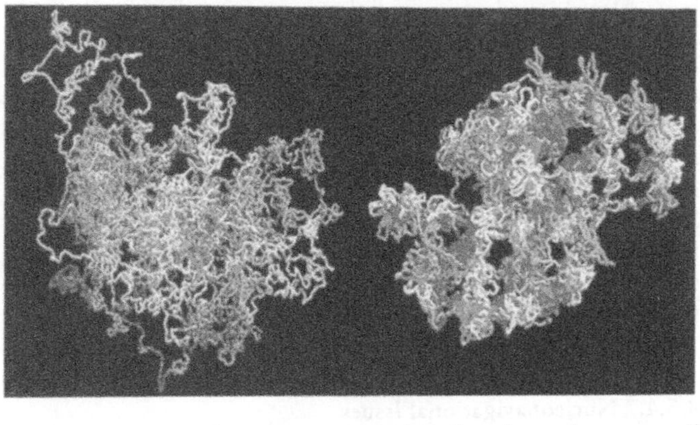

Fig. 8.51. Human chromosome 15 in its relaxed state between cell divisions. At left, RWGL model of chromosome 15 territory; at right, MLS model of chromosome 15 territory (courtesy of Tobias A. Knoch, Division of Biophysics of Macromolecules, German Cancer Research Centre, Heidelberg, Germany ©1999).[2465]

nuclear lamina or attaching to it by a pedicle. In nuclei having a centrally located nucleolus, the nuclear envelope is folded to form a nucleolar canal that is in direct contact with the nucleolus.[1141]

Most human nuclei contain only one nucleolus, except for liver cell nuclei which may contain more than one nucleolus[935] and cultured HeLa (cancer) cells which may have up to six.[1141] The number of nucleoli in a eukaryotic cell nucleus normally is determined by the number of chromosomes with secondary constrictions, or nucleolus organizer regions (NORs). The human genome contains five NORs per haploid chromosome set, or 10 NORs per diploid nucleus, each located near the tip of a chromosome. However, instead of 10 separate nucleoli, the typical human nucleus contains a single large nucleolus representing the fusion of loops of chromatin from the 10 separate chromosomes with NORs (Fig. 8.48). The DNA from the remaining diploid chromosomes is distributed in specific regions throughout the nucleoplasm (Fig. 8.47). During mitosis, the chromosomes condense into a more compact form and the nucleolus shrinks, then disappears altogether. A cell undergoing mitosis thus has no nucleolus and synthesizes no rRNA. Once mitosis is complete, the nucleolus reappears. As rRNA synthesis resumes, ten tiny nucleoli appear, one near the end of each of 10 different chromosomes; these enlarge, eventually fusing into the single large nucleolus characteristic of the interphase human nucleus.

8.5.4.6 Nuclear Matrix and Transcript Domains

Like the cytoskeleton of the cell, the nucleus is thought to possess a nuclear skeleton comprised of a network of insoluble protein fibers known as the nuclear matrix.[1134,3418-3423] This finely branched meshwork of superfine filaments attaches to the nuclear lamina or cortex (Section 8.5.4.3) and extends to the nucleolus. Assuming ~10^6 filaments each averaging ~50 nm long gives a total fiber length L_{fiber} ~ 50,000 microns, which for a D ~ 8 micron diameter nucleus implies a mean grid spacing of:

$$L_{grid} \sim \left(\frac{D^3}{L_{fiber}} \right)^{1/2} \sim 50 \text{ nm} \qquad \text{\{Eqn. 8.7\}}$$

Typical mesh spacings seen in electron micrographs do indeed range from ~50-100 nm.[1132] The filaments are constructed from a variety of nuclear matrix proteins (NMPs). More than a dozen NMPs have been identified, many of them cell-specific;[3421,3422] also, NMPs released by cancer cells differ from those released by normal cells of the same type.[3422,3423]

The nuclear matrix organizes thousands of DNA replication sites during mitosis, and provides architectural order during interphase for RNA metabolism (wherein mRNA molecules are synthesized, spliced, and made ready for export to the protein-synthesizing machinery in the cytoplasm).[1135] The regions where RNA metabolism occurs are called transcript domains.[1133,1135,2021] A human nucleus typically has 20-40 transcript domains, each ranging in diameter from ~0.5 to 3 microns and aligned in a planar horizontal array in the "lower" portion of the nucleus (Fig. 8.49); "lower" is toward the ventral surface of a cell that is adherent to the glass plate used in the microscopic study.[1135] A single nucleolus occupies the "upper" or "lower" portions of the nucleus with equal frequency; its position is established by sequence-specific DNA binding proteins.[1139] The outermost edge of a transcript domain lies an average of ~0.8 microns (range 0.5-1.2 microns) from the inside surface of the nuclear cortex or nuclear envelope. Located in the core of each domain is a protein called SC-35 that is required for the assembly of the molecular machinery that splices the introns out of mRNA,[3424] and each domain is surrounded by a discrete border of high-density chromatin—with a given chromosome always occupying the same general location in the nucleus at each mitotic phase. All 20-40 transcript domains collectively occupy ~5% of the total nuclear volume, whereas the specific RNA accumulations occupy no more than 1%.

However, nuclear matrix elements may not be necessary for physical support inside each chromosomal territory. Several theoretic descriptions of chromosome structure have been compared to experimental data, and one such description, the Random-Walk/Giant-Loop (RWGL) model,[2466,3416] proposes that huge 3-5 million base-pair (Mbp) loops are bound to a nuclear matrix that permeates the region. More recently, polymer dynamics simulations of chromosomal territories performed by Munkel, Langowski and Knoch[1013,2464,2465,3417] suggest that a Multi-Loop-Subcompartment (MLS) model is in better accord with experiment. In the MLS model, chromatin fiber is folded into ~120 Kbp sized loops which are organized into rosettes of 1-2 Mbp. The rosettes (which may be structural units for replication, etc.) are interconnected by a piece of chromatin of similar base pair content so that no protein matrix is needed for structural support. The MLS model agrees with the metaphase organization proposed by Pienta and Coffey.[2467] The MLS rosettes are clearly visible in Figure 8.50, which shows human chromosome 15 in its highly condensed metaphase state, as it might appear during mitosis. Figure 8.51 shows two polymer dynamics simulations of the 3-5 micron^3 territory of human chromosome 15 in its relaxed state between cell divisions, using the RWGL model (left) and the MLS model (right). The numerous apparently matrix-free voids up to ~0.5 micron in diameter that appear in the MLS simulation are presumably largely filled by another chromosome (not shown). (Sometimes the two copies of chromosome 15 are adjacent, but most of the time they are separated.) However, numerous ~0.1 micron voids do exist (c.f. 100-nm keyhole passage; Section 5.3.1.2), and dynamic processes may temporarily open still larger spaces possibly large enough for a medical nanorobot to seek slow, relatively safe and unobstructed passage, but the theoretical pathways of spheres, diffusion and percolation through territories remain to be studied [T. Knoch, personal communication, 1999].

8.5.4.7 Nucleonavigational Issues

Cytoplasmic medical nanorobots can perform many useful tasks without entering the nucleus. Such tasks might include:

1. physical mapping and compositional analysis of the nuclear envelope;
2. monitoring of nuclear pore traffic;
3. near-complete regulation of nuclear pore traffic using multiple manipulators or other devices;
4. monitoring, initiating, or modifying cytoskeletally-mediated mechanical signal transduction into the nuclear interior;
5. injection of enzymes, RNA or DNA fragments, or other bioactive materials through nuclear pores using hollow nanoinjectors; or
6. partial or complete nucleoplasmic replacement using artificial chromatin detachment enzymes dispensed by multiple injection and extraction nanorobots positioned at the nuclear pores, operated simultaneously and located antipodally around the nucleus to establish flowthrough.

Entering the nucleus is somewhat more difficult than entering the cytoplasmic space through the plasma membrane (Section 9.4.5.7). One reason is that the nucleus is almost completely surrounded by the membranes of the endoplasmic reticulum (Fig. 8.45), and the nearest of these membranes may lie only a few hundred nanometers from the outermost surface of the nuclear envelope (Fig. 8.46). The nuclear envelope is also a double-walled membrane. Another reason why nuclear entry is difficult is that physical forces applied to cytoskeletal elements in the immediate vicinity of the nucleus may trigger unwanted transcriptional, structural, or metabolic responses from within the nucleus. Additionally, the 10-100 nm grid size of the nuclear matrix filaments and the DNA rosette loops may allow little free maneuvering room for nanorobots, which may find it difficult to avoid tearing the nucleoskeleton during passage.

Given that the nucleus of a 20 micron human cell is only ~8 microns in diameter and thus encloses a volume of at most ~268 micron^3 (Table 8.17), there is precious little maneuvering room for a medical nanorobot that may be 1-30 micron^3 in size. Once inside the nucleus, a principle safety concern must be avoiding damage to the relaxed euchromatin strands that permeate the nucleoplasmic space. Only ~0.1 pN of force is required to move chromosomes around the nucleus at ~0.1 microns/sec during mitosis.[1463] DNA base pair hydrogen bonds may be pulled apart with 70-75 pN/bond of force,[1066] although the DNA backbone itself can withstand up to ~10 nN in tension; most conservatively, nanorobots should never apply tensile or shear forces greater than ~50 pN to chromatin strands during nucleoplasmic locomotion. Care should also be taken to design nanorobot exterior surfaces that are free of sharp edges and which possess electrochemical characteristics that tend to be nonattractive to DNA and to nucleosomal components. Since DNA is negatively charged and histones are positively charged (to bind the DNA), and since the lipid membranes are internally hydrophobic but polar on the surface, the ideal nanorobot exterior might require a surface of alternating charges which is nonhydrophobic and neutral with regard to DNA, histones, and lipid surfaces.

How can a nanorobot determine its intranuclear position? Chemonavigation is one crude approach. For example, a large number of stable RNA species—mostly the small nuclear ribonucleoproteins (snRNPs) essential for pre-messenger RNA splicing—are found in the nucleoplasm, the cytoplasm, or both. They range in size from 90-300 nucleotides and are present in 10^5-10^6 copies per cell (Table 8.19). snRNPs from HeLa (cancer line) cells contain ~40 proteins, 8 of which are shared by all snRNPs while the remaining ~32 proteins are snRNP-type specific.[1074] Nucleolus-specific proteins include UBF (94-97 kD), Ki-67 (345-390 kD), fibrillarin (34 kD), numatrin or B23 (38 kD), and nucleolin (100-110 kD);[1141] different nucleolar markers appear during mitosis. Detection of these species via chemosensors allows a nanorobot to distinguish cytoplasmic, nucleoplasmic, and nucleolar spaces, and possibly may permit even finer localizations. Various nucleic and protein products are continuously being transcribed from various chromosomes, whose distinct territories within the nucleus are relatively fixed during interphase (Sections 8.5.4.4 and 8.5.4.6). Detection of specific proteins and intermediate RNA transcription products in the nucleosol thus may allow chromosomal segment localization without having to actually sequence the segment (e.g., in early-generation medical nanorobotic systems).

Nanorobots requiring a 100-nm three-dimensional Cartesian navigation grid inside the nucleus may exploit the relatively uniform acoustic characteristics of the extranucleolar nucleoplasm by tethering a minimum of four small acoustic beacons tetrahedrally placed near the inside surface of the nuclear cortex at the antipodes of three transnuclear orthogonal coordinate axes. Each beacon emits brief ~1 GHz chirps in a distinguishable format unique to each beacon, at a very low duty cycle to avoid excessive energy consumption. From Eqn. 4.52, each chirp attenuates ~10^{-3} in amplitude per 100 nm of travel through the nucleoplasmic fluid. Hence an acoustic detector sensitive to 10^{-6} atm pressure changes can establish nanorobot position relative to each beacon to ~100 nm accuracy if the beacon output amplitude during the brief chirp is ~10^{-3} atm.

Table 8.19. Some Species of Stable RNAs and Their Localizations in Human Cells[996]

RNA Name	Length (# of Nucleotides)	Number of Molecules per Cell	Localization in Cell or Nucleus
U3	216	3 x 10^5	Nucleolus
U6	106	3 x 10^5	Perichromatin granules
U1	165	1 x 10^6	Nucleoplasm (heterogenous nuclear RNA)
U2	188	5 x 10^5	Nucleoplasm
U4	139	1 x 10^5	Nucleoplasm
U5	118	2 x 10^5	Nucleoplasm
7-3	300	2 x 10^5	Nucleus
4.5S	91-95	3 x 10^5	Nucleus and cytoplasm
7S	280	5 x 10^5	Nucleus and cytoplasm
7-2	290	1 x 10^5	Nucleus and cytoplasm

This should be low enough to avoid any possibility of cavitation damage to the chromatin or nuclear matrix. As a practical matter, additional beacons may be needed to reduce measurement uncertainties caused by nucleoplasmic nonuniformities and post-placement beacon positional shifts.

8.6 Ex Vivo Navigation

In this final Section of Chapter 8, we shall discuss ex vivo navigation—the task of navigating the spaces external to the human body. A comprehensive treatment is beyond the scope of this introductory text, so the following discourse is necessarily brief. From the nanomedical perspective, there are two distinct regimes in which ex vivo navigation may be necessary or useful: the epidermal regime and the exodermal regime.

8.6.1 Epidermal Navigation

Nanorobots traversing the epidermal regime (Section 9.5.2) must ascertain their position on the surface of the skin or in the hair. The epidermis averages ~100 microns thick but ranges up to 1000-1500 microns thick on the palms, soles, and other areas regularly subjected to rubbing or pressure. There are no blood vessels in the epidermis, so nanorobots may not be able to rely upon an internal microtransponder network or related navigational facilities.

The simplest solution to epidermal navigation is basic map-following. For example, the adult body has 2-4 million sweat glands (100-200/cm^2, mean separation ~800 microns). Most of these are saline- and urea-emitting eccrine glands ~20 microns in diameter, prevalent on the back, chest, forehead, palms, and soles. A smaller number of scent-secreting apocrine glands ~200 microns in diameter are concentrated at the underarms, nipples, genitals, and anus. Apocrine secretions are promptly broken down by skin bacteria to make odoriferous androstenone ("stale urine"), androstenol ("musky"), and isovaleric acid ("sweaty goatlike").[873] Sweat glands are persistent dermal landmarks that are readily mapped, along with their distinctive chemical secretions (including 0.028-0.4 mg/cm^3 glucose).[585] A positional or chemonavigational sweat gland map of the ~2 m^2 human skin surface to ~800 micron resolution requires ~3 million pixels or 24 megabits of data storage assuming 8-bit pixels.

An alternative or supplementary system is a follicular or crinal map of 50-100 micron diameter hair shafts that are irregularly distributed over the surface of the skin. Follicular map elements are reasonably stable due to subdermal anchoring. Hair follicles normally are most numerous on the scalp (~125,000 hairs or ~200/cm^2, with a ~700 micron mean separation between shafts and a mean natural life of 0.4-4 years), on the axillary (underarm), perineal and pubic regions, on the eyebrows and eyelids of both genders (each eyebrow has ~600 hairs with an average life of 112 days), and in a highly variable number density on the face, chest, arms and legs, most notably in males. An epidermal follicular map recording the locations of ~200,000 individual hair shafts using (700 micron)^2 8-bit pixels requires 4 million pixels and 32 megabits of data storage. Crinal navigation is readily accommodated as the nanorobot uses dead reckoning to track its position while traversing individually addressed hair shafts.

Epidermal map reliability is enhanced by noting numerous landmarks that may be regarded as "permanent" features on the timescale of nanorobotic actions. Such features might include scars, birthmarks, tattoos, warts, corns, cysts, nevi, small skin flaps, or dematofibromas. Stretch marks are found over the abdomen and breasts during pregnancy, over the abdomen in cases of obesity or fluid retention, on the necks of goiter patients, over the loins of patients suffering from disorders affecting the sacroiliac region, and over any distended organ. Epidermal maps are further enhanced using dermatoglyphics,[3425] the study of the patterns of ridges and lines on the skin of the fingers, palms, wrists, toes, soles, and neck. Many of these patterns are unique to a given individual (thus may be used to verify patient identity, e.g., fingerprints) and are persistent enough over time to serve as the basis for stable epidermal maps. Dermatoglyphics already plays a role in traditional diagnosis—Down's syndrome produces a characteristic mid-palm crease, and infant palm prints can reveal telltale signs of congenital heart defect.[3426-3428] Dermal ridges are also a sexually dimorphic trait—males have more ridges than females, and both sexes usually have more ridges on the right hand than on the left hand.[1052] In 1998, mole (nevi) photographic surveillance was a preventative skin mapping procedure to detect the onset of melanomas.

Less permanent but still useful epidermal landmarks include wounds, blisters, sunburns, eczematous or psoriatic regions, or chemical stains. Epidermal microbiotagraphic maps (Section 8.4.4) are also possible, but microbial populations usually cluster near apocrine glands and thus are unlikely to provide significant additional navigational information.

Skin temperature varies greatly across the epidermis (Section 8.4.1). The nonuniform number density of sweat glands in the skin produces highly localized periglandular temperature, moisture, and chemical compositional variations. However, these variations probably add little new information and are more difficult to interpret because readings may be strongly influenced by numerous complicating factors such as clothing and cosmetics, general physical activity level, localized physical activity (e.g., clapping hands), nonuniform sunlight-mediated heating, airflow and winds, immersion of body parts in water, and so forth. Nanorobots attempting to use this kind of information will need a very sophisticated global knowledge of somatic status.

Epidermal maps more accurate than ~1 mm might not prove particularly useful because natural movement of highly elastic dermal tissues may inject measurement errors of this magnitude into relative positional data used to locate adjacent glands, follicles or other epidermal landmarks.

8.6.2 Exodermal Navigation

Exodermal navigation encompasses an extremely broad range of operating environments. Most nanomedically relevant are nanorobots resident on or in droplets or boluses of sweat, saliva, mucus, epidermal flakes, hairs, ejaculate, urine or feces that are discharged from the body. Exodermal navigation also encompasses all medically relevant environments such as:

1. clothing or bedding;
2. the surfaces and interiors of furniture (upon which fingerprints typically stand ~5 microns tall), domiciles, vehicles, food, cosmetics, and refuse; and
3. all possible locales including land (e.g., sidewalks, roads, public buildings), water (e.g., drinking glasses containing beverage, bathtubs, swimming pools, rivers), air (e.g., exhaled nanorobots or airborne elements of nanorobotic personal defensive systems) and even vacuum (e.g., spaceborne nanorobots). Each environment poses unique navigational challenges, a complete treatment of which is quite beyond the scope of this book.

The airborne nanorobot (Section 9.5.3) is an interesting example of these unique challenges. Airborne nanorobots can identify their host patient by chemical signature, much like a bloodhound or mosquito following its quarry's scent.[3352] Such chemical signatures or "odortypes" may include:

1. naturally-produced "baseline" chemical scents;
2. behaviorally-related scents which may appear or intensify during specific events such as heavy exercise, fear reactions (e.g., emotional excitement alone can increase the sweat rate by ~50%), defecation or flatulence, sexual activity, intoxication, and the like;
3. artificial scents such as perfumes, colognes, cosmetics and deodorants; and
4. artificial molecular taggants specially designed to simplify the recognition task, as for instance an odorless, volatile, digitally-encoded messenger molecule emitted from an external facility that is controlled by the patient.

Airborne nanorobots can stationkeep in the vicinity of the host patient by acoustic homing on a coded ultrasonic beacon worn by the patient, all of whose emanations are inaudible to the human ear. From Eqn. 4.52 the amplitude of a ν = 100 KHz acoustic wave passing through STP air over a range of x = 1 meter only attenuates to ~25% of the original amplitude. Operational broadcast information is readily passed from patient to circumcorporeal aerial nanorobots using other similar acoustic channels (Section 7.4.8). Ex vivo nanorobots can also detect normal conversational speech at a range of ~2 meters using >2.4 micron^3 pressure sensors (Section 4.9.1.6).

Airborne nanorobots can navigate and avoid no-fly zones (Section 9.5.3.6) by various methods. For instance, a flying nanorobot approaching an infinite planar sheet of 308 K (35°C) human flesh would detect spatially anisotropic thermal emissions (peak wavelength λ_{max} = 9.35 microns, ν_{max} = 32 THz; Eqn. 6.20) in a response time of t_{meas} ~ 5 nanosec, assuming a photosensor area A_e = 1 micron^2, SNR = 2 (~7 photons per detection), and dermal radiative intensity[919] I_d ~ 30 W/m^2 (see Eqn. 4.59). (Mosquitos register a ~0.0006% temperature differential at a 1-cm distance from human skin in real time during flight; Section 4.6.1.)

As another example, all aerial nanorobots can continuously transmit relative skin-proximity data to their neighbors, allowing each device within a virtual "warning lattice" to estimate its rate of approach to the nearest prohibited surface. Consider a grid of 200 million nanorobotic acoustic buoys deposited on the ~2 m^2 dermal surface of a nude human body. The buoys are spaced 100 microns apart, and each device has a 10-micron-diameter acoustic radiator operating on a 16.7% duty cycle at 4.2 MHz, giving a ~10 microsec signal repeat time using 7-wave signal packets (SNR = 2). An aerial nanorobot with an acoustic receiver of equal size can detect a warning buoy signal at a distance of 100 microns from the skin-resident grid, assuming a continuous buoy broadcast power of ~35 pW/buoy through air at 298 K (25°C), giving a total grid emission power of 7 milliwatts. Note that a nanorobot flying at 10 m/sec travels 100 microns in 10 microsec. Monitoring Doppler shifts in received frequency allows only the largest changes in relative velocity to be measured over multiple packet cycles in a usefully short period of time. At 4.2 MHz, summing ~50 packets (~500 microsec receipt time) allows a relative velocity change of ~1 meter/sec to be detected (Section 4.3.2).

Direct acoustic air ranging by individual flying nanorobots (i.e., echolocation) is also feasible but should be combined with a "warning lattice" system to allow neighbors and prohibited surfaces to be efficiently distinguished.

Power requirements may be estimated using Eqn. 7.22 by doubling X_{path} in the exponential, multiplying P_{comm} by $(X_{path}/r_{antenna})^2$ to account for the doubled path length, and dividing P_{comm} by the coefficient of reflection at the air/skin interface (0.9995; Section 4.9.1.6). A 23.1% duty cycle at 3 MHz (again giving a ~10 microsec repeat time at SNR = 2) allows aerial nanorobots to detect an approaching skin surface from a distance of 100 microns, while consuming a continuous power draw of ~29,000 pW for a 10-micron diameter receiver or ~230 pW for a 20-micron receiver, in air at 298 K.

CHAPTER 9
Manipulation and Locomotion

9.1 Nanorobot Dexterity and Mobility

Manipulation and mobility are crucial basic capabilities in most classes of medical nanodevices. Manipulation includes handling fluids, biological objects such as tissue matrix fibers or cellular elements, and nanomachines or their components. Physicians must be able to direct tissue- or cell-repair nanorobots to travel to a specific site where treatment is required, and once there, to manipulate the local environment to achieve the desired results. Nanodevice mobility in vivo makes possible the rapid reconfiguration of nanomedical communication, navigation, and power systems, while ex vivo mobility allows the design of more robust diagnostic and personal defensive systems. In vivo locomotion also permits precise mapping of the internal regions of the human body across many size and time scales, both for diagnostic and for therapeutic purposes.

This Chapter opens with a discussion of adhesion forces at the molecular level and the performance of nanoscale fluid pumps and fluidic circuits (Section 9.2). Several useful classes of nanomanipulators are then presented, along with various tool tips and manipulator configurations such as massively parallel manipulator arrays (Section 9.3). Techniques of in vivo locomotion are next described in the context of biofluid and nanodevice rheology, including bloodstream swimming, cell walking and anchoring, tissue diving, cell penetration, intracellular mobility, and cytocarriage (Section 9.4). The Chapter concludes with a brief consideration of ex vivo locomotion (Section 9.5).

Our evaluation of the biocompatibility[3234] of various manipulation and propulsion systems for medical nanodevices is deferred to Chapter 15.

Finally, the reader should be aware that as of 1999, much of the available experimental data on cellular mechanics and forces in biomolecular systems was still very incomplete and ill-defined. There remained significant uncertainties in the reported numbers, many of which were of necessity compiled from large-area or bulk measurements, or for just one type of easily-studied cell, cell membrane, transmembrane protein, or receptor, and thus might prove inaccurate when applied to other, seemingly similar, cellular systems. Thus the calculations, estimates, and conclusions offered here are highly tentative and must be applied with great caution.

9.2 Adhesion and Fluid Transport

An understanding of surface forces is an essential preliminary to any study of mechanisms of manipulation or locomotion. Such adhesive forces become important at the submicron scale where nanorobotic parts are meshing with and sliding against one another. Surface adhesion forces may cause tools, parts or workpieces to stick together. Surface forces may cause airborne or solvent-immersed nanodevices to adhere to container walls, to other dry or humid surfaces, or to each other possibly causing clumping. For a 1-micron object, the adhesive forces may exceed gravitational and inertial forces by a factor of 10^6 or more. Capillary forces also are important in fluid transfers inside nanodevices, in fluid transfers between nanodevices or between nanodevices and their operating environment, and during nanodevice tasks requiring locomotion through, or limb/object manipulation in, a watery environment. Surface tension forces are especially relevant during locomotion missions requiring passage through air/water interfaces, as might occur in the lungs.

Bowling[1146] classifies adhesive forces between objects into three categories. The first category includes long-range attractive interactions that may bring a particle to a surface and establish the adhesion contact area, such as van der Waals forces (Section 9.2.1), electrostatic forces (Section 9.2.2), and magnetic forces (Sections 4.7.2 and 5.4.1). A second category of forces are the interfacial reactions that help to define the adhesion area, most importantly the capillary forces arising from the establishment of liquid or solid bridges between particle and surface (Section 9.2.3), but also including other effects such as sintering (diffusion and condensation), diffusive mixing, mutual dissolution and surface alloying, which will not be considered further here. In the third category are very short-range interactions that may strengthen adhesion after an adhesive contact area has already formed; such forces include chemical bonds of all types and various noncovalent bonds such as hydrogen bonds that have already been described in Section 3.5.1.

The rest of this Section is concerned with the transport and manipulation of fluids. After a brief discussion of capillarity theory and the unique problems associated with nanotubular fluid flow (Section 9.2.4), this Section presents basic aspects of continuum fluid flow (Section 9.2.5), describes the problems of effervescence and crystallescence during offloading (Section 9.2.6), and concludes by examining various design issues in submicron-scale fluid pumping, plumbing, mixing, and containerization (Section 9.2.7).

9.2.1 Van der Waals Adhesion Forces

In dry or vacuum environments, adhesion forces between <100 micron diameter particles and surfaces (nanorobot and other) separated by 100 nm or less are usually dominated by van der Waals interactions.[1149] Consider a spherical particle of radius r lying a small distance $z_{sep} \lesssim 100$ nm from a flat plate of surface area $A >> \pi r^2$. As a crude approximation, ignoring retardation effects that may become important in solution for $z_{sep} > 5$ nm,[10] the van der Waals adhesive force is approximated by:[1146]

$$F_{vdW} = \frac{H\,r}{6\,z_{sep}^2} \qquad \text{\{Eqn. 9.1\}}$$

for $z_{sep} << r$, where H is the Hamaker constant for the interaction. (Eqn. 9.1 also applies to two crossed cylinders of equal radius.[1152]) The Hamaker constants for the materials comprising the sphere, the plate, and the surrounding medium are H_s, H_p, and H_m, respectively (Table 9.1), giving:[1149]

$$H \sim (H_s^{1/2} - H_m^{1/2})\,(H_p^{1/2} - H_m^{1/2}) \qquad \text{\{Eqn. 9.2\}}$$

The adhesion separation distance z_{sep} is often taken as ~0.4 nm for particles in intimate (but chemically unbonded) contact with a surface.[1146,1148] Hence the force required to overcome the van der Waals adhesive attraction of a perfectly rigid r = 0.5 micron particle adhered to a diamond plate in vacuo (with z_{sep} = 0.4 nm, H = 340 zJ) is F_{vdW} ~ 180 nN.

Real particles are not perfectly rigid but deform under the influence of this adhesive force. If the adhesion surface area is increased from point contact to a circle of radius $r_{adhesion}$, then the van der Waals adhesion force increases to:[1146]

$$F_{vdW} = \left(\frac{H\,r}{6\,z_{sep}^2}\right) + \left(\frac{H\,r_{adhesion}}{6\,z_{sep}^3}\right) \qquad \text{\{Eqn. 9.3\}}$$

According to the JKR theory of adhesion mechanics[1155] for a sphere on a flat surface of the same material with a work of adhesion $W_{adhesion}$ (joined surface energy; Section 9.2.3) and elastic modulus K_e:[1149]

$$r_{adhesion} \sim \left(\frac{6\,\pi\,r^2\,W_{adhesion}}{K_e}\right)^{1/3} \qquad \text{\{Eqn. 9.4\}}$$

Assuming $W_{adhesion}$ ~10 J/m² and K_e ~ 10^{12} N/m² for smooth flawless diamond and r = 0.5 micron gives $r_{adhesion}$ ~ 36 nm. Taking z_{sep} = 0.4 nm contact with a flat diamond plate over a ~4100 nm² circular adhesion spot in vacuo, then F_{vdW} ~ 1300 nN, a mean surface pressure of $p_{mean} = F_{vdW} / \pi\, r_{adhesion}^2$ ~ 3200 atm over the contact circle and a peak pressure $p_{peak} = 1.5\, p_{mean}$ = 4800 atm at the center. As the sphere is pulled away, separation occurs abruptly when the contact radius falls to $r_{adhesion} / 4^{1/3}$ = (~63%) $r_{adhesion}$ = 23 nm.

Van der Waals forces also depend upon the roughness of the surface. If a smooth sphere approaches a surface having uniform rugosity or roughness b_{rug} with roughness feature size << r, then the van der Waals force is approximately:[1148]

$$F_{rug} = \left(\frac{z_{sep}}{z_{sep} + \frac{1}{2} b_{rug}}\right) F_{vdW} \qquad \text{\{Eqn. 9.5\}}$$

For z_{sep} = 0.4 nm and b_{rug} = 10 nm, F_{rug} = 2% F_{vdW} ~ 4 nN for the rigid sphere (in vacuo) in the examples given above. Surface dimpling is a common practice in MEMS fabrication, for example, to reduce adhesion between polysilicon layers and the substrate.[1382]

A few other geometries of rigid bodies approaching contact are useful as well. For example, the van der Waals adhesive force between two flat plates of equal interfacial area A and uniform separation z_{sep} is:[1152]

$$F_{vdW} = \frac{H\,A}{24\,\pi\,z_{sep}^3} \qquad \text{\{Eqn. 9.6\}}$$

Table 9.1. Hamaker Constant for Various Materials[10,1146,1149,1152,1162]

Material	Hamaker constant(zJ)
Vacuum or Air	~ 0
Cadherin-II coated surfaces[3547]	0.029
RBC plasma membrane[1162]	0.05-5
α-crystallin eye lens protein[3548]	0.26
Liquid helium	0.57
Methanol	36
Water	37
Polytetrafluoroethylene	38
Acetone	41
Ethanol	42
Hydrocarbons	~ 50
Hydrogen peroxide	54
Glycol	56
Fused silica (SiO_2 quartz)	65
Polystyrene	66
Glycerol	67
KBr crystals	76
Polyethylene	76
Polyvinyl chloride	78
Platelet surfaces[3545]	~100
Mica	135
Alumina (Al_2O_3, e.g., sapphire)	140
Germanium	252-290
Silicon	260-275
Graphite	275
Copper	325
Diamond	340
Silver	344
Metals (misc.)	300-500
Silicon carbide	440

Two (1 nm)² diamond plates separated by z_{sep} = 0.4 nm in vacuo require F_{vdW} ~ 0.07 nN (~7 atm) to overcome the van der Waals attractive force. Such plates are the same size as the contacting end surfaces of the logic rods employed in Drexler's mechanical computer design (Section 10.2.1); the design assumes a rod realignment force of 1 nN in the exemplar calculations.[10] This result suggests that forces on the order of 10-100 pN must be applied to mobile nanoscale components inside mechanical nanodevices in order to overcome static van der Waals adhesion that arises due to the contact proximity of parts within the structure.

For another example, two rigid spheres of radii r_1 and r_2, separated by a distance $z_{sep} << r_1, r_2$, have a van der Waals adhesive force of:[1152]

$$F_{vdW} = \frac{H\,r_{red}}{6\,z_{sep}^2} \qquad \text{\{Eqn. 9.7\}}$$

where the reduced radius $r_{red} = (r_1\, r_2) / (r_1 + r_2)$. A pair of 1-micron diameter rigid diamond spheres separated by z_{sep} = 0.4 nm in vacuo have a van der Waals mutual adhesive force F_{vdW} ~ 90 nN.

As one final example, the van der Waals force between two parallel cylinders of length L, radii r_1 and r_2, and separation z_{sep} is (differentiating V_{vdW} in Drexler[10]):

$$F_{vdW} = \frac{H\,L\,r_{sep}^{1/2}}{128^{1/2}\,z_{sep}^{5/2}} \qquad \text{\{Eqn. 9.8\}}$$

A pair of 1-nm diameter, 10-nm long rigid diamondoid cylinders lying exactly z_{sep} = 0.4 nm apart along their entire length in vacuo feel a van der Waals force of F_{vdW} ~ 1.5 nN. In all three examples, as before, the force rises slightly if the objects deform and declines significantly if surface rugosity is increased. (See also entropic packing, Section 9.4.2.3.)

9.2.2 Electrostatic Adhesion Forces

Two types of electrostatic forces may act to hold particles to surfaces. The first type of force is due to bulk excess charges present on the particle or surface which produce a classical Coulombic attraction known as the electrostatic image force. Consider two spheres of radii r_1 and r_2 located a distance z_{sep} apart, where $z_{sep} << r_1, r_2$. Then following Eqn. 4.40 the image force is given by:[1148]

$$F_{image} = \frac{q_1 q_2}{4 \pi \varepsilon_0 \kappa_e d_{sep}^2} = \frac{4 \pi \sigma_1 \sigma_2 r_{red}^2}{\varepsilon_0 \kappa_e} \qquad \text{\{Eqn. 9.9\}}$$

where q_1 and q_2 are charge on the two spheres (coul), σ_1 and σ_2 are the surface charge densities (coul/m^2), ε_0 = 8.85 x 10^{-12} farad/m (permittivity constant), κ_e is the dielectric constant of the medium, and d_{sep} ~ $r_1 + r_2$ is the distance between charge centers. Taking σ_1 ~ σ_2 = 10^{-5} coul/m^2 (~63 charges/micron^2; cf. ~1000 charges/micron^2 for "highly charged surfaces"[1151]), r_1 ~ r_2 = 0.5 micron and κ_e = 1 in vacuo, then F_{image} ~ 0.009 nN.

The electrostatic image force between two flat plates of equal interfacial area A, equal charge density σ, and uniform separation z_{sep} with $z_{sep} << A^{1/2}$, is:[727]

$$F_{image} = \frac{\sigma^2 A}{2 \varepsilon_0 \kappa_e} \qquad \text{\{Eqn. 9.10\}}$$

For σ ~ 10^{-5} coul/m^2 and A = 1 micron^2 in vacuo (κ_e = 1), F_{image} ~ 0.006 nN (~0.00006 atm). At larger z_{sep} and a voltage differential V_{plate} between the plates with capacitance C_{plate}, then:

$$F_{image} = \frac{C_{plate} V_{plate}^2}{2 z_{sep}} = \frac{\varepsilon_0 \kappa_e A V_{plate}^2}{2 z_{sep}^2} \qquad \text{\{Eqn. 9.11\}}$$

Thus if A = 1 micron^2, V_{plate} = 1 volt, and z_{sep} = 0.2 micron, then F_{image} ~ 0.1 nN.

The second and more important type of electrostatic force for very small particles is the electrostatic contact potentials, also known as induced electrical double layer forces.[1146] When two different initially uncharged materials with different local energy states and work functions are brought into contact, charge flows between them until an equilibrium is reached. The resulting potential difference is called a contact potential, $V_{contact}$, which typically ranges from ~0-1 volt. In the case of two metals, only the surface layer which is $x_{contact}$ ~ 1 nm thick (the gap for tunneling) carries contact charges; for semiconductors and insulators, these regions may extend into the bulk up to $x_{contact}$ ~ 1 micron or deeper.[1146] For a spherical particle of radius r at a distance z_{sep} from a surface, the induced charge density[1147] is $\sigma = \varepsilon_0 V_{contact} / z_{sep}$ and the contact force is:[1146]

$$F_{contact} = \frac{\pi \varepsilon_0 r V_{contact}^2}{z_{sep}} \qquad \text{\{Eqn. 9.12\}}$$

Taking r = 0.5 microns, $V_{contact}$ = 0.5 volts, and z_{sep} = 5 nm, then $F_{contact}$ ~ 1 nN (~0.01 atm). Induced charge densities vary experimentally from 2 x 10^{-7} coul/m^2 (~2 x 10^{-11} atm contact pressure) for polystyrene on polystyrene[1153] up to 2 x 10^{-2} coul/m^2 (~200 atm) for SiO_2 on mica.[1154] In this latter study, a pair of contact-adhered silica/silica sheets required a force of ~0.08 nN/nm to pull them apart and a mica/mica pair required ~ 0.11 nN/nm; however, due to contact electrification a silica/mica pair required 6.6-8.8 nN/nm to separate.[1154] Proper nanomechanical design can avoid or enhance these effects, as required.[10]

Double layer electrostatic contact forces usually predominate over electrostatic image forces for small particles; image forces are important only for materials that can carry high surface charges, such as polymers of poor conductivity or other extreme insulators. Because of their r/z_{sep} dependency, contact electrical forces are usually more important than van der Waals forces only for large particles and at separations wider than ~100 nm, although electrical forces can dominate in smaller particles if the surface asperities of the particles are significant enough to remove the bulk of the particle from the contact point, thus greatly reducing the van der Waals interaction.[1146] In either case, the total forces of adhesion far outweigh the force of gravity, given by:

$$F_{gravity} = \frac{4}{3} \pi r^3 \rho g \qquad \text{\{Eqn. 9.13\}}$$

For density ρ = 3510 kg/m^3 for diamond, acceleration of gravity g = 9.81 m/sec^2, and particle radius r = 0.5 micron, $F_{gravity}$ ~ 10^{-5} nN; for r = 1 nm, $F_{gravity}$ = 10^{-13} nN.

Entropic and electrostatic effects can sometimes interact to produce an apparent repulsion between opposite charges—as, for example, between positively charged bilayer surface and negatively charged colloidal particles.[3674]

9.2.3 Immersive Adhesion Forces

For hydrophilic particles exposed to high humidity, or immersed and then withdrawn from a fluid, a liquid film can form on the surface of the particle by capillary condensation or by capillary action between particle and surface. For a spherical particle of radius r linked by a liquid bridge to a planar surface of the same material with contact area A, separation z_{sep}, and liquid surface tension γ, then the capillary force between sphere and plane is $F_{capillary}$ ~ $2 \gamma A / z_{sep}$ for small contact angles between the liquid and the surfaces.[1147] Assuming hydrophilic (wettable) surfaces with wetting coefficient cos(θ) as defined in Section 9.2.4 and $z_{sep} << r$, the capillary force is given approximately by:[1146,1147,1149]

$$F_{capillary} = 4 \pi r \gamma \cos(\theta) \qquad \text{\{Eqn. 9.14\}}$$

which has been confirmed experimentally by direct measurement.[1149] For the water-air interface, cos(θ) ~ 1 and surface tension γ = 75.6 x 10^{-3} N/m at the freezing point (273 K), 72.75 x 10^{-3} N/m at room temperature (293 K), 70.05 x 10^{-3} N/m at human body temperature (~310 K), 58.90 x 10^{-3} N/m at the boiling point at 1 atm (373 K), and 110 x 10^{-3} N/m for ice at 273 K.[763,1149] Thus at room temperature, the capillary force on an r = 0.5 micron particle is $F_{capillary}$ ~ 460 nN; an r = 10 nm particle feels $F_{capillary}$ ~ 9 nN, a rather substantial force. Liquid bridges containing dissolved substances may evaporate and create solid crystalline bridges. Hydrophobic surfaces are generally unaffected by capillary forces.[1146]

Eqn. 9.14 also applies to nanorobots that are caught in an air-liquid interface such as the surface of a puddle of water, alveolar fluids in the lung, or an epidermal pool of sweat. However, adding capillary-active solute to a solvent may lower surface tension considerably. For dilute surface concentrations of a solute of molecular area A_{mol} in solvent of surface tension γ_0 at temperature T, the resulting surface tension of the solution drops to:[390]

$$\gamma = \gamma_0 - \frac{kT}{A_{mol}} \quad (N/m) \qquad \{Eqn. 9.15\}$$

For palmitic or stearic acid (e.g., soap), $A_{mol} \sim 0.21\ nm^2$;[2178] added to water ($\gamma_0 = 70.05 \times 10^{-3}$ N/m) at 310 K, surface tension falls to $\gamma = 49.70 \times 10^{-3}$ N/m. More concentrated solutions further reduce surface tension, nonlinearly with concentration. For example, $\gamma \sim 25 \times 10^{-3}$ N/m for a 0.1 M aqueous fatty-acid solution of hexanoic acid ($CH_3(CH_2)_4COOH$; MW = 116 daltons), a total of ~6 x 10^7 molecules, ~0.01 micron^3, or ~0.01 picograms of hexanoic acid per micron^3 of solution.[390] For the aqueous solution-air interface, inorganic electrolytes (e.g., NaCl), organic acid salts, low-MW bases, and certain nonvolatile nonelectrolytes such as glucose and glycerin are capillary inactive.[390]

Surface tension is reduced even more dramatically by biological surfactants. Lung surfactant, whose activity is largely attributed to the phospholipid palmitoylphosphatidylcholine,[996] produces a nonlinear change in surface tension with area. As the lungs fill with air, more-inflated alveoli have higher γ's than less-inflated alveoli, serving to stabilize alveoli of different sizes.[526] Aqueous solutions of surfactant from mammalian lung extracts show a surface tension reduction to as low as $\gamma \sim 0.7 \times 10^{-3}$ N/m at 20% of maximum film distension.[2179] Survanta, an intratracheal pulmonary surfactant commonly used in the treatment of respiratory distress syndrome (aka. hyaline membrane disease) in premature infants, lowers minimum aqueous surface tension to $\gamma \lesssim 8 \times 10^{-3}$ N/m.[2119]

Adhesion forces are greatly reduced for particles and surfaces that remain completely immersed in liquid. Surface tension effects are largely eliminated.[1146,1147] Electrostatic image forces (Eqns. 9.9 and 9.10), already quite small, are further reduced by a factor of $\kappa_e^{-1} \sim$ 1-2% (κ_e = 74.3 for pure water at 310 K, usually reduced to ~40 in a hydrophobic environment). Electrostatic contact forces may be greatly reduced because of sorption phenomena which tend to shield the charges (Sections 3.5.1 and 4.7.1). For particles and plates made of the same material, charges generally form the same double layers on both surfaces so that the double layer interactions are repulsive, thus reducing the net adhesive force, by an amount:[1146]

$$F_{shield} \sim 64\ \pi\ kT\ r\ c_{ion}\ x_{contact} \qquad \{Eqn. 9.16\}$$

where k = 0.01381 zJ/K (Boltzmann constant), T is temperature, r is particle radius, c_{ion} is the volumetric charge density of ions in the liquid, and $x_{contact}$ is the double layer thickness. Taking T = 310 K, r = 0.5 micron, $c_{ion} \sim 10^{26}$ ions/m^3 (~1% or 0.15M NaCl aqueous solution, ~human blood), and $x_{contact} \sim 0.8$ nm (~K_{dh}^{-1}; Section 3.5.1), then $F_{shield} \sim 34$ nN. (Effective double layer thickness $x_{contact}$ ~ 1 nm for a 0.1M solution of univalent electrolyte, ~10 nm for a 0.001M solution.[1162]) While different ions may collect in various alignments at unlike surfaces so that attractive (i.e.,contributing to adhesion) or repulsive shielding forces are possible, in most cases involving nanodevice surfaces that are fully immersed in human body fluids the electrostatic contact forces should be quite small.

The van der Waals force is also moderately reduced in fluids. For example, van der Waals adhesion between two diamondoid nanodevice surfaces fully immersed in water is only half of its vacuum value because the Hamaker constant (Eqn. 9.2) is reduced from 340 zJ to 153 zJ. Blood cells are subject to similar forces. It has been proposed that the ~15 nm gap frequently observed between the surfaces of aggregated red cells represents the position of the potential energy minimum where the forces of electrostatic repulsion (between negatively charged red cells) and the van der Waals attractive forces are equal.[1162] Taking H = 5 zJ, r_{red} = 3 microns and z_{sep} = 15 nm in Eqn. 9.7, the net attractive force between red cells is $F_{vdW} \sim 0.01$ nN.

Surface force experiments have demonstrated molecular control of adhesion at a fine level.[1152] According to the commonly-used JKR theory,[1155] the mechanical force needed to separate two elastic spheres each of radius r already adhered by molecular contact is:

$$F_{adhesion} = \left(\frac{3\pi}{4}\right) W_{adhesion}\ r \qquad \{Eqn. 9.17\}$$

where $W_{adhesion}$ is the Dupre reversible work of adhesion (energy per unit area). For example, hydrocarbon rubber spheres display $W_{adhesion} = 71 \times 10^{-3}$ J/m^2 in air but only 6.8 x 10^{-3} J/m^2 in water. When sodium dodecyl sulfate[1155] or dodecylammonium chloride[3546] is added to the water so the liquid can wet the surface, $W_{adhesion}$ actually becomes negative—the surfaces are pushed apart by the intervening fluid. Nonwetting liquids increase adhesion. For instance, polydimethyl siloxane rubber has $W_{adhesion} = 43.6 \times 10^{-3}$ J/m^2 to itself, in air. In water, a nonwetting liquid, adhesion nearly doubles to 74 x 10^{-3} J/m^2; in methanol, a wetting liquid, adhesion is almost eliminated, falling to 6 x 10^{-3} J/m^2.[1160] In nanomedical engineering applications where minimization of adhesive forces is an important design objective, adhesion of specific classes of materials may be virtually eliminated by surface modifications that reduce $W_{adhesion}$, as is commonplace in biological surfaces and in engineered capillary coatings designed to reduce electroosmotic drag force during capillary zone electrophoresis.[1229]

9.2.4 Capillarity and Nanoscale Fluid Flow

In vivo nanodevices will often find it necessary to inject or to extract small aliquots of fluid from organelles, cells, tissues, or the environment. Internal gas or liquid transfers will also be commonplace in fluidic tethers, hydraulic communication and power conduits, nanohydraulic pistons, manipulators and metamorphic bumper drivers, and in bulk transfers into sensor cavities or chemical reaction chambers inside nanofactories (Chapter 19). Nanopipes may also be used in biomimetic nanosystems such as artificial organs and artificial cell components such as tubulin substitutes (Chapter 21). Hence it is essential to examine the nature of fluid flows and "wicking" in nanocapillary vessels, and the likely behavior of fluids in nanomachines.

The theory of macroscale capillarity is well-studied.[1163] The concept of "wetting" is basic. Consider a fluid in a vessel. At the solid-liquid-gas interface (the vessel wall) there is a characteristic contact angle θ, the angle at which the meniscus contacts the container wall. This angle is indicative of the balance between the forces of (1) adhesion between the liquid and the solid wall and (2) cohesion within the surface of the liquid. A contact angle <90° means that adhesion is strong and the liquid is "wetting" the tube; an angle >90° implies that adhesion is relatively weak and the liquid is "nonwetting." In air against glass, the liquids alcohol, glycerol, and pure water have θ ~ 0°, while turpentine has θ ~ 17° and impure water has θ ~25°;[1164] all are wetting. On the other hand, mercury on glass has θ = 140° and water on paraffin has θ = 109°;[1164] both are nonwetting.

In the classical example of capillarity, one end of a narrow-bore open-ended tube is dipped vertically into a liquid. The liquid wets the tube, and the liquid rises until the force due to surface tension (F_{cap}) pulling the liquid upward equals the force of gravity (F_{grav}) pulling the column of liquid downward at some height h_{cap}, given by:[1163]

$$h_{cap} = \frac{2 \gamma_{lg} \cos(\theta)}{g\, r_{cap} (\rho_l - \rho_g)} \quad \text{\{Eqn. 9.18\}}$$

with wetting coefficient $\cos(\theta) = (\gamma_{sg} - \gamma_{sl}) / \gamma_{lg}$ (the Young equation[1163]) where γ is surface tension at the solid-gas (sg), solid-liquid (sl), or liquid-gas (lg) interfaces; ρ_l and ρ_g are liquid and gas density; g = 9.81 m/sec (acceleration of gravity) and r_{cap} is the inside diameter of the tube. Thus pure water with air at STP in a glass capillary with r_{cap} = 1 micron can rise h_{cap} = 15 meters against gravity, representing a mean pressure $p_{cap} = h_{cap}\, g\, (\rho_l - \rho_g)$ = 1.5 atm. A nonwetting liquid does not rise up the tube, but falls instead.

In the more general case of a linear capillary tube whose flow vector makes an angle φ_{grav} with the ambient gravity field (e.g., $\varphi_{grav} = \pi$ is a tube pointing straight up), then the force on the fluid column is:

$$F_{column} = F_{cap} + F_{grav} \quad \text{\{Eqn. 9.19\}}$$

$$F_{cap} = 2 \pi \gamma_{lg} \cos(\theta)\, r_{cap} \quad \text{\{Eqn. 9.20\}}$$

$$F_{grav} = \pi\, h_{cap} (\rho_l - \rho_g)\, g \cos(\varphi_{grav}) r_{cap}^2 \quad \text{\{Eqn. 9.21\}}$$

Taking the largest reasonable tube that might fit inside an in vivo nanorobot, h_{cap} = 1 micron, r_{cap} = 0.1 micron, $\rho_l - \rho_g \sim$ 1000 kg/m^3, $\gamma_{lg} \sim 72 \times 10^{-3}$ N/m for pure water, and taking $\cos(\theta) \sim \cos(\varphi_{grav}) \sim 1$, then $F_{cap}/F_{grav} \sim 10^8$, giving the familiar result that gravity can usually be ignored in nanoscale systems. For this example, $F_{column} \sim F_{cap}$ = 44 nN and column fluid pressure $p_{column} \sim 2\, \gamma_{lg} \cos(\theta) / r$ = 14 atm. Taking instead the smallest reasonable nanocapillary tube with h_{cap} = 20 nm and r = 2 nm, then $F_{cap}/F_{grav} \sim 10^{11}$, $F_{column} \sim$ 0.9 nN and $p_{column} \sim$ 700 atm, making a quite substantial wicking force. Of course, the frictional effect of the interface region requires that a finite pressure $P_0 \sim 2\, \alpha / r_{cap}$ must be applied before fluid motion will begin,[1188] where α = 0.01-0.1 N/m (experimental); taking $\alpha \sim$ 0.01 N/m, then $P_0 \sim$ 2 atm for r = 0.1 micron, or ~100 atm for r = 2 nm.

The capillary force may also be compared to the simple hydrostatic suction force:

$$F_{suck} = \pi\, r_{cap}^2\, \Delta p \quad \text{\{Eqn. 9.22\}}$$

A nanopipette with inside radius r_{cap} = 0.1 micron which is pressed against a plasma membrane surface and is then evacuated behind the attachment point sufficiently to create a surfacial pressure differential of Δp = 0.3 atm produces a purely hydrostatic suction force of F_{suck} = 1 nN.

Such classical continuum models assume, among other things, that the molecular graininess of the fluid can be ignored. This assumption fails when tube dimensions (e.g., r_{cap}) are comparable to the characteristic molecular length scale (λ) of the fluid.[10] In a gas, λ_{gas} is the mean free path between collisions. For T_{gas} = 310 K air with $n_{gas} = 2.4 \times 10^{25}$ molecules/m^3 at $p_{gas} = n_{gas}\, kT_{gas}$ = 1 atm pressure, the free path is given by:

$$\lambda_{gas} = (2^{1/2}\, \pi\, n_{gas}\, d_{gas}^2)^{-1} = (2^{1/2}\, \pi\, p_{gas}\, d_{gas}^2 / kT_{gas})^{-1} \sim 200 \text{ nm} \quad \text{\{Eqn. 9.23\}}$$

under ideal gas conditions, if we take the effective molecular diameter as $d_{gas} \sim$ 0.2 nm. At high pressure, van der Waals equation must be used (Section 10.3.2), but for p_{gas} = 1000 atm with $n_{gas} = 1.3 \times 10^{28}$ molecules/m^3, then $\lambda_{gas} \sim$ 0.4 nm. In a liquid, $\lambda_{liq} \sim d_{liq}$, the molecular diameter; for water molecules, $\lambda_{liq} \sim$ 0.3 nm.

A ratio of $r_{cap}/\lambda \sim 1$ marks an important transition because it implies that molecules are colliding with the walls about as often as they are colliding with each other. If $r_{cap} << \lambda$, then intermolecular interaction is rare, wall collisions are relatively frequent, and molecular motion is largely ballistic between wall impacts. But if $r_{cap} >> \lambda$, then molecule/wall interactions are relatively rare and intermolecular collisions are relatively frequent. In the latter situation the continuum flow relations should become valid, for example when r_{cap} >> 200 nm for gases at ~1 atm or when r_{cap} >> 0.4 nm for gases at ~1000 atm, or when r_{cap} >> 0.3 nm for liquids.

The range of non-continuum skin layer effects appears quite narrow in many cases. For instance, two smooth mica surfaces that are slowly brought together while immersed in various nonaqueous fluids display oscillating attractive and repulsive forces as a function of separation when the gap is less than 6-10 molecular diameters; periodic jump distances are about equal to the molecular diameter of the fluid.[1165] Oscillations become smaller between rough surfaces and in liquids that mix molecules of different sizes.[1149] Similar experiments in water with electrolyte produce similar behavior, but with ionic double layer repulsions superimposed—oscillatory solvent forces become significant only at z_{sep} < 2 nm.[1166] Elastohydrodynamic simulations suggest that flat gold surfaces separated by 2.3 nm with 0.9-nm asperities (the "near-overlap" case) should slide smoothly on a thin film of liquid lubricant molecules, albeit with nanometer-scale cavitated zones extending ~3 nm downstream persisting for ~0.1 nanosec at a sliding velocity of 10 m/sec.[1172] Solvation forces may also appear at separations below a few molecular diameters.[1149]

These results suggest that water-carrying nanocapillaries >2-4nm in internal diameter should function largely in line with continuum models. Early theoretical calculations predicted that open-ended carbon nanotubes as small as 0.8 nm in diameter might act as "nanostraws" and could wick in molecules from vapor or fluid phases.[1167] Subsequent experiments[1168-1170] confirmed that fluids with $\gamma_{lg} \lesssim 190 \times 10^{-3}$ N/m, including liquid sulfur, liquid selenium and nitric acid, are readily drawn into the inner cavity of carbon nanotubes with inside diameters of 4-8 nm through capillarity.[1169] This limit is sufficiently high to allow nanotube wetting by water ($\gamma_{lg} \sim 72 \times 10^{-3}$ N/m), most organic solvents ($\gamma_{lg} < 72 \times 10^{-3}$ N/m), and liquid acids (e.g., $\gamma_{lg} \sim 43 \times 10^{-3}$ N/m for HNO_3) which can then be used as low surface tension carriers to introduce dissolved solute into the nanotubes.[1170] Bulk nanotubes are readily wetted by water.[1168] Good wetting is favored when the polarizability of the tube material is higher than that of the liquid.[1171] Pure metals like molten lead or mercury with $\gamma_{lg} \gtrsim 190 \times 10^{-3}$ N/m do not wet carbon nanotubes and are not drawn in by capillarity. Such high-γ_{lg} liquids may be forced into the nanotubes by applying a hydrostatic pressure p_{force} given by the Laplace equation:[1168]

$$p_{force} \sim \frac{2\,\gamma_{lg}\cos(\theta)}{r_{cap}} \qquad \text{\{Eqn. 9.24\}}$$

Thus, liquid mercury with γ_{lg} = 490 x 10^{-3} N/m can be pushed into an r_{cap} = 0.5 micron tube by applying p_{force} ~ 20 atm to the fluid; p_{force} ~ 2000 atm for r_{cap} = 5 nm.

By 1998, detailed molecular dynamics simulation of fluid flow inside 1.3-1.6 nm diameter carbon nanotubes had been a subject of active research.[1173,1174] One major difference between macroscale and nanoscale fluidic systems is that in nanomachines the tube walls may be considerably less rigid* and may flex and resonate. Nanomachine designers must take into account the effects of these vibrations as they are transmitted through nanoscale structural elements attached to the tubes. Furthermore, tube wall motions are sometimes strongly size-dependent. The simulations confirmed that fluids flow faster through rigid tubes than through floppy tubes, as predicted by classical hydrodynamics theory (Section 9.2.5). At high flow velocities we may expect nanotubes to exhibit buckling modes, variable patency, progressive wave propagation, sluicing, flow-limiting flutter, and stall, by analogy to the fluid mechanics of compliant tube flow in human veins.[361] Carbon nanotubes may be rigidified by imposing a stretching tension, or possibly may be replaced by stiffer diamondoid tubes.[1173] If the fluid has more than one kind of atom, size-mass effects and differing interaction ranges or strengths may cause one or more species to segregate at the walls or to flow at different rates.[1174]

Material flow through nanotubes has been well-exploited by biology, including the bacterial sex pili[3549] (Section 5.4.2), bacterial anal pores and cytoprocts,[3550] cellular excretory canals (e.g., in the glandular cells of the pancreas), 10-100 nm intranuclear nucleolar canals (Section 8.5.4.5), the 20-40 nm wide hollow tubular fluid transport network that forms the smooth intracellular endoplasmic reticulum (Section 8.5.3.5), the 75-nm diameter nutrient-transporting tubovesicular membrane network of the human malaria parasite,[1183] the >100-nm wide fluid-carrying human bone canaliculi (Section 8.2.4), and prelymphatic tissue channels (Section 8.2.1.3).

The syringelike T4 bacteriophage tail assembly is perhaps the best-studied example of biological nanotube flow.[1179,1180] The 100-nm long, 20-nm wide cylindrical T4 tail assembly, made of 15 different proteins joined in 24 annular segments with an 8-nm inside bore, has a set of small fibers near the tip that attach to the plasma membrane of the host cell. After a lysozyme-like enzyme opens a breach in the host cell wall, the tail sheath thickens and contracts,[1181] inserting a ~2.8 megadalton hollow core protein nanotube (80 nm long, 7 nm wide, 2.5 nm inside bore) through the host cell integument. The protein nanotube is then uncorked in response to chemical signals, and a large-molecule (mostly putrescine and spermadine) pressure of ~30 atm ejects a single 70-micron long, 2-nm wide DNA thread (~50% of head volume) through the 2.5-nm nanotube aperture and out into the cell typically in ~3 seconds, a mean flow velocity of ~23 microns/sec.[1178] (DNA packing into the capsids of some phages is purely mechanical.[1723]) The double-stranded DNA thread rotates ~4000 times around its axis as it emerges.[1182] Under optimum conditions, initial injection velocity may start as high as 360 micron/sec with a minimum injection time of 0.23 sec.[1178]

The tensile strength of liquids may also be important in nanorobot internal fluid flows, even in the complete absence of capillarity. For instance, completely liquid-filled wetted tubes with no gas pockets make a continuous liquid column that can exhibit a large internal tensile strength K_{liquid} ~ 4 γ_{lg} / x_{molec},[1163] where x_{molec} ~ 10 nm is the approximate maximum range of intermolecular forces. Taking γ_{lg} ~ 72 x 10^{-3} N/m for water, K_{liquid} ~ 300 atm. There is experimental evidence that water saturated with air but denucleated by high pressures does exhibit a tensile strength on the order of ~300 atm.[1175] This tensile strength, and not capillarity, is credited for the ability of tall trees to pull sap up to 115 meters high,[1176] far exceeding the maximum 10.33 meters that water can be pulled vertically at the Earth's surface using a vacuum pump. M. Zimmermann[2031] reviews the sap transport system; the maximum pull recorded experimentally in trees is 120 atm.[2032]

9.2.5 Pipe Flow

Cellular and nuclear microinjection using fine glass pipette tips as small as 200 nm in diameter is commonplace in the experimental biological sciences.[1191] In small tubes or nanoinjectors with $r_{cap} >> \lambda$ (Section 9.2.4), nanoscale fluid flow behavior is approximated reasonably well by the classical continuum equations. Continuum flow[1390] is governed by the famous Hagen-Poiseuille Law (or more commonly, Poiseuille's Law), derived from the Navier-Stokes equations, which states that a pressure difference of Δp between the ends of a tube of radius r_{tube} and length l_{tube} will move an incompressible fluid of absolute viscosity η in laminar flow at a volume rate of:

$$\dot{V}_{HP} = \frac{\pi\, r_{tube}^4\, \Delta p}{8\,\eta\, l_{tube}} = \pi\, r_{tube}^2\, v_{flow} \quad (m^3/sec) \qquad \text{\{Eqn. 9.25\}}$$

The subsonic mean fluid velocity (v_{flow}), flow power dissipation (P_{flow}), and the flow time of an aliquot of fluid through the length of the entire tube (t_{flow}) then follow directly from Eqn. 9.25 as:

$$v_{flow} = \frac{r_{tube}^2\, \Delta p}{8\,\eta\, l_{tube}} \quad (m/sec) \qquad \text{\{Eqn. 9.26\}}$$

$$P_{flow} = \frac{\pi\, r_{tube}^4\, \Delta p^2}{8\,\eta\, l_{tube}} \quad (watts) \qquad \text{\{Eqn. 9.27\}}$$

$$t_{flow} = \frac{8\,\eta\, l_{tube}^2}{r_{tube}^2\, \Delta p} \quad (sec) \qquad \text{\{Eqn. 9.28\}}$$

Taking η= 0.6915 x 10^{-3} kg/m-sec for pure water at T = 310 K, a nanotube with r_{tube} = 10 nm, l_{tube} = 1 micron, and Δp = 1 atm passes fluid at $\dot{V}_{HP}$ = 0.6 micron^3/sec, v_{flow} = 2 mm/sec, with t_{flow} = 0.5 millisec. The incompressibility assumption generally holds in liquids and in gas flows where $\Delta p << p_{tube}$, where p_{tube} is the head pressure at the tube entrance.

The above equations describe the resistance to Poiseuille (laminar) flow in a pipe, which is the minimum of resistance of all possible flows in a pipe.[361] If the flow becomes turbulent, the resistance increases. The determinative parameter is a dimensionless quantity called the Reynolds number,[1187] N_R, which is the ratio of the inertial pressure (~ $\rho\, v_{flow}^2$) to the viscous pressure (~ $\eta\, v_{flow} / r_{tube}$) in the flow of a fluid of density ρ, or:

$$N_R = \frac{\rho\, v_{flow}\, r_{tube}}{\eta} \qquad \text{\{Eqn. 9.29\}}$$

For the example of the 10-nm nanotube in the previous paragraph, N_R ~ 10^{-5}. A large Reynolds number (Section 9.4.2.1) implies a

* *Approximately 100 nN of force are required to produce the first buckling[2659] of a carbon nanotube pressed perpendicularly onto a diamond surface. Nanotube compressive strength is ~1.5 x 10^{11} N/m^2 ~ 1.5 million atm, easily sufficient to penetrate any biological surface.*

preponderant inertial effect and the onset of turbulence; a small Reynolds number implies a predominant shear effect (e.g., viscosity) and the maintenance of laminar flow. Reynolds[1187] found that the transition from laminar to turbulent flow typically occurred at $N_R \sim 2000$-13,000, depending upon the smoothness of the entry conditions. The lowest value obtainable experimentally on a rough entrance appeared to be $N_R \sim 2000$. However, when extreme care was taken to establish smooth entry conditions (as is more likely in precisely structured nanotubes constructed using molecular manufacturing techniques) the transition could be delayed to Reynolds numbers as high as 40,000.

Even assuming the more conservative $N_R \sim 2000$ figure, it is clear that subsonic flow in nanoscale pipes will almost always be laminar. For a pipe with r_{tube} = 1 micron conveying water at 310 K (ρ = 993.4 kg/m^3), the onset of turbulent flow (taking $N_R \sim 2000$) occurs at v_{turb} (= v_{flow} in Eqn. 9.29) > 1400 m/sec, very nearly the speed of sound in water. In gases or liquids of lower density, or in pipes of narrower bore, or if a less conservative transitional Reynolds number is available due to superior design, then v_{turb} grows still larger. Thus turbulence is primarily a high-velocity, large-tube phenomenon.

In such turbulent flow situations with $N_R \gtrsim 1000$, a well-known empirical formula for the volume flow rate is:[363]

$$\dot{V}_{turb} \sim V_{HP} / Z \quad (m^3/sec) \qquad \text{\{Eqn. 9.30\}}$$

where the turbulence factor $Z = 0.005\, N_R^{3/4}$. Thus for N_R = 3000, $\dot{V}_{turb} \sim 0.5\, \dot{V}_{HP}$. Nevertheless, even in turbulent conditions of the general flow, fluid motion nearest the tube wall remains laminar in a thin layer of thickness x_{lam}, often estimated as:[1186]

$$x_{lam} \sim \eta \left(\frac{50\, l_{tube}}{\rho\, r_{tube}\, \Delta p} \right)^{1/2} \qquad \text{\{Eqn. 9.31\}}$$

For flowing water at 310 K and r_{tube} = 10 micron, l_{tube} = 100 micron, and Δp = 10 atm giving $v_{flow} \sim 200$ m/sec and $N_R \sim 3000$, then $x_{lam} \sim 0.5$ microns.

Poiseuille's Law assumes a rigid pipe, an assumption that may not hold for some nanotube designs and which certainly does not hold for human blood vessels, especially the veins. A complete treatment of fluid flow in elastic tubes is beyond the scope of this book. However, for steady laminar flow in an elastic tube with wall thickness h_{wall}, radius r_{tube}, length l_{tube}, p_0 and p_l the pressures at the entry and exit ends of the tube, and E_{wall} = Young's modulus of a Hookean (e.g., a linear force-distance relationship) wall material, then the volume flow rate through the tube may be approximated by:[361]

$$\dot{V}_{elastic} = \left(\frac{\pi\, c_h\, r_{tube}^4}{24\, \eta\, l_{tube}} \right) \left[\left(1 - \frac{p_l}{c_h}\right)^{-3} - \left(1 - \frac{p_0}{c_h}\right)^{-3} \right] \quad (m^3/sec) \qquad \text{\{Eqn. 9.32\}}$$

where $c_h = E\, h_{wall} / r_{tube}$. Taking $\eta = 0.6915 \times 10^{-3}$ kg/m-sec for water at 310 K, h_{wall} = 2 nm, r_{tube} = 10 nm, l_{tube} = 1 micron, p_l = (0.5 p_0) = 1 atm, and E = 10^7 N/m^2 (typical for human skin; Table 9.3), then $\dot{V}_{elastic}$ = 0.3 micron^3/sec. Care must be taken in applying this formula because many biological tube materials such as blood vessel walls are non-Hookean and exhibit a linear pressure-radius relationship instead. For small elastic deformations, the volume flow rate of such non-Hookean tubes may be approximated by:[361]

$$\dot{V}_{bv} = \frac{\pi\, r_{tube}^4}{20\, \alpha\, \eta\, l_{tube}} \qquad \text{\{Eqn. 9.33\}}$$

where α is the compliance constant, measured experimentally in feline pulmonary veins as 1.98-2.79 m^2/N for r_{tube} = 50-100 microns down to 0.57-0.79 m^2/N for r_{tube} = 400-600 microns.[1190] Other geometric nonuniformities such as regular and irregular tube tapers, embedded resonance chambers, tube bifurcations or multitube confluences have important effects on flow rate but are beyond the scope of this book. Poiseuille's Law also does not strictly hold for fluids seeded with polymers in concentrations as low as 10^{-4}-10^{-5} by weight, wherein drag may be reduced by a factor of 2-3.[2952,2953]

It bears repeating here that as pipes get very small, they can clog more easily due to van der Waals adhesive forces,[1152] so it becomes increasingly important to engineer interior vessel surfaces for minimum adhesivity with respect to all materials likely to be transported through the pipes (Section 9.2.3). Bursting strength of fluid-filled pressure vessels is addressed in Section 10.3.1.

9.2.6 Effervescence and Crystallescence

Diffusion-limited molecular inflow rates to nanodevices have already been discussed in connection with molecular transport (Section 3.2.2), chemical sensors (Section 4.2), chemical power sources (Sections 6.3.4.1 and 6.5.3), and chemical broadcast communication (Section 7.2.1). A related constraint applies when nanodevices attempt to offload endogenously produced or stored molecules into the local environment, whether by nozzled flow, reversible sorting rotors, or by simple bulk venting. If the excretion rate exceeds the solvation capacity of the surrounding solvent, offloaded gases may coalesce into bubbles and effervesce; offloaded solids may crystallize.

The inception of bubbles or crystals is a complex physical process whose detailed description is beyond the scope of this book. However, the diffusion-limited maximum offloading rate may be conservatively estimated by considering a point emission source releasing soluble gas molecules continuously into an aqueous environment at the constant rate $\dot{Q}$ (molecules/sec). Once emitted, molecules with diffusion coefficient D diffuse a distance $\Delta X \sim (2\, D\, \dot{Q}^{-1})^{1/2}$ (Eqns. 3.1 and 3.5), giving a minimum steady state concentration $c_{diffuse} \gtrsim (3 / 4\pi)\, (\dot{Q} / 2\, D)^{3/2}$ (molecules/m^3). As an approximation at pressures $\lesssim$100 atm for gases that do not chemically unite with the solvent, Henry's law gives the concentration of dissolved gas as $c_{solvated} = K_{henry}\, p_{gas}$ (molecules/m^3), where p_{gas} is the partial pressure of the solvated gas and K_{henry} is the Henry's law constant for the gas (Table 9.2). If the ambient concentration of the gas in the solvent is $c_{ambient}$, then the minimum offloading rate $\dot{Q}_{limit}$ necessary to enable the formation of bubbles occurs when $c_{diffuse} \gtrsim (c_{solvated} - c_{ambient})$, or:

$$\dot{Q}_{limit} \geq 2\, D \left[\left(\frac{4\pi}{3} \right) (c_{solvated} - c_{ambient}) \right]^{2/3} \quad (molecules/sec) \qquad \text{\{Eqn. 9.34\}}$$

Thus for oxygen dissolving in 0.15M saline (~human blood plasma), D = 2.0×10^{-9} m^2/sec (Table 3.3), $K_{henry} = 7.4 \times 10^{23}$ molecules/m^3-atm (Table 9.2), and $c_{ambient} = 3 \times 10^{22}$ molecules/m^3 (venous plasma; Appendix B), we have $\dot{Q}_{limit} \gtrsim 8 \times 10^7$ molecules/sec at p_{gas} = 1 atm, or $\dot{Q}_{limit} \gtrsim 2 \times 10^9$ molecules/sec at p_{gas} = 100 atm. Faster offloading rates than $\dot{Q}_{limit}$ may cause effervescence.

Table 9.2. Henry's Law Constants (gas solubility in water at 298 K)[390,526,2050]

Solvated Gas	Henry's Law Constant (molecules/m^3-atm)
He	~8 x 10^{22}
N_2 (0.15M saline)	3.5 x 10^{23}
N_2 (pure water)	3.8 x 10^{23}
H_2	4.7 x 10^{23}
CO	5.8 x 10^{23}
O_2 (0.15M saline)	7.4 x 10^{23}
O_2 (pure water)	7.6 x 10^{23}
CH_4	8.0 x 10^{23}
C_2H_6	1.1 x 10^{24}
C_2H_4	2.9 x 10^{24}
CO_2 (0.15M saline)	1.9 x 10^{25}
CO_2 (pure water)	2.0 x 10^{25}
C_2H_2	2.5 x 10^{25}
NH_3	1.5 x 10^{28}

For carbon dioxide in saline (ambient arterial plasma concentration), $\dot{Q}_{limit} \geq 7 \times 10^8$ molecules/sec (1 atm) or 1.5×10^{10} molecules/sec (100 atm). Once a gas bubble is formed and completely blocks a narrow pipe, the pressure required to dislodge it is approximately p_{force} as given by Eqn. 9.24, ~3 atm for an air bubble caught in a 1 micron wide tube carrying water at 310 K.

Similar considerations apply to solute releases which, if too rapid, may result in crystallization of the solid. In this case, Eqn. 9.34 may be used if $c_{solvated}$ is taken as the saturation concentration at the appropriate temperature and pressure. For example, a saturated 70% glucose solution has $c_{solvated} = 7.8 \times 10^{27}$ molecules/m^3; taking $D = 7.1 \times 10^{-10}$ m^2/sec and $c_{ambient} = 2.3 \times 10^{24}$ molecules/m^3 (~blood plasma; Appendix B), $\dot{Q}_{limit} \geq 1.4 \times 10^{10}$ molecules/sec.

Gas solubility almost always declines at warmer temperatures because gas-liquid solvation is exothermic, whereas the solubility of most solids (including glucose and most important electrolytes) usually rises at higher temperatures. (See also Section 10.5.3.)

9.2.7 Fluid Pumping and Plumbing

After reviewing specific requirements in nanomechanical systems for containing fluids within walls and seals, Drexler[10] concluded that nonbonded nanoscale interfaces could serve as seals to permit the relative motion of surfaces while hindering the flow of fluid between them. Such fluid-tight seals enable the construction of valves, pistons and cylinders, and hence fluid pumps. The following is a brief discussion of several useful classes of general-purpose nanopump designs. Molecule-specific nanopumps are described in Section 3.4; biocompatibility issues[3234] are deferred to Chapter 15.

9.2.7.1 Pressure Release Pumps

Some form of motive force must be applied to cause fluid to flow through a tube. The simplest possible motive force is pressurization. Consider a valved cylindrical nozzle of radius r_{tube} and length l_{tube} attached to a reservoir of volume $V_{reservoir}$ maintained at a constant pressurization $p_{reservoir}$ (even while being emptied). When the valve is opened, the fluid vents through the nozzle at a maximum velocity v_{max} into an external fluid environment having static pressure $p_{external} < p_{reservoir}$, emptying the reservoir in a time t_{empty}, both given by:

$$t_{empty} = \frac{8 \eta l_{tube} V_{reservoir}}{\pi r_{tube}^4 (p_{reservoir} - p_{external})} \qquad \{\text{Eqn. 9.35}\}$$

$$p_{reservoir} \lesssim p_{external} + \frac{8 \eta l_{tube} v_{max}}{r_{tube}^2} \qquad \{\text{Eqn. 9.36}\}$$

Taking $p_{external} \sim 1$ atm, $\eta = 0.6915 \times 10^{-3}$ kg/m-sec for water at 310 K, $r_{tube} = 10$ nm and $l_{tube} = 100$ nm, then holding $v_{max} \lesssim 10$ micron/sec (the velocity of random thermal intracellular hydrodynamic flows; Section 8.5.3.12) for intracellular discharges requires a driving pressure of $p_{reservoir} \sim 0.5 \times 10^{-3}$ atm, which takes $t_{empty} \sim 0.3$ sec to empty the reservoir at an energy cost (Eqn. 9.27) of $P_{flow}\, t_{empty} \sim 55$ zJ (~13 kT). As a practical matter, normal variations in physiological pressure due to ~1 Hz heartbeat pulse waves are 0.5-10 x 10^{-3} atm in the tissues and veins and up to 50-70 x 10^{-3} atm in the aorta (Section 4.9.1.2), so either valve aperture or $p_{reservoir}$ must be dynamically controlled if a steady exit velocity is required at such low discharge velocities. In addition, a minimum pressurization of ~p_{force} (Eqn. 9.24) must be used to overcome capillary forces and initiate the flow. Device cooling during rapid gas discharge is described in Section 5.3.3.

9.2.7.2 Positive Displacement Pumps

Mechanical energy may be converted to fluid flow using a side-mounted piston as a single-action reciprocating positive displacement pump. Consider a pipe of radius r_{tube} and length l_{tube}, with valves at either end and a piston mounted in a stub cylinder of radius r_{stub} mounted perpendicular to the pipe axis at the midpoint of the pipe length (Fig. 9.1). The valves may be purely passive, or may be actively controlled in synchronization with piston motions.

During a single pump cycle, the valve at one end of the pipe is opened and the piston in the stub cylinder is drawn out, sucking a fluid volume V_{cycle} from the external environment into the pipe through the open end. The first valve is then closed, the second valve at the other end is opened, and the piston is pushed back into the stub cylinder, forcing an equal volume V_{cycle} of fluid out through the opposite end of the pipe which is now open. Cycling this pump at a frequency ν_{pump} establishes a semicontinuous flow of $V_{pump} = \nu_{pump} V_{cycle}$, with pumped-fluid velocity v_{flow} and pump power P_{flow} given by:

$$v_{flow} = \frac{\nu_{pump} V_{cycle}}{\pi r_{tube}^2} \quad (\text{m/sec}) \qquad \{\text{Eqn. 9.37}\}$$

$$P_{flow} = P_{diss} + 8 \pi \eta l_{tube} v_{flow}^2 \quad (\text{watts}) \qquad \{\text{Eqn. 9.38}\}$$

where P_{diss} is the power dissipation due to piston wall friction, inertia, and fluid drag (Eqn. 6.13); for submicron pistons and $\nu_{pump} \lesssim 1$ MHz, $P_{diss} / \nu_{pump} << kT$ in good designs. From Eqn. 9.25, pumping pressure is given by $\Delta p = 8 \eta l_{tube} v_{flow} / r_{tube}^2$.

Operating frequency is restricted by at least four factors:

1. The mechanical response time of the fluid defines a maximum operating frequency of $\nu_{max} \lesssim v_{sound} / (l_{tube}/2)$; for l_{tube} = 100-1000 nm and v_{sound} ~ 1500 m/sec in water at 310 K, ν_{max} = 30-3 GHz. (Note also the requirements that $v_{max} << v_{sound}$ to avoid acoustic radiation losses, and that pressure and frequency must be sufficiently limited to avoid cavitation (Section 6.4.1).)

2. The maximum mechanical operating speed of nanoscale pistons is, conservatively, ν_{max} ~ GHz.[10]

3. The maximum acceptable flow velocity v_{max} defines a maximum operating frequency $\nu_{max} = \pi\, r_{tube}^2\, v_{max} / V_{cycle} = v_{max} / 4\, r_{tube}$ taking V_{cycle} ~ $(2\, r_{tube})^3$ (e.g., one full piston throw opens a volume equal to one cubic pipe diameter); taking v_{max} = 4 m/sec, then ν_{max} = 1-100 MHz for r_{tube} ~ r_{stub} = 1000-10 nm.

4. The maximum valving speed of v_{valve} = 0.01-1 m/sec (Sections 3.2.4 and 3.3.2) when applied to valves of radius r_{tube} defines a maximum valving frequency of $\nu_{max} = v_{valve} / r_{tube}$; for r_{tube} = 1000-10 nm, ν_{max} = 0.01-100 MHz.

These considerations suggest that as a conservative limit, ν_{max} ~ 1 MHz may be appropriate in nanomedical piston pump designs that are intended to interact with an aqueous or protoplasmic external biological environment. Nanorobot piston pumps transferring durable fluids internally may safely operate at frequencies up to ~GHz and pressures >1000 atm.

From Eqns. 9.37 and 9.38, and taking r_{tube} = 10 nm, l_{tube} = 100 nm, ν_{pump} = 1 MHz, η = 0.6915 x 10^{-3} kg/m-sec for 310 K water, and V_{cycle} ~ $(2\, r_{tube})^3$ = 8000 nm^3, then v_{flow} ~ 3 cm/sec, Δp = 1.6 atm, and P_{flow} ~ 1 pW assuming $P_{diss} << P_{flow}$, which will normally be the case. The mean pressure amplitude developed during each piston cycle is Δp_{piston} ~ $8\, \eta\, l_{tube}\, v_{flow} / r_{tube}^2$ ~ 1 atm. Reynolds number N_R ~ 0.0004 (Eqn. 9.29), giving laminar flow throughout the cycle; power losses due to differential compression of the streamlines as fluids curve through an elbow to enter and exit the piston stub should be negligible. If precise control of flow volume is not necessary, the active valves described above may be replaced by passive one-way check valves or flap valves analogous to those found in human veins (Fig. 8.3).

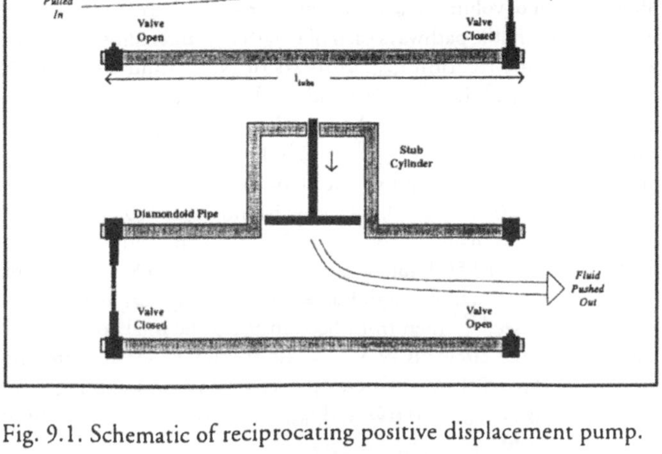

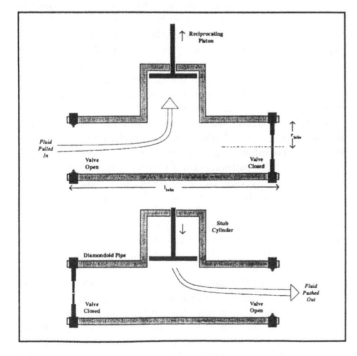

Fig. 9.1. Schematic of reciprocating positive displacement pump.

Many other mechanical positive displacement pumps are readily imagined—including diaphragm pumps, rotary pumps (valveless), hydraulic vane pumps (valveless), lobe pumps (valveless), screw pumps (valveless), reciprocating flap-valve or plunger pumps, bellows pumps, multiple piston pumps, continuous ciliary[2696] or peristaltic pumps (valveless),[1215,1216] and paddlewheel or waterwheel "gear" pumps (valveless)—all with similar scaling and performance parameters. The dominance of viscous forces over inertial forces in fluid flow at small scales favors the use of these positive displacement or static-type pumps over the use of rotodynamic or kinetic-type pumps such as centrifugal pumps (with impeller blades) and venturi or jet pumps (e.g., using a motive fluid, nozzle and diffuser).

9.2.7.3 Turbomolecular Gas Pumps

Drexler[10] has briefly reviewed the general design parameters of nanoscale turbomolecular gas pumps. Pump effectiveness depends on the ratio of the blade speed to the characteristic thermal speed of the lightest gas molecule to be pumped. If the blades are constructed of diamondoid materials, then blades may be as thin as ~1 nm and blade speed can exceed the velocities of the fastest gas molecules (e.g., 1960 m/sec for hydrogen at 310 K; Eqn. 3.3), providing a compression ratio of $\gtrsim$ 10 per blade row.[1204] Turbomolecular pumps are designed to operate under free-flow conditions involving essentially ballistic gas molecule trajectories of length λ_{gas} ~ 10 nm at 20 atm pressure, or λ_{gas} ~ 200 nm at 1 atm (Eqn. 9.23). Taking pump length per blade row ~10 nm for operating pressures up to ~20 atm, a pump assembly consisting of a stack of five blade disks achieves a compression ratio of ~10^5 in a ~50 nm pump length.

9.2.7.4 Nonmechanical Pumps

Nonmechanical pumps may induce fluid flow without using any moving parts in direct contact with the fluid. Electrohydrodynamic (EHD) pumps are one important class of these devices. Several different types of EHD micropumps have been fabricated.

For example, in the DC-charge injection pump[1205-1207] or ion drag pump,[1207-1209] ions are injected into the liquid at an emitting electrode under high field conditions and move under the influence of Coulombic forces toward a second collecting electrode where they are absorbed. Collisions between ions and fluid molecules transfer momentum from the ions to the fluid, producing fluid movement in the direction of ion flow. A prototype micropump has achieved a maximum pumping pressure of 0.01 atm (static) for ethanol flowing between two $(2500\ \text{micron})^2$ grids spaced 10 microns apart at 300 volts, producing a volumetric flow rate of $\dot{V}$ = 2.7 x 10^{-11} m^3/sec at a flow velocity of ~4 microns/sec.[1206] Static pump pressure p_{static} may be estimated[1208,1209] as:

$$p_{static} \sim c_{geom}\, \varepsilon_0\, \kappa_e \left(\frac{V}{d}\right)^2 \qquad \text{\{Eqn. 9.39\}}$$

where c_{geom} is a correction factor for electrode geometry of order unity, ε_0 = 8.85 x 10^{-12} farad/m (permittivity constant), κ_e = dielectric constant, V is electric potential and d is electrode separation. Taking V/d ~ 10^7 volt/m and κ_e ~ 74.31 for deionized water at 310 K, p_{static} ~ 0.7 atm. Pumping of different polar fluids with conductivities between 10^{-6}–10^{-12} $(\text{ohm-m})^{-1}$ such as propanol, acetone, deionized water, and many organic solvents including several oils has been demonstrated, but aqueous solutions of electrolytes could not be pumped due to their high ionic conductivity.

In the traveling wave electroconvection voltage pump,[1210-1212] phase-shifted rectangular voltages are applied across a series of parallel electrodes. Temperature induced conductivity gradients induce free electric charges which can interact with the traveling field due to charge relaxation processes in the volume of the fluid, causing fluid flow in a direction transverse to the electrodes. A small monotonic temperature gradient, which may be produced by the traveling waves themselves,[1212] is also required. Early prototype devices could pump only nonconductive fluids,[1211] but Fuhr et al[1212] have demonstrated EHD pumping of conductive fluids with conductivities between 0.0001-0.1 $(\text{ohm-m})^{-1}$ (e.g., up to ~0.01M NaCl aqueous solutions) using high frequencies and a low voltage waveform. Typically, volumetric flow rates of 10^{-10}–10^{-12} m^3/sec and flow velocities of 50-1000 micron/sec were achieved using traveling wave frequencies of 0.1-30 MHz at ~ 40 volts across 30 micron-wide electrodes spaced 30 microns apart in 50 x 70 micron square channels ~4000 microns in length.[1212] Flow velocity is a linear function of the square of the applied voltage and a complex function of the applied frequency. Further research is required to determine if unfavorable thermal scaling presents difficulties in submicron-size devices.

Other nonmechanical pumping methods have been studied. Electroosmotic pumping of electrolyte solutions has been observed in capillaries 50 microns in diameter or less, and separation of the components is also possible using electrokinetic phenomena with applied voltages up to 10,000 volts.[1213,1217] Electrowetting pumps using electrical control of the interfacial surface tension have produced ~0.1 atm flow pressures in 10 micron radius channels.[1221] Molecular flow can be induced by pulsed axial magnetic fields applied to carbon nanotubes placed in a transverse electric field. Ultrasonic pumps cause liquid to move in the direction of wave propagation with a speed proportional to the square of the acoustic amplitude;[1214,1215] speeds of 130 micron/sec have been observed in water at 3.5 MHz.[1214] Ferrofluids[1241] containing ~10 nm particles in suspension and electrorheological fluids[1242] allow electrostatic control of fluid flow via the Winslow effect,[1243] although early reports that blood flow could be electrostatically regulated have not yet been confirmed experimentally.[1244] Osmotic-pump motility across sugar gradients has been induced in micron-size phospholipid vesicles.[3269]

Optofluidic pumping is extremely energy inefficient and is feasible only at dangerously high beam intensities. Consider a beam of light of radius r_{beam} and intensity I_{beam} that exerts a photon-pressure force of $F_{beam} = \pi\, r_{beam}^2\, k_a\, I_{beam} / c$, where $c = 3 \times 10^8$ m/sec (speed of light) and $k_a = 0$ for total transmission, 1 for total absorption, and 2 for total reflection. Setting this equal to the Stokes law force (Eqn. 9.73) on a spherical target of radius r_{beam} in a fluid of absolute viscosity η gives the approximate magnitude of the fluid flow velocity as:

$$v_{flow} \sim \frac{k_a\, r_{beam}\, I_{beam}}{6\, \eta\, c} \qquad \text{\{Eqn. 9.40\}}$$

if we conservatively assume that dimensionless $k_a \sim r_{beam}\, \sigma_a$ where $\sigma_a \sim 300$ m^{-1} (optical absorption coefficient; Section 4.9.4). Taking $I_{beam} \sim 10^{11}$ W/m^2 (~optical tweezer intensity; compare maximum "safe" in vivo intensity of $\lesssim 10^5$ watts/m^2, Section 6.4.3.2) and $r_{beam} = 200$ nm giving $k_a \sim 6 \times 10^{-5}$ (almost complete transmission), then $v_{flow} \sim 1$ micron/sec but with a huge power dissipation of $\pi\, r_{beam}^2\, I_{beam} \sim 10$ milliwatts while developing a pumping pressure of only $p_{beam} \sim k_a\, I_{beam} / c = 2 \times 10^{-7}$ atm.

9.2.7.5 Fluid Mixing

In nanofluidic systems (e.g., pipes, chambers and junctions) of size $L \lesssim 100$ nm, even with strictly laminar flow, mixing of separate fluid streams is rapid because the small-molecule diffusion time $\tau \lesssim 10$ microsec (Eqn. 3.1 and Table 3.4). At the other extreme, systems of characteristic size $L \gtrsim 1000$ microns with $v_{flow} \gtrsim 1.4$ m/sec may readily establish a turbulent flow with $N_R \gtrsim 2000$ in water at 310 K (Eqn. 9.29), and again mixing of multiple fluid streams can be quite rapid.

However, for systems of scale 1000 microns > L > 100 nm, diffusion times range from 10^{-5}–10^3 sec for small molecules, and even longer for large molecules. Nonlaminar flow would demand unreasonably high fluid velocities, and diffusive stirring (Section 3.2.3.1) yields only modest improvements in mixing. To achieve rapid mixing in this intermediate size range, a micromixer chamber is first filled with one liquid, and then the other liquid is injected into the chamber volume simultaneously through a large number of very small nozzles. In the simplest micromixer designs the mixing nozzles form a regular coplanar array.[1219] In more complex designs, mixing nozzles will form a three-dimensional array possibly using a branching tree or fractal geometry with tip spacing ~1 micron to allow fully intimate mixing to be completed in ~1000 microsec; a ~100 nm tip spacing allows complete mixing in ~10 microsec.

9.2.7.6 Nanoplumbing and Fluidic Circuits

In fluid distribution systems that minimize total energy dissipation in laminar nonpulsatile flow, space-filling fractal networks of branching tubes are most efficient.[3242] At each branch point in such a network, where a single large tube of radius R bifurcates into N branches with each branch tube having radii $r_1, r_2, \ldots, r_N$, Murray[1220] found that shear stresses are equalized and flow impedance is minimized when:

$$R^3 = r_1^3 + r_2^3 + \ldots + r_N^3 \qquad \text{\{Eqn. 9.41\}}$$

In the special case where $r = r_1 = r_2 = \ldots = r_N$, which is quite common in biological systems, Murray's law reduces to $R^3 = N\, r^3$. For example, the human bronchial system typically has N = 2, so the ideal fractal network has $R/r \sim N^{1/3} = 1.26$; from Table 8.7, the actual value from trachea (generation 0) through the terminal bronchiole in generation 16 (after which alveoli begin to appear irregularly) is R/r = 1.24, in good agreement with Murray's law. In turbulent flow regimes, the exponent on Murray's law becomes 2.33, rather than 3.[1615] And in pulsatile flow through elastic tubes, which dominates the aorta and major arteries in the human circulatory system, the energy minimization principle requires area-preserving branching, or $R^2 = N\, r^2$ for the ideal network.[698]

Complex nanoscale fluidic logic devices are readily imagined. While fractal geometries are likely, for simplicity consider a three-dimensional fluidic circuit of volume $V_{circuit}$. A volume fraction f_{tube} consists of N_{tube} independent fluidic pathways each of length l_{tube} and radius r_{tube}, and a second volume fraction f_{valve} consists of N_{valve} fluidic gates each of volume L_{valve}^3. If each independent fluidic pathway is gated, on average, by a single valve, then $N_{tube} = N_{valve} = N = f_{valve}\, V_{circuit} / L_{valve}^3$ and $l_{tube} = (f_{tube} / \pi\, f_{valve})\, (L_{valve}^3 / r_{tube}^2)$. Ignoring reservoirs, inlet and outlet manifolds and support mechanisms, and taking $V_{circuit} = 1$ $micron^3$, $f_{tube} = 0.9$, $f_{valve} = 0.1$, $L_{valve} = 20$ nm, $r_{tube} = 10$ nm, and $\eta = 0.6915 \times 10^{-3}$ kg/m-sec for water at 310 K, then the fluidic circuit includes $N_{valve} = 12{,}500$ fluidic gates and $N_{tube} = 12{,}500$ independent fluidic pathways each of length $l_{tube} = 230$ nm. If typical flow velocity $v_{flow} = 1$ mm/sec,[1228] then from Section 9.2.5 the total volume flow rate through the circuit is $N\, \dot{V}_{HP} \sim 4000$ $micron^3$/sec at a pressure differential $\Delta p = 0.1$ atm. Circuit power dissipation (ignoring valve dissipation) is $N\, P_{flow} \sim 50$ pW and $t_{flow} \sim 0.2$ millisec assuming fully parallel operation (e.g., a path length l_{tube}), allowing a circuit operating frequency of t_{flow}^{-1} ~ 5000 Hz.

Capillary networks are readily gated by applying appropriate voltages, allowing valveless switching of liquid flow among various fluidic pathways. Purely electrical valving of fluid flows has been common practice in neurobiological research for decades. For example, the flow of acetylcholine from the open end of a micron-sized pipette (as it is inserted into tissue) is prevented by applying a negative bias or braking current of 3 nanoamps at the tip; flow resumes when the braking current is removed.[803] Constant-discharge flow-control valves using opposing polymer brushes with ~25 chains of ~40 monomers each[2902] and micron-scale electrorheological diodes[498] have been investigated. Macroscale fluidic NOR logic elements that can be used to construct arbitrary Boolean logic circuits* (for controlling materials flow) are widely available commercially,[1227] although these often employ the Coanda effect, vortices, or turbulence effects, which generally don't scale well to micron and submicron devices. In 1997, a microfluidic chip-based system for the integration of high-throughput drug discovery efforts was demonstrated by SmithKline Beecham and Orchid Biocomputer.[1222] This microfluidic chip incorporated microfabricated components for valving and pumping of organic solvents using electrokinetic transport within a three-dimensional fluidic network. The pumping and valving mechanisms had no moving parts, "making large scale integration feasible and inherently reliable." The study of microfluidic networks[1228,2697,2698] using hundreds of micron-wide channels was an active research area in 1998, and integrated chemical systems were being widely discussed.[121]

9.2.7.7 Containerized Flow

Once a block of fluid has passed into the interior of a nanodevice, it may be containerized or divergently subdivided and then transported at velocities far higher than diffusive flow (Eqn. 3.1) or Poiseuille flow (Eqn. 9.25) would otherwise permit. The velocities available in containerized flows are largely independent of fluid viscosity and total transport time (unlike diffusive flow), and are nearly independent of fluid pressure and flow channel length (unlike Poiseuille flow).

For easy comparison, consider a disk-shaped container of radius r_{block} and thickness h_{block} with useful fractional storage volume f_{block} (to account for container wall thickness and mechanism overhead). After loading with fluid, the container is transported through a channel of radius $r_{tube} \sim r_{block}$ and length l_{tube} at a velocity v_{block}, giving a volumetric flow rate of $\dot{V}_{block} = \pi\, r_{tube}^2\, f_{block}\, v_{block}$ (m³/sec) which is superior to the Poiseuille flow rate in a pressurized tube of equivalent size when:

$$v_{block} > \frac{r_{tube}^2 \Delta p}{8\, \eta\, l_{tube}\, f_{block}} \qquad \text{\{Eqn. 9.42\}}$$

Containerized transport thus may be preferred to Poiseuille flow in narrow, long transport channels, or in cases where fluid pressure is relatively low or fluid viscosity is relatively high, or where containers can be very thin-walled (e.g., high f_{block}) such as when strong diamondoid containers are used. For example, a containerized transport channel carrying water at 310 K with r_{tube} = 10 nm, l_{tube} = 1 micron, Δp = 1 atm, and f_{block} = 0.9 produces volume flow rates superior to Poiseuille flow if container transport velocity v_{block} > 0.002 m/sec. Container/channel sliding interfaces moving up to 1 m/sec have low frictional losses,[10] and speeds up to ~100 m/sec can probably be tolerated in internal mechanisms if flow speed (entirely inside nanodevices) is a more important design criterion than minimizing power dissipation in a particular application. An additional consideration is that subdividing a volume of fluid into many smaller blocks of fluid allows these smaller blocks to be transported independently through numerous spatially independent channels of much smaller bore, greatly increasing the number of flow design options and greatly increasing the relative advantage over Poiseuille flow through channels of similar size.

9.3 Nanomanipulators

Numerous simple actuators have been developed for microelectromechanical systems or MEMS.[1232,1253-1255,1267-1269] A few of these designs might possibly be useful in early nanomedical systems. All major components of an articulated micromanipulator having multiple degrees of freedom, workspaces on the order of 1 mm³, positional resolution up to ~10 nm, operating frequencies up to 10 KHz, and slewing speeds up to 4 mm/sec have been demonstrated experimentally; complete systems have even been proposed.[346,1253,1254]

Actuation and manipulation may be very broadly defined. For example, self-assembling and self-disassembling ~300 micron gold foil cubes have been fabricated and cycled repeatedly at ~1 Hz;[1251] "silicon origami" has also been described.[1382] Nonmechanical actuation has also been explored. In the Magnetic Stereotaxis System,[1256] a helmet with a cubic array of six superconducting coils is used to apply a 0.2 N force to a 3.2-mm wide, 4.7-mm long permanently magnetized cylindrical pellet that is embedded in brain material, causing stepped movement of the pellet through the brain material to a specified location with ~1 mm placement accuracy without any direct physical contact.

However, in the usual definition of a manipulator, an ergomechanical transducer (e.g., motors; Chapter 6) converts chemical, electrical, mechanical, acoustical, or some other form of energy into the mechanical energy of a manipulatory device which then exerts useful forces on objects or materials in the environment. In most cases a force-transmitting physical structure is required which may include both heavy load-bearing elements such as girders, struts, pneumatic tubes or rotary joints, and fine control elements such as stress cables, valves or switches (Section 9.3.1). An end-effector (e.g., gripper, cutter or molecular jig) is usually employed to focus and redirect the application of force at the distal end of the manipulation device (Section 9.3.2), or to perform specialized tasks. Sensors permit feedback control of manipulator motions as well as verification that the assigned manipulatory task has been properly executed (Section 9.3.3). Large numbers of manipulators can form ciliary arrays, allowing convenient mass transport of materials (Section 9.3.4); other classes of manipulators may be useful in bulk disassembly of materials (Section 9.3.5).

The diverse concepts outlined in this Section demonstrate the enormous range of possible nanomanipulator designs. These concepts are not intended as specific engineering proposals but rather as illustrations of certain useful classes of manipulators representing alternative design pathways that could provide the desired capability. No effort has been made to produce optimal systems that minimize energy dissipation, maximize speed, minimize parts count, or simplify manufacture. Biocompatibility issues[3234] will be addressed in Chapter 15.

* *In the 1950s, Marvin Minsky and Rollo Silver[289] built a "hydroflip computer" using hydraulic logic elements consisting of millimeter-wide grooves and holes in multiple layers of plastic sheets with small rods and balls inserted in some of the grooves. When the assembly was pressed together and connected to a water supply, it became a hydraulic computer powered by a 3-inch high column of water, operating at ~30 Hz.*

9.3.1 Nanoscale Manipulators

9.3.1.1 Biological Cilia

Biological cilia are motile, hairlike cylindrical processes typically 200-300 nm in diameter, 2-20 microns in length, and ~10^{-16}–10^{-15} kg in mass.[338,396,936,939,1394,1449] They are found in large numbers on some cell surfaces. Unicellular organisms use cilia both for locomotion and for food collection, while multicellular organisms use cilia primarily for mass transport of the environment past the cell.

Each cilium is bounded by an extension of the cellular plasma membrane (Fig. 9.2A), rising from a cytoskeletally-anchored centriole-like basal body consisting of an array of 9 triplets of common-walled microtubules ~150 nm in diameter and 300-500 nm in length. Sprouting upward from the basal body is the primary ciliary structure, called the axoneme. The axoneme is a cylinder of microtubules (Section 8.5.3.11) with 9 outer doublets of microtubules and two additional complete microtubules in the center, often called the central pair (Fig. 9.2B). The 9 outer doublets are extensions of two of the three microtubules comprising each of the nine basal body triplets. Each outer doublet of the axoneme consists of the A tubule (a complete 25-nm outer-diameter microtubule with the usual 13 protofilaments made of tubulin dimers), the B tubule (an incomplete microtubule with only 10-11 protofilaments), and a common wall containing the protein tektin (an intermediate-filament-like protein with high tensile strength) (Fig. 9.2C).

A set of 1-2 megadalton dynein side arms project outward from each of the A tubules, reaching clockwise toward the B tubules of the adjacent doublet (Fig. 9.2D). The dynein arms occur in pairs, one inner arm and one outer arm, spaced at regular ~30 nm intervals along the microtubule. Nexin protein interdoublet links at wider intervals join the outer doublets making circumferential rings, and radial spokes project inward from each of the 9 microtubule doublets. Microtubules do not change length during ciliary movement. Rather, the stalk of each dynein arm attaches to and detaches from the adjacent B tubule in an ATP-driven cyclic process,[3551-3554] pulling the stalk the length of one dimer along the tubule with a velocity of ~14 microns/sec.[1450] The maximum force generated by a dynein arm has been measured as ~1 pN.[452] The differential stress of adjacent doublet columns causes the axoneme to flex. Selective sidearm bonding and unbonding allows the cilium to generate a bend anywhere along its length.

In early experiments, bullfrog gullet ciliary surfaces developed a mechanical motive power of ~0.01 watts/m^2;[526] assuming 1-10 micron^2/cilium across the gullet surface gives an estimated mechanical power output P_{cilium} ~ 0.01-0.1 pW/cilium. Similarly, hair cell cilia of the human inner ear[446] respond to a minimum 2 x 10^{-5} N/m^2 (2 x 10^{-10} atm) pressure with a minimum 0.1 nm deflection at an applied force of ~10^{-3} pN, indicating a mechanical stiffness of ~10^{-5} N/m. (Axoneme bending moment is ~7 x 10^{-17} N-m.[1449]) Assuming a maximum D_p ~ 10^5 watts/m^3 power density in non-muscular working tissue (Table 6.8) and a ciliary volume of ~0.1-1 micron^3 also gives an estimated mechanical power output of P_{cilium} ~ 0.01-0.1 pW/cilium.

A simple cilium 12 microns long may beat at a frequency ν_{cilium} ~ 30 Hz with an angular velocity of 12 deg/millisec and a tip velocity of 2500 microns/sec in the effective stroke, while the bend in the recovery stroke propagates at ~350 microns/sec.[1394] (A 600-micron long compound cilium beats at ~20 Hz with angular velocity 10 deg/millisec and a 17 mm/sec recovery stroke.[1394]) Taking P_{cilium} ~ 0.05 pW and v_{cilium} ~500 microns/sec , then F_{cilium} ~ P_{cilium} / v_{cilium} ~ 0.1 nN.

9.3.1.2 Nanocilium Manipulators

Equally complex nanomechanical ciliary systems could probably be designed. But for simplicity, consider a nanociliary manipulator patterned more closely after the muscular trunk of the elephant or tentacle of the squid[1231] and based only loosely on the biological cilium. The model consists of a cylindrical central shaft of radius r_{shaft} and length l_{shaft}, the tip of which is bonded to one or more conduited shaft-attached control cables (radius r_{cable}) whose lengths and tensions can be predictably altered, causing the shaft to flex. A cable pulled with a force F_{cable} applies a transverse deflection force to the nanocilium shaft of approximate magnitude $F_{deflect}$ ~ (r_{cable}/l_{shaft}) F_{cable} for small deflections. The force required to deflect the terminus of a simple cantilevered rod is $F_{deflect} = 3\ E_{shaft}\ I_{shaft}\ d\ /\ l_{shaft}^3$, where E_{shaft} is Young's modulus and $I_{shaft} = \pi\ r_{shaft}^4\ /\ 4$ is the second moment of area (also known as the moment of inertia of the area) for a shaft of circular cross-section.[364] Solving for the deflection gives:

$$d = \left(\frac{4}{3\pi}\right)\left(\frac{r_{cable}\ l_{shaft}^2\ F_{cable}}{E_{shaft}\ r_{shaft}^4}\right) \qquad \text{\{Eqn. 9.43\}}$$

and a deflection angle $\theta_{shaft} = \tan^{-1}\ (d\ /\ l_{shaft})$. The shaft begins to buckle when F_{cable} exceeds the Euler force:[364]

$$F_{buckle} = \frac{\pi^2\ E_{shaft}\ I_{shaft}}{l_{cable}^2} = \frac{\pi^3\ E_{shaft}\ r_{shaft}^4}{4\ l_{shaft}^2} \qquad \text{\{Eqn. 9.44\}}$$

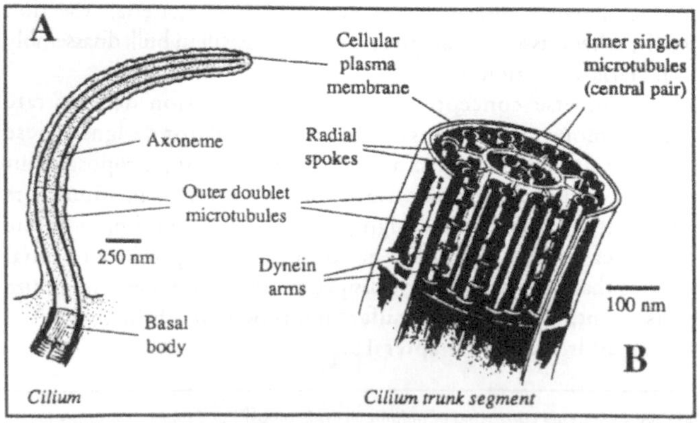

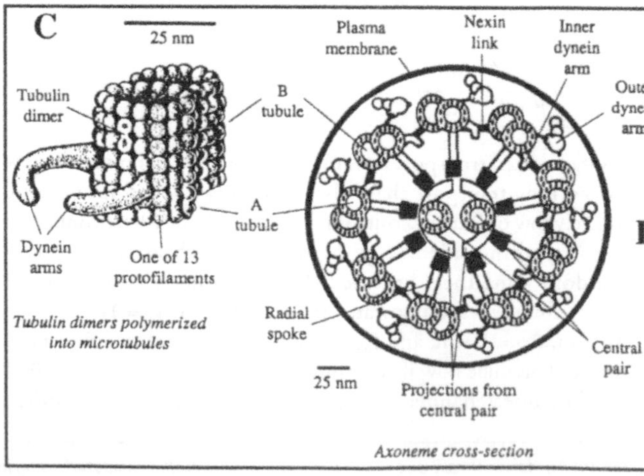

Fig. 9.2. Diagrammatic representation of the structure of a biological cilium (modified from Cormack[936] and Becker and Deamer[939]).

The maximum force that can be transmitted through a diamondoid cable of circular cross-section and tensile strength[536] $T_{str} = 1.9 \times 10^{11}$ N/m^2 with $r_{cable} = 1$ nm is $F_{max} = \pi\, r_{cable}^2\, T_{str} = 600$ nN. (For hollow cylinders of inside radius r and outside radius R, r_{shaft}^4 should be replaced by $(R^4 - r^4)$ in Eqn. 9.44.)

For a large nanocilium, we take $r_{shaft} = 50$ nm, $l_{shaft} = 1000$ nm, and $E_{shaft} \sim 10^8$ N/m^2 (~tendon strength[521]). At maximum deflection where $F_{cable} = F_{max} \sim 600$ nN, then d ~ 400 nm, $\theta_{shaft} \sim 22°$, and bending stiffness $k_{shaft} = F_{deflect} / d = (3\pi / 4)(E_{shaft}\, r_{shaft}^4 / l_{shaft}^3) \sim 0.001$ nN/nm. Maximum lateral force that may be applied by the nanocilium tip is $F_{deflect} \sim 0.6$ nN; setting this force equal to the Stokes law force (Eqn. 9.73) gives a maximum nanocilium velocity through water of ~10 cm/sec. If cable tension is uniformly distributed over a shaft endplate of radius r_{shaft}, the maximum mechanical pressure is $p_{shaft} = F_{max} / \pi\, r_{shaft}^2 = 8 \times 10^7$ N/m^2 < E_{shaft}. Shaft buckling commences at $F_{buckle} \sim 5$ nN with d = 3 nm and $\theta_{shaft} = 0.2°$; classical positional variance of the tip due to thermal noise[10] is $\Delta x = (kT / k_{shaft})^{1/2} \sim 2$ nm, very close to the minimum deflection at buckling. If the control cable may be moved at $v_{cable} \sim 1$ m/sec, then maximum nanocilium operating frequency $\nu_{max} \sim v_{cilium} / r_{shaft} = 20$ MHz; however, power dissipation is at least $P_{cilium} \sim F_{max}\, r_{shaft}\, \nu_{cilium} = 30$ pW at an operating frequency $\nu_{cilium} = 1$ KHz, plus up to ~60 pW of Stokes frictional dissipation (Eqn. 9.74) at the maximum ~10 cm/sec tip velocity.

For a very small nanocilium, we take $r_{shaft} = 10$ nm, $l_{shaft} = 100$ nm, and $E_{shaft} = 10^{10}$ N/m^2 where $F_{cable} = F_{max} \sim 600$ nN, then d = 25 nm, $\theta_{cable} = 14°$, $k_{shaft} = 0.2$ nN/nm, $F_{deflect} = 6$ nN, $p_{shaft} = 2 \times 10^9$ N/m^2 < E_{shaft}, $F_{buckle} = 78$ nN, $\Delta x = 0.1$ nm, maximum $\nu_{max} \sim 100$ MHz and $P_{cilium} = 6$ pW at $\nu_{cilium} = 1$ KHz. Maximum Stokes velocity in water is ~10 m/sec, but even at ~1 cm/sec the Stokes power dissipation is an additional ~6 pW.

Coiling the cable around the flexible shaft permits twisting motions to be imparted to the manipulator. Attachment of at least three control cables (at 120° circumferential intervals) allows full spherical angular coordinate steering of tip position. Adding additional control cable triplets on successive connection rings spaced along the length of the shaft allows independent addressing of intermediate shaft segments to permit the shaft to flex into a variety of sinuous shapes with some additional control of total radial extension. Two orthogonal pairs of tensioned cables attached on either side to ball joints separating each segment gives a more complex but highly redundant and highly controllable articulated manipulator (Fig. 9.3).

9.3.1.3 Pneumatic Manipulators

Differential tensions also can be applied to a nanomanipulator structure using gases (e.g., pneumatic actuators) or liquids (e.g., hydraulic actuators). Nanoscale pneumatic actuator elements must be of size L >> λ_{gas} (Eqn. 9.23) to ensure continuum flow. Thus for L ~ 1 micron, minimum pneumatic operating pressure p_{gas} >> 0.2 atm; for L = 10 nm, minimum p_{gas} >> 24 atm.

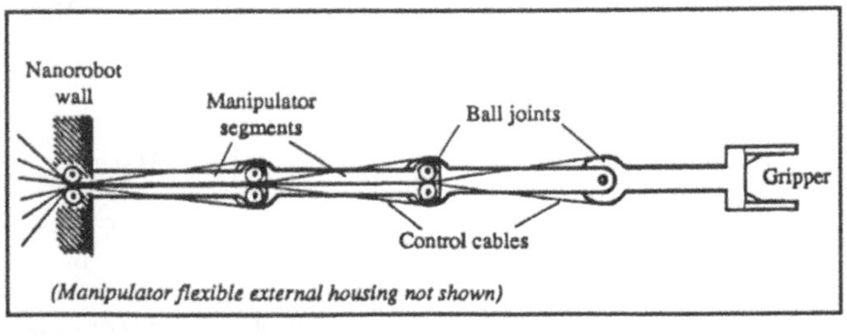

Fig. 9.3. Two-dimensional representation of segmented 3-D manipulator using ball joints (modified from Ma et al[1233]).

There are many examples of pressurized hydraulic tissue inflation in macroscale biology, including sea anemones, nematodes, echinoderm tube feet, spider legs, pupal butterfly wing extension, piscine swim bladders, and human sex organs. The pressurized pumping of DNA through a nanotube in the T4 bacteriophage has already been described (Section 9.2.4). As another possible example in nanobiology, the sperm of the sea cucumber *Thyone* rapidly elongates its ~700-nm wide spherical acrosomal vesicle into a 50-nm wide, 90-micron long tubular acrosomal process in less than 10 sec after a rapid influx of water doubles the volume of the 0.5 micron^3 acrosomal cup in which the vesicle is stored in 50-70 millisec (Fig. 9.4). This has led to the proposal that the elongation is at least partly hydraulically driven by a profilactin osmotic pressure of ~0.5 atm, because the speed of actin polymerization alone appears to be about an order of magnitude too slow.[1230]

Nanoscale manipulators may be constructed of simple orthotropic tubes with flexible ribbing and an elastic but nonextensible spine that allows manipulator flexure in only one direction when pressurized (Fig. 9.5). Experiments using compound manipulators constructed using centimeter-sized pneumatic orthotropic segments that were pressurized to 3-6 atm produced 90° flexures in 0.3-1 sec with 2-5 mm placement accuracy (0.4%-0.9%) and load-bearing strengths up to ~20 N at the tip.[1231]

Suzumori et al[1232] have constructed, tested and analyzed a simple but elegant pneumatic manipulator ~4 mm in diameter that should be readily adaptable to the microscopic scale. As shown in Figure 9.6, the manipulator consists of a flexible cylinder made of three separate 120°-sector longitudinal chambers that are permanently bonded together. Each chamber may be independently pressurized or depressurized through flexible tubes connected to pressure control valves. In the first configuration, purely circumferential reinforcing fibers (winding angle $\alpha = 0°$) allow the tri-chambered manipulator to easily deform in the axial direction, while resisting deformation in the radial direction. Pressure applied equally to the three chambers thus causes axial stretching. Pressure applied to only one chamber causes the manipulator to bend away from that chamber, so the device can be flexed in any direction by controlling the pressure in

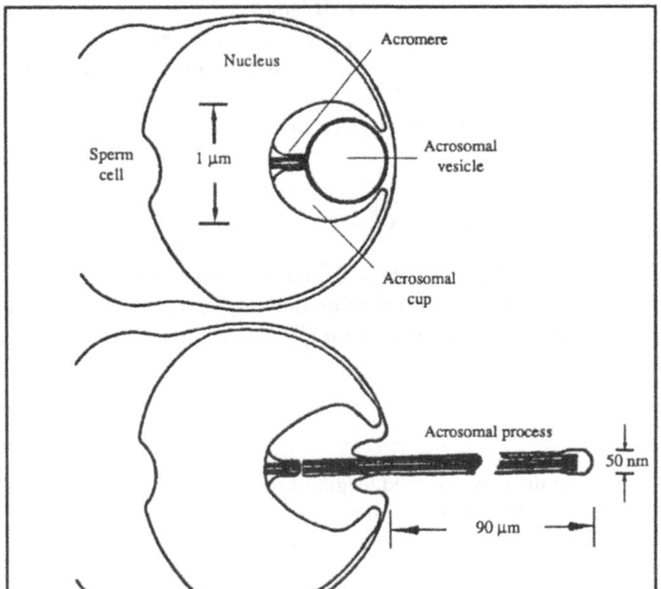

Fig. 9.4. Schematic of the acrosomal process in *Thyone* (modified from Oster and Perelson[1230]).

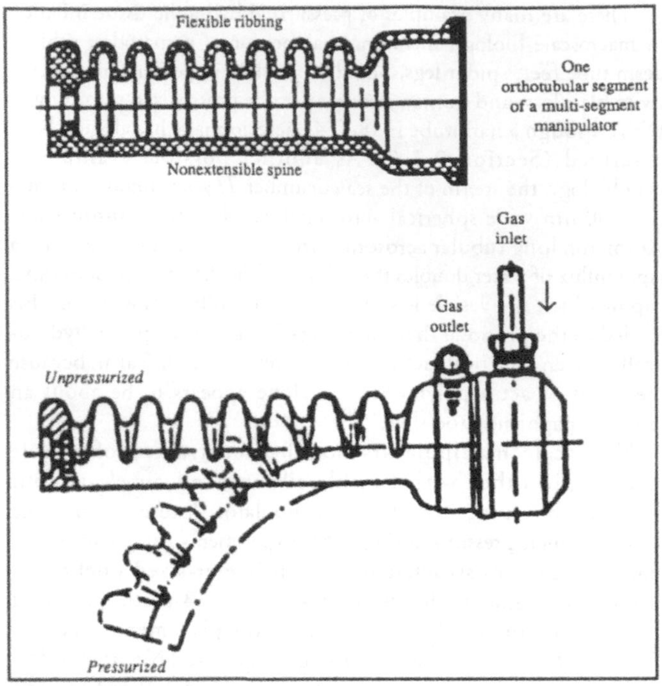

Fig. 9.5. Flexible ribbed orthotropic tube manipulator (modified from Wilson et al[1231]).

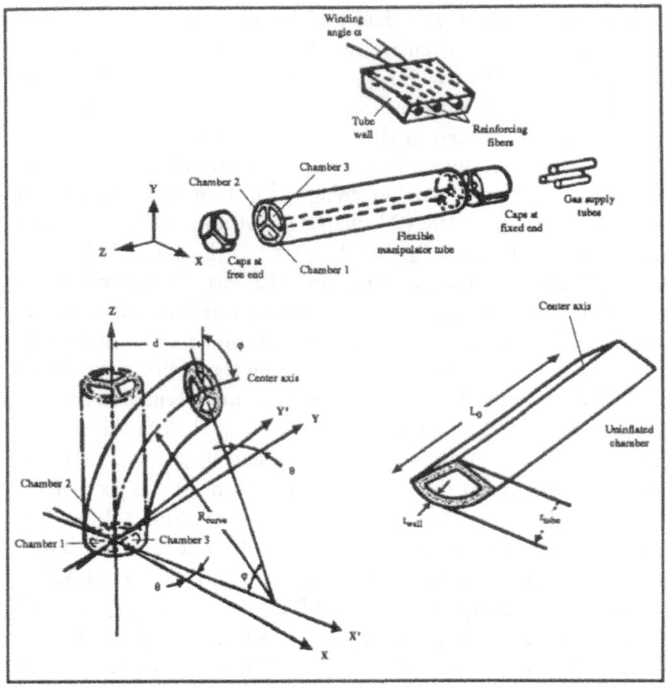

Fig. 9.6. Schematic design of tri-chambered pneumatic manipulator (modified from Suzumori, Iikura, and Tanaka[1232]).

the three chambers. In a second configuration, spiral reinforcing fibers ($\alpha = 5°$-$20°$) force a circumaxial rotation of the cylinder when chamber pressure is applied, allowing useful screwing motions to be generated at the tip. Thus the manipulator can achieve pitch, yaw, stretch, and rotation, although these four movements are not fully independent because there are only three independent control parameters.

Consider the tri-chambered pneumatic manipulator of Figure 9.6 with one end fixed, $\alpha = 0°$, tube radius r_{tube}, tube wall thickness t_{wall}, and chambers of equal relaxed length L_0 along the center axis that are then pressurized to p_1, p_2, and p_3, respectively. The fiber-reinforced tube wall material has Young's modulus E_{tube} in the transverse direction. Then the x-y projection of manipulator rotation around the vertical axis (θ) is given by:

$$\theta = \tan^{-1}\left(\frac{2p_1 - p_2 - p_3}{3^{1/2}(p_2 - p_3)}\right) \qquad \text{\{Eqn. 9.45\}}$$

For each of the three chambers, $\theta_1 = \theta$, $\theta_2 = \theta + (2\pi / 3)$, and $\theta_3 = \theta - (2\pi / 3)$. The angular deflection of the manipulator down from the vertical axis (φ) is the same for all three chambers, given as:

$$\varphi = \frac{L_{manip}}{R_{curve}} \qquad \text{\{Eqn. 9.46\}}$$

L_{manip} is the new stretched length of the manipulator at the center axis, R_{curve} is the radius of curvature of the manipulator, and the linear deflection from the vertical axis is:

$$d = (1 - \cos(\varphi))\, R_{curve} \qquad \text{\{Eqn. 9.47\}}$$

where:

$$L_{manip}^2 - (L_0)L_{manip} - \left(\frac{\pi\, r_{tube}\, L_0}{36\, E_{tube}}\right)\sum_i (p_i) = 0 \qquad \text{\{Eqn. 9.48\}}$$

$$R_{curve} \sim \left(\frac{9\, E_{tube}}{2\pi}\right)\left(\frac{\pi\, r_{tube} + 2\, L_{manip}}{\sum_i (p_i \sin(\theta_i))}\right) \qquad \text{\{Eqn. 9.49\}}$$

and Eqn. 9.48 is readily evaluated using the quadratic formula. Making a few simplifying assumptions, the bending stiffness of the manipulator is given approximately as:

$$k_{tube} \sim \frac{3^{1/2}\pi\, E_{tube}\, t_{wall}\, r_{tube}^3}{L_{manip}^3} \qquad \text{\{Eqn. 9.50\}}$$

and thus the maximum force that can be exerted at the tip is:

$$F_{tip} = k_{tube}\, d \qquad \text{\{Eqn. 9.51\}}$$

Finally, the lowest resonant frequency ν_{res} of a tri-chambered pneumatic manipulator of mean density ρ_{manip}, mass $M_{manip} \sim \pi\, r_{tube}^2\, L_0\, \rho_{manip}$, and carrying a tip load of M_{load} is given by:[1232]

$$\nu_{res} \sim \left(\frac{3\, E_{tube}\, I_{tube}}{4\pi^2\, L_{manip}^3\, (M_{load} + 0.236\, M_{manip})}\right)^{1/2} \quad \text{(Hz)} \qquad \text{\{Eqn. 9.52\}}$$

where the second moment of area $I_{tube} \sim (1/4)\,\pi\, r_{tube}^4 + (1/2)\, L_{manip}\, r_{tube}^3$. Manipulator power requirement in the absence of a viscous operating medium is:

$$P_{manip} \sim F_{tip}\, \nu_{manip}\, (L_{manip} - L_0) \quad \text{(watts)} \qquad \{\text{Eqn. 9.53}\}$$

where ν_{manip} is manipulator operating frequency.

As an example of a nanomedically useful pneumatic manipulator, consider a tri-chamber design with L_0 = 1200 nm, r_{tube} = 200 nm, t_{wall} = 50 nm, $E_{tube} = 10^8$ N/m^2, and maximum operating pressures up to ~1000 atm (pressure/volume relationships for air calculated using the ideal gas law are ~5% in error at 100 atm, ~50% in error at 1000 atm; Table 10.2). Application of a p_1 = 6 atm pressure pulse to one chamber of the manipulator produces an F_{tip} ~ 0.1 nN lateral force and a d ~ 1 nm tip displacement at zero load, costing ~3 kT/cycle at T = 310 K. Application of a 60 atm pulse produces ~1 nN and a 10 nm displacement (~300 kT/cycle); a 600 atm pressure step produces a 10 nN force and a 100 nm no load tip displacement at an energy cost of ~30,000 kT/cycle or P_{manip} ~ 100 pW continuous power draw at ν_{manip} = 1 MHz. Minimum driving pressure increments of ~6 atm (~3 kT/cycle) allow the manipulator tip to be reliably positioned in repeatable step sizes of ~1 nm, well above the classical positional variance of the tip due to thermal noise[10] which is $\Delta x = (kT / k_{shaft})^{1/2}$ ~ 0.2 nm, given a bending stiffness of k_{tube} ~ 0.1 N/m for this design.

Manipulator volume is ~0.15 micron^3 and manipulator mass M_{manip} ~ 0.1 picogram. At zero load in vacuo, ν_{res} ~ 30 MHz up to ~1000 atm; ν_{res} falls to ~5 MHz for a 1 picogram load (roughly the mass of a 1 micron^3 nanorobot) and to ~1 MHz for a ~30 picogram load, so up to ~MHz operating frequencies seem reasonable at modest loads. (For comparison, a 1 nN lifting force supports a 100,000 picogram mass against gravity.) At maximum cyclical tip displacement d = 100 nm and ν_{manip} = 1 MHz, mean tip velocity is $v_{tip} \sim d\, \nu_{manip}$ = 10 cm/sec. Maximum viscous drag power in vivo is P_{drag} ~ 140 pW using the formula for Stokes frictional dissipation (Eqn. 9.74) at a 10 cm/sec tip velocity and taking $r \sim (2\, r_{tube}\, L_0)^{1/2}$ for the manipulator and $\eta = 1.1 \times 10^{-3}$ kg/m-sec in tissue plasma at 310 K.

The pneumatic design outlined above is quite versatile. Manipulator tip displacement scales as $d \sim L_0\, p / E_{tube}$. Manipulator tip force scales as $F_{tip} \sim r_{tube}^3 / L_0^2$; tip force is nearly independent of E_{tube} down to $E_{tube} \sim 10^8$ N/m^2, below which F_{tip} falls rapidly. Pneumatic nanomanipulators using diamondoid wall materials (e.g., $E_{tube} \sim 10^{11}$ N/m^2) can have a stiffness on the order of k_{manip} ~ 10-100 nN/nm (comparable to the telescoping manipulator described in Section 9.3.1.4), although in such cases the maximum pneumatic tip displacement even at maximum operating pressures may be limited to ~1 nm or less. Longitudinal cables can be added to actively control the helical pitch (e.g., α) of the reinforcing fibers;[529] adding both circumferential and longitudinal reinforcing fibers allows deformation of compliant tube structures into multiply-coiled shapes.[1255] Adding tensioned control cables and additional layers of pneumatic chambers can give a full six degrees-of-freedom (DOF) manipulator, albeit with some increased complexity of the mechanism. Control of individual axial segments (e.g., selective locking/unlocking or differing Young's moduli of adjacent segments) allows arbitrary serpentine flexures through a three-dimensional work volume (Fig. 9.7). End effector control lines may be routed along the central axis.

Many interesting designs for "tentacle" or "snake" manipulators, also known as highly-redundant or hyper-redundant manipulators, have appeared in the literature.[1231,1233,1270-1273,1625,2387] These may be fabricated as stacks of multiple pneumatic segments connected coaxially. A biological snake may have ~200 separate jointed segments, though each joint has a pitch range of only ± 10°; snake robots having artificial joints with pitch ranges up to 135° have been built.[1625] Such designs are useful in nanomedical robotic systems because hyper-redundant manipulators can be made extremely fail-safe—if one joint fails (e.g., by locking tight, not falling limp, by design), the accessible work volume is not significantly diminished.

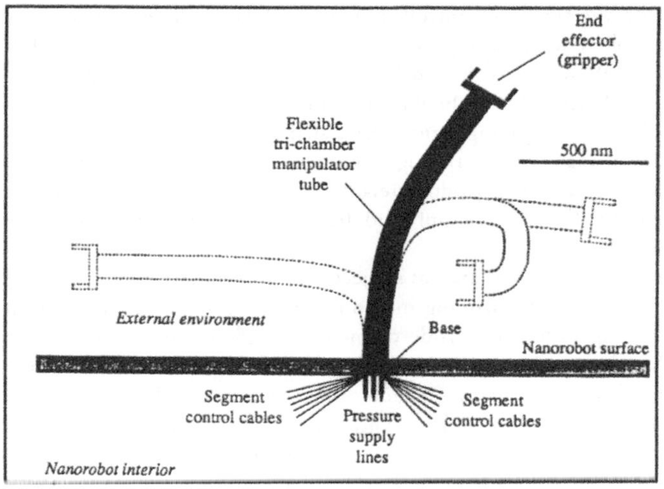

Fig. 9.7. Range of motion of "pneumatic snake" manipulator with direct segment control.

9.3.1.4 Telescoping Manipulators

Another useful class of manipulators is the telescoping design (Fig. 5.14), in which snugly fitted or threaded components extend or retract via sliding motions induced either pneumatically or by shaft-driven rotations of linked elements.

The best-known telescoping nanomanipulator design has been proposed by Drexler[10] in the context of a stiff mechanism that may be used for precision molecular positioning and assembly work. As depicted in Figure 9.8, the mechanism features a central telescoping joint whose extension and retraction is controlled by a 1.5-nm diameter drive shaft. The rapid rotation of this drive shaft (up to ~1 m/sec tangential velocity) forces a transmission gear to quickly execute a known number of turns, causing the telescoping joint to slowly unscrew or screw in the axial direction, thus lengthening or contracting the manipulator. Additionally, two pairs of canted rotary joints—one pair between the telescoping section and the base, the other pair between the telescoping section and the

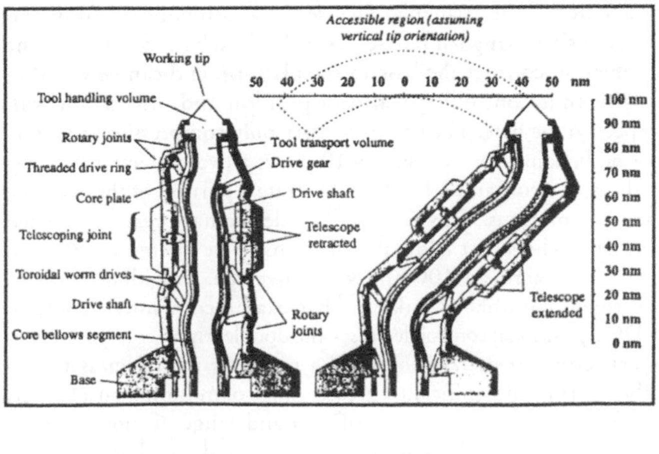

Fig. 9.8. Schematic cross-section of a telescoping nanomanipulator (adapted from Drexler[10]).

working tip—are controlled by toroidal worm drives. These joints enable a wide variety of complex angular motions and give full 6-DOF access to the work envelope (Fig. 9.9; isolated planetary gear (Section 2.4.1) shown at lower left, for comparison). By engaging and disengaging various drive shafts using clutches, these shafts can be made to turn through a known number of rotations between locked states giving odometer-like control of manipulator joint rotations. The power supply and drive shaft control systems originate outside the manipulator, thus are not subject to tight geometric constraints.

Drexler's telescoping manipulator is approximately cylindrical in shape with an outside diameter of ~35 nm and an extensible length from 90 nm to 100 nm measured from top of base to working tip. The manipulator includes a hollow circular channel 7 nm in diameter to allow tool tips and materials to be moved from below the manipulator through the base up to the working tip. At the tip, a slightly larger region is reserved for a mechanism to allow positioning and locking of tool tips. Device mass is ~10^{-19} kg, and the manipulator is constructed of ~4×10^6 atoms excluding the base and external power and control structures. Device stiffness (which scales roughly with arm length[10]) is k_s ~ 25 nN/nm, so that a force of 1 nN may be applied with an elastic deflection in the arm of only 0.04 nm. The classical positional variance of the manipulator at T = 310 K is $\Delta x \sim (kT / k_s)^{1/2} \sim 0.01$ nm, although with a manipulator tube segment thread pitch of 0.5 nm and drive shafts that execute ~700 turns to produce a single tube segment rotation, segment extension may be altered in ~0.001 nm steps. The workspace includes a 180° hemispherical-shell volume ~100 nm in diameter and ~10 nm deep. Conveyance of the tip through a full 100-nm arc requires ~10 microsec at a conservative ~1 cm/sec arm speed. Efficient task planning permits much smaller motion arcs, allowing ~MHz operating frequencies. The manipulator dissipates 0.1 pW of power (power density ~10^9 watts/m^3) while in motion under no-load conditions. Energy dissipated per unit mass of delivered payload is scale-invariant, and the design of telescoping manipulators generally becomes easier with increasing size.[10] Power dissipation scales roughly as the square of arm length and as the square of tip velocity;[10] power density scales inversely with arm length.

Like the ciliary and pneumatic designs, the telescoping manipulator is hermetically sealed, thus maintaining a controlled internal environment while allowing leakproof operation in vivo.

9.3.1.5 Stewart Platform Manipulators

Another class of simple manipulators is the 6-DOF Stewart platform.[1237,1238] The Stewart platform exploits the geometry of an octahedron—one triangular face serves as a mobile platform and the opposing triangular face serves as the fixed base. Six struts of the octahedron connect the base to the platform and can be varied in length, thus controlling platform position and orientation with respect to the base. The six struts carry only compressive or tensile, but no bending, forces. Figure 9.10 shows a two-dimensional analog with three struts and 3 DOF to illustrate a portion of the available range of motions. This 5×10^{-20} kg device has pressure-actuated vernier ratchets that allow strut lengths to be altered in ~0.1 nm increments across a 100-nm work envelope, providing excellent positional control.[10] Merkle[1239] has examined a novel family of 6-DOF positional control devices—the double tripod configuration—which offers greater stiffness for a given structural mass than a robotic arm and significantly greater range of motion than a Stewart platform. Tradeoffs between stiffness and range of motion in the double tripod can be continuously adjusted by altering simple design parameters.

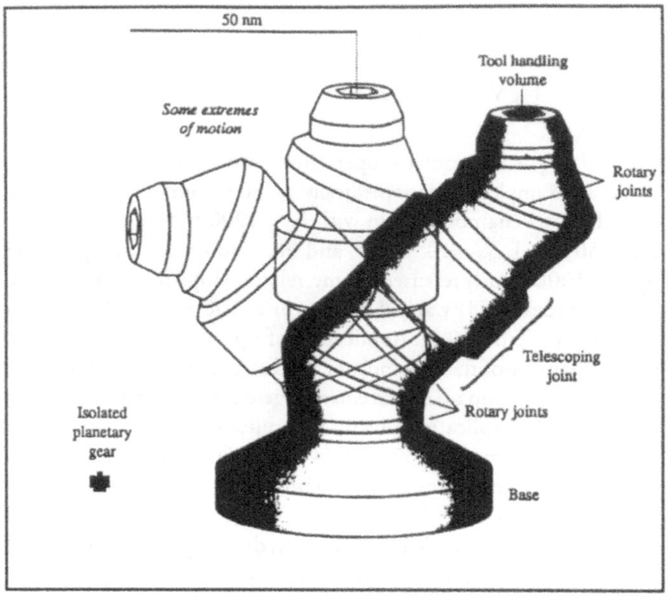

Fig. 9.9. External shape and range of motion of a telescoping nanomanipulator (adapted from Drexler[10]).

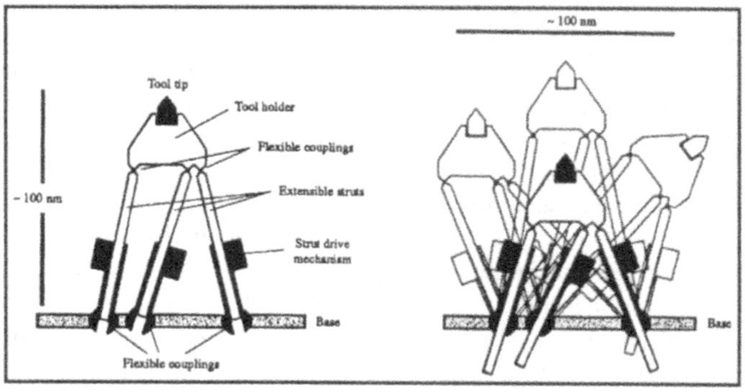

Fig. 9.10. Two-dimensional schematic of the range of motion of a Stewart platform manipulator (adapted from Drexler[10]).

Assembly of parts while immersed in a fluid eliminates electrostatic and surface tension effects.[1150] In the earliest, most primitive Stewart platform type nanomanipulators operating in aqueous suspension, R. Merkle suggests that leg extension and retraction may be controlled by manufacturing the legs using a repeating sequence of binding sites on the surfaces of two opposing struts. Chemical binding molecules are designed that can selectively link one strut to another, but only between one specific pair of binding sites (one site on each strut). Varying the linking agent controls which part of a strut links to the adjacent strut; cycling of link molecule types in solution forces the linking and unlinking in such a way as to move the struts along.[1303]

9.3.1.6 Metamorphic Manipulators

Metamorphic manipulators (Section 5.3.1.3) are fully reconfigurable manipulative or locomotive appendages that can be deployed from compact storage volumes. Surface area, contour, volume, length, and stiffness of the protuberance may be varied at ~KHz frequencies (Section 5.3.1.4). Metamorphic manipulators exuded from a nanorobot surface may temporarily assume many forms including arms/legs, hands/fingers, barriers and surrounds, grapples, bubbles, and a wide variety of geometric shapes, all under programmatic or stochastic control (Section 9.3.3).

Many examples of highly plastic protuberances are known in microbiology at many size scales, such as the pseudopods of fibroblasts and amoebas (an amoebic pseudopod can extend and engulf a 100-micron paramecium in ~10 sec,[1252] applying a stress force[1462] up to ~2900 N/m^2), blebbing and microspikes,[938] the ~40 nm import receptors (cytoplasmic filaments) ringing the mouth of the nuclear pore complex,[1264] cyclosis in giant green algae cells at velocities up to 100 microns/sec,[938] and the flexible plasma membrane extensions that occur during amoeboid locomotion (Section 9.4.3.7). Human axons elongate at ~10 nm/sec.[1240] The green plastid tubules of chloroplasts in plant cells are yet another example. These tubular projections arise initially as protuberances from the chloroplast surface that elongate and extend. They are dynamic in the living cell, continuously changing their shape, moving around, shrinking back, and sometimes connecting with other chloroplasts. Their width ranges from 350-850 nm, with lengths up to 15 microns. Plastid protuberances may extend at a velocity of 10-100 nm/sec and encircle another body, much like a finger curling around a sphere.[735] Metamorphic manipulators are expected to present significant, though probably not insurmountable, design challenges.

9.3.2 Nanoscale End-Effectors and Tool Tips

An end-effector is usually placed at the tip of a manipulator in order to focus and redirect the application of forces. Examples of simple force redirection include a screwdriver head or bolting socket, a cutting blade, a perforative needle, and levers, pry bars or wedges.

End-effectors can also be used to achieve very fine motion control at the tip. Perhaps the simplest task such an end-effector can perform is the grasping or gripping of target objects in the environment. Figure 9.11 offers a small sampling of the many possible schematic concepts for grasping end-effectors. Mechanical grippers as in (A) have been fabricated with a jawspan of ~10 microns, tines ~2 microns thick, and a ~5 KHz resonant frequency, and have been used to grasp individual 2.7-micron polystyrene spheres, dried red blood cells, and even various protozoa including a 7-micron diameter, 40-micron long *Euglena*.[1267] Pneumatic grippers (B) have been built and operated on a larger scale.[1232] Figure 9.11(C) illustrates how high-frequency acoustic point sources or ultrasonic resonance fields[1627] can be used to reversibly secure a small target object in a small space; electrodynamic fields, electrophoretic forces,[1628,1629] and optical tweezers[1247,1630,1631] employ similar principles. The suction gripper (D) works on any target immersed in a gas or liquid environment (Eqn. 9.22),[1619,1620] whereas the magnetic gripper (E) only works on magnetic materials. The electrostatic gripper (F) induces attractive Coulombic, image force, or dipole charge effects, and is helped by the increased breakdown field strength of very small gaps due to the Paschen effect. The van der Waals gripper shown in Figure 9.11(G) uses variable nanoscale surface roughness to regulate the van der Waals attractive force; fluid surface tension or related forces may be modulated to reversibly grip the target. Finally, any soft object in the environment can be impaled by a narrow articulating spike, which then drops anchor inside the object until the gripper is ready to withdraw (Fig. 9.11(H)).

Most of the end-effectors shown in Figure 9.11 involve direct physical contact with the target object. Undesired or accidental surface adhesivity (Section 9.2) of grippers and manipulators is a serious design issue that must be addressed with respect to all possible environments and target objects likely to be encountered by the manipulation mechanism during the performance of its mission. Complementary diamondoid surfaces in vacuo may adhere with a contact tensile strength up to ~10^4 atm, representing ~1 nN of contact

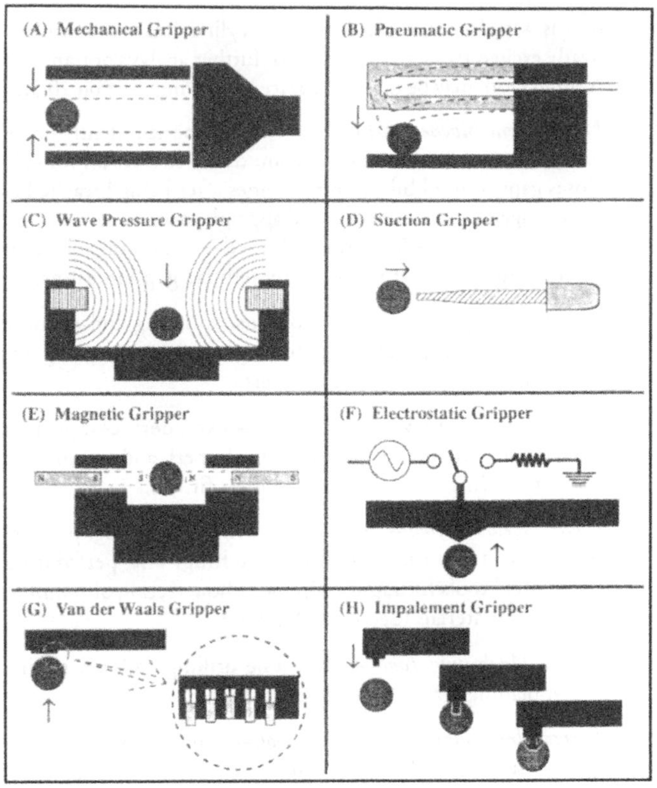

Fig. 9.11. Grasping effectors (schematic).

force per nm^2 of contact area and releasing ~5400 zJ/nm^2 of energy when the surfaces are joined.[10] However, noncomplementary surfaces in fluid environments can in theory be engineered to display almost any interfacial adhesivity desired—including negative adhesivity or repulsion (Section 9.2.3). Gripper/object adhesivity may vary according to many factors that are subject to design control. For example, all else equal, passivated diamond is 5-10 times more "sticky" in the van der Waals regime than glass or plastic (Table 9.1). Manipulator mechanism surfaces should in general be highly noncomplementary to container surfaces, biological surfaces, nanorobot surfaces, and the surfaces of adjacent manipulators. Contact electrification is minimized by using materials with a small contact potential difference between the gripper and the target object.[1147]

A wide variety of specialized complex nanomedical tool tips are readily imagined, although an exhaustive listing or description is beyond the scope of this book. Among the more interesting possible functions (offered without regard to specific implementation) are the following:

1. *Injectors*—pipettes, glue applicators, aerators/foamers, and compound grasper/fluid injectors.

2. *Adhesion Antennae*—partially selective binding tips that are swept through the environment, whereupon desired moieties or particles adhere and can be removed from the environment or drawn into the nanodevice (i.e., selective biochemical "dust mops"); transmembrane in cyto sensory appendages.

3. *Core Sampler*—a rapidly-spinning hollow cylindrical cutting tool that is driven into nearby tissue, whereupon suction is applied, an irising diaphragm closes at the distal end which separates the sample from the main tissue mass, and then the

tool is withdrawn, extracting a full cylindrical core sample of neatly excised tissue that is ready for further analysis or transport. A similar tool may be required for ice burrowing (Section 10.5.2).

4. *Noncovalent Biochemical Welders*—rejoins noncovalently linked biological structures that have become detached (Section 9.4.4.3); closes gaps in lipid bilayer membranes after being breached by the passage of an nanomechanical appendage or entire nanorobot device (Section 9.4.5.6); reattaches vesicles and organelles to microtubular tracks; reseals intercellular gap junctions.
5. *Joining and Spooling Tools*—bobbins, spinning and spooling tools; fiber manipulators including stitching, stapling and threading devices; rivet pin inserters.
6. *Compression and Compaction Tools*—extruders, compactors, compression rollers, beam benders, crimpers, and compression fitters including shrink fitters and press fitters.
7. *Coarse Shearing Tools*—microscale slitting, scissoring, piercing, punching, trimming, shaving, notching, and perforating; "eggbeater" tools for rapid pulping or liquefaction of semifluid biological materials (Section 10.4.2.5.3).
8. *Coarse Machining Tools*—microscale drilling, lathing, sawing, filing, planing, grinding and polishing.
9. *Pattern Impression and Coating Tools*—transfer molding, pantographic tracing; surface laminators, abstractors, decorators and other surfacing tools.
10. *Membrane Manipulation Tools*—cell and organelle lipid membrane bending, stretching, tearing, and joining; electric field-induced lipid bilayer membrane demixers;[1613] transmembrane channel inserters.
11. *Molecular Tools and Jigs*—tool tips designed to allow manipulation of individual molecules or molecular structures, perhaps using enzyme-like functionalizations for grasping (e.g., binding sites), cutting (e.g., pepsin, trypsin, collagenases, proteases, lipases, nucleases), joining (e.g., ribozymes, ligases), splicing (e.g., spliceosomes), folding (e.g., molecular chaperones,[466]), copying (e.g., DNA polymerase, reverse transcriptases), appending (e.g., transferases), and packing or pumping (e.g., hexagonal pRNA packs coiled DNA into viral capsids[1723]). The engineering of "wet" enzymes to accurately and reliably function when attached to stiff manipulators will be challenging because any attachment methods (multiple bonds) which will give the tip a high positional accuracy might also interfere with enzyme function. Enzymes generally require nanoscale movement to effect catalysis—the more tightly the tip is held, the less likely the enzyme will retain functionality.

Tool exchange ports and tool tip garages should lie within the accessible work volume of the nanomanipulator system, to allow convenient and watertight tool tip changeout, or else tool tips must be transferrable internally within the manipulator (e.g., Section 9.3.1.4).

9.3.3 Sensors and Manipulator Control

In addition to end-effectors, it will often be convenient to position various classes of sensors along the length of a manipulator, or at the tip. Monitoring control cable lengths, pneumatic chamber pressures, drive shaft rotations or strut lengths can allow a controller to know the position of a manipulator tip to the accuracy of one control increment, assuming no external forces and assuming regular recalibrations by periodically returning the arm to a precisely known "home" position. If low-stress stretch-inelastic metrological cables are embedded in the manipulator structure, then physical displacements of those cables in response to an applied load may be compared to no-load force/distance profiles, revealing the external force vector. Thus actual tip displacements are recorded directly by the metrological cables, and force feedback is continuously available. End effectors may include a wide variety of additional useful sensors, including gripper force and adhesion sensors, chemotactic sensors, vibration and acoustic sensors, electric or magnetic sensors, thermal or optical sensors, and so forth (Chapter 4).

Techniques for precise nanomanipulator control had received insufficient formal attention as of 1998. Pure open loop control (e.g., dead reckoning with no sensory feedback) could be sufficient in some molecular manufacturing operations. In this regard the inkjet printer might be a more suitable conceptual model than the robot arm, since a printer can build up considerable three-dimensional complexity during repeated passes over the workpiece following a simple linear chain of instructions in a raster pattern. Adding the ability to sense a fiducial structure near the workpiece can provide periodic checks on registration and reduce placement error, and Drexler[10] has described the use of sterically complementary probes or alignment pegs to help guide end-effectors precisely to their targets.

However, force reflection and other sensory feedback are likely to play important roles in nanomedical manipulator control. J.S. Hall, cited in Drexler,[10] points out that the ratios of the times and energies consumed by a typical nanomechanical computation to the times and energies consumed by a typical nanomanipulator motion are enormously greater than the corresponding ratios for microprocessor computation and macromechanical robotic arm motion. In other words, computation is relatively cheap for macroscale robotic manipulators while arm motion is relatively cheap for nanoscale robotic manipulators. Thus the moment-by-moment computer control of arm trajectories is the appropriate paradigm for macroscale robots, but not for nanoscale robots. For nanoscale robots, the appropriate manipulator control paradigm is often trajectory trial-and-error, also known as sensor-based motion control[1623,1638] or "groping."

Using trajectory trial-and-error, the nanomanipulator is moved generally in the direction of a desired endpoint, then is stopped and sensory feedback from the tip is obtained and examined for a match with the target destination profile. Given only a partial match, the arm is next moved in some direction and new sensory feedback is sampled. If the profile match has improved, another increment of motion is applied in the same direction; if the match has deteriorated, another direction is tried. Much like a blind man groping for his knife and fork by feeling around on the surface of a dinner table until he finds the utensils, the nanomanipulator is directed by trial-and-error progressively toward its goal, until the target is unambiguously located.

Efficient search algorithms for detecting and avoiding local maxima, identifying saddle points, rejecting outliers, and minimizing search times are well-known to mathematicians. In some cases, chemonavigational sensory readings may be taken using sensor pads (Section 4.2.5) at the manipulator tip to determine proximity to specific cellular processes or organelles. Unknown objects may be examined by haptic (tactile) exploration[1622] or by other means. Outside the cell, extracellular matrix (ECM) elements may be repeatedly chemotactically sampled to allow a nanomanipulator to feel its way toward a particular structure or node. Deployment of multiple nanomanipulators from a single device permits the simultaneous coordinated manipulation of several objects in the environment. In many cases, Brownian transport may suffice to bring a molecular target to the nanorobot arm.

If a nanomanipulator can be moved in minimum increments of ΔL at mean velocity v_{arm} throughout a typical work volume V_{work}, then an efficient search algorithm can locate any target volume of size ΔL^3 that lies within V_{work} in at most $N_{trial} \sim \log_2(V_{work}/\Delta L^3)$ trials, requiring a search time $t_{search} \sim N_{trial}\ \Delta t$ where the mean time per nanomanipulator motion is $\Delta t \lesssim V_{work}^{1/3} / v_{arm}$ assuming a reasonably smooth gradient in roughly cubical work volume. Taking $\Delta L = 1$ nm, $v_{arm} = 1$ cm/sec, and $V_{work} = 0.1$ micron^3 for a cell-repair type manipulator, then $N_{trial} \sim 27$ trials and $\Delta t \lesssim 46$ microsec, giving $t_{search} \lesssim 1$ millisec for the nanomanipulator arm to search for (and find) its intracellular target using the trial-and-error paradigm. This is consistent with the estimated time to search cell surfaces for specific markers (Eqn. 8.5). For the telescoping nanomanipulator to be used in molecular manufacturing as described by Drexler,[10] and taking $\Delta L \sim 0.25$ nm, $v_{arm} = 1$ cm/sec, and $V_{work} = 3$ nm^3, then $N_{trial} \sim 8$ trials and $\Delta t \lesssim 0.1$ microsec, giving $t_{search} \lesssim 1$ microsec.

Other control paradigms might also be useful in molecular manufacturing applications requiring high placement accuracy, possibly including full closed-loop operation in special cases.

9.3.4 Manipulator Arrays

Arrays of micron- or submicron-scale manipulator elements can be used to create 1-, 2-, or 3-dimensional programmable motion fields. In the simple 1-dimensional case, a single row of manipulators alternately grasp, transfer, and release a load, passing the payload down the line like a bucket brigade. In the 2-dimensional case, surfaces may be coated with closely-packed manipulators, allowing rapid and continuous transfers of multiple payload streams along multiple surface vectors simultaneously. In biology, ciliated epithelium is found in respiratory, excretory, digestive, circulatory, genital, and nervous systems of various animal groups, to drive fluid flow.[1617,1618] Examples in human physiology include the ciliated air passages of the bronchi (Section 8.2.2) and the villiated surfaces of the small intestine (Section 8.2.3). In these natural systems, payload transport speeds are typically 10-100 microns/sec. For instance, experiments with ciliated bullfrog gullet tissue show maximum transport efficiency when moving a load of ~5 grams/cm^2 at a speed of 27 microns/sec.[526] Ciliary arrays used by protozoa for locomotion also display time-synchronized wave patterns[3558] (Section 9.4.2.5.1), which may be analogous to the operation of submicron motion fields.

There are many possible applications of manipulator arrays in nanomedicine. Ciliary arrays inside hollow nanofactory workspaces can regulate throughput of physical materials for manufacturing (Chapter 19). Arrays can establish specified flows of environment fluids such as blood plasma across sensors, or may be used in device locomotion (both crawling and swimming; Section 9.4) or in self-cleaning activities. Medical nanosystems may incorporate complex three-dimensional manipulator arrays to control the transport of biocomponents in cell mills and organ mills (Chapter 21), to move chyme across an artificial stomach lining (Chapter 26), or to move fluids through artificial organs designed for chemical processing or filtration such as an artificial liver or kidney (Chapter 26). Ciliary transport systems may also support unique and highly sophisticated artificial whole-body nutrient transport systems such as the vasculoid-class devices described in Chapter 30. These nanomechanical arrays can be operated at transport speeds (1-100 cm/sec), flexure frequencies (up to 1 MHz), and power levels (0.1-100 pW per array element) characteristic of individual nanoscale manipulators (Section 9.3.1).

In 1998, the prototyping and testing of ciliary arrays in MEMS work was an active research area. Ataka et al[1274] fabricated and operated a 1 cm^2 array of 512 cantilever-type bimorph manipulators (each one 500 microns long, 100 microns wide, and 6 microns thick) and operated it at 10 Hz in a coordinated fashion to transport a 2.4 mg piece of silicon wafer at 27-500 micron/sec using ~100 micron strokes and a 4 milliwatt input power to each actuator. Bohringer et al[1639] fabricated a prototype array of 1024 cilia called the "cilia chip" that moves silicon chips at speeds up to 200 microns/sec with a placement accuracy of ~3 microns and a lifting capacity of 250 N/m^2. Individual ciliary pixel control allows movement of multiple components on different trajectories, enabling the performance of various assembly tasks. A larger manipulator chip (M-chip) consisting of ~10,000 micro-actuator "resonators" (5-micron tall cilia) has also been fabricated on a few cm^2 of silicon substrate and tested at ~5 KHz.[1645] A part dropped onto the array is propelled forward at a constant speed of ~800 microns/sec.[1646] Bohringer et al[1643,1644] also created a theory of programmable force fields to model the actions of a ciliary array; simulations have uncovered numerous important operational design issues.[1646] Analogously in experimental biology, an array of kinesin motors fastened to a fixed surface transported microtubules hand-over-hand when ATP was added.[2425,2426]

Peter Will et al[1640] developed a software toolkit to allow researchers to program Intelligent Motion Surfaces[1641,1642] to perform a variety of simple functions including centering parts, spiraling a part to center in a convergent field array, spiraling a part away from the center in a divergent field array, rotating a part about the center using four triangular fields, orienting a part in a programmable field array, and sorting two parts using a hole as a trap for a part being translated past it. Properly arrayed, such surfaces can form an assembly pipeline in which parts may enter at one end and be successively sorted, spaced (so parts flow through at a constant rate), centered, aligned and, ultimately, inserted into other parts.

9.3.5 Materials Disassembly for Disposal

From time to time, medical nanorobots will find it necessary to accept bulk materials of various sizes and types, and reduce those materials to smaller and simpler forms in preparation for analysis, transport, or disposal from the human body. For example, nanorobots may be required to mechanically excise unwanted tissue or mineral deposits from arterial walls. Disabled nanodevices or their component parts found freely floating in tissues may also require disposal. Both requirements are discussed below. A fuller treatment of the biocompatibility of in vivo refuse, and routes of final disposal thereof, is deferred to Chapters 15 and 16.

9.3.5.1 Morcellation and Mincing

Morcellation is the fragmentation of biological materials as they are excised from the body; mincing is the progressive reduction in size of tissue segments by mechanical means. Chunks of biological material may be excised from the body using a tool such as the core sampler described in Section 9.3.2. Cutting is required because many connective tissues have strengths on the order of 10-100 atm but the body is only pressurized to ~1 atm, so vacuum suction alone is insufficient to pull coherent tissues apart.

In the simplest design, morcellated material is passed through successive banks of fixed diamondoid cutting blades or rotating diamondoid cutting disks positioned at various angles with progressively more closely-spaced blade edges. The target material is minced into nanometer-sized bits. Each blade is geared for maximum force application at relatively slow speed and turns in a tightly fitted sleeve, providing an automatic self-cleaning action. More complex designs might include paddlewheeling-bucket or orthogonal-blade arrays whose interiors are cleared by pistons after completion of the mincing action on material compacted into the cutting chamber by a larger piston. Table 9.3 shows that diamond and other potential blade materials are far stronger than all forms of biological matter, including dental enamel which is the hardest natural substance found in the human body.

To quantify the mincing action, consider a blade of length L_{blade}, cutting edge width W_{edge}, and compressive strength T_{blade} (N/m^2) which applies a force F_{blade} to a biological sample of length L_{sample} and thickness x_{sample} and tearing strength T_{sample}. Assuming $L_{blade} = L_{sample}$, then the minimum force required to cut the sample is $F_{min} = T_{sample} L_{blade} W_{edge} \leq F_{blade}$, the chopping energy per full blade stroke is $E_{stroke} = F_{blade} x_{sample}$, and the continuous power requirement of the blade (neglecting drag during the return stroke) is $P_{blade} = E_{stroke} \nu_{blade}$ where ν_{blade} is chopping frequency in Hz. Taking L_{blade} = 1 micron, W_{edge} = 1 nm, x_{sample} = 1 micron, $T_{sample} = 10^8$ N/m^2, and ν_{blade} = 1 KHz, then F_{min} = 100 nN, E_{stroke} = 0.1 pJ, and P_{blade} = 100 pW.

Consider next an ideal morcellation system which accepts a cubic biological sample of volume $V_{sample} = L_{sample}^3$ and minces it by progressive halving into final pieces of volume $V_{minced} = L_{minced}^3$ in a minimum number of $N_{cut} = \log_2 (V_{sample} / V_{minced})$ cuts (analogous to "oct-trees" in computer science[3155]). The energy required to make the ith cut is $T_{sample} W_{edge} [V_{sample} / 2^{(i-1)}]^{2/3}$ and after the ith cut there are 2^i intermediate pieces, hence the total energy E_{minced} required to make all cuts down to the final pieces is:

$$E_{minced} = \frac{T_{sample} W_{edge} V_{sample}^{2/3} (2^{N_{cut}/3} - 1)}{(2^{1/3} - 1)} \qquad \{Eqn. 9.54\}$$

The minimum size of the final pieces depends on the character of the sample material, the edge sharpness and speed of the blades, and numerous other factors, but in most cases cannot be smaller than 1-10 nm—natural biomolecules like hemoglobin, insulin, or albumin are 5-10 nm in diameter (Fig. 3.15). A crude limit is $E_{stroke} \gtrsim E_{bond}$, where E_{bond} = 180-1800 zJ for individual covalent bonds (Section 3.5.1), which implies a minimum final piece size of $L_{min} \sim (E_{bond}/T_{sample} W_{edge})^{1/2}$ assuming $L_{blade} = x_{sample} = L_{min}$. Taking $E_{bond} \sim$ 1000 zJ, $T_{sample} = 10^8$ N/m^2 and W_{edge} = 1 nm, then $L_{min} \sim$ 3.2 nm.

Eqn. 9.54 may now be applied to a specific morcellator configuration. Taking V_{sample} = 1 micron^3, V_{minced} = 1000 nm^3 (L_{minced} = 10 nm), W_{edge} = 1 nm, $T_{sample} = 10^8$ N/m^2, and ν_{blade} = 1 KHz, then N_{cut} = 20 cuts, blade velocity $v_{blade} = \nu_{blade} V_{sample}^{1/3}$ = 1 mm/sec, total mincing time $t_{minced} = N_{cut} / \nu_{blade}$ = 20 millisec, volume mincing rate $\dot{V}_{minced} = V_{sample} / t_{minced}$ = 50 micron^3/sec, total energy to mince a single sample of volume V_{sample} is E_{minced} = 40 pJ, and continuous power dissipation while the morcellator is in operation is $P_{minced} = E_{minced} / t_{minced}$ = 2000 pW. Care must be taken to minimize sample adhesion in blade surface design (Section 9.2.3).*

Once reduced to multi-nanometer-scale chunks, biological refuse may be disposed of directly (Chapter 16) or may be further digested using inorganic acids, lysosomal enzymes (Sections 8.5.3.8 and 10.4.2), collagenases,[359] or even direct molecular mechanodecomposition (Section 9.3.5.3.5) which is the inverse of mechanosynthesis. A discussion of the biocompatibility of minced tissue and methods of final disposal is deferred to Chapters 15 and 16.

9.3.5.2 Disposability Engineering

Medical nanodevices should incorporate appropriate disposal pathways as explicit design criteria. For instance, morcellator wear during bulk materials processing will accumulate as a complicated function of ν_{blade}, T_{sample}/T_{blade}, and numerous other factors, until the blade fails. Proper morcellator design may include some ready means for blade replacement, recycling, or elimination, or else the entire subunit must be abandoned or discarded. Other internal nanorobotic structures such as diamondoid binding sites, sensor fittings, broken tool tips, or reconfigurable metamorphic drive elements also may require recycling if interior refuse storage volume is limited or if onboard fabrication materials are in short supply.

Additionally, disabled or malfunctioning whole nanodevices may require disposal. Drexler [personal communication, 1995] has suggested that nanodevices and their subassemblies could have frangible mechanical links incorporated into their structure to enable easy device disassembly for disposal. One can imagine a complex nanorobot comprised of strong and closely fitted subassemblies which are held in place by pins or tenons in the vacuum environment of the functional nanodevice interior. If the pins are soluble in water, or are readily unlocked by enzymatic agents, or are otherwise easily removable, then large strong devices may be rapidly dismantled into their constituent subassemblies with only modest effort, or automatically upon infiltration of the external environment. Of course, final disassembly or disposal of the subassemblies is still required to achieve complete biodegradability. Construction using special nonisotropic materials such as foamy diamond (containing patterned vacuum holes) or biodegradable fiber windings that are easily unraveled might also simplify this mode of disassembly (Chapter 11).

However, even setting aside biocompatibility issues, a major difficulty with the above-described "Chinese Puzzle Box" approach to disposability engineering is that no matter how clever the disposal design, there will always be some occasions when the "puzzle box" becomes jammed or sealed shut, or has been mechanically compromised, or is actively resisting normal disassembly procedures. Design for disposal thus must include provision of capabilities to allow the partial or complete dismantlement of disabled or uncooperative devices.

Finally, there is the problem of nonbiological waste disposal. Such wastes might include accidental releases into the in vivo environment (external to the nanorobot) of raw feedstock materials, specialized fuel elements, pressurized nanocontainers, or nanodevice components such as tool tips, sensors, integument plates, or hard-material work products in various stages of completion. All manner of nanorobot-related detritus might plausibly be found freely floating in the tissues or bloodstream, from the smallest diamondoid parts up to and including detached whole manipulator arms, major subassemblies following a major device breach, or debris resulting from the execution of a voluntary autodestruct protocol (Chapter 12). While reliable and clean operation is an essential design objective in nanomedical systems, it would be irresponsible to ignore the need for an explicit nonbiological materials waste scavenging and disposal capability (Chapter 16).

9.3.5.3 Diamondoid Decomposition

While most hard materials can be comminuted in approximately the same manner as biological materials (Section 9.3.5.1), the

** M. Krummenacker notes that mechanical bond cutting might leave behind reactive fragments, possibly including radicals, that could dehydrogenate the diamond blade surface via radical abstraction, leading to chemomechanical blade wear. A fluorine-passivated diamond blade might be more resistant to such wear, and hydrogen bonding with fluorine increases protein-diamond friction, possibly giving better cutting.*

Table 9.3. Mechanical Strength of Nanomedical Materials

Material	References	Young's Modulus E (N/m^2)	Failure Strength* (N/m^2)
Human Body Materials:			
Saphenous vein	362	$1.6-4.8 \times 10^{5}$	$\sim 2 \times 10^{5}$
Carotid artery	362	$<5.9 \times 10^{5}$	$\sim 2 \times 10^{5}$
Elastin	362,364	6×10^{5}	$\sim 2 \times 10^{5}$
Muscle tissue	362	--	$1-6 \times 10^{5}$
Elastic tissue	521	--	3×10^{5}
Thoracic aorta	521	$0.1-1.7 \times 10^{6}$	$0.1-1.7 \times 10^{6}$
Erythrocyte membrane	362,1325,1415	$\sim 0.001-1 \times 10^{6}$	$1-20 \times 10^{6}$
Axonemal microtubules	1449	$\sim 5 \times 10^{6}$	$\sim 1 \times 10^{6}$
Actin microfilaments	362,3210	$\sim 10^{10}$	$\sim 6 \times 10^{6}$
Soft tissues	(est.)	--	$\sim 0.01-10 \times 10^{7}$
Cartilage	364,521	$0.1-1.6 \times 10^{7}$	$0.12-2.5 \times 10^{7}$
Abdominal skin	521	$0.6-2.2 \times 10^{7}$	$0.4-1.4 \times 10^{7}$
Cancellous bone	364,585	$3-3.3 \times 10^{8}$	$0.4-5.0 \times 10^{7}$
Arterial plaque	1276	--	$0.1-1 \times 10^{8}$
Tendon	362,364,521	$1-9 \times 10^{8}$	$0.1-2.1 \times 10^{8}$
Collagen	362,364	$1-2 \times 10^{9}$	$0.2-1.4 \times 10^{8}$
Cornea	362	--	1×10^{8}
Intermediate filaments	364	4×10^{9}	2.5×10^{8}
Keratin (& wool)	364,3209	4×10^{9}	2.5×10^{8}
Wet compact bone	362,364,585	$0.5-2.7 \times 10^{10}$	$0.4-3.0 \times 10^{8}$
Dental enamel	364	7.5×10^{10}	8×10^{8}
Apatite	364	1.1×10^{11}	--
Bone hydroxyapatite	364	1.4×10^{11}	--
Bone fluoroapatite	362	1.7×10^{11}	--
Other Organic Materials:			
Resilin	362	1.8×10^{6}	3×10^{4}
Rubber	362,1280,1283	$1.4-2.5 \times 10^{6}$	1×10^{6}
Abductin	362,364	$1-4 \times 10^{6}$	--
Peptidoglycan, wet***	3149	1×10^{7}	3×10^{6}
Mature rat skin	521	4.4×10^{7}	1.34×10^{7}
Celluloid	1280	2.5×10^{9}	--
Cuticle (locust)	364	9×10^{9}	9.5×10^{7}
Wood	362,364,585,1280	$0.6-1.6 \times 10^{10}$	$0.02-2.2 \times 10^{8}$
Chitin	364	7×10^{10}	$0.2-7 \times 10^{8}$
Calcite shells	364	--	$0.5-1.0 \times 10^{8}$
Nautilus shell	364	4.4×10^{10}	$0.6-1.4 \times 10^{8}$
Peptidoglycan, dry***	3149	2×10^{10}	3×10^{8}
Cellophane	364	--	$0.6-3.8 \times 10^{8}$
Cellulose fibers	364,3209	$0.08-1.1 \times 10^{11}$	$2.0-9.2 \times 10^{8}$
Silk, *Bombyx mori*	364,3209	$0.5-1.6 \times 10^{10}$	$3.5-7.5 \times 10^{8}$
Silk, spider	362,364,1283	$0.06-1.0 \times 10^{10}$	$3-15 \times 10^{8}$
Nylon	364	4.5×10^{9}	7.5×10^{8}

Material	References	Young's Modulus E (N/m^2)	Failure Strength* (N/m^2)
Other Inorganic Materials:			
Water-ice (268-271 K)	1608-1609	$3.6-4.5 \times 10^{9}$	$0.05-1 \times 10^{7}$
Lead	460,1287	$1.4-1.5 \times 10^{10}$	1.4×10^{7}
Tin	460	$4.1-4.5 \times 10^{10}$	--
Concrete (unreinforced)	364	2.4×10^{10}	$0.3-3.6 \times 10^{7}$
Concrete with PMMA (+reinforcing fibers)	364	4.3×10^{10}	$1-16 \times 10^{7}$
Gold	460	$7.4-8.0 \times 10^{10}$	$\sim 2.0 \times 10^{7}$
Silver	460	$7.1-7.8 \times 10^{10}$	$\sim 2.1 \times 10^{7}$
Glass	1164,1280,1286	$4.5-7.4 \times 10^{10}$	$3-120 \times 10^{7}$
Granite	364	--	4×10^{7}
Copper	460,1164,1280,1288	$1.1-1.3 \times 10^{11}$	$1.1-3.9 \times 10^{8}$
Flint	364	--	$1.2-1.9 \times 10^{8}$
Cast iron (& wrought iron)	460,585,1280,1288	$0.8-3.0 \times 10^{11}$	$1-4 \times 10^{8}$
Mild steel (std. structural steel)	362,460,536,585,1164 1288	$1.7-2.1 \times 10^{11}$	$3.1-8.6 \times 10^{8}$
Aluminum	362,364,460,1164,1288	$6.9-9.0 \times 10^{10}$	$1.7-13 \times 10^{8}$
Platinum	460	1.5×10^{11}	$\sim 1 \times 10^{9}$
High carbon steel	460	1.9×10^{11}	3.9×10^{9}
Case hardened steel	460	$\sim 2.0 \times 10^{11}$	$2-7.8 \times 10^{9}$
Kevlar	1283	--	4×10^{9}
Tungsten	460,1281	$3.4-3.5 \times 10^{11}$	4×10^{9}
Silicon	10,460,763,1281	$1.1-1.8 \times 10^{11}$	$0.7-1.6 \times 10^{10}$
Boron	1281	4.4×10^{11}	1.3×10^{10}
Fused quartz	460,1282	$0.8-1.1 \times 10^{11}$	1.4×10^{10}
Silicon nitride	763,1281	3.9×10^{11}	1.4×10^{10}
Aluminum oxide	460,763,1281	5.3×10^{11}	$1.5-2.0 \times 10^{10}$
Sapphire	536,1602,1605	4.0×10^{11}	$1.0-2.0 \times 10^{10}$
Graphite whiskers	10,763,1281	6.9×10^{11}	2.0×10^{10}
Tungsten carbide	460,536	6.5×10^{11}	2.15×10^{10}
Boron carbide	460	--	2.2×10^{10}
Silicon carbide	460,763,1281	7.0×10^{11}	$1.8-3.9 \times 10^{10}$
Cubic boron nitride	460	--	4.4×10^{10}
Cubic carbon nitride	1284,1285	$\sim 1 \times 10^{12}$	$4.5-5.5 \times 10^{10}$
Graphite sheet (in plane)	1281,2280	6.9×10^{11}	2.0×10^{10}
Diamond	460,536,537,1281,1284	1.05×10^{12}	$0.5-1.0 \times 10^{11}$
Fullerenes**	10,1278,1279,1308	$1.3-1.8 \times 10^{12}$	$1.3-1.5 \times 10^{11}$

* Failure strength may differ significantly in tension, compression, bending, or torsion; value given is representative.
** Mechanical properties are a function of nanotube chirality.[2277]
*** *Bacillus subtilis*, bacterial cell wall.[3149]

onboard disassembly of diamondoid materials is clearly the greatest challenge. The six general approaches proposed in this Section are randomizing processes that destroy any atomic-level positional or compositional information contained within the structure that is being dismantled. Controlled information-preserving disassembly processes are described in Chapter 19.

9.3.5.3.1 Grinding

Two substances of nearly equal hardness can scratch each other, so a set of corrugated sacrificial diamond grinding elements can be used to mechanically grind or saw the target mass into nanometer-scale particulate waste. This process consumes a volume of grinder mechanism which is approximately equal to the volume of the target, hence is relatively energy inefficient because, in addition to the power dissipated by grinding, the sacrificial grinders must then be rebuilt which requires another expenditure of a similar magnitude of energy for fabrication. At least twice the volume of the original target in particulates is produced by this process. Alternatively, two or more diamond targets may be rubbed against each other destructively, most efficiently after the manner of a macroscale ball mill. Note that diamond detritus may be ground, though less efficiently, by sacrificial grinders comprised of materials of lesser hardness or strength—for example, cubic boron nitride or borazon, first synthesized in 1957, scratches diamond with ease.

9.3.5.3.2 Cleavage

Jewellers and diamond cutters have known for centuries that diamond has a "perfect cleavage" or "grain" in four directions, parallel to its octahedral crystal faces. After cutting a notch or "kerf" along the grain, a rather dull iron or steel edge is laid athwart the groove and a sharp ~20 microsec blow is struck, forcing apart the groove walls and causing the diamond sample to split along the cleavage plane of structural weakness. Large diamond crystals may be progressively fractured down to near-nanometer scale by this technique. A blade velocity of 500 m/sec should suffice for complete crack penetration through the crystal;[536] more energetic cleavage blows give higher fracture velocities which may produce rougher surfaces and even multiple fragmentation. Maximum crack propagation velocity is 1580 m/sec in glass, 4500 m/sec in sapphire, and 7200 m/sec in diamond.[536] A large impedance mismatch between the gripper mechanism and the diamond crystal target optimizes pulse reflection at the holding surfaces and maximizes fragmentation. A gripper mechanism made of nylon (failure strength ~10^9 N/m^2; Table 9.3) has an acoustic impedance of 2.9×10^6 kg/m^2-sec,[763] compared to 6.3×10^7 kg/m^2-sec for diamond,[536] a huge 22:1 impedance mismatch. A water bath also ensures acoustic reflection because of a large impedance mismatch with diamond (~1.5×10^6 kg/m^2-sec for water).

The weakest diamond cleavage plane with the lowest areal bond density is the {111} crystal plane which has a cleavage energy of 10.6 J/m^2.[536] Thus a single cleavage of a 1 micron^3 diamond cube requires 10.6 pJ; a striker blade 1 micron long and 10 nm in width must apply a pressure of ~10^9 N/m^2 (~10,000 atm) along the contact edge, well below the failure strength of the hardest steel (Table 9.3). As a crude estimate of total cleavage decomposition energy, the progressive fracture of a 1 micron^3 diamond cube into one million (10 nm)^3 cubes implies a thousandfold increase in surface area and the cleavage of 5.94×10^8 nm^2 of diamond plane, requiring a minimum energy expenditure of ~6300 pJ to perform the decomposition. The cleavage technique is most applicable to brittle solids and may be less useful in the fragmentation of composite diamondoid materials (Chapter 11).

9.3.5.3.3 Sonication

Multiple acoustic pulses applied simultaneously to the surfaces of a crystal may elevate the interior mechanical stress above the failure strength of the material, causing it to fracture. Consider six diamond hammers of facial area L^2 and failure strength ~1×10^{11} N/m^2 that simultaneously impact each of the six faces of a cubic diamond target of edge L, applying a non-self-fracturing peak pressure of 0.3×10^{11} N/m^2 at each face. The peak pressure rises to 1.8×10^{11} N/m^2 at the center of the cube where the plane waves converge, well exceeding the strength of diamond and shattering the target cube throughout its interior. Sonic pulverization is an analogous macroscale manufacturing process.

Single-walled fullerene nanotubes are cut by water-bath ultrasonication at 55 KHz,[1525] which is inferred to produce microscopic domains of high temperature[1523] following the collapse of cavitation bubbles, leading to localized sonochemistry that opens a hole in the tube side. Vigorous sonication of multi-walled fullerene nanotubes produces similar damage in a CH_2Cl_2 bath.[1590]

9.3.5.3.4 Thermal Decomposition

Since carbon burns readily in oxygen, simple incineration in a high-pressure oxygen-rich atmosphere seems an obvious approach to diamond decomposition. A sapphire inner wall coating provides a flameproof combustion chamber with a ~200,000 atm failure strength (Table 9.3), and an externally insulated electrodynamic vacuum suspension (Section 6.3.4.4) prevents rapid thermal conduction and allows maintenance of high operating temperatures. The combustion temperature of diamond in air at 1 atm is usually given as 870-1070 K,[691] and higher oxygen pressures should lower this range considerably. Evans[1277] has studied the noncombustive oxidation of diamond in pure oxygen atmospheres as a function of temperature and pressure. Using data from Evans' oxidation rate/pressure and Arrhenius oxidation/temperature plots, the etch rate (in meters/sec) for the {111} diamond crystal face (which oxidizes most readily) may be crudely approximated as:

$$v_{etch} \sim k_1 \, p_{oxy} \, e^{-k_2/T} \quad \text{for: } T \lesssim 1050 \text{ K} \qquad \text{\{Eqn. 9.55\}}$$

$$v_{etch} \sim k_3 p_{oxy} \quad \text{for: } 1050 \text{ K} \lesssim T \lesssim 1600 \text{ K} \qquad \text{\{Eqn. 9.56\}}$$

where p_{oxy} is oxygen pressure (atm), T is diamond temperature (K), $k_1 = 3.6 \times 10^6$ m/sec-atm, $k_2 = 2.68 \times 10^4$ K, $k_3 = 3 \times 10^{-5}$ m/sec-atm, and the time required to completely oxidize a diamond cube of edge L is $t_{decomp} = L / v_{etch}$. For p_{oxy} = 100 atm, a 100 nm diamond cube is consumed in 1 second at T ~ 750 K; a 1 nm cube heated to T ~ 660 K decomposes to oxide in 1 second, or in ~1 hour at 530 K. Although not modeled using high-pressure data, Eqn. 9.55 hints that a pure oxygen atmosphere at p_{oxy} ~ 1000 atm might support active combustion at an ignition temperature as low as ~700 K. Oxygen ions at 100-1000 eV can machine the diamond {100} face at a rate of ~0.01 (nm/sec) / (ion/sec-nm^2) that saturates at a gas pressure >10^{-7} atm.[2708]

Extremely high temperatures are required to initiate and to sustain pure graphitization—the transformation of hard diamond into relatively soft (and more easily disposable) graphite by simple heating. In vacuo, unstressed polished hydrogenated diamond surfacesremain chemically and mechanically stable up to ~1275 K, at which temperature the passivating hydrogens are removed and crystallographic surface reconstruction begins.[1291] Drexler[10] estimates the characteristic thermal cleavage time for unstressed 556-zJ C-C bonds in diamond as ~10^{85} sec at 300 K, ~10^{12} sec at 700 K, and ~10^4 sec at 1000 K. At 1300 K, a shear stress ≳0.18 nN/bond initiates plastic flow,[1292] but diamond remains chemically stable up to ~1800 K in an inert atmosphere. Heating above 1800 K can result in extensive graphitization,[1290] an autocatalytic process that spreads outward from nucleation centers. The experimental graphitization rate of the {111} diamond crystal face at zero pressure is approximated by Evans[1277] as:

$$v_{graphite} = k_4 \, e^{-E_a/kT} \quad \text{(m/sec)} \qquad \text{\{Eqn. 9.57\}}$$

where the activation energy E_a = 1760 zJ/atom, k = 0.01381 zJ/K (Boltzmann constant), T = temperature (K), and $k_4 = 5.4 \times 10^{16}$ m/sec. At 1800 K, graphitization is very slow, about 1 nm/day; $v_{graphite}$ ~ 1 nm/sec at T = 2150 K, ~1 micron/sec at T = 2440 K, well above the 2070 K softening point and the 2310 K melting point of sapphire.[1602] Catalytic graphitization by Ni and Fe has been observed at ≳ 1070 K.[1596] But because of the high temperatures involved, thermal decomposition of diamond by graphitization is impractical in vivo.

9.3.5.3.5 Molecular Mechanodecomposition

Molecular mechanosynthesis can be used to construct nanoscale objects, using either precise moiety-by-moiety placement or mechanical part-by-part placement of individual nanoscale parts (Chapters 2 and 19). Following the same process in reverse, diamondoid objects may be decomposed atom by atom into their constituent elemental components. This molecular mechanodecomposition may proceed rapidly using many tools working simultaneously, if no attempt is made to preserve or record the encoded structural pattern information.

Many of the radical-based reaction mechanisms for diamond mechanosynthesis described by Drexler[10] may be reversible with the application of mechanical energy, since at elevated temperatures surface groups and radical vacancies apparently can migrate after placement on growing diamond surfaces.[1293] M. Krummenacker [personal communication, 1997] suggests a speculative mechanochemical decomposition process in which a few surface hydrogen atoms are first abstracted from an edge or corner of the diamond surface to minimize steric congestion at the disassembly site. Then a radical-based tool, possibly with an oxygen radical at the tip, bonds to an exposed carbon atom and pulls it upward far enough to insert another reactive moiety such as a nitrene (an analog to carbene) into the gap, replacing another C-C lattice bond and allowing the first carbon atom to be pulled further out of the matrix. This process is repeated on an adjoining carbon atom, resulting in a two-carbon unit with four bonds to the manipulator tool, which can then be pulled the rest of the way out by mechanically disrupting the two remaining C-C bonds to the diamond lattice without exceeding the tensile strength of the tool tip. (A great deal of sensing and chemical inference remains to be described in this scenario.) Krummenacker's process might also be used to record structural information, if required (Chapter 19).

Evans[1277] estimates that 1760 zJ/atom of energy are required to break three C-C bonds and detach a single carbon atom from the {111} diamond crystal surface into the gas phase. With 176 carbon atoms/nm^3 in diamond, mechanodecomposition of bulk diamond would require ~300 nJ/micron^3. Generously assuming only ~5 manipulator arm motions to remove each carbon atom and a manipulator operating frequency of ~1 MHz, a single manipulator can mechanically disassemble diamond at a volumetric rate of ~1000 nm^3/sec-manipulator. The volume of each mechanosynthetic manipulator described in Section 9.3.1.4 is ~10^5 nm^3, so ~1000 manipulators disassembling in parallel occupy ~10% of a 1 micron^3 work space and can collectively mechanically decompose ~0.001 micron^3/sec of diamond crystal while drawing a total of ~300 pW of continuous power. Actual power usage may be far less, since in any reasonable decomposition process some energy will be recovered when the liberated carbon atom forms new bonds; high energies will only be encountered in the transition state, as in any chemical reaction.

9.3.5.3.6 Chemical and Microbial Decomposition

Four issues are considered briefly here. First, can diamond or sapphire be chemically solvated? Second, does any microbe likely exist which is capable of attacking a diamond or sapphire surface? Third, could such a microbe evolve naturally? Fourth, could such a microbe be artificially engineered? (The author thanks R. Bradbury, M. Krummenacker, R. Merkle, and J. Soreff for helpful discussions and important contributions to this Section.)

I. *Can diamond or sapphire be chemically solvated?* Although carbon is soluble in molten Fe (e.g., >1808 K at 1 atm),[763] Co, Mn, Ni, and Cr, there is no known room temperature solvent that dissolves pure crystalline diamond. Intact diamond and fullerene surfaces are extremely inert. For example, after facet-cutting, gem diamonds are boiled in concentrated sulfuric acid for cleaning, leaving the gem surface unaffected. The outer faces of natural hydrophobic diamond may be terminated partly by hydrogen and partly by bridging oxygen, with a significant proportion of carbonyl groups and a small number of -OH and carboxyl (-COOH) groups as well.[1596]

Diamond is almost completely resistant to attack by room-temperature ground-state molecular oxygen (see Eqn. 9.55), although oxidative erosion by atomic oxygen has been shown at rates of ~0.04 nm/min[1599] and ozone or various radicals might also be effective. Molecular fluorine only fluorinates the surface,[1598] producing a "Teflon" coat (stable up to ~1120 K)[1596] while not disturbing the underlying C-C bonds because F makes only single bonds; chlorine is also taken up by diamond surfaces.[1600] Molten sodium nitrate attacks diamond at ≳700 K.[1597] At high temperature or pressure, carbon from diamond can migrate and form a metal carbide phase in carbide-forming metals including W, Ta, Ti, and Zr,[1597] and metal oxides of Cu, Fe, Co, and Ni are reduced to the metal (a redox reaction with the carbon escaping as oxide) upon heating in vacuo.[1596]

Non-intact diamondoid surfaces may be more susceptible to chemical attack. For instance, open-ended single-walled fullerene nanotubes are consumed by a 3:1 mixture of sulfuric (98%) and nitric (70%) acids at 343 K at a rate of ~130 nm/hour even in the absence of sonication;[1525] the same mixture intercalates and exfoliates graphite.[1524] A 4:1 mixture of sulfuric acid (98%) and hydrogen peroxide (30%) at 343 K also etches the exposed ends of open nanotubes at ~200 nm/hour, "much like the burning of a fuse."[1525] Etch rate may vary with the chiral indices (n, m) of the nanotubes.[1525] COCl-derivatized single-walled carbon nanotubes will solvate in organic solvents,[2164] and high-strain sites such as the outer fold of a kinked nanotube are subject to attack by nitric acid.[2954]

Sapphire is primarily corundum or α-Al_2O_3, the oxide ions forming a hexagonally close-packed array and the Al ions distributed symmetrically among the octahedral interstices.[691] The solubility of α-Al_2O_3 in ~neutral water at room temperature is given variously as 10^{-7} - 10^{-5} M (~60-6000 atoms/micron^3) at equilibrium,[1602,1603] but solubility rises sharply below pH 4 and above pH 9 in an almost U-shaped curve.[1603] (Human blood pH normally ranges from 7.35-7.45).[1604] Aluminum oxide is amphoteric, forming hydrated Al^{+++} ions in acidic solutions (pH < 4) and $Al(OH)_4^-$ ions in alkaline solutions (pH > 9).[1603] Corundum dissolves slowly in boiling nitric acid and in orthophosphoric acid to 570 K, and dissolves well in potassium bisulfate at 670-870 K, or in borax or sodium fluoaluminate (cryolite) at 1070-1270 K.[1602]

Air-exposed Al metal is protected by a thin[1601] (~5 nm) adherent oxide layer having a defect rock-salt structure[691] easily compromised by amalgamation or halogens, or by alkali hydroxides (e.g., NaOH) with the generation of hydrogen in seconds at room temperature. Complex-forming reagents such as Cu^{++} + Cl^- also react with oxide-coated aluminum metal in less than 1 minute.

II. *Does any existing microbe possess the natural ability to attack a diamond or sapphire surface?* Extensive tests have not yet been performed, and negatives cannot be proven, but the prospects are poor. Most organisms develop the means for attacking materials in their environment because these materials are abundant and provide essential molecules or elements that are needed for energy production or important biochemical functions.

For diamondophagy to evolve naturally, a microbe probably must occupy a niche in which diamond is more abundant than competing carbon sources. This is unlikely except many kilometers below the natural oil/coal deposits in the Earth's crust, though the possibility cannot be definitely ruled out because deep-crustal-dwelling bacteria and other archaic biota have been found in rocks at depths of at least 2.7 kilometers, a field of study now known as geomicrobiology.[1592,3096] However, far more abundant nonpolymeric carbon sources are usually available. Highly polymeric molecules including long-chain hydrocarbons, cellulose, and starches tend to be fairly resistant to enzymatic degradation—nature has found it relatively difficult to devise an attack strategy for cellulose (e.g., wood) and chitin (e.g., crab and insect shells). With their crystalline arrays, diamond and sapphire would seem to fall into this category as well.

A microbe naturally evolved to attack sapphire would probably be seeking to extract the aluminum (sapphirophagy), since oxygen is plentiful elsewhere. However, Al is generally considered toxic,[752,3278-3281] and reports of microbes that feed on Al-rich minerals are extremely infrequent and remain unconfirmed, though microbial aluminum tolerance is well-known.[3282,3283] Organisms use +1/+2/+3 metal ions (mostly Cu, Fe, Mn, and more rarely Mo and Co) in enzymes to catalyze specific difficult reactions. Yet in seawater, Al is ~10-1000 times more abundant than Cu, ~50-500 times more abundant than Fe, ~100-1000 times more abundant than Mn, ~500-3000 times more abundant than Mo, and ~10,000 times more abundant than Co,[763] suggesting that Nature has gone to great lengths to avoid the use of aluminum in biological systems. Natural sapphire also contains ~0.1% iron atoms (Fe^{++} and Fe^{+++}), and natural ruby has traces of chromium (Cr^{+++}), biologically useful atoms more conveniently available from alternative sources.

III. *Could a microbe capable of attacking diamond or sapphire evolve naturally?* There are $>10^{23}$ bacteria living inside Earth's human population alone. While most of these microbes (>99%) are harmless or beneficial, up to $\sim 10^{21}$ may be undesirable pathogens possibly subject to attack by medical nanorobots. Could this large "natural laboratory" population of bacteria evolve diamondophagy or sapphirophagy as a defense against artificial nanomachines?

In the case of sapphire, most biological metal absorption is initiated by secretion of acids strong enough to dissolve the metal-containing material. Evolving an acid production capacity isn't difficult because most bacteria use H^+ ion gradients as power sources. Common bacteria normally create a mildly acidic environment. Typical energy sources (e.g., glucose) are oxidized to increase the external H^+ ion concentration. The flow of the H^+ ions back into the cell through the ATPase enzyme generates ATP (as in mitochondria). Blocking or minimizing ATP production and limiting external H^+ diffusion could produce fairly high local H^+ concentrations. Bacteria such as *Thiobacillus ferrodoxians*, found in environments where better energy sources are lacking, oxidize metal sulfides to generate energy.[3559,3560] These result in the generation of sulfuric acid and environmental pH values of 2-3. Extremozymes that can work at a pH below 1.0 have been isolated from the cell wall and underlying cell membrane of some acidophilic bacteria;[1591] some acids (e.g., HF) that dissolve oxides (e.g., SiO_2) may be safely stored in purely organic vessels (e.g., wax or plastic). As noted earlier, sapphire is also attacked by strong alkali (but see below).

Natural evolution of a diamondophagic capability is even more arduous. Acids such as HF, HCl and H_2SO_4 will not harm either H-terminated diamondoid surfaces or cellular lipid membranes which generally also have hydrogenated surfaces. While high H^+ concentrations should remove oxygens from SiO_2 or, with more difficulty, from Al_2O_3, a more efficient attack strategy for H-terminated diamondoid might be an extremely alkaline environment, although the most alkaliphilic bacteria (such as the *Natranobacterium gregoryi* normally found in soda lakes and high-carbonate soils)[3561] only reach a pH of 10-11. High OH^- environments can destroy lipid bilayers, RNA, and standard proteases and lipases.[1591] Also, the biochemistries of acidophiles and alkaliphiles are so tuned to their natural environments[3562] that the predominantly neutral pH found in the human body might prove toxic for these microbes.

Most human-pathogenic bacteria likely to be attacked by medical nanodevices are not extremophiles. Consequently, as R. Bradbury observes, Nature's design challenge is for non-extremophiles to evolve systems of creating very high local H^+ concentrations,[3563] having the energy resources available to drive this pathway and to minimize ATP production which utilizes the H^+ ions. Such evolution seems unlikely. Only if medical nanodevices were constructed of an essential material that is in short supply, such as iron, or could provide a better energy source than the surrounding plasma or cytosol, could bacteria be selected which have the potential of attacking nanomachinery. Whether extremophiles might subsequently repopulate the vacated microecological niches currently occupied by natural pathogenic bacterial species is an open issue worthy of future study.

IV. *Could a microbe capable of attacking diamond or sapphire be artificially engineered?* Almost certainly the answer is yes. In the simplest case using conventional biotechnology, a bacterium would be designed to produce and secrete an appropriate acid or alkali, creating a highly corrosive environment local to the target material by binding to the surface and secreting the acid (or ions) into sequestered adherent pockets.

J. Soreff suggests other approaches that may employ locally far-from-equilibrium states which are harder to get (at least with fast kinetics) in normal chemistry. One strategy is to engineer artificial enzymelike structures that can bind to the target surface at one end while catalyzing the local production of molecules in excited states (e.g., by crude analogy to luciferase in bioluminescence)[3564] at the other end. Enzymes like catalase and superoxide dismutase already handle locally powerful oxidants, and in the presence of light and oxygen, C_{60} can pass its superfluous excitation energy onto nearby O_2 molecules, creating singlet oxygen. An enzyme might be designed to catalyze $HOCl + H_2O_2 \rightarrow HCl + H_2O + O_2^*$ (singlet state oxygen)[3565,3566], other singlets,[3567,3568] triplets,[3569-3572] quartets,[3573] or other electronically-excited oxidizers.[3574] However, survival of such an enzyme over multiple cycles is problematical. Another strategy is to design novel mechanochemical tools into the bacterium. Proteins can convert ATP hydrolysis into mechanical motion. Such motion, perhaps combined with a "snap-action" elastic energy storage mechanism to allow tool release speeds comparable to vibrational times, could be used to mechanically hammer an oxidant into a diamond surface, thus reducing the chemical energy required to be released at the point of action.

9.4 In Vivo Locomotion

One of the most important basic capabilities a medical nanorobot may possess is the ability to move about inside the human body. At its most simple, this movement may be purely statistical, with nanodevices carried along with the natural ebb and flow of bodily fluids. At the other extreme, nanorobot locomotion may be highly deterministic, including powered drive mechanisms, mapping and active navigation, and traverses of diverse histological territories having markedly different mechanical and chemical characteristics. The subject matter is huge and quite impossible to cover fully in a single Chapter. As a result, the discussion here is merely a preliminary survey of the most important issues and challenges of in vivo locomotion, suggesting promising new areas for future research.

Section 9.4.1 opens with an overview of fluid viscosity generally and the rheology (flow characteristics) of nanorobot-rich biofluids that might be associated with passive nanorobot locomotion. Aspects and techniques of active swimming through the bloodstream, or sanguinatation, are described in Section 9.4.2. This is followed by discussions of cytoambulation (cell surface walking and anchoring) in Section 9.4.3, histonatation (tissue diving including diapedesis, ECM transit, and intercellular passage) in Section 9.4.4, cytopenetration (entering individual cells) in Section 9.4.5, locomotion inside the cell (Section 9.4.6), and finally cytocarriage (nanorobotic pilotage of natural motile cells) in Section 9.4.7. The biocompatibility of motive mechanisms is discussed in Chapter 15.

9.4.1 Rheology of Nanorobot-Rich Biofluids

The study of biofluid flow, or biorheology, is useful in nanomedicine because it is necessary to understand the flow characteristics of fluids through which nanorobots must navigate—whether a nanorobot is actively swimming or is simply drifting with the flow, or whether the nanorobot is traveling in an ordinary Newtonian fluid such as water or in more complex viscoelastic biofluids such as mucus or saliva. Additionally, the presence of large numbers of nanorobots may dramatically alter bloodstream viscosity (depending on nanorobot number density and shape), with important medical consequences. The following discussion examines biofluid and whole-blood viscosities (Sections 9.4.1.1 and 9.4.1.2), the radial distribution of blood elements in blood vessels (Section 9.4.1.3), viscosity and bloodstream velocity profiles of nanorobot-rich blood (Sections 9.4.1.4 and 9.4.1.5), and hematocrit reduction in narrow blood vessels (Section 9.4.1.6).

9.4.1.1 Biofluid Viscosity

Viscosity is a measure of the resistance of a fluid to shearing when the fluid is in motion. Consider a plate of surface area A moving parallel to a fixed plane surface with constant velocity v, being pushed laterally by a constant force F. A fluid of viscosity eta fills the volume between the two surfaces, which are separated by a distance d. The fluid layer nearest the moving plate also moves at velocity v and the layer nearest the stationary plane remains stationary. In between the two surfaces, the velocity increases linearly with distance, establishing a constant gradient. This gradient is usually called the shear rate (essentially a size-normalized velocity), or $\dot{\gamma} = v/d$ (m/sec-m, or sec^{-1}). The absolute viscosity may then be defined by:

$$F/A = \eta \dot{\gamma} \quad (N/m^2) \qquad \{Eqn.\ 9.58\}$$

where η has MKS units of N-sec/m^2, Pascal-sec, or, more simply, kg/m-sec. In a Newtonian fluid, the shear stress F/A (N/m^2) increases linearly with shear rate $\dot{\gamma}$, so that viscosity η is constant over a wide range of shear rates. Many common fluids such as air, water, saline and blood serum closely approximate the ideal Newtonian fluid. The viscosity of solutions of molecules is related to the diffusion coefficient; see Eqn. 3.5.

The viscosities of some common materials are given in Table 9.4. The viscosity of an ideal gas is independent of density and independent of pressure between 0.01-10 atm; at higher pressures, intermolecular interactions lead to higher viscosities.[390] Theory predicts that gas viscosity ~ $T^{1/2}$ (e.g., rises with the square-root of temperature T), but a somewhat larger temperature exponent is obtained experimentally for real gases. In contrast, the viscosity of liquids increases with rising pressure (typically by a factor of 2-3 after moving from 1 atm up to 1000 atm for organic liquids) and decreases with rising temperature. In normal liquids the temperature dependence is approximated by Andrade's formula which gives:

$$\eta \sim k_v \, e^{E_v / kT} \qquad \{Eqn.\ 9.59\}$$

where for example the activation energy for viscosity E_v ~ 25 zJ and the constant k_v ~ 2.1 x 10^{-6} kg/m-sec for pure water at 1 atm. Nonelectrolytes dissolved in water generally cause viscosity to rise, while solvation of electrolytes may increase or decrease viscosity (the effect is typically ~10% or less for a 1M solution). Large asymmetric solute molecules increase viscosity more than an equal mass of small spherical molecules. The threshold between solid and liquid is generally taken as η ~ 10^{14} kg/m-sec.[364]

Most biofluids are viscoelastic and non-Newtonian, with apparent viscosity η_a varying with shear rate and displaying other nonlinear characteristics such as hysteresis, relaxation, and creep.[362] Saliva behaves more like an elastic body than like water. Because of its high molecular weight, DNA solution is viscoelastic even at low concentrations. Sex glands produce viscoelastic fluids, including semen and uterine cervical mucus[1392] (η_a varies ~20% during the menstrual cycle).[3575-3577] Human synovial fluid becomes increasingly incompressible at higher pressures, with η_a ~ 10 kg/m-sec at $\dot{\gamma}$ ~ 0.1 sec^{-1} (e.g., knee flexion during very slow walking) declining to η_a ~ 0.1 kg/m-sec at $\dot{\gamma}$ ~ 10 sec^{-1} (very fast running), and to η_a ~ 0.001 kg/m-sec at $\dot{\gamma}$ ~ 10,000 sec^{-1} (experimental).[362] Viscoelasticity is also an important property of respiratory tract mucus, which typically shows an η_a ~ 1 kg/m-sec at low shear rates near $\dot{\gamma}$ ~ 0.1-1 sec^{-1}, falling to η_a ~ 0.01 kg/m-sec at high shear rates near $\dot{\gamma}$ ~ 100-1000 sec^{-1}.[362] Even ice is a viscoelastic material, with η_a ~ 10^{10}–10^{13} kg/m-sec (estimated as maximum shear stress divided by shear rate from data in Sinha et al[1609]) for $\dot{\gamma}$ ~ 10^{-3}-10^{-7} sec^{-1} at 262 K; ice viscosity varies with temperature (Table 9.4) as described by Andrade's formula, with E_v ~ 110 zJ as determined experimentally for pure ice,[1609] and taking k_v ~ 6.3 x 10^{-4} kg/m-sec at high shear rate.

Cytoplasm is a complex viscoelastic material having a continuous liquid phase (the cytosol) plus various suspended particles, granules, and membranous structures. More precisely, the cytomatrix is a mixed-phase body composed of a fibrillar network penetrated by a solution.[1408] As a result, viscosity is different in the various phases. From flow behavior, the viscosity of *E. coli* protoplasm was estimated as ~1000 kg/m-sec; from measured diffusion rates of sucrose, dextran, and β-galactosidase, the apparent viscosity was 3-4 x 10^{-3} kg/m-sec.[1407] Cytoplasm is inhomogeneous and anisotropic at many levels of organization.

9.4.1.2 Viscosity of Whole Blood

Human blood is a suspension of cells, in plasma (an aqueous solution of electrolytes and nonelectrolytes; Appendix B). The plasma is ~90% water by weight, 7% plasma proteins, 1% inorganic materials, and 1% other organic substances. The cellular component (Appendix B) is essentially all erythrocytes, or red blood cells (RBCs; Figure 8.43), with white cells of various categories comprising less than 1/600th of the total volume of cells and platelets less than 1/800th.

Pure blood plasma is a Newtonian viscous fluid, with η_{plasma} = 1.1 x 10^{-3} kg/m-sec at 310 K. Blood plasma is the environment

Table 9.4. Absolute Viscosity of Some Common Materials[362,386,389,585,763,1081,1325,1328,1407,1458,1505,1609,3166,3306-3314,3611]

Material (Gas, Liquid, Solid)	Viscosity (kg/m-sec)	Material (Gas, Liquid, Solid)	Viscosity (kg/m-sec)
Water @ 0°C (273 K)	1.787×10^{-3}	Earth's mantle (geological)	$\sim 10^{21}$
@ 20°C (293 K)	1.002×10^{-3}	Pitch (room temperature)	$\sim 10^{14}$
@ 37°C (310 K)	0.6915×10^{-3}	Glass @ 720-920 K (anneal)	2.5×10^{12}
@ 50°C (323 K)	0.5468×10^{-3}	Glass @ ~1300 K (blowing)	$\sim 1 \times 10^{6}$
@ 100°C (373 K)	0.2818×10^{-3}	Glass @ 1500-1700 K (furnace)	$\sim 1 \times 10^{2}$
Ice @ -11°C (262 K)	$\sim 10^{10}$-10^{13}		
@ -82°C (191 K)	$\sim 10^{15}$ est.	Glucose (295 K)	9.1×10^{12}
@ -109°C (164 K)	$\sim 10^{18}$ est.	Glucose (310 K)	1.4×10^{9}
@ -129°C (144 K)	$\sim 10^{21}$ est.	Glucose (373 K)	2.5×10^{1}
Squid axoplasm	$1\text{-}10 \times 10^{6}$	Golden syrup (285 K)	$140{,}000 \times 10^{-3}$
Pulmonary macrophage cells	$0.12\text{-}0.27 \times 10^{6}$	Glycerin (273 K)	$12{,}110 \times 10^{-3}$
Chick fibroblast cells	$\sim 0.01 \times 10^{6}$	Corn syrup (294 K)	$\sim 5{,}000 \times 10^{-3}$
Human feces, range (est.)	$\sim 10^{-2}$-10^{5}	Glycerin (303 K)	629×10^{-3}
E. coli cytoplasm	$>1{,}000{,}000 \times 10^{-3}$	Castor oil (310 K)	297×10^{-3}
Mucus and sputum (310 K)	$10\text{-}750{,}000 \times 10^{-3}$	Machine oil, heavy (310 K)	130×10^{-3}
Erythrocyte membrane (310 K)	$\sim 100{,}000 \times 10^{-3}$	Machine oil, light (310 K)	35×10^{-3}
Plasma membrane (~310 K)	$10{,}000\text{-}100{,}000 \times 10^{-3}$	Oleic acid (303 K)	25.6×10^{-3}
T-cell cytoplasm (298 K)	$27{,}300 \times 10^{-3}$	Sulfuric acid, 100% (293 K)	25.4×10^{-3}
Leukocyte, adhered cell (310 K)	$66{,}800 \times 10^{-3}$	Ethylene glycol (310 K)	10.7×10^{-3}
Human fibroblast cytoplasm	$5000\text{-}8000 \times 10^{-3}$	Lead, liquid (623 K)	2.58×10^{-3}
Leukocyte, free cell (310 K)	4500×10^{-3}	Iron + 2.5% C, liquid (1673 K)	2.25×10^{-3}
Amoeba cytoplasm	$1000\text{-}30{,}000 \times 10^{-3}$	Propanol (310 K)	1.5×10^{-3}
Human chyme, normal (est.)	$100\text{-}30{,}000 \times 10^{-3}$	Mercury, liquid (310 K)	1.465×10^{-3}
Human semen	9.4×10^{-3}	Acetic acid (310 K)	1.01×10^{-3}
Saliva (310 K)	$4\text{-}10{,}000 \times 10^{-3}$	Ethanol (310 K)	0.885×10^{-3}
Synovial (knee) fluid (298 K)	$1\text{-}10{,}000 \times 10^{-3}$	Methanol (310 K)	0.472×10^{-3}
Whole blood, low shear rate:		Acetone (310 K)	0.285×10^{-3}
Hct = 45%	$\sim 100 \times 10^{-3}$	Diethyl ether (310 K)	0.202×10^{-3}
Hct = 90%	$\sim 1000 \times 10^{-3}$	Air, liquid (81 K)	0.172×10^{-3}
Whole blood, high shear rate:		Carbon dioxide, liquid (303 K)	0.053×10^{-3}
Hct = 45%	$\sim 10 \times 10^{-3}$	Neon, gas (310 K)	0.032×10^{-3}
Hct = 90%	$\sim 100 \times 10^{-3}$	Oxygen, gas (310 K)	0.021×10^{-3}
RBC contents (Hb solution)	$6\text{-}13 \times 10^{-3}$	Air, gas (310 K)	0.01894×10^{-3}
Human blood plasma (310 K)	$1.1\text{-}1.2 \times 10^{-3}$	Nitrogen, gas (310 K)	0.018×10^{-3}
Serum/Interstitial fluid (310 K)	$1.0\text{-}1.1 \times 10^{-3}$	Carbon dioxide, gas (310 K)	0.0157×10^{-3}
Bile fluid (probably liver)	$0.84\text{-}2.3 \times 10^{-3}$	Hydrogen, liquid (~20 K)	0.011×10^{-3}
Human tears (310 K)	$0.73\text{-}0.97 \times 10^{-3}$	Hydrogen, gas (310 K)	0.0091×10^{-3}

normally encountered by micron-sized bloodstream-traversing nanorobots as they move between blood cells.

On the other hand, "whole" blood is the complete natural mixture of blood plasma and blood cells. In blood vessels whose diameters are much larger than the size of blood cells, or in the case of mechanical systems with dimensions much larger than the characteristic sizes of blood cells, whole blood must be treated as an homogenous non-Newtonian fluid. The bulk viscosity of whole blood decreases with rising shear rate and increases with rising hematocrit (Hct), the percentage of blood volume occupied by red cells. (The human male hematocrit has a normal range of Hct = 40%-52%, average Hct = 46%,[743] which optimizes oxygen transport.[1325]) As an example, for whole blood at a low shear rate of $\dot{\gamma} \sim 0.1$ sec^{-1}, then $\eta_a \sim 0.001$ kg/m-sec at Hct = 0%, ~0.1 kg/m-sec at Hct = 45%, and ~1 kg/m-sec at Hct = 90%. At a high shear rate of $\dot{\gamma} \sim 100$ sec^{-1}, then $\eta_a \sim 0.001$ kg/m-sec at Hct = 0%, ~0.01 kg/m-sec at Hct = 45%, and ~0.1 kg/m-sec at Hct = 90%.[362] At still higher shear rates $\dot{\gamma} > 100$ sec^{-1}, whole blood behaves almost like a Newtonian fluid with a nearly constant η_a (Fig. 9.12). Viscosity also varies with disease state (if any) and slightly with temperature. For whole blood at normal Hct and $\dot{\gamma} = 0.1$ sec^{-1}, then $\eta_a \sim 0.10$ kg/m-sec at 310 K and ~0.15 kg/m-sec at 283 K; for $\dot{\gamma} = 100$ sec^{-1}, then $\eta_a \sim 0.010$ kg/m-sec at 310 K and ~0.015 kg/m-sec at 283 K.[362]

For large blood vessels, the effect of hematocrit on viscosity for Hct $\lesssim$ 45% has been modeled experimentally by Cokelet et al[1318] as:

$$\eta_a/\eta_{plasma} = (1 - \mathrm{Hct})^{-2.5} \qquad \text{\{Eqn. 9.60\}}$$

with Hct expressed as a fraction. This formula, which also gives good results for RBC-sized oil/water emulsions in the same volume fraction range,[1316] is only useful up to volume fraction of ~10% in the case of rigid-particle suspensions, whose viscosity behaves markedly differently from that of RBC suspensions (see below).

It has long been known[1313] that human red blood cells can form aggregates known as rouleaux, in which the discoid RBCs adhere loosely in a "stack of coins" configuration at shear rates <100 sec^{-1}.[1314] Formation of linear and branched chain aggregates (rouleaux) depends on the presence of the cell-surface cross-linking proteins fibrinogen and globulin in the plasma. The lower the shear rate (e.g., the slower the blood velocity), the more prevalent (larger size and number density) are the aggregates. As the shear rate goes to zero, it is speculated that human blood becomes one big aggregate, which then may behave as a viscoelastic or viscoplastic solid.[362]

As shear rate increases, the rouleaux tend to break up. Individual red cells also deform slightly, elongating and lining up with the streamlines. These two effects combine to reduce blood viscosity with rising shear, as illustrated by Figure 9.12 which shows the relative viscosity η_a / η_{plasma} for human blood at Hct = 45% as a function of shear rate. Note that for rigid particles (including hardened red cells, normal leukocytes, and nondeforming nanorobots), bulk viscosity is essentially independent of shear rate.

Normal blood vessel wall (peripheral zone) shear rates in physiological bloodflow range from 50-700 sec^{-1} in the larger arteries to 250-2000 sec^{-1} in the smallest arteries and capillaries, and 20-200 sec^{-1} in large and small veins.[386] At shear rates >100 sec^{-1} where RBC aggregation ceases to be important, pure whole blood remains fluid even up to 98% RBC concentration by volume (e.g., Hct = 98% volume fraction).[1319]

9.4.1.3 Radial Distribution of Blood Elements

At low shear rates, red cells aggregate into rouleaux and migrate inward, forming a network of aggregates in the core of the tube. Individual rouleaux may incorporate 10-20 red cells, or more, creating by far the largest cellular elements normally present in the blood. At the highest shear rates, the rouleaux break up entirely into single red cells, and the red cells then distribute themselves more uniformly in the radial direction.

The radial distribution of white cells is also a function of flow conditions.[1325,1333-1336] At low shear rates, under conditions allowing red cell aggregation, the white cells are displaced to the periphery of the flow by the much larger red cell rouleaux. At the highest shear rates, white cell concentration is highest along the tube axis, displacing some red cells, since most white cells are larger than individual red cells.

The radial distribution of the local platelet concentration during blood flow in tubes has also been investigated.[1337,1338] In plasma containing only platelets, the platelet distribution is radially uniform. However, in whole blood flow under all shear conditions, the platelet concentration is highest near the vessel wall. In arterioles, the platelet number density is about two times higher near the wall than in the center of the vessel.[1342] Platelets are much smaller than either red cells or white cells, thus tend to be crowded out of the center whenever red cells or white cells are present.

These experimental observations are consistent with the general principle that during blood flow in a vessel, the largest particles, or "flow units," move toward the axial region, leaving the smallest particles more concentrated at the periphery.[1332] In most cases, bloodborne medical nanorobots will be ~2 microns in diameter or smaller. As such, they will normally constitute the smallest particles in the bloodstream. More than any other blood element, free-floating nanorobots should tend to migrate nearest the blood vessel walls, although at high shear rates the radial diffusivity is significantly increased due to local fluid motions generated by red cell rotations (Section 3.2.2). Small molecules and complexes such as lipoproteins are less subject to erythrocyte-induced diffusivity enhancement, hence may migrate toward the walls.

9.4.1.4 Viscosity of Nanorobot-Rich Blood

The presence of large numbers of relatively rigid nanorobots dramatically alters bloodstream viscosity. Figure 9.13 shows the relative viscosity η_a / η_{plasma} for human blood at 298 K with shear rate >100 sec^{-1} as a function of particle volume fraction, compared to the relative viscosity of suspensions of latex rigid spheres, rigid disks, emulsion droplets, and sickled erythrocytes (which are virtually nondeformable), as determined experimentally.[1312] Figure 9.13 reveals that a 50% suspension of micron-sized rigid nanorobots will increase blood viscosity by a factor of ~350, seriously impeding flow especially in the smaller vessels. However, a plasma suspension of microspheres at a ~10% particle volume fraction has a relative viscosity indistinguishable from Hct = 10% whole blood. This suggests a conservative 10% volume-fraction limit for the maximum bloodstream concentration of medical nanorobots (e.g., a maximum "nanocrit" or Nct = 10%), a limit that may also ensure free flow of the fluid (see also Sections 9.4.1.5 and 9.4.2.6).

Relative viscosity also depends on particle size, though the effect due to the presence of medical nanorobots is usually minor. As a conservative upper limit in the smallest vessels:[1315]

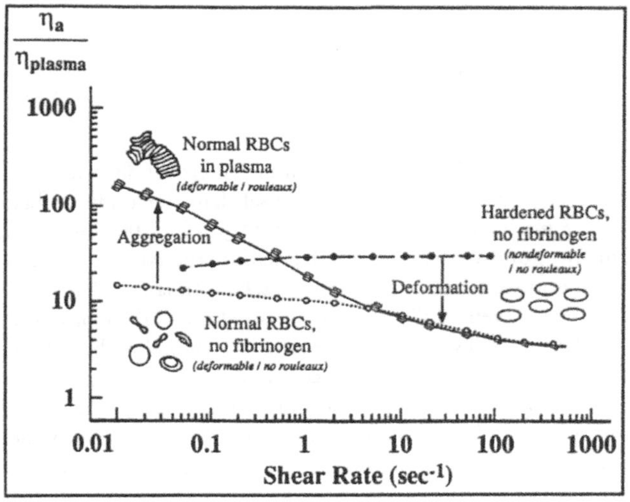

Fig. 9.12. Viscosity of human blood as a function of shear rate, at Hct = 45% (relative apparent viscosity at 310 K, redrawn from Chien[1314]).

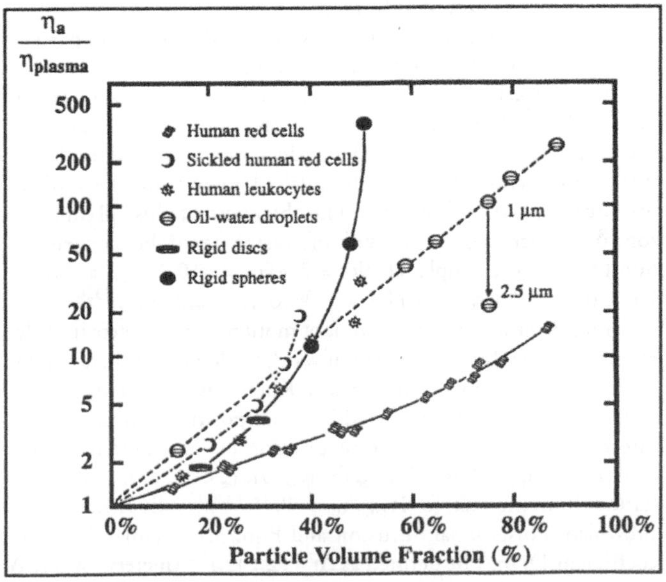

Fig. 9.13. Viscosity of nanorobot-rich human blood at high shear rate (relative apparent viscosity at 298 K, shear rate > 100 sec^{-1}; redrawn from Goldsmith and Mason,[1312] Cokelet and Lichtman[1402]).

$$\eta_a/\eta_{plasma} = \left[1 - \left(\frac{D_{nano}}{d_{tube}}\right)^4\right]^{-1} \qquad \text{\{Eqn. 9.61\}}$$

where D_{nano} (= 2 R_{nano}) is the maximum nanorobot diameter (radius) and d_{tube} (= 2 r_{tube}) is the blood vessel diameter (radius). Taking d_{tube} = 8 microns (capillaries), then η_a / η_{plasma} = 1.0002 for D_{nano} = 1 micron, or 1.07 for D_{nano} = 4 microns (the largest bloodborne nanorobot; see Sections 5.2.1 and 8.2.1.2). In larger blood vessels, this effect is even smaller for micron-sized medical nanorobots.

Relative blood viscosity also depends on nanorobot shape. Chien's measurements[1314] of effective viscosity as a function of particle shape in dilute suspensions found that minimum viscosity is achieved by hard spheres or by 1:1 hard cylinders. Thin disks or long cylinders have higher viscosity. For example, 10:1 rods (10 times longer than wide) produce a suspension with ~10 times higher viscosity than a suspension containing an equal volume of spheres; for 100:1 rods, viscosity increases ~2500-fold. The implication for nanodevice design is that a large population of bloodborne medical nanorobots will have the minimum impact on blood viscosity if each nanorobot is closest to spherical in shape. Long rod or flat disk shapes will greatly increase blood viscosity, in comparison to spheres, although at the lowest nanodevice number densities the total impact on blood viscosity may be negligible.

Chien's results[1314] also suggest that metamorphic nanorobots capable of continuous surface deformations in response to flow conditions (like RBCs) may further reduce their contribution to blood viscosity by at least a factor of 2-6, depending on shear rate (Fig. 9.12). Goldsmith and Turitto[386] show that at shear rates over 200 sec^{-1}, typical in physiological blood, the optimum shape for red cells is ellipsoidal, positioned at an angle to the flow, with the surface rotating in the direction of flow in a tank-tread-like motion. In experiments with flowing emulsions, the deformation of a liquid droplet results in its migration across the streamlines away from the tube wall. Thus in physiological blood over the whole range of normal hematocrits and typical flow rates, there is a plasma-rich (blood-cell-rare) or "plasmatic" zone δ_{plasma} ~ 2-4 microns deep at the walls of vessels whose diameters exceed 100 microns.[362,1319]

Such lateral migration is not observed with small rigid particles of any shape at high concentrations and at low Reynolds numbers (Section 9.4.2.1) $N_R \lesssim 10^{-3}$ (e.g., arterioles and smaller vessels; Table 8.2).[1319] However, for vessels with $N_R \gtrsim 1$ (e.g., arteries and veins; Table 8.2), inertial effects do come into play and rigid free-floating nanorobots will be pushed away from the wall to produce a particle-free zone. The thickness of this "plasmatic" zone δ_{nano} decreases sharply with increasing nanorobot concentration (Nct). For example, at Nct = 2%, δ_{nano} ~ 0.3 r_{tube}; at Nct = 10%, δ_{nano} ~ 0.1 r_{tube}; at Nct = 30%, δ_{nano} ~ 0.01 r_{tube}.[1320]

In terms of individual nanorobot motion, a rigid sphere initially placed near the tube wall migrates inward, while a rigid sphere placed near the tube axis migrates outward. Known as the "tubular pinch effect,"[1321] rigid spheres started in either position converge to an intermediate equilibrium radius position (as measured from the tube axis) of r_{eq} ~ (0.6-0.7) r_{tube} for R_{nano}/r_{tube} << 1, or r_{eq} ~ 0.5 r_{tube} (farther from the wall) for R_{nano}/r_{tube} ~0.25.[1320,1321] By analogy with Brownian translational diffusion and Eqn. 3.1, a radial dispersion coefficient D_r may be defined as $\Delta r = (2\,\tau\,D_r)^{1/2}$ (meters), where Δr is the RMS radial displacement of a bloodborne object in an observation time τ. The analogy is imperfect because these radial motions are not random, but are due to multibody collisions determined by the local velocity gradient, particle concentration, and surface deformations of the objects. At any given concentration, displacements are greatest at radial distances between 0.5-0.8 r_{tube}. For local shear rates of 5-20 sec^{-1} and volume concentrations from 20%-70%, D_r = 1-20 x 10^{-12} m^2/sec both for red cells and for rigid 2-micron diameter microspheres,[386] and 3-86 x 10^{-11} m^2/sec for platelets in whole blood,[1398] as determined experimentally.[1358] Thus the mean time for a nanorobot (R_{nano} = 1 micron) to migrate a radial distance Δr ~1 micron is τ ~25-500 millisec—about an order of magnitude faster than simple Brownian diffusion (Section 3.2.1).

9.4.1.5 Bloodstream Velocity Profiles

Consider a Newtonian fluid of viscosity η flowing through a cylindrical tube of length l_{tube} and radius r_{tube} with pressure differential Δp between the ends. The average fluid velocity (v_{flow}) for laminar or Poiseuille flow* is given by Eqn. 9.26, but imposing a no-slip condition at the vessel wall produces a radius-dependent parabolic velocity profile:[362]

$$v_{Pois}(r) = k_p(r_{tube}^2 - r^2) \quad \text{(m/sec)} \qquad \text{\{Eqn. 9.62\}}$$

where r is radial distance from the tube axis and $k_p = \Delta p / 4\,\eta\,l_{tube} = 2\,v_{flow} / r_{tube}^2$. Maximum flow velocity $v_{max} = 2\,v_{flow}$, and occurs at the centerline (r = 0).

Of course, as fluid enters a tube from a large reservoir, there is an entrance region called the inlet length (l_{inlet}) which lies between the entrance and a point downstream, where the parabolic profile is in the process of being established asymptotically (Fig. 9.14). For $N_R \lesssim 1$, l_{inlet} ~ 1.3 r_{tube}, while for $N_R \gtrsim 30$, l_{inlet} ~ 0.16 N_R r_{tube}, producing, post-inlet, a <1% deviation from an ideal Poiseuille (parabolic) profile.[361,1331] Inlet conditions prevail throughout the entire length of the aorta and most of the major arteries, but entrance effects are minimal in the smaller vessels.

Now suppose that red blood cells are added to the plasma. Due to the inward migration of red cells and other factors, the velocity profile of whole blood is affected by flow rate and hematocrit, particularly in vessels <500 microns in diameter, becoming blunted (Fig. 9.15). The degree of blunting decreases with increasing flow rate and increases with rising hematocrit. But the ability of RBCs to

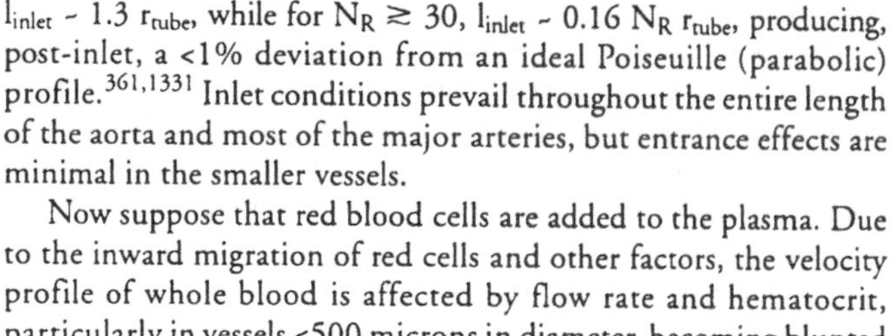

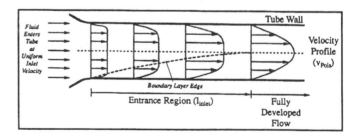

Fig. 9.14. Establishment of parabolic velocity profile in Poiseuille tube flow (redrawn from Goldsmith and Turitto[386]).

* *For well-developed turbulent flows, the velocity profile may be expressed as* $v_{turb} = v_{max}\,(1 - (r / r_{tube}))^{(1/m)}$ *away from the laminar sublayer near the wall, where m ~ 7 for a wide range of Reynolds numbers.*[1390]

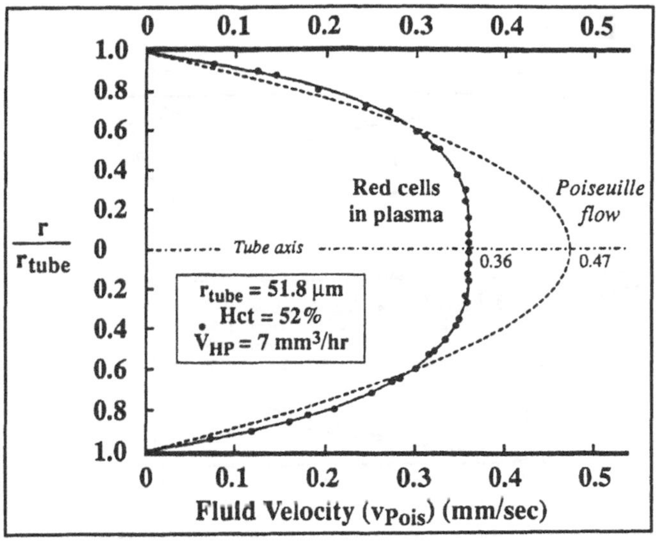

Fig. 9.15. Blunted velocity profile in whole blood flow (modified from Goldsmith and Turitto[386]).

deform under the influences of cell crowding and fluid stresses in shear flow allows whole blood to continue to flow up to Hct ~ 98%.[1319] It is theoretically possible that metamorphic nanorobots could approach this level of performance, though this issue has not yet been studied extensively.

What if rigid spherical nanorobots are added to the plasma instead of red cells? At small R_{nano} and low Nct, the flow profile remains parabolic. Onset of velocity profile blunting generally occurs either when Nct $\gtrsim$ 20% or when $R_{nano} \gtrsim 0.05\ r_{tube}$.[1322] Such blunted flow is sometimes called partial plug flow. Partial plug flow was not observed experimentally when (Nct R_{nano}/r_{tube}) $\lesssim$ 0.6%. Thus, non-plug, purely Poiseuille flow can probably be maintained for 2-micron diameter bloodborne nanorobots even while passing through the smallest d_{tube} = 4 micron human capillary by holding Nct $\lesssim$ 1.2%.

Figure 9.16 shows the experimentally-determined effects of Nct, R_{nano}/r_{tube}, and fluid flow rate on the velocity profile of suspensions of rigid spheres and disks.[1317,1322] As Nct and R_{nano}/r_{tube} continue to rise, complete plug flow eventually ensues (Fig. 9.16(B)), wherein the entire mass of fluid moves stiffly at constant velocity, like toothpaste squeezed from a tube. Plug flow requires much higher pumping power (and pumping pressure) than laminar flow. Complete plug flow was observed at Nct = 38% and $R_{nano} = 0.112\ r_{tube}$, that is, when (Nct R_{nano} / r_{tube}) $\gtrsim$ 3.8%. If complete plug flow can be avoided by holding R_{nano}/r_{tube} < 0.38 at our assumed maximum Nct ~ 10% (Section 9.4.2.6), then for the smallest d_{tube} = 4 micron human capillary, R_{nano} < 0.76 microns, allowing up to D_{nano} = 1.5 micron diameter for bloodborne nanodevices at the maximum nanocrit.

Further analysis that might consider the effects (on bloodborne nanorobot velocity profiles) of vessel geometry (including bifurcations, nozzling, and curved paths), vessel wall elasticity (including collapsible tubes), pulsatile flow, and adding nanorobots of various mixtures of sizes and shapes to whole blood rather than plasma, would be useful but is beyond the scope of this book.

9.4.1.6 Hematocrit Reduction in Narrow Vessels

Fahraeus[1313] found that when blood of a constant hematocrit Hct is allowed to flow from a large feed reservoir into a small tube, hematocrit in the tube (Hct_{tube}) decreases as the tube diameter decreases; Fahraeus and Lindqvist[1323] found a decrease in apparent viscosity when tube diameter is reduced to below 300 microns (Fig. 9.17). Barbee and Cokelet[1324] crudely approximated the experimental data using the following (slightly modified) empirical formula:

$$Hct_{tube} \sim (a\ \ln(d_{tube}) + b)\ Hct \quad (\%) \qquad \{Eqn.\ 9.63\}$$

where a = 0.196, b = -0.117, and d_{tube} is expressed in microns. Given a normal human male hematocrit of Hct = 46%, in smaller vessels this falls to Hct_{tube} = 36% at d_{tube} = 100 microns, 25% at 30 microns, and 13% at 8 microns. Surveying the literature, Gaehtgens[1329] concludes that minimum hematocrit Hct_{tube} generally occurs at d_{tube} ~ 15-20 microns, which Cokelet[1327] suggests marks the transition from multi-file flow to single-file flow among the red cells. Gaehtgens[1330] also showed that the relative viscosity of human RBC suspensions reaches a minimum at about 5-7 microns.

Hematocrit decreases in small blood vessels for several reasons. First, a cell-free layer approximately equal to RBC radius exists near the wall, so the smaller the vessel, the larger the fraction of volume occupied by this layer, hence the lower the hematocrit.[362] Second, a vessel side branch that draws mainly from the cell-free layer produces a lower hematocrit in that side branch (an effect called plasma skimming.[1326]) Third, red cells are elongated and oriented along the direction of shear flow, making it less likely that they will enter a side branch aligned perpendicular to the direction of flow (an effect at $d_{tube} \lesssim 29$ microns,[1327] sometimes called screening or steric hindrance.[1328]) All three factors should be less important for near-spherical rigid nanorobots that are smaller than RBCs, hence any reduction in nanocrit during passage through narrow blood vessels should be quite modest.

The velocity of a cell or nanorobot located on the axis of a small vessel is greater than the mean velocity of the suspending fluid,[1328] but is always slightly less than the fluid in the immediate vicinity on the axis (Section 9.4.1.5). The simplest model is the stacked-coins model discussed by Whitmore,[1315] wherein the nanorobot velocity v_{nano} is given by:

$$\frac{v_{nano}}{v_{flow}} = 2\left[1 + \left(\frac{D_{nano}}{d_{tube}}\right)^2\right]^{-1} \qquad \{Eqn.\ 9.64\}$$

Taking d_{tube} = 8 microns and v_{flow} = 1 mm/sec for a typical capillary (Table 8.2), a nanorobot with diameter D_{nano} = 2 microns has v_{nano} = 1.88 mm/sec, which is faster than v_{flow} but is slower than v_{max} = 2 mm/sec.

9.4.2 Sanguinatation

Medical nanorobots will often be called upon to travel from place to place within the human body by actively swimming through the bloodstream, a process called sanguinatation. This Section describes the general nature of the process in terms of the Reynolds number (Section 9.4.2.1), rotations and collisions with vessel walls and cellular blood components likely to be experienced by free-floating or powered nanorobots (Section 9.4.2.2), nanorobot hydrodynamics (Section 9.4.2.3), general force and power requirements for submersive swimming (Section 9.4.2.4), various specific natation mechanisms (Section 9.4.2.5), and some additional considerations regarding sanguinatation (Section 9.4.2.6).

9.4.2.1 Reynolds Number

Consider an object of characteristic dimension L moving at velocity v through a fluid of density ρ and viscosity η. The object's

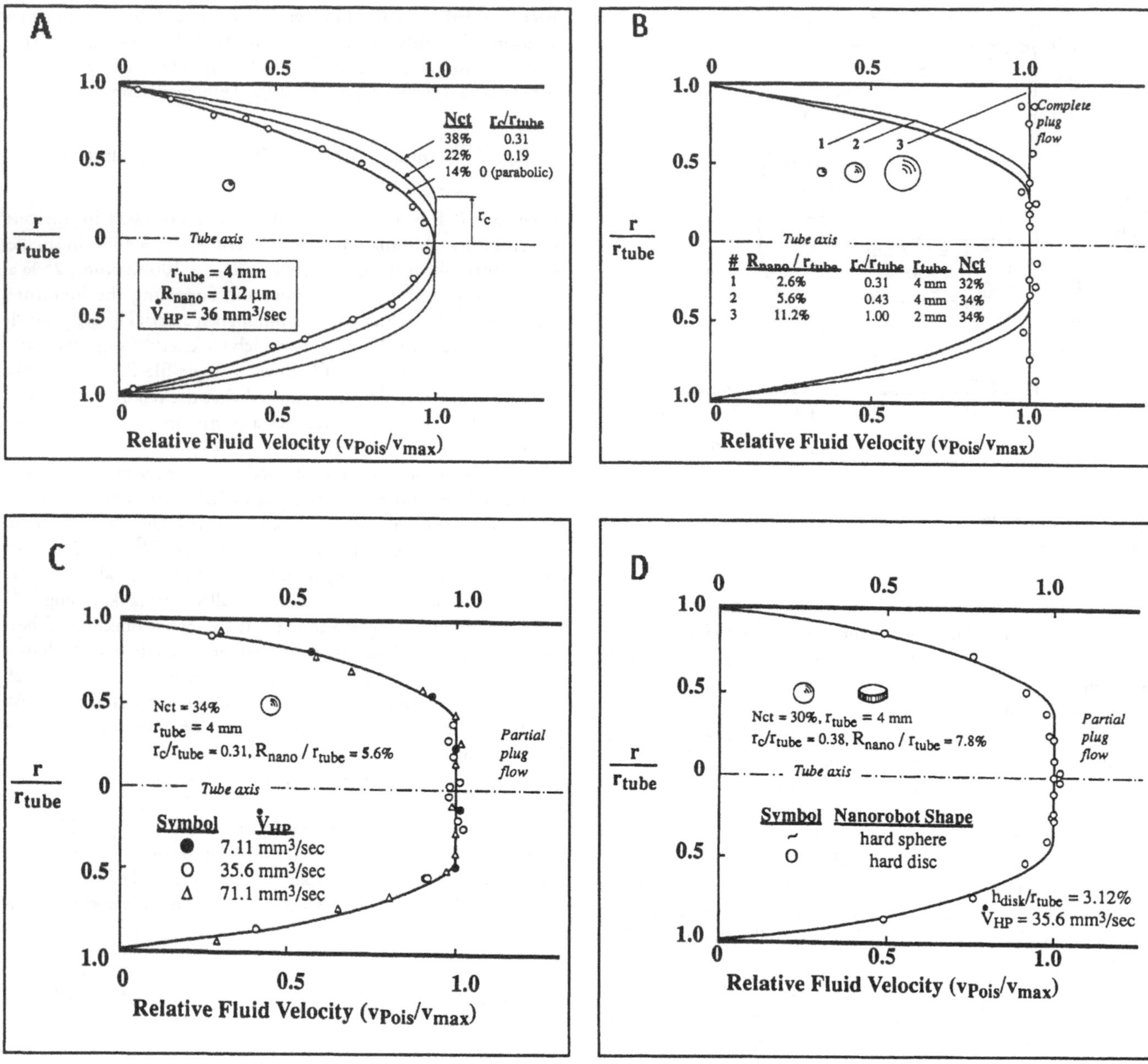

Fig. 9.16. Dimensionless velocity profiles in flowing aqueous nanorobot suspensions (rigid spheres and discs in rigid tubes; modified from Karnis, Goldsmith, and Mason[1322]). A) Effect of concentration (Nct = % nanocrit). B) Effect of particle size (R_{nano}/r_{tube}). C) Effect of fluid flow rate ($\dot{V}_{HP}$). D) Effect of nanorobot shape.

movement is resisted by two forces—inertia and viscous drag. The inertial force on the object is of order $F_{inertial} \sim \rho\, v^2\, L^2$; the viscous drag force is of order $F_{viscous} \sim \eta\, v\, L$. Thus a slow human underwater swimmer with $L \sim 1$ meter, $v \sim 0.1$ m/sec, $\rho \sim 1000$ kg/m^3, and $\eta \sim 10^{-3}$ kg/m-sec must apply $F_{inertial} \sim 10$ N plus a minor additional $F_{viscous} \sim 10^{-4}$ N of motive force in order to keep moving forward. Clearly, the human swimmer lives in a world of predominantly inertial forces.

A bacterial swimmer faces entirely different challenges.[389,1386,1387] A bacterium of size $L \sim 1$ micron and velocity $v \sim 10$ micron/sec must apply $F_{inertial} \sim 10^{-4}$ fN (femtonewtons; 1 fN = 10^{-15} N) but also a much larger $F_{viscous} \sim 10$ fN of motive force in order to keep moving forward. The ratio of the two forces is still 10^5:1, but the roles have reversed. The bacterium (or any micron-scale medical nanorobot) lives in a world dominated by viscosity, where, as an example, the phenomenon of "coasting" essentially ceases to exist. For instance, if motive power to a swimming nanorobot with radius $R_{nano} = 1$ micron and velocity $v_{nano} = 1$ cm/sec is suddenly stopped, then the nanorobot will "coast" to a halt in a time $t_{coast} = \rho\, R_{nano}^2 / 15\, \eta = 0.1$ microsec and in a distance $x_{coast} \sim v_{nano}\, t_{coast} = 1$ nm.[1395] If the nanorobot is rotating at a frequency $\nu_{nano} = 100$ Hz when its rotational power source is suddenly turned off, ν_{nano} decays exponentially to zero in a time $t_{coast} \sim 0.1$ microsec and stops after turning $\theta_{coast} = 2\,\pi\,\nu_{nano}\,\rho\, R_{nano}^2 / 15\,\eta \sim 40$ microradians.

The ratio of inertial to viscous forces is called the Reynolds number N_R, or:

$$N_R = \frac{F_{inertial}}{F_{viscous}} \sim \frac{\rho\, v\, L}{\eta} \qquad \text{\{Eqn. 9.65\}}$$

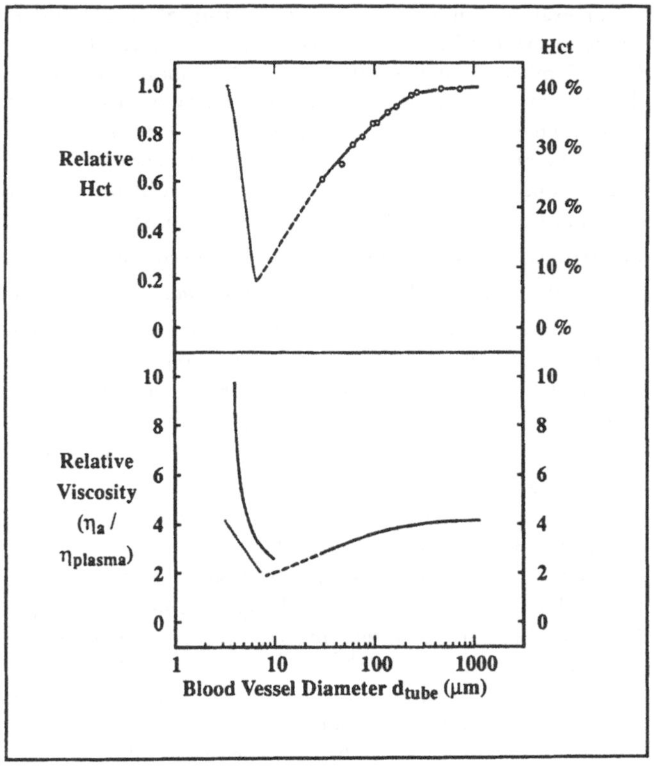

Fig. 9.17. Reduction of hematocrit (Hct) and blood viscosity in narrow blood vessels[1313,1324,1325] (redrawn from Chien[1325]).

which is a dimensionless number. In the examples given above, $N_R = 10^5$ for the human swimmer and $N_R = 10^{-5}$ for the bacterium. Purcell[389] notes that for a man to be swimming at the same Reynolds number as his own sperm, he would have to be placed in a swimming pool full of molasses and then be forbidden to move any part of his body faster than 1 cm/min, roughly the speed of the minute-hand of a large wall clock.

The Reynolds number has already been introduced in connection with laminar tube flow (Section 9.2.5), and elsewhere it has been noted that N_R = 100-6100 in the arteries, 200-900 in the veins, 0.0004-0.003 in the blood capillaries (Table 8.2), and $\sim 10^{-6}$–1 for lymph vessels (Table 8.5). However, these figures are relevant only when considering flow phenomenon on a scale large enough such that the cellular graininess of human blood may be ignored. In the case of microscopic motile cells and medical nanorobots, this assumption is not valid.

On the contrary, nanorobotic sanguinatators will find themselves negotiating a viscous Newtonian-fluid plasmatic environment, punctuated by numerous closely-spaced free-floating cellular obstacles. Powered sanguinatation thus may involve traversing opportunistic clear volumes of blood plasma between red cells, then altering course to take advantage of the next available open space further along, following a zig-zag path generally in the desired direction. While the sizes and shapes of these clear volumes are strongly time- and position-dependent, their characteristic size is $x_{clear} \sim (MCV\ (100\%\text{-}Hct)\ /\ Hct)^{1/3}$. Taking the Mean Cell Volume MCV = 94 micron^3 for red cells (Section 8.2.1.2), then $x_{clear} \sim 5$ microns in the arteries where Hct ~ 46% and $x_{clear} \sim 10$ microns in the capillaries where Hct = $Hct_{tube} \sim 10\%$ (Section 9.4.1.6). If paths taken through clear volumes at a mean velocity v_{nano} average an angle θ_{path} relative to the desired direction of travel, then the net forward velocity in the desired direction is $v_{net} = v_{nano} \cos(\theta_{path})$. Taking $v_{nano} \sim 1$ cm/sec giving $N_R = 10^{-2}$, then $v_{net} \sim 0.5$ cm/sec through heavy traffic in the vessel lumen assuming $\theta_{path} \sim 60°$. Brownian displacements of RBCs are negligible by comparison—$v_{brownian} \sim \Delta X / \tau \sim 0.1$ micron/sec for $\Delta X \sim 1$ micron (Eqn. 3.1)—while shear velocities in small arteries are typically ~1 mm/sec (Section 9.4.2.2). For powered trajectories exclusively confined to the cell-free "plasmatic" zone near the blood vessel wall (the vascular "express lane" for the fastest-moving nanorobot traffic; Section 9.4.2.6), x_{clear} is largely independent of Hct, $\theta_{path} \sim 0°$, and $v_{net} \sim v_{nano}$.

9.4.2.2 Rotations and Collisions in sanguo

From Eqn. 9.62 describing the axial fluid velocity v_{Pois} as a function of radial distance r in laminar tube flow, the velocity gradient, or shear rate $\dot{\gamma}$, is seen to increase linearly with r, as:

$$\dot{\gamma} = \left(\frac{\Delta p}{2\,\eta\, l_{tube}}\right) r = \left(\frac{4\, v_{flow}}{r_{tube}^2}\right) r \quad (sec^{-1}) \qquad \text{\{Eqn. 9.66\}}$$

When a suspending liquid is subjected to laminar flow, the fluid stresses on the surface of suspended rigid bodies cause those bodies to rotate as they travel down the tube.[1319] Rigid free-floating spherical nanorobots will rotate with uniform angular velocity, or, more specifically, with a rotational frequency of:

$$\nu_{nano} = \frac{\dot{\gamma}}{4\pi} = \left(\frac{\Delta p}{8\,\pi\,\eta\, l_{tube}}\right) r = \left(\frac{v_{flow}}{\pi\, r_{tube}^2}\right) r \quad (Hz) \qquad \text{\{Eqn. 9.67\}}$$

For example, a rigid free-floating spherical nanorobot traveling in an artery with r_{tube} = 500 micron and v_{flow} = 100 mm/sec (Table 8.2) rotates at $\nu_{nano} \sim 63$ Hz at r = 495 microns (very near the vessel wall), which is much faster than the random ~0.1 Hz Brownian rotation typical for micron-scale nanorobots (Section 3.2.1). Non-spherical rigid particles[1343] and red cells[1344] display variable angular velocity but spend more time in each orbit aligned with the direction of flow. Platelets can be seen tumbling in arterioles, especially near the vessel wall,[1340] but they tend to align with the flow, a tendency which is strongest nearest the wall.[1341]

Gyroscopic effects are present in every rotating body, with pitch, roll, yaw, and turning producing torques which cause precessions, giving periodic increases in bearing pressures and stresses. Fortunately, these stresses remain modest in most nanomechanical designs. For example, consider a rapidly spinning component inside the tumbling spherical nanorobot described in the previous paragraph. This internal component is a diamondoid disk of radius r_{disk}, thickness h_{disk}, and density ρ_{disk}, spinning at an angular velocity ω_{disk} around an axis oriented in the plane of the nanorobot tumble (tumbling is at frequency ν_{nano}), and supported by two coaxial bearings located a distance $x_{bearing}$ apart. The gyroscopic reaction force on the bearings is given by:

$$F_{bearing} = \frac{\pi^2\, r_{disk}^4\, h_{disk}\, \rho_{disk}\, \omega_{disk}\, \nu_{nano}}{x_{bearing}} \qquad \text{\{Eqn. 9.68\}}$$

Taking r_{disk} = 100 nm, h_{disk} = 20 nm, ρ_{disk} = 3510 kg/m^3, $\omega_{disk} \sim \omega_{max} \sim 10^{10}$ rad/sec (Eqn. 4.17), ν_{nano} = 63 Hz, and $x_{bearing} \sim h_{disk}$, then $F_{bearing} \sim 2$ pN.

In general, if two micron-scale objects are translating at the same mean speed, more energy is dissipated by the one that produces the larger amount of vorticity—that is, an axisymmetric object that rotates as it swims is less efficient than the nonrotating swimmer.[1389] The tangential force required to neutralize the hydrodynamic torque acting on a rigid sphere of radius R_{nano} and tumble frequency ν_{nano} is torque divided by radius, or:[1396]

$$F_{tumble} = 16\,\pi^2\,\eta\,R_{nano}^2\,\nu_{nano} \qquad \text{\{Eqn. 9.69\}}$$

For R_{nano} = 1 micron, ν_{nano} = 63 Hz, and $\eta = 1.1 \times 10^{-3}$ kg/m-sec for plasma at 310 K, then F_{tumble} = 11 pN. Application of such small forces may be controlled using measurements of absolute orientation taken from an onboard nanogyroscope (Section 4.3.4.1). Given that $F_{bearing}$ and F_{tumble} are of similar magnitude, direct anti-tumble gyrostabilization and gyroscopic rotational locomotion (gyrorotation) may be possible in some nanorobot applications.

The velocity gradient often brings suspended particles into close proximity. Kinetic theories of flowing suspensions have been developed from experiments on model systems involving two-body collisions between rigid and deformable spheres[1345] and between rigid cylinders.[1343] Goldsmith and Mason[1312] estimate that the per-object collision frequency K for equal-sized rigid spheres of volume concentration c flowing at velocity v at a radial distance r from the center of a tube of radius r_{tube} is:

$$K = \frac{32\,v\,r\,c}{\pi\,r_{tube}^2} \quad \text{(collisions/sec)} \qquad \text{\{Eqn. 9.70\}}$$

However, no complete theory yet exists to describe all the interactions of multiple classes of rigid bodies and deformable cells in blood vessels.

As a crude approximation, consider the laminar flow of a fluid suspension of two types of spherical objects (i = 1, 2) of radius R_i, density ρ_i (kg/m^3), number density n_i (m^{-3}), and volumetric concentration $c_i = (4\,\pi\,/\,3)\;n_i\;R_i^3$ expressed as a fraction. Each object occupies a cubic fluid volume of dimension $L_i \sim n_i^{-1/3} = (4\,\pi\,R_i\,/\,3\,c_i)^{1/3}$, and in laminar flow, two radially-adjacent boxes move past each other (a "collision") at a mean relative velocity of $v_{ij} \sim \dot{\gamma}\,(R_i + R_j)$ when R_i, $R_j \ll r_{tube}$, and interact for a time $t_{ij} \sim L_i\,/\,v_{ij}$ (j = 1, 2). From the viewpoint of object i, the probability that after $N_{coll\,ij}$ collisions at least one object j has been encountered is $p_j = 1 - (1 - c_j)^{N_{coll\,ij}}$. Taking $p_j \sim 0.9$ (the final result is relatively insensitive to the exact threshold selected), and multiplying by 2 because there is a concentric layer on either side of object i, then the mean collision rate experienced by each object i with an object j also present in the suspension is $K_{ij} \sim 2\,(N_{coll\,ij}\,t_{ij})^{-1}$, which, at a radial distance r in the tube, may be written as:

$$K_{ij} \sim 2\left(\frac{48}{\pi}\right)^{1/3}\left(\frac{v_{flow}\,c_i^{1/3}}{r_{tube}^2}\right)\left(\frac{R_i + R_j}{R_i}\right) r\,\log_{10}\,(1 - c_j)^{-1} \quad \text{(collisions/sec)} \qquad \text{\{Eqn. 9.71\}}$$

and the mean free path ($\bar{l}_{ij}$) between an object i and an object j in the suspension (neglecting all velocity profile and margination effects) is given approximately by:

$$\bar{l}_{ij} \sim \left(\frac{\pi}{6}\right)^{1/3}\left(R_i\,c_i^{-1/3} + R_j\,c_j^{-1/3}\right) \qquad \text{\{Eqn. 9.72\}}$$

For example, in a suspension consisting of R_i = 1 micron nanorobots with volume concentration c_i = 0.10 (Nct = 10%), and $R_j \sim 1.5$ micron platelets with c_j = 0.0035 (mean physiological plateletocrit), flowing through a small artery with r_{tube} = 500 microns at mean velocity v_{flow} = 100 mm/sec, and at a radial distance r = 495 microns (near the tube wall), then for nanorobot/platelet interactions, $K_{ij} \sim 2$ collisions/sec, mean collision velocity $v_{ij} \sim 2$ mm/sec, and $\bar{l}_{ij}$ = 9.7 microns. For nanorobot/nanorobot interactions, $K_{ij} \sim 40$ collisions/sec (cf. K = 200 collisions/sec using Eqn. 9.70), $v_{ij} \sim 1.6$ mm/sec, and $\bar{l}_{ij}$ = 3.5 microns. These figures are crude estimates at best, since they ignore many possible complicating factors such as aggregation and margination, collision inelasticities and n-body collisions (n > 2), nonspherical object shapes, the presence or absence of specific macromolecules, receptor interactions, pulsatile flow, ionic strength of the medium, and cell surface electrostatics.[1325,3545]

Free-floating nanorobots that collide with blood vessel walls produce negligible shear forces, given the no-slip condition at the wall. Powered nanorobots of radius R_{nano} that impact a vessel wall at velocity v_{nano} may apply a maximum shear stress of $p_{shear} \sim \rho_{nano}\,v_{nano}^2$; taking $\rho_{nano} \sim 1000$ kg/m^3 and $v_{nano} \sim 1$ cm/sec, then $p_{shear} \sim 0.1$ N/m^2. By comparison, the time-averaged shear stress for blood circulation in normal vessels[362,1346,1347,1352] is 1-2 N/m^2 (range 0.5-5.6 N/m^2)[386], reaching up to 10-40 N/m^2 when small arteries and arterioles are partially occluded as by atherosclerosis or vascular spasm.[1348,1349] This may also be compared to the threshold limit for shear stress-induced platelet aggregation of 6-9 N/m^2,[1346,1349-1351] the shearing stress of 5-100 N/m^2 acting at the interface between a leukocyte and an endothelium when the leukocyte is adhering to or rolling on the endothelium of a venule,[366] and the critical shear stress of 42 N/m^2 known to initiate major changes in the endothelial cells in the arteries.[365]

9.4.2.3 Disturbed Flows, Hydrodynamic Interactions, and Entropic Packing

Two kinds of fluid flow have already been described—laminar or Poiseuille streamline flow, and turbulent or random flow. However, in branching or nonuniform-diameter blood vessels, nanorobots may also be required to negotiate an additional flow regime that is not observed in straight tubes of uniform diameter. This third regime, called "disturbed flow," involves secondary fluid motions in directions away from that of the primary flow, often with separation of the streamlines from the vessel walls to form a vortex or a recirculation zone between the forward flowing mainstream and the wall.[1358] Disturbed flow is most common in the larger blood vessels.

Studies have been conducted to observe the flow patterns in various vessels of simple and complex geometries, using flow visualization and cinemicrographic techniques.[1358-1366] In one extensive series of experiments,[1359] tracer polystyrene microspheres were photographed at various flow rates as they traveled through glass tube models or through chemically-transparentized natural blood vessels. The developed movie films were then projected on a drafting table and analyzed frame by frame. Figure 9.18 illustrates some results for progressively higher-angle blood vessel bifurcations. The cross-streamline and vortex patterns are quasi-stable; in pulsatile flow, vortices vary periodically in size and intensity, with the axial location of the vortex center and reattachment point oscillating in phase with the upstream fluid velocity between maximum and minimum positions about a mean.[1361] A model study using red cells[1361] found that over time periods long in comparison with the orbital period, single cells and small aggregates <20 microns in

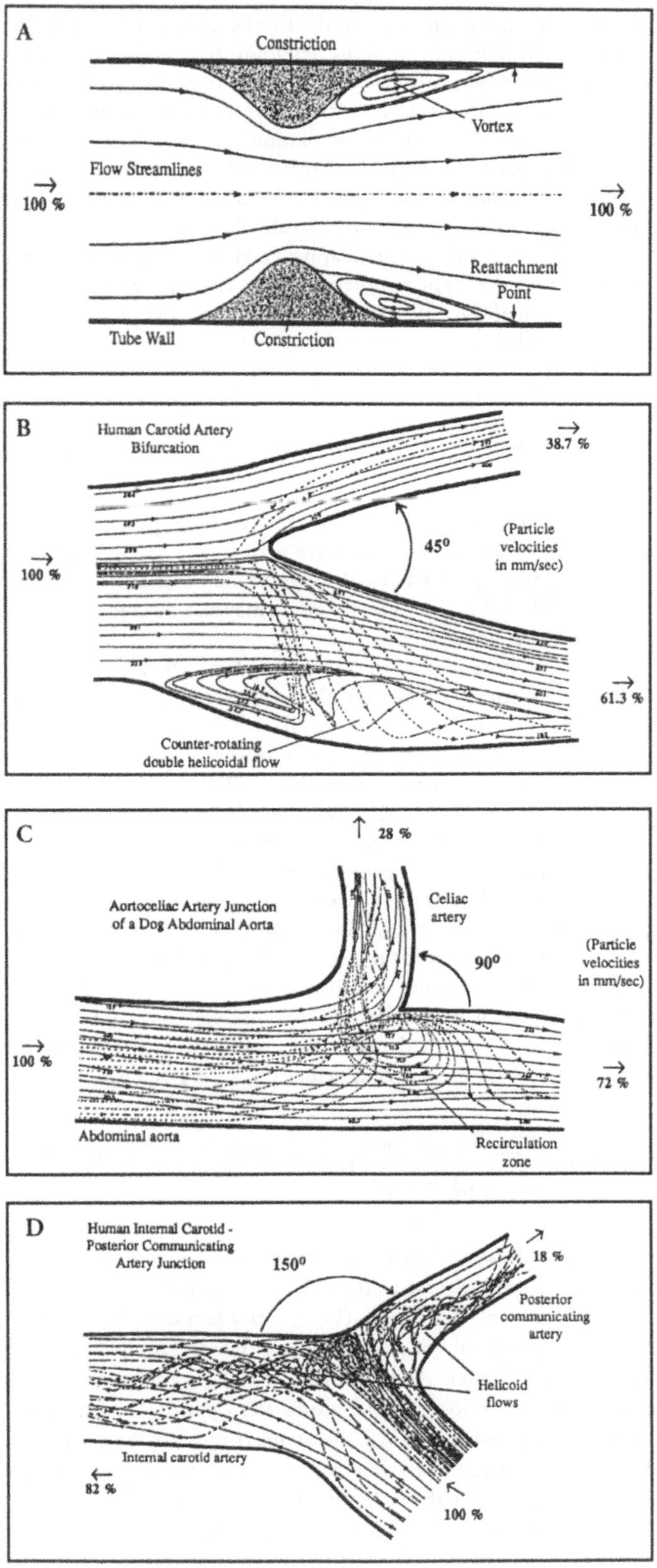

Fig. 9.18. Disturbed flow streamlines in progressively higher-angle blood vessel bifurcations. A) Axisymmetric-constricted tube with no bifurcation (redrawn from Karino et al[1359]). B) 45° bifurcation (redrawn from Motomiya and Karino[1364]). C) 90° bifurcation (redrawn from Karino, Motomiya, and Goldsmith[1404]). D) 150° bifurcation (redrawn from Karino et al[1359]).

diameter migrate outward across the closed streamlines and exit the vortex after describing a series of spiral orbits of continually increasing diameter until rejoining the mainstream. Erythrocyte rouleaux >30 microns in size remain trapped within the vortex, either assuming equilibrium orbits or staying at the center. The vortex also provides favorable conditions for the spontaneous aggregation of normal human platelets through shear-induced collisions of particles circulating in their orbits.[1362] An intimate knowledge of disturbed flow patterns in all human blood vessels will be essential in any nanomedical mission design requiring sanguinatating nanorobots, but further detailed discussion is beyond the scope of this book.

A variety of early studies attempted to model the hydrodynamics of micron-scale swimmers, including descriptions of the hydrodynamics of an individual swimming cell,[1367,1368,3583] the hydrodynamic interaction of two magnetotactic bacteria,[1369] and the interaction of two parallel swimming cells.[1370] Wall effects are well-known.[1393,3584,3585] For instance, the velocity of a flagellar swimmer decreases as it moves closer to a solid boundary; the boundary effect is strong at low N_R, with speed reduced 5% even at 10 object radii from the wall.[1391] Flagellates swim in curved paths near a solid boundary.[338] Another effort to model the hydrodynamic interaction of pairs of flagellar-driven 1-micron diameter bacterial swimmers found that cells are attracted toward each other when they are swimming side by side and are repelled when swimming one behind the other.[336] The researchers also modeled two microswimmers approaching each other from opposite directions along parallel but non-coaxial paths.[336] As the two cells pass, they move closer together, causing mutual cell rotations which lead to a significant change in swimming orientation. Eventually the cells move away from each other along a straight, now-coaxial path whose deflection angle to the original path is determined by the initial off-axis separation of the two cells (Fig. 9.19)—a motion vaguely reminiscent of the "planetary slingshot" maneuver often performed by NASA spacecraft to change direction. This unusual cell-cell hydrodynamic interaction has now been

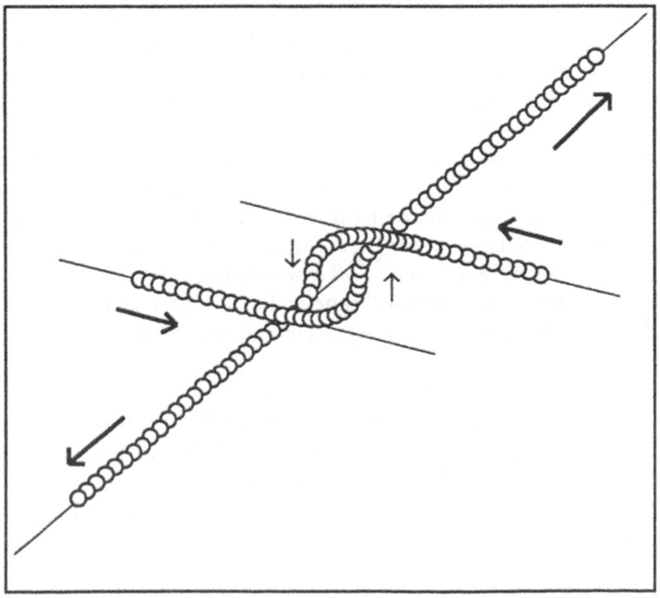

Fig. 9.19. Hydrodynamic interaction of approaching flagellates (redrawn from Dillon, Fauci, and Gaver[336]).

observed experimentally in *E. coli* traversing fluid in a glass microcapillary.[1371] Hydrodynamic interactions among bacterial flagellar swimmers are greatest when cell separation distances are less than the overall length of the cells including the length of the flagella, or $\lesssim$ 10 microns.[336]

In 1998, relatively little was known about the likely hydrodynamic behavior of nanorobots in the close company of large numbers of other nanorobots and natural blood cells. Differing sizes, shapes, and surface characteristics may lead to subtle and unexpected hydrodynamic interactions. For example,[846,3579] leukocyte axial velocity in capillaries is slightly lower than that of erythrocytes because the white cell surface undergoes a smaller deformation during flow due to the higher stiffness and larger volume of a leukocyte—e.g., the relative velocity ratio is 0.88 in a 6.8-micron diameter capillary, is somewhat closer but still under 1.00 in larger vessels, and differs among leukocyte types.[1353] This small velocity differential causes an axial redistribution of a train of erythrocytes in the presence of a white cell. Upstream from the leukocyte, red cells bunch up, forming a region of elevated hematocrit; downstream, a plasma gap develops, increasing linearly with time and with the velocity differential between the white cell and the next red cell down the line.[1354,1356] Upon entering a postcapillary venule, the configuration breaks up as the erythrocyte immediately upstream of the leukocyte passes the white cell and pushes it laterally against the vessel wall, often causing the white cell to attach to the endothelial surface of the venule. (Without red cells, leukocytes make no regular attachment to the venous endothelium[1356,1357]). The remaining red cells then close up the gap in the flow.[1356] Medical nanorobots may exhibit equally unusual flow behaviors.

Self-organizing spatial patterns may also arise in mixtures of nanorobot-size particles of different shapes and sizes, a process which minimizes entropy.[2168] Entropic forces become significant at scales of a few tens of nanometers to several microns.[2168] For example, micron-diameter spheres mixed with micron-long, 10-nm thick rods in water solidify into two arrangements as water is removed—one a "cake" with layers of vertical rods alternating with a thin frosting of balls (a stacked, lamellar arrangement akin to cell plasma membranes) and the other a lattice of vertical columns of clustered spheres embedded in a horizontal sea of parallel rods (a columnar arrangement often found in glues).[2169] Other less-stable patterns such as ropes with lamellar order and chains of rod packets interspersed with spheres are also observed. In another series of experiments, small spheres $\lesssim$ 100 nm in diameter were mixed with large spheres ~500 nm in diameter in a ~1000:1 ratio, and the small spheres pushed the larger ones against the hard, flat container walls. Large balls were also forced against the most curved sections of the inner walls of pear-shaped rigid vessels.[2170] These entropic forces are attractive at low concentrations of small spheres, but at higher concentrations the force alternates between repulsion and attraction.[2170]

9.4.2.4 Force and Power Requirements

Consider a spherical nanorobot of radius R_{nano} that is falling at uniform velocity v_{nano} through an incompressible (Newtonian) fluid of viscosity η. If the Reynolds number $N_R << 1$ (Eqn. 9.65), then Stokes[1373] found that the total force of resistance imparted on the sphere by the fluid is given by:

$$F_{nano} = 6 \pi \eta R_{nano} v_{nano} \quad \text{(newtons)} \qquad \text{\{Eqn. 9.73\}}$$

also known as Stokes law. This result applies only in the case of a single sphere in an infinite expanse of homogeneous viscous fluid, and neglects all inertial terms. If the fluid container is finite in size, or if there are other spheres in the neighborhood, or if inertial forces cannot be entirely ignored because $N_R \gtrsim 1$ (e.g., R_{nano} = 1 micron, v_{nano} > 1 m/sec in water), then the equation must be corrected.[1374] Dynamic effects due to sphere oscillation, sudden release from rest, or variable speed also require corrections,[1374] and there are other corrections for neighboring spheres.[1375] Most of these corrections are of order near-unity for micron-scale objects.

Eqn. 9.73 provides a useful approximation of the motive force required to drive a spherical nanorobot through blood plasma. Assuming a perfectly efficient drive mechanism, the power requirement[337] is at least:

$$P_{nano} = F_{nano} v_{nano}$$

$$= 6 \pi \eta R_{nano} v_{nano}^2 \quad \text{(watts)} \qquad \text{\{Eqn. 9.74\}}$$

For example, a force of F_{nano} = 200 pN and a power of at least P_{nano} = 2 pW are required to drive a R_{nano} = 1 micron spherical nanorobot at v_{nano} = 1 cm/sec through blood plasma at 310 K with $\eta = 1.1 \times 10^{-3}$ kg/m-sec. These formulas may also be used to estimate nanodevice velocity, given F_{nano} or P_{nano}.

Of course, drive mechanisms are not perfectly efficient. Propulsion efficiency is often poor for objects that swim at low Reynolds numbers (e.g., typically $N_R \sim 10^{-3}$ for flagellates).[3578] A sphere driven by a helical propeller (e.g., flagellar propulsion; Section 9.4.2.5.2) of arbitrary length may have a propulsion efficiency as low as e% ~ 0.01(1%).[389] Propulsive efficiency for organisms with spherical heads 10-40 times larger than their flagellar radius (optimum shape), using helical flagellar beats, ranges from e% = 0.10-0.28 (10%-28%),[1377] requiring a propulsive input power of ~P_{nano}/e% ~ 7-20 pW in the previous example. Other drive mechanisms may prove more efficient.

Force requirements for nonspherical nanorobots are similar in magnitude. For example, consider a cylinder of radius R_{nano} and length L_{nano} translating uniformly in a direction normal to its axis. Lighthill[1367,1376] shows that the force (applied at the midpoint) required to move this object at velocity v_{nano} is given by:

$$F_{nanoN} = \frac{8 \pi \eta L_{nano} v_{nano}}{1 + \ln\left(\frac{L_{nano}^2}{R_{nano}^2}\right)} \quad \text{(newtons)} \qquad \text{\{Eqn. 9.75\}}$$

for $L_{nano} >> R_{nano}$.[363] (If the perpendicular force is applied at a distance c from one end of the cylinder, then the L_{nano}^2 term in Eqn. 9.75 is replaced by 4 c (L_{nano} - c) when c >> R_{nano}.) Eqn. 9.75 does not hold for a perpendicular force applied near the ends of the cylinder. Also, a constant F_{nano} actually produces a slowly varying velocity field along the cylinder length; for a midpoint-applied force, v_{nano} is at maximum at the midpoint, but the percentage variation over most of the cylinder is not large.[363] Experiments show that needle-shaped bodies fall in viscous media about half as fast sideways as they do end-on;[1378] that is, the force on a long cylinder translating parallel to its axis is $F_{nanoP} \sim (1/2) F_{nanoN}$. The power requirement is then calculated as in Eqn. 9.74.

Interestingly, there seems to be a sharp minimum size limit of ~0.6 microns for free-swimming foraging microbes, below which size locomotion has no apparent benefit.[3581] This theoretical conclusion is supported by the observation that the smallest 97 genera of motile bacteria have a mean length of 0.8 microns, whereas 18 of 94 nonmotile genera are smaller.[3581]

9.4.2.5 Nanomechanisms for Natation

Swimming motions consisting purely of reciprocal deformations (e.g., shape A deforms into shape B, then retraces the same motion back to shape A) cannot produce forward progress in a viscosity-dominated environment.[389,1386] For example, in the macroscale world, a scallop may open its shell slowly, then close it rapidly to squirt out water, relying upon inertia and "coasting" to carry it forward a little bit each cycle. At the low Reynolds numbers of most medical nanorobots, such single-hinge deformations yield only back-and-forth motion. Indeed, Fukuda et al[1385] estimate that a vibrating-fin-driven water-swimming robot shorter than ~6 mm can no longer overcome viscous drag.* Purcell[389] notes that the simplest possible mechanical swimmer may require at least two hinges and a cyclical deformation loop traced out in a two-dimensional configuration space.

At least four distinct classes of mechanisms for natation are readily distinguished, as described below.

9.4.2.5.1 Surface Deformation

The use of flexible or metamorphic surfaces (Section 5.3) allows natative structures to deform asymmetrically. For example, it is impossible to "row a boat" that is fully submerged in a viscous fluid, because the stiff oars are simply reciprocating. But if the structures are flexible, then the oar can bend one way during the first half of the stroke and the other way during the second half, providing an asymmetry that permits the object to advance (Fig. 9.20). If the oar is metamorphic and can also vary its total surface area throughout the cycle, then this asymmetry can be enhanced.

Another example is the metamorphic doughnut-shaped nanorobot (Fig. 9.21A). An invaginating torus (e.g., a "smoke ring" motion) can swim along a vector normal to the torus plane because its outer surface is larger and moving faster than its inner surface (in the doughnut's "hole"), giving rise to a differential viscous force in the same direction as the inner surface is moving—the opposite travel direction from what might be expected in an inertia-dominated environment. Differential rotation of circumaxial surface segments allows steering.

Yet another example proposed by Purcell is a single device constructed as two reversibly-adhered continuously-rotating spheroids (Fig. 9.21B). The spheroids stick together but are free to roll all over each other's surfaces, by selectively binding and releasing mateable surface elements. A differential viscous force arises because the outermost surface of the pair is always fully bathed in viscous fluid but the inner contact surface is partially shielded from the fluid. By altering speeds and rotational axes, the pair can establish a velocity vector in any direction in three-dimensional space. A similar locomotive method is provided by Solem's "viscous-lift helicopter" design (Fig. 9.22). Viscous drag on each of the four rotating wheels is $F_{wheel} \sim (16 \pi / 3)\ \eta\ \nu_{wheel}\ R_{wheel}^2$ for wheels of radius R_{wheel} turning at frequency ν_{wheel} (Hz) in a medium of viscosity η, and device mass is $m_{nano} \sim 2\ \pi\ \rho_{nano}\ R_{wheel}^3$ for a device of density ρ_{nano}.[1982] Taking ν_{wheel} = 10 KHz, R_{wheel} = 1 micron, ρ_{nano} = 2000 kg/m^3, and $\eta \sim 10^{-3}$ for water, then $F_{wheel} \sim$ 170 pN per wheel, or ~0.7 nN for the whole device. There is a vast range of possibilities, according to Purcell:[389] "Turn anything—if it isn't perfectly symmetrical, you'll swim."

While incompressible tangential surface deformations alone are not propulsive, even single-sphere swimmers can translate or rotate using specific cyclic, nonreciprocal, compressible surface distortions (i.e.,traveling waves). Such waves have been suggested as the mode of locomotion employed by appendageless spheroidal cyanobacteria,[1388] and surface undulations passing backward from the advancing edge of the cell have been observed in mammalian fibroblasts.[1467] Swimming speed for an object of radius R_{nano} is ~10 R_{nano} per second using a radial deformation of $\varepsilon \sim 0.05$ (5%); with n = 10 surface ripples, energy efficiency is approximated by $e\% \sim (3\ \pi^2\ n / 128)\ \varepsilon^2 = 0.006$ (0.6%) for $\varepsilon << 1$.[1388] (If the waves are not shallow, and $(n\ \varepsilon) > 1$, then the peak-to-peak spacing becomes less

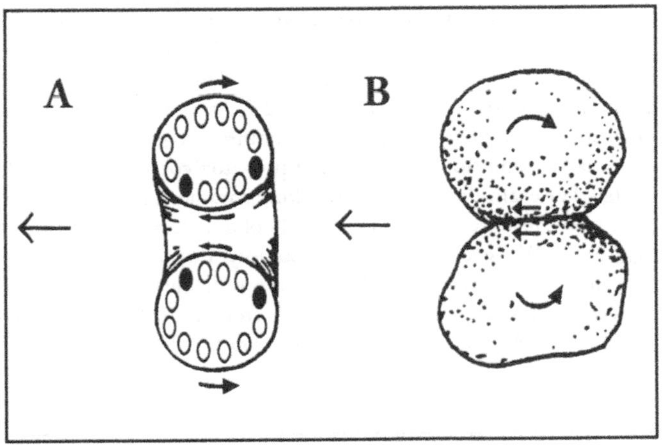

Fig. 9.21. (A) Invaginating torus; (B) Sticky spheroids; redrawn from Purcell[389]).

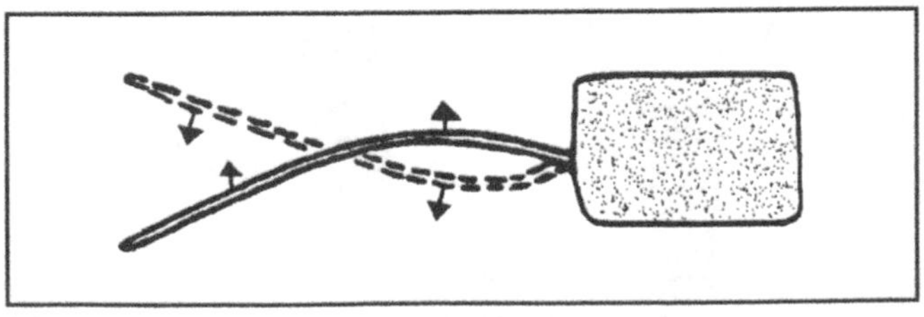

Fig. 9.20. Flexible oar (redrawn from Purcell[389]).

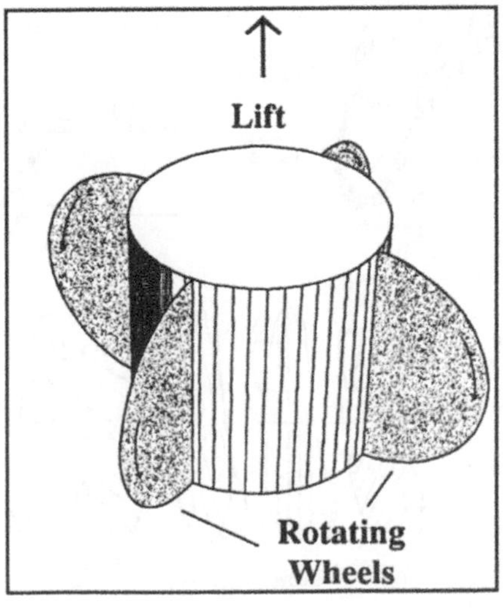

Fig. 9.22. Viscous-lift helicopter design (modified from Solem[1982]).

* *The smallest known swimming fish is the dwarf pygmy goby (*Pandaka pygmaea*), measuring 7.1-9.7 mm long in the adult form.*[739]

than the peak-to-valley depth, whereupon friction from the vertical movement of the waves' walls should dominate energy consumption.)

A more familiar example of a deformable natation structure is the simple cilium (Section 9.3.1.1). In ciliate protozoa, cilia are typically much shorter than body length and are arranged in large numbers in rows on the body surface. Individual cilia have a regular beat pattern, typically including a rapid forward power stroke at full extension, followed by a slower return or recovery stroke with the cilium bent close to the body surface. Ciliary arrays (Section 9.3.4) may also display metachronism, or time-synchronized wave patterns, that can be used for precision steering and speed control, as, for example, by a 60 micron x 220 micron (~600,000 micron^3) *Paramecium caudatum*, which rotates as it progresses forward in its path (Fig. 9.23) using the ~2500 cilia on its outer surface.[526] Metachronal waves traveling in the same direction as the power stroke are symplectic; such waves are antiplectic if they travel against the power stroke, and are dexioplectic or laeoplectic (or, more generally, diaplectic) when the power stroke is to either side of the line of wave propagation.[1405,3555] The swimming paramecium may adjust its wave patterns while negotiating a liquid medium of varying viscosity.[1406,3558] These and similar results should be generalized and extended to the case of nanorobotic ciliary propulsion.

For a medical nanorobot coated with propulsive cilia with wave velocity v_{cilium}, then v_{nano}/v_{cilium} = 0.125-0.25 and e% = 0.125-0.30 (12.5%-30%).[1379,1380] If v_{nano} = 1 cm/sec, then v_{cilium} ~ 4-8 cm/sec giving p_{shear} ~ 2-6 N/m^2 (Section 9.4.2.2), well within the normal range for human blood and probably nonthrombogenic to platelets.

Ciliary propulsion even by large protozoa costs relatively little energy. For example, a 220-micron long paramecium swimming at ~1 mm/sec in water experiences ~1 nN of drag force and consumes P_{drag} ~ (1 pW / e%) of power to locomote, but the animal can be very inefficient because ~10,000 pW are available to a paramecium with power density ~10^4 watts/m^3 (est. from Table 6.8). Observed propulsion velocities of paramecia range from 0.2-2.5 mm/sec.[1460,3586]

9.4.2.5.2 Inclined Plane

Another class of mechanisms for natation makes use of the inclined plane, a basic mechanical device that can convert viscous forces into forward motion. The simplest example is a threaded screw. In standard propeller theory at high Reynolds number, forward thrust is proportional to the rate at which a mass of fluid can be ejected out the rear (e.g., inertial forces). However, at low Reynolds number, the fluid that is pushed backwards by the rotating tilted planes does not provide thrust primarily by its inertial movement, but rather serves as a resistive medium against which the device can push itself forward. In the world of the nanorobot, the environment is very thick and viscous. The motive effect is not unlike the forward motion achieved by a threaded screw as it is screwed into a piece of wood using a screwdriver.[3580]

The motive force and power consumption of a microscale screw drive (Fig. 9.24) with pitch angle φ and mean radius R_{screw} may be very crudely approximated as follows. Consider a helical ribbon of width w_{thread} and total length l_{thread} that is wrapped around an axially-translating cylindrical body, making a pitch angle φ as measured from normal to the direction of travel of the screw body. From Stokes law (Eqn. 9.73), a square element of that ribbon with area w_{thread}^2 experiences a maximum drag force of ~$6 \pi \eta w_{thread} v_{thread}$. There are $n_{element} = l_{thread}/w_{thread}$ square elements in the entire ribbon; neglecting flow field interactions of the elements and of the solid center for this approximation, the maximum laminar drag force on the entire ribbon is F_{max} ~ $6 \pi \eta l_{thread} v_{thread}$. Viscous drag is lowest at φ = 0° (edge on) and highest at φ = 90° (face on); a factor of $(3\text{-}\cos(2\varphi))/4$ captures the experimental behavior of needle-shaped bodies which fall in viscous media about half as fast sideways as they do end-on (Section 9.4.2.4), with periodicity of π. The number of threads around the screw is $N_{thread} = l_{thread} \cos(\varphi)) / (2 \pi R_{screw})$ and the screw rotates at a frequency $\nu_{screw} = v_{thread} / (2 \pi R_{screw})$, hence the total force required to turn the screw is:

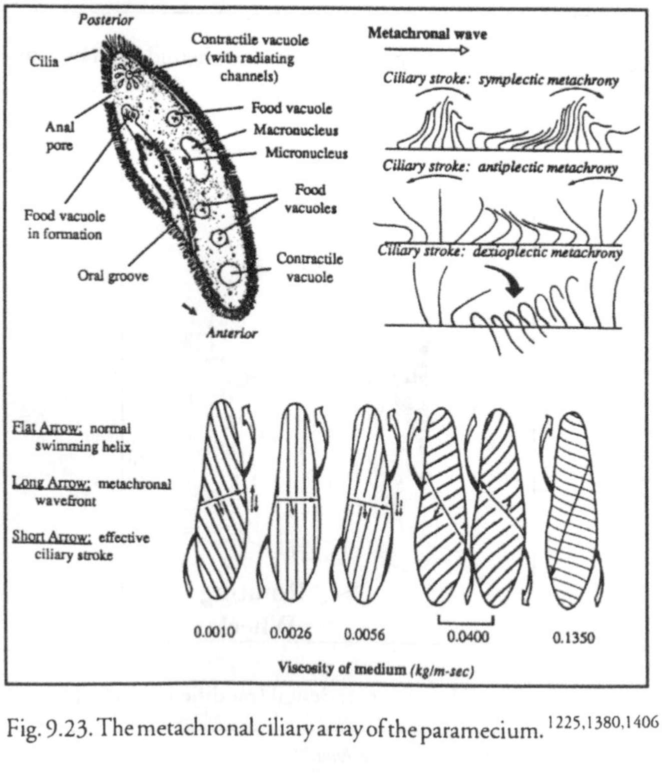

Fig. 9.23. The metachronal ciliary array of the paramecium.[1225,1380,1406]

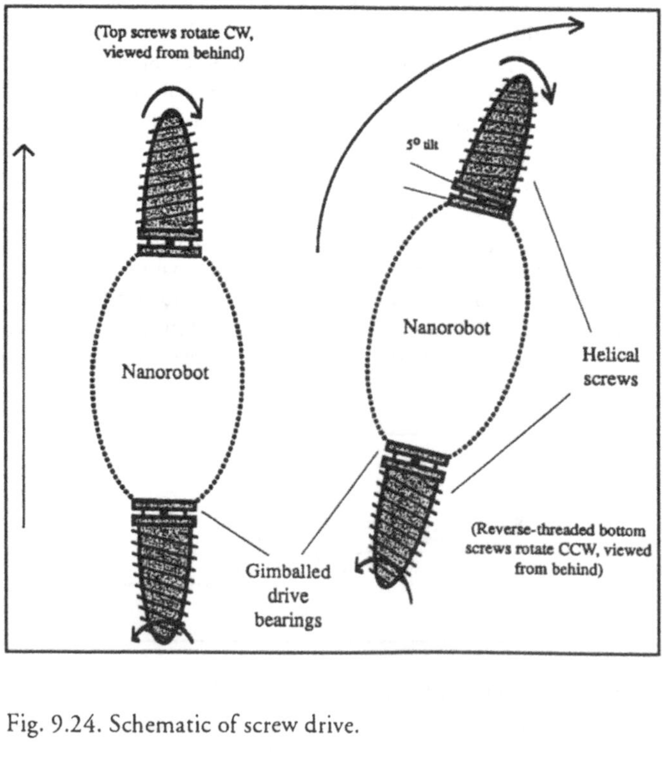

Fig. 9.24. Schematic of screw drive.

$$F_{screw} = \frac{6\pi^3 \eta v_{screw} N_{thread} R^2_{screw}(3-\cos(2\varphi))}{\cos(\varphi)} \quad \text{\{Eqn. 9.76\}}$$

with total drag power $P_{screw} \sim F_{screw} v_{thread} = 12\pi^4 \eta v_{screw}^2 N_{thread} R_{screw}^3 (3-\cos(2\varphi)) / \cos(\varphi)$. To further simplify the calculation, we assume a "no slip" condition such that each complete revolution of the screw carries the nanorobot forward by a distance $\sim 2\pi R_{screw} \tan(\varphi)$, although more slip may occur as the thread becomes looser (e.g., at high φ and low N_{thread}). To avoid turbulence in fluid passing through the threads, from Eqns. 9.29 and 9.65, we must require $v_{thread} << 2000\ \eta / \rho L$, a condition easily met for $L \sim 1$ micron devices. Under "no slip" conditions, the velocity of forward translation is approximated by $v_{nano} \sim 2\pi R_{screw} v_{screw} \tan(\varphi)$, giving from Stokes law a net forward towing force of $F_{nano} \sim 6\pi\eta R_{screw} v_{nano}$ and a net mechanical efficiency $e\% \sim 2\cos(\varphi)\tan^2(\varphi) / [\pi N_{thread} (3-\cos(2\varphi))]$.

Taking R_{screw} = 1 micron, w_{thread} = 0.1 micron, N_{thread} = 1 turn, φ = 60°, $\eta = 1.1 \times 10^{-3}$ kg/m-sec for plasma at 310 K, and v_{screw} = 920 Hz, then v_{nano} = 1 cm/sec, $F_{nano} \sim$ 200 pN, v_{thread} = 0.6 cm/sec, total power requirement is $P_{screw} \sim$ 7.6 pW, efficiency is $e\% \sim 0.27$ (27%), and the pressure at the screw thread surface is $p_{thread} = F_{screw} / (l_{thread}\ w_{thread}) \sim 10^3$ N/m^2 << ~5 x 10^5 N/m^2 (required to induce transient cavitation in water at this frequency; Section 6.4.1). The outside edge of the screw thread is blunted to minimize energy transfer to impacted biological blood elements. A second counterrotating reverse-threaded screw mounted coaxially doubles the motive force while reducing net viscous torque on the natator to zero. If each screw of the screw-pair is mounted on gimbals, the nanorobot can achieve controlled translation and rotation in any direction in three-dimensional space; changing leading screw rotation from clockwise (CW) to counterclockwise (CCW) enables the nanodevice to reverse direction or to undertake more complex motions.

Another well-known instance of the inclined plane in locomotion is the corkscrew drive (Fig. 9.25), of which the bacterial flagellum is the most familiar biological example.[216,581,1395,1397] The flagellum works because of the differential viscous forces felt by thin cylinders passing through fluid at various angles of attack (e.g., because $F_{nano_N} \neq F_{nano_P}$; Section 9.4.2.4). The typical bacterial flagellum is a closely-packed rigid helix ~20 nm in diameter (with a ~3 nm flagellin protein core), and its length is almost always more than 100 times its thickness,[338] up to 10 microns long. The bacterial flagellum is turned by a ~0.0001 pW motor that rotates up to 300 Hz at 310 K (~15 Hz under load) and can reverse its direction of rotation in ~1 millisec (Section 6.3.4.2). The bacterium typically uses about 0.1% of its available metabolic energy (under growth conditions) to run the flagellum.[581] Forward motion may be achieved using either planar waves or (more efficient) spiral/helical waves. The highest swimming speed attainable by a flagellate (body length up to 50 microns with flagella >100 microns long in eukaryotes) is ~50% of the front-to-back wave speed of its flagellum,[1380] although ~20% is more typical.[1401] Measured swimming speeds are up to 100-200 microns/sec in various sperm species.[1449] The flexural rigidity of the bull sperm flagellar tail is 30 x 10^{-21} N-m^2 in the rigor state, and 2 x 10^{-21} N-m^2 in the more flexible state in the presence of ATP;[1451] see Eqn. 8.6. Energy efficiency may vary widely (Section 9.4.2.4).

9.4.2.5.3 Volume Displacement

Locomotion may also be achieved in a high-viscosity medium by physically removing fluid from the path ahead, then occupying the void before it closes up, and filling the volume behind with the vacated fluid—a process not unlike a tunneling mole. Forward velocity is largely determined by the speed at which blocks of fluid can be transferred from one end of the nanorobot to the other, whether along internal or external pathways.

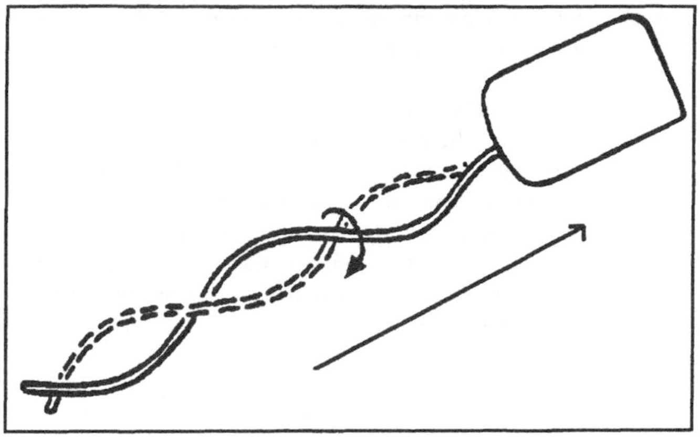

Fig. 9.25. Flagellar corkscrew (redrawn from Purcell[389]).

Fluid pumping (Section 9.2.7) provides the simplest means of volume displacement. Consider a tube of radius r_{tube} = 100 nm and length l_{tube} = 1 micron installed across the diameter of a 1-micron wide spherical nanorobot (R_{nano} = 0.5 micron), along with a single positive displacement piston pump of single-cycle displacement volume V_{cycle} = 0.008 micron^3 (Fig. 9.1). From the relations given in Section 9.2.7.2, operating the pump at v_{pump} = 1 MHz produces a time-averaged fluid flow velocity of v_{flow} = 26 cm/sec, a volume flow rate of $\dot{V}_{pump}$ = 8000 micron^3/sec, a nanorobot velocity of $v_{nano} = \dot{V}_{pump} / \pi R_{nano}^2$ = 1 cm/sec, and a power draw of $P_{flow} \sim$ 1800 pW. From Eqn. 9.25, $\Delta p \sim$ 2 atm across the nanorobot diameter, though this might be reduced to ~0.02 atm by flaring the entry and exit portals. Power usage, operating pressure, and the risks of clogging or fouling are relatively high, but this system has the virtue of simplicity, occupies less than 8% of total device internal volume, and can be expanded to three-dimensional motility by adding orthogonal entry portals. Jet propulsion is energy inefficient at small sizes and high speeds.[2022]

9.4.2.5.4 Viscous Anchoring

By extending ahead of it a structure whose surface area is capable of being expanded, a nanorobot can set an anchor forward along its path, then winch itself towards the anchor. In a typical cycle, the deflated anchor is thrust forward. Then the anchor is expanded tenfold in area (thus increasing its viscous resistance to backwards movement by approximately tenfold). The nanorobot pulls itself forward by attempting to reel in the anchor. The anchor is then deflated, and the cycle is repeated. The anchor mechanism may resemble an umbrella that is opened and closed, or a balloon that is inflated and deflated, at the end of a telescoping rod. A second anchor placed aft and countercycled with the first permits continuous motion by alternating pushing with pulling; noncoaxial anchor settings allow arbitrary rotation and access to all headings in three-dimensional space.

Energy efficiency can be good because less fluid may be sheared during nanorobot movement, although in 1998 this method had not been widely studied. If the forward anchor is pushed many diameters ahead before inflation, then even the expansion of an anchor much larger than the nanorobot might prove less energy-expensive than anything except a device with skin than could flow backwards to match laminar streamlines (Section 5.1).

9.4.2.6 Additional Considerations

The need for safe shear stresses (Section 9.4.2.2), and nanorobot power requirements for swimming (Section 9.4.2.4), both suggest that the maximum sanguinatation velocity to be employed by nanorobots in the human body in normal circumstances should be $\lesssim$ 1 cm/sec. Also, from Eqn. 9.65, a 1-micron nanorobot in water has a Reynolds number $N_R \sim v$; hence, to remain in the purely viscous regime, v << 1 m/sec. The following analysis provides additional support for this speed limit.

Consider a spherical nanorobot of radius R_{nano} swimming at velocity v_{nano} in the bloodstream, that impacts a passing blood cell. Virtually all cells encountered in this way will be erythrocytes. The elastic modulus for the viscoelastic red cell plasma membrane is $E_{cell} \sim 10^3$ N/m^2 for isoareal deformation (pure shear), $\sim 10^5$ N/m^2 at low areal strain (elastic area compressibility modulus), and the rupture strength is $\sim 10^6$ N/m^2.[1325] The force that is driving the sphere F_{nano} (Eqn. 9.73) may be distributed over the smallest possible impact area $\sim \pi R_{nano}^2$, and the resulting stress must be less than the rupture strength or elastic modulus to prevent significant damage or deformation of the cell surface, hence:

$$v_{nano} < \frac{R_{nano} E_{cell}}{6\eta} \quad \text{(m/sec)} \qquad \text{\{Eqn. 9.77\}}$$

Taking $\eta \sim 7 \times 10^{-3}$ kg/m-sec (Table 9.4) for the red cell contents ($\sim$0.33 gm/cm^3 hemoglobin solution) and R_{nano} = 1 micron, then the impacted erythrocyte deforms slightly with no change in surface area when $v_{nano} \lesssim 2$ cm/sec, deforms significantly with some change in surface area when $v_{nano} \sim 2$ m/sec, and finally ruptures when $v_{nano} \gtrsim 20$ m/sec. This suggests a conservative maximum velocity of $\lesssim$ 2 cm/sec for medical nanorobots traversing the human bloodstream, consistent with our proposed $\sim$1 cm/sec speed limit.

Nanorobot biocompatibility[3234] is an issue of crucial importance in nanomedicine (Chapter 15). Consider a fleet of $N_{nano} = 3 V_{blood} Nct / 4 \pi R_{nano}^3$ nanorobots uniformly deployed in a blood volume V_{blood} populated by red blood cells of typical length L_{RBC}. Each nanorobot swims past $\sim v_{nano}/L_{RBC}$ red cells per second, of which some small fraction κ_x are injured as a result of the encounter. If the iatrogenic injury rate is conservatively set equal to the natural rate of erythrocyte loss in the human body, or $K_0 \sim 3 \times 10^6$ sec^{-1}, then:

$$\kappa_x \lesssim \frac{4 \pi R_{nano}^3 K_0 L_{RBC}}{3 V_{blood} Nct\, v_{nano}} \qquad \text{\{Eqn. 9.78\}}$$

Taking v_{nano} = 1 cm/sec, $L_{RBC} \sim 7$ microns, V_{blood} = 5400 cm^3, and a 1 cm^3 therapeutic dose of R_{nano} = 1 micron medical nanorobots (which implies $N_{nano} \sim 2 \times 10^{11}$ nanorobots and Nct $\sim$ 0.02%), then $\kappa_x \lesssim 10^{-8}$. This amounts to a net erythrocyte injury rate of only $L_{RBC} / (v_{nano} \kappa_x) \sim 1$ cell/day per nanorobot—a challenging but probably attainable goal. ($K_0 \sim 2 \times 10^6$ sec^{-1} for platelets, 0.3-2 x 10^6 sec^{-1} for blood leukocytes.) Higher rates of red cell damage in theory could be accommodated by administering compensatory erythropoietin to stimulate RBC production (Chapter 22), but this approach would violate the general nanomedical design principle of avoiding iatrogenic harm whenever possible (Chapter 11).

Another velocity-related consideration involves the largely cell-free plasmatic zone (the "nanorobot freeway") that extends 2-4 microns from noncapillary blood vessel walls (Section 9.4.1.4), with the larger width occurring at higher shear rates.[362] Even in very narrow capillary blood vessels, moving red cells never come into solid-to-solid contact with the endothelium of the blood vessel. There is always a thin fluid layer in between, that serves as a lubrication layer.[362] In experiments with glass capillaries 7.6-8.5 microns in diameter, the apparent plasma layer thickness $\delta_{plasma} \sim 0.6$ microns for a red cell velocity $v_{RBC} \sim 0$ mm/sec, $\delta_{plasma} \sim 1.0$ microns at $v_{RBC} \sim 0.5$ mm/sec, and $\delta_{plasma} \sim 1.4$ microns at $v_{RBC} \sim 1.5$ mm/sec.[1399] This layer will usually be wide enough to accommodate most bloodborne nanorobots, which are expected to be 2 microns or smaller in diameter.

Note that a 1 cm^3 therapeutic dose of 1 micron^3 nanorobots includes $\sim 10^{12}$ devices, each of cross-sectional area $\sim$1 micron^2. Such a fleet would occupy $\sim$1 m^2 if spread out uniformly on a surface, adjacent and one layer thick. The total surface of the entire human vascular system is $\sim$313 m^2, but the summed area of all large veins and main arterial branches alone totals $\sim$1 m^2 (Table 8.1). Thus, small therapeutic doses of medical nanorobots may safely travel the cell-free plasmatic "freeway" at somewhat higher speeds than previously estimated, though possibly at the expense of significantly greater power consumption (Section 9.4.2.4) and possibly, at the highest number densities, interfering with the lubrication effect normally provided by the plasmatic layer, especially in the capillaries.

The need to maintain moderate viscosity of nanorobot-rich blood (Section 9.4.1.4) and to avoid complete plug flow in the narrowest human capillaries (Section 9.4.1.5) implies that the maximum nanocrit to be employed by nanorobots in the human bloodstream in normal circumstances should be Nct $\lesssim$ 10%. The following simple analysis provides another constraint that is consistent with this estimate, and is valid for rigid and metamorphic nanorobots alike.

The frequency of close encounters and collisions among nanorobots may be taken as a conservative metric of the likelihood of physical jamming, mission interference, and other pathological effects of crowding. Consider a spherical nanorobot of radius R_{nano} and volume $V_{nano} = (4/3) \pi R_{nano}^3$, and a second spherical nanorobot of identical size that approaches the first until the two are in contact, defining a "collision" event. If the number density $n_{nano} = 3\, Nct / [4 \pi R_{nano}^3 (1\text{-}Hct)]$ of a uniformly distributed population of such nanorobots exceeds 2 devices within a spherical volume of radius $2R_{nano}$, then, on average, all devices are in collision. This defines a maximum upper bound for nanocrit of $Nct_{maxHi} \gtrsim (1\text{-}Hct) / 4$, representing the onset of a highly collisional state; Nct_{maxHi} = 13.5% for Hct = 46% in the arteries, 22.5% for Hct $\sim$ 10% in the capillaries. Similarly, if the nanorobot number density is less than 1 device within a spherical volume of radius $2R_{nano}$, then each device, on average, is surrounded by a nanorobot-free zone the width of a single nanorobot radius, and collisions in a uniformly distributed population are relatively infrequent,* defining $Nct_{maxLo} \sim (1\text{-}Hct) / 8$. For Nct $\gtrsim Nct_{maxLo}$, the nanorobot population begins transitioning to an increasingly collisional state; Nct_{maxLo} = 6.8% for Hct = 46% in the arteries, 11.3% for Hct $\sim$ 10% in the capillaries. Thus in the arteries, an Nct < 6.8% is relatively noncollisional,* an Nct > 13.5% is highly collisional, and a 6.8% < Nct < 13.5% (midpoint Nct $\sim$ 10%) is transitional.

9.4.3 Cytoambulation

Many applications of medical nanorobots will require the ability to "walk" across biomaterial-embedded cellular tissues, packed-cell blocks, or vascular surfaces, a process called cytoambulation.

* *But only "relatively"—for example, the multi-body collision frequency is appreciable among red cells even at hematocrits as low as 5%.*[1358]

Cytoambulation may involve treading the surfaces of blood or lymph vessel walls which are lined with endothelial cells; negotiating flexible surfaces such as the walls of the urinary or gall bladders; traversing interior synovial or bursal surfaces such as the articular cartilage inside skeletal joints; and walking the walls of various excretory ducts, bulbs, tubes, and glands. Cytoambulating nanorobots may be required to cross various classes of tissue and cellular membranes. Tissue membranes are typically composed of epithelial and connective tissues and include:

a. serous membranes lining the cavities of the body and surrounding the various organs (e.g., the pericardium, pleura, peritoneum, and meninges);

b. mucous membranes lining the alimentary, respiratory, and genito-urinary tracts; and

c. fibrous membranes composed entirely of connective tissues (e.g., perichondrium, periosteum, and synovial membranes).

Traversing such tissue membranes will often involve crossing the individual plasma membranes of tissue-embedded cells of various classes. Nanorobots also may cytoambulate across the surfaces of motile or free-floating cells, including individual erythrocytes and red-cell rouleaux, leukocytes, fibroblasts, platelets, large protozoa, and even some bacteria.

A comprehensive survey of all possible cytoambulatory modes and requirements is beyond the scope of this book. This Section is restricted to a discussion of basic cell-surface walking, including the single footpad contact event (Section 9.4.3.1), cell plasma membrane elasticity (Section 9.4.3.2), anchoring and dislodgement forces (Section 9.4.3.3), the physical limits of contact event cycling (Section 9.4.3.4), and examples of a few specific physical nanomechanisms for cytoambulation (Sections 9.4.3.5-9.4.2.8). The reader is encouraged to review Section 8.5.3 on cell structure before proceeding further.

9.4.3.1 Ambulatory Contact Event

Stripped to its fundamentals, the act of ambulation requires that a mobile surface (e.g., a footpad) is brought into adhesive contact with a fixed surface to be traversed. After the contact event has occurred, the point of adhesion becomes a fulcrum allowing mechanical leverage to be applied against the fixed surface, thus permitting forward motion of a mass attached to a lever. The mobile surface may then be detached from the fixed surface and the cycle repeated.

Consider a footpad approaching the extracellular surface of a cell. The footpad first encounters 5-8 nm thick strands of the circumcellular glycocalyx at a number density of ~10^5 strands/micron^2, typically at a distance of 10-100 nm from the plasma membrane surface (see Section 8.5.3.2). A reversible binding site embedded in the footpad contact area (Section 4.2.8) can recognize glycocalyx chains unique to specific cell types or tissues, or more generally any glycoprotein chain, and then securely bind to such chain until mechanically released. If cell-type specificity is not an important design requirement, then a simple reversible mechanical grappling system may be employed. Each carbohydrate chain may be up to 100-200 nm in length, so a footpad adhering to a cell surface in this fashion may experience up to ~100 nm of horizontal or vertical free play in its anchorage. This can seriously degrade the efficiency of motive levers (e.g., nanorobot legs) $\lesssim$1 micron in length, and can make ambulatory locomotion nearly impossible for motive levers $\lesssim$100 nm in length. (If the footpad adheres to many chains, free play is substantially reduced.)

Alternatively, footpads may employ spikelike structures and glycophobic coatings to penetrate the glycocalyx without injuring it. At 10-20 nm above the plasma membrane surface, these footpad structures will encounter the extracellular polar regions of integral proteins that are embedded in the cellular plasma membrane. Integral proteins, typically ~100,000 daltons, are present in RBCs at a number density of ~10^5/micron^2; however, ~100 different integral protein types are present, reducing the number density of any one common type (e.g., red cell glycophorins) to 10^3-10^4/micron^2. Free-floating integral proteins (constituting 20%-70% of the total number[1435]) exhibit considerable lateral diffusion but can provide adequate anchorage if the dwell time is brief enough. Transmembrane proteins are often immobilized by links to protein networks located near the cytoplasmic side of the plasma membrane, possibly reducing free play to ~20-30 nm, although many transmembrane proteins are required to be unattached to the internal cytoskeleton, permitting them to circulate so they can mediate multi-receptor signal transduction.

Penetrating still further to the plasma membrane surface, reversibly-hydrophilic footpads may bind with the polar phospholipid heads of the ~650 dalton molecules comprising the lipid bilayer, with number density ~2.5 x 10^6/micron^2 in each of the two layers. (The erythrocyte plasma membrane contains well over 100 different lipid species,[1430] in much lesser concentrations.) Adjacent phospholipid molecules generally are not bound covalently, so individual molecules may be extracted from the lipid bilayer with a modest vertical force (taking ~10 zJ/nm^2 interlipid hydrophobic binding energy (Section 3.5.1) and lipid-lipid contact area ~4 nm^2/lipid divided by single-layer extraction distance ~4 nm implies a single-lipid, single-layer extraction force F_{lipid} ~ 10 pN, comparable to the estimate by Evans[1415]) and hence provide relatively weak anchorage in the vertical direction. Although such anchorage may suffice in many applications, artificial amphipathic transmembrane anchored structures (Section 9.4.3.3) can provide an even more secure bond for locomotion and parking.

After the contact event has occurred, the adhesion structure is used as a fulcrum to apply mechanical leverage against the cell plasma membrane surface, giving rise to tensile or shear forces at the point of attachment. How large are these forces?* As a minimal estimate, we assume that each transmembrane protein is anchored to the internal cytoskeleton by only a single actin microfilament. An actin microfilament has a failure strength of ~2.2 x 10^6 N/m^2 (Table 9.3) and a cross-sectional area of ~30 nm^2 (Section 8.5.3.11), thus requiring a tearing force of ~108 pN for detachment.[362] A glycoprotein molecule consisting primarily of a chain of C-C covalent bonds may have a rupture strength on the order of ~10,000 pN (Section 3.5.1).

When mechanical leverage is applied against the cell surface, plasma membrane components feel a force in the direction opposite to the direction of travel of the ambulating nanorobot. Since the plasma membrane is a fluid, components within the membrane may be free

** J. Hoh emphasizes that a large thermal contribution exists for forces in the piconewton range; the smaller the force, the larger the time-dependent contribution. Normal biomolecular interactions, such as antibody-antigen interactions at $\gtrsim$100 pN, have finite lifetimes and will unbind on a timescale of hours or days in the absence of any force. Even a very small loading force may shift the unbinding timescale significantly downward. As a result, the binding forces for nanorobot footpads will be critically linked to the speed at which the nanorobot is moving. Hoh believes these variations in force may span orders of magnitude; additional research on nanorobot footpad mechanics is clearly needed.*

to slip backwards, reducing traction. For simplicity of analysis, consider a spherical nanorobot of radius R_{nano} that inserts a spherical footpad of radius R_{foot} into a lipid bilayer membrane, at the end of each of N_{leg} legs each of a width that is small in comparison with R_{foot} (so that the contribution from the legs may be ignored). The viscosity of the plasma membrane that resists the backward movement of the footpad is approximately $\eta_{membrane} \sim 10$ kg/m-sec and the viscosity of the extracellular fluid is $\eta_{extra} \sim 10^{-3}$ kg/m-sec (Table 9.4). The nanorobot ambulates across the cell surface through the extracellular fluid at a velocity v_{nano} against a "headwind" of $v_{headwind}$ (the fluid speed relative to plasma membrane surface), during which movement the footpad slips backwards at a velocity v_{foot}. Equating the forces on the nanorobot and the footpad from Eqn. 9.73 gives:

$$v_{nano} \sim (\kappa_{traction} N_{leg} v_{foot}) - v_{headwind} \quad \text{(m/sec)} \quad \{\text{Eqn. 9.79}\}$$

where the coefficient of traction $\kappa_{traction} = \eta_{membrane} R_{foot} / \eta_{extra} R_{nano}$. Taking $N_{leg} = 2$, $R_{nano} = 1$ micron and $R_{foot} = 10$ nm, then $\kappa_{traction} = 200$. Thus with $v_{headwind} = 0$, the footpads of a bipedal nanorobot traveling forward at $v_{nano} = 1$ cm/sec slip backward within the lipid bilayer membrane at only $v_{foot} = 50$ microns/sec. This process is functionally similar to the tracked system modeled by kinesin microtubule transport (Section 9.4.6) wherein productive steps are directed by protein-protein interaction affinities.

Repeated application of physical forces across a cell surface may activate mechanical signal transduction pathways mediated by specific transmembrane proteins such as the integrins and cadherins (Sections 8.5.2.2 and 8.5.3.11). These signals can trigger major changes in cell behavior and in cellular protein expression. Microfilaments readily transduce 0.01-2 Hz mechanical signals throughout the cell.[1202] In 1998, it was not yet known whether much higher frequencies, such as might be employed in cytoambulation, also induce a significant cellular response, except, of course, in specialized mechanoreceptor cells such as the cochlear stereocilia.[3597,3598] Footpad target proteins, motions, and operating frequencies should be selected with the objective of minimizing mechanical signal transduction effects.

9.4.3.2 Cell Plasma Membrane Elasticity

Does the temporary attachment and passage of a cytoambulating nanorobot across a cell surface have a significant mechanical effect on that surface? Cell and plasma membrane deformation can be quite complex. However, taking the plasma membrane to be a two-dimensional, incompressible elastic solid, a deformation will always consist of one or more of three fundamental independent deformations: expansion without bending or shear (characterized by the area expansion modulus K, in N/m), elongation (shear) without expanding or bending (shear modulus μ_{shear}, in N/m), and bending without shear or expansion (bending modulus B, in N-m). Each mode is discussed briefly, below.

9.4.3.2.1 Plasma Membrane Areal Expansion Elasticity

A nanorobot with a footpad of width $L_{foot} = 10$ nm that applies a pressure of $P_{nano} = 10 \text{ pN} / L_{foot}^2$ across a span L_{foot} of plasma membrane surface (and normal to it) creates an isotropic tension of $T \sim P_{nano} L_{foot} = 1 \times 10^{-3}$ N/m within the membrane, causing the plasma membrane under the nanorobot to expand uniformly without shearing or bending. For comparison, the tension required to smooth out the thermal undulations or "Brownian motion" of the outer membrane of artificial phospholipid vesicles 10-20 microns in diameter (typical cell size) was determined experimentally to be $0.01\text{-}0.1 \times 10^{-3}$ N/m.[368] At the other extreme, osmotically swollen red cells will instantaneously lyse* at a plasma membrane tension of $T_{lyse} = 10\text{-}20 \times 10^{-3}$ N/m[1415,1421] or at an elastic modulus with respect to area dilation of $T_{lyse} / h_{cell} \sim 3 \times 10^6$ N/m^2,[1422] where red cell wall thickness $h_{cell} = 8$ nm.

The relative area expansion of the plasma membrane under the nanorobot footpad is $\Delta A / A = T / K$,[1415] where the experimentally-determined area compressibility modulus is $K = 0.45$ N/m for red cell plasma membrane at 298 K[1412,1413,3171,3172] (change in area compressibility modulus with temperature is -6×10^{-3} N/m-K)[3172]; $K = 1.7$ N/m for certain cholesterol-lipid mixtures.[1414] This gives $\Delta A / A \sim 0.2\%$ or 0.06% for the nanorobot footpad of size L_{foot} described above (2%-4% areal expansion produces lysis[1415]), or a mean linear strain of $\varepsilon = (\Delta A / A)^{1/2} \sim 0.04$ (4%) or 0.02 (2%). For $\varepsilon << 1$, the footpad depresses the surface by $\Delta x \sim L_{foot} (\varepsilon/2)^{1/2} \sim 1.5$ nm into the red cell's interior. This deflection represents only ~15% of lipid bilayer membrane thickness and must be considered modest in most circumstances. For leukocyte plasma membranes, measured $K = 0.636$ N/m.[846]

The design of cytoambulation mechanisms should attempt to minimize the activation of sodium-ion (and many other) stretch-activated channels—gated transmembrane channels that are activated by simply stretching the plasma membrane, or by tension or stress development in cytoskeletal elements associated with the cell membrane.[362,1506] Such channels have already been implicated in the maintenance of cell volume.[491,1416] Biochemical transduction of mechanical strain has also been investigated in bone cells during normal loading. Linear strains of $\varepsilon < 0.05\%$ were nonstimulative; those between 0.05%-0.15% maintained normal bone mass, and strains of $\varepsilon > 0.15\%$ stimulated osteoblasts to increase bone mass.[1417-1419] Linear strains >1% induced osteoblasts to alter morphology, becoming fibroblast-like,[1420] and red cells lyse at $\varepsilon \gtrsim 20\%$.[362] A limit of $\Delta A / A \sim 0.05\%$ for a 10 nm footpad on a red cell surface would give an estimate of ~2 pN for the activation threshold. However, a force of 1 pN across a protein stretch sensor of cross-sectional area ~1 nm^2 represents an energy density of 10^6 joules/m^3, or 10 zJ (~2 kT) for a ~10 nm^3 sensor volume, which is probably close to the limit for biological force detection consistent with earlier estimates of nanosensor detection limits (Section 4.4.1).

From these comparisons, it appears that a biological response, stimulated by plasma membrane areal expansion due to the passage of nanorobot footpads across the cell surface employing forces typical in cytoambulation (e.g., ~20 pN; Section 9.4.3.5), cannot be ruled out. However, in 1998 it was not yet known how efficiently mechanical pressures cycled at 10-100 KHz are transduced by plasma membrane stretch sensors, since most mechanical cell stimulation experiments have been conducted at frequencies between 0.05-5 Hz.** Energy coupling may be poor due to a large mechanical impedance mismatch. Looser glycocalyx anchorages also could minimize stretch activation effects.

** $T \sim 6 \times 10^{-3}$ N/m produces red cell plasma membrane lysis after ~10 sec; time of lysis is a stochastic function that increases to ~120 days (maximum red cell lifetime) at $T \sim 3\text{-}4 \times 10^{-3}$ N/m.[1415]*

***Specifically: 0.05 Hz,[3599] 0.1 Hz,[3600] 0.25 Hz,[3601] 0.33 Hz,[3600,3602] 0.5 Hz,[3603,3604] 1 Hz,[3604-3609] 1.67 Hz,[3609] 2 Hz,[3604] and 5 Hz.[3610]*

9.4.3.2.2 Plasma Membrane Shear Elasticity

A plasma membrane surface can deform by "shear"—elongation in one dimension while narrowing in another dimension—without bending or increasing surface area. If a deforming force normal to a plasma membrane surface is suddenly removed, the membrane surface will recover its normal unstressed shape in a characteristic time $t_{snapback} = \eta_{surface} / \mu_{shear} \sim 0.1$ sec,[3171] where elastic shear modulus μ_{shear} = 6.6 x 10^{-6} N/m for the red cell plasma membrane at 298 K,[3172] as determined experimentally, and the measured coefficient of surface viscosity $\eta_{surface} \sim 10^{-6}$ N-sec/m,[3171] is the product of plasma membrane viscosity (~100 kg/m-sec for RBC; Table 9.4) and plasma membrane thickness (~8 nm for RBC), with measured $\eta_{surface}$ = 0.6-1.2 x 10^{-6} N-sec/m for the red cell plasma membrane.[371] (The change in elastic shear modulus with temperature is -6 x 10^{-8} N/m-K.[3172]) Shape recovery is dominated by plasma membrane viscosity, not cytoplasm viscosity, in some systems, particularly RBCs;[362] however, J. Hoh [personal communication, 1999] notes that this does not hold for all cells, and that for most cell types it is the cytoplasm that dominates the rheological properties, as experimentally measured, for example, by indentors or piezo controlled microplates.[3611] The time required for a leukocyte to enter a capillary is ~1000-2000 times longer than the time required by red cells,[846] suggesting $t_{snapback} \sim 100$ sec for white cells.

With nanorobot legswing frequency $\nu_{leg} >> t_{snapback}^{-1}$, a section of plasma membrane distorted by the passage of one nanorobot footpad may not be able to resume its fully relaxed state before the arrival of another footpad in the same spot as the first. If a traverse through a narrow passage of cell-rich tissue by large numbers of ambulating nanorobots is contemplated for a particular application, then footpad placements should be randomized as much as possible to avoid repeat-deformation grooving, rutting, or other persistent indentation features in the plasma membrane surface.

9.4.3.2.3 Plasma Membrane Bending Elasticity

The bending stiffness (bending modulus) of the red cell plasma membrane at room temperature is B ~ 1.8 x 10^{-19} N-m.[371,1203,1411,3171] The energy required to bend the plasma membrane into a hemispherical cap is ~4 π B ~ 2300 zJ.[1203] A nanorobot footpad of size L_{foot} that exerts a backward force F ~ 10 pN against the plasma membrane may cause the membrane surface behind the footpad to fold into a ripple with radius of curvature $r_{curve} \sim B / F \sim 20$ nm. The dynamic resistance to RBC plasma membrane folding appears to be limited by viscous dissipation in the cytoplasmic and external fluid phases.[3171] The plasma membrane has only a very weak resistance to bending.

9.4.3.3 Anchoring and Dislodgement Forces

A footpad which is noncovalently bound only to a single lipid[1481] or unanchored protein[1482,1483] molecule embedded in the plasma membrane will slowly move as the membrane molecule(s) to which it is attached experiences translation diffusion according to the well-known Einstein-Smoluchowski equation:

$$\Delta X = (2\, D\, \tau)^{1/2} \quad \text{(meters)} \qquad \text{\{Eqn. 9.80\}}$$

which is readily obtained by combining Eqns. 3.1 and 3.5. For lipidic probes, translational diffusion coefficients in artificial fluid bilayer systems generally range from D = 1-10 x 10^{-12} m²/sec;[1430] for plasma membrane lipids in human fibroblasts, D = 1.6 x 10^{-12} m²/sec at 310 K.[1431] Proteins reconstituted in phospholipid bilayers show diffusion coefficients from D = 0.7-8 x 10^{-12} m²/sec. LDL receptors in human fibroblasts have D = 0.2 x 10^{-12} m²/sec at 310 K; MHC Class I (HLA) antigens in human neutrophils, lymphocytes and fibroblasts have D = 0.05-0.07 x 10^{-12} m²/sec, or 0.15-0.30 x 10^{-12} m²/sec in human endothelial cells.[1482] There is a weak dependence on protein molecular size[1430]—according to Monte Carlo simulations, a plasma membrane lattice covered up to 82% with impermeable (protein) domains diminishes D by only a factor of 20 in comparison to the zero concentration limit.[1436] In erythrocyte plasma membranes, spectrin-anchored proteins such as the anion transport protein band 3 have D ~ 0.0045 x 10^{-12} m²/sec, while D = 0.25 x 10^{-12} m²/sec in spectrin-depleted cells where the same proteins are no longer anchored;[1432,1434] in either case, D = 0.8-1.5 x 10^{-12} m²/sec for RBC plasma membrane lipids.[1432,1433] A few covalently glycolipid-linked proteins show exceptionally stable anchorage,[1485] such as the sperm antigen PH-20 with D = 0.00001 x 10^{-12} m²/sec.[1482]

Taking $\tau \sim \nu_{leg}^{-1} \sim$ 10-100 microsec (Section 9.4.3.5) as the duration of the anchoring event during legged ambulation, then attachment to a lipid or an unanchored protein (D ~ 10^{-12} m²/sec) gives a footpad wander of ΔX ~ 4-14 nm, which is probably acceptable in most applications. Footholds on transmembrane proteins that are mechanically linked to the submembrane cytomatrix will require a force of at least 100 pN/molecule to dislodge, and will have even less free play, given the lower D. Additionally, for a cylindrical protein of radius R ~ 3 nm traversing a plasma membrane of thickness h ~ 10 nm, the rotational diffusion coefficient D_{rot} is given by:[1483]

$$D_{rot} = \frac{kT}{4\,\pi\,\eta_{membrane}\,R^2\,h} = 380 \text{ sec}^{-1} \qquad \text{\{Eqn. 9.81\}}$$

taking $\eta_{membrane} \sim 10$ kg/m-sec at 310 K, which gives a diffusional rotation of $\Delta\alpha = (2\, D_{rot}\, \tau)^{1/2}$ = 0.1-0.3 radian taking τ ~ 10-100 microsec.

For much longer parking times (e.g., τ ~ 1 sec), in the classical fluid mosaic model of the cell plasma membrane (Section 8.5.3.2), ΔX ~ 1 micron for footpads attached to lipids or unanchored proteins. However, recent work by Kusumi and Sako[1476] has demonstrated that a substantial fraction of unanchored proteins are transiently confined to domains somewhat smaller than this. According to their membrane-skeleton fence model, a spectrin-like meshwork (Fig. 8.43) closely apposed to the cytoplasmic face of the plasma membrane sterically confines transmembrane proteins to regions on the order of the cytoskeletal mesh size. The fences appear elastic, because, for example, transferrin receptors rebound after they strike barriers, and a small fraction of these receptors seem to be fixed to the underlying cytoskeleton by spring-like tethers.[1477] For cadherins, transferrin receptors, and epidermal growth factor receptors, the domains (e.g., the barrier-free path or BFP) are 300-600 nm in diameter and confinement lasts 3-30 sec.[1476-1478] BFPs for the lipid-linked and membrane-spanning isoforms of the MHC (Section 8.5.2.1) antigens are ~1700 nm and ~600 nm, respectively, at a temperature of 296 K.[1479] Confinement was also found for a lipid-linked isoform of neural cell adhesion molecules (NCAMs) in muscle cells (which cannot be directly trapped by the cytoskeletal network), with BFP domains ~280 nm in diameter and a mean trapping time of ~8 sec.[1480] Still, footholds to well-anchored proteins may be preferred for the longest parking times.

An annular footpad of radius R_{foot} = 10 nm firmly attached around its circumference to a ring of plasma membrane-surface lipid molecules, taking each molecule of area A_{lipid} ~ 0.4 nm²/molecule and assuming a single-lipid extraction force F_{lipid} ~ 1 pN (Section 9.4.3.1), achieves an anchorage force $F_{anchor} = 2 \pi R_{foot} F_{lipid} / A_{lipid}^{1/2}$ ~ 100 pN (~3 atm); somewhat more compact anchor geometries are possible. Equally strong footholds may be gained using artificial amphipathic transmembrane anchors terminated with ~20-nm-diameter expansible submembrane compartments (analogous cytosolic "anchor domains" are common in cytochemistry; see Figs. 8.33 and 8.34), or using amphipathic transmembrane anchors which are directly but reversibly secured to the cytomatrix. Taking the membranolytic limit as 3 x 10^6 N/m²,[1422] then a 100 nm² footpad can apply up to 300 pN of anchoring force without tearing the plasma membrane.

A cluster of ten 100-pN anchors can resist at least ~1000 pN of dislodgement force applied to a medical nanorobot. Most in vivo dislodgement forces will be considerably smaller than this. For example, mean shear stress at blood vessel walls due to normal blood flow is ~2 N/m² (Section 9.4.2.2), giving a typical dislodgement force of F_{dis} ~ 2 pN on a 1-micron² nanorobot. (The net attractive force of ~70 pN between red cells in a rouleaux is also ~2 N/m²; Section 9.2.3.) Shear stress in partially occluded arteries produces a maximum F_{dis} ~ 40 pN, and shearing stresses between venule endothelium and a rolling leukocyte may reach 100 N/m² (Section 9.4.2.2), giving F_{dis} ~ 100 pN if a white cell bumps or rolls over an anchored nanorobot. Impact by a rapidly sanguinatating nanorobot moving at 1 cm/sec (Section 9.4.2.4) produces a dislodgement force of at most F_{dis} ~ 200 pN.

For comparison, the adhesion strength for the protozoan *Amoeba proteus* has been measured as ~100-1000 nN,[1456] giving an adhesion force of 100-1000 pN/micron² over a focal contact area of ~1000 micron².[1454] The tension force exerted by a single fibroblast during locomotion has been measured as ~165 nN,[1461] or ~1000 pN/micron² (1000 N/m²). Cell-cell adhesion of T cells and target cells is ~1500 pN/micron².[1458]

Cytoambulatory dislodgement forces elsewhere in the human body are equally modest. For example, taking Eqn. 9.58 and crude estimates using data from Table 9.4 and Section 8.2, shear stress is ~0.001-0.1 N/m² along the walls of the small intestine and ~0.01-1 N/m² in the large intestine; at the rectal wall, ~1-100 N/m² during normal defecation and ~10-100 N/m² during explosive defecation; on the walls of the male urethra, shear stress is ~1 N/m² during urination and up to ~10-100 N/m² during ejaculation; on the esophageal walls, shear stress is ~0.001 N/m² when swallowing water, ~1 N/m² while swallowing food, and ~10-100 N/m² during emesis; on the corneal surface of the eye, ~0.1 N/m² during eyelid flapping; and on the tracheal and nasal surfaces, ~0.001 N/m² during a sneeze.

9.4.3.4 Contact Event Cycling

How fast can ambulatory contact events be cycled? Molecular receptors ~10 nm² in size can bind large (5-10 nm), "common" (~10^{-2}/nm³) molecules in t_{EQ} ~ 0.2 microsec (Section 4.2.1). With ~10^5/micron² glycocalyx strands and a similar number of integral proteins near the cell surface (Section 9.4.3.1), there are ~10 strands and ~10 proteins under each 100 nm² footpad. For either glycocalyx strands or integral proteins, mean separation is ~3 nm giving a concentration of ~4 x 10^{-2}/nm³ > 10^{-2}/nm³, thus qualifying as "common" molecules in the footpad environment. (There are also ~250 bilayer lipid heads directly beneath a 100 nm² footpad, of which ~100 are phospholipids, ~50 are cholesterols, 10-75 are glycolipids, and the remaining 25-90 are other lipids.) Alternatively, mechanical grippers that close and open on a 5-nm wide molecular target using a 1 cm/sec jaw speed require ~1 microsec per gripping cycle.

Finally, a mechanical manipulator appendage traveling at a conservative ~1 cm/sec (Section 9.3.1) can transit the 10-100 nm glycocalyx, reaching the plasma membrane surface, if necessary, in 1-10 microsec. A similar amount of time must be allowed for the limb to be retracted from the cell surface. These figures are all consistent with a maximum legswing frequency ν_{leg} ~ 100 KHz.

9.4.3.5 Legged Ambulation

Consider a 1 micron³ nanorobot cytoambulating using legs tipped with appropriate footpads to traverse a vascular wall. Each leg is assumed to be similar in size and function to the 100-nm long, 30-nm wide cylindrical telescoping nanomanipulator described in Section 9.3.1.4. Each nanorobot has a total of 100 legs, occupying 7% of the 10^6 nm² underside area of the device. To allow tenfold redundancy, at any one time only N_{leg} = 10 legs are deployed and in use. The remainder are stowed as spares.

Ignoring ≲ 1% traction losses (Section 9.4.3.1), the total force that must be supplied by all N_{leg} working legs is:

$$F_{total} = F_{dis} + N_{leg} F_{leg} + F_{nano} \qquad \text{\{Eqn. 9.82\}}$$

The maximum dislodgement or "headwind" force normally encountered along blood vessel walls is F_{dis} ~ 40 pN (Section 9.4.3.3). The viscous force on each leg is approximated by Eqn. 9.75 as F_{leg} ~ F_{nanoN} ~ 6 pN, taking L_{leg} = 100 nm, R_{leg} = 15 nm, and v_{leg} = 1 cm/sec. From Eqn. 9.73, F_{nano} ~ 100 pN, taking $\eta = 1.1 \times 10^{-3}$ kg/m-sec for plasma at 310 K, R_{nano} ~ 0.5 micron, and v_{nano} = 1 cm/sec. F_{total} = 200 pN, easily within the capacity of a single leg (Section 9.3.1.4), giving an allocation of F_{total}/N_{leg} = 20 pN per leg. Maximum safe towing force is ≲ 300 pN/leg, assuming 100 nm² footpads and a 3 x 10^6 N/m² membranolytic limit for plasma membrane.[1422]

Many N-podal gaits are possible.[3499-3507] In the most conservative gait, only 1 leg is moved at a time while the remaining (N_{leg}-1) legs stay anchored at their footpads. Given a full center-to-center working arc of X_{arc} ~ 80 nm, each leg must travel $X_{swing} = X_{arc}/N_{leg}$ = 8 nm in a time $t_{swing} = X_{swing} / v_{leg}$ = 0.8 microsec at a velocity v_{leg} = 1 cm/sec, with a per-leg duty cycle of $f_{duty} = N_{leg}^{-1}$ = 10% and an operating frequency of $\nu_{leg} = f_{duty}/t_{swing}$ ~ 100 KHz. From Eqn. 9.74, nanorobot motive power is $P_{nano} = F_{total} v_{nano} / e\%$ ~ 10 pW, taking e% ~ 0.20 (20%). Conservatively taking each footpad binding event as costing E_{bind} ~ 100 zJ (Section 4.2.1), then footpad binding power requirement is $P_{bind} = N_{leg} \nu_{leg} E_{bind}$ ~ 0.1 pW, a negligible contribution.

For the least conservative gait, only 1 leg stays anchored while the remaining (N_{leg}-1) legs are in motion. In this case, $X_{swing} = X_{arc}$ = 80 nm giving t_{swing} = 8 microsec and ν_{leg} ~ 10 KHz, but motive power, nanorobot velocity, and leg duty cycle are unchanged. Doubling leg length to L_{leg} = 200 nm while holding R_{leg}, v_{leg}, and v_{nano} unchanged decreases operating frequency to ν_{leg} ~ 5 KHz while increasing F_{total} to 230 pN and P_{nano} to 12 pW. Doubling the velocities doubles force and operating frequency, and quadruples the power demand. Perhaps counterintuitively from common macroscale experience,[1486] for small ambulators traveling in viscous-dominated media (e.g., low Reynolds number ambulators), shorter legs may produce the highest motive velocity for the lowest power requirement and applied force.

As a biological analog, tiny extensible hydraulic tube feet specialized for burrowing and stepping locomotion, often with terminal suckers, have been extensively described in echinoderms.[1472-1475]

9.4.3.6 Tank-Tread Rolling

When an injured cell "calls for help" from leukocytes, the cell secretes cytokines such as IL-1 and TNF, causing nearby vascular endothelial cells to express P-selectin and E-selectin on their luminal surfaces.[415] Passing white cells adhere to these protruding molecules because their carbohydrate coat contains complementary structures. When a leukocyte touches a venule wall, its rate of movement slows because of the stickiness between the cell and the wall, but the force of the circulating blood keeps the cell moving with a tank-tread motion in what is called a rolling interaction (Fig. 9.28). The average white cell rolling velocity is only $<$4% of the mean blood flow velocity in the venule,[361] typically ~10-40 microns/sec.[1027,1484,1507]

This form of locomotion is easily implemented by rigid medical nanorobots. A primitive example would be a spherical device with numerous flexible knobs projecting radially from its surface, located a distance Δy apart. A mechanical gripper or binding pad located at the tip of each knob is switched on or off, depending on the direction the nanorobot desires to go. Anchored with one knob, Brownian or hydrodynamic forces cause the device to bounce around until one of the active knobs contacts the surface, whereupon that knob binds, and the previous anchor knob releases. The device has now progressed a distance Δy in the desired direction. A micron-size nanorobot could achieve v_{nano} ~ 1 micron/sec in a quiet environment or up to v_{nano} ~ 1 mm/sec in blood vessels, at a near-negligible power cost ($\ll$ 1 pW) because only footpads must be operated. In the limit of a flexible knob-dense surface, a nanorobot with ~1 micron^2 of continuous contact surface could, in theory, tow up to 3,000,000 pN of load before reaching the ~3 x 10^6 N/m^2 membranolytic limit.[1422]

9.4.3.7 Amoeboid Locomotion

The most common cells exhibiting amoeboid locomotion[3613] in the human body are white cells, having moved out of the blood into the tissues in the form of tissue microphages or macrophages. Fibroblasts and normally sessile germinal skin cells can move into damaged areas to assist in wound repair. Embryonic cells in the fetus such as neurons often migrate long distances to their final location by amoeboid movement, after which they become fixed in tissue as sessile cells. The 200-600 micron carnivorous *Amoeba proteus* also displays this form of locomotion and was the subject of the earliest studies, hence the name.

Amoeboid movement is associated with two properties—cytoplasmic streaming, and the extension and retraction of pseudopods—the motive effects of which could be simulated by medical nanorobots using metamorphic exterior surfaces (Section 5.3). As shown in Figure 9.26, the monopodial amoeboid cell progresses by establishing a series of attachment points or focal contacts with the surface it is traversing. Viewed from the side, the amoeba steps forward on new pseudopods that make adhesive contact with the surface, with the tail region and retracting pseudopods lifted clear of the surface.[1464] The plasma membrane with its mucus coat is a relatively permanent structure that plays a passive role during locomotion,[1465] rotating forward during locomotion something like a water balloon rolling across a tilted tabletop.

Inside the plasma membrane are two regions of cytoplasm with varying viscosity—the actin microfilament-rich outer portion, called the ectoplasm or cell cortex, and the inner portion called the endoplasm. To move forward, the ectoplasm at the front end becomes thin, causing a pseudopodium to bulge forward; the ectoplasm at the tail end contracts, pushing endoplasm into the pseudopodium and extending it further.[1466] Actin monomers in the pseudopods are gelated to actin polymers in the pseudopods, then solated back to monomers in the tail. (Gels depolymerize when Ca^{++} activates gelsolin protein, which severs actin; actin repolymerizes into gel when Ca^{++} concentration is reduced.) The surface for new pseudopod formation is unfolded from the sink of convoluted surface in retracted pseudopods and in the tail. In each pseudopod, the surface rolls forward over the stationary ectoplasmic tube on a lubricating layer of hyaloplasm dispersed from the hyaline cap.[1380] Isolated amoebic cytoplasm, when injected with ATP, streams spontaneously at up to 160 microns/sec.[1394]

The formation of a focal contact between fibroblast and surface is a biphasic process in which the fast (~1 sec) initial phase of establishing small (~0.25 micron^2) immature contacts at large separation distances is followed by a slower (~15 sec) phase of widening mature contacts with narrowing separation distances.[1457] Leukocyte pseudopodia are ~1 micron in length with a typical extension velocity of ~0.08 microns/sec,[846] so white cells and fibroblasts readily cytoambulate at ~0.05-0.1 micron/sec;[359,1513] chemotactically-stimulated leukocytes can locomote at up to ~0.7 microns/sec.[1516] An individual fibroblast has a towing strength of ~165 nN,[1461] giving an implied low-load motive power demand of only ~0.02 pW (force x velocity). Measured motive force of a whole amoeba (~towing force) is 50-290 nN,[1462,1469] or ~100 nN per 50-micron pseudopod; internal hydrostatic pressures have been estimated from 10-100 N/m^2 [1470,1471] up to ~10^5 N/m^2.[1453] Ambulatory velocity ranges from 1-50 microns/sec, but averages ~10 microns/sec.[1394] A nanorobot using metamorphic pseudopods spaced ~1 micron apart and cycling its adhesive contacts at 10 KHz

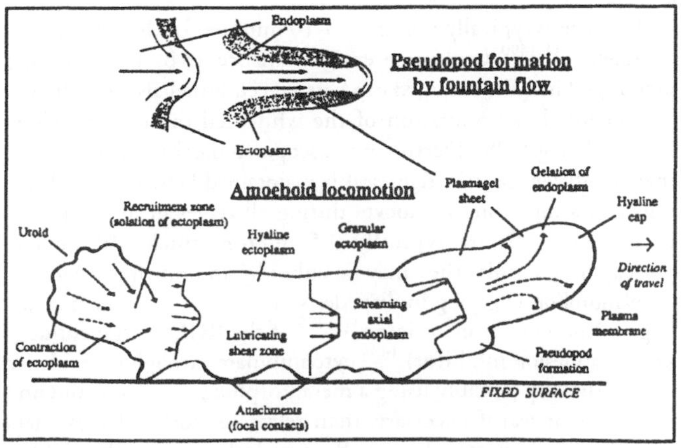

Fig. 9.26. Protoplasmic streaming in a monopodal amoeba with velocity profiles at three loci (modified from Holberton[1380]).

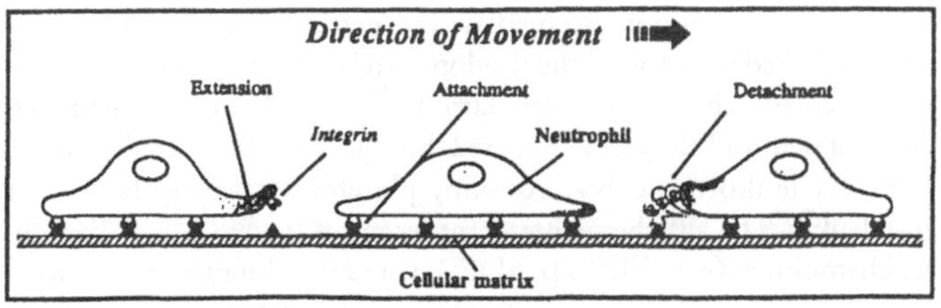

Fig. 9.27. Schematic of neutrophil cytoambulation (redrawn from Horwitz[1511]).

could achieve v_{nano} ~ 1 cm/sec within a ~10 pW motive power budget (Section 5.3.1.4).

Neutrophils walk from one site to another by forming and breaking integrin-mediated attachments to a matrix (Fig. 9.27). Integrin receptor surface density is ~2000/micron^2 on neutrophils,[1510] with each fibrinogen attachment having a detachment strength of ~2 pN.[1508]

9.4.3.8 Inchworm Locomotion

Another ambulatory strategy that has been investigated for medical robots is inchworm locomotion.[1632,3086] In this mode, the tail end of a flexible tubular nanodevice is anchored. The front end extends in the desired direction across the cell surface by pushing against the anchor. Once fully extended, the front end sets anchor. The rear end unlocks, slides itself forward toward the front anchor across the cell surface, then resets in preparation for the next cycle. Inchworm mobility may be particularly applicable to environments with extremely rough, uneven terrain.[3083] A related strategy is "Slinky" locomotion,[3084,3085] which is similar to the inchworm except that each end temporarily loses contact with the cell surface while it is extending or retracting by pushing or pulling against the anchor point.

9.4.4 Histonatation

Histonatation, or swimming through biological tissues, will be necessary for medical nanorobots that need to reach a specific histological or cellular target to begin diagnostic or repair work. Each tissue that must be traversed has its own unique set of biochemical, immunochemical, mechanical, electrokinetic, and other characteristics that will affect the precise mode and manner of locomotion. A complete survey of all possible tissue types is beyond the scope of this book. This Section briefly considers a few important issues in the following general circumstances—exiting endothelial-cell-lined blood vessels to enter the tissues (Section 9.4.4.1), passage through largely acellular tissue (Section 9.4.4.2), passage through cell-dense tissue (Section 9.4.4.3), and tissue-resident nanorobot conjugation and partition (Section 9.4.4.4).

9.4.4.1 Nanorobot Diapedesis

The passage of formed blood elements, especially white cells, through the intact walls of blood vessels, is called transendothelial migration or diapedesis (Fig. 9.28). Diapedesis is a stereotyped behavior of certain motile cells that may occur everywhere in the human body except (usually) through the brain-blood barrier.

Normally, ~75% of circulating neutrophils are adherent to the endothelium at any time.[1491] Following its rolling interaction (Section 9.4.3.6), a leukocyte may abruptly attach to the wall of a venule and leave the bloodstream by squeezing between adjacent endothelial cells. Prior to attachment, the leukocyte does not stop rolling until certain binding events occur between the vessel wall and the white cell plasma membrane. Rapid triggering (e.g., in a few seconds) of integrin-mediated adhesion is required for the arrest of bloodborne lymphocytes and neutrophils at sites of leukocyte recruitment from the blood. This adhesion is also mediated by pertussis toxin-sensitive $G\alpha_1$ protein-linked receptors of the rhodopsin-related seven-transmembrane or serpentine chemoattractant family.[982,1027] β2 integrin-mediated arrest of neutrophils can be triggered through stimulation of the formyl peptide, leukotriene B4, eotaxin, platelet activating factor, or interleukin-8 (IL-8) chemoattractant receptors in vivo.[982,1484] Particular chemokines (e.g., MIP-2β, SDF-1α, and 6-C-kine) induce flowing lymphocytes to decelerate and adhere to an integrin target protein within ~500 millisec.[1484] Adhesion is then followed by diapedesis, the final step in extravasation (exiting the blood vessel), given the presence of

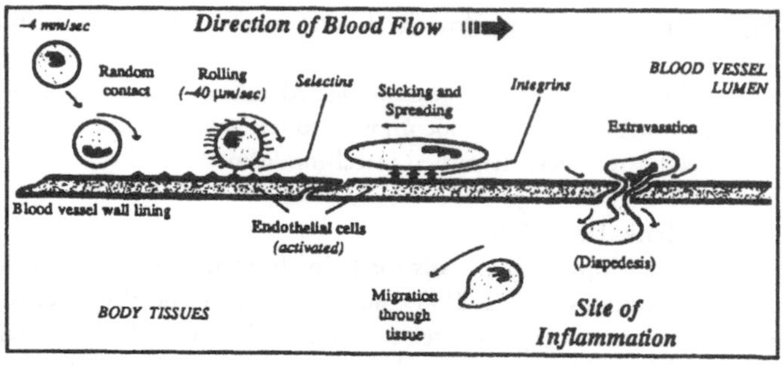

Fig. 9.28. Schematic of leukocyte diapedesis.

appropriate haptotactic (adhesion-gradient) or chemoattractant (0.0001-1 nanomolar[1512,1515] concentration-gradient) signals.

The same β_2 and α_4 integrins involved in lymphocyte arrest, in conjunction with other adhesion receptors, trigger the final steps in transendothelial migration.[1027] The junctions between adjacent endothelial cells in capillaries and venules are normally very narrow, with parallel plasma membranes forming an intercellular cleft of ~10-20 nm.[361,1493] The discontinuous-type endothelium found in the liver, spleen, and bone marrow (whose functions include the addition or extraction of whole cells from the blood) have resting gaps ~150 nm wide.[1492] In the final step of diapedesis, biochemical mediators acting on capillary endothelial cells cause those cells to loosen their attachments to their neighbors.[531] The wall gaps in the capillaries open more widely, allowing diapedesis of white cells into the tissues.[71] A wide range of pharmacologically active compounds (including prostaglandins, angiotensins, serotonin, histamine, epinephrine, and nicotine) have been observed to encourage the splitting of endothelial junctions along their symmetry plane, followed by cell separation and the appearance of gaps large enough to allow passage of whole cells—especially in the postcapillary venules.[1493] It also appears that the emigration of neutrophils and monocytes from the vasculature is normally regulated by at least three distinct molecular signals—selectin-carbohydrate, chemoattractant-receptor, and integrin-Ig interactions—acting in sequence, not in parallel. This establishes a three-digit "area code" for cell localization in the body, "as if leukocytes carr[ied] cellular phones."[1495] The sequence in which these signals act on neutrophils and lymphocytes may differ. (A neutrophil surface typically has 5 x 10^5 Mac-I integrin receptors and 2-4 x 10^4 selectin receptors).[1509,1510] Properly configured medical nanorobots can undoubtedly read these "area codes" as well (Section 8.4.3).

Diapedesis typically requires ~3-10 minutes for the white cell to complete.[1488,1490] Leukocyte emigration occurs by insertion of a pseudopod into the enlarged gap between endothelial cells, followed by amoeboid-like migration of the white cell through the blood vessel wall (Fig. 9.28). Electron microscopic studies have demonstrated that an efficient protein-tight seal is maintained between endothelial cells and a migrating leukocyte during all stages of its escape.[1489] Endothelial cells are typically 0.5 microns thick, although in postcapillary venules they may be cuboidal and much thicker.

Nanorobots engaging in diapedesis may release a minute quantity (e.g., ~0.0005 micron^3/micron^3) [1496] of the RGDS tetrapeptide (a known adhesion inhibitor),[1494] cytoambulate through the widened endothelial gap possibly using a metamorphic surface to maintain a protein-tight seal if necessary, then release endothelial movement inhibitors such as cytochalasin B or endothelial growth inhibitor protein (EGIP)[1494] to encourage endothelial reattachment, returning the gap to its normal size. (Active chemokine concentrations are typically ~10 molecules/micron^3; Section 7.4.5.2.) The actual transit of the gap should require only milliseconds assuming ~mm/sec ambulation velocities, but a time on the order of seconds could be required for biochemically-mediated endothelial cell gap width management. Physical force may be used to spread or to close a temporary gap much faster (Section 9.4.4.3) but may be inconsistent with endothelial cell homeostasis. As already noted in Section 8.2.1.3, the lymphatic endothelium can probably open gaps at least ~22.5 microns wide,[851] so micron-sized nanorobots should also find easy passage into and out of the lymphatic system.

9.4.4.2 ECM Brachiation

Taking the standard reference male human body volume of 60,000 cm^3 and subtracting ~16,000 cm^3 (27%) for fluids, digestive contents, and expandables (Section 8.2.5), then subtracting another ~27,000 cm^3 (45%) for the volume of all tissue cells (Section 8.5.1), leaves ~17,000 cm^3 (28%) which comprises the intercellular tissue volume. This volume is thoroughly penetrated by the extracellular matrix or ECM, a fibrous scaffolding that helps organize cells into tissues. The ECM contains both protein and carbohydrate components. (Matrical water is not in the form of a dilute aqueous solution but is strongly influenced by the macromolecules that are present; diffusion of small molecules is much slower in matrix water than in bulk water.)

Nanorobots with at least two appendages can alternately grasp and release a succession of adjacent ECM elements, brachiating[1621] "hand over hand" through tissue in a manner crudely analogous to a scuba diver pulling himself along an underwater rope mesh ladder. Similarly, fibroblasts migrating through tissue toward the site of a wound move toward a chemotactic distress gradient by extending lamellipodia toward the stimulus while their opposite poles remain firmly bound until released (haptotaxis). ECM fibrils strongly influence the direction of migration since cultured fibroblasts tend to align and migrate along discontinuities in substrata to which they are attached (contact guidance), and only along, but not across, fibronectin fibrils.[1537]

ECMs are composed of different collagen types, elastin, large glycoproteins (e.g., fibronectin, laminin, entactin, osteopontin), and proteoglycans that contain large glycosaminoglycan side chains (e.g., heparan sulfate, chondroitin sulfate, dermatan sulfate, keratan sulfate, hyaluronic acid).[938,985,1511] While all ECMs share these components, the organization, form, and mechanical properties of ECMs vary widely in different tissues. For example, interstitial collagens (e.g., Types I & III) self-assemble into a three-dimensional lattice which binds fibronectin and proteoglycans. This type of ECM hydrogel forms the backbone of loose connective tissues such as dermis.[985] In contrast, basement tissue membrane collagens (Types IV & V) assemble into planar arrays. When these collagenous sheets interact with fibronectin, laminin, and heparan sulfate proteoglycan, the result is a planar ECM scaffolding. The ability of tendons to resist tension, and of cartilage and bone to resist compression, similarly results from local differences in the composition and organization of the ECM.[985]

Tissues are dynamic structures that exhibit continual turnover of all molecular and cellular components. The ECM helps to maintain tissue pattern integrity, allowing cells that are lost due to injury or aging to be replaced in an organized fashion. For instance, when tissue cells are killed by freezing or poisoning, all of the cellular components may die and be removed, but the basement tissue membrane often remains intact. These residual scaffoldings ensure correct repositioning of cells (e.g., cell polarity) and proper restoration of different cell types to their correct locations (e.g., muscle cells in muscle basement tissue membrane, nerve cells in nerve sheaths, endothelium within vessels). Conversely, loss of ECM integrity during wound healing may cause permanent disorganization of tissue patterns, producing dermal scars.[985] The ECM also plays a role in controlling cell function and morphology. Hepatocytes cultured upon fibronectin or laminin at low fiber surface density (1-50 ng/cm^2) exhibit differentiation, but switch to growth at high fiber surface density (1000 ng/cm^2).[1501] Capillary-like tube formation by endothelial cells can be induced by purely mechanical means (simulating mechanical stresses in the natural ECM).[1502] Cells cultured on substrates containing adhesive islands (mimicking spatial patterns of ECM adhesivity) change shape to match the shape of the islands.[718]

The mesh size of the fibrous components of the ECM varies widely according to tissue type, but a few generalizations and specific examples can be given. For instance, the matrical function of collagen and elastin is mostly structural, while the function of fibronectin and laminin is primarily adhesive. Yet collagens are also adhesive for cells and other macromolecules, and fibronectin provides the major matrical support in clot and early granulation tissue formation (the first stages of wound repair).[985]

Collagens are the major proteins of the ECM and comprise ~25% of total mammalian protein mass.[396] The collagen family currently contains 19 members.[971,1497,1498,3614] The collagen molecule is a long (~300 nm), thin (~1.5 nm) fiber, the center of which is a characteristic triple helix running ~95% of the length.[938] Micrographs of endothelial cells cultured on a disorganized collagen-rich gel show that the cells quickly remodel the substrate into a network of collagen pads, cords, cables and bridges with grid sizes ranging from 100-1000 microns.[1499] Photomicrographs of excised tissue samples show a gap of 4-12 microns between adjacent collagen fibrils in skin tissue and in tendons.[938] Cartilage (which contains much collagen) has large aggregates of proteoglycans, with as many as 100 molecules attached to a single hyaluronic acid, giving a length of ~10 microns and a diameter of 500-600 nm; a tissue micrograph of fibrous cartilage in the disks between the vertebral bodies shows gaps of 10-30 microns between adjacent fibrils.[938]

Fibronectin is usually formed as a disulfide-linked dimer consisting of two 220-250 kilodalton peptide subunits, each containing binding sites for collagen, for heparin, for the clotting protein fibrin, and for several other ECM molecules, along with cell surface receptors.[938] The main function of laminin (a 50 nm x 70 nm cross-shaped molecule[938]) is to mediate the binding of cells to Type IV collagen. Fibronectins or laminins may be present in ECM at low density (<1 ng/mm^3) or high density (>5 ng/mm^3),[985] giving, from Eqn. 8.7, an estimated typical intermolecular spacing of L_{grid} ~ 10 microns at low density and L_{grid} ~ 4 microns at high density.

Although the matrix grid can be as narrow as 0.3-3 microns in special cases such as the ECM between the epidermis and the somites of the axolotl embryo, or between the highly flexible elastin fibers in the walls of the aorta,[938] in most cases the gaps between ECM elements should be wide enough for micron-size nanorobots to slip through without much difficulty. Even quite large rigid objects should be able to negotiate the ECM. Experimentally, teflon particles up to 80 microns in diameter were injected extravascularly and migrated to distant locations around the body including lymph nodes, lungs, and kidneys.[946]

From Eqn. 9.75, an isolated cylindrical ECM element ~1 micron long and ~0.1 micron wide could be shoved aside at a lateral velocity of ~1 mm/sec in plasma with a force of ~5 pN, easily within the strength limits of medical nanorobots having the appropriate manipulatory and motive appendages. Chemosensor pads also will allow the nanorobot to identify fiber type and tissue type (having unique chemical signatures) as the device crawls or brachiates through the ECM forest. For example, only two kinds of carbohydrate are found attached to the hydroxylysines of collagen. Elastin lacks the amino acid methionine. The family of integrins binds fibronectin, and fibronectin has lots of binding sites. Proteoglycans typically have a long core protein to which are attached up to 100 very large glycosaminoglycan (GAG) chains, with each population of core proteins having many different carbohydrates, varying in size, charge, and even composition.[938] Sensor pads can make a cell-type or tissue-type determination in as little as 2 millisec (Section 8.5.2.2), suggesting an upper limit on nanorobot ECM brachiation of ν_{brach} ~ 500 Hz if chemopositional validation is required at every step.

What is the maximum safe nanorobot brachiation speed through the ECM? In theory, a dibrachial armswing of ~1 micron repeated at ~100 Hz allows an ECM transit speed up to 100 microns/sec through clear fluid lanes in the matrix. From Eqn. 9.73, the force required to pull a 1 micron spherical object through 310 K interstitial fluid (Table 9.4) at 100 microns/sec is ~2 pN, somewhat less than the ~10 pN likely to stimulate a mechanically-transduced cellular response (Section 9.4.3.2.1). (One study found that the force required to break individual integrin bonds to fibrinogen is ~2.1 pN;[1508] another study found ~1000 cell adhesion proteoglycan molecules on each marine sponge cell surface, with pairs on adjacent surfaces having an experimentally measured adhesion of 40-400 pN per pair, depending upon Ca^{++} concentration.[1248]) Assuming a pair of 1 micron long, 0.1 micron thick cylindrical nanorobot arms and applying Eqn. 9.75, an additional ~0.5 pN is required to move each arm forward, giving a total power requirement of only ~0.0003 pW for brachiation at ~100 microns/sec. For comparison, a proposal to drive a millimeter-size "seed" through human brain parenchyma using external magnetic forces, while maintaining what was believed to be an adequate margin of safety, was tested experimentally at a net tissue transit speed of ~8 microns/sec.[1256,1257]

Natural movement of biological entities through ECM is much slower. The ECM provides a handhold-rich scaffold for fibroblast migration.[359] Leukocyte and fibroblast amoeboid motion through extracellular tissue is typically ~0.050-0.7 microns/sec (Section 9.4.3.7), although white cell diapedesis through the blood vessel walls (~0.005 microns/sec; Section 9.4.4.1) is much slower. Chain migration of neuronal precursor cells across a restricted pathway in the brain, through a complex parenchyma between two regions separated by several millimeters, occurs at ~0.008 microns/sec.[947] The migratory speed of cultured smooth muscle cells taken from coronary and peripheral arterial walls is also only ~0.006-0.015 microns/sec.[1503] Epithelial cells migrate over a wound surface in a sheet at ~0.035 microns/sec, while wound contraction proceeds at 0.007-0.009 microns/sec.[359] Osteoclasts tunnel through old bone, remodeling it, advancing at a rate of only ~0.0006 microns/sec.[531] However, inside cytomatrix-rich cells, membrane-bound vesicles undergo axonal transport at a typical speed ~2-4 microns/sec,[938,939] pigment granules in chromatophores move at 2-10 microns/sec,[938] and mitochondria (~micron-sized organelles) are shuttled around the cellular interior at up to ~10 microns/sec,[453] so faster ECM transit speeds up to ~100 microns/sec are probably safe.

9.4.4.3 Intercellular Passage

With just a few notable exceptions, virtually all tissue cells lie within ~2-3 cell widths of a capillary, or ~50 microns.[71,531] Thus a bloodborne nanorobot may reach any tissue cell by rapidly traveling most of the way by capillary, then exiting the capillary and crossing at most 1-2 cells to arrive at a given target cell. In cell dense tissue, it may become necessary to crawl between adhering cells.

Tissue cells are not packed so tightly that adjacent cell surfaces are in direct contact with each other. There is usually a space of at least 20 nm between the opposing plasma membranes of adjacent cells, wide enough to admit a slender nanorobot manipulator arm (Section 9.3.1). This space is filled with extracellular fluid and provides a pathway for substances to pass between cells on their way to and from the blood in nearby capillaries. Most tissues employ desmosome or gap junctions[2922] wherein the opposing plasma membranes come within 2-4 nm of each other over a space of ~5 nm on the membrane surface, with these junctions spaced ~20 nm apart across the plasma membranes and opposing plasma membranes, retaining a fluid-filled 25-35 nm gap between them. Tight or "occluding" junctions (as in the endothelial blood-brain barrier and certain epithelial surfaces comprised of intestinal cells, bladder cells, and some exocrine cells) have <2.5 nm wide intermembrane gaps.[361] None of these spaces is wide enough to allow passage of whole (even metamorphic) medical nanorobots. To pass between cells in cell-rich tissue, it is necessary for an advancing nanorobot to disrupt some minimum number of cell-to-cell adhesive contacts that lie ahead in its path. After that, and with the objective of minimizing biointrusiveness, the nanorobot must reseal those adhesive contacts in its wake, after passage, crudely analogous to a burrowing mole.

A full treatment of all types of cell-cell contacts and anchoring mechanisms is beyond the scope of this book, but a few specific examples can be given. For instance, spot desmosomes (Section 5.4) are ~30-nm-long "spot weld" molecules linking neighboring cells, spaced ~8 nm apart across the apposed cellular surfaces. A force of 6-10 pN is required to separate each connexin-32 hepatic cell gap junction unit (Section 5.4.2). Integrins may average ~20 nm separation, and require ~2.1 pN to separate from a fibronectin molecule in the ECM,[1508] although direct cell-ECM connections are relatively scarce inside cell-cell junctions.

As a crude estimate, assume that intercellular adhesion molecules h_{adhes} ~ 30 nm in length are spaced X_{adhes} ~ 10 nm apart across the cell surfaces and require F_{adhes} ~ 10 pN to pull apart,[1223] and that an L_{nano} ~ 1 micron wide nanorobot wishes to pass through by dynamically clearing a path ahead that is L_{nano} wide and L_{nano} long. Along the leading edge, L_{nano}/X_{adhes} adhesive joints must be detached one by one, requiring a detachment energy of $E_{detach} \sim L_{nano} F_{adhes} h_{adhes} / X_{adhes}$ ~ 30,000 zJ to advance a distance X_{adhes}. This gives a power requirement of $P_{travel} \sim E_{detach} v_{travel} / X_{adhes}$ ~ 0.003 pW if the velocity of forward travel through the cell-cell junction is v_{travel} ~ 1 micron/sec, allowing transit between two adhered 20-micron cells in ~20 sec. Adding manipulator arm energy dissipation raises the total to ~0.01 pW (viscous drag power is ~10^{-5} pW; Eqns. 9.74 and 9.75). Total detachment rate is $v_{detach} \sim L_{nano} v_{travel} / X_{adhes}^2$ ~ 10,000 detachments/sec, a burden which can be shared by more than one manipulatory appendage, each equipped with appropriate lytic end-effectors (e.g., trypsin-like tool tips; Section 9.3.2). Rejoining the parted cell junctions astern requires, at worst, a similar energy expenditure; in the case of noncovalent bonds, unassisted rejoining may be energetically favorable if the edges have been left in relative proximity. Reattachment may be facilitated using a metamorphic nanorobot integument, together with a surfacial hydrophilic solvation wave drive system (Section 9.4.5.3), to establish a teardrop-shaped cross-section that can slowly adduct the separated plasma membrane faces and maneuver the detached stubs of parted anchor macromolecules into close proximity. Traffic density and frequency should be locally restricted to minimize mechanical stimulation of unwanted ECM and cytomatrical responses (Sections 9.4.3.2.1 and 9.4.4.2), and especially detachment-triggered apoptosis (Section 10.4.1.1), perhaps by restricting intercellular passage to nanorobots traveling single-file through a relatively small number of channels.

9.4.4.4 Nanorobot Conjugation and Partition

Occasionally it may be necessary for two or more motile nanorobots to dock, or conjugate,[3617-3632] during histonatation (e.g., Section 8.3.3). Assuming the existence of in vivo communication and navigation networks (Sections 7.3 and 8.3), two nanorobots that are attempting to dock can exchange positional information until the two devices are within a range of ~3 microns. Once within such close range, the devices switch to ~GHz chirps which, from Eqn. 4.52, attenuate ~0.001%/nm in 310 K plasma. Using an acoustic receiver sensitive to 10^{-6} atm pressure changes, and 0.01-atm transmitted pulses, and assuming that no other nanorobots are present and chirping in the immediate vicinity at the same time, the two nanorobots can locomote up the attenuation gradient to within ~10 nm proximity, approximately the minimum scale of the docking mechanism (e.g., metamorphic bumpers; Section 5.4). Conjugating microbes employ chemical communications to similar effect.[3628,3629]

Once physical contact is made, nanomechanical communication at ~1 GHz transfers ~1000 bits during a ~1 microsec contact event (Section 7.2.4), sufficient to mutually validate identity. A universal clamp may be used for unrestricted docking among devices of any machine species that meet in any orientation. Device shape or surface features can be used to control docking orientation (Section 5.4.1). Docking clamps can also be designed to connect in only one way if the spatial or rotational positioning of the conjugated pair is an important mission requirement; from Eqn. 3.1, Brownian motion provides ~4000 random docking trials per second for two 1-micron nanorobots maintaining a mean 10-nm separation in 310 K interstitial fluid. Docking clamps may serve a purely adhesive function,[3630-3632] or may additionally provide communicating junctions that transfer fluids, power, or data between conjugated devices. Similar procedures permit three or more nanorobots to conjugate in vivo, and may allow a growing nanorobot aggregate to sequentially add new members to the collective at specific locations in the developing structure.

Partition,[3617-3619] or separation of linked nanorobots, requires a defined procedure in which all transtegumental openings in nanorobots are sealed or valved shut prior to release of docking clamps and physical separation. Once separated, and depending upon their mode of locomotion and the timing of their release, partitioned nanorobots must temporarily observe a dense-traffic protocol involving slower and lower-amplitude motions of motive appendages or rotating elements in order to:

1. avoid mechanical conflict among such appendages or elements between neighbors;
2. avoid potentially chaotic hydrodynamic interactions (Section 9.4.2.3); and
3. clear a sufficient interdevice distance to preclude significant error in positional readings from the navigation grid (Section 8.3.3), due to spurious acoustic refraction and attenuation effects if there is a large number density of nanorobots in the vicinity.

9.4.5 Cytopenetration

Upon arriving at a target tissue cell, a cellular repair nanorobot may require entry into the cytosol. The following is a necessarily brief and incomplete discussion of several techniques and issues involved in penetrating the plasma membrane, and by extension, in penetrating other intracellular membrane structures including the doubled-walled nuclear envelope and the multilayer outer membranes of Gram-negative bacteria (Section 10.4.2.5). Micron-size siliceous diatoms and "nanobacteria" with calcium shells[2149,3096] and will require additional penetrative mechanisms that are not described here. This discussion also is applicable to the insertion of sensory appendages or manipulatory devices through cell or organelle lipid membranes.

9.4.5.1 Transmembrane Brachiation

One simple approach to cytopenetration is to insert a narrow manipulator arm through the plasma membrane, perhaps assisted by a wall-breaching tool tip analogous to the T4 lysozyme enzyme that opens a hole in bacterial cell peptidoglycan walls,[3150-3152] or the T4 DNA-injection system that is specifically designed for lipid bilayer penetration.[1179,1180] The terminus of the manipulator firmly attaches to an actin or microtubular fixed component of the interior cytoskeleton, then retracts, towing the nanorobot through the lipid bilayer surface. Metamorphic reshaping of the nanorobot aspect minimizes the total number of noncovalent lipid bilayer bonds that must be disturbed during transit. Cell surfaces tolerate forces up to ~1 nN per 100 nm^2 before breaking, so a ~1 nN arm tip smaller than 100 nm^2 in cross section should be able to push itself through the cellular plasma membrane and into the interior of the cell. As a very crude estimate of the penetration energy required, taking the membranolytic limit as 3×10^6 N/m^2, then a 1-micron long, 1-nm wide tear can be opened up by applying ~3000 pN of force through a distance of ~10 nm (typical plasma membrane thickness) costing ~30,000 zJ of energy, a ~0.003 pW power demand during a ~10 millisec transit time at a ~100 micron/sec transit speed. It may also be possible to reduce entry forces by inducing lipid bilayer membrane demixing using a tangentially-applied electric field.[1613]

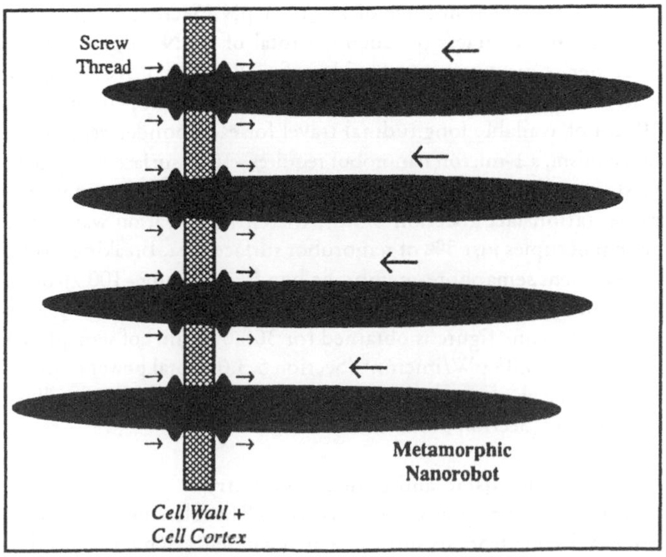

Fig. 9.29. Schematic of metamorphic screw drive for cytopenetration.

9.4.5.2 Metamorphic Screw Drive

A nanorobot with a hydrophobic (e.g., diamondoid) metamorphic surface may locally reconfigure its prow in the shape of a screw having two traveling raised ridges, with a thread width at least as wide as the plasma membrane plus the plasma membrane skeleton or cell cortex, perhaps 30-50 nm thick (Section 8.5.3.11). After the screw has initially penetrated the surface and the first thread course is locked in place (Section 9.4.5.1), the thread pattern may then be translated toward the rear of the nanorobot, allowing the device to screw itself into the cell's interior (Fig. 9.29). A ~100 micron/sec transit speed requires <0.001 pW for a 1 micron^2 cross-section nanorobot to overcome viscous drag (Section 9.4.2.4) and ~0.01 pW to operate a 100-nm wide section of metamorphic surface assuming ~0.35 micron^2 of surface dissipating ~0.03 pW/micron^2 (Sections 5.3.1.4 and 5.3.6). Cell entry is completed in ~10 millisec.

9.4.5.3 Solvation Wave Drive

The lipid bilayer membrane is hydrophilic on the outermost and innermost surfaces, and lipophilic in the interior (Fig. 8.37). Much like the physical screw described in the previous Section, the hydrophilicity of the nanorobot exterior surface may also be manipulated to produce a traveling helical solvation wave that establishes temporary noncovalent bonds with elements of the plasma membrane, allowing the nanorobot to pull itself through the lipid bilayer (Fig. 9.30). The plasma membrane is typically 6-10 nm thick (Section 8.5.3.2). The cholesterol-poor lipid membranes of the mitochondria and the endoplasmic reticulum have a 2.5 nm inner hydrophobic region, while cholesterol-rich lipid membranes like those of the plasma membrane and the endosomes have a 3.1 nm wide hydrophobic region.[1113-1115] Each contact point may be envisioned as a semaphore-like mechanism (Section 5.3.6) by which lipophilic or hydrophilic moieties are rotated into an exposed position (facilitating noncovalent bonding with a particular lipid bilayer phase), then moved a short distance relative to the nanorobot body (transmitting force to the nanorobot), then rotated back into a nonexposed position (breaking the bond to the lipid membrane).

From Eqn. 9.73, a 1-micron nanorobot traveling at ~100 microns/sec must generate ~2 pN of motive force in order to overcome the viscous resistance of plasmalike fluid at 310 K. Given a single-lipid extraction force of F_{lipid} ~ 1 pN (Section 9.4.3.1), ten simultaneous contacts producing a total of 2 pN reduces applied force per contact to a reasonably safe ~20% F_{lipid}. Assuming 10 simultaneous contacts spaced around the nanorobot perimeter and 10 nm of available longitudinal travel for each bonded semaphore mechanism, a 1-micron nanorobot requires ~1000 surface semaphores in staggered configuration. Allowing ~300 nm^2 per semaphore presentation face (Section 5.3.6), the entire solvation wave drive system occupies just 5% of nanorobot surface area. Breaking ~1000 noncovalent semaphore-membrane bonds, assuming ~100 zJ/bond (Section 3.5.2), during a 10 millisec transit requires ~0.01 pW of power; the same figure is obtained for 300,000 nm^2 of semaphores dissipating ~0.03 pW/micron^2 (Section 5.3.6).Total power required to overcome viscous resistance is ~0.0002 pW during the ~10 millisec transit time (Section 9.4.2.4).

9.4.5.4 Vesicle Fusion and Endocytotic Entry

A nanorobot may also gain entry to a cell by releasing amphipathic lipid molecules from its surface, which will self-assemble into a thin lipid bilayer coat, enveloping the entire nanorobot. Natural viruses[1721] and synthetic carriers[1722] use similar methods to convey extracellular DNA across outer cell plasma membranes and nuclear membranes. The materials comprising a 10-nm thick lipid bilayer surrounding a spherical object ~1 micron in radius can be stored in a ~0.1 micron^3 internal tank, occupying only ~3% of total internal device volume. The fusion of two distinct lipid bilayers is energetically unfavorable in the absence of specialized proteins.[1530] Thus after approaching the target plasma membrane, the enveloped nanorobot must emit specialized plasma membrane fusion proteins, known as fusogens,[1587,3658] similar to the sperm protein PH-30α–β that allows sperm and egg to merge,[1082] the HIV virus envelope protein gp120-gp41 with a typical contact area of ~8 nm^2,[1531,1587] the envelope glycoprotein H employed by the herpesvirsuses,[3657] and the hemagglutinin protein found on the surface of influenza virus.[1532] (Nonprotein fusogens also are well-known, including lipids such as N-acyl phosphatidylethanolamines (NAPEs),[3659] fatty acids such as arachidonic acid,[3660] carbohydrates such as polyethylene glycol,[3661] and simple solvents such as dimethyl sulfoxide (DMSO).[3662])The nanorobot lipid bilayer, now fusion active, can join with the plasma membrane layer and unfold, bringing the

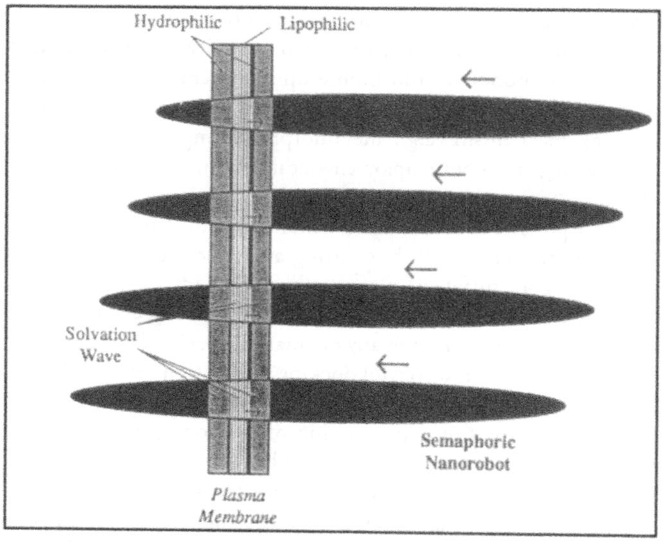

Fig. 9.30. Schematic of solvation wave drive for cytopenetration.

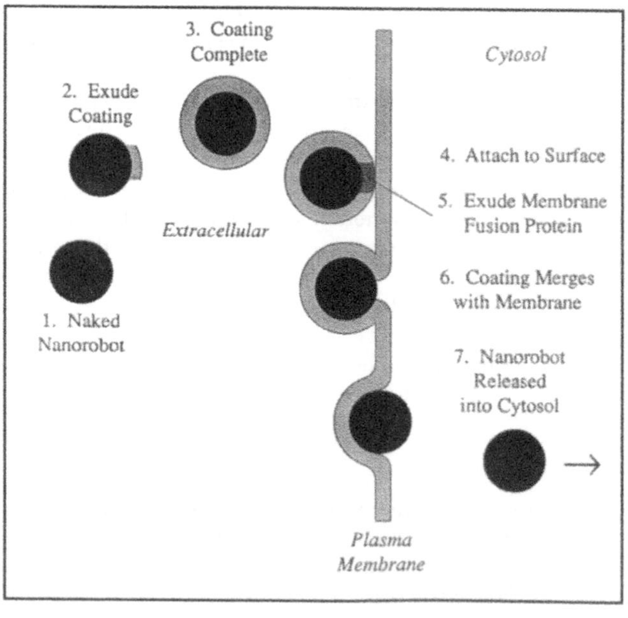

Fig. 9.31. Schematic of vesicle fusion for cytopenetration.

formerly fully enclosed nanorobot into direct sealed contact with the cytosol with a negligible energy expenditure (Fig. 9.31). This process will add 0.5%-1.0% new lipid, by volume, to the existing ~14-24 micron^3 plasma membrane volume (Table 8.17) of a 20-micron tissue cell. Added lipids that don't exactly match the native lipids of the cell might disrupt the normal protein/lipid membrane ratio and modify membrane fluidity, possibly altering signal timing and other cell behaviors. If this is a problem, nanorobots employing this entry technique could be designed to reabsorb and recycle the foreign lipid, once inside the cell.

Other means of cell entry, such as "induced uptake," are well known. Like bacterial invaders, a nanorobot may emit cytochemical "entry mediator" signals (e.g., the outer wall membrane protein invasin, in *Yersinia* bacteria) to induce the target cell to form an endocytotic vacuole around the device and suck it into the interior of the cell. A membrane fusion-type tool may subsequently be used to escape from the resulting endosome. Macrophages ingest up to ~25% of their volume per hour,[996] a volume equivalent to hundreds of micron-sized nanorobots. Many bacteria[1012,1561] and viruses[1530,1533] gain entry to cells by this means, and phagocytosis is mechanically similar. Both are initiated by ligand-receptor interactions that activate host signaling, with the actin cytoskeleton providing the necessary force to internalize the particle into a membrane-bound vacuole.[1012] Invasive bacteria utilize two major types of induced uptake:

1. a "zipper" type mechanism involving direct contact between bacterial ligands and cellular receptors that sequentially encircle the organism (e.g., *Yersinia*, *Listeria*); and;
2. a "trigger" mechanism in which bacterial signals to the cell induce dramatic plasma membrane ruffling and cytoskeletal rearrangements resulting in macropinocytosis with virtually passive entry of the bacterium (e.g., *Salmonella*, *Shigella*) into the cell.[1012,1561,3191]

9.4.5.5 Cytosolic Leakage During Transit

If the nanorobot-membrane interface is not tight, some leakage of material into or out of the cell (depending upon relative hydraulic and osmotic pressures) may occur during nanodevice transit. For example, from Eqn. 3.1 the Brownian diffusion distance during a $t_{transit}$ ~ 10 millisec transit time is ~3 microns for small molecules like amino acids (MW ~ 100 daltons), ~1 micron for large protein molecules (MW ~ 100,000 daltons). An annular leakage ring of width h_{leak} ~ 10 nm around the circumference of a nanorobot of radius R_{nano} ~ 1 micron may pass $V_{leak} \sim 2 \pi R_{nano} h_{leak} v_{leak} t_{transit}$ ~ 0.006 micron^3 of cytosolic fluid during each transit (~0.00008% of cell volume), assuming v_{leak} ~ 10 microns/sec for random hydrodynamic flows induced by thermal fluctuations inside a cell (Section 8.5.3.12). Alternatively, modeling the leak as a ring of $N_{pipe} = 2 \pi R_{nano} / r_{tube}$ = 1257 nanopipes each of radius $r_{tube} \sim h_{leak}/2$ and length l_{tube} ~ 10 nm, and taking Δp ~ 0.001 atm for the interstitial/cellular pressure differential (Section 4.9.1.2), then from Eqn. 9.25 the total leakage volume from the ring of nanopipes is $V_{leak} \sim N_{pipe} \dot{V}_{HP} t_{transit}$ ~ 0.03 micron^3 of cytosolic fluid during each transit, or ~0.0004% of cell volume. Leakage may be reduced by encouraging a tighter seal during transit using a dynamic ring pattern of lipophilic semaphores at the nanorobot surface (Section 9.4.5.3) that tracks the device's passage through the plasma membrane. In some cases such as nerve cells, significant ionic leakage could produce depolarization and thus should be avoided.

9.4.5.6 Breach Sealing and Intrusiveness

Some cytopenetration techniques involve tearing the lipid bilayer. This breach must be resealed after transit. A fractured lipid membrane presents two "greasy" surfaces to water; it is thermodynamically favorable for these two cut surfaces to fuse together so as to eliminate the unfavorable water-fat interface.[27,2316] Such fusion may be encouraged mechanically by the passing nanorobot (Section 9.4.4.3), although the edges of the tear will attempt to round off and self-seal, without rejoining.

Nevertheless, it is not uncommon to observe rapid natural resealing of plasma membranes with little loss of intracellular contents, a useful property given the many transient plasma membrane disruptions that commonly occur in cells that experience significant mechanical stress, such as gut, skin, endothelium, and muscle.[1534,3665] In one experiment, tissue cell plasma membranes were punctured using 2-3 micron diameter micropipettes and a 300 millisec transit (wounding) time, and the torn plasma membrane spontaneously resealed in 10-30 sec with relatively little visible loss of injected dye.[1534] Exocytosis-based resealing[3666-3668] of a microneedle puncture through the fibroblast plasma membrane occurs in 5-10 sec,[3667] but a second puncture at the same site heals faster than the initial wound[3668]—at first wounding, the cell uses existing endocytotic compartment to add membrane necessary for resealing, but Ca^{++} entry at the first wound stimulates vesicle formation from the Golgi apparatus, resulting in more rapid resealing of the second membrane disruption.[3668]

Watertight breach sealing might even be possible for nanorobots trailing narrow, untensioned tethers with lipophilic coatings, although such tethers may cause other problems (Sections 6.4.3.6 and 7.3.3); 0.1-micron optical fiber tips have been poked through a cellular plasma membrane to measure the pH of the cytoplasm inside, in single cells and in single rat embryos, without ill effect on these large cells.[577] In small cells (2-15 micron diameter), "stab" microinjection at high pressure (0.1-0.2 atm) is problematic because the nucleus-to-cytoplasm ratio is higher so the nucleus is more likely to be damaged during the stab. In one experiment, less than 5% of neutrophils survived the high-pressure stab intact, but a low-pressure (~0.01 atm) injection through a lipid bridge produced a ~100% survival rate.[2346]

How many nanorobots (or other pieces of exogenous matter) can safely squeeze into a living cell? This question is addressed further in Chapter 15, but an extremely conservative volumetric injection limit is ~50-100 micron^3 per tissue cell (0.5-1% of typical cell volume) without any significant observed effect on cell viability[1192]—equivalent to ~3-100 bloodborne nanorobots, depending upon object size. Individual lymphocytes (~200 micron^3)[777] have also been observed circulating for hours inside large living cells, with no evident ill effect (Section 8.5.3.12).

In some nanorobotic system configurations and applications, it may be useful to deploy smaller intracellular probes tethered to larger extracellular command centers. For example, axonal "cleanout" could be an important anti-aging activity, given the evidence that axonal transport slows with age presumably due to debris accumulation or a decline in energy supplies; yet full-size nanorobots might not conveniently fit inside some neural axons. Transmembrane tethers (tipped with relatively small unfurlable mechanisms) may be passed into the cell's interior by threading them through an anchored transmembrane sleeve device. Fluid leakage between tether and inner sleeve wall, either into or out of the cytosol, can be minimized if both surfaces are hydrophobic. There are, of course, many important drawbacks to the use of tethered systems generally (Sections 6.4.3.6 and 7.3.3).

9.4.5.7 Nuclear Membrane Penetration

Most of the methods proposed for plasma membrane penetration can also be applied to the nuclear membrane, with several important differences. First, the entry procedure should proceed at a much slower velocity, to preclude any possibility of damaging the chromatin (Section 8.5.4.7). Second, chromatin is attached to the nuclear cortex away from the nuclear pores, and also in specific chromosomal territories, so special care must be taken to avoid disturbing these configurations. Third, the region to be traversed is much deeper—two lipid bilayer membranes separated by a perinuclear space, and lined on the nucleoplasmic side by a nuclear cortex of varying width (Fig. 8.46)—which may require a somewhat different design than systems used for single-membrane bilayer penetration.

9.4.6 In Cyto Locomotion

Once inside a cell, a motile nanorobot must navigate a cluttered and highly viscous cytomatrix-rich environment (Section 8.5.3). (When microscopic iron particles are introduced into the cytoplasm, they move erratically (rather than smoothly) under the influence of external magnetic fields.[938]) Any of the methods described for cytoambulation (Section 9.4.3), histonatation (Section 9.4.4), or cytopenetration (Section 9.4.5) may also be employed in modified form within the cell. From Eqn. 9.65 and the data in Table 9.4, and assuming a top speed of v ~ 10 microns/sec (Section 9.4.4.2), then the Reynolds number of an L ~ 1 micron object inside a red blood cell (a nucleus-free floppy bag filled with hemoglobin solution) is $N_R \sim 10^{-6}$. For a nanorobot inside a free leukocyte, $N_R \sim 10^{-9}$; inside an *E. coli* bacterium, $N_R \sim 10^{-11}$, taking the higher viscosity into account.

There are many natural transport mechanisms inside cytomatrix-rich cells which may serve as analogs for in cyto nanorobot locomotion. For example, vesicles and granules ~100 nm in diameter or larger are carried at a peak speed of up to ~2 microns/sec (although mean unloaded kinesin motor speed is usually 0.5-0.8 microns/sec) on the back of a 60-nm kinesin transport molecule (Fig. 9.32) that takes 8-nm ATP-powered steps along microtubule tracks running throughout the cell[1535,1536,3202-3204] with a stall force of 5-7 pN;[3201,3202] typically kinesin takes ~100 steps along a microtubule, then lets go. Nanorobots could be designed to brachiate along these tracks as well. Inside giant amoebas, mitochondria measuring 1-3 microns in length are carried along microtubules at speeds up to 10 microns/sec,[453] and the pseudopods of fibroblasts (and amoebas) can also extend at ~10 microns/sec.[1252] Faster speeds may be possible for well-designed nanorobots, but an upper limit of ~10 microns/sec through fluid-rich intracellular clear channels seems reasonably conservative.

It is well-known that several pathogenic bacterial species, once free in the cytoplasm of a human cell, propel themselves through the cytosol using a continuous actin polymerization process that takes place at one pole of the bacterium.[1012] Actin assembly is visible as a tail of polymerized F-actin that remains stationary in the cytosol while the bacterium moves ahead. The polymerizing tail rectifies the random thermal motions of the bacterium, preventing it from diffusing backwards while permitting forward diffusion; thus the tail doesn't actually "push" the bacterium forward.[1203] Actin-based motility is mediated by a single bacterial protein—ActA (610 amino acids) in *Listeria* and IcsA/VirG (120,000 daltons) in *Shigella*—localized in the polar regions of the bacterium.[1012] Actin microfilaments (and tubulin) typically self-assemble at ~0.1-1 micron/sec;[942] actin polymerization gives a stall force of ~10 pN per fiber, sufficient to drive a 1-micron object at ~1.5 micron/sec against a ~1 pN load in free fluid cytoplasm.[1203] This probably defines the top speed for actin-based bacterial mobility.

To progress through dense cytomatrical regions, motile nanorobots of similar size to bacteria must cut or detach cross-bridged cytoskeletal elements lying across the path ahead, then attempt to reattach or reconstruct those elements after the nanorobot has passed through the breach, because these elements lack sufficient elasticity (and grid sizes are too small) to be pushed completely out of the way. Such cytoskeletal elements will most commonly include intermediate filaments and actin-based microfilaments. This procedure is crudely analogous to the process employed by fibroblasts transiting the ECM during wound repair. Fibroblast movement into cross-linked fibrin blood clots or tightly woven ECM requires an active proteolytic system that cleaves a pathway for migration; known enzymes serving this purpose include plasminogen activator, interstitial collagenase (MMP-1), the 72 kilodalton gelatinase A (MMP-2), and stromelysin (MMP-3).[1537]

For an average filament grid size of $L_{grid} \sim 100$ nm for the cortical actin cytogel[1203] and a nanorobot of radius $R_{nano} \sim 1$ micron, a minimum of two long diagonal cuts each of length 2 R_{nano} (simplistically, making four triangular flaps) to allow passage requires $N_{cut} = 4\ R_{nano}\ /\ L_{grid} = 40$ transected grid segments in order to advance a distance L_{grid}, or $\nu_{cut} = 4\ R_{nano}\ v_{nano}\ /\ L_{grid}^2 = 400$ cuts (or reattachments) per second at $v_{nano} \sim 1$ micron/sec. This compares favorably with the $\nu_{brach} \sim 500$ Hz estimated earlier for a manipulator arm used for ECM brachiation, where chemopositional validation is required at every step (Section 9.4.4.2), and is well below the $\nu_{detach} \sim 10$ KHz estimated for intercellular passage where such validation is not required (Section 9.4.4.3). An important additional design issue for in cyto brachiation systems is to minimize accidental mechanical

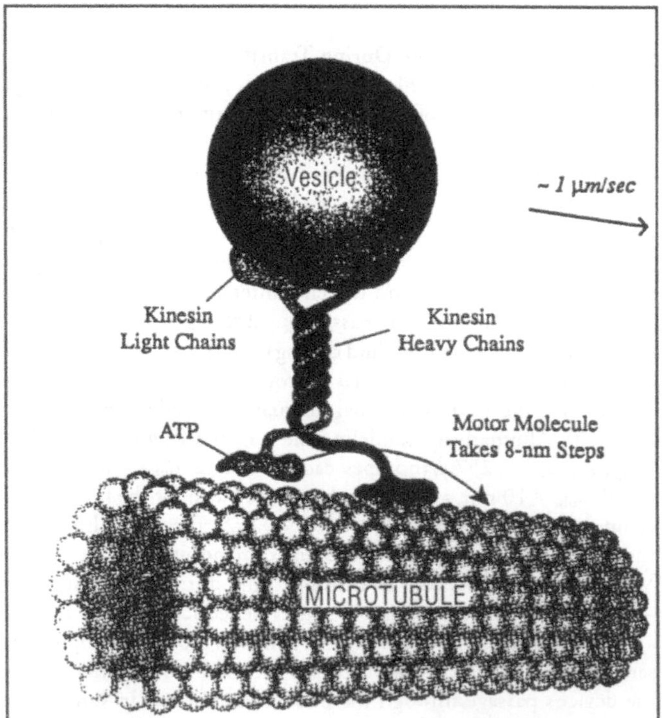

Fig. 9.32. Vesicle carried along microtubule track by kinesin transport molecule (schematic only, modified from Travis[1535]).

signal transduction into the nucleus, which may trigger unwanted cytological responses.

Power requirements for intracellular mobility are typically modest but vary widely, depending mainly upon velocity, the type of cell, and the path chosen. In highly fluidic clear channels, viscosity should more closely resemble that of the red cell interior ($\eta \sim 10^{-2}$ kg/m-sec), so from Eqn. 9.74 and taking R_{nano} = 1 micron and $v_{nano} \sim$ 10 microns/sec, then $P_{nano}/e\% \sim$ (0.00002 pW)/e% for pure cytonatation. Nanorobots traversing pathways through filament-rich regions of the cell will experience much higher effective viscosities, on the order of $\eta \sim$ 10-1000 kg/m-sec (Table 9.4), but will also travel more slowly (e.g., $v_{nano} \sim$ 1 micron/sec), giving a viscous resistance power requirement for the nanorobot body of $P_{nano}/e\% \sim$ (0.0002-0.02 pW)/e%, from Eqn. 9.74. A telescoping manipulator arm measuring 500 nm in length, performing the filament cuts and joins at $v_{cut} \sim v_{join} \sim$ 400 Hz with ~2.5 microns of tool-tip travel per cycle, moves at a tip speed of ~1 mm/sec, producing ~0.025 pW of mechanical losses under no-load conditions (Section 9.3.1.4); there are at least two operational arms, one fore and one (or more) aft. Multiple arms may be needed in a dense filament network. Another ~0.025 pW is required to overcome the viscous resistance against each moving arm (using Eqn. 9.75), giving a total power cost of 0.1-0.3 pW for transfilamentary intracellular locomotion at $v_{nano} \sim$ 1 micron/sec assuming locomotive efficiency e% = 0.10 (10%).

Some of the difficulties and limitations of in nucleo locomotion have already been mentioned in Sections 8.5.4.7 and 9.4.5.7. The most important constraint is to observe a maximum speed limit that avoids mechanical chromatin damage. Although a 500 kilodalton protein would diffuse from one side of a 5-8 micron nucleus to the other in only ~5-6 sec (~1 micron/sec average), normal chromosomal movements during interphase have been estimated by observing the motions of individual centromeres, typically 0.002-0.003 microns/sec,[1529] and peak chromosome transport speeds during mitosis are ~0.1 micron/sec.[1463] A strict in nucleo speed limit of ~0.1 micron/sec on all nanorobot bodies and most exposed appendages appears prudent. A force limit of ~50 pN for intranuclear locomotion should also be observed (Section 8.5.4.7)—a 1-micron nanorobot picking its way through a filament-rich medium of net viscosity ~10 kg/m-sec requires the application of ~20 pN to overcome viscous drag at a travel speed of ~0.1 micron/sec.

9.4.7 Cytocarriage

The commandeering of natural motile cells by medical nanorobots, known as cytocarriage, offers an alternative mode of in vivo transport. During cytocarriage, one or more medical nanorobots may enter a motile cell, ride or steer the cell to a desired destination inside the human body, then vacate the cell upon arrival. The discussion here is a necessarily brief overview of the objectives of cytocarriage (Section 9.4.7.1), cytovehicle selection (Section 9.4.7.2), initiating cytocarriage (Section 9.4.7.3), steering and control during the journey (Section 9.4.7.4), cytocarriage navigation and sensing (Section 9.4.7.5) and cytovehicular behavioral control (Section 9.4.7.6).

9.4.7.1 Objectives of Cytocarriage

One of the most important utilities of cytocarriage is the "cell herding" function.[9] Nanorobots can marshall significant resources drawn from the body's natural immune and wound repair systems, and redirect them to particular sites that are in urgent need of assistance. In this role, medical nanorobots may act as immune system or wound repair homeostatic accelerants, regardless of the nanorobots' own additional inherent reparative functions, which may be considerable. Nanorobots may also seize control of pathogen and parasite mobility systems, then guide them to natural disposal sites within the body.

While nanorobot control of the natural motility apparatus might slightly improve its performance, as a practical matter the maximum speed of cytovehicles being driven through tissues is probably limited to near the maximum observed natural speeds of in vivo progression of uncontrolled cells (e.g., ~1-10 microns/sec). This will normally be considerably slower than the maximum transtissue speeds available to self-propelled medical nanodevices (e.g., 100-1000 microns/sec). Also, cytocarriage is usually energetically inefficient compared to self-propelled medical nanorobots. However, in some circumstances a strategy of cytocarriage may avoid the need to include certain propulsive mechanisms in the nanorobot design for some segments of the mission pathway, thus reducing nanodevice design complexity and freeing up scarce onboard storage volume for additional consumables or mission-critical machinery. Cytovehicles (e.g., leukocytes) engineered to display organ-specific tissue homing could be preloaded with passenger nanorobots prior to injection into the patient. Once injected, the nanorobots would be delivered to the intended destination with acceptable reliability. Of course, surface-placed antigen semaphores (Section 5.3.6) may directly confer a similar homing ability on bloodborne nanorobots, with equal or superior reliability.

Due to the small size of most readily available cytovehicles, conservatively only one or at most a few nanorobots may be able to safely enter and occupy the interior of each commandeered motile cell without triggering unwanted cellular responses (Chapter 15). However, additional nanorobot passengers may adhere to the exterior of the plasma membrane of the cytovehicle (after disabling certain natural haptotactic reactivities), or may be towed by the motile cell, allowing the motile cell to serve as a "pack animal" or "biological tractor." Interestingly, protozoa called mixotrichs that are present in the termite gut are propelled by several thousand bacterial spirochetes attached to the protozoan as obligate symbiotes;[2025-2027] S. Vogel observes that "the protozoa have adopted bacteria as engines the way a human might use a team of horses."[2022]

Even heavily burdened cytovehicles operate at very low Reynolds numbers (Section 9.4.2.1), so the total mass of passengers (M_{pass}, determining the inertial load) is relatively unimportant compared to the total surface area of the passengers (A_{pass}, determining the viscous load); $M_{pass} \sim N_{pass}$ (the number of passengers per cell), but $A_{pass} \sim N_{pass}^{2/3}$ for efficiently packed passengers. Given a towing strength of 165 nN for the human fibroblast,[1461] a properly harnessed single fibroblast cell traversing interstitial fluid at a speed of 10 microns/sec can in theory tow behind it a 20-micron wide, 1000-micron long cylindrically-packed aggregate of $N_{pass} \sim$ 300,000 1-micron^3 nanorobot passengers with a towing force of only F_{nanop} = 0.01 nN (Eqn. 9.75). (A fibroblast pulling 165 nN at 10 microns/sec consumes ~2 pW of power.)

9.4.7.2 Cytovehicle Selection

Which motile human cells may be the most appropriate cytovehicles? Since almost all cells exhibit migratory behavior at the embryonic stages of development, in theory all cells can probably be mobilized, given access to the nuclear chromatin and the ability to manipulate it (Chapter 20). However, it is a safer and simpler matter to choose cells which are exclusively or at least facultatively motile in the human adult. The obvious candidates include white cells (e.g., neutrophils, monocytes, dendritic cells, eosinophils, basophils), lymphocytes (up to ~0.5 microns/sec[848]), macrophages, and fibroblasts—the speediest and most widely distributed cytovehicles—as well as Kupffer cells, osteoblasts and osteoclasts, endothelial cells, smooth muscle cells, sperm cells, malignant tumor cells (after safing), neuronal cells, and some migratory epithelial (e.g., Langerhans' cells) and mesenchymal cells. Motions analogous to crawling transform blood platelets from smooth disks into spiny spheres to plug vascular leaks after injury.[1564] Most bacteria are too small for whole-device entry, although their motility could be controlled by spoofing the external chemosensors, perhaps making them useful for piggybacking or towing (Section 9.4.7.1), or for steering to disposal sites. Other possibilities include parasites such as *Entamoeba histolytica* (found in the gut during amoebic dysentery, the liver during hepatic amebiasis, the bloodstream, and elsewhere), *Giardia lamblia* (an intestinal parasite), *Plasmodium* (a bloodstream parasite producing malaria), and so forth.

Erythrocytes are a special case. Though not motile, red blood cells are plentiful in the body, flow to within ~50 microns of virtually every tissue cell in the body, and have a tough, floppy outer plasma membrane. Experimentalists often replace the hemoglobin solution of red cells with an isotonic aqueous solution, producing "ghost cells" that mechanically behave much like the original cells minus the respiratory functions. In theory, nanorobots could enter an erythrocyte ghost cell and erect an artificial internal cytoskeleton to control cell shape, rotation, and possibly simulate amoeboid motions. However, naturally motile cells such as white cells already possess hardwired programs for creeping, diapedesis, object engulfment, etc. that can be triggered mechanically or biochemically with a minimum of effort (Section 9.4.7.6), hence these cells are much more attractive cytovehicles.

Passive cytocarriage is widely practiced in the microscopic world. Dengue-2 virus enters macrophages and B lymphocytes, hitching a ride;[3082] bacteria stably associated with human cells (e.g., *E. coli* in the intestinal mucosa) are well known. Larger microbes such as the tuberculosis bacterium also employ opportunistic cytocarriage.[1558] These bacteria are specially adapted to recognize and lock on to the large macrophages distributed throughout pulmonary tissue, and then to induce these cells to ingest them. Once inside the macrophages, the microbes get a free ride into the blood or the lymphatic system, enabling them to reach destinations all over the human body.[384]

9.4.7.3 Cytocarriage Initiation

There are ~7000 leukocytes/mm^3 in adult human blood (Appendix B) with a mean separation of ~50 microns, providing numerous and readily-available cytovehicles. A white cell that is cytoambulating at ~10 microns/sec moves only ~0.02 micron during the ~2 millisec required to establish identity (Section 8.5.2.2), and another ~0.1 micron during the ~10 millisec required for the piloting nanorobot to penetrate the plasma membrane (Section 9.4.5). Nevertheless, it may be desirable to temporarily halt the progression of the cytovehicle during the period in which nanorobot control is being established. This is readily accomplished by biochemical means. For example, when leukocytes are placed in an isotonic solution containing EDTA, active spontaneous movement stops and the cells respond passively to external loads.[362] Excess zinc immobilizes macrophages.[359] Integrins respond to intracellular messages, altering both selectivity and binding strength: the $\alpha_2\beta_1$ integrin can be inactive, a receptor for collagen, or a receptor for both collagen and laminin, depending on the type of cell that produces it and the signals received from inside the cell.[1511]

Once inside a 10-micron diameter leukocyte, a nanorobot traveling at ~1 micron/sec may require ~5 sec to migrate to an appropriate location near the center of the cell and establish control. Leukocyte towing harnesses may be quite simple in design but must be non-destructive. A required towing force of 0.01 nN (Section 9.4.7.1) requires only ~5 noncovalent bonds (breaking strength ~2 pN/bond; Section 9.4.4.2) to the glycocalyx or plasma membrane; a single 100 nm^2 footpad (Section 9.4.3.3) can provide up to 0.3 nN of harness anchoring force.

9.4.7.4 Steering and Control

A complete understanding of motile cell mobility biological control systems is not yet available. However, present knowledge[1564] is sufficient to support the conclusion that virtually complete command of cellular mobility systems by in cyto medical nanorobots should be feasible. Such control may be effected by either biochemical or mechanical means.

The "amoeboid" movement (Section 9.4.3.7) of leukocytes and fibroblasts relies primarily upon temporary extensions of the cell surface rather than major movements of cytoplasm. These temporary extensions, such as the small filopodia and the larger lamellipodia, are surface evaginations involving bundles of actin filaments or microtubules* in parallel array, often comprising a large fraction of the total surface area of the cell. Motion is made possible by an internal system of bracing which is built or modified according to the needs of the cell. Immediately below the plasma membrane is a region of densely packed and interconnected actin microfilaments called the cell cortex (Section 8.5.3.11). A leukocyte moves by breaking down actin filaments and rebuilding them in the proper orientation, pushing the cell in a new direction and allowing the posterior regions to retract.[312]

Fiber bundles isolated by microlaser surgery from a glycerinated fibroblast have been shown to contract with the addition of ATP.[938] Focal attachments between substrate and cell are modulated both by external chemotactic gradients on the substrate and by internal biochemical regulatory pathways (second messenger molecules; Section 7.4.5.1); similar signal transduction pathways control the polymerization and disassembly of filaments and microtubules comprising the podial extensions. Regulatory proteins that bind actin monomers and filaments, some of which function in response to transmembrane signaling, include ADF, adseverin, caldesmon, cap Z, cap 100, cofilin, gelsolin, MCP, phospholipase C-γ, profilin, and severin.[1564] Manipulation of the internal concentrations and spatial distributions of appropriate intracellular messenger molecules and ATP should permit in cyto medical nanorobots to command these biochemical pathways and to regulate localized polymerization processes,[1943] thus controlling the speed and direction of motile cell locomotion.

As another example of an intracellular mediator system that may be subject to direct nanorobotic control, consider the Ras superfamily of small guanosine triphosphatases (GTPases). One member of this superfamily, known as Rho, can be activated by the addition of extracellular ligands (such as lysophosphatidic acid), leading to the assembly of contractile actin-myosin filaments (stress fibers) and associated focal adhesion complexes.[1538] Rho acts as a molecular switch to control a signal transduction pathway linking plasma membrane receptors to the cytoskeleton.[1539] Rac, another member of the Rho subfamily, can be activated by a distinct set of agonists

* *Treadmilling and dynamic instability control microtubule length in vivo.*[1560]

** *PDGF concentration in human serum is 50 ng/cm^3 (Appendix B); optimum concentration is 1-20 ng/cm^3,*[3153] *or ~1 molecule/micron^3, for chemotactic response of neutrophils and monocytes during wound repair (Chapter 24). Fibroblasts need the higher concentration in this range (~20 ng/cm^3); PDGF stimulates a full mitogenic response.*[1554]

such as platelet-derived growth factor (PDGF)** or insulin, leading to the assembly of a meshwork of actin filaments at the cell periphery to produce lamellipodia and plasma membrane ruffles.[1540] Activation of Cdc42, another Rho subfamily member, induces actin-rich filopodial surface protrusions that are also associated with distinct integrin-based adhesion complexes.[1541,1542] There is significant cross-talk between GTPases of the Ras and Rho subfamilies—Ras can activate Rac (thus Ras induces lamellipodia), Cdc42 activates Rac (thus associating filopodial and lamellipodial formation), and Rac can activate Rho.[1540,1541] Members of the Rho GTPase family appear to be key regulatory molecules linking surface receptors to the organization of the actin cytoskeleton.[1539] By 1998, about 10 GTPase-activating proteins and 3 guanine nucleotide dissociation inhibitors (both potential down-regulators of GTPase activity), and at least 20 cellular effector targets with relevant protein-protein interaction domains, had been described.[1539] Local cytoplasmic injections or extractions of nanomolar concentrations of these second-messenger substances should permit full control of cytovehicular direction and speed.

Less subtle biochemical methods of cytoskeletal manipulation are also available to nanorobotic pilots. For example, the drugs colchicine and taxol disrupt microtubule function in distinctly different ways. Colchicine binds to tubulin, strongly inhibiting its further assembly into microtubules and fostering the disassembly of existing microtubules;[939] two other alkaloids, vinblastine and vincristine, also reversibly inhibit microtubule assembly.[936] (Microtubules are always losing and reacquiring tubulin dimers, and these three drugs prevent reassembly, so eventually the tubules would disappear entirely.) Colchicine diminishes neutrophil migration into inflammatory foci.[936] By contrast, taxol binds tightly to microtubules, stabilizing them and causing much of the free tubulin in the cell to assemble into microtubules.[939] Similarly, the drug phalloidin (e.g., ~5 nanomoles/cm^3)[1557] blocks the depolymerization of actin, thereby stabilizing microfilaments, whereas cytochalasin B inhibits the polymerization of actin microfilaments.[939] Drug molecule diffusion time over ~1 micron ranges is ~1 millisec, consistent with ~KHz cycling. S. Smith notes that the use of oncogene products like members of the Ras supergene family, coupled with cytotoxins and genotoxins like phalloidin and vinblastine for steering, could transform a leukocyte. The risk of generating a leukemia must be avoided, perhaps by implanting a timed self-destruct signal in the cytovehicle before initiating cytocarriage.

Cytovehicles may also be piloted by palpating the cytoskeleton mechanically—for instance, by applying tension to selected parts of the cytoskeleton using nanorobot manipulators. ECM-mediated mechanical forces can pull cells into square and rectangular shapes with sharp 90° corners.[718,1555] Mechanical manipulation may also be needed to drive cells into places they will not normally go. For instance, cells parked on experimentally-created micropatterned adhesive islands surrounded by nonadhesive (PEG-coated) boundaries cannot be induced to step off the islands even when stimulated with high concentrations of soluble growth factors.[1555] Mechanical signals are transduced into biochemical signals via mechanosensory plasma membrane channels[1506] and by other means.

How fast can cytovehicles be driven? Even using supranormal concentrations of biochemical control molecules combined with close placement to active sites in order to minimize diffusion time delays, a purely biochemically-mediated control system is probably limited to the maximum speeds of actin polymerization or osmotic inflation, or ~1-10 microns/sec. However, purely mechanical cytovehicular control systems can be cycled at much higher speeds, at least in tension. Individual actin microfilaments will tolerate a maximum tensile stress of ~108 pN (Section 8.5.3.11); the binding force between cytoskeleton and cell cortex at focal adhesions is of similar magnitude. Let us assume that the piloting nanorobot manipulates just a single fiber to drive each ~1 micron diameter lamellipodium, and that this single fiber is not driven beyond 10% of its theoretical failure strength, a very conservative limit. Using Eqn. 9.73 to crudely approximate the viscous drag force on the protuberance as it moves through interstitial fluid, each lamellipodium can be flexed at speeds up to ~500 micron/sec. Manipulating more fibers adds to the margin of safety. (Cyclosis in mature plant cells such as *Nitella* and *Chara* produces circular motions of some cell components as fast as 100 microns/sec.[938]) Similar manipulation of the much stronger intermediate fiber (IF) cytoskeleton (Section 8.5.3.11) would in theory permit speeds up to ~0.1 m/sec, but such aggressive forces might rip the IF fibers loose from their intracellular moorings. Another potential concern is that rapid cycling will stimulate unwanted peripheral actin polymerization or depolymerization reactions unless they are actively suppressed.

Electric fields may also drive leukocyte motion (Section 4.9.3.1). For example, a mild electric current induces lymphocytes to travel in the same direction of the current ("electrotaxis") at speeds up to ~0.3 microns/sec.[848] Small electric gradients have been shown experimentally to stimulate leukocyte diapedesis (Section 4.9.3.1),[690] though multiple nanorobots would probably be required to generate the necessary currents.

9.4.7.5 Navigation and Sensing

The nanorobotic pilot can directly access the high-resolution extracellular acoustic navigational grid (if such has been installed in the patient; Section 8.3.3) to establish absolute position and orientation of the cytovehicle within the human body, or may employ alternative positional or functional navigational cues as may be provided by the attending physician (Chapter 8). Chemosensory data (including tissue- and cell-recognition events) reaching the exterior surface of the piloted cell trigger natural internal biochemical cascades which are readily monitored and interpreted by in cyto nanorobots. Extracellular and ECM-related mechanosensory data and plasma membrane stretch sensor data produce similar recognizable internal biochemical and cytomechanical effects.

Eavesdropping on natural chemotactic signals is particularly effective. For instance, after leaving the blood vessels, neutrophils recognize biochemicals produced by bacteria and migrate toward a rising concentration. Laboratory demonstrations of neutrophil chemotaxis often use a concentration gradient of fMLP (n-formyl methionine-leucine-phenylalanine), a peptide chain produced by some bacteria, at ~0.1 nanomole/cm^3.[1554] Chemotaxis also occurs among human T-lymphocytes in the presence of a 0.01-1 picomole/cm^3 gradient of Met-enkephalin or β-endorphin.[1512] Chemotactic cytokines for leukocytes, macrophages, and fibroblasts—many of which are tissue-specific (and thus additionally serve as an aid to navigation) or condition-specific (e.g., inflammation)—are well-studied.[767,1516,1565-1570]

Similarly, *E. coli* has chemosensory receptors (three different transmembrane methyl-accepting chemotaxis proteins or MCPs[531] located mostly in clusters at one pole of the cell.[1544] At least two cytoplasmic signaling proteins, CheA and CheW, are known to interact with chemosensors in vitro.[1544,1545] Various intracellular mediator protein molecules convey chemoreceptor signals by diffusion (across one cell length in ~200 millisec)[1546] to the flagellar motors, which drive the bacterium forward in 20-40 micron/sec bursts.[437]

MCPs respond to attractants and repellants in the extracellular environment. All these signals can be detected in cyto by an eavesdropping "piggybacking" nanorobotic pilot equipped with appropriate (membrane-penetrating) cytoplasmic chemosensors.

The nanorobotic pilot may also deploy loosely-tethered nanosensor remotes and insert them into the cytovehicle's plasma membrane, during or after cytopenetration. These nanosensors may employ simple mechanical plasma membrane locking (Section 9.4.5.2) or a stationary solvation wave pattern (Section 9.4.5.3) to straddle the plasma membrane, mimicking natural transmembrane integral proteins (Fig. 8.37), or could anchor one end of their transmembrane structure to the underlying cellular cortex. Such sensors could gather whatever extracellular thermal, mechanical, acoustic, chemical, or electromagnetic data might be required by the pilot for proper navigation and steering. The nanosensors are retrieved when the nanorobotic pilot exits the cytovehicle at the destination.

When macrophages and other leukocytic cells become infected, they express B7 (a co-stimulator molecule) on their plasma membrane surface which can be recognized by a T-cell CD28 receptor protein, triggering an immunologic response in the presence of surface-displayed antigen.[1556] Nanorobotic pilots should inspect the cell surface of all prospective cytovehicles for B7 and similar pathogenic flags prior to cytopenetration, so as not to unintentionally choose an infected cell for cytocarriage which could then spread the infection or become subject to immunosystem attack. If the cell subsequently becomes infected and begins expressing B7 or other warning substances during the journey, the nanorobotic pilot should abort the mission and steer the cytovehicle to a nearby disposal site, or implement immediate cytotherapeutic measures. Failing this, the pilot should abandon the vehicle at once.

9.4.7.6 Cytovehicular Behavioral Control

Besides simple steering and chemotaxis, many stereotypical cell behaviors may be triggered biochemically as well. Diapedesis, ECM brachiation with a preference for a particular ECM ligand, particle engulfment, transitions between migratory and profibrotic phenotypes in fibroblasts,[1537] cell volume and shape changes, cell cycling and growth, and epithelial-mesenchymal transformations[1547] may be initiated, amplified, or suppressed by regulating the flows and distributions of various cytoplasmic signal molecules which may include proteins or nonproteins (such as Ca^{++} or GTP). Motility-stimulating factors such as autocrine stimulating factor[1548] and migration stimulating factor[1549] are produced by fibroblasts and act in an autocrine (Section 7.4.5.1) fashion. Leukocytes keep rolling over vascular endothelium until a neutrophil activator (e.g., a selectin) is encountered, whereupon they stick tightly and undergo the shape change characteristic of neutrophil diapedesis[978]—a process that nanorobotic pilots should be able to monitor and control. Mammary epithelial cells receive mechanical signals from the ECM via a tyrosine kinase (biochemical) signal transduction pathway through the β_1 integrin receptor leading to the activation of elements in the promoter region of the β-casein gene.[1550] Release of Sr^{++} inside cytolytic T lymphocytes induces degranulation—the emission of cytotoxic granules containing granulysin that can inhibit growth in a broad spectrum of pathogens, including bacteria, fungi, and parasites, and can directly kill the tuberculosis bacterium.[2165]

Most integrins bind to their ECM ligands via the tripeptide RGD (Arg-Gly-Asp), so the nanorobotic pilot can release RGD as an antagonist to moderate or to prevent cell-ECM interactions.[1551] Alternatively, ECM-integrin binding can be enhanced by specific cytoplasmic molecules such as the cell adhesion regulator (CAR), a myristoylated protein that can connect the plasma membrane to the cytoskeleton.[1552] ECM molecules interact with their receptors at the cell surface, transmitting signals directly or indirectly to second messengers which in turn unravel a cascade of events leading to the coordinated expression of a variety of genes involved in cell adhesion and release, migration, proliferation, differentiation, and death.[1553] By intercepting and regulating specific second messenger pathways, or by artificially triggering them mechanically, the pilot can exercise considerable control over cell behavior.

The nanorobotic pilot must inhibit certain natural cell behaviors that might distract the cytovehicle from its imposed mission. For example, emission of Rap1-GTP protein into the cytoplasm of a Jurkat T cell renders the cell anergic (unresponsive) and incapable of transcribing the gene encoding interleukin-2 when stimulated with antigen.[1562] Intracellular kinesin molecular motors (Fig. 9.32) are inhibited by adociasulfate-2 (AS-2; MW = 738 daltons), a molecule that targets the kinesin motor domain.[1563] Activated macrophages themselves secrete chemoattractant factors that may draw a crowd of leukocytes, fibroblasts, and other macrophages toward the flight path, impeding mobility and possibly triggering a natural granulomatous (encapsulation) reaction. These processes may be desirable to stimulate at the destination, but they should be suppressed en route.

Unwanted cytovehicular responses due to nanorobot intrusion should also be suppressed, much as pathogens such as *M. tuberculosis* resist or inhibit oxidative killing, attack by defensins, phagosome-lysosome fusion, and formation of the electron-transparent zone that impairs lysosomal enzyme diffusion, thus ensuring their survival inside macrophages for long periods of time.[1558,1559]

Cell behavior can also be mechanically regulated by altering cell shape, because cells can detect when a mechanical strain is placed upon them.[942,1020] In one experiment, stretching a fibroblast by 1% for 180 sec triggered large-scale changes in cell shape, including retraction of pseudopods and cell elongation.[1557] Other experiments show that very flat cells, with their cytoskeletons stretched, sense that more cells are needed to cover the surrounding substrate (as in wound repair) and that cell division is needed. A rounded shape indicates that too many cells are competing for space on the matrix and that cells may be excessively proliferating; some must die to prevent tumor formation. Normal tissue function is established and maintained between these two extremes.[1021] Certain mechanical stresses on cells, such as might be generated by a nanorobotic pilot inside the cytovehicle or dense cytovehicular traffic near the destination, may trigger unwanted reactions that should be avoided.

9.5 Ex Vivo Locomotion

In this final Section of Chapter 9, our attention turns to locomotion across, through, and around the external surfaces of the human body. The most important of such surfaces are the teeth (Section 9.5.1) and the skin (Section 9.5.2). Another important consideration is aerial locomotion near the human body (Section 9.5.3). These discussions are necessarily incomplete; more comprehensive treatments are beyond the scope of this introductory text.

9.5.1 Dental Walking

The exposed surfaces of natural dentition consist of a ~500 micron thick layer of enamel coating the exposed crown of each tooth inside the mouth. Enamel is a composite structure containing ~96% inorganic material similar to hydroxyapatite, a dense bone mineral, embedded in an organic matrix of glycoprotein and a keratin-like protein. The mineral forms crystallites oriented into hexagonal cylinders with a horseshoe-shaped cross-section wrapping around the dentin, forming enamel prisms ~5 microns in diameter stacked in parallel congeries.[646,854,1571] These prismatic columns are directed vertically at the summit of the crown and horizontally along the sides of the tooth, pursuing a generally wavy course. There are no nutritive channels permeating the enamel and leading into the dentinal layer below, although dentinal tubules (nutritive channels) do extend from the pulp chamber into the dentin which may get extremely close to the occlusal (enamel) surface of the tooth, and may be exposed by receding gums. However, ~0.4-micron-wide fissures separating enamel prisms are filled with an interprismatic substance of much higher organic content. The entire enamel surface is pockmarked by numerous micropores of irregular but generally oval shape, ranging from 0.1-2 microns (average ~0.5 micron) in diameter and spaced ~1-2 microns apart. Thus a dental-walking micron-size nanorobot encounters a spongelike topography with holes and fissures comparable in size to the nanorobot diameter, and with gently rolling hills ~2 device diameters in height and ~5 diameters across. (There is also a thin layer of salivary proteins coating the tooth enamel surface.)[3669,3670]

Nanorobots may traverse tooth enamel using ambulatory techniques previously described in other contexts (Section 9.4), including legged walking, rolling, or amoeboid locomotion using footpads for anchorage. Teeth may be clenched with a force up to 300-500 N,[1296,3671-3673] although forces of ~50 N are more common during normal mastication of soft foods. Assuming ~1 cm^2 of dental contact surface, shear forces at that surface during chewing or clenching are 0.5-5 x 10^6 N/m^2, close to the limit for noncovalent anchorage (Section 9.4.3.3). Nanorobots seeking further refuge from shear forces may congregate in the valleys between enamel prisms or can seat themselves in the irregular micropores. E. Reifman notes that ~90% of U.S. adults have multiple occlusal surface restorations composed of many different materials such as resin composites of various hardness coefficients, porcelain or gold crowns, amalgam fillings, composites, and the relatively newer but very popular glass polymer crowns, representing a substantial percentage of all exposed dental surfaces with which oral nanodevices must cope; yield strength of these materials at 0.1% strain deformation typically ranges from 110-10,000 atm.[3271]

Are the forces of dental grinding sufficient to crush medical nanodevices? Tests of sized jeweler's grinding powders by the author confirm that even irregularly-shaped diamondoid particles ~3 microns and smaller apparently roll smoothly out of the way when ground between the teeth, whereas particles larger than ~3 microns cannot roll sufficiently and retain a sensible grittiness. In the case of a trapped nanorobot-size diamond block slowly being squeezed between opposed enamel surfaces (static force), the Young's moduli for enamel and diamond are 7.5 x 10^{10} N/m^2 and 1.05 x 10^{12} N/m^2, respectively (Table 9.3), so the enamel deforms ~14 times more than the diamond. Crystalline diamond can deform at least ~5% before fracturing, diamond composites (Chapter 11) much more; a 50% strain in each enamel surface (an indentation equal to the entire diamond block radius, probably causing the enamel to fail) produces a 3.6% deformation across the diameter of the block, slightly below the conservative tolerance limit for diamondoid fracture strain. In the case of a 50-gram jaw moving at the maximum 0.1 m/sec clenching velocity that is suddenly brought to a halt via enamel deformation to a depth equal to a ~1 micron nanorobot radius across a 1 cm^2 enamel contact area, the jaw decelerates at ~1000 g's producing a kinetic force of ~500 N and a contact force of 5 x 10^6 N/m^2 (~50 atm), well below the ~10^{11} N/m^2 failure strength of solid diamond.

However, nanorobot crushing strength is an explicit design parameter which is normally significantly lower than for solid diamond if the device has large unbraced internal voids or diameters that are weak in compression. Such nanorobots may not be regarded as solid diamond structures as assumed above. For example, the Euler buckling force for a solid cylindrical rod of outer radius R is proportional to R^4 (Eqn. 9.44), but for a hollow cylinder with inner radius r the buckling force is proportional instead to (R^4-r^4) during axial compressions.[364] Hence a trapped, thin-walled cylindrical nanorobot of radius R with r/R = 0.90 buckles at only ~34% of the force needed to buckle a solid rod of radius R, and thus could probably be crushed by static compression of the teeth. The oral cavity appears to be the only place in the human body where thin-walled medical nanorobots might plausibly be destroyed by mechanical grinding. Such destruction is avoided by nanorobots with composite diamondoid shells $\gtrsim$10% R thick at a maximum allowable strain $\lesssim$ 10%, or by nanodevices possessing maps of mastication contact spots that actively avoid those spots during nanorobotic perambulations.

9.5.2 Epidermal Locomotion

The epidermis is a modified cellular surface, so most of the techniques described for cytoambulation (Section 9.4.3) are applicable to epidermal locomotion as well. There are so many special situations and obstacles to motility on skin that we can only mention a few of them here:

A. *Flaky Corneum*—Desiccated stratified epidermal cells crack, chip, or flake off entirely when rubbed or jostled with too much force. Nanorobots traversing a dead cell could find themselves flaked off into the air or onto the floor, especially if the surface is rubbed by the patient.

B. *Steep Topography*—Many physical features of the skin are huge in scale compared to a micron-size nanorobot and thus must be carefully circumnavigated. Dermal fingerprint ridges are ~500 microns wide and 20-50 microns deep. Hair follicle shafts are 50-100 microns in diameter. Scent-secreting apocrine glands are ~200 microns in diameter; eccrine (sweat) glands are only 20 microns wide. Skin-dwelling fungi (e.g., athlete's foot) grow into irregular globs 5-20 microns in size. The tongue surface includes taste buds ~150 microns wide and tiny papillae measuring 30 microns wide and 80 microns long. Other surface features are described in Section 8.6.1. At the micron scale, the topmost layer of the epidermis is littered with obstacles and protrusions, with electron micrographs showing a surface that closely resembles a flaky puff pastry in appearance.[1571]

C. *Constant Motion*—The skin is almost always in motion at size scales up to ~1000 microns, folding and unfolding, stretching and tightening, twisting and curving, with normally distant surfaces being brought into and out of contact as the patient moves about normally.

D. *Dust Mites and Bacteria*—In eyelashes and eyebrows, the hairs of the upper lip, in the ears, and elsewhere on the body, dust mites measuring 150 microns x 300 microns survive by chewing up dead skin cells. Epidermal-walking nanorobots must be able to identify mite surfaces, and avoid climbing aboard them by mistake. Everyone inhales a few mites now and then; mite excrement (to which some patients are allergic) is concentrated into fecal packets so small and light that they float in the air and may settle back onto the skin. Many other surface-dwelling ectoparasites and microfauna similarly must be avoided.[3253] Bacterial density over most of the body surface is quite low, ~$10^3/cm^2$; the count ranges from ~$10^2/cm^2$ on the palms and dorsa of the hands, up to 10^4-10^5/cm^2 on the hairy axilla, scalp, perineal regions, and beneath the distal end of the nail plate.[360]

E. *Obstructions*—The skin may be covered with dirt, or grease, or cooking oils and fats, or sebaceous gland oils, which may be many tens or even hundreds of microns thick. Another potential obstacle is the sweat wash—the skin can pour out up to 2 liters/hour of perspiration. Nanorobots can easily crawl underneath the tightest-fitting clothing or rubber gloves, although a patch of superglue stuck to the skin could provide a formidable obstacle requiring overpassage.

F. *Itching/Crawling Sensations*—Tickling sensations attributable to isolated nanorobots traversing the skin are unlikely. Skin-crawling ~2-mm ants are readily detected; ~100-micron mites are not. Absolute epidermal pressure stimulus thresholds, as measured by a laboratory esthesiometer, range from a low of 2000 N/m^2 at the tongue- and finger-tip, up to 12,000 N/m^2 on the back of the hand, 26,000 N/m^2 on abdomen, 48,000 N/m^2 on the loin, and a high of 250,000 N/m^2 on the thickest part of the sole of the foot.[773] By comparison, the weight of a (100 micron)^3 nanorobot, if distributed across a (100 micron)^2 contact surface, is only ~1 N/m^2, quite undetectable on the skin. At a velocity of 1 cm/sec, the inertial force required to propel a 100-micron nanorobot is ~1 nN (Section 9.4.2.1). This additional force, if distributed over 10 footpads each of area 100 micron^2, gives a shear pressure of ~1 N/m^2 across all contact surfaces, also undetectable; the sensible threshold velocity for such a nanorobot is ~45 cm/sec. Skin sensor frequency response is << KHz (Table 7.3), whereas skin walkers $\lesssim$ 10 microns in size may employ ν_{leg} $\gtrsim$ KHz leg motions; the weight of a 1 micron^3 nanorobot produces only ~0.01 N/m^2 of contact pressure.

Nanorobots of large size can also step over most of the obstacles described above. Consider an R_{nano} = 50 micron walking nanorobot with N_{leg} = 10, L_{leg} = 100 microns, R_{leg} = 15 microns, and v_{leg} = 1 cm/sec as defined for Eqn. 9.82, with $\nu_{leg} \sim v_{leg} / 2\, L_{leg}$ ~ 50 Hz. From Eqn. 9.75, the viscous force per leg is $F_{leg} \sim F_{nano_N}$ ~ 5 nN in a 20°C water bath, 0.1 nN in 20°C air. From Eqn. 9.73, F_{nano} ~9 nN in water, 0.2 nN in air. Thus the total driving force F_{total} = 59 nN in water, 1.2 nN in air, assuming a still medium.

Another way to avoid obstacles is to hop over them in the manner of a jumping flea, an insect that subjects itself to an acceleration of ~200 g's while leaping ~130 times its own dimension.[739] Diamondoid saltators could tolerate much higher accelerations, although it is important not to disturb the takeoff surface; also, airborne ex vivo trajectories may be only poorly controlled. The approach is interesting[1982,2385,2386] but will not be considered further in this book.

What about dislodgement forces? Assuming a headwind of v ~ 1 m/sec and a d ~ 10 micron boundary layer, then from Eqn. 9.58 the shear stress (and shear force) on a 100-micron wide nanorobot is F/A ~ 100 N/m^2 (1000 nN) in water, 2 N/m^2 (20 nN) in air. A single 10 micron^2 footpad with a conservative adhesive pressure of 10^5 N/m^2 (Section 9.4.3.3) provides a 1000 nN anchorage force, allowing the nanorobot to remain adhered to the skin even in the strongest water currents (e.g., white water rapids, showers, or spas at ~1 m/sec per anchored footpad used) and air currents (e.g., up to ~50 m/sec (~110 mph) winds per anchored footpad used). A finger rubbed hard against the skin with the objective of dislodging adhered epidermal-resident nanorobots may apply up to 10 N of force over a ~1 cm^2 area, giving a ~10^5 N/m^2 shear force (~ 1,000,000 nN) which may be resisted by ten 100 micron^2 footpads each having a maximum adhesive pressure of ~10^6 N/m^2 (Section 9.4.3.3).

What about epidermal penetration? Complex and subtle low-speed methods are readily imagined (Section 9.4.4), but let us consider here a simple brute-force approach. Failure strength of human skin is ~10^7 N/m^2 (Table 9.3), so a 1 micron^2 rod may be driven through the skin with a force of ~10,000 nN. A 100-micron long telescoping manipulator arm with stiffness ~25,000 nN/nm can apply 10,000 nN to the rod at 1 cm/sec producing an elastic deflection in the arm of less than 1 nm, drawing ~100,000 pW of power (manipulator arm power density ~10^6 watts/m^3) at the moment of penetration (Section 9.3.1.4). Bruising and other biocompatibility issues related to dermal penetration are deferred to Chapter 15.

The surfaces of toenails and fingernails have 2-20 micron features and longitudinal striations with 10-15 micron valleys, and are usually littered with dirt, bits of skin, and other surface debris as small as 1-2 microns in size. The nail surface is heavily keratinized, with a failure strength about 20 times higher than that of skin (Table 9.3). Similar considerations apply as with the skin, in regard to nanorobot locomotion.

What happens if the nanorobot falls off, or is otherwise removed from, the epidermal surface? Solem[1982] has analyzed the case of nanorobots walking on walls and ceilings. Setting the electrostatic image force (Eqn. 9.11) equal to the gravity force $\rho_{nano}\, L_{nano}{}^3\, g$ for a cubical conducting-surface nanorobot of edge L_{nano}, the voltage required to cling to the ceiling without falling off is:

$$V_{plate} = z_{sep} \left(\frac{2\, \rho_{nano}\, L_{nano}\, g}{\varepsilon_0\, \kappa_e} \right)^{1/2} \quad \text{(volts)} \qquad \{\text{Eqn. 9.83}\}$$

Taking z_{sep} = 0.5 microns, ρ_{nano} = 2000 kg/m^3, g = 9.81 m/sec^2, ε_0 = 8.85 x 10^{-12} farad/m, κ_e = 1, and L_{nano} = 10 microns, then V_{plate} ~ 0.1 volt. Similarly, the largest nanorobot that can cling to the ceiling using an adhesive contact surface of strength S has a characteristic dimension:[1982]

$$L_{max} \sim \frac{S}{\rho_{nano}\, g} \qquad \{\text{Eqn. 9.84}\}$$

For S = 10-100 N/m^2 (typical for weak adhesives such as Post-It notes), then L_{max} ~ 500-5000 microns. By wetting the contact area with water having surface tension γ ~ 73 x 10^{-3} N/m at room temperature (Section 9.2.3), a cubical nanorobot clinging to the ceiling may have a maximum characteristic dimension of:[1982]

$$L_{max} \sim \left(\frac{4\gamma}{\rho_{nano}\, g} \right)^{1/2} \sim 3900 \text{ microns} \qquad \{\text{Eqn. 9.85}\}$$

9.5.3 Nanoflight

Perhaps surprisingly, aerobotics has many useful applications in nanomedicine. Examples include monitoring and diagnostic systems, since flying nanorobots can transit the length of a patient's body in ~1 sec or less (Chapter 18); sterile fields (Chapter 19); personal defensive systems (Chapter 21); and accident recovery systems (Chapter 24). Unfortunately, in 1998 the aerodynamics of micron-scale flight systems was only lightly studied[347,348,1573-1576,1982] and aerial robotics was still considered an exotic sport[2995] or a military curiosity.[3175]

9.5.3.1 Nanoflight and Reynolds Number

It has been observed that a 30-cm paper airplane will glide slowly and stably, but a 3-cm paper airplane made from thinner paper requires a much higher velocity/size ratio to remain airborne, and with a noticeable lack of stability—sometimes the plane flies well, sometimes not. If size is further reduced into the millimeter range, the plane almost cannot fly.[1573]

As in the case of swimming, this transition can be explained in terms of the Reynolds number N_R (Section 9.4.2.1), the ratio of inertial to viscous forces acting on a body that is passing through a fluid such as air. Generally speaking, microscopic organisms (e.g., $N_R \sim 10^{-5}$) or flying nanorobots with $N_R << 1$ move by utilizing viscosity, while macroscopic objects such as aircraft (e.g., $N_R \sim 10^8$) with $N_R >> 1$ use inertia to generate lift. Millimeter-size airfoils with $N_R \sim 0.1\text{-}100$, as typified by flying insects, occupy a transitional regime. Insects make use of both inertial and viscous forces, often employing unusual wing flapping patterns[1577,1578,1585] and elastic energy storage systems[1578,1582] to remain aloft. The smallest known flying insect[1579] that can make any use of aerodynamic lift (inertial) forces is the four-winged parasitic chalcid wasp *Encarsia formosa*, which has a total wingspan of ~1.4 mm.[1578] Aerobotic machines with wingspans smaller than ~100 microns probably must make almost exclusive use of viscous propulsive forces.[363]

A nanorobot of dimension L flying at velocity v through 20°C sea-level dry air (ρ_{air} = 1.205 kg/m^3, absolute viscosity η_{air} = 0.0183 x 10^{-3} kg/m-sec)[763] has a Reynolds number N_R = 66,000 v L (Eqn. 9.65). Viscous forces dominate when $N_R < 1$, or when:

$$v < \frac{15}{L_{micron}} \quad (m/sec) \qquad \{Eqn. 9.86\}$$

where L_{micron} is characteristic nanorobot size expressed in microns. Thus a 1-micron nanorobot remains in the viscous regime up to ~ 15 m/sec flight velocity (34 mph), a sufficient speed for most medical applications. Note that formulas involving viscous forces may not apply to aerobotic airfoils with $L \lesssim \lambda_{gas}$ (Eqn. 9.23), indicating transitional or ballistic flow (Section 9.2.4).

The main implication of Eqn. 9.86 is that conventional aeronautics technologies such as rigid wings and jets are usually inappropriate for micron-size flyers. Instead, aerial nanorobots may more profitably employ natation mechanisms as described in Section 9.4.2.5, including surface deformations (e.g., flexible oars or wings, cilia, invaginating doughnuts, rotating spheroids, traveling waves), inclined planes (e.g., screw drives, corkscrews, flagella), volume displacement, and viscous anchoring. Specific aeromotive mechanisms are of great interest but will not be considered further in this Volume. In many cases, a viscous-regime nanorobot may exit the bodily fluids and enter the atmosphere,* or vice versa, using the same propulsive mechanisms, though operated at a modified speed or pitch angle.

9.5.3.2 Nanoflight and Gravity

In addition to forward progression through the medium, atmospheric flight requires active and continuous support against the pull of gravity. For small spherical objects of radius $R = R_{nano}$ in the laminar flow (low N_R) regime, the rate of fall in a still medium is approximated by Stokes Law for Sedimentation (Eqn. 3.10).** For nanorobots near the Earth's surface that are falling in air, with g = 9.81 m/sec^2, $\rho_{particle} \sim 1000$ kg/m^3, $\rho_{fluid} = \rho_{air}$ and $\eta = \eta_{air}$, then terminal velocity $v_t = 1.2 \times 10^8 R_{nano}^2$ (m/sec). An R_{nano} = 1 micron nanorobot falls at v_t = 120 microns/sec; an R_{nano} = 10 micron nanorobot falls at v_t = 1.2 cm/sec, requiring a rather modest power expenditure of only P_{nano}/e% = (0.5 pW)/e% to remain aloft (Eqn. 9.74).

Note also that in free atmosphere only the largest particles ever settle out by gravity alone. Thermal and dynamic turbulence keeps most of the smaller particles in suspension long beyond the period indicated by Eqn. 3.10. For example, nanorobot thermal velocity $v_{thermal}$ (Eqn. 3.3) exceeds nanorobot terminal velocity v_t (Eqn. 3.10) for a nanorobot radius $R_{nano} \lesssim 2$ microns in sea level air at 20°C with $\rho_{nano} \sim 1000$ kg/m^3. The energy required to raise a 1-micron nanorobot a height of ~1 micron in a 1 g gravity field equals ~kT. Random indoor atmospheric eddies of 1-10 cm/sec caused by the movements of people, animals, doors, and heating and air conditioning systems equal or exceed the Stokes terminal velocity for particles of $R \lesssim$ 10-30 microns.

9.5.3.3 Buoyant Nanoballoons

Gravity may also be overcome by reducing density relative to the surrounding medium. An object has neutral buoyancy when its density equals that of the medium in which it is suspended, becoming "weightless" within that medium. For example, a nanorobot whose interior volume consists 90% of vacuum has a v_t ~10 times smaller than a completely solid object of equal size.

What is the tiniest possible lighter-than-air balloon? J.S. Hall notes that for a one-atom-thick graphene shell the out-of-plane bending stiffness of the C-C bond is much lower than the in-plane stretching stiffness. This is why hollow fullerenes of submicron diameter are experimentally observed to collapse (and remain collapsed due to van der Waals forces) even when their interiors are not evacuated. Simple internal bracing sufficient to stabilize an evacuated structure outweighs the lift. For example, applying the Euler buckling formula (Eqn. 9.44) to three diamondoid orthogonal diametral stiffening rods inside a spherical evacuated nanoballoon gives a scale-invariant total beam mass ~6 times the mass of the displaced air, hence net lift is impossible for any device radius using this minimal crossbeam design although macroscale geodesic trusswork-stabilized vacuum balloons cannot be ruled out. (See also Section 10.3.5.)

Hall also observes that pressurizing nanoballoons to atmospheric pressure removes most shell stress. This strategy also eliminates the need to thicken the single-atom shell walls, up to a nanoballoon radius of at least $\sigma_w t_{wall} / \Delta p \sim 100$ microns, taking wall thickness t_{wall} = 0.17 nm, a conservative diamondoid wall working stress σ_w = 10^{10} N/m^2 (Table 9.3), and allowing a maximum environmental pressure fluctuation of $\Delta p \sim 0.17$ atm (vs. ~0.002 atm for 140 dB sound waves (Section 4.9.1.5), ~0.1 atm normal barometric variation (Section 4.9.1.6), and ~2 atm maximum sound pressure in air). Bursting strength of pressure shells is briefly treated in Section 10.3.1.

The smallest atmospheric-pressurized atomic-walled nanoballoon that can achieve neutral buoyancy has radius $R_{min} = 3 \rho_{wall} t_{wall} / (\rho_{air} - \rho_{gas})$, where ρ_{wall} is wall density, ρ_{air} is air density (ρ_{air} = 1.2929 kg/m^3 for dry air at STP), and ρ_{gas} is the density of the filling gas. Thus R_{min} = 1.6 micron for hydrogen gas with ρ_{gas} = 0.0899 kg/m^3; R_{min} = 1.7 micron for STP helium gas (ρ_{gas} = 0.1785 kg/m^3) which, in conjunction with a slightly thicker nondiamondoid (e.g., sapphire)

* *From Eqn. 9.14, the capillary force will restrain a 1-micron diameter nanorobot with a force of ~440 nN in pure water at the liquid-air interface due to surface tension, but this attraction may be reduced at least to ~4 nN by discharging small aliquots of the appropriate surfactants into the local aqueous environment; Section 9.2.3.*

** *In sea level pressure dry air, particles of 100 nm diameter will fall about twice as fast as estimated by Eqn. 3.10; 10-nm diameter particles fall about 12 times as fast as Stokes' sedimentation formula predicts.*[1572]

shell, eliminates flammability concerns at all device number densities. Diffusion leakage must also be addressed (Section 10.3.4).

Nanoballoons of radius $R > R_{min}$ can carry payloads of mass:

$$M_{payload} = \frac{4}{3}\pi\,\rho_{air}\,R^3\left(1 - \frac{\rho_{gas}}{\rho_{air}}\right) - 4\,\pi\,\rho_{wall}\,t_{wall}\,R^2$$

{Eqn.9.87}

For instance, a helium-filled R = 2.2-micron fullerene sphere can lift a $\sim 10^{-17}$ kg payload mass, representing a payload volume of ~0.01 $micron^3$ at $\rho_{payload} \sim 1000\ kg/m^3$. Expanding nanoballoon radius to R = 6.8 microns increases payload volume to ~1 $micron^3$. Pressurized buoyancy-based lift systems may be useful either in early-generation aerial nanodevices that must rely upon primitive energy supplies, or in default-float applications. However, the modest power expenditure needed to overcome gravity in micron-size devices (Section 9.5.3.2) suggests that nonbuoyant active-propulsion designs will normally be preferred.

9.5.3.4 Nanoflyer Force and Power Requirements

What forces must be applied, and what power must be expended, in order for a flying nanorobot to maintain continuous and controlled progression through the air? An exact calculation requires a detailed knowledge of the mode of locomotion, the shape and dimensions of wing or body, airfoil surface characteristics, and many other factors. However, the force needed to drive a spherical flyer of mass m_{nano} through the air at a velocity v_{nano} may be approximated by summing the three drag components of skin friction ($F_{viscous}$), pressure drag ($F_{inertial}$), and induced drag due to lift ($F_{induced}$), as:

$$F_{nano} = F_{viscous} + F_{inertial} + F_{induced} \quad \text{(newtons)}$$ {Eqn. 9.88}

$$F_{viscous} \sim 6\,\pi\,\eta_{air}\,R_{nano}\,v_{nano}$$ {Eqn. 9.89}

$$F_{inertial} \sim C_D(\pi R^2_{nano})(\rho_{air}\,v^2_{nano})/2$$ {Eqn. 9.90}

while conservatively taking the dimensionless coefficient of drag $C_D \sim 2$. Induced drag, associated with the shedding of transient vortexes from each wing tip, is an important consideration in macroscale winged vehicles but may be ignored here (e.g., $F_{induced} \sim 0$) for microscale flyers operating in the viscous or transitional flight regimes.

The nanorobot aeromotive energy plant, of efficiency e%, must develop a continuous power of:

$$P_{nano} \sim \frac{v_{nano}\,F_{nano}}{e\%} \quad \text{(watts)}$$ {Eqn. 9.91}

giving a whole-device power density of:

$$D_{nano} \sim \frac{3\,P_{nano}}{4\,\pi\,R^3_{nano}} \quad (\text{watts/m}^3)$$ {Eqn. 9.92}

These formulas give somewhat conservative results (e.g., overestimates of required force and power) because they do not take into account special body shapes, dynamic wing motions (e.g., delayed stall, rotational circulation, and wake capture[3268]), virtually complete pressure recovery in creeping flow, and so forth that may be used to improve flight efficiency in an optimized design. On the other hand, flight efficiency may be reduced by the accretion of water molecules and other environmental substances on working surfaces, and by the power expended in shearing air (dominant at the micron scale) or in imparting net kinetic energy to the air (at higher Reynolds numbers).

Table 9.5 shows force, power, and power density for spherical flying nanorobots of various sizes and airspeeds, computed using the above relations. Note that power scales as $\sim v_{nano}^2$ in the viscous regime, $\sim v_{nano}^3$ in the transitional regime. (The maximum sustainable velocity for transitional-regime insects is ~11 m/sec*.)

For an R_{nano} = 1 micron aerial nanorobot, taking $\eta_{air} = 0.0183 \times 10^{-3}$ kg/m-sec and $\rho_{air} = 1.205\ kg/m^3$ in dry air at 20°C and at 1 atm, with $r_{nano} \sim 1000$ kg/m and e% = 0.10 (10%), a v_{nano} = 1 cm/sec airspeed requires $F_{nano} \sim 4$ pN and a $P_{nano} \sim 0.4$ pW powerplant ($D_{nano} \sim 82{,}000\ watts/m^3$). At v_{nano} = 1 m/sec, then $F_{nano} \sim 350$ pN and $P_{nano} \sim 3500$ pW powerplant ($D_{nano} \sim 8 \times 10^8\ watts/m^3$). A much larger R_{nano} = 1 mm nanorobot flying at v_{nano} = 1 m/sec requires $F_{nano} \sim 4\ \mu N$ and $P_{nano} \sim 41\ \mu W$ ($D_{nano} \sim 10{,}000\ watts/m^3$). Again, an optimized design might reduce some of the power figures by a factor of 10 or more.

Aerobot power density D_{nano} scales as $\sim v_{nano}^2$ and $\sim R_{nano}^{-2}$ in the viscous regime. In the transitional regime, power density scales as $\sim v_{nano}^3$, and as $\sim R_{nano}^{-2}$ at low velocities and $\sim R_{nano}^{-1}$ at high velocities. Thus, to minimize power density and therefore conserve energy, circumcorporeal clouds of aerial nanorobots may coalesce into progressively larger but fewer tightly-packed clumps as the collective velocity of the cloud moves to higher airspeeds, assuming that the aeromotive mechanism design is largely scale-invariant over the full size range of the progressive aggregations. This strategy is most effective in the viscous regime.

For example, consider a cloudlet consisting of 1 million nanorobots, each of size R_{nano} = 1 micron. With individual nanorobots traveling at $v_{nano} \sim 30$ cm/sec, the cloudlet consumes ~0.4 milliwatts and operates at a power density of $\sim 10^8\ watts/m^3$. Now assume that the cloudlet must speed up to 10 m/sec to track a fast-moving object around which it is stationkeeping, or to compensate for a heavy wind. If the individual nanorobots comprising the cloudlet simply increase their airspeed to 10 m/sec, then power density in each nanorobot increases to $\sim 10^{11}\ watts/m^3$ and cloudlet power consumption rises to ~400 milliwatts (a 1000-fold increase). However, if the nanorobots temporarily aggregate into a single collective approximating a single device of R_{nano} = 100 microns, then the power consumption of the collective can be held to the original 0.4 milliwatts and power density remains constant at $\sim 10^8$ $watts/m^3$. Facultative aggregation may permit stationkeeping over a wide range of velocities without significantly increasing power. (Other power-conserving behaviors, such as preferential migration into the downwind slipstream of a rapidly-moving tracked object, are not considered further here but may be useful.)

How fast can nanoflyers accelerate? The answer is highly design-dependent but a crude generalization may be made. Consider a spherical nanorobot of radius R_{nano} that uses circumferential wings of similar size to impart momentum to a nearby mass of air by speeding up that mass of air to a higher velocity. The wings sweep

---

* *The first well-documented report of maximum insect flight speed was by Tillyard,[3157] who used a stopwatch to time the flight of the dragonfly* Australophlebia costalis *along a downhill slope at 27 m/sec; Hocking[3158] subsequently calculated that the maximum speed of* A. costalis *would only be 16 m/sec on a level surface. Unpublished slow-motion cinematography research by Butler[3159] reported an unconfirmed 40 m/sec burst of speed by the male* Hybomitra hinei wrighti *during an Immelmann Turn maneuver[3160] at the beginning of female pursuit.*

Table 9.5. Conservatively Estimated Force, Power, and Power Density for Hovering and Flying Spherical Nanorobots as a Function of Size and Velocity

(R_{nano}) Nanorobot Radius	$(v_{terminal})$ Terminal Velocity	(Force) (Power) (Density)	Nanorobot Airspeed: (0 mph) At Hover	(~0.02 mph) 1 cm/sec	(~0.2 mph) 10 cm/sec	(~2 mph) 1 m/sec	(~20 mph) 10 m/sec
VISCOUS FLIGHT REGIME:							
0.1 μm	1.2 μm/sec	F_{nano} (N)	4.1×10^{-17}	3.5×10^{-13}	3.5×10^{-12}	3.5×10^{-11}	3.5×10^{-10}
		P_{nano} (W)	5.0×10^{-22}	3.5×10^{-14}	3.5×10^{-12}	3.5×10^{-10}	3.5×10^{-8}
		D_{nano} (W/m^3)	1.2×10^{-1}	8.2×10^{6}	8.2×10^{8}	8.2×10^{10}	8.3×10^{12}
1 μm	120 μm/sec	F_{nano} (N)	4.1×10^{-14}	3.5×10^{-12}	3.5×10^{-11}	3.5×10^{-10}	3.8×10^{-9}
		P_{nano} (W)	4.9×10^{-17}	3.5×10^{-13}	3.5×10^{-11}	3.5×10^{-9}	3.8×10^{-7}
		D_{nano} (W/m^3)	1.2×10^{1}	8.2×10^{4}	8.2×10^{6}	8.3×10^{8}	9.1×10^{10}
10 μm	1.2 cm/sec	F_{nano} (N)	4.2×10^{-11}	3.5×10^{-11}	3.5×10^{-10}	3.8×10^{-9}	7.2×10^{-8}
		P_{nano} (W)	5.0×10^{-12}	3.5×10^{-12}	3.5×10^{-10}	3.8×10^{-8}	7.2×10^{-6}
		D_{nano} (W/m^3)	1.2×10^{3}	8.2×10^{2}	8.3×10^{4}	9.1×10^{6}	1.7×10^{9}
TRANSITIONAL FLIGHT REGIME:							
100 μm	68 cm/sec	F_{nano} (N)	4.1×10^{-8}	3.5×10^{-10}	3.8×10^{-9}	7.2×10^{-8}	4.1×10^{-6}
		P_{nano} (W)	2.8×10^{-7}	3.5×10^{-11}	3.8×10^{-9}	7.2×10^{-7}	4.1×10^{-4}
		D_{nano} (W/m^3)	6.6×10^{4}	8.3×10^{0}	9.1×10^{2}	1.7×10^{5}	9.9×10^{7}
1 mm	3.2 m/sec	F_{nano} (N)	4.0×10^{-5}*	3.8×10^{-9}	7.2×10^{-8}	4.1×10^{-6}	3.8×10^{-4}
		P_{nano} (W)	1.3×10^{-3}*	3.8×10^{-10}	7.2×10^{-8}	4.1×10^{-5}	3.8×10^{-2}
		D_{nano} (W/m^3)	3.0×10^{5}*	9.1×10^{-2}	1.7×10^{1}	9.9×10^{3}	9.1×10^{6}
1 cm	10 m/sec	F_{nano} (N)	---*	7.2×10^{-8}	4.1×10^{-6}	3.8×10^{-4}	3.8×10^{-2}
		P_{nano} (W)	---*	7.2×10^{-9}	4.1×10^{-6}	3.8×10^{-3}	3.8×10^{0}
		D_{nano} (W/m^3)	---*	1.7×10^{-3}	9.9×10^{-1}	9.1×10^{2}	9.0×10^{5}

* aerodynamic lift forces available for hovering at this size scale

air from a circular cross-section of radius $2R_{nano}$. The nanoflyer accelerates with constant acceleration $a_{nano} = v_{nano}^2 / 2 X_{accel}$ from a standing start to a final velocity v_{nano} in a time $t_{accel} = v_{nano}/a_{nano}$ and a running distance X_{accel}. The mass of the swept-out air is $M_{air} = 4 \pi \rho_{air} X_{accel} R_{nano}^2$ and the mass of the nanorobot is $M_{nano} = (4/3) \pi \rho_{nano} R_{nano}^3$. To conserve momentum, $M_{air} v_{air} = M_{nano} v_{nano}$, hence $v_{air} = \rho_{nano} v_{nano} R_{nano} / 3 \rho_{air} X_{accel}$; $v_{air} < v_{sound} = 343$ m/sec in dry air at 20°C and 1 atm to remain subsonic (Section 9.5.3.5). The kinetic energy imparted to the swept-out air is $KE_{air} = (1/2) M_{air} v_{air}^2$ and to the nanorobot is $KE_{nano} = (1/2) M_{nano} v_{nano}^2$, with $KE_{total} = KE_{air} + KE_{nano}$. Neglecting drag losses (e.g., ~3500 pW for R_{nano} = 1 micron and v_{nano} = 1 m/sec; Table 9.5) and assuming negligible losses within the air-accelerating mechanism itself and any drag on the air used as reaction mass, then propulsive efficiency is $e\% \sim KE_{nano} / KE_{total}$ and total power consumption is $P_{nano} \sim P_{drag} + (KE_{total} / e\% \; t_{accel})$. In the examples below we take R_{nano} = 1 micron, v_{nano} = 1 m/sec, P_{drag} ~ 3500 pW (Table 9.5), ρ_{air} = 1.205 kg/m^3 for dry air at 20°C and 1 atm, and ρ_{nano} = 1000 kg/m^3; here the Reynolds number is near unity.

A 1 micron^3 high-density (~10^{12} W/m^3; Chapter 6) powerplant develops P_{nano} ~ 1 million pW. At this high power level, a nanorobot can accelerate at a_{nano} ~ 12,000 g's for t_{accel} ~ 9 microsec, reaching v_{nano} = 1 m/sec after crossing a running distance of X_{accel} ~ 4.4 microns with an efficiency of e% ~ (0.016) 1.6% and v_{air} ~ 64 m/sec. As an alternative approach, note that a 5-microsec gas discharge from a simple pressure-release pump (Section 9.2.7.1) of volume $V_{reservoir}$ ~ 0.1 micron^3 having a pressure differential of 1000 atm (storing ~10^8 J/m^3; Section 6.2.2.3) produces a mean discharge power of P_{nano} ~ 2 million pW, which allows a_{nano} ~ 15,000 g's of acceleration with e% ~ (0.01) 1% for a maximum gas exit velocity of v_{max} ~ 70 m/sec using a nozzle of length l_{tube} = 1 micron and radius r_{tube} ~ 10 nm (Eqn. 9.36).

At a more modest P_{nano} ~ 4500 pW, the nanoflyer accelerates at a_{nano} ~ 1100 g's for t_{accel} ~ 96 microsec, reaching v_{nano} = 1 m/sec after crossing a running distance of X_{accel} ~ 48 microns with an efficiency of e% ~ 0.15 (15%) and v_{air} ~ 6 m/sec.

Attitude control of flying machines is a problem often mentioned in MEMS aerobotics work;[1576] airborne nanorobots may employ gravity-based dynamic stabilization (Section 8.3.3), gyrostabilization (Section 9.4.2.2), or other means. In 1998, the energetics and control of steering maneuvers in highly-maneuverable insects was being investigated.[1581,1582]

9.5.3.5 Hovering Flight

In large helicopters, thrust is produced by imparting a downward velocity to the mass of air flowing through the rotor, with lift proportional to the change in momentum. In 1997, engineers at the Institute for Microtechnology in Mainz, Germany, constructed a 3-cm long, 1-cm tall mini-helicopter weighing 0.3 gm with two blades turning at ~1700 Hz, and flew it to a hovering altitude of

13 cm, then landed it safely. I. Kroo at Stanford University has built and flown a "mesicopter" whose motor is 3 mm in diameter and 5 mm long, weighing ~0.3 gm, that turns the oddly-shaped rotors at ~50,000 rpm.[3246]

As helicopter size shrinks through the transitional regime, drag grows at the expense of lift and the rotorblade microhelicopter becomes increasing inefficient. However, the viscous-lift helicopter (Fig. 9.22) is estimated to be able to hover by rotating its four wheels at a frequency of $\nu_{wheel} \sim 3\, \rho_{nano}\, g\, R_{wheel} / 32\, \eta_{air} \sim 1$ KHz, taking $\rho_{nano} = 2000$ kg/m^3, g = 9.81 m/sec^2, and R_{wheel} = 10 micron.[1982]

In the general case, the terminal velocity $v_{terminal}$ of a compact nonaerodynamic body of any size falling through fluid may be approximated by setting:

$$F_{viscous} + F_{inertial} = \frac{4}{3}\,\pi\, R^3_{nano}\, g\, (\rho_{air} - \rho_{nano}) \qquad \text{\{Eqn. 9.93\}}$$

and solving the resulting quadratic for $v_{terminal}$ (= v_{nano}), using $F_{viscous}$ and $F_{inertial}$ for spherical bodies from Eqns. 9.89 and 9.90. This velocity may then be used in Eqns. 9.88 through 9.92 to conservatively estimate F_{nano}, P_{nano}, and D_{nano} for hovering. Representative values are given in Table 9.5, assuming flight in dry sea-level air and powerplant efficiency e% = 0.10 (10%). Hovering power P_{hover} scales as $\sim R_{nano}^5$ for $R_{nano} \lesssim 10$ microns and as $\sim R_{nano}^{3.5}$ in the R_{nano} ~ 0.1-1 mm range; for $R_{nano} \gtrsim 1$ mm, aerodynamic lift forces are available, the computation of which is beyond the scope of this book. For R_{nano} = 1 micron in air, $v_{terminal}$ = 120 microns/sec (Section 9.5.3.2) and P_{hover} ~ 0.00005 pW (e% = 0.10 (10%)); for R_{nano} = 10 microns, $v_{terminal}$ = 1.2 cm/sec and P_{hover} ~ 5 pW (e% = 0.10 (10%)).

In the special case of flapping winged aerobots in the transitional flight regime (e.g., 100 microns $\lesssim R_{nano} \lesssim$ 10 cm) during steady-state hovering, T. Weis-Fogh[1578,1583] calculates that the average aerodynamic power needed for small winged objects to remain airborne is:

$$P_{hover} = \frac{2}{3}\pi^2\, \rho_{air}\, \tau\, C_D\, \nu^3_{wing}\, \varphi^3_{wing}\, w_{wing}\, L^4_{wing} \quad \text{(watts)} \qquad \text{\{Eqn. 9.94\}}$$

where ρ_{air} = 1.205 kg/m^3 at 1 atm and 20°C, τ is a shape factor that equals 0.5 for a rectangular wing, 0.1 for a triangular wing attached at the base, and 0.4 for a triangular wing attached at the apex; C_D = 0.07-0.36 for bats, birds, and insects with wing length of L_{wing} = 0.25-13 cm and wing width (chord) of w_{wing} = 0.7-55 mm (flight mass M = 0.001-20 gm); wingstroke frequency ν_{wing} ranges from 15 Hz at L_{wing} = 13 cm (large hummingbird) to 600 Hz at L_{wing} = 0.25 cm; and stroke angle φ_{wing} is the angle subtended by each flapping wing in the flapping plane during a complete stroke cycle, typically 2-3 radians (120°-180°).

Thus for example, the common honeybee *Apis mellifera* (N_R ~ 1900) has M = 100 milligrams, L_{wing} = 1.0 cm, w_{wing} = 0.43 cm, τ = 0.27 (half-ellipse), C_D = 0.09, ν_{wing} = 240 Hz, and φ_{wing} = 2.09 rad, giving P_{hover} = 1 milliwatt with a dynamic efficiency of e% = 30%*; during level flight at peak speeds near ~6 m/sec,[739] experimentally-measured honeybee metabolic demand is 20-60 milliwatts.[1580] Honeybees can also carry a ~40 milligram payload of honey. At the lower extreme of the transitional flight regime, the parasitic chalcid wasp *Encarsia formosa* (N_R ~ 15) has M = 25 μg, L_{wing} = 620 microns, w_{wing} = 230 microns, τ = 0.50 (rectangle), C_D = 3.20, ν_{wing} = 400 Hz, and φ_{wing} = 2.36 rad, giving P_{hover} = 0.4 microwatt. Wingspeed v_{wing} > 1.5 m/sec during the downstroke.[1578] From the conservative assumption that biological wing muscles are limited to ~200 watts/kg (~300,000 watts/m^3), Weis-Fogh[1577] estimates than no flying animal with a mass larger than ~100 grams can hover continuously by means of wing flapping and wing twisting alone.

For artificial nanorobotic flyers near the edge of the design envelope, maximum wingbeat frequency $\nu_{max} \lesssim v_{wing} / L_{wing}$. To avoid supersonic turbulence, $v_{wing} < v_{sound}$ ~ 343 m/sec in air at 20°C and 1 atm, giving $\nu_{max} \lesssim$ 10-100 MHz for L_{wing} = 3-30 microns and $\lesssim$100 KHz for L_{wing} = 3 mm. For each small-wing cycle at 100 MHz, the boundary layer after an impulsive start is at most (modified from Prandtl[1584]) $\delta_{layer} \sim (\eta_{air} / \rho_{air}\, \nu_{max})^{1/2} \sim 0.4$ micron ~ λ_{gas} ~ 0.2 microns, the mean free path of air molecules at 1 atm (Eqn. 9.23); faster cycling would allow insufficient time for mechanical coupling to the medium. Note also that v_{sound} is significantly slower than the torsional deformation propagation velocity $v_{torsion} \sim (G / \rho_{wing})^{1/2} \sim$ 12,000 m/sec along the wing structure, taking G ~ 5 x 10^{11} N/m^2 and ρ_{wing} ~ 3510 kg/m^3 for diamondoid materials. For comparison, the slowest insectile wingbeat frequency is ~5 Hz for the swallowtail butterfly (*Papilo machaon*); the fastest is ~1046 Hz for the tiny midge *Forcipomyia* in natural conditions, up to ~2200 Hz at 310 K in laboratory experiments with truncated wings.[739,2033]

9.5.3.6 No-Fly Zones

Most circumcorporeal aerial nanorobots should take care to avoid certain well-defined zones near the human body. Perhaps the most important medical issue is that particles under 5 microns in diameter are dangerous to inhale. Concentrations of >10^8 m^{-3} of free silica particles <5 microns in size are usually considered hazardous.[1572] Airborne nanorobots may be deployed in number densities of ~10^{12} m^{-3} or higher (Section 7.4.8), so anti-inhalation, inhale-safe, and post-inhalation extraction protocols are essential in this application. (Particles larger than 2-5 microns that are inspired through the nose become trapped on the nasal mucus membrane and do not reach the lower airway; Section 8.2.2.)

At rest, inhalation velocity at the trachea is $v_{inhale\ rest}$ ~ 0.3 m/sec. During the heaviest exercise, turbulent airflow into the trachea peaks near ~3.3 liters/sec at a maximum inhalation airspeed of $v_{inhale\ max}$ ~ 5 m/sec (Section 8.2.2 and Eqn. 9.30). Nanorobots capable of flying at $v_{nano} \gtrsim v_{inhale\ max}$ can outrun even the fastest inspired air by simply reversing course. Nanorobots restricted to slower speeds can also avoid inhalation by promptly initiating lateral motion immediately upon entering either of two hemiellipsoidal no-fly zones which are very conservatively estimated to be of major-axial radius:

$$R_{clear} \sim \frac{R_{oral}\, v_{inhale\ max}}{2\, v_{nano}} \quad \text{(meters)} \qquad \text{\{Eqn. 9.95\}}$$

centered on the vestibule of the mouth and on the anterior nares of the nose, where R_{oral} ~ 2.5 cm is the radius of the oral orifice. Thus a nanorobot with maximum airspeed v_{nano} = 1 m/sec must observe a perifacial no-fly major-axial radius of R_{clear} ~ 6 cm.

The second most important no-fly zone is the surface of the skin, including (in special circumstances) the oral mucous (tissue) membrane, tongue, soft palate, larynx, trachea, and nasal passages. It is theoretically possible for diamondoid nanorobots with rigid protrusions that accidentally impact the epidermis at high speeds to irritate or even tear the skin. Consider a nanorobot of density ρ and dimension L with a rigid appendage of dimension q L, that impacts

* *A few other dynamic efficiency figures for hovering flight include the hornet wasp (31%), hummingbird (51%), mosquito (70%), fruit fly (95%), and butterfly (97%).*[1578]

an epidermal surface of tearing strength σ_{tear} at a velocity v, coming to a halt in a distance $X_{scratch}$. If the impact energy is transferred exclusively through the appendage, then the skin tears if:

$$X_{scratch} \lesssim \frac{\rho L v^2}{2 q^2 \sigma_{tear}} \quad \text{(meters)} \qquad \text{\{Eqn. 9.96\}}$$

Taking ρ = 2000 kg/m^3, L = 100 microns, v = 10 m/sec, q/L = 0.1, and σ_{tear} = 10^7 N/m^2, then $X_{scratch} \lesssim$ 100 microns—potentially leaving up to a 100-micron long, 10-micron deep scratch on the skin. Long scalp hair, which often waves randomly in the wind, should also be avoided (or actively managed; Chapter 28) by the aerial nanorobot cloud. Nanorobots with 10-100 micron-long wings operated at 0.1-1 MHz (avoiding subharmonics to ensure buzzless performance) can have transverse wingtip velocities up to 1-10 m/sec, which could damage soft tissues upon impact.

Another possible no-fly zone is the interior of the auditory canal, especially immediately adjacent to the tympanic membrane. In theory (Section 7.4.8), a very dense nanorobot cloud using acoustic communications at high bandwidth could generate a pressure intensity at the eardrum that exceeds the threshold of pain, although this is unlikely in practice. (More interestingly, such a cloud could enter the ear canal and emit coordinated audible subharmonics in the 100-1000 Hz range, thus "speaking" directly to the user; Section 7.4.6.3.)

Optical communication intensities are equally unlikely to exceed safe limits in the vicinity of the human eye (Section 7.4.8). However, entirely aside from the epidermal no-fly zone (above), general-purpose aerial nanorobots should especially avoid all contact with the surface of the cornea, the conjunctiva, and the inner surfaces of the eyelid, in order to prevent irritation, or serious scoring and gouging (e.g., corneal ulcer, conjunctivitis, or superficial punctate keratitis), or embedment in these much softer, exposed mucosal tissues.

CHAPTER 10

Other Basic Capabilities

This final Chapter describes a miscellany of important technical capabilities that may prove useful in some or all medical nanodevices, in various scenarios or theaters of operation. Any one of these subjects deserves an entire chapter to itself, but unfortunately there is only space in this introductory text for a brief survey of each area. The most important of these topics is computation (Section 10.2), including nanomechanical, nanoelectronic, and biological computing, as well as nanoscale data storage technologies. However, the fields of organic and fullerene nanoelectronics, biocomputing, and quantum computing are advancing so fast that whatever is written here will quickly become obsolete. Thus our coverage in this Volume is limited to a broad overview. Interested readers are strongly advised to consult the current literature for the latest results.

Other important basic capabilities covered in this Chapter include timers and nanoclocks with long-term nanosecond stability (Section 10.1); high-pressure materials storage (Section 10.3); defensive cytocidal and antiviral weaponry to allow the efficient destruction of pathogenic intruders and unrepairable tumor cells (Section 10.4); and the effects of very hot or very cold temperatures on nanorobot materials and operations (Section 10.5).

10.1 Nanochronometry

Nanorobots will use clocks in many applications. Computer gating,* navigation, and high-speed sensor applications may require repeatable timing in the 1-1000 nanosec range, or 1-1000 microsec for lower-speed chemical and chemotactic sensing, although long-term clock stability is not especially critical for computing. Neuron-mediated signals and muscle motions are monitored and controlled on a 1-1000 millisec timescale, while conscious human action and most human biorhythms occur in the 1-10^5 sec range.

This Section briefly introduces human chronobiology (Section 10.1.1), then describes possible nanoscale oscillator systems that could be useful in nanorobotic clocks (Section 10.1.2), basic principles of pre- and post-infusion nanorobot chronometer synchronization (Section 10.1.3), and dedicated chronometer organs (Section 10.1.4).

10.1.1 Human Chronobiology

The human body incorporates numerous biological clocks.[1665,1666] The best-known and most-studied example is the daily (24-hour) endogenous circadian oscillator.[1665] This internal clock is normally reset by natural sunlight, which is much brighter than indoor lighting. The clock, in turn, sets the cadence for most of the other 24-hour body rhythms—for example, sleep/wakefulness cycles (e.g., melatonin[1676]), urine production,[1677] body temperature, blood cortisol and ACTH cycles[1677] (Appendix B), and the diurnal rhythm of mitosis in epidermal epithelium (e.g., greatest during sleep or inactivity, least during wakefulness or activity).[359] The circadian clock stability (variation in free-running period) is ~1% in *Drosophila*[1683] and ~0.2% in humans.[3434]

Mammalian circadian rhythms are regulated by a master pacemaker within the suprachiasmatic nuclei (SCN) of the hypothalamus (just above the point at which the optic nerves from each eye cross in mid-brain).[1678] In humans, the SCN is comprised of ~10,000 special cells that send out electrochemical signals in a 24-hour timing pattern. Entrainment of the clock to light-dark cycles is mediated by photoreceptors in the retina,[1679] with light information conveyed directly from ganglion cells of the retina to the SCN via the retinohypothalamic tract.[1680] Mammals and other vertebrates have another independent circadian clock in each retina, possibly driven by the retinal cryptochromes CRY1 (also made in the SCN) and CRY2, producing rhythms in local physiology[1676] such as the diurnal renewal cycles of rods and cones.[1664] CRY1 is also abundant in skin tissues. Clock-resetting photoreceptors have been found in the human popliteal region (behind the knees),[1675] and such photoreceptors may exist in many different tissues throughout the human body.[1673,1675]

The current model for a core circadian oscillator comprises, in part, a transcription/translation-based negative feedback loop in which clock genes are rhythmically expressed, giving rise to cycling levels of clock RNAs and proteins (negative elements). The proteins then feed back, after a lag, to depress the level of their own transcripts, perhaps by interfering with positive elements that increase transcription of the clock genes.[1681] In 1998 this genetic network was still in the discovery process.[1667-1672] One ~100,000-base-pair gene, aptly named "clock," was known to produce an 855-residue protein (mCLOCK in mice, 115.7 kD) that serves as a major regulator of the ~10 other, still unidentified, genes thought to affect circadian rhythm.[1671,1672] (One portion of mCLOCK is the same as in a related 1023-residue clock protein, dCLOCK, found in *Drosophila* fruit flies[1672]). Circadian rhythms will almost certainly be made up of many interconnected feedback loops that interact with the CLOCK-related core pathway.[1681] It is believed that this interconnected

* *Clocks are not strictly required for computation. D.E. Muller pioneered attempts[1880,1881] in the late 1950s to eliminate all time dependencies in digital logic circuits, including fundamental mode circuits,[1882] speed-independent circuits and delay insensitive circuits (generally considered the most difficult, expensive and elusive circuits to design[1883]). Traditional asynchronous control designs[1884] employ considerably more circuitry than is required by a functionally equivalent clocked Boolean logic circuit; K.M. Fant and S.A. Brandt[1885] have devised a more parsimonious and theoretically complete approach to delay insensitive circuits called Null Convention Logic.*

ensemble will ultimately determine all of the classical circadian properties—period length,[1665,1666] temperature compensation,[1682,1683] and resetting by light or temperature.[1684,1685,1963] In 1998, most chronobiologists believed that many of these outer loops would be organism specific and that only the core loop would be more universal.[1681]

In addition to the 24-hour circadian oscillator, many other biological clocks have been identified in humans. For example, the 28-day menstrual cycle is timed by two ovarian clocks, each delimiting a period of 14 days.[1686] One of these two clocks is the Graafian follicle and its production of estradiol, while the other clock is the corpus luteum and its secretion of progesterone. Both are obligatorily dependent upon the proper functioning of a third clock located in the arcuate region of the hypothalamus, known as the GnRH pulse generator,[1687,3675-3678] which ensures the rhythmic production and release of the gonadotropic hormones into the peripheral circulation with a cyclical period of ~1 hour (±25% stability), coincident with a 1-hour cycle of hypothalamic electrical activity (±12% stability).[1686,1687] A 90-minute clock paces the development of the somites, blocks of tissue that form in regular arrays along the spinal cord of vertebrate embryos. One regulatory gene, named "chairy," undergoes repeated 90-minute activity cycles and is known not to require protein synthesis; gene expression follows the repeating pattern even when protein synthesis is biochemically blocked.[1688] A much longer half-weekly (circasemiseptan) pattern has been observed in mitotic activity in cancer patients.[3326]

Other biological clocks abound. The stomach produces rhythmic contractions of ~3/minute during digestion. Rhythmic segmentation contractions of the bowel at ~0.2 Hz (Section 8.2.3) are driven by a thin layer of specialized pacemaker cells called the intestinal cells of Cajal, which demonstrate electrical oscillations at about the same rate as the contractions.[1725] Cardiac pacemaker cells in the sinoatrial node emit a cyclical pulse that triggers a heartbeat at a ~1 Hz basal rate. The respiratory centers in the medulla oblongata produce an autonomic contraction cycle of the diaphragm at ~0.3 Hz. The human eye produces many spontaneous rhythmic dilations and constrictions, including high-frequency ocular microtremors present in all people (mean frequency ~84-88 Hz),[3679] accommodation microfluctuations (~1-2 Hz)[3681-3683] with the pupil varying <300 microns in diameter,[3680] and low-frequency pupillary oscillations (e.g., ~0.2 Hz "hippus").[3683-3685] Electrical rhythms generated by the brain that are detectable by an electroencephalograph include alpha waves predominantly in the occipital region at 8-13 Hz, beta waves in the frontal and central areas at 18-30 Hz, delta waves at <4 Hz during deep sleep or abnormal function, and theta waves in the temporal and parietal areas at 4-7 Hz.[1689]

Individual cells display a number of oscillatory biochemical pathways as well, including calcium ion oscillations, cyclic AMP signalling, and various other cell cycles.[1666] For instance, the glycolytic enzyme oscillator, controlled primarily by phosphofructokinase, may mediate various rhythmic physiological behaviors such as slow waves of contraction in smooth muscle, electrical activity in neurons, and insulin release from β islet cells of the pancreas. In one experiment,[1690] this oscillator mediated a 55 mV voltage change in guinea pig cardiomyocytes at 0.010 Hz (±10% stability) in an almost perfectly sinusoidal pattern, although a few cells displayed oscillations with irregular phase, amplitude, or both. In another experiment, fluorescently-labeled puffs of tumor-cell cytoplasm were observed being released through plasma membrane ruptures, regularly at ~0.05 Hz during a neutrophil-mediated cytolytic attack, matching the nicotinamide-adenine dinucleotide phosphate and superoxide release periods for neutrophils.[3663] By 1998 there was a growing belief that many, if not most, of the cells in an animal may possess individual biological clocks;[2015] fruit flies were already known to have clocks distributed throughout their wings, legs, and abdomen.

The human brain also possesses an interval timer[1691,3686-3688] that allows a person to gauge the passage of seconds or minutes to a mean accuracy of ±15%. The interval timer functions like a stopwatch and resides in the basal ganglia, a region of the brain that coordinates voluntary muscle movements. A population of neurons in the substantia nigra releases regular pulses of dopamine into an accumulator, called the caudate-putamen, a major part of the basal ganglia. These pulses are then read via neural pathways to the cerebral cortex which are known as striato-cortical loops. Other internal "alarm clocks" that reliably allow waking from sleep at desired times* have been described.[2693]

In vivo nanorobots should be able to eavesdrop on most of these active chronobiological channels, gaining complete knowledge of the oscillator frequencies and phase settings of virtually all of the human body's biological clock systems. For example, blood plasma cortisol typically peaks in the morning (e.g., 6-23 x 10^{-8} gm/cm^3 at 8 AM), then declines throughout the day (e.g., 3-15 x 10^{-8} gm/cm^3 at 4 PM, then ~50% of 8 AM value at 10 PM). Melatonin (also detectable in saliva) cycles in the opposite direction, normally peaking at 6-7 x 10^{-11} gm/cm^3 at night and then falling to 1.4 x 10^{-11} gm/cm^3 during the day (Appendix B). Longer cycles are easily tracked too. For instance, blood viscosity in healthy young women shows the rhythmic variation of the menstrual cycle, probably due to changes in serum fibrinogen and globulin levels which can be measured more directly.[1325] These nanorobot-accessible readings may be used either to measure "body time" or to control it, and in some cases can recalibrate relevant onboard nanochronometers.

Environmental time cues may also be detected by in vivo nanorobots (e.g., temporal macrosensing), such as the level of illumination penetrating the epidermis (sometimes permitting inference of day or night) or the all-pervasive 60/50 Hz (U.S./Europe) electromagnetic hum generated by alternating current electrical supply systems in common use throughout the world, a crude frequency standard whose voltage can sometimes display time-of-day load-related fluctuations.[3026]

10.1.2 Artificial Nanoscale Oscillators

Nanorobot clocks must perform at least two critical functions: (1) Interval timing (measuring elapsed time between two or more sequential events) and chronometry (maintaining an onboard calendrical "standard time" in good calibration with an external time standard such as Coordinated Universal Time[3027,3302]). Complete clock design, including clutches, feedback mechanisms and governors, dampers and filters, triggers and strikers, amplifiers and mixers, phase detectors and counters, regenerative frequency dividers and frequency multipliers, and antivibration housings, is very complex and quite beyond the scope of this text. However, both timing and chronometry require a high-frequency oscillator of known and stable frequency, whose oscillations can then be counted for clocking purposes. If frequency multipliers can be built, then the primary oscillator need not be high frequency; the requirement for frequency stability is more fundamental. Timing accuracies of 1-1000 nanosec are typically needed for sensor (Chapter 4), navigation (Section 8.3.3), and

*Long ago, native American Indians of the Sioux tribe learned, after carefully controlled experiments, that they could use a full urinary bladder as a kind of alarm clock. By drinking a certain amount of water at bedtime, they found they would awaken in a specific number of hours—drink more fluid, and they would awaken earlier from the urge to urinate; drink less, and they would awaken later.[2223]

computational (Section 10.2) applications, with operating frequencies up to $\nu_{osc} \sim 1$ GHz and durations ranging from 1 microsec up to 10^5 sec (~1 day) between timed events or between clock recalibrations (Section 10.1.3). This Section presents a brief survey of several useful nanoscale oscillator systems.

10.1.2.1 Mechanochemical and Photochemical Oscillators

A chemical oscillator involves transitions between two well-defined chemical, energetic, or conformational states. For example, repetitive room-temperature protein folding such as α-helical coiling may occur in $\sim 10^{-6}$ sec (e.g., $\nu_{osc} \sim 1$ MHz).[467] Turnover number (molecules of substrate converted to product per active site per unit time) for catalase, one of the fastest known enzymes, is $k_{cat} = \nu_{osc} = 40$ MHz.[759] Reversible gas phase reactions may occur at up to 5 GHz.[390] However, chemical-based clocks are expected to display poor frequency stability. Most chemical reactions display $\sim e^{-1/T}$ rate dependence, giving a frequency stability of $\Delta\nu / \nu \sim 1\%$ for a ~1 K temperature (T) variation in the oscillator near 310 K. Chemically-driven mechanical oscillators such as biological cilia display a similar temperature dependency and frequency stability.[1695] Time measurements that depend on the rates of thermally activated bulk reactions also suffer Poisson noise in the reaction rate from the statistics of interaction of many random independent molecules.

Some molecular transitions are even faster. Molecular dynamics simulations of carbonmonoxy-myoglobin show periodic openings and closings of internal voids on a time scale of ~100 picosec,[1693] giving $\nu_{osc} \sim 10$ GHz. The torsional isomerization of the retinal chromophore in rhodopsin from the 11-cis to the 11-trans structure, a ~0.5 nm physical motion detectable by displacement nanosensors (Section 4.3.1), occurs within ~0.2 picosec of the absorption of the 500 nm photon (~420 zJ/molecule), potentially allowing event timing at $\nu_{osc} \sim 5$ THz. The frequency of decomposition of activated complexes in classical reaction rate theory is given by Eyring[1694] as $\nu_{active} \sim kT / h \sim 6$ THz, approximately the characteristic timescale for molecular vibrations. The frequency stability of these transitions is unknown.

10.1.2.2 Mechanical Oscillators

The most accurate macroscale mechanical clock was the Shortt pendulum clock, the primary timekeeper at the Greenwich and U.S. Naval observatories until the late 1940s. The Shortt clock consisted of a pendulum swinging freely in near-vacuum at constant temperature, driven by another identical clock slaved to the first; frequency stability was $\Delta\nu / \nu \sim 4 \times 10^{-8}$.[1696]

In the nanoscale realm, Drexler[10] proposes a $\nu_{osc} \sim 1$ GHz mechanical clock intended to drive a nanomechanical computer CPU (Section 10.2.1). In this clock, a DC electrostatic motor (Section 6.3.5) turns a crankshaft that converts rotary motion into sinusoidally oscillating linear motions of a drive rod. A cam surface on the drive rod forces a follower rod into up or down positions, generating regular clock pulses with intervals determined by the position of the follower with respect to the mean position of the ramp on the cam surface. Clock stability is limited by the stability of the crankshaft rotation rate. The proposed DC electrostatic motor has radius $R_{motor} = 195$ nm, rim speed $v_{rim} = 1000$ m/sec, and output power $P_{motor} = 1.1$ microwatt, giving a developed torque of $\tau_{motor} \sim 2 \times 10^{-16}$ N-m. From Eqn. 4.23, the minimum detectable force (e.g., to establish feedback control, such as a Watt governor) for a 195-nm force sensor with 99% reliability is at most ~0.4 pN, giving a minimum detectable torque of $\tau_{min} = 8 \times 10^{-20}$ N-m. At constant torque, variation in crankshaft angular velocity $\Delta\omega / \omega$ (= $\Delta\nu / \nu$) $\sim \tau_{min} / \tau_{motor} = 4 \times 10^{-4}$.

Numerous alternative mechanical oscillators are readily conceived:

A. *Tuning Fork* — A diamondoid tuning fork with tines of length $L_{fork} = 100$ nm, half-thickness $R_{fork} = 10$ nm, density $\rho_{fork} = 3510$ kg/m^3 and Young's modulus $E_{fork} = 1.05 \times 10^{12}$ N/m^2 has a natural vibrational frequency of:[1697,1698]

$$\nu_{osc} = \frac{R_{fork}\, E_{fork}^{1/2}}{\pi\, \rho_{fork}^{1/2}\, L_{fork}^2} \sim 6 \text{ GHz} \qquad \text{\{Eqn. 10.1\}}$$

In 1998, Sandia National Laboratories began offering a product line of electrostatically-driven ~1 MHz polysilicon "tuning fork" microresonators.

B. *Helical Spring* — A helical spring with spring constant $k_s = 10$ N/m and mass $m_{spring} \sim 2 \times 10^{-19}$ kg (~40-nm-edge diamond cube) has a natural vibrational frequency of:

$$\nu_{osc} = \frac{1}{2\pi}\left(\frac{k_s}{m_{spring}}\right)^{1/2} \sim 1 \text{ GHz} \qquad \text{\{Eqn. 10.2\}}$$

ignoring gravity and spring mass.

C. *Circular Membrane* — A flexible, thin circular membrane of radius $R_{membrane} = 100$ nm, uniform density $\rho_{membrane} = 3510$ kg/m^3, and thickness $h_{membrane} = 10$ nm, if clamped at its boundary and stretched by a tension $F_{membrane}$ (the force per unit length anywhere in the membrane), has characteristic frequencies of vibration of:[1698]

$$\nu_{osc} = \frac{\beta\, F_{membrane}^{1/2}}{2\, R_{membrane}\, h_{membrane}^{1/2}\, \rho_{membrane}^{1/2}} \sim 8 \text{ GHz} \qquad \text{\{Eqn. 10.3\}}$$

where $F_{membrane} \sim 100$ N/m for a 10-nm thick diamondoid sheet stretched to near a conservative working stress of $\sim 10^{10}$ N/m^2, and β is a constant of order unity, derived from the roots of Bessel functions for various diametral and circular vibrational nodes.

D. *Torsional Pendulum* — Another oscillator is the torsional pendulum, wherein a diamondoid rod of radius $R_{rod} = 35$ nm, length $L_{rod} = 1900$ nm, density $\rho_{rod} = 3510$ kg/m^3, and shear modulus $G_{rod} = 5 \times 10^{11}$ N/m^2, is clamped at one end and the other end twists around the longitudinal axis in vacuo at a characteristic oscillation frequency:[1164]

$$\nu_{osc} = \left(\frac{G_{rod}}{4\pi^2\, L_{rod}^2\, \rho_{rod}}\right)^{1/2} \sim 1 \text{ GHz} \qquad \text{\{Eqn. 10.4\}}$$

If the end of this rod twists through an amplitude ΔX, then the time averaged power loss due to shear radiation[10] is $P_{rad} = \pi R_{rod}^6 \Delta X^2 G_{rod}^{3/2} / 256 L_{rod}^6 \rho_{rod}^{1/2} \sim 26$ pW for $\Delta X \lesssim 95$ nm, a rod strain of $\Delta X / L_{rod} \lesssim 5\%$ and an oscillator power density of $D_{rod} = P_{rad} / \pi R_{rod}^2 L_{rod} \sim 4 \times 10^9$ watts/m^3. The stored torsional energy is $E_{rod} = (1/2)\, k_{torsion}\, \theta^2 = \pi G_{rod} \Delta X^2 R_{rod}^2 / 4 L_{rod}$, so the characteristic decay time for the oscillation in the exemplar system is:

$$t_{decay} \sim \frac{E_{rod}}{P_{rad}} = \frac{64\, L_{rod}^5\, \rho_{rod}^{1/2}}{R_{rod}^4\, G_{rod}^{1/2}} \sim 0.1 \text{ sec} \qquad \text{\{Eqn. 10.5\}}$$

giving plenty of access time for clock resonance driver mechanisms. Aside from exogenous noise sources, which can be considerable in magnitude but may be filtered out by good design, one important endogenous source of uncertainty in ν_{osc} is the elastic longitudinal displacement (ΔL) for the end of a thermally excited rod that randomly alters rod length, slightly changing the frequency. For bulk diamond at T ~ 300 K, and ignoring entropic contributions which become important only in longer, narrower rods than in this example, $\Delta L \sim 10^{-16}\ L_{rod}^{1/2}\ /\ 2\ R_{rod}$ (Tables 5.8 and 5.16 in Drexler[10]). Since $\nu_{osc} \sim L_{rod}^{-1}$, then $\Delta\nu\ /\ \nu \sim \Delta L\ /\ L_{rod}$ and so:

$$\frac{\Delta\nu}{\nu} = \left(\frac{k_{elast}}{L_{rod}\ R_{rod}^2}\right)^{1/2} \sim 1 \times 10^{-6} \qquad \{\text{Eqn. 10.6}\}$$

for $k_{elast} \sim 2.5 \times 10^{-33}\ m^3$, L_{rod} = 1900 nm, and R_{rod} = 35 nm. Another systemic source of uncertainty is rod length variation due to the slowly temporally- and spatially-varying ambient human body temperature. Given a coefficient of volume expansion $\beta = 3.5 \times 10^{-6}\ K^{-1}$ for diamond,[567] a typical variation of $\Delta T \sim 3$ K per $t_{circ} \sim 60$ sec circulation time for bloodborne nanorobots, and a thermal recalibration time of $t_{recalib} \sim 1$ sec (to correct for temperature dependence), then $\Delta\nu\ /\ \nu \sim t_{recalib}\ \Delta T\ \beta\ /\ t_{circ} \sim 2 \times 10^{-7}$. J. Soreff notes that yet another limitation on oscillator accuracy is the 1/Q resonance width, which is a function of the design details.

Clock accuracy may be defined by a time measurement error over a single observation cycle (N_{obs} = 1) of $\Delta t_{error} = t_{actual} - t_{clock}$, where $t_{actual} = (\nu_{osc})^{-1}$ and $t_{clock} = (\nu_{osc}\ (1 + \Delta\nu\ /\ \nu))^{-1}$. Time measurement errors over multiple cycles (e.g., $N_{obs} = \nu_{osc}\ t_{obs} > 1$), spanning a total observation time t_{obs} between clock recalibrations, are randomly distributed around zero but do not sum to zero, constituting instead a random walk with a maximum excursion of:

$$t_{error} \sim N_{obs}^{1/2}\ \Delta t_{error} = \left(\frac{t_{obs}}{\nu_{osc}}\right)^{1/2} \left(\frac{\Delta\nu/\nu}{1 + \Delta\nu/\nu}\right) \qquad \{\text{Eqn. 10.7}\}$$

This assumes that the errors are uncorrelated—e.g., for thermal fluctuation errors, individual observation times must lie at least t_{EQ} apart, where t_{EQ} is the time required for thermal equilibration with the environment (Eqn. 10.24). For the exemplar oscillator with $\Delta\nu\ /\ \nu \sim 10^{-6}$ at ν_{osc} = 1 GHz, accumulated $t_{error} \sim 1$ nanosec during a continuous (uncalibrated) observation time of $t_{obs} \sim 1000$ sec.

10.1.2.3 Acoustic Transmission Line Oscillators

Drexler[10] describes a diamondoid acoustic transmission line in which a ~2 nN force pulse is initiated at one end, travels to the far end at $v_{sound} \sim 17{,}300$ m/sec, then is received by a mechanical displacement probe, possibly with significant energy recovery. Such lines may also be used to generate precisely delayed acoustic signal sets suitable for clocking applications. Consider a "starter" pulse applied to a short feeder line that symmetrically bifurcates into a set of n_{line} = 10 lines each of length l_n = (1730 n) nm (n = 1, 2, ..., n_{line}), requiring a total length $L_{line} = (1730)\ n_{line}\ (n_{line} + 1)\ /\ 2$ = 95,150 nm of transmission line to obtain a set of lines having all n_{line} time delays. The bifurcated pulses arrive at the end of each line in 0.1 nanosec (n = 1), 0.2 nanosec (n = 2), ..., 1.0 nanosec (n = 10); any of these pulses may be drawn off and used for diverse clocking purposes, or may be fed back into the initiation mechanism and used either to trigger the next starter pulse or to achieve more robust error correction. If acoustic lines have a cross-sectional area of ~30 nm^2, then the total volume of all ten lines is ~3,000,000 nm^3, which may be coiled into ~0.3% of the volume of a 1 micron^3 nanorobot. Such diamondoid acoustic power transmission lines are essentially lossless (Section 7.2.5.3). If a complete set of lines containing all n_{line} delays is not required, any desired single delay time may be obtained by connecting up to n_{line} segments end to end, or by bouncing a pulse off of the ends of a single line up to n_{line} times.

Aside from the many potential frequency instabilities inherent in pulse detection, signal re-initiation, and acoustic interferometry mechanisms, two fundamental sources of frequency instability include:

1. changes in the velocity of sound due to thermal variations, and;
2. changes in acoustic path length due to elastic longitudinal displacements of thermally excited transmission rods.

First, the speed of transverse sound waves in an isotropic elastic medium having Poisson's ratio $c_{Poisson}$ (~0.1 for diamond) is given by:[10]

$$v_{sound} = \left(\frac{E}{\rho}\right)^{1/2} \left[\frac{1 - c_{Poisson}}{(1 + c_{Poisson})(1 - 2\ c_{Poisson})}\right]^{1/2} \sim 17{,}300\ \text{m/sec}$$

{Eqn. 10.8}

where Young's modulus E = 1.05×10^{12} N/m^2 and density ρ = 3510 kg/m^3 for diamond. In addition to the thermal dependency of E, ρ varies as $(1 + \beta_{thermal}\ T)^{-1}$ where T is temperature, because volume changes according to the volume coefficient of thermal expansion $\beta_{thermal} = 3.5 \times 10^{-6}\ K^{-1}$ for diamond, $1.56 \times 10^{-5}\ K^{-1}$ for sapphire. In an uncorrected oscillator system, $\Delta\nu\ /\ \nu \sim \Delta v_{sound}\ /\ v_{sound} \sim (1/2)\ \beta_{thermal}\ \Delta T \sim 10^{-5}$ for diamondoid transmission lines, assuming that $\Delta T \sim 6$ K temperature variations are typically encountered inside the human body (Table 8.11). Correcting oscillator timing using independent temperature sensors accurate to $\Delta T_{min}\ /\ T \sim 10^{-6}$ (Section 4.6), and ignoring other possible sources of frequency instability (which may be significant), could reduce measurement ΔT to ~310 microkelvins at T ~ 310 K, thus improving $\Delta\nu\ /\ \nu$ significantly for this source of frequency instability.

Second, longitudinal displacements $\Delta L\ /\ L_{rod} \sim 10^{-4} - 10^{-5}$ at 300 K for rods of length L_{rod} = 1.73-17.3 microns and cross-section $A_{rod} \sim 30$ nm^2 (Figure 5.8 in Drexler[10]); J. Soreff observes that $\Delta L\ /\ L_{rod} \sim (kT\ /\ E\ L_{rod}\ A_{rod})^{1/2} \sim 10^{-6}$ for ~0.01 micron^3-volume systems. For the zeroth longitudinal vibrational mode,[10] these displacements occur on a timescale $\nu_{osc}^{-1} = 4\ L_{rod}\ (\rho\ /\ E)^{1/2}$ = 0.4-4 nanosec, comparable to signal transit times, taking ρ and E for diamond as above and L_{rod} = (1730 n) nm with n = 1, 2, ..., n_{line}. This may restrict $\Delta\nu\ /\ \nu$ to ~ 10^{-6} unless transmission lines can be further rigidized by end-clamping, sheathing, or latticed bracing at intervals, all of which, in effect, enlarge A_{rod}.

10.1.2.4 Quartz Resonators

Piezoelectric quartz crystals, when cut in a predetermined manner and mounted so that two opposing faces have electrical contacts, will compress or expand when an oscillating electric field is applied across the faces.[1701,1702] The amplitude of crystal vibration falls off very rapidly as the applied electric field frequency deviates from the resonant frequency of the crystal. (Cyclical mechanical compressions at the resonant frequency also induce oscillating electric fields of maximum amplitude.) In 1998, most high-precision timing devices were based on quartz crystal resonators, with ~2 billion resonators manufactured annually worldwide for oscillator, clock, and filter applications.[1699] Commercially-available off-the-shelf GHz devices (e.g., Micro Networks' M101 resonator) typically displayed ~10 ppm stability, or $\Delta\nu / \nu \sim 10^{-5}$, readily improved to $\sim 10^{-7}$ in temperature-controlled ovens.

The fundamental mode resonant frequency of a quartz crystal plate of thickness $d_{quartz} \sim 1$ micron (~2000 molecular layers thick), density $\rho_{quartz} \sim 2650$ kg/m^3,[763] and elastic (Young's) modulus $E_{quartz} \sim 1.1 \times 10^{11}$ N/m^2 (Table 9.3) vibrating in thickness mode is:[1699]

$$\nu_{osc} = \left(\frac{1}{2\, d_{quartz}}\right)\left(\frac{E_{quartz}}{\rho_{quartz}}\right)^{1/2} \sim 3 \text{ GHz} \qquad \text{\{Eqn. 10.9\}}$$

The resonant frequencies of the highest-quality, lowest-noise quartz macroresonators can be measured with a precision of 14 significant figures,[1699] e.g., the noise is $\Delta\nu / \nu \sim 3 \times 10^{-14}$ at the optimum measurement times.[1700] However, each variable in Eqn. 10.9 is temperature dependent. For instance, the thermal expansion of quartz (affecting density) and the temperature coefficients of E_{quartz} (ranging from positive to negative values) are highly dependent on the angles of cut of the plate relative to the crystallographic axes. Quartz resonator frequency may vary monotonically with temperature at 10^{-5} - 10^{-4} K^{-1}; the noise floor (i.e., the Allan deviation floor[1702]) for quartz microresonators has been estimated[1699] as $\Delta\nu / \nu \sim (1.2 \times 10^{-19}$ Hz$^{-1}) \nu_{osc} \sim 10^{-10}$ for $\nu_{osc} \sim 1$ GHz. Atomistic simulation of submicron quartz oscillators by Broughton[2669] suggests that such oscillators must have at least ~10^6 atoms to display bulk elastic constants, and that differences from continuum mechanical frequency predictions are observable for 17-nm (or smaller) devices, and that nanoscale devices with even a single defect may exhibit dramatic anharmonicity.

10.1.2.5 Atomic Frequency Standards

The most accurate oscillators are the Atomic Frequency Standards (AFS) used in "atomic clocks." In these "clocks," an atom flips between two slightly different configurations—one in which the electron spin and the nuclear spin point in the same direction, and another configuration in which the two spins point in opposite directions. In its original form,[3028,3029] a beam of cesium (Cs^{133}) atoms is emitted from an oven and passes through an evacuated (~10^{-11} atm) chamber, where the atoms are focused by one fixed magnet, then defocused by a second fixed magnet. Between the two fixed magnets, the beam passes through a microwave field. When the frequency of this oscillating field exactly matches a natural atomic resonance ground-state hyperfine transition frequency of Cs (~9.192,631,770 GHz), the spin energy state can switch polarity, allowing "flipped" atoms to focus, rather than defocus, at the second fixed magnet. Atoms arriving at the focus are ionized by a hot-wire ionizer target, then directed onto an electron multiplier by a mass spectrometer to be counted. The microwave frequency is adjusted until the electron multiplier output current is maximized, constituting the measurement of the atoms' resonance frequency.

Early cesium AFSs were used to recalibrate a quartz oscillator about once a day, achieving $\Delta\nu / \nu \sim 3 \times 10^{-11}$. In 1998, the best non-cryogenic laboratory Cs or Rb (rubidium) AFS had $\Delta\nu / \nu \sim 2 \times 10^{-14}$, with a temperature stability of ~10^{-13} K^{-1} between 263-313 K and a magnetic stability of ~10^{-12}/gauss.[1703] The smallest non-cryogenic Rb AFS was a space-qualified system with mass of 1.3 kg and power consumption of 11 watts (~10^4 watts/m^3), achieving $\Delta\nu / \nu \lesssim 5 \times 10^{-13}$. Another system that achieved $\Delta\nu / \nu \lesssim 5 \times 10^{-14}$ had mass ~5.5 kg and drew 39 watts.[1703] Laser-cooled low-temperature clocks using Bose-Einstein condensates were expected eventually to demonstrate $\Delta\nu / \nu \sim 10^{-18}$.

In 1998, the miniaturization of rubidium AFS for space applications was being actively studied,[1704,1705] along with newer approaches such as optically-pumped cesium AFS using solid state diode lasers (thus eliminating the bulky magnets),[1706] diode laser-pumped rubidium AFS in which the Rb discharge lamp is replaced with a ~100% efficient diode laser tuned to the correct transition frequency,[1707,1708] and Hg^+ "optical clocks."[1709] Optical pumping methods using diode lasers defined the NIST-7 atomic-beam standard of $\Delta\nu / \nu \lesssim 5 \times 10^{-15}$, starting in 1993.

A detailed analysis of micron-size atomic clocks is beyond the scope of this book. The possibility cannot be ruled out, but in 1998 the feasibility was unknown. From Eqn. 4.50, the minimum sensor capable of detecting a spin transition requires $N_{min} \sim 7 \times 10^6$ Cs atoms (~0.001 micron^3 of Cs), taking transition frequency ν_L = 9.192,631,770 GHz and electron spin angular momentum $L_{electron} = L_{proton}$. However, many problems must be overcome including interactions involving spontaneous decay, measurement-induced transitions, phase changes due to gas molecule collisions, spatial confinement effects, the use of symmetries and cancellation of couplings. J. Soreff [personal communication, 1998] suggests consideration of an oscillator structure in which a phosphorus atom is covalently bound to a tetrahedral support of carbyne rods extending to the ends of an evacuated chamber. The fifth valence electron on the phosphorus atom should have a hyperfine interaction with the P^{31} nucleus, but it is presently unknown how tightly coupled the thermal vibrations in the rods are to the hyperfine state transition, since many coupling modes may vanish by symmetry.

10.1.3 Nanorobot Synchronization

Ideally, the clocks of all nanorobots present in a patient's body will be synchronized to some universal time. This time setting may be defined by the patient, by the physician, or by reference to some external standard. As part of a chronometry-critical nanorobot installation procedure prior to infusion, an initializing signal can be transmitted throughout the infusate volume, allowing each individual nanorobot present therein to receive the signal and set its clock.

Acoustic synchronization pulses are appropriate if ~microsec precision will suffice. Sound waves passing at v_{sound} = 1500 m/sec through an L_{vial} = 1.5 cm wide container of well-stirred aqueous-suspended nanorobots restricts synchronization error to $\Delta t_{error} \sim L_{vial} / v_{sound}$ = 10 microsec; from Eqn. 10.7, repetition of N_{obs} = 100 synchronization pulses can reduce synchronization error to ~1 microsec.

For the highest pre-infusion synchronization accuracy, optical (Section 4.7.3) or rf (Section 4.7.1) pulses will be employed. Electromagnetic energy travels at $c \sim 3 \times 10^8$ m/sec across the container volume until intercepted by a nanorobot optical sensor, giving $\Delta t_{error} \sim L_{vial} / c$ = 0.05 nsec. Allowing 100 green photons (360 zJ/photon at 550 nm) per nanorobot at a nanorobot number density of 10^{12} cm^{-3}, the flash injects ~40 J/m^3 of energy into the container, raising the water temperature by ~10 microkelvins after this energy is fully thermalized. A 1-nsec flash produces a peak intensity of ~4×10^{10} watts/m^2, comparable to monochromatic optical tweezers which are tolerated by biological macromolecules.[1630,1631] Some nanorobots inevitably will miss the signal and may later synchronize, prior to infusion, via close or direct physical contact with others who received the signal, or else multiple synchronization pulses can be used.

Onboard nanorobot clocks can also be synchronized post-infusion. For example, a pressure cuff inflated around the patient's arm can administer acoustic synchronization pulses to ~microsec precision as bloodborne nanorobots pass through the blood vessels within; after signaling for several mean blood circulation times (e.g., a few minutes), most bloodborne nanorobots should be properly synchronized. Whole-body acoustic transmissions at 0.1-1 MHz may be generated by operating tables, vibrating chairpads, wristwatch transmitters and the like (Section 6.4.1). Such methods may produce synchronization errors of ~100 microsec over 15-cm anteroposterior path lengths, reducible to ~1 microsec error using N_{obs} = 10,000 repetitions of the calibration signal (Eqn. 10.7). For higher precision, the physician transmits ~MHz radio wave pulses into the body; such pulses may be detected by appropriate onboard receivers (Section 6.4.2). Such waves have only ~75% attenuation over 15-cm anteroposterior path lengths (Eqn. 6.32), producing 0.5 nsec synchronization accuracy. Optical photons applied to the skin surface are subject to scattering, producing signal pulse broadening which increases synchronization error, and to absorption, which makes signal reception difficult or impossible beyond tissue depths of a few centimeters (Section 4.9.4).

Another approach is to inject a relatively small number of chronocytes—mobile communicytes (Section 7.2.6) modified to include an onboard nanoclock of high precision (e.g., a portable frequency standard) and the ability to transmit clocking synchronization signals to calibrate neighboring nanorobots. These signals may be transmitted acoustically at close proximity to the nodes of a mobile communications network (Section 7.3.2), subsequently allowing all nanorobots within 100 microns of a calibrated node to synchronize to within ≤67 nsec. Averaging algorithms can be employed to synchronize uncalibrated nodes in the system that were not recently visited by a chronocyte. Bloodborne chronocytes will normally be carried from the capillary vasculature to within ~100 microns of most tissue locations, thus allowing ≤67 nsec single-pulse acoustic synchronization even in the absence of an installed communications network (Section 7.3).

10.1.4 Dedicated Chronometer Organs

Just as the hypothalamus is the physical locus of the natural circadian clock (Section 10.1.1), it may be convenient to establish artificial chronometer organs inside the human body for various purposes. Dedicated nano-organs have been described previously in connection with power (Section 6.4.4), communication (Section 7.3.4), and navigational (Section 8.3.6) systems.

Chronometer organs, which would likely be millimeter-scale or smaller, could be used as endogenous clocks to regulate the precise administration of time-release substances or devices. Such organs could serve as highly accurate timers to improve the natural human interval timing sense from ±15% accuracy in biological systems (Section 10.1.1) to parts per million accuracy, or better, using artificial systems. If linked to the patient or user through various outmessaging channels (Section 7.4.6), chronometer organs can provide a continuously-available, consciously-accessible unfailing "time sense" of extraordinary precision for time of day, calendar date, and other time-related information.

Dedicated chronometer organs can be used to synchronize chronocytes or mobile communication networks at the nodes (Section 7.3.2). For example, chronocytes with lower-stability crystal oscillators could be repeatedly recalibrated as they passed near larger embedded chronometer organs during each blood circulation cycle (e.g., once per minute). Such chronometer organs might incorporate higher-stability onboard atomic frequency standards. Alternatively, chronometer organs could serve as transdermal data ports through which timing synchronization signals can be injected into fiber-based in vivo communication networks (Section 7.3.1) from external timing sources, similar to the autoclock pulse (containing time and date information) that is added to most contemporary television broadcast signals. Hard connectors, centimeter-scale rf wireless antennas, and other types of links are possible (Sections 6.4.2 and 7.2.3). In 1998, a desk clock could be purchased for $50 that automatically recalibrated itself by picking up WWVB radio signals anywhere in North America, several times a night, using a few centimeters of rod antenna.[1711] WWV's carrier frequency is regulated to $\Delta\nu / \nu \sim 5 \times 10^{-12}$, ultimately providing a time synchronicity at the receiver of ~100 microsec/day. With a slightly larger in vivo antenna, satellite GPS signals may be received, providing ≤20 nanosec time error.[1711] If buildings and vehicles are rewired to permit dissemination of time synchronization pulses and other useful information via continuous rf or IR channels, chronometer organs could employ smaller in vivo antennas and still achieve very precise results.

Although it has been informally speculated[3025] that nanorobots could use biological nerve fibers as rf antennas to receive electromagnetic time recalibration signals from outside the human body, such as from WWV, this concept is probably unworkable for several reasons. First, the axoplasm is only ~10^{-7} as electrically conductive as a metal wire of equivalent size, because axoplasmic charge carrier density and mobility are much lower than for electrons in a wire.[799] Second, passively conducted axonal currents are quickly attenuated by leakage through ion channels in the membrane, which is a very poor insulator. From cable theory applied to neurons,[799,3022] the length constant λ_n is defined as the distance over which an applied potential depolarizes to 1/e (~37%) of its maximum value; $\lambda_n = (d_{neuron}\, r_{mem} / 4\, r_{axo})^{1/2} \sim (0.04\, d_{neuron})^{1/2}$, where d_{neuron} is axonal diameter in meters, r_{mem} is the specific membrane resistance (~0.2 ohm-m^2 in human neurons) and r_{axo} is the specific resistance of the axoplasm (~1.25 ohm-m in human neurons). For a typical human axon with d_{neuron} ~ 1 micron, then λ_n ~ 200 microns (~internodal distance between nodes of Ranvier) and an external signal is >99% attenuated in ~1 mm of longitudinal travel. Third, short pulses (e.g., rapidly-oscillating rf signals) are severely distorted and attenuated by the electrical capacitance of the cell membrane. The capacitive time constant in human nerves and muscle cells ranges from 1-20 millisec,[799] thus limiting any possible electromagnetic reception to frequencies under 50-200 Hz, although pulsed microwaves directed through the brain can induce auditory effects in animals and humans.[3473-3481]

10.2 Nanocomputers

Many important medical nanorobotic tasks will require computation during the acquisition and processing of sensor data, the control of tools, manipulators, and motility systems, navigation and communication, and during the coordination of collective activities with neighboring nanorobots. Ex vivo computation has few theoretical limits, but computation by in vivo nanorobots will be subject to a number of constraints such as physical size, power consumption, onboard memory and processing speed.

The memory required onboard a medical nanorobot will be strongly mission dependent. Recognizing and manipulating molecules is fundamental. A very simple mission might demand only the identification or handling of perhaps ~10 different molecules. For example, basic respiratory gas transport nanorobots such as respirocytes[1400] (Chapter 22) may require the operation of fixed-shape receptors that bind simple molecules such as O_2, CO_2, H_2O, and glucose. Identifiers for such receptors may need only a few bits, hence this memory requirement should be negligible. A toxin removal device (Chapter 19) similarly may require keeping track of only a few types of fixed-shape receptors. On the other hand, a survey or assay mission might need to recognize N = 100-1000 distinct proteins. A spherical

1-micron nanorobot can have >10^4 fixed-shape receptors on its surface; if these will suffice, then we require N $\log_2$ (N) ~ 10^4 bits to identify each of N = 1000 different receptor types. This seems more efficient than using more advanced reconfigurable receptors (Section 3.5.7.4), which might need >10^4 bits per receptor-pattern to specify each binding site geometry to the necessary atomic-scale resolution (Section 3.5.7.5), thus imposing a total memory requirement of >10^7 bits for an onboard library of N = 1000 different receptor types. Consequently, simple missions involving basic process control with limited motility may require no more than ~10^5-10^6 bits of memory, comparable to an old Apple II computer (including RAM plus floppy disk drive). At the other extreme, a complex cell repair mission might require the onboard storage of a substantial fraction of the patient's genetic code, representing ~10^9 bits of memory including perhaps ~0.2 x 10^9 bits of linear sequence data for all 100,000 protein types found in the human body, again assuming 300 amino acids per protein. (Most amino acids are folded into the protein's interior and are not readily accessible to surface probing unless the protein is unfolded, which usually is not desirable or convenient. On the other hand, binding sites for large molecules should be physically easier to construct than small-molecule receptors; Section 3.5.9.) An onboard memory of 10^9-10^{10} bits would be in the same range as the 1985 Cray-2 (2 x 10^{10} bits) or the 1989 Cray-3 (6 x 10^8 bits) supercomputers.[1]

Computational speed will also be strongly mission dependent. However, extremely simple process control systems in basic factory settings may only require speeds as slow as 10^4 bit/sec (Chapter 12). Individual natural biocomputational devices (as opposed to multiple such biodevices operating in parallel) generally do not exceed this speed. Examples include mRNA translation during protein manufacture at ~15 Hz (~75 bits/sec assuming 5 bits/protein);[997] transcription from DNA by RNA polymerase at ~40 Hz (~80 bits/sec at 2 bits/nucleotide);[997] DNA replication at ~800 Hz (~1600 bits/sec at 2 bits/nucleotide);[997] typically 5-100 Hz (bits/sec) for neural electrical discharges (Section 4.8.6); ~1000 Hz (bits/sec) for excitory cholinergic synapses, and gated ion channels at ~10^4 Hz (bits/sec) (Section 7.4.5.6). At the other extreme, a processing speed of 10^9 bits/sec allows a ~10^9 bit genomic information store to be processed in ~1 sec, the small-molecule diffusion time across an average 20-micron wide cell. In 1998, personal desktop computers capable of ~10^9-10^{10} bits/sec (~10^8 operations/sec) were commonly available.

This Section describes possible nanomechanical (Section 10.2.1) and nanoelectronic (Section 10.2.2) computers, biocomputers (Section 10.2.3), and briefly examines the ultimate limits to computation including reversible and quantum computing (Section 10.2.4). Computer architectural issues are not explicitly addressed here. (For example, advanced architectures, especially large CPU systems, may employ distributed clocks and a distributed computing network.)

10.2.1 Nanomechanical Computers

Electronic computers were evolutionarily preceded by purely mechanical computational devices, starting with the venerable abacus (hand-operated movable beads on rods) in ~3000 BC,[1726,1727] the Pascaline (the first hands-on algorithm-executing machine) in 1642,[1728] and the Difference Engine (the first hands-off algorithm-executing machine) designed in 1821 by Charles Babbage.[1728-1731,1744] A 2000-part working subsection of the brass-geared Engine was demonstrated in 1832; an entire working Difference Engine was reconstructed by historians in 1991, proving that Babbage's design was sound.[1732] In the 1840s, Thomas Fowler built and exhibited a calculating device using sliding rods made of wood instead of metal.[1733] Whereas Babbage's engines used the familiar 0-9 decimal system with each number represented by a discrete position of a rotating gear wheel, Fowler's machine was more fully digital, using as its active element not rotating wheels but sliding "trinary" rods which could occupy only one of three positions at any time, the first known example of "rod logic." (By reducing the number of distinct physical states, parts could be made less precisely.)

By 1834, Babbage had also conceived detailed plans for his Analytical Engine, intended as a general-purpose programmable computing machine but based entirely on 19th century mechanical technology. The Analytical Engine was to have a random-access memory consisting of 1000 words of 50 decimal digits each (~175,000 bits), with separate memory and central processing unit (CPU), stored program control, data entry via punched metal cards, and even an output printer.[1728,1730,1732] This ambitious device, though well specified, was never built.

The mechanical computing tradition was not entirely abandoned. Vannevar Bush built his analog mechanical computer, the Differential Analyzer, in 1930 at MIT.[1736] In 1954, M. Minsky and R. Silver[289] used hydraulic logic elements to build a mechanical "hydroflip computer" which was operated at ~30 Hz and powered by a 3-inch high column of water. (Section 9.2.7.6 describes the basis for a mechanical fluidic computer operating at ~5000 Hz.) In 1975, D. Hillis and B. Silverman[1738] built a special-purpose all-mechanical computer ~2 meters in size, entirely out of Tinkertoys, and powered by a hand crank, that was able to play tic-tac-toe. In 1990, University of Minnesota engineers[1734] fabricated a complete family of micromechanical digital logic devices, including electrostatically-actuated linear-sliding ~30-micron mechanical logic elements confined to a one-dimensional track, forming NAND and NOR gates suitable for low-speed radiation-hard digital functions "in environments hostile to electronic devices." Sandia's pin-in-maze microlocks[2356] could also be used to make a mechanical computer, albeit at the above-micron scale. In 1996, J. Gimzewski and colleagues[1735] at IBM Zurich used a scanning tunneling microscope (STM) probe to repeatedly reposition spherical C_{60} fullerene molecules ~1 nm in diameter along a terraced copper substrate that constrained the buckyballs to move only in a straight line, operating the mechanical array like beads on an abacus. In 1997, Stoddart's group[2540] described a mechanical XOR gate based on their "molecular shuttles."

Perhaps the best-characterized (though not yet built) mechanical nanocomputer is Drexler's rod logic design.[10,2282] In this design, one sliding rod with a knob intersects a second knobbed sliding rod at right angles to the first. Depending upon the position of the first rod, the second may be free to move, or unable to move. This simple blocking interaction serves as the basis for logical operations. Figure 10.1 shows a nanomechanical implementation of a Boolean NAND "interlock" gate, using clock-driven input and output logic rods 1 nm wide which interact via knobs that prevent or enable motion, all encased in a housing, allowing ~16 nm^3/interlock. (Any logic function, no matter how complicated, can be built from NAND or NOR gates alone.[1736]) Figure 10.2 is an exploded diagram of the moving parts of a thermodynamically efficient class of register capable of mechanical data storage, using rods ~1 nm in width with 0.1-nanosec switching speeds, allowing ~40 nm^3/register. The activity sequence depicts a simplified version of Drexler's register, omitting the reading mechanism.[1743] Initially the register shows a 0 (black ball position in A) or a 1 (B). Then the barrier is lowered and the ball wanders freely (C); entropy increases. The register is then reset to 0 by spring-rod compression, converting ~kT ln(2) joules of work into heat (D). To write a 0, the barrier is raised (E). To write

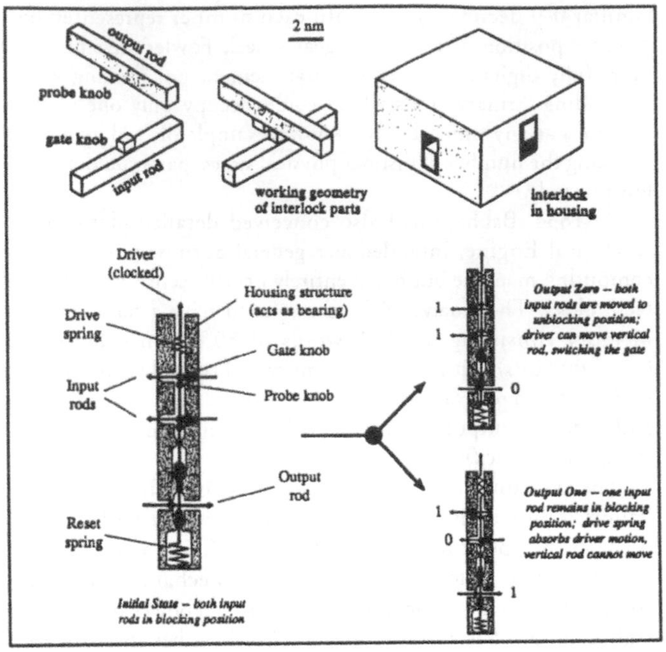

Fig. 10.1. Schematic of nanomechanical rod logic NAND gate (modified from Drexler[10]).

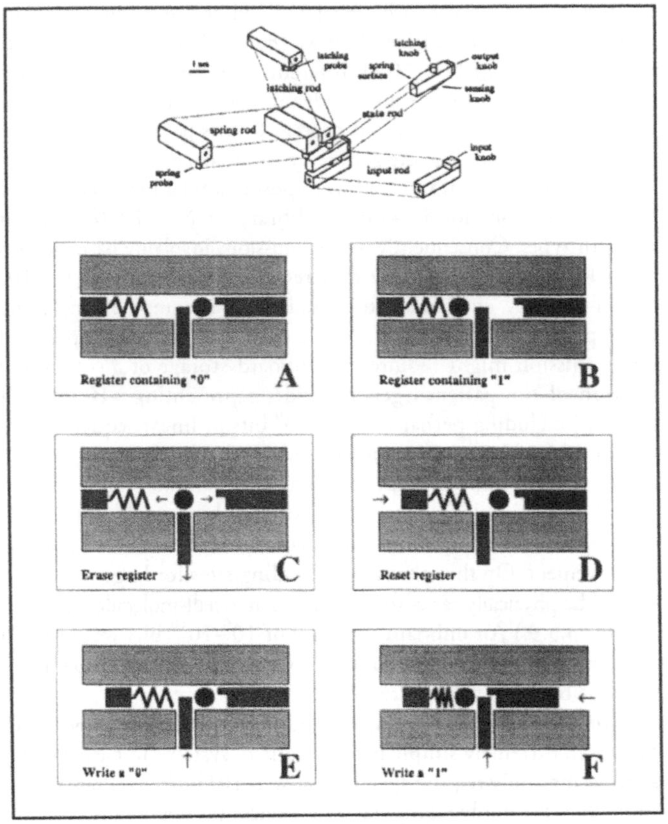

Fig. 10.2. Schematic of nanomechanical rod logic data storage registers (modified from Drexler[10] and Hall[1743]).

a 1, the input rod at right is first extended and then the barrier is raised (F); the input rod does work compressing the ball into the spring, but this energy can be retrieved when the spring rod is retracted. Finally, the spring rod is retracted, returning the device to state (A) or (B).

Figure 10.3 illustrates a programmable logic array (PLA) using knobbed rods (omitting several drive and spring systems for clarity) to implement nanomechanical logic, which, in combination with rod-based registers, can be used to build much of the control circuitry for a CPU in a ≳1 GHz clocked computer system. For details of operation, see Drexler.[10] While a PLA system requires three successive rod displacement cycles to compute a set of Boolean functions, the functions AND, OR, and NOT can also be computed in a single displacement cycle by employing a linkage in which any input rod can displace the output rod without displacing any other input rod; Figure 10.4 illustrates this alternative approach for an asynchronous-input OR gate.

Drexler's benchmark mechanical nanocomputer design has 10^6 interlock gates, 10^5 logic rods, 10^4 registers, an energy-buffering flywheel and other components with total cubic volume (~400 nm)^3, mass ~10^{-16} kg, and total power ~ 60 nW, giving a power density of ~10^{12} watts/m^3.[10] Power dissipation per logic operation is ~0.013 zJ per gate per cycle, giving (including register dissipation) ~2 x 10^4 operations/sec-pW.[10] Processing speed is ~10^9 operations/sec (~1 gigaflop) or ~10^{28} operations/sec-m^3; assuming one bit per register, processing speed is ~10^{13} bits/sec or ~10^{32} bits/sec-m^3. In 1998, the typical desktop PC operated at ~10^8 operations/sec. Cooling is provided by a refrigerant fluid flowing through an integral fractal plumbing system at near the speed of sound.[10]

The most primitive 4-bit Intel 4004 microprocessor, introduced in 1971 for early-generation pocket calculators, had 2300 transistors. A comparably simple early mechanical nanocomputer with 2000 interlock gates, 100 registers, and a 1 KHz clock speed could have a volume as small as 36,000 nm^3, a (~33 nm)^3 cube, assuming 16 nm^3/gate and 40 nm^3/register, and could process ~10^5 bits/sec.

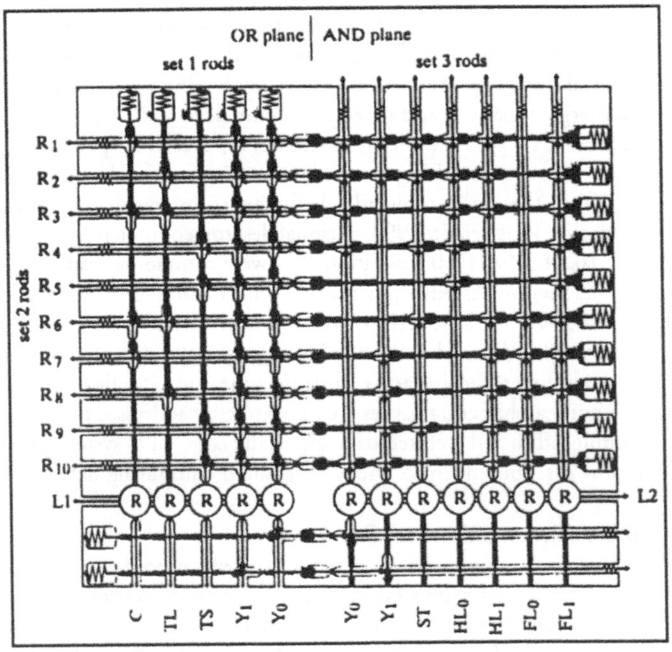

Fig. 10.3. Schematic of programmable logic array (PLA) finite state machine implementing rod logic for a nanomechanical central processing unit (modified from Drexler[10]).

One major disadvantage of mechanical nanocomputers is that they will almost certainly be slower than nanoelectronic systems,

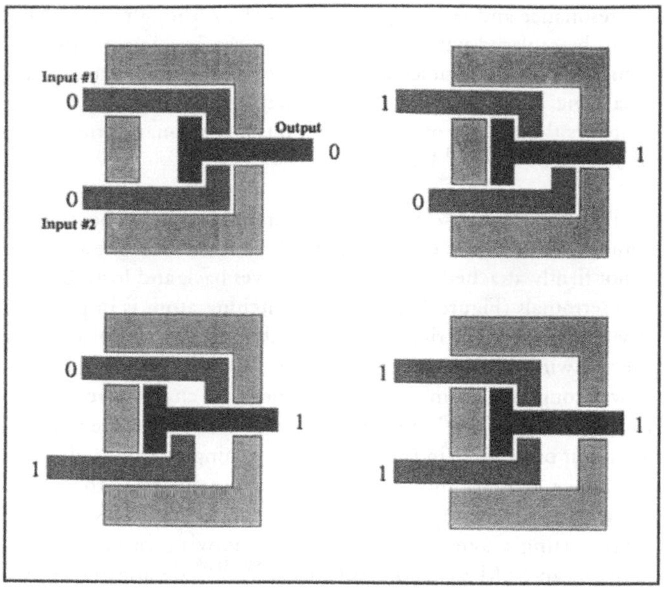

Fig. 10.4. Schematic diagram of a single displacement cycle asynchronous-input nanomechanical OR gate (redrawn from Drexler[10]).

because a device that depends on moving heavy nuclei (~10^{-27} kg) will necessarily be slower than a device that depends on moving less-massive electrons (~10^{-30} kg).[280] Mechanical signals travel near the speed of sound (~10^4 m/sec in diamond), whereas electronic signals may travel near the speed of light (~10^8 m/sec). Thus while nanomechanical computers may be limited to switching speeds of ~50 picoseconds, electronic devices may be ~10^3-10^4 times faster. On the other hand, mechanical computers are more EMP (electromagnetic pulse) resistant, conceptually easier to understand and to model, and mechanical designs scale readily from the macroscale to the nanoscale, unlike most nanoelectronic designs. In 1996, a ~50 nm reversible mechanical latch was fabricated and physically cycled using an AFM; the similarity to Drexler's mechanical OR gate (Figure 10.4) was explicitly noted in the paper.[1737]

What about mechanical data storage? In the MEMS world, Halg[1742] fabricated a nonvolatile microelectromechanical memory cell consisting of a longitudinally-stressed surface-micromachined ~10 micron bridge that mechanically buckles into one of two states, making a bistable storage device. Moving to the nanoscale, data could be mechanically stored using compact three-dimensional arrays of diamondoid register rods (~10^7 bits/micron^3, ~10^{10} bits/sec access speed; Figure 10.2, Section 7.2.6, and Drexler[10]). Another theoretical mechanical storage medium is spooled hydrofluorocarbon memory tape (~10^{10} bits/micron^3, ~10^9 bits/sec access speed; Sections 7.2.1.1 and 7.2.6 and Drexler[10]), or polymer or diamond surface-bound patterns of H and F atoms that could be read using an optimized $(CH_3)_3PO$ scanning probe tip with a maximum raw error rate of 6×10^{-8} per read.[1200] (Linear DNA molecules achieve ~10^9 bits/micron^3 data storage, by comparison.) Direct AFM reading and recording of 10-nm pits on a polycarbonate surface (~10^6 bits/micron^2, up to ~10^7 bits/sec access speed)[1739] and other means of directly reading and writing data at the atomic level[1749,2182] have been studied, and the fullerene abacus[1735] described earlier is one of the first experimental efforts to mechanically store numerical information using individual molecules at room temperature.

It has been speculated that individual atoms or atomic vacancies could serve as information units.[278,1200,1739,1745,2711] For example, Y. Mo[1741] used an STM to store information in the reversible rotational states of individual antimony dimers deposited on a silicon substrate. In theory, a block of diamond with data encoded as single-atom lattice vacancies could store up to ~176 bits/nm^3, or nearly ~2×10^{11} bits/micron^3, although cryogenic temperatures might be required to reduce diffusion effects and structural lability to acceptable levels consistent with long-term information storage. Phonon probes or other nondestructive means of lattice interrogation could be employed for readout.

10.2.2 Nanoelectronic Computers

In 1998, the metal-oxide-semiconductor field-effect transistor (MOSFET) was still the most common type of transistor in general use. These solid-state devices are characterized by an electrical source, an electrical drain, and a gate that controls the flow. Since its inception, the FET has scaled well to lower sizes. Individual working transistors with 40-nm gate lengths have been demonstrated in silicon,[1751] and 25-nm gate-length transistors have been fabricated in gallium arsenide.[1752] However, as feature sizes shrink below ≲100 nm, a number of obstacles to stable operation begin to appear and the cost-effective downscaling of dense circuitry may not persist.[1753-1757] A number of solid-state replacements for the bulk-effect semiconductor transistor have been suggested that could overcome these obstacles by taking advantage of nanometer-scale quantum mechanical effects.[1813] Such replacements include quantum dots (QDs),[1784-1787] resonant tunneling devices (RTDs),[1787-1791,1747] electron turnstiles,[2709] and single-electron transistors (SETs).[1794-1799,1855] However, while hybrid RTD-FET circuits[1791] and SETs[1814,1815] have been successfully switched at room temperature, many of these devices must be operated at cryogenic temperatures[1830] and other practical challenges remain;[1747,1784,1791-1794] such top-down approaches to nanoelectronics are not considered further here.

In contrast, molecular nanoelectronics uses primarily covalently bonded molecular structures, electrically isolated from a bulk substrate, producing wires, switches and devices composed of individual molecules and nanometer-scale supramolecular structures.[1747] While it is relatively difficult and expensive to sculpt trillions of identical nanoscale structures in bulk materials (e.g., using 2-nm resolution electron-beam lithographic techniques[1816]), individual molecules are natural nanometer-scale structures that can be manufactured to be exactly the same in near-mole quantities.[1867] The great versatility of organic chemistry offers more options for designing and fabricating nanoelectronic devices than are available in silicon.[1773-1778] Investigators are designing, modeling, fabricating, and testing individual molecules[1760-1769,1871] and nanometer-scale supramolecular structures[1811,1817] that act as electrical switches and even exhibit some of the same properties as small solid-state transistors.[1768] For example, three- and four- terminal devices with ~0.3-nm feature sizes have been examined computationally.[1879]

Molecular electronics is a rapidly growing area in the literature.[1769-1776,1832,1924] J.M. Tour expects experimental demonstration of molecular-sized transistor devices by 2000-2001, and commercial high-level computers using molecular electronics by 2008-2013.[1517] A current list of major research groups is maintained by the International Society for Molecular Electronics and Biocomputing. Some of the following discussion is appreciatively drawn from an extensive 1997 review by MITRE Corporation.[1747]

10.2.2.1 Molecular Wires

Before one can seriously discuss molecular electronic devices embedded in single molecules, it must be asked whether a small single molecule can be made to conduct electrical current at all. A series of difficult and sensitive experiments[1765,1767,1800] and theoretical investigations[1758-1761] during the 1990s answered this question affirmatively. Single molecule conduction was demonstrated by Tour[1766,1767] using a conducting molecule characterized by repeating structures—in this case, a series of benzene-like rings connected by acetylene linkages—each part of which is linked to the next by bonds including many π-electrons above and below the plane of the structure. These electrons in the π orbitals[1818] conjugate with each other, or interact, to form a single large orbital throughout the length of the wire to permit mobile electrons to flow.[1778,1831] Thiol (-SH) functional groups at either end adsorb well to gold surfaces and act as "alligator clips" for attaching molecular electronic units to metal substrates.[1819,1764,1867-1870] Tour's polyphenylene wires can carry ~nanoampere currents. Such molecular wires also have the desirable property that they can be made quite long, if necessary, because they can be lengthened systematically using chemosynthetic methods.[1766,1820] Another experiment using a single benzene ring attached between two gold electrodes through thiol groups across a 0.846-nm gap found a single-ring threshold resistance of ~20 megohm and a capacitance on the order of ~0.1 e^2 / kT ~ 10^{-19} farad.[1811,1812,1837]

Fullerene carbon nanotubes (Section 2.3.2) or "buckytubes"[1821] are hollow cylindrical tubes, essentially rolled-up sheets of graphite, measuring ≳1 nm in diameter that (in many chiral and compositional forms; Section 10.2.2.4) can conduct electricity. For instance, both individual 10-20 nm diameter carbon nanotubes[1822,1844] and atomic wires pulled from an unraveling carbon nanotube[643] can conduct currents of ~1-10 microamps (vs. nanoamps via tunneling). Maximum nanotube current density is ~10^{10}-10^{11} amp/m^2 over a 0.2-6.0 volt range,[1844,1857] superior to the ~10^9 amp/m^2 typically achieved in superconductors. Nanotube resistivity measures ~8-20 ohm-m for straight tubes, ~38-49 ohm-m for slightly curved (5-30°) tubes, and >100 ohm-m for highly curved (65-80°) tubes.[1844] Interestingly, electronic transport in carbon nanotubes is ballistic (e.g., like electron waveguides, permitting only a few propagating modes[1308]), with all waste heat being dissipated in the leads to the nanotube element and none in the nanotube itself.[1857] Buckytubes are stiff enough to serve as supports for molecular circuit elements, and if filled with conducting metal can create one of the structurally strongest nanowires that is chemically possible. (See also Section 10.2.2.4.)

Other 0.6-3 nm molecular wires,[1767,1801,1802,1864] 3-20 nm semiconductor wires,[1843] and nanoscale metallic wires[1740,1862,1863] have been studied as well.

10.2.2.2 Electromechanical Molecular Switching Devices

In 1998, the best-studied category of molecular electronics device is probably the electromechanical molecular switch. This class of switch employs electrically or mechanically applied forces to turn a current on and off, either by changing the conformation of the molecule[1768] or by moving a switching molecule or group of atoms in the manner of a gate.[1805,1806] These switches are promising because they could be laid down in a dense network on a solid substrate, or in some cases in three-dimensional arrays; unfortunately, no integrated CPU-scale designs have yet been attempted, although plans for a half-adder[1769] and a molecular shift register[1750] have been published. Some examples:

A. *Electromechanical Amplifier* — Joachim and Gimzewski[1768] measured conductance through a single buckyball held between an STM tip and a conducting substrate. By pressing down harder on the STM tip, the buckyball deforms, tuning the conduction off-resonance and reducing current ~50%. Although the STM tip could be replaced with a small in-situ piezoelectric gate, the ideal actuator would be a molecular-scale electromechanical actuator akin to a logic rod; the major fundamental limit to the speed of this switch is the natural mechanical vibrational resonance frequencies of a buckyball, ~10^{13} Hz.

B. *Linear Atomic Relay* — Researchers at Hitachi Corporation[1823] simulated a two-state electronic switch wherein a mobile atom that is not firmly attached to a substrate moves back and forth between two terminals (Figure 10.5). If the switching atom is in place, the device conducts electricity; if the switching atom is displaced from the two wires, the resulting gap greatly reduces the current that can flow through the atom wire. A small negative charge placed on the third atom wire "gate" near the switching atom moves the switching atom out of its place in the wire; the switching atom is pulled back into place by a second "reset" gate after each use of the switch. Actual experiments approximating this design created a bistable atom switch using a xenon switching atom moving back and forth between an STM tip and a substrate,[1807,1808] demonstrating that the movement of a single atom can be the basis of a nanometer-scale switch. In a more mature device, relays could be ~10 nm^2 in size with a speed limited only by the intrinsic vibrational frequency of atoms, typically ~100 THz, but it seems likely that atom relays could only operate at very low temperatures because not much energy would be required to evaporate a switching atom off the substrate and out of the plane of the atom wires, destroying the switch.[1747]

C. *Rotational Molecular Relay* — A more reliable two-state device based on atom movement uses the rotation of a molecular group to affect an electric current. The switching atom is part of a rotating group, or "rotamer,"[1824] which itself is part of a larger molecule, perhaps affixed to the same surface as the atom wires. Figure 10.6 is a conceptual diagram illustrating this approach,[1747] wherein the electric field of a nearby gate forces the switching atom to rotate in or out of the atom wire. When the switching atom is "in," wire conductance is high and the switch is "on"; when the switching atom is "out," a second group takes its place, hindering current flow and turning the switch "off." A third large group may provide resistance to thermal free rotation. Alternatively, hydrogen bonding might provide enough rotational resistance to stop the rotamer in the conducting position, but not so much that reversing the gate voltage would be insufficient to turn the rotamer. Controlled rotational state switching of a Pt-adsorbed oxygen molecule by STM using 0.15-volt 20-microsec pulses was demonstrated in 1998.[1874]

While a rotating switch with a methyl-like rotamer group has three distinct switch positions, a hinging switch that rotates back

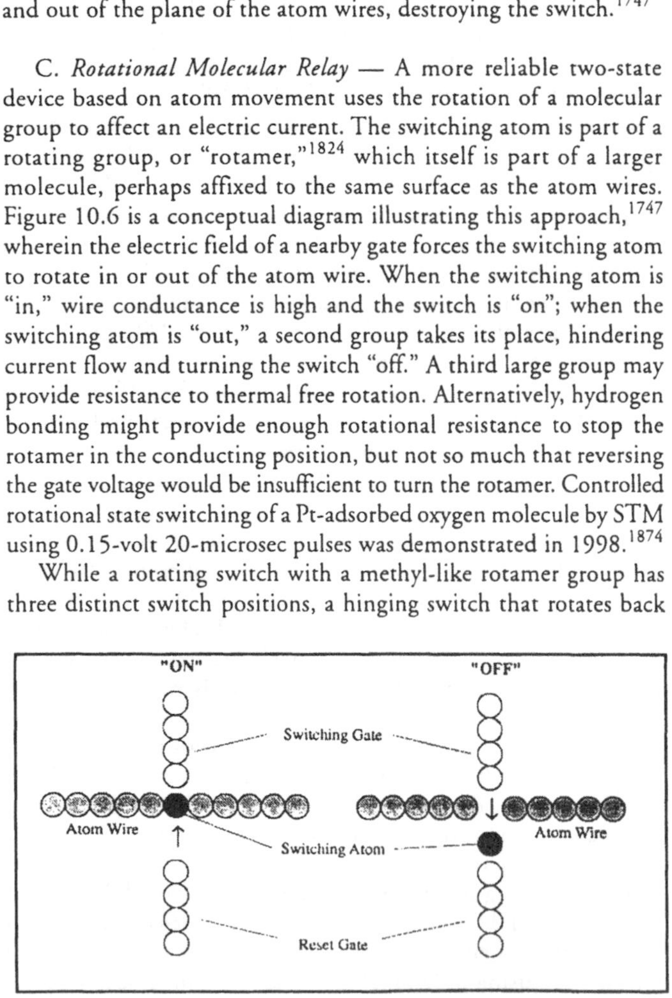

Fig. 10.5. Linear atomic relay switch.[1747]

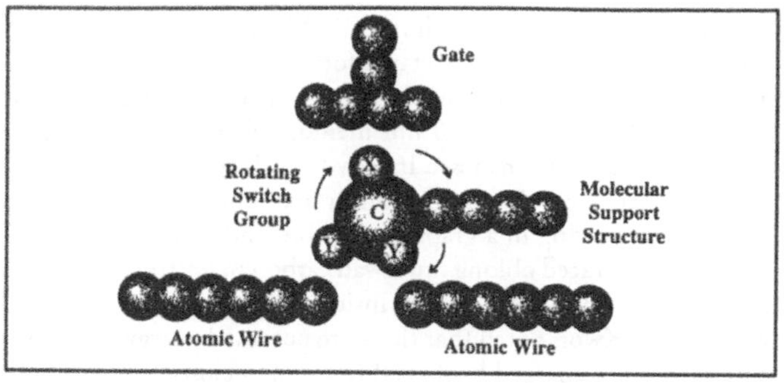

Fig. 10.6. Rotational molecular relay switch.[1747]

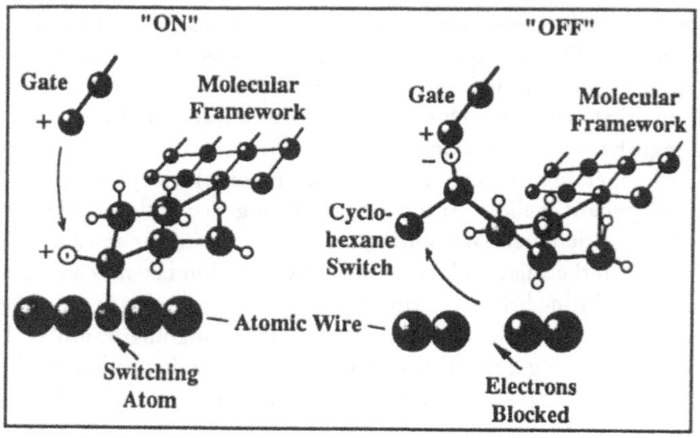

Fig. 10.7. Hinging molecular relay switch.[1747]

and forth between two distinct states might be preferable. Cyclohexane, a simple example of this kind of molecule, can bend into two different forms, commonly known at the "boat" and "chair" conformations.[1809,1810] As shown schematically in Figure 10.7, a voltage on a nearby gate might force the cyclohexane switch into one of its two conformations, affecting the conductivity of a nearby atom wire. The cyclohexane-type molecule attaches to a molecular framework while the remaining ring carbons are replaced by groups tailored to use steric repulsions or van der Waals attractions to reduce undesired switching caused by thermal energy. Switch speed is limited by molecular rotational and torsional frequencies, typically ~1-1000 GHz, which is slower than the atom relay but more reliable. Also in contrast to the atom relay, molecular relays could be packed in three dimensions, possibly up to ~1 nm^{-3} densities.

D. *Molecular Shuttle Switch* — A rotaxane "shuttle switch" has been synthesized by F. Stoddart's group[1805] that consists of one ring-shaped molecule that encircles and slides along a shaft-like chain molecule (Figure 10.8). Two large terminal groups at either end of the shaft prevent the shuttle ring from slipping off the shaft. The shaft contains two other functional groups, a biphenol group and a benzidine group, that serve as natural stations between which the shuttle moves. The shuttle molecule contains four positively charged functional groups that cause it to be attracted to shaft sites with extra negative change, so the shuttle spends 84% of its time at the benzidine station, which is a better electron donor than the biphenol station. Removing an electron from the benzidine station forces the shuttle to switch to the other station; switching may be controlled chemically or electrochemically.[1805] A charged gate could be added at one or both ends to force the shuttle to move between stations, with switch state probed by arranging for the ring to complete an electric circuit in one of its two positions.[1747] Switching speed is slow, limited by the speed of electron transfer to and from the benzidine station and the sluggish motion of the ring which is ~10^6 times heavier than an electron, but three-dimensional packing densities of ~0.01 nm^{-3} appear plausible. Other rotaxane shuttle systems have been studied.[1845,1846,2487,2522,2529,2530] In 1999, the first chemically-assembled rotaxane-based logic gate was demonstrated,[3541] although the gates could be opened only irreversibly.

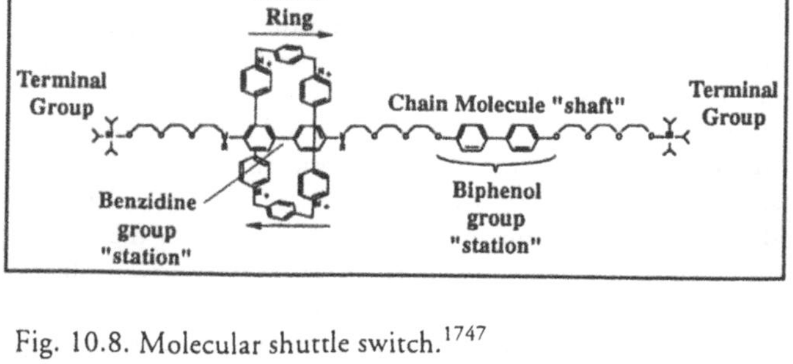

Fig. 10.8. Molecular shuttle switch.[1747]

10.2.2.3 Field-Controlled Molecular Switching Devices

A second category of molecular electronics device that appears promising for the development of molecular nanoelectronic digital computers is the electric-field controlled molecular switching devices, including molecular quantum-effect devices. These are most closely descended from the solid-state microelectronics and nanoelectronic devices described earlier, and promise to be the fastest and most densely integrated among all of the current alternatives. A group at Purdue University has used self-assembly to fabricate and demonstrate functioning arrays of molecular electronic quantum confinement structures connected by molecular wires.[1811,1812] As another example, J.M. Tour proposes embedding a quantum well in a molecular wire by inserting pairs of barrier groups that break the sequence of conjugated π-orbitals (Figure 10.9), forming a two-terminal molecular RTD;[1747] other structures for three-terminal molecules have been suggested.[1825] (In February 1999, Tour reported the demonstration of RTD effects in the manner proposed above; at press time, the paper was still in review [J.M. Tour, personal communication, 1999].) Nondissipative (adiabatic) Thouless electron pumping has also been described at 0.33 K.[3189]

Merkle and Drexler[1097] consider a hypothetical "helical logic" device in which a single electron can switch another single electron,

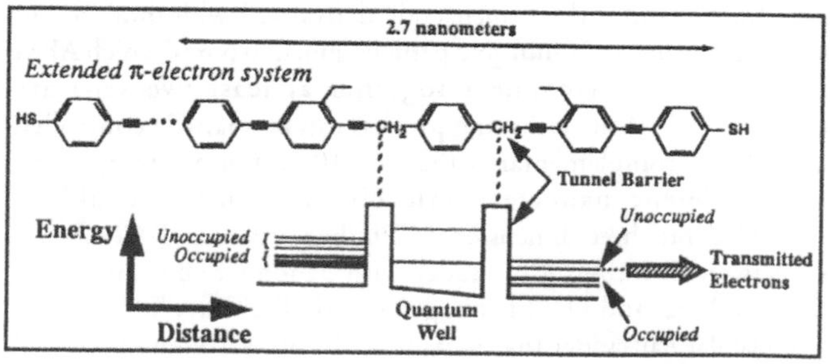

Fig. 10.9. Two-terminal molecular resonant tunneling device (RTD).[1747] Proposed RTD: Insulating barrier groups generate a potential well for quantum confinement, creating a resonant tunneling effect when molecule is subjected to voltage bias, permitting a current of electrons to be transmitted through the device.

with 1 or 0 represented as the presence or absence of individual electrons. The electrons are constrained to move along helical paths, driven by a rotating immersive electric field (normal to the helical axis) that confines each charge carrier to a fraction of a turn of a single helical loop, moving it like water in an Archimedean screw. A logic operation involves two helices, one of which splits into two "descendant" helices. At the point of divergence, differences in the electrostatic potential resulting from the presence or absence of a carrier in the adjacent helix control the direction taken by a carrier in the splitting helix; the sequence is reversible, allowing two initially distinct helical paths to merge into a single outgoing helical path without forcing a dissipative transition. Energy dissipation at ~10 GHz is ~10^{-6} zJ/gate-cycle at an operating temperature of 1 K.

10.2.2.4 Other Molecular Electronic Devices

Other classes of molecular electronic devices have been studied, including picosecond photoactive or photochromic molecular switching devices[1777-1783,1835,1836] using light, and electrochemical molecular devices[1803,1805] using electrochemical reactions, to change the shape, orientation, or electron configuration of a molecule in order to switch a current. However, photoactive devices in a dense network would require an NSOM-like emitter (Section 4.8.4) to switch individually, since optical photon pathways are not easily confined at length scales very much below optical wavelengths of ~500-1000 nm; electrochemical molecular devices might require immersion in solvent to operate.[1747]

Fullerenes exhibit a wide range of quantized conductivities that may be useful in nanoelectronic computers.[1821,2120] For example, chemisorption alters properties: 3 alkali dopant atoms per C_{60} buckyball gives high conductivity, while none or 6 dopant atoms gives an insulator.[1826] Buckytube conductivity also varies with mechanical stress and torsion,[1844,1872] tube diameter, and other geometrical parameters.[1852-1854,1821] Depending upon the direction of the nanotube chiral vector, carbon nanotubes may be either metallic or semiconducting.[1847,1848] Suitably-sized, doped, flexed, stressed, or chiralized fullerenes could be nested to make insulated wires[1829] or joined to make nanoelectronic computer components[1821,1858-1861,1876-1878] including resistors with quantized "staircase" resistance of $nh/2e^2$, n = 1, 2, ... (e is electronic charge, h is Planck's constant),[1857] two-terminal devices such as diodes,[1838,1873] three- or four-terminal devices such as heterojunction,[1828,1849,1858] TUBEFET,[1875] or thin-film[1827] transistors, and gates that introduce electric fields.[641,1850] A single-molecule transistor using semiconducting buckytubes has been demonstrated experimentally at room temperature.[2276]

Carbon nanotubes have been cut to length, size-sorted by field flow fractionation, their open ends derivatized with thiol groups and then tethered to 10-nm gold particle "junction boxes" which AFM images show can connect together at least two separate tubes.[1525,2713] If the tethering process can be spatially controlled using DNA complementarity (Section 10.2.3) or by other means, then fullerene nanoelectronic circuit elements could be assembled into three-dimensional CPU-like structures. P. Collins[1873] expects an all-carbon 8-bit adder with nanometer dimensions by the year 2002, and J.C. Ellenbogen of MITRE Corp. has designed a molecular half-adder that measures ~10 nm x 10 nm in size.[2275] This research area was extremely active in 1998.

Fullerenes may also allow compact memory devices. For example, it has long been speculated that a ~1 nm buckyball encapsulated in a ~1 nm diameter nanotube segment may glide freely back and forth, trapped weakly in each end cap by van der Waals forces. An external voltage could nudge a charged C_{60} molecule to one end of the other, creating a two-state "buckyshuttle RAM" storage device.[1308,2849] Such a device could store one bit of information in a ~10 nm^3 volume, a storage density of ~10^8 bits/$micron^3$; the C_{60} thermal velocity of ~100 m/sec at 310 K inside a ~10 nm memory element gives a typical read/write time of ~0.1 nanosec. In early 1999, Kwon and colleagues[2951] reported that finely dispersed 4-6 nm diamond powder thermally annealed by heating in a graphite crucible under argon at 1800°C for 1 hour produced oblong multiwall carbon nanostructures which in some cases could move around inside each other, like C_{60} trapped within C_{480}. Kwon noted that there are potential energy minima at either end, so a charged buckyball (e.g., an enclosed ion) could be shuttled with an applied electric field, which could be used for memory storage. Computational simulation of writing a bit showed that the interior buckyball neatly shuttled to the correct end, then gently bounced to rest in ~0.01 nanosec (i.e., ~100 GHz operation) dissipating only ~10 kT in the C_{480}. Kwon proposed a high density memory board using aligned buckyshuttles in a hexagonal lattice with addressing wires above and below, not unlike a ferrite core memory; the memory would likely be nonvolatile at room temperature, with mass production based on self-assembly.

10.2.2.5 Molecular Electrostatic Field Computers

In 1998, bulk semiconductor technology typically required ~16,000 electrons to transfer one bit of information.[1981] SET and related techniques described above promise to reduce this to ~1 electron per bit. But a "traditional" molecular electronics nanocomputer with a mean gate density of ~1 nm^{-3} operating at ~10 GHz and using single electrons to transport, indicate, fetch, or represent a binary digit would move ~1 coul/sec of electrons (~1 amp at ~1 volt, or ~1 watt) through a 1 $micron^3$ CPU, producing an untenable ~10^{18} watt/m^3 power density, compared to ~10^{12} watts/m^3 for the nanomechanical CPU described in Section 10.2.1.

In order to reclaim this factor of 10^6, Tour and Seminario[1879,1981] conclude that a molecular CPU must operate by electrostatic interactions rather than by electron currents, using intermolecular "talk" to efficiently transfer a bit using only ~10^{-6} electron.[1517] This charge-density approach is already well-known in biology, where enzyme-ligand recognition is mediated by hydrogen bonding or van der Waals interactions, working through the electric fields of the molecules even though no formal charge transfer occurs. Similarly, in an electrostatic nanocomputer the input signal is initiated by bringing up a charge to one end of the molecular device, thus reshaping the local charge density. That molecular device, in turn, perturbs the electrostatic field of an adjacent molecular device, rearranging its electron density in <10^{-15} sec,[1981] and so the electrostatic field perturbation is propagated without charge transfer: "These movements of electrons (wave-particle entities) in the molecular orbitals (or circuits) are performed without any dissipation of energy (stationary states)."[1981] Perturbation pulses may have an energy magnitude similar to those of van der Waals interactions (Section 3.5.1). The hypothetical electrostatic molecular logic device shown in Figure 10.10 serves as an OR gate if the output is active (as a potential) or as a NOR gate if the output is passive (as an impedance) if positive logic is used, or an AND or NAND gate if negative logic is used.[1879]

Gates at input/output interfaces must still be able to receive or to drive signals from standard electronic circuits, but the vast majority of molecular gates would lie within the molecular CPU and could process information by controllably affecting the electrostatic potential of neighboring molecules. Such devices would likely shift the hardware/software equilibrium towards hardware, with massively wired-logic supplanting programmed-logic computing,

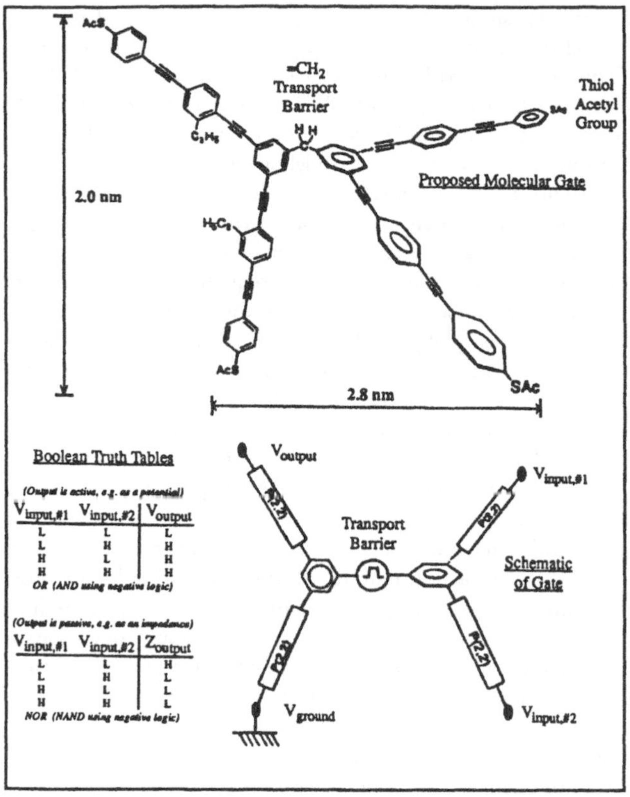

Fig. 10.10. Molecular electrostatic logic device (modified from Tour, Kozaki and Seminario[1879]).

and with large molecular arrays allowing computation to take place inside the CPU with minimal need for main or auxiliary memories.[1981] Tour expects the first laboratory demonstration of electrostatic field information transfer by 2001-2003.[1517] J.C. Ellenbogen [personal communication, 1998] notes that a charge density nanocomputer achieves low dissipation by operating very close to equilibrium at all times, but notes that clock speeds of at least 1-10 KHz should still be obtainable with this approach; Tour [personal communication, 1999] claims that 1-10 THz switching is possible. Current-free polarization gates have also been proposed[3216] and fabricated.[3217]

10.2.3 Biocomputers

Biocomputers use natural organic materials, thus offer the possibility of self-assembly or construction by natural or engineered biological organisms. At least three classes of biocomputers are distinguishable—biochemical, biomechanical, and bioelectronic.

10.2.3.1 Biochemical Computers

The Systron-Donner Analog Computer familiar to engineering students in the 1960s and 1970s used potentiometers and high-gain DC amplifiers, called operational amplifiers, to allow the creation of electrical circuits comprised of adders, multipliers, and integrators arranged in feedback loops capable of solving complex time-dependent differential equations modeling actual physical systems. In 1998, Motorola and others were producing programmable analog chips containing arrays of operational amplifiers and other analog components. Related control systems are commonplace in human physiology.[71]

Biochemical feedback loops exemplified by enzyme activity in the living cell exhibit similar analog computational functionality.[2695,3509,3543,3544] To start with, the net flow of carbon through an enzyme-catalyzed reaction may be influenced by

1. the absolute quantity of enzyme present,
2. the pool of nonenzyme reactants and products available, and
3. the catalytic efficiency of the enzyme.[996]

All three influences may themselves be subject to recursive enzymatic control. For instance, the absolute quantity of enzyme present is determined by competing rates of synthesis and degradation; both of these processes are controlled by other enzymes. Product synthesis may be triggered by an inducer, or may be repressed by an end product. Local concentrations of coenzymes or metal ions can regulate catalytic efficiency. Inhibited activity of an enzyme in a biosynthetic pathway by an end product of that pathway, such as the much-studied inhibition of aspartate transcarbamoylase by cytidine triphosphate (CTP),[3689-3691] is called feedback inhibition.[3689-3693] Typically the feedback inhibitor, acting as a negative allosteric effector, binds to the sensitive enzyme at an allosteric site that is spatially distinct from the catalytic site. Further fine control is provided by additional multiple feedback loops, exhibiting such features as cumulative feedback inhibition (e.g., the inhibitory effect of two or more end products on a single regulatory enzyme is strictly additive),[3694-3696] multivalent feedback inhibition (e.g., complete inhibition occurs only when two or more end products both are present in excess),[3697,3698] and cooperative feedback inhibition (e.g., single end product present in excess inhibits the enzyme, but inhibitory effect of two or more end products present in excess is "multiplicative").[3699,3700] Similarly, parallel chemical computers consisting of open, bistable coupled reaction systems[3542] capable of pattern storage and pattern recognition have been proposed and simulated to model a neural network,[1911] and experiments have been performed with a system of 16 coupled bistable chemical oscillators using the chlorite-iodide reaction.[1912]

Networks of interacting enzymatic reactivities can also be used to create biochemical digital computers.[2851] An enzymatic Turing machine was first proposed by C.H. Bennett,[296] and Liberman[3471] described the living cell as an analog-digital molecular stochastic parallel computer. More recently, T. Knight of the MIT Artificial Intelligence Laboratory suggested that normal cellular activities can be co-opted to implement digital logic gates, a process he calls "cellular gate technology."[1962,3544] In this scheme, protein concentrations are used as binary signals. The signal is "1" if the marker protein is being synthesized, thus reaching some detectable threshold equilibrium value where the rates of synthesis and degradation are equal. The signal is "0" if the synthesis of the marker protein is being inhibited by some other protein, and thus the concentration is trending toward zero.

This principle may be used to make logical circuit elements. For example, an inverter system consists of two different proteins, one of which is inhibiting the synthesis of the other. A NOR gate requires a system in which either of two proteins can inhibit the synthesis of a third protein; multivalent feedback inhibition in which two proteins are both required to inhibit production of a third makes a NAND gate. This is sufficient to implement any Boolean function, given enough gates and signals. Two NORs crossed in a loop makes a bistable multivibrator, or flip-flop, a fundamental component in data registers, shift registers, rectangular pulse generators, or pulse delay elements. The logic circuitry (the arrangement of "gates" and "wires") comprises a set of designed DNA sequences that determine which proteins are being synthesized and which combinations of proteins can inhibit the synthesis of others.

In the most optimistic case, we assume operation near concentrations of $c_{prot} \sim 10^{-4}$ gm/cm^3 (similar to most complement factors and some clotting factors in human blood; Appendix B), marker proteins and gating enzymes of mass $MW_{prot} \sim 10$ kilodaltons, and a minimum of $N_{prot} \sim 100$ protein molecules per gate, giving a typical logic element size of $V_{gate} \sim N_{prot}\, MW_{prot} / N_A\, c_{prot} \sim 0.02$ micron^3/gate where N_A is Avogadro's number. Flip-flop registers may store ~50 bits/micron^3. In theory, the DNA specifications for this computer could be grafted onto the genome of an animal cell (~20 micron^3 = up to 1000 gate volumes) or a bacterial cell (~2 micron^3 = up to 100 gate volumes), taking care to avoid any unwanted interactions with natural biochemical pathways. Minimum diffusion-limited gating time across a biochemical gate of characteristic dimension $\Delta X \sim V_{gate}^{1/3}$ is given by Eqn. 9.80 as $\tau = \Delta X^2 / 2D \sim 0.3$ millisec assuming protein marker diffusivity $D \sim 10^{-10}$ m^2/sec (Table 3-3), consistent with ~KHz maximum operating frequencies when DNA is localized near the gates. For nucleoplasmic DNA with cytoplasmic computation, diffusion-limited maximum switching frequency falls to ~0.1-1 Hz. For comparison with natural systems, genes controlling the fibroblast cell proliferation program have been observed to switch states in ~900 sec,[2683] implying computation at ~0.001 Hz.

Other classes of biochemically-modulated biomolecular switches have been investigated. For example, Matthews[1929] incorporated an artificial molecular on-off switch into an enzyme by adding a pair of thiol groups into the active site of native lysozyme, replacing two amino acids on opposite side of the active site with cysteine, an amino acid with a thiol-containing side chain. Thiols may form covalent bridges (-SS-) or broken bridges (-SH HS-) under suitable chemical conditions. Cycling the solution composition causes the cysteines to form a bridge across the active site (inactivating the enzyme) or to break the bridge (activating the enzyme); the process is completely reversible. Another experiment[1930] involved genetic modification to the bacterial phage lambda, a virus with two behavioral states called lytic (replication-active) and lysogenic (replication-inactive). The NIH researchers installed a synthetic molecular switch[1976] in lambda that allows the virus to be biochemically toggled between its lysogenic and lytic phases by the introduction of active HIV-1 protease. The genetic circuit that controls the phage lambda lysis-lysogeny decision has been flowcharted in detail using Boolean logic operators.[223] The immunological synapse[3453]—the specialized junction between a T cell and an antigen-presenting cell—acts as a kind of biochemical logic gate with a ~0.06 Hz switching rate.[3453-3455]

In 1998, the DNA molecule also was being actively investigated for biochemical computers. DNA-based Turing machines were first proposed by C.H. Bennett and R. Landauer.[296,1894] In 1994, L. Adelman demonstrated the first DNA computer[1895,1896] using fragments of DNA to compute the solution to a simple graph theory problem. Adleman used short DNA sequences to represent vertices of a network, or graph. Combinations of these sequences were then synthesized randomly by massively parallel chemical reactions in aqueous solution using a combination of the copying and combination reactions applied to the artificial DNA strands, comprising all possible random paths through the graph, after which a sequence representing the designed result was biochemically extracted from the stew.

Initially it was thought that DNA computing would be limited to the solution of combinatorial problems,[1897] but subsequent research has shown that the approach can be applied to a much wider class of digital computations.[1898-1902] The well-known problem of combinatorial explosion (e.g., even a small protein of 300 amino acids has a sequence space of 10^{390}) leading to huge-volume DNA libraries during a complex computation may be avoided using a recursive selection approach[1899] crudely analogous to genetic algorithms. Some work has been done using plasmids and restriction endonucleases to implement a DNA-based Turing machine, using only commercially available restriction enzymes and ligases for every operation with states represented as sequences of bases around a plasmid,[1886] and Warren Smith has another Turing machine design using the chemistry of guide RNAs in *Trypanosome* kinetoplasts.[3701] Practical challenges include finding fast, efficient, and low-noise input and output techniques.[1902,2331]

DNA computation is in theory energetically efficient, requiring only ~12 kT per ligation operation at room temperature, with massively parallel operations although each ligation reaction requires ~1 sec to complete.[1896] DNA data representation allows up to ~1 bit/nm^3 storage density.[1895] However, a practical mass storage device would probably require 10-100 nucleotide-long words to avoid ambiguities during the recall process,[1903] thus reducing maximum density to 10^7-10^8 bits/micron^3, though of course some of this reduction could be offset by reducing read rate requirements (e.g., by using multiple read heads with majority logic).

10.2.3.2 Biomechanical Computers

Components of mechanical computers could be constructed entirely of biologically-derived materials which in theory might be fabricated using synthesis pathways accessible to engineered microbiota. For example, Drexler's mechanical nanocomputer [10] assumes diamondoid logic rods with a Young's modulus of $E = 5 \times 10^{11}$ N/m^2, but the Young's modulus for human bone hydroxyapatite and fluoroapatite crystals is almost as high, with $E \sim 1\text{-}2 \times 10^{11}$ N/m^2 (Table 9.3). Ignoring the significant problems inherent in noneutactic rod logic systems, apatite-based mechanical computer structures might be laid down using engineered osteocytes, perhaps assisted by chemotactic or contact guidance techniques. Failure strength of apatites is ~100 times poorer than for diamond, so apatite logic rod force and acceleration should be reduced by ~100 and rod vibrational energy by ~10^4, increasing minimum switching time by a factor of ~10 (to ~1 nanosec) and decreasing maximum rod speed to ~1 m/sec.

N. Seeman has constructed molecular building blocks from unusual DNA motifs (Section 2.3.1), using stable-branched DNA molecules with the connectivity of a cube[1914] or a truncated octahedron.[1915] E. Winfree[1919] has proposed using arrays of DNA crossover molecules[1920] in DNA-based computing, requiring the ability to build periodic backbones with bases differing from one unit cell to another. In addition to branching topology, DNA also allows control of linking topology. DNA-based topological control has led to the construction of Borromean rings which could be used in DNA-based computing applications.[1916-1918] In Borromean rings, the linkage between any pair of rings disappears in the absence of the third. Rings can be designed with an arbitrary number of circles; the integrity of a link could represent the truth of each of a group of logical statements.[1916]

DNA structural transitions could be used to drive nanomechanical devices via branch migration.[1916] Application of torque to a cruciform leads to the extrusion or intrusion of a cruciform.[1921] A synthetic branched junction with two opposite arms linked can relocate its branch point in response to positive ethidium-induced supercoiling, representing the first experimental step in developing DNA structural transitions that can achieve a nanomechanical result.[1922] The possible use of the B-Z transition (e.g., from right-handed B-DNA to left-handed Z-DNA) in nanomechanical devices is being explored.[2409]

In 1998, Winfree and colleagues in Seeman's laboratory[1970] described a simple, predictable, highly precise technique for arranging DNA molecules into two-dimensional crystals. At the same time, a paper by Heath and others[1980] described a defect-tolerant computer architecture called the Teramac, a massively parallel experimental computer which apparently could operate normally with at least half of its most critical components failed. The authors claimed this architecture showed it would be "feasible to chemically synthesize individual [molecular] electronic components with less than a 100% yield, assemble them into systems with appreciable uncertainty in their connectivity, and still create a powerful and reliable data communications network."

One can also imagine a network of interlocking enzymelike conformational switches, possibly embedded in a semirigid two- or three-dimensional scaffolding of DNA[1904,1913-1916] or protein[1905,1913] molecules. Enzymes may display multivalent feedback inhibition (making a NAND gate; Section 10.2.3.1) or may have multiple metal-ion binding sites influencing enzymatic action;[1928] an enzyme requiring two conformational changes to inhibit its action could serve as a biomechanical NAND gate if tethered to other similar enzymes in an appropriately structured protein array.[1905] Single-device error rates will be high but might be reduced to acceptable levels by employing short multiply-redundant pathways for each digital computational operation, or a sufficiently parallel architecture.[1980] Site-directed mutagenesis optimization of antibodies has shown that natural proteins can be made significantly stiffer and more stable by the mutation of just a few amino acids. Systems of reciprocating actomyosin molecular motors (e.g., as found in muscle fibers; Section 6.3.4.2) might serve as interdigitating components of a push-pull mechanical logic architecture resembling rod logic or a three-dimensional loom. In early 1999, Viola Vogel (University of Washington Center for Nanotechnology) and colleagues discovered, via computer simulation, a tension-activated fully-reversible biomechanical switch comprised of a single strand of fibronectin protein—like untying a shoelace, a slight mechanical tug unravels a folded segment, switching off the protein's biochemical activity.[3249]

Mechanical coupling of intracellular Ca^{++} ion release channels allows coordinated voltage gating across the surface membrane of the sarcoplasmic reticulum inside muscle cells.[1964] R. Bradbury [personal communication, 1999] suggests that site-directed mutagenesis could produce a family of proteins that could be activated by the release of various mono- (e.g., K^+), di- (e.g., Ca^{++}), and tri-valent (e.g., Al^{+++}) ions. This would allow multivalued logic (e.g., K = 1, Ca = 2, Al = 4), or increased parallelism or bandwidth (e.g., Ca = !(K & K), Al = !(Ca & Ca), etc.); once a protein exists that can be activated by a single ion, then varying its architecture to allow substitution of an ion of different size or charge is a relatively straightforward engineering exercise. A biomechanical Turing machine design has also been reported by Shapiro.[3247]

10.2.3.3 Organic and Bioelectronic Computers

Many organic materials may be useful in electronic computing. Electrical conduction in synthetic organic molecules is well known[1761,1906-1909,3125-3128] and already exploited in liquid-crystal displays of laptop computers.[1925] Doped polyacetylene is a conducting plastic with a carbon backbone; undoped, it is an insulator. There are many other known families of conducting polymers such as polyaniline, which includes nitrogen atoms in the backbone, and polythiophene, which includes sulfur.[1833] Three-dimensional interconnect arrays of organic conducting polymers have been fabricated;[1839] conductivity is higher along a chain than between chains, so sheets of oriented chains can produce relative conductivity anisotropies as high as 100-1000.[1927] An all-plastic transistor has been built.[1935] Organic transistors have been used as the active semiconducting element in thin-film transistors fabricated with organic-material thicknesses ranging from 5-150 nm,[1842] and organic microscale transistors and other organic devices may exploit bulk-effect electron transport just like silicon-based semiconductor devices.[1923] Conjugated polymer poly(1,6-heptadiester) was employed to make an optical correlator with a peak processing rate of 3×10^{16} operations/sec.[1841] Spin-transition polymers could serve as thermal sensors or memory devices with the theoretical ability to store one bit in a ~4 nm cube (~2×10^7 bits/micron^3 storage density) with ~GHz addressing speeds at room temperature.[1840] Other organic polymers possibly useful in logic circuits have been investigated.[2899]

Natural biological materials may also be useful in electronic computing,[1777,1925,3129] particularly because of the ability of biological materials to self-assemble. Biomolecular electronics is a subfield of molecular electronics that investigates the use of native as well as modified biological molecules (chromophores, proteins, etc.) in place of the organic molecules synthesized in the laboratory.[1777] In theory, a three-dimensional DNA or protein scaffolding could be self-assembled, with bacteriorhodopsin, ferritin and magnetite, or related bioelectromagnetic molecules inserted into precise locations within the structure to produce a crystal lattice bioelectronic or biooptoelectronic nanocomputer. DNA already has been used as an atomic scaffold upon which to build silver wires ~100 nm in diameter[1961] and has been decorated with fullerenes.[3024] Self-assembly can generate membrane-based[1931,1932] and biotubule-based[1926] devices, and site-directed mutagenesis is a valuable tool for high-resolution protein device engineering.[1933] Nucleotide sequence-specific electron transfer between metallic electron donor and acceptor complexes covalently or noncovalently intercalated into strands of B-DNA has been demonstrated.[1934]

Perhaps the best-known bioelectronic (and biochemical) computer is the neuron cell and its congeries—the ganglia, nerve trunks, and brains. In 1997, David Stenger (NRL) and James Hickman (SAIC) were attempting to culture and link together neuronal cells to build a bioelectronic cell-based sensor "computer" for performing complex pattern-recognition tasks.[1966,1967] In early 1999, W.L. Ditto at Georgia Tech announced the creation of a biological computer comprised entirely of leech neurons, that was capable of perfoming simple sums.[3245] We can certainly imagine large numbers of cultured neurons arranged in artificial three-dimensional spatial patterns to produce a synthetic bioneural computer, but such a computer would operate at only ~KHz frequencies and would be very energy inefficient since each neuron consumes ~10^{10} kT per discharge (Section 4.8.6.2)—thus offering few advantages.

10.2.4 Ultimate Limits to Computation

A nanosystem designer quickly discovers that total nanorobot power demand (Section 6.5) is often dominated by computational heat dissipation, rather than by energy dissipation from chemical or mechanical processes. Thus important design objectives are to:

1. minimize onboard computation,

2. maximize algorithmic efficiency (e.g., super-Turing computers),[1910,3176] and
3. minimize power dissipation per computation operation, an objective which may be met using reversible computing.

It is also interesting to consider the maximum possible information density in physical matter as a calibration for current and projected achievements.

10.2.4.1 Reversible Computers

Computers may be thought of as engines for transforming free energy into waste heat and mathematical work.[296] Early pioneers of computing theory[1984,1985] believed that each step in a a computer's binary computation required a minimum energy expenditure of ~kT ln(2) ~3 zJ/bit at T = 310 K. In 1961, R. Landauer[1986] argued that it was the erasure of information, not computation per se, that generates waste heat. It is now known that computers can in principle do an arbitrarily large amount of reliable computation per kT of energy dissipated.[296] Following Landauer's insight, Fredkin and Toffoli[1987] suggested an idealized "ballistic computer" that could, in theory, compute at finite speed with zero energy dissipation and zero error. A more pragmatic family of models are the "Brownian computers"[296] in which thermal noise pushes system elements in a random walk throughout the entire accessible portion of the computer's configuration space; in these models, energy dissipation trends to zero only in the limit of zero speed. Both ballistic and Brownian computers require that all computations are logically reversible, with no irreversible bit erasures and no machine state having more than one logical predecessor—that is, the output uniquely specifies the input.[10]

One simple implementation of reversible computing is the retractile cascade.[10,296,1743] In a retractile cascade, all inputs and all intermediate states leading to a result are retained during the course of a computation. After the computation is complete, the final result is copied to an output register, requiring the irreversible erasure of only enough bits in the output register to hold a copy of the final result, which need cost no more than kT ln(2) per erased bit. The computation is then reversed, step by step, culminating with the original inputs; the slower the reversible steps are performed, the less energy they may dissipate (but the longer the computation takes). Schematics for a retractile AND gate, adder, shifter, and programmable logic array have been published,[1743] and in 1998 a reversible processor based on a modern RISC architecture was being designed.[1994] A conventional computer architecture, implemented without regard to reversibility, may perform 0.1-1 bit erasures/gate-cycle; by comparison, a retractile computer might average $<10^{-4}$ bit erasures/gate-cycle.[1743] During the reversible portion of the computation, Drexler's exemplar rod logic design (Section 10.2.1) employs a retractile cascade that reduces room-temperature energy dissipation from the "classical" minimum of ~0.7 kT down to ~0.003 kT per gate-cycle. In the limit of slow motion, all identified energy dissipation mechanisms in combinatorial rod logic systems approach zero.[10] The Tour-Seminario electrostatic field switch might attain $\sim 10^{-5}$ kT per gate-cycle at room temperature; low-temperature helical logic (Section 10.2.2.3) could achieve $\sim 10^{-7}$ kT per gate-cycle. Feynman[1996] notes that the minimum free energy required for a reversible computation may be made independent of the complexity or number of steps in the calculation, and may be as small as ~kT per bit of the output answer.

J.S. Hall[1743] suggests two principal design rules for efficient nanocomputers:

1. erase as few bits as possible, and
2. eliminate entropy loss in operations that do not erase bits.

Many reviews of reversible computing have been published.[296,713,1097,1743,1988,1989]

10.2.4.2 Quantum Computers

Digital computers manipulate discrete units of information, with data strings stored as binary digits, or bits. Any two-state physical system (e.g., high or low voltages in semiconductor circuits) can represent these bits. Similarly, a quantum computer would use quantum states of atomic or molecular systems to store data. For example, the states of a hydrogen atom could be assigned such that a wavefunction corresponding to a state of hydrogen would represent a bit of data. Shining laser light on the atoms would trigger processing the data by inducing transitions between electronic states.

Quantum systems, however, exhibit a peculiar phenomenon known as superposition, in which several discrete states can be processed by a single physical system at once, crudely analogous to the musical effect of a single note being made up of many different harmonics.[1259] Superposition gives quantum systems the potential to be enormously more powerful than conventional computers. Since more than one state can be supported, quantum bits, or qubits, may store a mixture of many bits of data at the same time. A superposition of N qubits can store 2^N binary digits. An operation on these mixtures is massively parallel, effectively performing many calculations simultaneously. For example, photons interacting with an atom in a superposition of states drive all the states in the superposition, producing another superposition corresponding to all solutions of the original states. The advantage over conventional computers is not merely linear, but exponential: A conventional processor operates sequentially on 64-bit numbers, but a quantum computer with 64 qubits would simultaneously operate on the full set of 2^{64} ($\sim 10^{19}$) binary values. An N-qubit quantum computer could model an N-body system in real time[6]; in contrast, the number of operations required by a conventional computer to perform such a simulation increases exponentially with the number of bodies.

Since the early 1980s, theoretical interest in quantum computing has developed rapidly.[6,1996-2004,2013] Many groups have begun designing quantum computational architectures and constructing physical quantum gates and devices. In 1995, one group at NIST made a controlled NOT gate of two qubits from a cooled beryllium ion in a radio-frequency trap,[2005] while a French group used single photons trapped in quantum cavities to control cesium atom states.[2006] In 1999, experiments began on an analog quantum computer using electrons floating on liquid helium.[3276] Others work with NMR techniques,[2007,2008,2014] storing data not in electron states but in nuclear spins, which are less susceptible to perturbations.[2002] Resonance effects between proton and electron spins in hydrogen atoms can make AND and NOT gates, hence NAND gates, from which all Boolean computers can be made. It has been suggested that by encoding the amplitudes of a couple of thousand electron states in a superposition, large amounts of data could be written onto a single atom (see Section 10.2.4.3). The discovery of certain error-correcting procedures,[2003] since verified experimentally,[2141] was another important breakthrough. Unlike conventional devices, it is not possible to simply check that qubits are in the right states, because the act of measuring destroys the coherence. But Shor[2009] proved that information can be reliably stored and read from a several qubit system even if one of the bits is corrupted, and it has been shown that error correction can be applied during the computation process itself.[2010] This opens the door to many-qubit systems; by 1998, two groups had already performed 4-bit sums, and one group had demonstrated a 2-qubit device.[2329] Quantum game theory has also been investigated.[2867]

10.2.4.3 Bekenstein-Bounded Computation

A fundamental upper limit on the number of possible quantum states in a bounded region (e.g., the maximum number of bits that can be coded in a bounded region)—is given by the Bekenstein Bound[1990] as:

$$I_{Bek} = \frac{2 \pi E R}{\hbar c \ln(2)} \quad \text{(bits)} \qquad \text{\{Eqn. 10.10\}}$$

within a spherical region of radius R containing energy $E = mc^2$ where m is the enclosed mass, $c = 3 \times 10^8$ m/sec (speed of light), and $\hbar = h / 2\pi$ where $h = 6.63 \times 10^{-34}$ joule-sec (Planck's constant). Maximum processing speed $\dot{I}$ is then bounded by the minimum time for a state transition, which cannot be less than the time required for light to cross the region of radius R, or:

$$\dot{I}_{Bek} = \frac{\pi E}{\hbar \ln(2)} \quad \text{(bits/sec)} \qquad \text{\{Eqn. 10.11\}}$$

Thus in theory, a single carbon atom of mass $m = 2 \times 10^{-26}$ kg and radius R ~ 0.15 nm could be impressed with up to $I_{Bek} \sim 10^8$ bits and could process information up to $\dot{I}_{Bek} \sim 10^{26}$ bits/sec in an optimally-designed quantum computer. For a 1 micron^3 computer of mass ~10^{-15} kg, $I_{Bek} \sim 10^{22}$ bits maximum storage capacity and $\dot{I}_{Bek} \sim 10^{37}$ bits/sec maximum processing capacity. These values are not the least upper limits; Schiffer and Bekenstein[1991] estimate that the Bekenstein Bound probably overestimates I and $\dot{I}$ by at least a factor of 100, but Likharev[1992] and Margolus and Levitin[2319] have derived similar limits. In 1998, proposed reversible quantum computer systems would perform significantly below the Bekenstein Bound.[1993,1994]

10.2.5 Dedicated Computational Organs

Nanostructured artificial organs specializing in control, information processing, or data storage could be permanently embedded within the human body. Such organs could provide a user-accessible computational facility, or help coordinate and control (or even subsume) the activities of in vivo medical nanorobots or other dedicated nano-organs, including energy (Section 6.4.4), communications (Section 7.3.4), navigation (Section 8.3.6), or chronometer (Section 10.1.4) systems. Computational organs could also serve as embedded data repositories (library nodules), including personal medical and experiential records,[2958,2959] customized calendars and personal data banks, or as communications encryption and security interfaces.

In 1998, microchips glued to honeybees[3727] or implanted under the skin of livestock and household pets contained owner/address information that could be retrieved by passing a reading wand over the animal (e.g., Pet Trac, manufactured by A.V.I.D. Identification Systems; Norco, California). Read-only microchips with identification numbers for individual cattle were encased in acid-resistant porcelain and inserted into an animal's stomach ten days after birth. These chips could be read by a handheld computer or a stationary reader; Shearwell Data, which sold the chips for $6 each, planned to adapt them to communicate with global positioning satellites so that farmers could remotely track herd movements.[3037] Peter Cochrane[2958] notes that a colleague (Kevin Warwick) has had a computer chip embedded under his skin,[3324] bearing such personal information as medical records and bank account and passport numbers. There were also unconfirmed rumors of a subdermally-implanted bio-powered (4 milliamp) 16 mm^2 transmitter chip called Sky-Eye, sold by Gen-Etics for $7,500 as kidnap deterrence for "the rich and famous," that supposedly emitted a personal tracking signal detectable by satellite.[3702]

10.3 Pressure Storage and Ballasting

Storage of gases at high pressure is useful for nanorobots that must perform physiological gas transport functions[1400] (Chapters 22 and 26) or emergency reactive functions (Chapter 24), for devices which employ gases in onboard energy systems (Chapter 6), or for devices which require gaseous chemicals for onboard materials processing (Chapter 19). Pressurized gases are useful in buoyancy maintenance to facilitate device exfusion from the human body (Section 10.3.6), and possibly in the deactivation of toxic biochemicals or microbial pathogens (Table 10.3). Keeping a eutactic environment[10] inside nanodevices requires the ability to draw and to maintain a vacuum (Section 10.3.5). This ability also may assist in metamorphic bumper (Section 5.4) and buoyancy control.

10.3.1 Fluid Storage Tank Scaling

The ability of a vessel to store fluids at high pressure is determined by the rupture strength of the valve and pipe systems and by the tensile strength of the tank walls. A symmetric structural shell transmitting only normal stresses in orthogonal directions may employ either a stressed skin or a ribbed design. The stressed skin is more efficient because the same material carries stress in both directions and there is integral resistance to secondary torsional and bending loads.[2023] For a stressed skin spherical pressure vessel of radius R with wall material of density ρ_{wall} and working stress σ_w, containing fluid at pressure differential p_{fluid}, the required wall thickness t_{wall} is given by:[2023]

$$t_{wall} = \frac{p_{fluid} R}{2(\sigma_w - g \rho_{wall} R)} \qquad \text{\{Eqn. 10.12\}}$$

where $g = 9.81$ m/sec^2 (acceleration of gravity). For all but the most enormous macroscale tanks, the second term in the denominator is negligible and so the maximum pressure differential that can be restrained by a spherical microscale tank without bursting is:

$$p_{max\,sph} = \frac{2 t_{wall} \sigma_w}{R} \qquad \text{\{Eqn. 10.13\}}$$

Thus a tank of radius R = 1 micron made of diamondoid walls which are $t_{wall} = 5$ nm (~30 carbon atoms) thick with $\sigma_w = 10^{10}$ N/m^2 (~0.2 times the failure strength of diamond; Table 9.3) can store fluids up to a maximum pressure differential of $p_{maxsph} = 1000$ atm. Empty tank mass is $M_{tank} \sim 4 \pi \rho_{wall} t_{wall} R^2 = (4 \pi \rho_{wall} / 2 \sigma_w) p_{maxsph} R^3$, for $t_{wall} << R$. A spherical fullerene nanotank with defect-free single-carbon walls ($t_{wall} \sim 0.34$ nm thick), pressurized to $p_{maxsph} \sim 1000$ atm differential, must have $R \lesssim 67$ nm or it may burst.

Similarly, for a cylinder or pipe of radius R:

$$p_{max\,cyl} = \frac{t_{wall} \sigma_w}{R} \qquad \text{\{Eqn. 10.14\}}$$

Note that a hemispherical-capped cylindrical tank, pressurized until it explodes, will usually split its sides before blowing off its ends because $p_{maxsph} = 2\, p_{max\,cyl}$. Wall stress for a cylindrical tube with Young's modulus E, inside radius R and wall thickness t_{wall} upon which is imposed a pressure differential of p_{cyl} is ~ $p_{cyl} R / t_{wall}$,[362] giving a wall strain of $S \sim p_{cyl} R / t_{wall} E$; hence a single-walled carbon nanotube with R = 20 nm, $t_{wall} \sim 0.2$ nm, and $E \sim 10^{12}$ N/m^2 pressurized to p_{cyl} = 1000 atm stretches by S ~ 1%. (For comparison, aluminum soda pop cans are pressurized to ~2 atm differential, beer cans ~1 atm.)[3703]

For a toroid tank of small meridional radius r and large circumferential (hoop direction) radius R, the burst pressure in the meridional ($p_{max\ merid}$) and hoop ($p_{max\ hoop}$) directions are:[2023]

$$p_{max\ merid} = \frac{t_{wall}\ \sigma_w}{r} \qquad \text{\{Eqn. 10.15\}}$$

$$p_{max\ hoop} = \frac{2\ t_{wall}\ \sigma_w}{r} \qquad \text{\{Eqn. 10.16\}}$$

Hence as pressure is raised, the toroidal tank fails first in the meridional direction, much like the capped cylinder.

Spherical pressure vessels are the most efficient. The maximum mass of gas that can be contained within a spherical tank at ideal gas pressures (Section 10.3.2) is $M_{gas} \sim (4 \pi N_A m_{gas} / 3 R_{gas} T_{gas}) p_{max} R^3$, where $N_A = 6.023 \times 10^{23}$ molecules/mole (Avogadro's number), m_{gas} is the mass per gas molecule, R_{gas} = 8.31 J/mole-K (universal gas constant), and T_{gas} is gas temperature. Thus we observe that the ratio of gas mass to structural mass (M_{gas}/M_{tank}) at a given pressure is constant and independent of the size of the tank. This ratio reaches a maximum value at maximum pressurization; the maximum value is independent of both tank size and the maximum pressure selected (within the ideal gas range). In particular, $M_{gas}/M_{tank} \sim 2 \sigma_w N_A m_{gas} / 3 R_{gas} T_{gas} \rho_{wall} \sim 21$ for nitrogen gas molecules ($m_{gas} = 4.65 \times 10^{-26}$ kg/molecule) stored at temperature T_{gas} = 310 K. That is, the tank can store up to ~21 times its weight of gas.

Other important microtank design constraints include diffusion leakage and vessel flammability (Section 10.3.4), vapor pressure of tank materials at high temperatures (Section 10.3.5), thermal cycling during filling and discharging operations (Section 5.3.3), resistance to mechanical crushing, and susceptibility to acoustic resonances (e.g., the natural frequency of an $r_{sph} \sim 1$ micron hollow diamondoid sphere is of order $\sim v_{sound} / r_{sph} \sim 20$ GHz, fortunately much higher than most nanomedically useful frequencies).

10.3.2 The Van der Waals Equation

The compressibility of gases is most simply described by the well-known ideal gas law:

$$p_{gas}\ V_{gas} = n\ R_{gas}\ T_{gas} \qquad \text{\{Eqn. 10.17\}}$$

where p_{gas}, V_{gas} and n are gas pressure, volume, and number of moles, respectively. However, all real gases deviate to some extent from the ideal gas law, even at STP. Most real gases obey the ideal gas law to within a few percent at low densities—that is, at low pressures (e.g., $\lesssim$ 1 atm) and at temperatures well above their condensation points. For real gases at high pressure, finite molecular volumes and intermolecular attractions cause significant deviation from the ideal gas law. In 1873, J.D. van der Waals deduced an empirical equation of state (subsequently derived from statistical mechanics using suitable approximations[1031]) that reproduces the observed behavior of real gases with moderate accuracy:

$$\left(p_{gas} + \frac{A\ n^2}{V_{gas}^2}\right)\left(V_{gas} - B\ n\right) = n\ R_{gas}\ T_{gas} \qquad \text{\{Eqn. 10.18\}}$$

where A is a measure of intermolecular attraction and B is a measure of finite molecular volumes. The van der Waals gas "constants," given in Table 10.1 for various gases, are known to vary slightly with temperature. Nevertheless, while Eqn. 10.18 is only one of several expressions commonly employed to represent real gas behavior, it is the simplest to use and to interpret. The van der Waals equation remains approximately valid even at temperatures and molar volumes so low that the gas has become a liquid.[1031] Note that the critical temperature T_{crit}, the highest temperature at which gas and liquid may exist as separate phases at any pressure, is approximated by $T_{crit} = 8 c_1 A / 27 B R_{gas}$, where $c_1 = 1.01 \times 10^5$ J/m^3-atm and R_{gas} = 8.31 J/mole-K; critical pressure $p_{crit} = A / 27 B^2$.[390] For example, in the case of water, at temperatures and pressures above T_{crit} = 647.3 K and p_{crit} = 218.3 atm,[763] the vapor and liquid phases become indistinguishable.

The boiling point of a pure liquid as a function of pressure may be approximated by:[2036]

$$\ln\left(\frac{p_2}{p_1}\right) = \frac{\Delta H_{vap}}{R_{gas}}\left(\frac{1}{T_1} - \frac{1}{T_2}\right) \qquad \text{\{Eqn. 10.19\}}$$

where T_1 and T_2 are the boiling points (in K) at pressures p_1 and p_2, respectively, ΔH_{vap} is the molar heat of vaporization for the liquid (Table 10.8), and R_{gas} = 8.31 J/mole-K. (This formula assumes that ΔH_{vap} is constant over the temperature range from T_1 to T_2.) Taking T_1 = 373.16 K, ΔH_{vap} = 40,690 J/mole, and p_1 = 1 atm for water, then at p_2 = 6.4 atm the boiling point has risen to T_2 = 435 K. Boiling point also is altered by the presence of solute (Section 10.5.3).

Table 10.2 shows the molecular number density achieved inside gas storage vessels maintained at various pressures at T_{gas} = 310 K. Note that there are significant (near-linear) gains in gas molecule packing density up to 1000 atm, minor (non-linear) gains up to 10,000 atm, and no significant gain at >100,000 atm as density approaches a limiting value for the liquid or solid state. Table 10.2 also shows that pressures calculated using the ideal gas law vary from pressures calculated using the van der Waals equation by ~5% at 100 atm and ~50% at 1000 atm.*

One early experiment provided evidence of stably trapped (Section 10.3.4) room-temperature gases at ~1300 atm pressure inside carbon

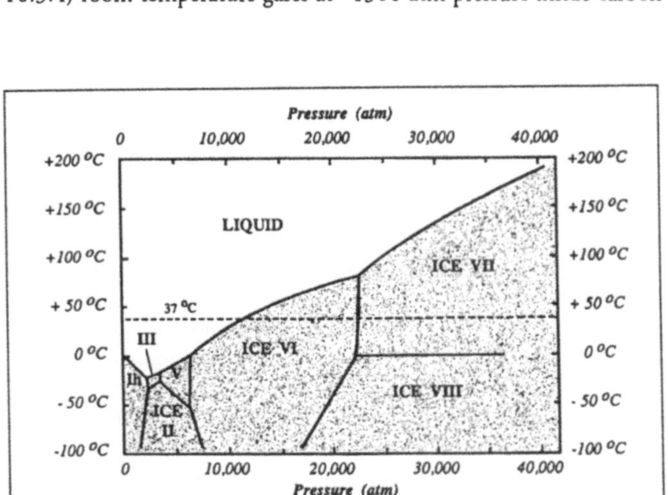

Fig. 10.11. Phase diagram for water and ice (stable phases only).[2053,2054]

Table 10.1. Van der Waals Equation Gas Constants[763]

Gas Molecule	Chemical Formula	A (m^6-atm/mole^2)	B (m^3/mole)
Acetic acid	CH_3COOH	1.759×10^{-5}	1.068×10^{-4}
Acetone	$(CH_2)_2CO$	1.391×10^{-5}	9.940×10^{-5}
Acetylene	C_2H_2	4.390×10^{-6}	5.136×10^{-5}
Ammonia	NH_3	4.170×10^{-6}	3.707×10^{-5}
Argon	Ar	1.345×10^{-6}	3.219×10^{-5}
Benzene	C_6H_6	1.800×10^{-5}	1.154×10^{-4}
n-Butane	C_4H_{10}	1.447×10^{-5}	1.226×10^{-4}
Carbon dioxide	CO_2	3.592×10^{-6}	4.267×10^{-5}
Carbon monoxide	CO	1.485×10^{-6}	3.985×10^{-5}
Chlorine	Cl_2	6.493×10^{-6}	5.622×10^{-5}
Chloroform	$CHCl_3$	1.517×10^{-5}	1.022×10^{-4}
Diethyl ether	$(C_2H_5)_2O$	1.738×10^{-5}	1.344×10^{-4}
Ethane	C_2H_6	5.489×10^{-6}	6.380×10^{-5}
Ethanol	C_2H_5OH	1.202×10^{-5}	8.407×10^{-5}
Ethylene	C_2H_4	4.471×10^{-6}	5.714×10^{-5}
Helium	He	3.412×10^{-8}	2.370×10^{-5}
n-Hexane	C_6H_{14}	2.439×10^{-5}	1.735×10^{-4}
Hydrogen	H_2	2.444×10^{-7}	2.661×10^{-5}
Hydrogen chloride	HCl	3.667×10^{-6}	4.081×10^{-5}
Methane	CH_4	2.253×10^{-6}	4.278×10^{-5}
Methanol	CH_3OH	9.523×10^{-6}	6.702×10^{-5}
Naphthalene	$C_{10}H_8$	3.974×10^{-5}	1.937×10^{-4}
Neon	Ne	2.107×10^{-7}	1.709×10^{-5}
Nitric oxide	NO	1.340×10^{-6}	2.789×10^{-5}
Nitrogen	N_2	1.390×10^{-6}	3.913×10^{-5}
Nitrous oxide	N_2O	3.782×10^{-6}	4.415×10^{-5}
n-Octane	C_8H_{18}	3.732×10^{-5}	2.368×10^{-4}
Oxygen	O_2	1.360×10^{-6}	3.183×10^{-5}
Phosphorus	P_4	5.294×10^{-5}	1.566×10^{-4}
Propane	C_3H_8	8.664×10^{-6}	8.445×10^{-5}
Water	H_2O	5.464×10^{-6}	3.049×10^{-5}

Table 10.2. Gas Molecules Packed into a Pressure Vessel: Number Density as a Function of Pressure at 310 K, using the Van der Waals Equation

Applied Pressure	O_2 Molecules per m^3	CO_2 Molecules per m^3	N_2 Molecules per m^3	He Atoms per m^3	Ideal Gas Law, No. per m^3
(Solid)	268×10^{26}	214×10^{26}	221×10^{26}	---	---
(Liquid)	215×10^{26}	151×10^{26}	174×10^{26}	184×10^{26}	---
≥100,000 atm	189×10^{26}	141×10^{26}	153×10^{26}	---	$23,700 \times 10^{26}$
10,000 atm	177×10^{26}	134×10^{26}	145×10^{26}	---	2370×10^{26}
1000 atm	126×10^{26}	111×10^{26}	106×10^{26}	123×10^{26}	237×10^{26}
100 atm	25.5×10^{26}	68.9×10^{26}	24.5×10^{26}	21.7×10^{26}	23.7×10^{26}
10 atm	2.38×10^{26}	2.47×10^{26}	2.38×10^{26}	2.34×10^{26}	2.37×10^{26}
1 atm	0.237×10^{26}	0.238×10^{26}	0.237×10^{26}	0.237×10^{26}	0.237×10^{26}
0.1 atm	0.0237×10^{26}	0.0237×10^{26}	0.0237×10^{26}	0.0237×10^{26}	0.0237×10^{26}
Molecular mass:	5.32×10^{-26} kg	7.31×10^{-26} kg	4.65×10^{-26} kg	6.64×10^{-27} kg	---

nanotubes.[1169] Single-walled carbon nanotubes have been experimentally charged with trapped hydrogen gas up to 5-10% by weight,[2024] and with argon gas at ~600 atm.[2034]

10.3.3 Pressure-Altered Physical Properties

It is only possible here to briefly mention the many pressure-mediated changes of physical properties that may be relevant in nanomedical systems. Perhaps the most familiar is phase change, as illustrated by Figure 10.11 in the case of water.[2039,2040] Note that as pressure rises from 1 atm to 2054 atm, the temperature at which water remains liquid dips from 273.2 K to 251.2 K (the Ice I/III/water triple point,[2962]), but then the liquidity threshold returns to higher temperatures as pressure rises further and a different ice phase forms; D_2O shows similar behavior.[2960] At a constant 310 K (37°C),

* *For comparison, pressures of ~1000 atm occur naturally in the deepest part of the ocean (the Marianas Trench), ~10,000 atm at the crust-mantle interface (the Mohorovic discontinuity), 3.64 million atm at the Earth's core, and ~10^9 atm at the center of the Sun.*

isothermal static compression of pure liquid water causes crystallization from the liquid to solid Ice VI near ~11,500 atm. Unlike water, most materials contract upon freezing, thus freezing point is normally raised by higher pressure. For example, the melting point of paraffin wax is 319.8 K at 1 atm but rises to 323.1 K at 100 atm.[1697]

At 273 K, gaseous carbon dioxide compressed to 35 atm suddenly liquefies; at 300 K, pressurized CO_2 remains liquid up to ~4500 atm, whereupon it solidifies.[2035] However, T_{crit} = 304.2 K for CO_2, so if the gas is stored in pressure vessels at 310 K (human body temperature) > T_{crit}, the physical properties change continuously, showing no sign that the gas has condensed to a liquid, although over ~200 atm the fluid behaves like carbon dioxide liquid.[2036] CO_2 compressed to 400,000 atm at 1800 K forms a translucent quartzlike extended covalent solid that is metastable down to ~room temperature at pressures >10,000 atm.[3181] Other gases of nanomedical interest such as oxygen (T_{crit} = 154.4 K), nitrogen (T_{crit} = 126.1 K), hydrogen (T_{crit} = 33.3 K), and helium (T_{crit} = 5.3 K) show a similar continuous progression of gas/liquid properties at 310 K with rising pressure. Helium solidifies to ~1000 kg/m^3 crystals at 115,000 atm at 297 K.[2037] Room temperature isopropyl alcohol solidifies into a glassy state at ~44,000 atm, while a 4:1 methanol/ethanol mixture remains hydrostatic up to 104,000 atm.[2051] Hydrogen solidifies at 57,000 atm at 298 K, making 600 kg/m^3 crystals;[568] solid deuterium at 300 K compacts from ~620 kg/m^3 at 100,000 atm to ~1400 kg/m^3 at 1 million atm.[2038]

Vessel wall materials also are subject to pressure changes. Diamond crystal plastically deforms at a pressure of only ~1 atm at ~1773 K, but at ~1300 K, ductile flow in diamond requires pressures >60,000 atm.[2041] At room temperature the diamond {111} surface compressed in the {110} direction is indented by pressures $\gtrsim$880,000 atm; compression of the {001} surface requires 560,000-1 million atm for indentation, depending upon the direction of the applied load.[1597] Colorless diamond takes on a light brown coloration between 1.0-1.7 million atm, a probable crystallographic phase transition.[2043] The equilibrium phase diagram for the carbon system suggests that graphite could begin to be converted to diamond at room temperature as low as 20,000 atm, although pressures of 50,000-65,000 atm at 1600-2000 K are employed for commercial diamond production in combination with Group VIII metal catalysts,[537,2042] and experiments show that graphite transforms to a transparent (but nondiamond) phase at ~180,000 atm at room temperature.[2856] Fullerenes are also susceptible to allotropic change at high pressure—nonhydrostatic compression of C_{60} molecules induces a transformation to diamond above ~150,000 atm,[2044] and bulk C_{60} converts into two different metastable structures (e.g., face-centered cubic at 600-700 K and rhombohedral at 800-1100 K) at 50,000 atm.[2045] Computer simulations suggest that an "armchair" carbon nanotube can tolerate ~10^6 atm for ~10 years before failing.[2957] As for sapphire and ruby (primarily corundum or Al_2O_3), no structural transformations were observed in an x-ray diffraction study of ruby compressed to 1.75 million atm at room temperature,[2046] a similar study found a polymorphic phase transformation at pressures as low as 850,000 atm when the ruby was heated above ~1000 K.[2047] Finally, while negative volume compressibility is thermodynamically forbidden, lanthanum niobate crystals and several other materials display negative linear or areal compressibilities—that is, they expand in one or two directions (while maintaining constant volume) when hydrostatic pressure is applied.[1297]

The solubility of gases in liquids strongly increases with pressure (Section 9.2.6), but the effect of pressure on solubility of crystalline or liquid substances in liquids is usually very small and may be predicted by Le Chatelier's principle since it depends on the relative volumes of the solution and the component substances.[2048] For example, raising the pressure from 1 atm to 1000 atm only increases the 298 K aqueous solubility of sodium chloride from 359 gm/liter to 370 gm/liter.[2036] Room temperature liquid carbon dioxide at ~200 atm pressure (~753 kg/m^3 at 310 K) has been used for decades as a nontoxic solvent in chemical processing, such as the process for extraction of caffeine from coffee pioneered by General Foods; a microemulsion of aqueous micelles in liquid carbon dioxide extends solvation to proteins which are normally insoluble in pure CO_2.[2049]

There are many other effects of elevated pressures. For example, the speed of sound generally increases with higher pressure (e.g., by ~0.25 (m/sec)/atm in water near 1 atm; Section 4.5.1). As another example, very highly compressed materials may enter a metallic (electrically conducting) state (e.g., room temperature cesium iodide becomes metallic at ~1.15 million atm[2052]).

There are also significant effects of elevated pressures on biology.[3218] The summary in Table 10.3 suggests that the largest biological cells are harmed by pressures under 1000 atm; small cells and viruses may be inactivated at a few thousand atm; antigens, toxins, enzymes, and other proteins are deactivated or denatured near ~10,000 atm of pressure.[585] (See also Section 10.4.2.3.) Microbial death at >2000 atm is considered to be due to changes in the permeability of cell membranes.[3106] Protein denaturation occurs at higher pressures because noncovalent bonds are destroyed or formed as system volume declines.[3107] Proteins, carbohydrates and nucleic acids, whose tertiary structures are composed of noncovalent bonds, change their structures at pressures between 2000-10,000 atm, leading to denaturation, coagulation, or gelatinization; covalent bonds in pure substances usually do not undergo changes at these pressures.[3106] Irreversible effects on biological materials are generally observed at pressures >1000-2000 atm.[3106] Most of the challenges presented by very high pressures as described in this Section can be avoided by conservatively restricting nanomedical storage vessels to a maximum operating pressure of ~1000 atm.

10.3.4 Vessel Leakage and Flammability

Drexler[10] estimates that valve, gasket or seal mechanisms with opposing faces at an equilibrium separation of 0.3 nm should experience a negligible fluid leakage rate at elevated pressures for all atoms or molecules except helium. In the case of helium at 300 K, the estimated leakage rate of ~10^{-15} atoms/nm-sec through a seal opposing a ~10^{-5} atm head pressure (~10^{20} atoms/m^3) rises to ~10^{-7} atoms/nm-sec at a ~1000 atm head pressure (~10^{28} atoms/m^3)[10]. Thus at 1000 atm, the mean waiting time for a seal of length 100 nm to pass a single He atom is ~10^5 sec (~1 day), which is an extremely slow leakage rate given that a 1 micron^3 pressure vessel at 1000 atm contains ~10^{10} helium atoms (Table 10.2). Positive ions such as Li^+ and Be^{++} have smaller radii than helium atoms and thus could in theory pass more easily than helium through a seal, but these ions will rarely be found in large numbers outside a solvating liquid environment.[10]

Gases might also leak out by diffusion through pressure vessel walls. Hydrogen has the highest coefficient of diffusion of all the gases (Table 3.3). H_2 readily diffuses through porous substances such as clay, rubber, and even quartz and silica at elevated temperatures. Gases may diffuse through conventional metals, which have numerous defects, dislocations and grain boundaries, and through silicate glasses, which have open irregular structures that permit substantial diffusion of helium.[10] Hydrogen also dissolves in and diffuses through the metals of the nickel, palladium and platinum groups. For example, Pd may dissolve ~900 volumes of H_2 at 293 K and 1 atm, and diffusion through a palladium thimble

Table 10.3. Biological and Biochemical Effects of High Pressure[585,3106,3112,3401]

Biological Material	Pressure (atm)	Results of Compression to Very High Pressures
Cell Division:		
Eggs (*Arbacia*)	100-400	Progressive reversible solation of gelated cortical cytoplasm
Eggs (annelid, echinoderm, vertebrate)	100-500	Cleavage-inhibiting pressure, increases with temperature (5-30°C)
Eggs, misc. marine	200-400	Reversible inhibition of cleavage
Eggs (*Urechis*)	300-400	Reversible solation of spindles and asters; chromosome movement stopped
Eggs (*Arabacia*)	400	Reversible regression of cleavage furrows and cortical plasmagel solation
Eggs (*Ascaria*)	800	Exceptionally resistant to pressure; division not inhibited
Cell Physiology:		
Amoeba population growth	136-340	Severely depressed; reversible after >1 day at top pressure
Ciliary movement	200-400	Reversible increase in beat frequency with rise in pressure
Contraction of pigment cells (fish)	200-400	Contraction phase reversibly inhibited; totally inhibited at higher pressures
Protoplasmic streaming (*Elodea*)	200-400	Solation of cytoplasm; streaming slowed, stopped at 400 atm; reversible
Protoplasmic streaming (*Pelomyxa*)	200-400	Solation of plasmagel; streaming stopped
Amoeboid movement (*A. proteus*)	200-500	Reversible plasmagel solation; pseudopodia collapsed; movement stopped
Heart rate (cultured tissue, frog)	300	Retardation at lower temperatures; acceleration at higher temperatures
Cells/Tissues:		
Erythrocytes	500-3000	Rounded
Carcinoma (Brown-Pearce)	1000	Resistant
Chick heart (embryonic tissue)	1000-1850	Reduction of subsequent growth in culture
Sarcoma transplants (rat)	1800	Inactivated
Carcinoma (Brown-Pearce)	1800	Transplantability destroyed
Erythrocytes	5000	Disintegrated
Bacteria/Fungi:		
Staphylococci and colon bacteria	3000	Unaffected
Bacillus anthracis	3000	Partial loss of virulence; death of vegetative cells
Streptococci	3000	Killed or retarded in growth
E. coli	3800	Inactivated after 10-minute exposure
Yeast cells	4000-6000	Death, preceded by cytoplasmic flocculation or coagulation
Bacteria (various species)	5000	Vegetative cells killed
Bacterial spores	12,000	Killed
Viruses:		
Rous sarcoma, Shope papilloma	1800	Tumors delayed
Staphylococci bacteriophage	2000	Inactivated
Yellow fever (monkey)	3000	Slightly attenuated
Herpes (rabbit)	3000	Inactivated
Tobacco necrosis	3000-5000	Inactivated
Rabies (rabbit)	4000	Attenuated
Papilloma Sarcoma filtrate	4000	No tumors
Avian pest (fowl plague)	4000	Inactivated, but retained antigenicity
Foot and mouth disease	4000	Inactivated
Vaccimia (rabbit)	4500	Inactivated
Rabies (rabbit)	5000	Inactivated
Bacteriophage (*B. megatherium*)	7000	Inactivated
Bacteriophage (*B. subtilis, B. typhosa*)	7000	Inactivated
Encephalomyelitis (rabbit)	7000	Inactivated
Tobacco mosaic virus	7500	Inactivated; coagulated
Antigens/Antibodies:		
Tuberculin, Cobra venom	13,500	Not destroyed; lethality unchanged
Equine tetanus antitoxin	13,500	Gelated; partially inactivated
Diphtheria toxin	13,500	Partially destroyed
Tetanus toxin	13,500	Greatly attenuated or inactivated
Diphtheria toxin	17,600	Mostly destroyed
Enzymes:		
Ribonucleode polymerase	6000	Reversible diminution in activity
Pepsin, Rennin	6000-7600	Inactivated or largely inactivated
Chymotrypsinogen, Trypsin	7600	Partially inactivated
Amylase, Lipase, Sucrase, Lactase	8000-15,000	Some completely, others partially inactivated
Proteins:		
Gelatin	2000	Gelation accelerated
Gelatin gel	3000	Water squeezed out
Equine serum globulin	3000-13,000	Gelated
Soy protein	4000	Completely coagulated
Egg albumin	5000	Slight stiffening
Egg albumin	7000	Completely coagulated
Egg albumin	7500	Denatured and coagulated; SH groups exposed
Carboxyhemoglobin	9000	Coagulated
Insulin	10,000	Coagulated, but not physiologically inactivated

is often used in the laboratory to purify hydrogen gas. H_2 diffusion through bulk metals has been widely studied.[2056,2057]

However, diffusion leakage through defect-free pressure vessel walls comprised of diamond, graphene, or corundum should be negligible. "It is difficult to see how a molecule can pass through these materials without undergoing a reactive transformation." [10] The energy required to move atomic hydrogen from free space into a minimum-energy site in diamond is thermally prohibitive ($\gtrsim$800 zJ),[2055] and the required energy is even higher for molecular hydrogen. Room temperature gases at ~1300 atm[1169] and argon gas at ~600 atm[2034] have been stably trapped inside carbon nanotubes, and confirmed by computer simulations,[3212-3215] and helium atoms at energies up to ~5 eV (~800 zJ) cannot penetrate a graphene sheet. Ruby (corundum) is commonly used in diamond anvil experiments in which hydrogen is compressed to pressures $>10^6$ atm with no apparent leakage.[2043] Thus it appears that essentially leakproof pressure vessel walls can be constructed, although no computational studies of diamond/sapphire interfaces had been performed by 1998 [D.W. Brenner, personal communication, 1999]. Double-walled structures with an intervening space containing either getter materials or a pumped vacuum may be used, if necessary, for added safety.[10]

Microscopic pressure vessels comprised of diamond and filled with compressed hydrogen or oxygen are potentially flammable, even explosive. However, the chemical energy contained within a volume scales as $\sim L^3$ while the dissipation of that energy during an explosive event (e.g., pressure, heat, light) occurs across a surface which scales as $\sim L^2$, hence energy dissipation per unit area (and thus the relative impact of an explosion on the local environment) scales as $\sim L^{-1}$ which implies declining severity at smaller device sizes (Chapter 17). For example, a liter of nitroglycerine produces a blast intensity of $\sim 10^8$ J/m^2, while a spherical 1 micron^3 of nitroglycerine gives only $\sim 10^3$ J/m^2 upon decomposition.

Heat from operating valves is small and is rapidly conducted away in a diamondoid structure. Corundum employed at all structure/oxidant interfaces virtually eliminates device combustibility. Even for bulk diamond in contact with pure oxygen gas at 1000 atm, the time required to etch a single layer of carbon atoms of thickness ~0.17 nm at 310 K may be crudely estimated from Eqn. 9.55 as $\sim 10^{11}$ years; at 400 K, the atomic-layer etch time is still ~400 years. Further discussion of possible nanodevice combustibility is deferred to Chapter 17.

10.3.5 Vacuum Pumping and Storage

It will frequently be necessary to establish and maintain vacuum conditions inside nanorobots. Vacuum-enclosing shells were briefly considered in Section 9.5.3.3 and were found incapable of providing sufficient buoyant lift in normal air due to buckling instabilities. However, nanoscale pressure hulls capable of retaining vacuum may be surprisingly thin-walled. In the simplest case, consider a circular cylindrical diamondoid tube of inside radius r_{tube}, wall thickness h_{tube}, Young's modulus $E = 1.05 \times 10^{12}$ N/m^2 and Poisson's ratio $c_{Poisson} \sim 0.1$.[10] When the relative external pressure on the hull is so large that the cylinder becomes neutrally unstable, a small deformation into an elliptical cylinder is possible. The critical pressure of buckling is given by:[361]

$$p_{crit} = \frac{E\, h_{tube}^3}{4\, r_{tube}^3 (1 - c_{Poisson}^2)} \qquad \text{\{Eqn. 10.20\}}$$

Taking r_{tube} = 500 nm and $p_{crit} \lesssim 1$ atm for a vacuum vessel surrounded by normal atmospheric pressure, a hull thickness of $h_{tube} \gtrsim 3.7$ nm will not buckle. Such a hull has a mass ~60 times greater than the mass of the displaced air.

How fast can the vacuum be established? Consider a cubical vessel of volume $V_{box} = L_{box}^3$ = 1 micron^3 containing gas at molecular number density n_{gas}, which is to be evacuated. Molecular sorting rotors (Section 3.4.2) are embedded in the six walls, with each rotor mechanism of area A_{rotor} = 100 nm^2 having at least one binding site of area $A_{receptor}$ = 0.1 nm^2 always exposed to the box interior. There are $N_{rotor} = (6\, L_{box}^2 / A_{rotor})$ = 60,000 sorting rotors in the box walls. Gas molecules of thermal velocity $v_{thermal}$ (Eqn. 3.3) nearest the walls travel one mean free path λ_{gas} (Eqn. 9.23) and impact a rotor mechanism. On average, after $A_{rotor}/A_{receptor}$ impacts a binding site is hit; after $n_{encounter}$ = 10 independent hits, the molecule is finally captured by the receptor. Thus the time required for a receptor to capture a gas molecule is $t_{bind} \sim n_{encounter}\, \lambda_{gas}\, A_{rotor} / v_{thermal}\, A_{receptor}$ and the time required to evacuate the box is approximately:

$$t_{vac} \sim \frac{n_{gas}\, V_{box}\, t_{bind}}{N_{rotor}} = \frac{n_{gas}\, n_{encounter}\, \lambda_{gas}\, L_{box}\, A_{rotor}^2}{6\, v_{thermal}\, A_{receptor}} \qquad \text{\{Eqn. 10.21\}}$$

At 1 atm and 310 K, $n_{gas} = 2.4 \times 10^{25}$ molecules/m^3 (Table 10.2) and λ_{gas} = 200 nm; for pressures <0.2 atm, $\lambda_{gas} \sim L_{box}$ in the ballistic regime. Taking $\lambda_{gas} \sim 1$ micron and $v_{thermal}$ = 490 m/sec for O_2 at 310 K gives $t_{bind} \sim 20$ microsec and the box is evacuated in $t_{vac} \sim 10$ millisec. Note that for microscale vessels at atmospheric pressure, t_{vac} scales as $\sim L_{box}^2$.

Tank wall material sublimates into the vacuum, the solid establishing equilibrium with its vapor at a temperature-dependent vapor pressure. However, this process produces negligible effluent at moderate temperatures for likely nanorobot building materials. A volumetric number density of one wall-material atom per micron^3 of vacuum, representing a minimum detectable contamination in a ~1 micron^3 box, equals a contaminant partial pressure of 4×10^{-8} atm. To reach this vapor pressure, carbon must be heated to 2480 K, aluminum to 1040 K (liquid), silver and corundum (e.g., ruby, sapphire) to 800 K, and even zinc (a soft, low melting point, metal) to 500 K.[763] At 310 K, the vapor pressure of tank-wall carbon is only $\sim 10^{-116}$ atm, aluminum $\sim 10^{-39}$ atm, corundum $\sim 10^{-19}$ atm, and zinc $\sim 10^{-16}$ atm. Many organic materials evaporate or sublimate more readily. At a vapor pressure of 0.001 atm, ethanol (C_2H_5OH) vaporizes at or above 241.9 K, vs. 253 K for water-ice, 259.2 K for octane (C_8H_{18}), 313.1 K for phenol (C_6H_5OH), but 426.8 K for palmitic acid ($CH_3(CH_2)_{14}COOH$), a typical fatty acid.[763] A water-ice surface exposed to hard vacuum sublimates at the rate of 6.5 nm/day at 134 K, 1.4 microns/day at 152 K, and 1.2 mm/day at 183 K.[2320]

10.3.6 Buoyancy Control and Nanapheresis

Another design issue that may arise when operating in an aqueous medium is buoyancy, which can readily be controlled by loading or unloading ballast. At the extremes, a diamondoid sphere of radius 500 nm and wall thickness 5 nm may range in density from ~100 kg/m^3 if filled with vacuum to ~3000 kg/m^3 if densely packed with diamondoid machinery. Placed in blood plasma, these spheres would rise at ~0.5 micron/sec or fall at ~1 micron/sec, respectively, relative to the local gravity field, according to Stokes' Law for Sedimentation (Eqn. 3.10), taking ρ_{plasma} = 1025 kg/m^3 and plasma absolute viscosity as $\eta_{plasma} = 1.1 \times 10^{-3}$ kg/m-sec at 310 K. This range of speeds lies near the low end of cytonatation velocities (0.1-10 microns/sec; Section 9.4.6) and well below the maximum sanguinatation velocity (~10,000 microns/sec; Section 9.4.2.6), which suggests that buoyancy control is unlikely to play a significant role during routine in vivo nanorobot locomotion. By comparison, the small difference in density between individual red blood cells (1100 kg/m^3) and blood plasma at 310 K causes them to settle out of suspension at a slightly faster 1-3 microns/sec depending on hematocrit (the volumetric percentage of blood occupied by red cells, typically ~46% in humans; Section 9.4.1.2) and degree of RBC aggregation. Free-floating natural erythrocytes appear unhandicapped by their faster settling rate, so active ballast management for free-floating artificial nanorobots is probably unnecessary in normal operations.

However, once a therapeutic purpose is completed it may be desirable to extract artificial devices from circulation. Active ballast control may be extremely useful during nanorobot exfusion from the blood, particularly in the case of simpler devices which are incapable of removing themselves from the body (Chapter 16). Blood to be cleared may be passed from the patient to a specialized centrifugation apparatus analogous to an apheresis circuit such as a cytapheresis or plasmapheresis system. In nanapheresis, acoustic transmitters command passing nanorobots to establish neutral buoyancy. No other solid blood component can maintain exact neutral buoyancy, hence those other components precipitate outward during the gentle centrifugation and are drawn off and added back to filtered plasma on the other side of the apparatus. Meanwhile, after a period of centrifugation, the plasma, containing mostly suspended nanorobots but few other solids, is drawn off through a simple filter, removing the devices as residue. Plasma filtrate is then recombined with centrifuged solid components and returned undamaged to the patient's body.

10.4 Cytocide and Virucide

The objective of nanomedical treatment is often cell repair or replacement (Chapter 21). However, it will frequently be necessary for medical nanorobots to destroy foreign viruses and pathogenic bacteria, protozoa, or metazoan parasites. It may also become necessary to eliminate native human tissue cells that have grown too numerous in a local region, cells that have adopted or developed major pathological, teratological or other undesirable patterns, or which have been too severely traumatized to permit efficient repair.

There are at least two classes of nanomedical cytocidal instrumentalities that may be employed to rid the human body of unwanted cells. The first may be termed the biochemical approach (Section 10.4.1), including methods which may take up to hours or days to proceed to completion with acceptable reliability. Biochemical methods can require relatively modest technological sophistication to implement—an important consideration in the early years of nanomedical device development. The second method may be termed the mechanical approach (Section 10.4.2), which may require only seconds or minutes to proceed to completion with very high reliability, but which involves more sophisticated nanomechanisms that might only be available in a mature nanomedical technology environment.

10.4.1 Biochemical Cytocide and Virucide

Biochemical cytocide involves the killing of pathogenic cells using biochemical, cytochemical, or other means which cause the cell to die a "natural," though perhaps highly accelerated, death. Any agent or set of conditions that stresses the metabolism or normal response mechanisms of a cell may trigger the process of apoptosis, or programmed cell death, but the level of stress is crucial.[2060]

At high stress levels, including sharp pH changes or high toxin levels (Section 10.4.1.4), or high agitation rates,[2061] cells may die instantly by necrosis,[2291,2292] largely because they have no time to respond to the stimulus. In necrotic cytocide, neighboring cells are showered with cellular debris as the necrotic cell swells and lyses, an event likely to cause wider injury and a process to be avoided in nanomedical situations wherever possible.

At intermediate levels of cell stress, the cell is injured but not killed, and so has time to activate its own suicide program.[2060] The contents of the dying cell are retained within sealed vesicles until removed through phagocytosis, thus the cell dies in a controlled and tissue-friendly way.

At low levels of environmental stress, cells can, for example, switch on the production of heat shock proteins which helps them to survive until the stress is removed,[2060] largely by accelerating the refolding of proteins which have been damaged by heat and some other insults. Similarly, UV radiation activates a DNA damage response, cell starvation activates the proteasome protein-recycling response, and glucocorticoids might activate responses to eliminate all non-essential functions.

Of course, once a certain stress threshold is passed and survival is deemed impossible, death by apoptosis ensues. Nanomedical bio-cytocidal instrumentalities should seek to dispose of cells by apoptotic methods (Section 10.4.1.1), or by functionally equivalent techniques such as phagocytic flagging (Section 10.4.1.2) or cell division arrest (Section 10.4.1.3).

10.4.1.1 Apoptosis

It is believed that all nucleated (eukaryotic) cells of all multicellular life on Earth incorporate an evolutionarily conserved self-destruct mechanism called programmed cell death, cell suicide, or simply apoptosis. Scattered reports on cell death have appeared in the literature (and were initially disbelieved) for more than a century, but advances in cytochemistry in the 1980s and early 1990s stimulated an explosion of interest in apoptosis, with ~2500 papers published during 1989-1994[2062] and ~20,000 publications during 1994-1998.[2065]

Exactly what is apoptosis? Programmed cell death is the outcome of a programmed intracellular cascade of genetically determined steps. During apoptosis, the eukaryotic cell disassembles its DNA and breaks up its contents into membrane-wrapped packets which can then be cleared away without causing inflammation. Animals use apoptosis to eliminate extraneous, virus-infected, or otherwise dangerous cells.[2075] Apoptosis plays a central role both in development and in homeostasis of metazoans. Cells die by apoptosis in the developing embryo during morphogenesis or synaptogenesis, and in the adult animal during tissue turnover in the skin or gut or at the end of an immune response. Tight coupling of cell death and cell multiplication ensures in some tissues a constant, controlled flux of fresh cells which are crucial to the preservation and optimal functioning of the adult organism.[2065] Such tissues include those which are environmentally exposed, inside or outside, primarily epithelial tissue and severely insulted liver tissue, plus cells involved in reproductive function.

Apoptosis requires specialized machinery. The central component of this machinery is an irreversible proteolytic system involving a family of protein-chopping enzymes now called "caspases" from "cysteine-containing aspartate-specific proteases" (aka ICE or Interleukin-1β-Converting Enzyme). Caspases are expressed as 30-50 kD proenzymes with an NH_2-terminal domain, a large ~20 kD subunit, and a small ~10 kD subunit.[2068] These enzymes participate in a cascade that is triggered in response to proapoptotic signals and culminates in cleavage of a set of proteins, ultimately resulting in an orderly disassembly of the cell.[2068]

Such complex proteolytic systems involve a combination of regulatory proteases, cofactors, feedbacks, and thresholds that converge to control the activity of an effector protease, which in turn carries out the function of the whole process.[2071] These systems keep the effector protease inactive but are able to rapidly activate large amounts of it in response to minute quantities of an appropriate inducer.[2068] Survival signals from the cell's environment and internal cellular integrity sensors normally hold a cell's apoptotic machinery in check.

Four kinds of events can trigger a suicidal cascade in a eukaryote.[2069] First, if a cell loses its normal contact with its surroundings or sustains irreparable internal damage, then that cell initiates apoptosis. Second, a cell that simultaneously receives conflicting signals driving or attenuating its division cycle also undertakes apoptosis.[2074] Third, the immune system can actively direct individual cells to self-destruct, an event called "instructive" apoptosis.[2076-2078] Fourth, perhaps a majority of all apoptosis occurs during gestation and development, probably in response to external signal molecules or to a lack of sufficient levels of molecular signal gradients involved in biostructural development regulation.

Death receptors[2069]—cell surface receptors that transmit apoptosis signals initiated by specific death ligands—play a central role in instructive apoptosis. Death receptors can activate death caspases within seconds of ligand binding, causing the apoptotic demise of the cell within hours.[2069] Death receptors belong to the tumor necrosis factor (TNF) receptor gene superfamily. (TNF is produced mainly by activated macrophages and T cells in response to an infection.[2079]) The death receptors contain a homologous cytoplasmic sequence termed the "death domain."[2080,2081] Death domains enable death receptors to engage the cell's apoptotic machinery, and mediate functions that are distinct from or even counteract apoptosis.[2069] In 1998, the best characterized death receptors were CD95 (aka Fas[2066] or Apo1) and CD120a (aka TNFR1, Tumor Necrosis Factor Receptor 1, or p55), but others were known including avian CAR1, Death Receptor 3 (DR3; aka Apo3, WSL-1, TRAMP, LARD), DR4, and DR5 (aka Apo2, TRAIL-R2, TRICK-2, KILLER).[2069]

When a caspase cascade is triggered, the first task is to inactivate proteins that protect living cells from apoptosis.[2068] This accomplished, caspases next begin the direct disassembly of cell structure. One example is the destruction of the nuclear lamina (Section 8.5.4.3), the rigid structure underlying the nuclear membrane that is involved in chromatin organization. Lamina is formed by head-to-tail polymers of intermediate filament proteins called lamins (Section 8.5.3.11). During apoptosis, lamins are cleaved at a single site by caspases, causing the lamina to collapse, contributing to chromatin condensation.[2082,2083]

Caspases also reorganize cell structures indirectly by cleaving several proteins involved in cytoskeletal regulation, including gelsolin,[2084] focal adhesion kinase (FAK),[2085] and p21-activated kinase 2 (PAK2).[2086] Cleavage of these proteins results in deregulation of their activity.[2068] Dissociation of regulatory and effector domains is another hallmark of caspase function. For example, they inactivate or deregulate proteins involved in DNA repair (such as DNA-PK_{cs}), mRNA splicing (such as U1-70K), and DNA replication (such as replication factor C).[2087,2088]

In 1998, 13 mammalian caspases—named caspase-1 to caspase-13—were known.[2067,2068] Caspases cut their substrate proteins at tetrapeptide sites with high specificity and with characteristic motifs.[2089] For example, caspase-3 recognizes DEVD sequences and, during apoptosis, cleaves and inactivates several significant cellular proteins in the cytosol, nucleus and cytoskeleton.[2090-2092] Caspases participate in apoptosis "in a manner reminiscent of a well-planned and executed military operation;"[2068] they:

1. cut off contacts with surrounding cells, so the cell balls up;
2. import calcium,[2075] strongly complexing phosphates;
3. shut down DNA replication and repair, interrupt splicing, disrupt the nuclear structure and condense the chromatin;
4. induce the loss of microvilli;[2093]
5. destroy cellular DNA by mobilizing apoptotic-unique nucleases[2091,2092] to cleave the double helix at regular intervals in an orderly fashion, first into large fragments of 300-750 kilobases, followed by fragments of ~50 kilobases, then finally oligonucleosomal length DNA fragments of ~200 base pairs[2062-2064] (giving a characteristic pattern by gel electrophoresis called "DNA laddering"[2094]);
6. reorganize the cytoskeleton;
7. induce the cell to display signals in the outer membrane that mark the cell for phagocytosis by neighboring cells or macrophages;[2095]
8. induce downstream blocking of mitochondrial respiratory chain components, resulting in mitochondrial malfunction (via transcriptional induction of redox related genes, the formation of reactive oxygen species, and finally the oxidative degradation of mitochondrial components[2072,2073] including dissipation of mitochondrial inner transmembrane potential and the release of cytochrome c through the outer mitochondrial membrane[2162]), with lysosomal involvement;[2293]
9. initiate membrane blebbing (surface blisters) and cell shrinkage; and finally
10. disassemble the cell into multiple membrane-enclosed vesicles called apoptotic bodies without destroying organelle membranes.

In vivo, this process culminates with the engulfment and phagocytization of apoptotic bodies by other cells, preventing inflammation and other complications that would result from a release of intracellular contents. These changes occur in a predictable, reproducible sequence and can be completed within 30-60 minutes.[2068]

Many different ways of activating the apoptotic process are known or suspected.[2096] Simple detachment of tissue cells from all contacts with the ECM[1553] or manipulation of cell shape[718] have been shown to induce apoptosis experimentally. Apoptosis can also be indirectly initiated by a variety of cellular insults that can damage DNA, including ultraviolet- and x-irradiation, hypoxia, and chemotherapeutic neoplastic drugs (e.g., alkylating agents such as nitrogen mustard derivatives, antimetabolites and plant alkaloids) which inflict cell damage that is then translated via the Bcl-2 protein family[2097] through several poorly understood steps into activation of caspase-9.[2068] Proteins that sense DNA damage and help trigger apoptosis also affect the cell cycle—stopping cell division so the damage can be repaired or making the decision (with the activation of tumor suppressor p53) that the damage has gone too far and the cell must die.[2074] B and T lymphocytes undergo apoptosis in response to anti-IgM antibodies and dexamethasone (a glucocorticoid), respectively.[2098] The cell death program can also be activated by inhibition of proteasome function,[2099] or by infection with a wide variety of viruses.[2118]

Caspases can be directly activated by two distinct intracellular mechanisms that interact with the death receptor complexes. First, because all caspases have similar cleavage specificity, the simplest way to activate a procaspase is to expose it to a previously activated caspase molecule. This caspase cascade is used extensively by cells for the activation of the downstream effector caspases: caspase-3, caspase-6, and caspase-7.[2068]

A second method for activating caspases is the use of apoptotic chaperones, which herd together inactive proenzymes to increase their local concentration and ease them into conformations that promote their activation. This "induced proximity" was first observed in caspase-8 (aka FLICE, MACH), an initiator caspase that acts downstream of the CD95 death receptor.[2069] Upon trimeric ligand binding, CD95 receptor molecules are aggregated into a membrane-bound complex. This signaling complex recruits, via the receptor-bound adaptor protein FADD (Fas-Associated protein with Death Domain; aka Mort-1[2100]), several procaspase-8 molecules, resulting in a high local concentration of procaspase-8. Under these conditions, the low protease activity inherent to procaspases is sufficient to drive intermolecular proteolytic activation of the receptor-associated procaspase-8 molecules.[2068] Proximity-induced activation may also be used to activate caspase-9.[2101] Procaspase-9 activation involves a complex with the cofactor Apaf-1 through the CARD (Caspase Recruitment Domain), but activation of caspase-9 also requires cytochrome c (released into the cytosol by mitochondria[2073]) and deoxyadenosine triphosphate, indicating that caspase activation may require multiple cofactors.

Death receptors can be expressed on both normal and cancerous cells in the human body, so the challenge for conventional drug-based therapy is to find some way to activate death receptors selectively on cancer cells only.[2068,2069] For medical nanorobots, such selectivity should be simple and routine using multiple chemosensors (Section 4.2), a benefit that is characteristic of most nanorobot-based therapeutics. If caspase cascade amplification is sufficient to permit single-site activation of the cascade, then in theory an extracellular nanorobot intending cytocide could press onto the outer surface of a target cell an appropriate ligand display tool. This tool might contain suitably exposed trimeric CD95L (aka FasL[2066]) ligand (binds to the extracellular domains of three CD95 death receptors), TNF or lymphotoxin α (binds to CD120a), Apo3L ligand aka TWEAK (binds to DR3), or Apo2L ligand aka TRAIL (binds to DR4 and DR5).[2069,2070] The binding event would then activate a single death receptor complex, potentially triggering the entire irreversible cytocidal cascade. If necessary, multiple display tools could be employed. This technique avoids the storage requirement for bulky consumables onboard the medical nanorobot.

As another approach, molecular sorting rotors could be used to selectively extract from the cytoplasm specific crucial molecular species of IAPs (Inhibitors of Apoptosis[2102]) that can hold the apoptotic process in check. Examples include survivin, commonly found in human cancer cells [2058], the transcription factor NF-κB [2142], and Akt, which delivers a survival signal that inhibits the apoptosis induced by growth factor withdrawal in neurons, fibroblasts, and lymphoid cells [2103]. Conversely, decoy receptors (DcRs) that compete with DR4 and DR5 for binding to Apo2L[2104-2106] could be saturated with intrinsically harmless but precisely engineered intracellular "chaff" ligands. With IAPs removed or DcRs blockaded, apoptosis may be free to proceed.

Multicellular plants and animals,[2074,2075] human fibroblasts,[2107] and even slime molds show various forms of apoptotic cell death. Other processes of programmed cell death that may be distinct from either apoptosis or necrosis have been reported in lung fibroblasts,[2108] the caspase-free yeast *Saccharomyces cerevisiae*,[2097] and other cells.[2109-2112] In 1998, apoptosis had not yet been reported in any bacterial species, nor was it expected because conventional evolutionary logic does not favor the emergence of cell suicide in the case of obligate single-celled organisms.[2073,2074] Autolysis has been reported in bacteria in specialized circumstances,[2113-2115,3704] including addiction modules[3318-3320] and phage exclusion,[3320-3322] though these cases, while sometimes termed "programmed cell death,"[2113,3705-3709] all involve a (messy) necrotic cytocidal outcome or self-damage short of cell death, rather than a (clean) apoptotic cytocidal outcome. Apoptosis also is not found in viruses.

It is theoretically possible that an artificial plasmid could be designed that embodies an engineered self-contained apoptotic system capable of unleashing a non-necrotic cell death process inside a prokaryote. A single such proapoptotic artificial plasmid (similar to artificial chromosomes,[2432] already in use by 1998) could then be injected into the target bacterium, giving the desired clean cytocidal outcome. R. Bradbury suggests the following useful components:

1. a restriction enzyme to fragment the bacterial DNA, that is effective against that specific bacteria;
2. DNase to digest the DNA entirely, if not already present;
3. RNase to digest the RNA entirely; if not already present;
4. one or more proteases such as trypsin, to digest internal proteins; and
5. one or more lipases to digest any lipids.

A lambda-phage container holding an engineered vector with only the first two capabilities could still effectively "neuter" the bacterium. Such a biorobot could be relatively harmless to eukaryotic cells, assuming its enzymes lacked nuclear localization targeting sequences; cleanup could be effectively handled by the immune system. Bradbury also suggests another approach—using a DNA replication blocker such as antisense DNA polymerase, in combination with a mitotic promoter, to induce the cell to attempt to divide forever while lacking any DNA in the progeny. Essential biomolecules would eventually be diluted to such a low level that growth would radically slow and perhaps even death would result. This second approach might yield a faster decline in bacterial activity than simple neutering, due to the diversion of bacterial resources in an attempt to regain intracellular molecular balances. In either approach (as with mechanical approaches; Section 10.4.2), it is necessary to avoid fragmenting the bacterium in a way which allows release of superantigen molecules such as LPS which could cause an immune system overreaction, leading to toxic shock.

10.4.1.2 Phagocytic Flagging

Target cells may be flagged with biochemical substances capable of triggering a reaction by the body's natural defensive or scavenging systems. For example, novel recognition molecules are expressed on the surface of apoptotic cells. In the case of T lymphocytes, one such molecule is phosphatidylserine, a lipid that is normally restricted to the inner side of the plasma membrane (Section 8.5.3.2) but, after the induction of apoptosis, appears on the outside.[2117] Cells bearing this novel surface molecule are then capable of being recognized and removed by phagocytic cells. Seeding the outer wall of a target cell with phosphatidylserine or other molecules with similar action could activate phagocytic behavior by macrophages which had mistakenly identified the target cell as apoptotic. Loading the target cell membrane surface with B7 costimulator molecules permits T-cell recognition, allowing an immunologic response[1556] via what has been termed the immunological synapse.[2930,2931,3453] This tagging operation should work well against cells which have an apoptotic response which can be triggered by cytotoxic T cells—such as human cancer cells and cysts.

Aside from false apoptosis, removal or destruction of cell-surface MHC class I receptors might convince the immune system that the target cell was not native (e.g., "self"), making the target susceptible to attack by natural killer NK lymphocytes.[2130] (Macrophages should be able to engulf a eukaryotic cell, as they are large enough to absorb protozoa.[531]) Alternatively, the target cell's surface would be salted with a non-self antigen-containing MHC Class I molecule, or with self MHC Class I molecules with foreign peptide attached (particularly one for which the patient has already been vaccinated), with the expectation that the cell would mistakenly be identified as foreign, and thus be phagocytosed. Other methods of engineering chemical reactivity by cell surface remodeling[2127] are readily envisioned, such as flagging with lymphokines or oligohistidine-tagged fusion proteins.[2274] But the best approach may be to seed the target cell with antigens for which the patient already has a high titer of circulating antibodies, which then will bind to the antigens and attract the immune system. Antibodies occur in higher concentrations than B/T cells and therefore would presumably trigger a faster response. As a general rule, cells with bad MHC molecules are targeted for apoptosis, while cells with antibodies attached are targeted for phagocytosis.

10.4.1.3 Cell Division Arrest

In some circumstances it may be useful to eliminate a target cell's ability to replicate via cell division, thus rendering it incapable of further growth. For example, many prokaryotic microorganisms respond to starvation by entering growth-free stationary phases[3710-3712] or by forming dormant spores;[2116] nanorobot manipulation of cellular biochemical states possibly could induce stasis in bacteria, though spore formation should be avoided. The Bcl-2 protein family can modulate eukaryotic cell cycle progression; under suboptimal growth conditions, Bcl-2 promotes exit into quiescence and retards reentry into cycle.[2097] A gene fragment on human chromosome 4, called mortality factor 4 (morf4), when added to cancerous (eukaryotic) cells in vitro converts proliferating cells into senescent cells that have stopped dividing.[2128] Ceramide, the breakdown product of sphingomyelins, can drive a eukaryotic cell either to cycle arrest, or to apoptosis, depending upon other conditions within the cell,[2062] and p16 and p27 are known eukaryotic cell cycle inhibitors.[2059] Cytochalasins, which are derived from molds, interfere with the division of cytoplasm, inhibit cell movement, and can cause extrusion of the interphase nucleus.[3718]

Eukaryotic mitosis has four distinct stages (prophase, metaphase, anaphase, telophase) and interphase (between divisions), each associated with distinct biochemical and cytoarchitectural states. Thus it is not surprising that specific biochemical agents have been found that are capable of selectively halting, accelerating, or altering mitosis at any of the many stages; a few examples are in Table 10.4. Cell cycle control is discussed further in Chapter 12.

Many chemotherapeutic agents function by eliminating the cell's ability to undergo mitosis. For example, plicamycin (mithramycin) is believed to form a complex with DNA which inhibits DNA-dependent or DNA-directed cellular RNA and enzymatic RNA synthesis—48-hour lethal dose in human HeLa cancer cells is ~1 part/million by weight or ~10^5 molecules/cell.[2119] Eukaryotic cell cycling may be interrupted by inhibitors of RNA polymerases I, II, and III (which produce RNAs specific to different functions in the cell), or by inhibitors of uracil synthesis or other steps in general RNA base production which would interfere with RNA synthesis overall. Vincristine applied at similar dosage (e.g., ~10^{-18} kg/cell) inhibits microtubule formation in the mitotic spindle, resulting in an arrest of dividing cells at the metaphase stage.[2119] Large doses lead to necrotic cytocide; a smaller dose may trigger apoptosis.

A theoretical enzyme capable of selectively lysing DNA telomeres in the nucleus would prevent cell replication, but would probably trigger apoptosis due to massive chromatin damage because TTAGGG sequences are scattered throughout the chromosome.[383] Telomere length affects eukaryotic cell division only indirectly, either because short telomeres activate a DNA damage response that blocks cell division or because genes near the ends of chromosomes which are essential for cell division may be lost or misregulated. Telomerolytic enzymes would be useless against common bacteria (e.g., *E. coli*) and viruses (e.g., SV40) which have circular DNA chromosomes, or viruses such as the adenoviruses that cause bronchitis and pneumonia which have linear DNA locked with a terminal protein—but no telomeres in either case.[383] Alternatively, R. Bradbury suggests the introduction of DNA (or RNA) for antisense sequences, for genes essential for cell cycle progression or for proteases which cut or digest these same proteins, as for instance an antisense gene for cyclin or one of the many cdc genes—if phosphorylation or dephosphorylation of the cyclins or cdc genes is occurring, the introduction of a phosphatase or kinase could easily block the entire cell division process.

10.4.1.4 Chemical Poisoning

There are a great many (often inefficient) ways to poison a cell or virion simply by releasing chemical agents near, on, or within it, but if done incautiously this approach may lead to necrotic, rather than apoptotic, cell death. Here are a few examples of some well-known classes of biocidal agents, many of which may be inappropriate for use by in vivo medical nanorobots:

1. *Phagosomal Biochemicals* — Both types of phagocytic cells (e.g., neutrophils and macrophages) contain specialized organelles that fuse with newly formed phagocytic vesicles (phagosomes), exposing phagocytosed microorganisms to a barrage of enzymatically produced, highly reactive molecules of superoxide (O_2^-) and hypochlorite (HOCl, the active ingredient in bleach), called the "oxidative burst" that punctures cell walls, and to a concentrated mixture of lysosomal hydrolases.[531] Human neutrophils also use antimicrobial peptides such as the serprocidins (e.g., proteinase 3, azurocidin, and cathepsin G, a metabolic inhibitor) against fungi and bacteria.[2132]

2. *Cytolytic Enzymes* — Lysozymes, present in tears, nasal mucus and sputum, destroy the cell walls of many airborne Gram-positive bacteria by catalyzing the hydrolysis of β-1,4 linkages between N-acetyl muramic acid and N-acetyl glucosamine (peptidoglycan degradation) in bacterial cell walls[996]—causing the bacteria to burst open, spilling their contents. Lysozyme, zymolase, glucalase and lyticase are frequently used with bacteria and yeast cells to dissolve coats, capsules, or capsids. Granulysin released by cytolytic T lymphocytes directly kills intracellular *Mycobacterium tuberculosis* by altering the membrane integrity of the bacillus.[2165]

Table 10.4. Organic Compounds Affecting Eukaryotic Cell Division at Specific Phases of Mitosis [585,760]

Organic Substance	Cell/Tissue	Specific Mitotic Cycle Effect
Prophase:		
Aureomycin	Onion root	Membrane dissolution delayed
Glutathione	*Amoeba proteus*	Prophase accelerated
Nitrophenols	Sea urchin egg	Prophase blocked
Purines	*Arbacia* egg	Reversion to interphase
Trypan blue	Rabbit fibroblast	Spindle formation slowed
Urethan	Rabbit fibroblast	Prophase accelerated
Metaphase:		
Alcohol, DDT	Onion root	Nucleolus neoformation
Benzene	Mammal marrow	Mitotic poison—blocking agent
Colchicine (0.00001 M)	*Chortophaga* neuroblast	Mitotic poison—blocking agent
Diphenyl, Indoleacetic acid	Wheat root	Spindle rotation
Epinephrine (0.01%)	Chicken fibroblast	Mitotic poison—blocking agent
Methyl naphthohydroquinone diacetate	Onion root	Multipolar spindle induced
Morphine (0.0001 M)	Chick epithelium	Mitotic poison—blocking agent
Nicotine (0.0001 M)	Rabbit fibroblast	Mitotic poison—blocking agent
Phenylurethan	Sea urchin egg	Monopolar mitotic figure induced
Podophyllotoxin (10^{-7} M)	*Echinarachnius* egg	Mitotic poison—blocking agent
Streptomycin	Onion root	Reversion to interphase
Sulfanilamide	*Paracentrotus* egg	Mitotic poison—blocking agent
Testosterone, Estrone	Rabbit fibroblast	Abnormal chromosome orientation
Anaphase:		
Caffeine	Onion root	Incomplete chromosome separation
Ryanodine	Sand dollar egg	Incomplete chromosome separation
Trypaflavine	Rabbit fibroblast	Incomplete chromosome separation
Telophase:		
Aureomycin	Chicken fibroblast	Cytoplasmic division suppressed
Carbamate	Sea urchin egg	Cytoplasmic division suppressed
Chloroacetophenone	Chicken osteoblast	Nuclear reconstruction retarded
Nicotine	Pea seedling	Spindle remnant persists
Rotenone	Sea urchin egg	Cytoplasmic division suppressed
Thiourea	Chicken fibroblast	Nuclear reconstruction retarded
Interphase:		
Acridines	Chicken fibroblast	Initiation of prophase inhibited
Azaguanine	Mouse tumors	Initiation of prophase inhibited
Dyes	Frog sperm	Initiation of prophase inhibited
Hypoxanthine	Chicken osteoblast	Interphase shortened
Glucose	Mouse epidermis	Division stimulated
Nitrogen mustard	Rat corneal epithelium	Initiation of prophase inhibited
Trypaflavine	Onion root	Destruction of interphase nucleus
Multiple Phases:		
Aminobenzoate, Coumarin	Onion root	Chromosome breaks
Cysteine	Protozoan	Chromosome reduction induced
Dyes, N-butyl gallate	Onion root	Chromosome adhesion
Ethoxycaffeine	Onion root	Chromosome rearrangements
Mustards	Spiderwort mother cell	Centromere misdivision
Urea	Fruit fly salivary gland	Chromosome dispersion/despiralization

3. *Organelle Poisons* — Certain drugs and other substances, if injected into the cytoplasm, may interfere with the workings of specific organelles or cell subsystems. For example, the fungal metabolite drug brefeldin A disrupts the Golgi, causing it to collapse back into the ER.[2347,3441,3442] Colchicine,[939] vinblastine and vincristine[936] bind to tubulin, causing microtubules to disassemble, griseofulvin (an antifungal agent) prevents microtubule assembly,[996] and taxol inhibits microtubule depolymerization, while cytochalasin B inhibits the polymerization of cytoskeletal actin microfilaments.[939] Adociasulfate-2 is a kinesin motor inhibitor.[2390] High concentrations of vitamin A weaken the lysosomal membrane. Proteasome inhibitors such as vinyl sulphone[2911] are usually lethal for the eukaryotic cell. Oligomycin inhibits the F_0F_1-adenosine triphosphatase (ATPase) proton pump of the mitochondrial inner membrane, and cyanide poisons mitochondrial oxidative phosphorylation.[2073] Nitric oxide (conc. ~60 nanomolar) inhibits mitochondrial respiration,[2918,2919] specifically by inhibiting cytochrome oxidase by outcompeting oxygen at the oxygen binding site;[2920] NO also prevents viral replication by inactivating a crucial protease.[2969] Antipsychotic drugs such as chlorpromazine, thioridazine, and fluphenazine are potent peroxisome inhibitors.[3067] The nucleus of an oocyte is ejected from a cell treated with etoposide and cycloheximide (chemical enucleation),[3719,3720] microtubule poisons such as colchicine, colcemid and vinblastine cause extrusion of nuclei,[3721] and EDDF is involved in erythroid

Table 10.5. Inhibitors of Protein or RNA Synthesis[531,2119,2180]

Biochemical Inhibitor	Specific Molecular Inhibitory Effect
Acting Only on Prokaryotes:*	
Chloramphenicol	Blocks the peptidyl transferase reaction on ribosomes (MIC ~8-14 μg/cm^3)
Erythromycin	Blocks the translocation reaction on ribosomes (MIC ~1-2 μg/cm^3)
Rifamycin	Blocks initiation of RNA chains by binding to RNA polymerase (prevents RNA synthesis) (MIC ~1 μg/cm^3)
Streptomycin	Prevents the transition from the initiation complex to chain-elongating ribosome and causes miscoding (MIC ~2-10 μg/cm^3; 800-4000 molecules/cm^3)
Tetracycline	Blocks binding of aminoacyl-tRNA to A-site of ribosome (MIC ~2-4 μg/cm^3)
Acting on Prokaryotes and Eukaryotes:	
Actinomycin D	Binds to DNA and blocks the movement of RNA polymerase (prevents RNA synthesis)
Pyromycin	Causes the premature release of nascent polypeptide chains by its addition to growing end chain
Acting Only on Eukaryotes:	
α-Amanitin	Blocks mRNA synthesis by binding preferentially to RNA polymerase II
Anisomycin	Blocks the peptidyl transferase reaction on ribosomes
Cycloheximide	Blocks the translocation reaction on ribosomes

* The ribosomes of eukaryotic mitochondria (and chloroplasts) often resemble those of prokaryotes in their sensitivity to inhibitors
MIC = Minimum Inhibitory Concentration

cell denucleation;[3722] there is at least one report of nuclear extrusion in lymphocytes.[3723] Selected organelle populations (e.g., mitochondria) could also be ubiquinitized.

4. *Antibiotics* — Drugs that prevent bacteria from multiplying (bacteriostatic) or that kill bacteria outright (bactericidal) are called antibiotics; in 1998, ~100 such drugs were FDA approved for U.S. use. Major groups include the aminoglycosides, cephalosporins, macrolides, penicillins, polypeptides, quinolones, sulfonamides, and tetracyclines;[2119] many are naturally-derived products. All act by interfering with protein synthesis, cell wall construction, or DNA replication. For example, gonococci isolated in the preantibiotic (pre-resistance) era were inhibited by benzylpenicillin ($C_{16}H_{18}N_2O_4S$, MW = 334 daltons) in concentrations as low as ~7 molecules/micron^3;[2135] in the 1990s, some highly resistant bacterial isolates required ~1000-fold higher concentrations. Vancomycin derivatives are active against Gram-positive bacteria at 10-100 molecules/micron^3.[3227] Antibiotics are available with protein/RNA synthesis inhibition activity against either prokaryotic or eukaryotic cells (Table 10.5).

5. *Bactericidal Phages* — Bacteriophages (viruses that infect bacteria) are capable of penetrating bacterial membranes and delivering foreign DNA which can take control of all metabolic processes; in ~700 sec after penetration, the first complete virion particles begin appearing in the cytoplasm; at ~1500 sec, the bacterium bursts, necrotically liberating ~200 virus particles. These viruses are often very host-specific. Still, it may be possible to design artificial general-purpose bacteriophages that are capable of disabling or destroying all bacterial DNA, or are capable of replicating more bacteriophage particles to which only the targeted bacterial cells are susceptible (see also Section 10.4.1.1). Engineered macrophages or artificial neutrophils might also be deployed to achieve targeted bacterial digestion. Reaching intracellular parasites such as mycoplasmas and rickettsias might be one of the biggest challenges for such biorobots.

6. *Bacteriocins* — Probably 99% of all bacteria generate at least one bacteriocin, small proteins that function as narrow-spectrum antibiotics that may have developed as poisons to kill competing bacteria.[2121,3724-2726] In 1998, ~80 bacteriocins were known, most of them produced by fermentation microbes, including nisin which is used in 45 countries including the U.S. as a commercial food additive for pasteurized egg products. Bacteriocins seem to work by entering the outer membrane of a susceptible bacterium, congregating in groups, and forming pores that allow the unregulated outflow of essential ions. The target bacterium begins breaking down ATP in a vain attempt to produce enough new protons to recharge the membrane, a futile cycle that quickly results in exhaustion of bacterial ATP. Bacteriocins are most effective in acid and least effective in salty environments. Bacteriocins of Gram-positive bacteria such as *Listeria* and *Clostridium botulinum* are ineffective against Gram-negative bacteria such as *E. coli* and *Salmonella* which have a protective double-walled outer membrane. In 1998, several Gram-negative bacteriocins were known. One example is the colicins, water-soluble cytotoxins secreted by and active against *E. coli*, that form voltage-sensitive ion channels in the bacterial inner membrane that kill the cell by selectively siphoning out key cell nutrients[2150,2151] and inhibit protein synthesis.[3190]

7. *Porins and Superporins* — C. Sublette notes that it should be possible to design and insert into a cell a piece of RNA or DNA designed to produce high levels of a "superporin" protein that migrates to the cell membrane, then self-assembles into a large

channel in the membrane several orders of magnitude larger than an ion channel, allowing a large, lethal ion influx or outflux. For example, normal cytosolic Ca^{++} concentration ranges from 60-3000 ions/micron^3;[531] blood plasma concentration is ~10^6 ions/micron^3 (Appendix B), but even cytosolic concentrations as low as ~10^4 ions/micron^3 may be toxic (Section 7.4.5.3). (See also Section 10.4.2.1.) Possible templates for such subunits are the bacterial porins,[2133] minus their charged amino acid residues lining the inner passage which produce nonspecific aqueous diffusion channels across the outermost LPS bacterial membrane, and granulysin,[2165] perforin and members of the amoebapore family[2166,2167] which are thought to damage target cell membranes by inducing formation of microscopic pores.

8. *Ionophores* — Ionophores are small hydrophobic molecules that dissolve in lipid bilayers, thus increasing ion permeability of cell membranes.[531] Most are synthesized by microorganisms, presumably as biological weapons to weaken their competitors. There two classes of ionophores—(highly temperature-sensitive) mobile ion carriers, and channel formers—both operating by shielding the charge of the transported ion so that it can penetrate the hydrophobic interior of the lipid bilayer.[531] (Ionophores permit net movement only down their electrochemical gradients, since no energy sources are available.) Valinomycin, a ring-shaped polymer that increases K^+ permeability of membranes, is an example of a mobile ion carrier. Another example is A23187, which acts as an ion-exchange shuttle, carrying two H^+ out of the cell for every divalent cation (such as Ca^{++} and Mg^{++}) carried in. Transport rates through a mobile carrier are ~2×10^4 ions/sec.[531] A channel-forming ionophore is gramicidin ($C_{148}H_{210}N_{30}O_{26}$, MW = 2822 daltons), a 15-residue linear polypeptide with all hydrophobic side chains. Two such molecules come together in the bilayer to form a transmembrane channel that selectively allows monovalent cations (most readily H^+, K^+ somewhat less readily, Na^+ still less readily) to flow down their electrochemical gradients at a rate of ~2×10^7 cations/sec.[531] The dimers are unstable, constantly forming and dissociating, with average channel open time ~1 sec.[531] Gramicidin is produced by *Bacillus brevis* and is active against Gram-positive cocci and bacilli. A 5 microgram dose kills, in vitro, 10^9 *pneumococci* or group A *streptococci* in 2 hours at 30°C,[751] giving a fatal dose of ~1000 molecules/micron^3 assuming a ~1 cm^3 culture volume in this experiment.

9. *Channel Blockers* — Cells import and export nutrients, ions, water, and wastes through variety of gated channels (Section 3.3.3) and transporter molecular pumps (Section 3.4.1). If these channels or pumps are permanently blocked, cytocide may ensue. Blocking the ~10^3/micron^2 cellular transport systems embedded in a typical eukaryotic cellular membrane requires ~10^3/micron^2 "steric plugs" that permanently jam in the throat of critical ion channels or pumps. For example, the acetylcholine receptor channel narrows to ~0.65 nm at its waist, so an efficiently designed steric plug could have a volume of ~1 nm^3 or ~10^{-21} gm. (By comparison, a single molecule of 318 dalton tetrodotoxin, or puffer fish toxin, has mass ~0.53×10^{-21} gm; apparently, saxitoxin (shellfish toxin, human IV lethal dose ~68 micrograms) and palytoxin are slightly smaller, whereas botulin toxin is a fairly high-mass zinc metalloprotease protein that inhibits release of acetylcholine at the neuromuscular junction.) Plugging all channels in the surface of a (2 micron)^3 bacterial cell (~10 micron^2) or a (20 micron)^3 tissue cell (~1000 micron^2) requires ~10^4 or ~10^6 plugs, respectively, a nanorobot-dispensed ~10^{-5} micron^3 or ~10^{-3} micron^3 dosage of plugs at the target cell, assuming ~100% efficiency. A mean migration distance per plug of ~1 micron gives a Brownian diffusion time of ~1 millisec, so a micron-scale nanorobot with 0.1 micron^3 of onboard storage carries sufficient plug-doses to incapacitate ~10^4 bacterial cells in ~10 sec or ~10^2 tissue cells in ~0.1 sec, ignoring cell-to-cell travel time. Assuming a mean interbacterial separation of ~100 microns (an implied pathogen number density of ~10^6/cm^3 in the tissue) and a maximum nanodevice intercellular travel speed of ~100 micron/sec (Section 9.4.4.2), a nanorobot spends ~1 sec in transit between neighboring bacterial cells, ~0.002 sec in cell-type recognition (Section 8.5.2.2), and ~0.001 sec killing the bacterium once the nanorobot arrives.

10. *Channel Destroyers* — Some smaller number (perhaps as few as one) of an enzyme-like toxin molecule capable of destroying either the steric or the electrochemical specificity of each ion channel by permanently altering the physical structure of that channel. For example, in the case of the acetylcholine receptor channel, an artificial enzyme possibly could be designed to alter the ring of negatively charged residues at the entrance to the receptor, allowing anions to enter the pore and ultimately depolarizing the cell. Enzymes typically operate at ~1000 Hz and the diffusion time across ~20 nm between adjacent ion channels is ~0.5 microsec, so a single enzyme neutralizes all 10^4 channels in a bacterial cell in ~10 sec and ~1000 artificial enzymatic molecules would incapacitate the cell in ~10 millisec.

11. *Complement* — The complement system is a group of ~20 soluble serum-resident proteins acting in combination with specific cytolysin antibodies in amplification cascades along two separate pathways to initiate reactions to foreign antigens (Chapter 15). Complement proteins are enzymes that act on foreign cells by punching holes in their membranes by inserting lipid-soluble pores (the membrane attack complex, C5-C9), causing necrotic osmotic cytolysis. In addition, complement plus antibody designates cells to be engulfed by phagocytic cells.

12. *Animal Venoms and Toxins* — The bufagin from the *Bufo arenarum* toad of Argentina (arenobufagin, $C_{25}H_{34}O_6$, MW = 430 daltons) has a mean lethal toxicity of 92 microgram/kg,[585] the equivalent of ~10^6 bufagin molecules per 20-micron tissue cell (~100 molecules/micron^3). Most reptile venoms have lethal toxicities of 200-1000 micrograms per kg of body weight.[585] Sea anemone granulitoxin (4958 daltons) has a mouse LD50 of 400 micrograms/kg (~49 molecules/micron^3);[3458] another sea anemone protein extract has a mouse LD50 of 40 micrograms/kg.[3459] Maurotoxin, a 34-residue scorpion venom (*Scorpio maurus*), has an intracerebroventricular mouse LD50 of ~80 nanograms,[3460] or ~0.4 molecules/micron^3. The LD50 value to mice of *Vespa luctuosa* hornet venom is 1600 micrograms/kg, the most lethal known wasp venom.[3457] Venoms and toxins may not be cytocidal against all cell types—some act by interfering with nerve transmission or by paralyzing muscles.

13. *Plant and Microbial Toxins* — A variety of microbes manufacture neurotoxins or neurolysins that destroy the ability of human ganglion and cortical neural cells to function.[3461] A single molecule of some neurotoxins can incapacitate a cell, though the rate of action tends to be very slow. For example, botulin toxin is the second deadliest poison known (e.g., median human lethality ~5-50 nanograms/kg).[3462] The toxin acts at cholinergic nerve terminals to prevent acetylcholine release, a permanent physiologic denervation that causes muscle paralysis, often resulting in death by respiratory system failure in 2-8 days. Recovery requires the sprouting of new axon twigs and the formation of new myoneural junctions,[2122] which is

why the recovery time for sub-lethal botulin poisoning is very long, several months to a year or more. Botulin is a ~150,000-dalton protein comprised of 1285 amino acid,[2171,3462] which implies a lethal concentration of 0.2-2 molecules per 20-micron tissue cell. Other toxins are capable of killing a cell outright with just a few molecules, such as ricin: mouse and rabbit IV LD50 ~400-4000 nanograms/kg or 30-300 molecules per 20-micron tissue cell,[3463-3465] possibly due to lower specificity in binding to cells and other pharmacokinetic effects). Ricin is a phytotoxic enzymatic 65,750-dalton protein[3466] taken from the seeds of the castor oil plant that cleaves the ribosome complexes, shutting down protein manufacturing. This damage is normally irreversible, killing the organism in ~4 days at minimum dosage and ~8 hours at the highest dosages, so a reasonable lower limit for killing an individual cell is probably ~10^4 sec.

14. *Antifungals* — Antifungal agents such as amphotericin B or fluconazole are fungistatic. For example, the growth of *Candida* and many other fungi is inhibited by amphotericin B ($C_{47}H_{73}NO_{17}$, MW = 924 daltons) concentrations of 30-1000 micrograms/cm^3 in vitro.[2119] A number of natural antimicrobial peptides are induced in epithelial cells at sites of inflammation; for example, lingual antimicrobial peptide (LAP), a member of the b-defensin class, has been isolated from bovine tongue and exhibits both antifungal (e.g., *Candida*) and antibacterial (e.g., *E. coli*) activity[2129] at concentrations as low as ~16 microgram/cm^3. In 1998, antifungals were known to target membrane function, metabolism, cell wall synthesis, protein and ergosterol synthesis, nuclear division, and nucleic acid synthesis and function.[2131] In those circumstances where fungal cells have learned to communicate to effect mating or cooperative behaviors, such communication may be disrupted to their detriment. If the genetic pathways involved in these behaviors include primitive forms of apoptosis, these could be exploited as well.

15. *Antivirals* — Antiviral drugs may work by interfering with viral replication processes, including cell attachment, cell uptake, viral coat removal, and viral DNA or RNA replication by the cell, and are primarily virostatic. For example, acyclovir (MW = 225 daltons) in concentrations of 0.01-13.5 micrograms/cm^3 inhibits by 50% the growth of *herpes simplex* virus in vitro.[2119] In 1998, ~20 antivirals were FDA approved for U.S. use. Antibodies may also serve a virostatic function. For example, the rabies-like vesicular stomatitis virus (VSV) rhabdovirus has a surface envelope with ~1200 identical glycoprotein molecules that form a regular and densely ordered pattern of spike tips.[2139] Rhabdoviruses are neutralized if they cannot dock with their cellular receptors; this requires a minimum of 200-500 IgG antibody molecules bound per virion.[2140] Another challenge for medical nanorobots will be the retroviruses, which insert their genome into the host DNA, thus will require chromosomal editing or replacement (Chapter 20) to remove.

16. *Iodine-Based Microbicides (iodophors)* — In tincture of iodine, all of the iodine is in the free form at ~10% by weight and is readily available for instantaneous reaction and killing of bacteria in a few seconds.[360] The minimum lethal iodine dose for a 2-micron bacterium (assuming complete exhaustion of a 0.1-micron perimicrobial iodophor layer) may be of order ~0.001 picomoles or ~0.1 picogram iodine (~10^8 molecules), which is ~3% of the mass of a bacterium—not terribly efficient, as expected for a broad-spectrum agent. Iodoacetate inactivates most cytoplasmic enzymes and blocks anaerobic metabolism, or glycolysis (fluoride is also a glycolytic poison).[758] Yodoxin (64% organically bound iodine) is amoebicidal.[2119] Thebroadest-known spectrum iodine-based microbicide is betadine (povidone-iodine) 10% solution,[2119] employed in surgical scrub and many other general antiseptic uses. Betadine kills most bacteria in 15-30 sec, and also kills viruses, fungi, yeasts and protozoa; no bacterial resistance has been reported.

17. *Silver* — Silver foil has been used in bacteriocidal wound dressings,[2158] and silver metal has been employed for centuries to purify water. In 1998, there were more than 600 silver-based antibacterial products available in Japan including silver-impregnated pens, floppy disks, calculators, ATM machines, floor tiles, plastic food wrap, socks, shirts, public park sand, and toilet seats.[2126] At least 20 companies in the U.S. offer silver/copper-based systems for swimming pool sanitation and commercial air conditioning cooling towers. The passive dissociation of silver from the metallic phase into a wound with antimicrobial results[2123] and the antiseptic action of silver compounds[2124] are well known. A quantitative study of the metal's antimicrobial properties in vitro found that a silver ion concentration of ~25 micrograms/cm^3 (~10^5 ions/$micron^3$) reduced the number density of *Staphylococcus* and *Pseudomonas* bacterial cells and *Candida* fungal cells by a factor of 1-10 million relative to microbial control aliquots.[2125]

18. *Platinum, Bismuth, and Other Elements* — Platinum-based cisplatin ($PtCl_2H_6N_2$, MW = 300 daltons) is an antitumor and bacteriostatic drug that interacts with tumor-cell DNA by forming a Pt-GG intrastrand crosslink as the critical lesion leading to cytotoxicity.[2136] A typical ~100 mg whole-body dose[2119] produces a mean concentration of ~2000 molecules/$micron^3$. Colloidal bismuth subcitrate exerts a direct antimicrobial effect against *H. pylori* (gastritis) at concentrations of 4-25 micrograms/cm^3 (6000-38,000 molecules/$micron^3$), with treated bacteria showing deposits of bismuth on their surface and internally.[2137] Mercury (chronic toxicity in blood ~600 atoms/$micron^3$), lead (toxic in blood at ~2900 atoms/$micron^3$), and arsenic (toxic in blood at ~4800 atoms/$micron^3$) are general poisons (Appendix B) that have been used for medicinal purposes. Indirect poisons such as iron and copper catalyze free-radical formation. Interestingly, bacterial growth is constrained by essential nutrients, and human immune cells scavenge and sequester iron when faced with a bacterial threat; nanorobotic "deferritization" of a bacterium could kill the organism.

19. *Sugar* — Medical lore has it that sugar, and especially honey[2158,2334] (Section 1.2.1.2), makes an excellent antibacterial disinfectant. Blood glucose levels of 0.01-0.07 M in untreated diabetics cause tissue and cellular damage, at least partly via osmotic cellular dehydration (honey and NaCl salt have a similar effect), and protein glycosylation and Maillard reaction (Section 6.3.4.4) which diminish enzyme function; ~15% cytosolic glucose concentrations are toxic.

20. *Hydrogen-Bond and Disulfide-Bond Breaking Agents* — At high concentrations, guanidine hydrochloride disintegrates the bacterial S-layer coat which is held together only by noncovalent forces.[525] Local heating (hyperthermia; Section 10.4.2.3) also disrupts H-bonds. Other agents are available to break disulfide bonds, disrupting many classes of proteins.

21. *Nuclear Alkalination and Other Nucleic Disruption* — RNA breaks down in slightly alkaline environments (e.g., pH $\gtrsim$ 8.0;[1591] to increase the pH of a typical cellular nucleus from 7.2 to 8.0 would require the injection of ~10^5 OH^- ions. RNA is also broken down by RNases; DNA is broken down by DNases, or by using restriction enzymes.

22. *Tissue Liquefaction* — A 2-hour exposure to 0.25% trypsin enzyme solution digests and breaks up the extracellular matrix,[570] turning an organized tissue into a jumble of individual cells.

23. *Other Poisons* — Cyanide causes cells to swell and lyse at concentrations of ~0.002 M (~1 x 10^6 ions/micron^3).[758] Assuming serum reference levels, ethanol should be cytotoxic at ~0.09 M (~50 x 10^6 molecules/micron^3).[1604] Ethylene oxide (C_2H_4O) gas is a microbial sterilant and fumigant; chlorine dioxide (chlorite ion) is an antimicrobial sometimes found in mouthwashes. Chlorine and bromine are used as antibacterials in swimming pools and hot tubs. Most chemotherapy agents also kill cells. Common lab detergents such as Triton X-100 and tributyl phosphate readily destroy bacteria and the majority of viruses sheathed in protein envelopes.[3252]

Nanorobot biocidal delivery vehicles can be used to present the chemical agent on a cell-by-cell basis. For example, a major whole-body infection involving ~10^{12} pathogens (e.g., ~10^6 bacteria/cm^3) with each microbe capable of being killed by ~10^5 precisely-delivered biocidal molecules each of molecular weight ~1000 daltons requires a minimum treatment dose of ~10^{17} biocidal molecules or ~0.1 mm^3 of material. This dose could be carried and dispensed in ~1000 sec by one billion ~1 micron^3 "pharmacyte" nanorobots (total volume of therapeutic nanorobots ~0.001 cm^3) assuming each nanorobot has ~0.1 micron^3 of internal storage for the biocidal agent and assuming as before a mean ~1 sec cell-to-cell transit time.

10.4.2 Mechanical Cytocide and Virucide

Mechanical cytocide involves the killing of biological cells or the destruction of virion particles partially or primarily by mechanical, rather than by strictly biochemical, means. Such means may include disablement, partial physical destruction of critical components, or even complete disassembly of the target cell, bacterium, or viral particle.

10.4.2.1 Transmembrane Siphonation and Ionic Disequilibration

A number of rigid diamondoid tubes with membrane-locking lipophilic external coatings and hydrophilic end rings may be inserted through the target cell membrane, preventing self-sealing of the breach (Section 9.4.5.6) and resulting in drainage of internal fluids and disruption of ionic balances, probably triggering apoptosis in eukaryotic cells after ~10^4 sec.

What magnitude of siphonage may be required to achieve cell lethality? A cytosolic concentration of $\gtrsim 10^4$ Ca^{++} ions/micron^3 is believed to be toxic (Section 7.4.5.3) and there are ~10^6 Ca^{++} ions/micron^3 present in blood plasma (Appendix B) or interstitial fluid, so replacing ~1% of cell volume (e.g., ~0.1 micron^3 for a bacterium, ~80 micron^3 for a tissue cell) with raw extracellular fluid should be lethal. Macrophages can ingest up to ~25% of their volume per hour,[996] or ~10% of their volume in ~1000 sec, but the paramecium, a large protozoan, excretes through its contractive vacuole a quantity of water equal to 100% of its volume in 15-20 minutes,[758] or ~10% in ~100 sec.

Conservatively assuming that a ~10% target cell volume influx of extracellular fluid in 1 sec will cause serious cell damage or induce apoptosis, the size and number of passive transmembrane siphons may be crudely estimated. Mean interstitial fluid pressure is ~0.0002 atm (Section 8.4.2). Thus from Eqn. 9.25, the total volume flow rate through water-bearing transmembrane tubes of length l_{tube} = 300 nm with pressure differential Δp ~ 0.0002 atm is $\dot{V}_{HP}$ = 4 x 10^{10} N_{tube} r_{tube}^4 (m^3/sec) for N_{tube} tubes each of inside radius r_{tube}. To exchange 10% of the volume of a ~2 micron diameter bacterium by siphonation with extracellular fluids in ~1 sec ($\dot{V}_{HP}$ ~ 1 micron^3/sec) requires one tube of radius r_{tube} ~ 70 nm. For a ~20 micron tissue cell, $\dot{V}_{HP}$ ~ 1000 micron^3/sec which requires one tube of radius r_{tube} ~ 400 nm or 15 tubes of radius r_{tube} ~ 200 nm.

It is important that passive siphon tubes should be employed in minimum numbers and never be left unattended. They should be tethered to the nanorobot during use and retrieved after each use. Left unattended in the plasma membrane of a dying cell, diamondoid siphon tubes could become serious systemic poisons. For example, macrophages phagocytosing apoptotic siphon-studded cells would be unable to digest the tubes and might themselves become accidentally siphoned, or might pass the lethal tubes to other innocent cells in the liver, spleen, or elsewhere.

Death by siphonation may be hastened if the nanorobot actively pumps extracellular fluids (or cations directly) into the target cytosol. A pressure differential of ~1 atm applied along a simple bulk fluid injector with r_{tube} = 50 nm and l_{tube} = 300 nm gives $\dot{V}_{HP}$ ~ 1000 micron^3/sec and draws ~76 pW of power during the transfer.

Artificial cytocidal cation inflows must surpass the net natural cellular outpumping rates of those cations. For instance, there are at least five known Ca^{++} concentration-maintenance mechanisms in eukaryotic cells:

1. a cell membrane ATP-driven Ca^{++} exporting pump,
2. a cell membrane $3Na^+/Ca^{++}$ exchange transporter,
3. a Ca^{++} transporter into the mitochondria,
4. a $2Na^+/Ca^{++}$ exchange transporter into the mitochondria, and
5. an ATP-driven Ca^{++} pump into the endoplasmic reticulum.[3146]

What is the maximum natural outflow rate? Normal cytosolic Ca^{++} concentration ranges from 60 ions/micron^3 for a resting cell up to 3000 ions/micron^3 for an activated cell (Section 7.4.5.3). From Eqn. 3.4, the diffusion-limited ion current through the surface of a 20-micron tissue cell is ~2 x 10^7 ions/sec for a resting cell and ~10^9 ions/sec for an activated cell. Taking the extracellular concentration of ~10^6 Ca^{++} ions/micron^3 gives a minimum lethal extracellular bulk fluid inflow rate of ~1000 micron^3/sec to defeat the maximum possible pumping rate of an activated 20-micron cell, consistent with the previous estimate. (The diffusion limit for a nanorobot pumping Ca^{++} from the interstitial fluid into the cytosol is ~3 x 10^{11} ions/sec, far higher than the maximum rate at which the cell can outpump.) Similarly, Na^+/K^+ transporters present in the eukaryotic membrane at 1000/micron^2, each device transporting 500 ions/sec (Section 3.4.1), move at most ~10^9 ions/sec through the ~2400 micron^2 (Table 8-17) plasma membrane. The Na^+/K^+ pumping cost is ~16 zJ/ion (Section 3.4.1); devoting the entire 30 pW power budget of the typical cell (Section 6.5.1) to such pumping would allow the transport of ~2 x 10^9 cations. Thus, >1000 molecular sorting rotors each operating at ~10^6 ions/rotor-sec (Section 3.4.2)—the entire array transporting >10^9 ion/sec—should allow an attacking nanorobot to defeat a cell's attempts to resist ionic disequilibration.

10.4.2.2 Mechanical Cytoskeletolysis and Monkeywrenching

It may have occurred to the alert reader that a simple way to kill a eukaryotic cell might be to cytopenetrate and then motor around inside the cytoplasm at higher-than-recommended velocities, thus indiscriminately bursting lysosomes, shredding the thin membranes of the endoplasmic reticulum (ER) and the Golgi, and trashing other delicate cellular structures, depending upon the motility mechanism employed (Section 9.4). Such a course would almost certainly result in an unwanted necrotic cellular lysis.

Rupture of lysosomes (Section 8.5.3.8) should especially be avoided because lysosomal lipases and other corrosive enzymes would be released into the cytosol, possibly provoking some autolysis, local disintegration of the plasma membrane, and inflammation. Peroxisome (Section 8.5.3.9) rupture may produce similar effects, since these organelles catalyze some of the fatty acid breakdown in the cell. Selective destruction of ribosomes (Section 8.5.3.4), the ER (Section 8.5.3.5), the Golgi complex (Section 8.5.3.6), the mitochondria (Section 8.5.3.10), or the nucleus (Section 8.5.4) will more slowly kill the cell but again this may be a nonapoptotic death if the transcription, protein synthesis, or energizing mechanisms necessary to sustain the apoptotic cascade are disabled. Loss of power due to mitochondrial destruction eliminates the cell's ability to maintain long-term membrane recycling; the cell will eventually come apart due to the accumulated damage in the membrane.

However, elements of the cytoskeleton probably can be safely destroyed without disabling apoptosis, while simultaneously severely reducing the chances of post-attack cell survival, particularly in cells that are incapable of further division. Chemical cytoskeletolysis by caspases (Section 10.4.1.1) and various mitotic inhibitors such as the microtubule inhibitor vincristine (Sections 9.4.7.4 and 10.4.1.3) have been described earlier. We can speculate that mechanical cytoskeletolysis may trigger apoptosis in eukaryotic cells because the entire cytoskeletal structure per se does not appear to be a crucial operational component of the apoptotic cascade.

How best to perform the cytoskeletolysis? Microtubules in cyto preferentially absorb light at ~350 nm,[1070] so in theory a sufficiently intense laser source at this frequency could selectively disrupt the microtubule network. However, proteolytic or mechanical chopping should be more energy efficient (especially if used to activate a few of the molecules at the upstream end of the cascade). For example, p56 severs microtubules slowly in an ATP-independent manner;[3147] katanin is a heterodimeric protein that severs and disassembles microtubules in an ATP-dependent manner.[3148] Human elongation factor 1α (EF-1α, ~48 kilodaltons) rapidly severs taxol-stabilized fluorescent microtubules in vitro, and induces rapid fragmentation of cytoplasmic microtubule arrays when microinjected into fibroblasts, at concentrations of $\gtrsim$15 microgram/cm^3 ($\gtrsim$200 molecules/micron^3).[1083] In theory, a pair of fiber cleavage tools modeled after EF-1α operating at ~500 Hz (Section 9.4.6) would lyse ~1000 fibers/sec. If the cytoskeleton of a typical tissue cell has a total of ~10^6 intermediate filament segments (Table 8.17), then 10% of all such filaments can be mechanochemically cleaved by a single tool pair in ~100 sec, ignoring travel time.

The cytoskeleton can also be mechanically cleaved. Individual microfilaments have a tensile tearing strength of ~0.1 nN, microtubules ~1 nN, and intermediate filaments (IFs) ~100 nN. Consider a cutting blade of length 50 nm rotating at ~1 KHz (blade tip speed ~ 0.3 mm/sec). The energy required to cut a single 10-nm thick IF is ~ 0.001 pJ (Section 9.3.5.1); the power required to cut 10% of all cellular IFs in ~100 sec is ~1 pW. The continuous drag power of the freely rotating blade in plasma during the 100-sec cytoskeletolysis program is ~0.1 pW (Eqn. 9.75). A 1-micron^2 cross-section nanorobot traversing the entire 8000 micron^3 volume of a 20-micron tissue cell traces an 8000-micron path, a 100-sec travel time at a mean ~80 microns/sec velocity; continuous nanorobot drag power at this velocity even in a cytoskeleton-rich cytoplasm of viscosity ~10 kg/m-sec (Section 9.4.6) is ~1 pW (Eqn. 9.73).

Another simple technique for mechanical disruption of the cell may informally be termed "monkeywrenching." As examples, active DNA cutters (e.g., restriction enzymes), or in situ manufactured H_2O_2 along with some iron borrowed from local ferritin molecules, could be injected into the eukaryotic nucleus, rapidly generating enough double-strand breaks to activate the fatal DNA damage response. R. Bradbury notes that a nanorobot could seize a single mitochondrion (~0.4% of nuclear volume; Table 8.17), transport it to the nuclear envelope and then forcibly insert it into the nucleus—if there are sufficient oxygen and other small reactant molecules present, the mitochondrion would probably produce enough local free radicals to initiate the DNA-damage (apoptotic) cascade. Methods for synthesizing superoxide, hydrogen peroxide, and hypochlorite from locally available materials are described in Chapter 19. In the case of prokaryotes, medical nanorobots could introduce restriction enzyme molecules that are alien to the target strain of bacterium, followed by some DNase (in case the strain has none). R. Bradbury believes that ribonucleases and peptidases may be unnecessary because some endogenous ribonucleases should always be present and the remaining lipid bag of proteins would not represent much of a threat.

10.4.2.3 Gross Cellular Disruption

A number of crude cytocidal techniques have been proposed which for the most part are inadvisable. For instance, simple lancing or "harpooning" of cells (e.g., Feynman's "stab the paramecium"[355]) would likely be followed by self-sealing or a messy necrosis, depending on the duration and severity of the penetration.* Acoustic shock waves would cause random mechanical damage, ending in necrosis. Bulk pressurization (see Section 10.3.3) can be lethal to biology—high pressure treatment to kill bacteria was first described in 1895 by Royer,[3102] and by Hite and colleagues[3105] in 1899 in connection with the high pressure preservation of milk. Cells are generally inactivated between 2000-5000 atm, bacteria and viruses above 5000 atm, antibodies and enzymes over 10,000-20,000 atm (Table 10.3). Bacterial spores are killed at ~6000 atm and 45°C - 60°C.[3103,3104] A pressure-initiated apoptotic response might be difficult to control because the apoptosis-inducing and necrosis-inducing pressure thresholds are not widely separated and may vary among cell types, physiological states, external conditions, and even among cells of apparently similar characteristics. Bulk pressurization followed by release would almost certainly permanently inactivate viruses (Table 10.3), but could lead to inflammation if large populations of deactivated viruses are set adrift in the tissues.

Some fragmentation of DNA molecules in aqueous solution by ~1 MHz ultrasound irradiation has been reported at intensities as low as ~2000 watts/m^2 for >15-min exposures, but 10-min exposures to 50,000 watts/m^2 completely fragment the DNA, due to shearing forces acting on the large molecules rather than cavitation (which requires higher intensities).[730] Plant cell chromosomal damage occurs at 10^4-10^5 watts/m^2, and red blood cell suspensions suffer increased membrane permeability but no membrane disruption up to 30,000 watts/m^2, although platelets in aqueous suspension may be disrupted by >2000 watts/m^2 at 1 MHz for >5 min.[730]

Local hyperthermia can selectively destroy cancer cells in vivo,[505] presumably with an apoptotic outcome. Temperatures of 42.5°C or higher for 20-30 minutes appear necessary for tumoricidal effects, and several sessions are needed for significant tumor regression.

*Self-sealing of ruptured neurons is inhibited by administering cysteine protease inhibitors or calmodulin inhibitors.[3664]

Focused 1 MHz ultrasound beams produce brain lesions, with in situ spatial-peak intensities at 2 megawatts/m^2 for 10 sec causing purely thermal damage and higher intensities up to 0.2 gigawatts/m^2 for 300 microsec adding a contribution from direct mechanical effect, possibly cavitation.[505] Large numbers of nanorobots in a small tissue volume could produce significant localized or cell-wide heating for extended durations that might be difficult or impossible for individual nanorobots to achieve.

Very high intensity laser light (>10^{11} watts/m^2) can necrotically "optocute" biological cells;[1630,1631] bioparticle optical trapping pioneer A. Ashkin notes that during his experiments, "if the power got too high, the bacteria would just explode."[2145] Threshold laser ablation rates are ~1 nJ/micron^2 for a 248-nm KrF excimer laser photoablating organic material[2146] and 0.5 nJ/micron^2 for ablative etching of corneal tissue at 193 nm (probably as a result of photodecomposition of the peptide bonds).[645] At 193 nm, a single 20-nanosec, 20 nJ/micron^2 (~10^{12} watt/m^2) pulse ablates 2.4 microns of bile duct tissue;[645] hard biomaterials like tooth dentine and dental enamel ablate 0.5-1.9 microns at 248 nm and a fluence of ~10^{13} watts/m^2. Microlasers are an established technology,[497] but such methods produce necrosis and require far too much power to be practical for in vivo cytocide.

However, ultraviolet UVC band photons (190-290 nm) induce cell destruction[645] much more selectively and energy-efficiently. For example, nucleic acids have an optical absorption maximum near ~260 nm[508,997] that is characteristic for each base;[997] the absorption of DNA itself is ~40% less than would be displayed by a mixture of free nucleotides of the same composition, known as the hypochromic effect.[997] The primary mode of UV damage is the formation of thymine dimers in the DNA, which block both transcription and replication until repaired. In sufficient numbers, these defects probably activate the DNA damage response (repair or apoptotic) pathways. At higher-energy shorter wavelengths (e.g., 193 nm), the UV photons don't penetrate the cell far enough to reach the nucleus.[645] Lower-energy longer-wavelength UV photons can still damage DNA by producing oxidizing chromophores and decreasing enzyme synthesis, which has the effect of reducing the repair and regrowth properties of DNA;[645] protein containing the aromatic (chromophoric) amino acids tryptophan and tyrosine have maximum absorption near 275 nm[508,996] and phenylalanine more weakly near 260 nm,[996] and peptide bonds absorb strongly at wavelengths under 240 nm.[508] Thus photons of a precise wavelength can cause very selective damage. Suspensions of *Streptococcus*, *Lactobacilli* and *Actinomyces* bacteria stained with toluidene blue experienced millionfold kill rates after 60-sec exposure to helium-neon laser photons at an intensity of only 5600 watts/m^2.[2147] Viral genetic material is also strongly susceptible to UV damage.[328]

Particulate radiation is another poor choice for inflicting selective damage to individual cells in a controlled manner. It is true that Co^{60} irradiation is used to sterilize sutures,[359] and antitumor radiation treatments have been commonplace in 20th century medicine. However, the range of natural-emission α-rays in protoplasm is >20 microns, raising the likelihood of some collateral damage, and an accelerator capable of generating artificial lower-energy alpha beams would be energetically and geometrically prohibitive in most in vivo nanomedical contexts.

10.4.2.4 Mechanical Virucide

Viruses are acellular bioactive parasites that attack virtually every form of cellular life. Viruses have diameters[2148] ranging from 16-300 nm—for example, poliomyelitis ~18 nm, yellow fever ~25 nm, influenza ~100 nm, herpes simplex and rabies ~125 nm, and psittacosis ~275 nm.[751] Their shape is either pseudospherical with icosahedral symmetry, as in the poliomyelitis virus, or rodlike, as in the tobacco mosaic virus (TMV). Viruses consist of a core of RNA (most plant viruses and animal viruses such as the rhinoviruses, polio and flu viruses, and all retroviruses) or DNA (most bacterial and some animal viruses), but never both. This nuclear material is surrounded by a protein coat called a capsid, a quasi-symmetrical structure assembled from one or only a few protein subunits called capsomeres. A virus surrounded only by capsid is a naked virus; some viruses acquire a lipid membrane envelope from their host cell upon release, and are called enveloped viruses. Attached to the capsid are other protein structures necessary for host infection, especially attachment or docking proteins. The interior capsid volume is usually only slightly larger, and never more than twice as large, as the volume of the enclosed nuclear material.[997] For instance, the adenovirus (one family of viruses that causes the common cold in humans) is an icosahedral particle ~70 nm in diameter (~180,000 nm^3) containing one double-stranded DNA molecule ~11 microns (~35,000 bases or ~10^7 daltons) in length (~15,000 nm^3), giving a composition of approximately 92% protein and 8% DNA by volume. By comparison, the TMV has 5% nucleic acid, the bushy stunt virus 17%, and the tobacco ringspot virus has 40%.[751]

There are at least two methods by which such viruses may be eliminated from the human body, as follows.

10.4.2.4.1 Sequester and Transport (ST)

Nanorobots may extend chemosensory pads (Section 4.2.8) which will selectively and reversibly adhere to the capsid coat of a nonenveloped viral target. For enveloped viruses, the nanorobot must carefully pick over the camouflage lipid membrane to find viral-specific antigens. R. Bradbury suggests that such lipid-coated viruses might also be distinguishable from host cells by measuring their membrane curvature (viruses are much smaller than eukaryotic cells) or local ion concentrations (viruses emit no metabolic effluents).

Once the virus is bound to the pad, the nanorobot packs the whole virus particle into an internal storage cannister. When the cannister is full, the nanorobot ceases operations and either delivers its cargo to a dedicated biodisposal organ or other in vivo facility, or eliminates itself from the body (Chapter 16). A nanorobot with a 1.8 micron^3 cannister can warehouse up to ~10,000 compacted adenovirus particles. With viral infections reaching ~10^{10} particles/cm^3 localized in the upper respiratory mucosal tissues, mean distance between free-floating particles is of order ~5 microns, or ~100 millisec travel time at ~100 micron/sec, probably dominating the exclusive antigenic identification time of ~2 millisec (Section 8.5.2.2). As part of a nanomedical treatment for viral infection[3233] (Chapter 23), a minimum therapeutic dosage of ~10^8 nanorobots/cm^3 can extract and sequester the entire adenovirus population from infected human tissue in ~1000 sec (~17 minutes); larger doses can clear the tissues even faster, and may also assist in the cytoplasmic and nucleoplasmic clearance of viral DNA.

10.4.2.4.2 Digest and Discharge (DD)

After virion acquisition as previously described, the particle is placed in a leakproof transfer chamber. The virus is then pistoned into a morcellation chamber (Section 9.3.5.1) where it is chopped by orthogonally traveling diamondoid blades into ~10 nm pieces, greatly increasing the reactive surface area of the virus material. The morcellate is then pistoned into a reaction chamber. Capsid-specific proteinases and peptidases are introduced, reducing all virus proteins to amino acids, which are removed from solution by molecular sorting rotors (Section 3.4.2) and discharged. Lipases are required for digesting enveloped viruses. Deoxyribonuclease and ribonuclease enzymes are also introduced, reducing viral DNA or RNA to nucleotides which are themselves removed from the solution by a second set of molecular sorting rotors and discharged. The enzymes remaining in solution are pumped back into storage vessels via sorting rotors, and the reaction chamber is ready for the next cycle.

For example, a 70-nm adenovirus particle containing 8% DNA by weight is reduced to 1.7×10^{-16} gm (~10^6 molecules) of amino acids and 1.4×10^{-17} gm (~30,000 molecules) of nucleotides. Natural bloodstream concentrations of all amino acids are typically ~5×10^{-5} gm/cm^3 (~3×10^{11} adenovirus equivalents per cm^3), and ~10^{-6} gm/cm^3 (~7×10^{10} adenovirus equivalents per cm^3) for nucleotides (Appendix B), so the maximum "safe" viral material discharge rate appears nucleotide-limited to ~10^{11} virus particles per cm^3, which is at or above the typical virion particle density in serious infections. Hence, digested-virus material discharges should not significantly augment natural serum concentrations of amino acids or nucleotides.

Energy costs are minimal. Single-virus mincing costs ~0.1 pW of power for a duration of ~8 millisec (Eqn. 9.54). Representative enzyme operating frequencies (turnover numbers) range from 1-2 KHz for lactate dehydrogenase and penicillinase to 15-100 Hz for DNA polymerase and chymotrypsin,[759] giving digestion times on the order of 1-100 millisec when an excess of enzyme is present. Out-rotoring all final-product amino acids costs at most ~ 20 pW for at most ~10 millisec duration using ~100 sorting rotors per each of the 20 essential amino acid types. Pumping a generous ~100 virus-volumes of enzyme-rich solution through a 1-micron length of 60-nm diameter pipe at 1 atm pressure costs 2 pW for ~ 1 millisec duration (Section 9.2.5). Hence virion processing time is of order ~100 millisec and requires at most ~30 pW during processing.

10.4.2.5 Mechanical Bacteriocide

Bacteria are unicellular microorganisms capable of independent metabolism, growth, and replication. Their shapes are generally spherical or ovoid (cocci), cylindrical or rodlike (bacilli), and curved-rod, spiral or comma-like (spirilla). Bacilli may remain associated after cell division and form colonies configured like strings of sausages. Bacteria range in size from 0.2-2 microns in width or diameter, and from 1-10 microns in length for the nonspherical species; the largest known bacterium is *Thiomargarita namibiensis*, with spheroidal diameters from 100-750 microns.[3225] Spherical bacteria as small as 50-500 nm in diameter have been reported,[2149] but it has been theorized that the smallest possible cell size into which the minimum essential molecular machinery can be contained within a membrane is a diameter of ~40-50 nm.[527] Many spherical bacteria are ~1 micron in diameter; an average rod or short spiral cell is ~1 micron wide and 3-5 microns long. Each bacterial cell consists of a mass of protoplasm enclosed within the usual thin lipid bilayer plasma membrane. Most Gram-positive bacteria are surrounded by a thick, mechanically strong but porous peptidoglycan cell wall. Gram-negative bacteria like *E. coli* surround themselves with an additional two-layer coat atop the peptidoglycan layer. This coat has an unsaturated inner lipid layer but a more rigid outer leaflet composed of an unusual lipid, called lipopolysaccharide (LPS), in which fatty acid chains are all saturated and 6-7 chains are covalently linked in a single LPS molecule.[2134]

Bacterial cells have no internal membranous surfaces and no internal organelles, although some functional compartmentalization does exist.[3616] Bacteria possess small internal vacuoles, ribosomes, and granules of stored food, and usually one or more externally-attached flagella (Section 9.4.2.5.2). Some rod-shaped bacteria can form tiny spherical or oval endospores that survive when conditions become inhospitable for metabolism, such as extreme heat (>100°C) or desiccation (for up to 60 years).[1225] As prokaryotes, bacteria have no distinct nucleus. However, a single circular chromosome is organized into one or more compact aggregates, called nucleoids, that may occupy about one-third of cell volume.[997] *E. coli*, a well-studied cylindrical bacterium measuring 0.65 microns wide and 1.7 microns long (cell volume ~ 0.6 micron^3), has one double-stranded DNA chromosome ~1.3 mm (~4.2 megabases or ~10^9 daltons) in length (strand volume ~ 0.002 micron^3), organized in ~40 kilobase loops.[997] Chromosomes spilled from lysed bacteria show ~80% DNA content, suggesting loop stabilization by proteins and at least a primitive membrane-associated cytoskeleton.

Table 10.6 gives the approximate mean composition of a 4 micron^3 bacterium. There are at least three methods for eliminating an unwelcome microbe from the human body, described below. An additional serious problem in bacterial infections is that many microbes release toxins into the bloodstream that can wreak havoc even if all the bacteria are killed. Toxin cleanup (Chapter 19) is a necessary component of any comprehensive antibacterial treatment strategy.

10.4.2.5.1 Desiccate, Sequester and Transport (DST)

After the target bacterium has been identified by chemosensory pads binding, the nanorobot secures itself to the cell exterior. The first objective is to desiccate the bacterium. An efficiently designed molecular sorting rotor for water may require ~30 nm^2/receptor of exposed surface with 600 nm^3/rotor which includes 50% volume overhead for housings and other mechanical elements, and transports ~10^6 molecules/sec at a cost of ~0.01 pW/rotor (Section 3.4.2). Of total bacterial water, ~2/3 is freely diffusible as bulk water and ~1/3 is loosely bound as hydration water (Section 8.5.3.3). Thus to accomplish the desiccation, the nanorobot inserts a 0.3-micron wide, 2-micron long cylindrical water extraction probe into the cell interior. Taking the experimentally measured[3149] failure strength of the wet peptidoglycan wall as ~3×10^6 N/m^2 (Table 9.3), a probe tip configured as a core sampler tool (Section 9.3.2) with an annular cutting edge of thickness W_{edge} = 1 nm (Section 9.3.5.1) can penetrate the bacterial wall by applying a force of ~3 nN perpendicular to the surface; a rotating serrated cutting edge requires even less force. In the alternative, a chemical or enzymatic cutting tool may be employed.[3150-3152]

The extraction probe is tiled with ~66,000 sorting rotors of volume ~0.04 micron^3. Extraction probe volume is ~0.14 micron^3, which leaves ~0.10 micron^3 for probe structure, probe plumbing manifold, pipes and pumps, and probe control mechanisms. All bulk water is extracted from the bacterium in ~1 sec, shrinking the cell by half from ~4 micron^3 to a volume of ~2 micron^3. (Sorting rotors covering ~2 micron^2 remove ~3×10^{10} molecules/sec-micron^2, far outpacing possible backflows which may be crudely estimated from maximum macrophage water-ingestion rates (Section 10.4.2.1), suggesting at most ~10^7 molecules/sec-micron^2 across a ~13 micron^2 bacterial surface.) Engulf formations of metamorphic nanorobots (Section 5.3.4) could be especially useful in this application.

Its volume halved, the bacterium is packed into a nanorobot storage cannister of volume ~2 micron^3 and is delivered to an appropriate dedicated biodisposal organ or other biodisposal facility (Section 10.4.2.4)—one dead bacterium per nanorobot. (A rigid wet hollow peptidoglycan sphere of diameter ~2 microns and thickness ~20 nm can be compacted into a 2-micron wide storage cylinder by a 2-micron piston by applying an Euler buckling force

Table 10.6. Summary of Biochemical Composition and Net Digestion Breakdown Products of a Representative 4 μm³ Bacterium (modified from Becker[313] and Lewin[997])

Cell Component	Cell Mass %	Avg. Molecular Weight (daltons)	Cell Mass (gm)	Number of Molecules
Inorganic:				
Water	70.0%	18	3.0×10^{-12}	1.0×10^{11}
Salts	1.0%	~55	4.3×10^{-14}	4.7×10^{8}
Organic:				
Carbohydrates	3.0%	~180	1.3×10^{-13}	4.3×10^{8}
Amino Acids	0.5%	~100	2.1×10^{-14}	1.3×10^{8}
Nucleotides	0.5%	~308	2.1×10^{-14}	4.2×10^{7}
Large Molecules:				
Proteins	14.5%	~30,000	6.2×10^{-13}	1.2×10^{7}
Lipids	2.0%	~700	8.5×10^{-14}	7.3×10^{7}
Polysaccharides	2.0%	~1000	8.5×10^{-14}	5.1×10^{7}
RNA	6.0%	$\sim 10^{6}$	2.6×10^{-13}	1.5×10^{5}
DNA	0.5%	$\sim 10^{9}$	2.1×10^{-14}	~1
TOTALS:	100.0%	---	4.3×10^{-12}	1.01×10^{11}

Net Digestion Products	Digestion Product # of Molecules	Digestion Product Mass (gm)	Natural Blood Conc. (gm/cm³)	Blood/Bacterium Equivalents (#/cm³)
(Water)	1.0×10^{11}	3.0×10^{-12}	~0.94	3.1×10^{11}
Inorganic Salts	4.7×10^{8}	4.3×10^{-14}	$\sim 7 \times 10^{-3}$	1.6×10^{11}
Fatty Acids	2.0×10^{8}	8.5×10^{-14}	$\sim 4 \times 10^{-3}$	4.7×10^{10}
Simple Sugars	7.1×10^{8}	2.1×10^{-13}	$\sim 2 \times 10^{-3}$	9.4×10^{9}
Amino Acids	3.9×10^{9}	6.4×10^{-13}	$\sim 5 \times 10^{-5}$	7.8×10^{7}
Nucleotides	5.8×10^{8}	3.0×10^{-13}	$\sim 1 \times 10^{-6}$	3.3×10^{6}
TOTALS	1.1×10^{11}	4.3×10^{-12}	---	---

(Eqn. 9.44) of ~1540 nN, or ~5 atm; a dry peptidoglycan sphere of this size would require ~10,000 atm to crush.) Serious infections of $\sim 10^7$ bacteria/cm³ (mean separation ~50 microns) thus require a minimum therapeutic dose of $\gtrsim 10^7$ nanorobots/cm³. Bacterial clearance time for infected tissue at minimum dosage is dominated by entry and withdrawal times (Chapter 16) for single-cell-payload nanorobots, which may require several blood circulation times, but is certainly less than 1000 sec.[3233] An alternative suggestion is that a desiccated bacterium could be "shrink-wrapped," possibly using a tightly wound surface webbing consisting of polymerized glucose (e.g., cellulose or "string"), then flagged for phagocytic removal (Section 10.4.1.2) and released, with the objective of improving the microbe-processing speed of nanorobots. Unfortunately this incautious approach allows bacterial DNA to remain intact. If the wrapping is easily digestible, the prokaryote might escape confinement prior to disposal, and reinflate; if not easily digestible, blockade of the macrophage system could result.

Note that cellular RNA synthesis and protein synthesis stop below 70%-80% hydration. All metabolism of small molecules, lipid synthesis, amino acid synthesis, and CO_2 fixation into organic molecules ceases below ~35% hydration.[941]

10.4.2.5.2 Neuter and Release (NR)

After identification and docking, the nanorobot extends an adhesion antenna tool (Section 9.3.2) into the bacterial interior and sweeps it around inside. The antenna recognizes DNA and RNA material including chromosomes, plasmids, and ribosomes. Any such material found during antenna sweeps through the protoplasm adheres to reversible binding sites on the antenna. The antenna of diameter d_{ant} is then rotated $N_{rot} \sim L_{DNA} / \pi\, d_{ant}$ turns which is sufficient to randomly enspool a chromosome strand of maximum length L_{DNA}; taking $d_{ant} = 0.1$ micron and $L_{DNA} = 1.3$ mm for ~4.2 Mb *E. coli*, $N_{rot} = 4100$ turns which probably may be executed in ~1 sec without strand breakage because the bonding between chromosome and cellular matrix is likely noncovalent. The mean thickness of the bolus of DNA that is tightly spooled around the antenna is $\Delta X = ((V_{DNA} / \pi\, L_{bolus}) + (d_{ant}^2 / 4))^{1/2} - (d_{ant}/2) = 12$ nm, where DNA volume $V_{DNA} \sim 4.2 \times 10^6$ nm³ at ~1 nm³/bp and $L_{bolus} \sim 1$ micron is the bolus length.

The adhesion antenna* is retracted, with patching lipids ejected from the tip as it clears the hole, thus auto-sealing the hole. The adhered genetic material is pushed into a reaction chamber (Section 10.4.2.4.2), whereupon deoxyribonuclease enzymes are introduced to reduce bacterial DNA to nucleotides which are then removed from the solution by molecular sorting rotors and discharged. Ribonucleases and peptidases are also present to reduce RNA and ribosomes to dischargeable effluent, leaving the cell with no genetic or transcription capability, effectively neutering the bacterium. After minor surface modifications to enhance immune system recognition (Section 10.4.1.2), the cell is abandoned to allow natural phagocytic processes to run their course.

** R. Bradbury suggests that a DNA-binding grappling hook mounted on a cable sliding inside a nanotube sheath could be inserted less disruptively through a bacterial cell wall. The interior DNA strands are snagged and then pulled into the nanorobot through the sheath by retracting the cable.*

10.4.2.5.3 Liquefy, Digest and Discharge (LDD)

After identification and docking, the nanorobot extends a retractible, self-cleaning, flexible diamondoid filament rotating "eggbeater" tool (Section 9.3.2) into the bacterial interior and sweeps the tool around inside the cell. A mechanical sensor that serves as a registration bumper detects the presence of cell wall, allowing the rapidly rotating mechanism to avoid damaging the bacterial outer perimeter. A beater with four tines of length 500 nm, tine width 50 nm, and forward cutting edge 10 nm, bowed to a 200 nm diameter and rotating at ~100 Hz has an equatorial velocity of ~60 micron/sec and can cut material having tearing strength ~10^8 N/m^2 (~maximum for soft biological materials; Table 9.3) while consuming ~30 pW (Eqn. 9.75) in continuous operation in highly viscous *E. coli* cytoplasm (absolute viscosity η ~ 1000 kg/m-sec; Table 9.4). As liquefaction proceeds, the protoplasm may become less viscous, allowing rotation rates to be increased and input power to be reduced.

After 1-10 sec, the appropriately liquefied material is pumped from the exemplar 4 micron^3 bacterium interior into the 1 micron^3 enzymatic reaction chamber in ~0.01 micron^3 aliquots and is processed as described earlier in ~100 millisec cycles consuming ~30 pW (Section 10.4.2.4.2). However, the LDD chamber also includes lipases to digest lipids, amylases and related enzymes to digest carbohydrates, and molecular sorting rotors able to transport and discharge fatty acids, sugars, and inorganic ions. A few specialized additional enzymes may be required to fully digest unusual or rare metabolites that might already be present or might appear during processing. Processing time for ~400 cycles is ~40 sec. Finally, the bacterial coat, plasma membrane, and flagella (another ~0.3 micron^3 plus ~0.001 micron^3/flagellum) are sectioned, drawn into the reaction chamber, processed in like fashion, and then discharged in an additional 30 chamber cycles or ~3 sec. Care should be taken not to fragment the coat until nearly all of the cell contents are evacuated, thus minimizing contamination of the extracellular environment. A few additional sorting rotors and special processing may be required for endotoxins, native cellular enzymes, indigestible bacterium-resident poisons and heavy metals, and so forth. Operating simultaneously and in parallel, all 10^{11} water molecules are discharged in ~50 sec by 2000 sorting rotors drawing 20 pW. Thus, total processing time is ~50 sec, consuming ~50 pW.

Table 10.6 also compares the composition of bacterial digestion products to natural bloodstream concentrations of those same products (Appendix B), and shows that the (extremely conservative) maximum "safe" bacterium material discharge rate is nucleotide-limited to ~10^7 microbes/cm^3, which is near the typical microbial number density in serious infections. Digested-bacterium material discharges should not significantly augment natural serum concentrations of most of these substances.

Processing 20-micron tissue cells may proceed by similar, but more cautious, means, and will require on the order of one nanorobot-day to digest and discharge each such cell. A cooperative group of ~100 LDD nanorobots occupying ~10% of a tissue cell surface can perform a complete disassembly and discharge in ~1000 sec, employing a group power draw of ~5000 pW for the duration.

10.4.2.6 Cytocarriage Disposal

Unwanted bacterial or other motile cells may be piloted to natural disposal sites in the human body via cytocarriage (Section 9.4.7), a potentially efficient pathogen-clearing technique that is elaborated in greater detail in Volume II.

10.5 Temperature Effects on Medical Nanorobots

Will medical nanorobots retain functionality at unusually high or low operating temperatures? This is an important question for nanodevices at work in human limbs that may be subjected to hot scalding, combustion, explosion, or other burn traumas, or, at the cold temperature extreme, to severe frostbite or exposure of the extremities whether in space or in arctic conditions, accidental ice burial after an avalanche, or in situations requiring the repair and resuscitation of cold-vitrified or cryogenically-preserved tissues, organs, or whole organisms.

A complete review of the many effects of environmental temperature on the operations of medical nanodevices is beyond the scope of this text. This Section can only briefly mention a few of the many design issues that may arise if nanorobot operations are contemplated significantly above or below normal human body temperatures.

10.5.1 Dimensional Stability and Strength

At high applied stress, covalent bonds cleave much more readily at higher temperatures. For example,[10] at an applied stress of 8 nN/bond a C=C double bond cleaves in ~10^{27} sec at 0 K, ~10^4 sec at 300 K, and ~10^{-3} sec at 500 K. The positional uncertainty is somewhat less problematic in design—the mean classical thermal longitudinal displacement of a diamondoid logic rod varies only as ~$T^{1/2}$.[10] The endpoint of such a rod 1 nm wide and 100 nm long displaces ~0.05 nm at 77 K (liquid N_2), ~0.10 nm at 300 K, and ~0.14 nm at 600 K (liquid lead). Mechanical elements thus become more reliable at lower temperature—e.g., the probability of error in a force sensor (Section 4.4.1) scales as ~exp(1/T), so a 1% error in a sensor at 310 K increases to a 10% error at 600 K, but falls to just 10^{-6} % error at 77 K.

Most materials contract when cold and expand when hot (although zirconium tungstate is a well-known exception[2938]). Thus a 1000-nm long diamondoid rod at 310 K contracts to ~999 nm at 77 K and expands to 1001 nm at 600 K. However, the coefficients of thermal expansion and various other thermophysical parameters are themselves temperature-dependent. The coefficients of volumetric thermal expansion at ~298 K (~25°C) are 3.5 x 10^{-6} K^{-1} for diamond, 15.6 x 10^{-6} K^{-1} for sapphire, 1.2 x 10^{-6} K^{-1} for vitreous silica and 36 x 10^{-6} K^{-1} for crystalline silica or quartz.[567]

Young's modulus (modulus of elasticity) and the other moduli are also temperature-sensitive, especially and most obviously near phase changes—e.g., sapphire melts at 2310 K but "softens" at 2070 K.[1602] At ~1773 K, diamond plastically deforms at just ~1 atm pressure, but >60,000 atm are required to deform diamond at ~1300 K.[2041] At the cold extreme, anyone who has seen the hammering of a nail using a piece of banana cooled in liquid N_2 has witnessed the temperature sensitivity of materials strength.

10.5.2 Viscosity and Locomotion in Ice

The viscosity of liquids generally declines with rising temperature following Andrade's formula (Section 9.4.1.1); water is ~6 times more viscous at 273 K (near freezing) than at 373 K (near boiling) (Table 9.4). Viscosity affects internal fluid transfers but also locomotion. Natation in liquid nitrogen should require relatively less power than in water, since liquid air (at 81 K) is only one-quarter as viscous as liquid water at 310 K (Table 9.4).

An equally relevant but far more serious challenge is locomotion through solid water ice. Just below freezing, crystalline ice viscosity is

~10^{10} kg/m-sec, requiring a 1-micron nanorobot to expend on the order of ~200,000 pW to creep forward at 1 micron/sec (Eqn. 9.73) by viscoplastic flow in which ice crystals are deformed without breaking. Just halfway from freezing to liquid nitrogen temperature, at 164 K, viscosity has already risen to ~10^{21} kg/m-sec, roughly equivalent to solid mantle rock, and the power requirement has increased 100-billionfold, clearly prohibitive. (Microdroplets of pure water may be supercooled in the liquid state to 235 K at 1 atm, or 181 K at ~2000 atm.[2965]).

One solution that avoids this problem at temperatures near the melting point is baronatation, which depends upon the fact that water, almost uniquely, is less dense as a solid than a liquid (i.e., ice floats), suggesting a freezing point depression effect with increasing pressure that is visible as the short downleg from 0°C to −16°C in the phase diagram for Ice Ih (Figure 10.11). This is confirmed experimentally by suspending two heavy weights from a wire stretched across a block of ice. The wire passes slowly through the block, the wire exerting a pressure that melts a thin layer of water ahead of it, allowing the wire to progress; as the water passes behind the wire to the lower pressure region, it refreezes, a process known as regelation.[1697] The melting ice ahead of the wire absorbs the heat of fusion while the refreezing water gives up the heat of fusion, with heat steadily transferred by the wire, hence a good conductor cuts better than a poor one.[1697] The barostatic freezing point depression constant for ice is 134 atm/°C[390,2050] up to ~2100 atm. By exerting a higher pressure (force per unit area) ahead of it than behind it, a baronatating nanorobot of roughly conical geometry can progress slowly through ice that is no colder than −16°C.

Taking the heat of fusion for water ice as ΔH_{fus} = 306 pJ/micron^3 (334 J/gm at 0°C) and assuming at least ~3 micron^3 of ice must be melted to allow 1 micron of forward progress, then baronatation power requirement is very conservatively estimated as $P_{baro} \sim 3\, \Delta H_{fus}\, v_{nano} \sim 900$ pW for v_{nano} = 1 micron/sec. (This is energy flow, which is not necessarily energy dissipation, since most of the heat loss will come from water refreezing at the rear of the nanorobot and only the losses from finite thermal conductivity must be made up.) Below −16°C the ice would have to be heated to that temperature before melting can occur, requiring a probably prohibitive additional power dissipation $P_{heat} \sim L_{nano}\, K_t\, \Delta T$ ~22,000,000 pW to produce a ΔT = 10°C warming of size L_{nano} = 1 micron in ice assuming thermal conductivity of K_t ~ ~2,200,000 pW/micron-°C at -24°C. Bejan and Tyvand[2961] have analyzed gravity-induced pressure-melting of ice due to the passage of solid bodies having square, disklike, or cylindrical contact surfaces. The details of compression-driven phase transitions in ice are also being studied computationally using the tools of molecular dynamics.[2966,2967]

The freezing point depression effect (Section 10.5.3) in which solute molecules are released ahead and recovered behind might serve as the basis for a similar drive system concept at temperatures just below the melting point.

Burrowing by progressive voids is yet another alternative that will work over a wider range of cold temperatures. The binding energy per hydrogen bond in the ice ahead is E_{HBond} = 33 zJ/bond (4.6 Kcal/mole,[2036]), there are two hydrogen bonds per water molecule, and $n_{water} = 3 \times 10^{10}$ water molecules/micron^3 in ice at 273 K, so H-bond-breaking power is at most $P_{HBond} \sim 2\, E_{HBond}\, n_{water}\, L_{nano}^2\, v_{nano}$ = 2000 pW for a nanorobot of dimension L = 1 micron and velocity v_{nano} = 1 micron/sec. (Again, this is a conservative estimate because it may be possible to recapture some of the energy that is liberated as the water molecules are returned to an ice lattice at the rear of the nanorobot.)* Additionally, a molecule handling device of an efficiency comparable to the telescoping manipulator arm (~10 zJ/nm per molecule; Section 3.4.3) that moves ice molecules a total distance ~10 nm to and from a conveyor device of efficiency ~10^{-6} zJ/nm per molecule (Section 3.4.3) running a ~1 micron course consumes $E_{transport}$ = 100.001 zJ/molecule, so molecule-moving power is at most $P_{move} \sim E_{transport}\, n_{water}\, L_{nano}^2\, v_{nano}$ = 3000 pW, hence total motive power for a 1-micron ice-burrowing nanorobot moving at 1 micron/sec is at most ~5000 pW. Moving ice in small chunks may be another energy-saving alternative.

10.5.3 Solubility and Solvents

Gas solubility always declines, while the solubility of most solids rises, with higher temperature (Section 9.2.6). Liquid solutes behave as solids in this regard, but note that unit volumes of miscible fluids are not precisely additive. For example, if one liter of ethanol is added to 1 liter of water, the result is only 1.93 liters of solution.[2036]

A solution of a nonvolatile nonelectrolyte solute (e.g., glucose) has a boiling point T_{boil} that is elevated above the boiling point of pure solvent by $\Delta T_{boil} = n\, k_b\, Ml$, where Ml is the molality of the solution (moles solute per kilogram of solvent), k_b is the boiling point constant for the solvent (Table 10.7), and n = 1. The presence of solute also slightly lowers solvent freezing point T_{freeze} by $\Delta T_{freeze} = n\, k_f\, Ml$, where k_f is the freezing point constant for the solvent (Table 10.7). Both effects are a direct consequence of the lowering of solvent vapor pressure by a solute. The constants may be estimated as:[390]

$$k_f = \frac{R\, T_{freeze}^2\, MW}{1000\, \Delta H_{fus}} \quad (°C/\text{molal}) \qquad \{\text{Eqn. } 10.22\}$$

$$k_b = \frac{R\, T_{boil}^2\, MW}{1000\, \Delta H_{vap}} \quad (°C/\text{molal}) \qquad \{\text{Eqn. } 10.23\}$$

where R = 8.31 J/mole-K (universal gas constant), MW is molecular weight in gm/mole or daltons, T_{freeze} and T_{boil} in K, and ΔH_{fus} and ΔH_{vap} are the heats of fusion and vaporization, respectively (Table 10.8).

In the case of electrolyte solutes (e.g., KCl) in dilute solutions (e.g., Ml ≲ 0.01 molal), n is approximately the moles of ions per mole of solute (e.g., n ~ 2 for KCl). In more concentrated solutions, experimental values of n are slightly lower, as explained by Debye-Huckel theory due to ion-ion and ion-solvent interactions. For example, with KCl in water, n = 1.94 at Ml = 0.01 molal but n = 1.80 at Ml = 0.50 molal.[2050] The most concentrated salt solution (e.g., 6.2 molal NaCl) depresses the freezing point of water by ~20°C.

At still lower temperatures, solvents with much lower melting points may be employed to avoid solvent freezing. In general, substances dissolve in liquids that are chemically similar. Water (itself a polar solvent) and many organic compounds including

* *An additional complication is that the uppermost molecular layers of ice may not be fully frozen. Experiments by Van Hove and Somorjai[2699] show that even as cold as 90 K, the amplitude of vibrational motions in the topmost surface water monolayer is several times that of the water molecules buried deeper in the bulk ice. The second molecular layer also has enhanced vibrational motion, but far less than the top monolayer. This excess motion is attributed to a lack of water molecules above the monolayer, hence the monolayer molecules have fewer motion-restricting hydrogen bonds to other water molecules than those of the layers beneath the surface. At 200 K, the amorphous film becomes thicker; above 230 K, the film becomes a quasi-liquid layer measured as ~12 nm thick at 249 K and ~30 nm thick at 268 K, rising to ~70 nm thick at 272.5 K.*[2701]

Table 10.7. Molal Freezing and Boiling Point Constants[390,763,2036,2050]

Solvent	Freezing Point (°C)	k_f (°C/molal)	Boiling Point (°C)	k_b (°C/molal)
Acetic acid	16.6	3.90	118.5	2.93
Acetone	-95.4	---	56.2	1.71
Benzene	5.5	5.12	80.1	2.53
Camphor	176.0	40.0	209.0	5.95
Chloroform	-63.5	4.73	61.2	3.63
Cyclohexane	6.5	20.2	81.0	2.79
Diethyl ether	-116.2	---	34.6	2.11
Ethanol	-117.3	1.85	78.5	1.19
n-Hexane	-95.0	1.75	68.0	2.75
Methanol	-97.8	2.58	65.0	0.83
Naphthalene	80.2	6.85	217.9	---
n-Octane	-56.5	2.14	125.5	4.02
Phenol	43.0	7.27	182.0	3.56
Water	0.0	1.86	100.0	0.512

Table 10.8. Molar Heats of Fusion and Vaporization at 1 atm[390,763,1164,2036,2048,2050,2161]

Substance	ΔH_{fus} (J/mole)	ΔH_{vap} (J/mole)
Acetic acid	11,700	24,400
Aluminum	10,500	230,000
Ammonia	5,660	23,400
Argon	1,110	6,540
Benzene	9,850	30,800
n-Butane	4,670	22,400
Carbon monoxide	---	6,080
Chlorine (Cl_2)	6,410	20,100
Chloroform	9,220	29,500
Diethyl ether	---	26,000
Ethane	2,860	14,700
Ethanol	5,030	38,600
Fluorine (F_2)	1,590	6,320
Helium	21	84
n-Hexane	13,000	28,900
Hydrogen (H_2)	117	905
Iodine	16,800	44,000
Iron	1,290	380,000
Lead	5,080	170,000
Mercury	2,300	56,600
Methane	943	8,190
Methanol	3,170	35,300
Nitrogen (N_2)	721	5,580
n-Octane	20,800	35,000
Oxygen	444	6,830
Platinum	22,200	520,000
Sapphire/Ruby	109,000	(decomp.)
Silver	9,520	250,000
Sodium Chloride	28,900	180,000
Water	6,017	40,690

glucose are soluble in ethanol, which remains a liquid to -117°C (156 K).[763] Sodium chloride is slightly soluble in ethanol, and also in liquid ammonia which melts at -78°C (195 K).[763] Some natural enzymes are known to retain their function in liquid ammonia, and others in supercritical carbon dioxide; artificial enzyme systems based on natural peptides, or other polymers with protein-like conformational properties, could in principle operate in cryogenic solvents such as tetrafluoromethane,[261] carbon monoxide (a polar solvent, liquid from -191.5°C to -199°C) or liquid nitrogen (a nonpolar solvent, liquid -195.8°C to -209.9°C). Lactate dehydrogenase enzyme found in cold water Antarctic fishes operates as fast as the related enzyme in animals with higher body temperatures, even though enzyme action normally halves for every 10°C temperature drop (Section 4.6.4). The Antarctic fish enzyme compensates for the cold with modifications near the enzyme's active site that increase flexibility and mobility, in effect "greasing the hinges so that the enzyme can move more quickly."[2152]

10.5.4 Heat Conductivity and Capacity, and Refrigeration

Thermophysical characteristics of various materials at 310 K are given in Table 8-12, but what is the temperature dependency? Heat capacity (C_V) generally rises with temperature. For example, the heat capacity of ice rises from 0.63 x 10^6 J/m^3-K at -196°C (liquid N_2) to 1.7 x 10^6 J/m^3-K at -30°C.[763] Thermal conductivity (K_t) may have a more complicated relationship with temperature. For example, the thermal conductivity of liquid water rises with temperature, from 0.561 W/m-K at 0°C to 0.681 W/m-K at 100°C.[763] The thermal conductivity of sapphire normal to the optical or c-axis also rises from 2.3 W/m-K at 310 K to 6.0 W/m-K at 900 K, according to one source;[2153] however, in the direction parallel to the optical axis, the thermal conductivity of sapphire rises from 0.3 W/m-K at 3 K to a peak of ~200 W/m-K near 70 K, then falls to ~30 W/m-K at 310 K and ~6 W/m-K at 1000 K;[2154] conductivity for ruby falls from ~20 W/m-K at 310 K to ~6 W/m-K at 1000 K.[2154] In the case of diamond, thermal conductivity rises from ~10 W/m-K at 3 K to a peak of 12,500 W/m-K at 69 K, then falls to ~2000 W/m-K at 300 K.[2154]

Is it possible to build micron-scale refrigerators? Refrigerators serve to maintain a temperature differential between an enclosed volume and the external environment. Leaving aside vacuum isolation levitation techniques (Section 6.3.4.4), thermal equilibration of a volume of size L by conduction* requires an equilibration time of approximately:

$$t_{EQ} \sim \frac{L^2 C_V}{K_t} \quad \text{(sec)} \qquad \text{\{Eqn. 10.24\}}$$

For water at 310 K, C_V = 4.19 x 10^6 J/m^3-K and K_t = 0.623 W/m-K,[763] hence t_{EQ} ~ (6.7 x 10^6) L^2 (sec) for in vivo medical nanorobot refrigerators. Thus a cold box 1 mm wide requires t_{EQ} ~ 7 sec, but a 1 micron^3 box equilibrates in only ~7 microsec. Diamond is far more conductive; a 1 micron^3 cold box embedded in a surplus of diamondoid structure (C_V = 1.8 x 10^6 J/m^3-K) inside a nanorobot has a t_{EQ} ~ (900) L^2 = 0.9 nanosec equilibration time (giving a ~10^{11} kelvin/sec cool rate, assuming ΔT ~ 100 K). Thus in order to avoid thermal re-equilibration with the surroundings, a ~1 micron^3 refrigeration mechanism must circulate working coolant fluid at a velocity v_{fluid} ~ L / t_{EQ} ~ 1000 m/sec, very near the speed of sound in most fluids, hence sub-ambient refrigerators smaller than ~1 micron^3 are not feasible using this method.

Drexler[10] proposes a working fluid consisting of encapsulated submicron water ice particles with surface structures preventing aggregation and flexible enough to allow repeated expand/contract

* *Also, the nature of radiative transfer (Section 6.3.4.4(E)) changes drastically as the size of the box gets close to the wavelength of the peak of the distribution, e.g., 3-30 microns (100-1000 K; Eqn. 6.20) with heat transfer rates enhanced by up to several orders of magnitude,[652,653] making sub-ambient cooling much more difficult.*

cycles as the contained ice alternately freezes and thaws, combined with a low-viscosity, low-melting point carrier such as a light hydrocarbon. The heat absorbed by a substance that melts at constant temperature (the melting point) is the heat (or enthalpy) of fusion; the much larger heat required to boil a liquid is the heat (or enthalpy) of vaporization (Table 10.8); the heat of sublimation is simply the sum of the two.[390,2050] Phase changes provide the most efficient cooling—ice absorbs 306 pJ/micron^3 of heat when it melts at 0°C, and water absorbs 2170 pJ/micron^3 when it boils at 100°C, but water at 37°C absorbs only 42 pJ/micron^3 when it warms by 10°C. The exact temperature of a reversible phase transition in a refrigerant working fluid can be precisely controlled by judicious selection of operating pressures and fluid materials. Thermal-driven phase-change microactuators have been tested.[545]

Many other possible refrigeration technologies are known but have yet to be investigated in the context of nanorobot refrigeration, including "magnetic cooling" by adiabatic demagnetization[1031] or magnetocaloric refrigerators,[2159] Seebeck effect or Peltier effect electronic cooling,[1034,1035,2160,2933] thermoacoustic refrigeration (Section 6.3.3), optical refrigerators,[549] chemomechanical turbines operated in reverse,[597] heat of solvation cooling mediated by molecular sorting rotors (e.g., $KMnO_4$ cools solvent water by 44,000 J/mole, which is ~750 pJ/micron^3 or ~73 zJ/molecule, as it dissolves,[763]) heat of allotropic-transition cooling (e.g., transition from red α-HgI_2 to yellow β-HgI_2 absorbs ~13,000 J/mole or ~180 pJ/micron^3,[2036]) and acoustic, polymeric, or mechanical prevention of ice crystallization during supercooling of working fluid.

10.5.5 Other Temperature-Dependent Properties

There are a great many temperature-dependent materials properties of nanomedical relevance, but there is only space here to mention just a few:

1. *Denaturation and Combustion* — Protein denaturation and reduced receptor-ligand fidelity may occur at temperatures as low as 50-100°C. It is true that not much happens to a block of diamond dropped into boiling water,[280] but the maximum combustion point for diamond in air is ~800°C,[691] and carbon nanotubes start to burn in air at ~700°C.[1857] At low temperatures, receptor-ligand binding may occur with greater fidelity but more slowly, and there are various unusual biological effects that occur at low temperature—for example, the lens of the human eye becomes opaque when cooled to below freezing [G. Fahy, personal communication, 1997].

2. *Speed of Sound* — Acoustic waves travel at different speeds in cold and hot media, potentially affecting medical nanorobot sensing, energy transmission, communication and navigation. In general, the speed of sound (v_{sound}) in liquids depends upon the adiabatic bulk modulus B and density ρ, both of which are temperature-dependent, as $v_{sound} = (B/\rho)^{1/2}$ (Eqn. 4.30). The temperature dependence of the speed of sound in pure water at 1 atm has been carefully studied and is approximated fairly well by:[2155]

$$v_{sound} \sim 1557 - (0.0245)(347 - T)^2 \qquad \text{\{Eqn. 10.25\}}$$

where T is temperature in K. Thus the speed of sound increases with rising temperature up to a peak at 347 K (74°C), then decreases thereafter. For practically all other liquids, v_{sound} decreases with rising temperature over the entire range in which the material remains a liquid.[2156] (In most liquids, v_{sound} increases linearly, though only very slightly, with pressure. For example, v_{sound} in benzene rises ~17% when pressure is increased from 1 atm to 500 atm;[2156] see also Section 10.3.3.) The speed of sound in water-ice just below the freezing point, estimated from Eqn. 4.30, is ~1000 m/sec. The speed of sound in dry air at 1 atm increases with rising temperature and is approximated by:[1164]

$$v_{sound} \sim 332\,[1 + (0.003366)(T - 273)]^{1/2} \qquad \text{\{Eqn. 10.26\}}$$

3. *Energy Absorption* — Acoustic absorption and attenuation coefficients change with temperature, affecting the efficiency of acoustic power transfer. Absorption per unit of radio frequency (rf) energy in tissue during diathermic heating also varies with temperature.

4. *Surface Tension* — The surface tension of liquids at the air-liquid interface tends to decline as temperature rises, falling to zero at the boiling point. For instance, the air-liquid surface tension for a 48% volumetric ethanol-water mixture (96 proof, U.S. spirit) is 30.10 x 10^{-3} N/m at 20°C but 28.93 x 10^{-3} N/m at 40°C;[763] values for pure water are given elsewhere (Section 9.2.3).

5. *Dielectric Constant* — The electrical properties of materials may be temperature-dependent. For example, the dielectric constant of water declines with rising temperature and is crudely approximated by:[2157]

$$\kappa_{water} \sim 80 - 0.4\,(T - 293) \qquad \text{\{Eqn. 10.27\}}$$

for temperatures in kelvins from T = 273-373 K (0-100°C), for rf frequencies up to 100 MHz, and at 1 atm pressure. The dielectric constant of ice at 0°C is virtually the same as that of water (88.0), but decreases rapidly with decreasing temperatures below 0°C, and with increasing frequency; by 0.1 MHz, κ_{ice} ~ 2-4 with little influence of temperature.[2157] Relative permittivity decreases by a large factor for many other substances as they change state at the freezing point; for example, κ falls from 35 for liquid nitrobenzene at 279 K to 3 for solid nitrobenzene at 279 K.[727] In general, nonpolar liquids have a small dielectric constant (e.g., 1.5-2.5) that is nearly independent of the temperature, whereas polar liquids have a larger value that declines rapidly as temperature rises.[2036]

AFTERWORD

Ralph C. Merkle, Ph.D.
Xerox PARC

Introduction

One of life's pleasures is writing an afterword for a classic-in-the-making. Not only will some of the glory inevitably rub off, there's also the illicit pleasure of having peeked at the future, like peeking at the Christmas presents before Christmas. A few of the possibilities of this new field of nanomedicine have been hinted at, a few more have been sketched in some research papers, but only with the publication of *Nanomedicine* have we started to see the full richness of it.

Like cresting the top of a hill and beholding, for the first time and in one sweep, the whole of a new land, our minds are both captivated by the prospects and at another level churning with plans and ideas and tasks. For at the same time we see what is possible, we are also aware of the work that remains to be done to convert this vision into reality. *Nanomedicine* is more than just a description of what might be, it is a call to action. While it will take decades to convert the possible to the actual, that is what we are called upon to do—not only for the good of all, not only to advance our knowledge, not only to help future generations, but to help ourselves as well.

The Long View

While planning beyond a decade is rare in this society, our lives can span over a century. We should not be shortsighted or timid about this. When I was a child, my sister was wise and very old: all of twenty years in age! My parents, in their 40's, were old beyond concepts of antiquity. Like the sky above and the ground beneath, they had existed since the beginnings of time—at least, of my time. Yet somehow I am now 47, and when I protest my age I am laughed at by my grandmother-in-law who views me, from her 90's, as a mere youth.

The field of nanomedicine will take decades to develop, but those decades will pass and that future will arrive. Most of us will find we are still here: a bit older, a bit slower, perhaps a bit wiser, yet still filled with the excitement of life and the joy of living. Think of yourself on that future day, looking back on what was and looking forward to what will be. Will the future still be bright, still be open, and still be filled with uncharted possibilities?

That depends on what we do today. If we ignore the future, if we dismiss the decades ahead and focus narrowly on the next few weeks or months, then the future will catch us by surprise, unprepared. But if we start now, if we raise up our eyes from the distractions of the moment and prepare for the future that we know will come, then when that future arrives we will look back and be pleased with what we did, and will look forward and be pleased with the even greater possibilities of what we can do.

The Tasks Ahead

Perhaps the first task is to decide whether the capabilities described so well in *Nanomedicine* are indeed possible. If they are, then developing this new technology is a matter, quite literally, of life and death for many of us, our children, and future generations. Making this decision is harder than it might seem. As a society, we deal with new ideas poorly if we deal with them at all. Most people do not have the intellectual resources to directly evaluate new proposals, and so must rely on the statements of others. But those who in principle might be able to evaluate a new idea and so help our collective understanding often get it wrong. Looking back at a few historical examples, we can begin to see the magnitude of the difficulty.

John Aubrey, a contemporary of William Harvey, wrote this account of the response to the publication in 1628 of Harvey's book *De Motu Cordis* in which Harvey described his discovery of the blood's circulation:

> *"...I heard Harvey say that after his book came out, he fell mightily in his practice. 'Twas believed by the vulgar that he was crack-brained, and all the physicians were against him. I knew several doctors in London that would not have given threepence for one of his medicines."* [1]

In 1873 Sir John Erichsen offered this grim assessment of the future of surgery:

> *"There cannot always be fresh fields of conquest by the knife; there must be portions of the human frame that will ever remain sacred from its intrusions, at least in the surgeon's hands. That we have already, if not quite, reached these final limits, there can be little question. The abdomen, the chest, and the brain will be forever shut from the intrusion of the wise and humane surgeon."* [1]

Nanomedicine, as *Nanosystems*[2] before it, is based on the laws of physics which describe our world with phenomenal accuracy. Both books advance arguments grounded on those laws, and both can therefore be evaluated with respect to the accuracy of their conclusions with respect to those laws. *Nanosystems* was published in 1992, and no significant flaws have been found. Given the volume of public debate and the number of people who have read the book, the simplest explanation for this absence of reported errors is that its logic is basically correct and its conclusions are basically sound. Today, these conclusions are working their way into our collective decision making processes and guiding our next steps. Research is being focused on how best to develop this new technology, companies are being formed to achieve the goals that we now accept as possible, and people are beginning to grapple with the potential consequences.

Nanomedicine, working from the foundations laid by *Nanosystems*, develops the consequences of nanotechnology for medicine. These consequences are extraordinary, and must be both explained and publicly examined. We must firstly encourage the early review and more rapid acceptance of *Nanomedicine*, for the next steps will only be taken after concluding that its reasoning is largely sound and its conclusions mostly correct—the same pattern we saw with *Nanosystems*.

An Immediate Concern

Actually, there is one thing we must do even earlier: ensure the completion of this exceptional series of books. What you are reading is only Volume I. Volumes II and III, and the popular book to follow, do not yet (as of 1999 when this is being written) exist, except in Freitas' head.

We need to support him, in order to move this first and most critical series to completion. This is always the hardest time for a new idea—before it has been codified and laid out, before it has been clothed in words, when it exists only as thoughts. The work of making it solid and substantial is great, and yet this work is given the least support.

What funding committee will agree to fund a book describing an entire new field that has never before been dreamt of? Committees base their conclusions on a shared understanding of a common body of knowledge. Their members are drawn from an existing society of experts to evaluate the next incremental improvement. What do you do when there are no experts? Who lays claim to expertise in nanomedicine? Who has spent their life in this field which is just being conceived? No one. The committee process breaks down when we move into truly new terrain. It fails us just when failure is most expensive: at the beginnings of new things. Here we must fall back on individuals—individuals who are bold enough to believe in themselves when there are no experts to turn to for help and support. Individuals who are willing to back up their own beliefs with action, who will nurture the truly new and the truly groundbreaking without having to first seek the approval of others. For there are no others! On the far frontiers there are very few, and sometimes there is only one.

The Research That Must Be Done

What happens later, when some significant part of society agrees that nanomedicine will happen? Research.

- Research to clarify the goals and objectives. Just because people agree it will happen doesn't mean they agree about how it will happen, or when, or which sub-objectives should be given higher priority, or....
- Research to persuade more people that nanomedicine is feasible. Don't forget that this society runs on majority rule. If 20% of a committee thinks an idea is worthwhile and should be pursued, it still gets voted down.
- Research to identify early applications. The sooner we can identify profitable opportunities that move us closer to the long-term objectives, the sooner we can establish support that doesn't require persuading committees.
- Research to advance our experimental capabilities. This accomplishes two purposes: it moves us closer to the goal, and it makes it easier for people to understand that the goal is feasible.

Broadly speaking, the research that must be done can be divided into theoretical and experimental. The theoretical work includes both traditional paper-and-pencil methods, and also the newer methods of computational modeling and "digital experiments" made possible by the computer. Theoretical and computational methods can be applied to the proposals advanced in *Nanomedicine* both to check feasibility and to provide more detailed understanding of the performance and capabilities. Computational models in particular, especially when they are based on detailed descriptions of physical interactions, force a very thorough treatment of the design and bring into the light any hidden assumptions.

Backward Chaining

Theoretical and computational methods can also be applied to near-term and intermediate-term proposals. Achieving a long-term objective often requires taking many steps, and all of those steps except the first one are (pretty much by definition) not experimentally accessible. While experimental work is focused on taking the next step, the theoretical and computational work should be focused on clarifying the whole pathway from today's technology to the future applications. This feeds back into the experimental work in two ways. First, it provides information about which approaches are more likely or less likely to succeed. Second, it provides a reason for supporting the experimental work. The value and feasibility of the long-term objectives makes experimental progress more valuable, and as this understanding spreads it becomes easier for experimentalists to get funding for work that moves us closer to those long-range objectives.

Consider one example: Freitas' respirocyte[3] is based on the observation that a red blood cell stores very little oxygen when compared with a tank of similar size which holds oxygen compressed to ~1,000 atmospheres. The design calls for strong materials (to hold oxygen at high pressure) and very finely detailed structural components (to control the release and storage of the oxygen). On a theoretical and computational front, sub-components that are composed of not-too-many atoms can be modeled in great detail. The position of each atom and the forces between the atoms can be modeled using techniques that provide remarkable accuracy and simultaneously impose a discipline and rigor on the designer. Compelling the designer to account for the location of every atom, and to propose a design that fully satisfies the physical laws incorporated into the computational model—a model that has been checked and verified against countless other molecular structures—prevents the designer from sidestepping awkward issues that might cause the design to fail.

Such a design then feeds back important constraints on earlier steps in the development process. For example, we must be able to make very precise, very detailed, and very strong structures. The material often proposed for this (and other nanotechnological) applications is typically diamond and variants on diamond (structures with a stiff hydrocarbon backbone and surface terminations that are chemically stable; hydrogenated diamond surfaces are common, as are the use of oxygen on (100) surfaces, nitrogen on (111) surfaces, and the like). If stiff hydrocarbons are important, then we must have good PEFs (Potential Energy Functions) for such structures in order to perform molecular mechanics and molecular dynamics calculations that are accurate. The use of Brenner's potential for modeling hydrocarbons is common today, and extensions to this potential to incorporate elements other than hydrogen and carbon, as well as to improve its accuracy, are clearly of great importance to the computational research aimed at developing nanotechnology.

The requirement for highly detailed structures made of stiff hydrocarbons in turn implies we must analyze chemical reactions able to synthesize such materials. The chemical reactions involved in the growth of diamond are reasonably well understood, and many reaction pathways have been proposed by which such growth can occur. We can adopt reaction pathways similar to those seen in the chemical vapor deposition (CVD) growth of diamond, but provide finer control over where they occur by positioning the reacting compounds using positional devices. Better computational methods for analyzing individual reactions are possible using ab initio methods, which can also provide accurate descriptions of the interactions of small numbers of atoms which then feed into the design of better PEFs. Better understanding of reactions relevant to the growth of diamond can also be pursued experimentally, and particular reactions of interest can be looked at in the laboratory as well as on a computer.

The need to position molecular components in its turn implies we must consider positional devices—both improvements to today's SPMs (Scanning Probe Microscopes) and future molecular scale versions that are faster, more accurate, and have a greater range of tip configurations. This implies a strong interest in experimental and theoretical work on positioning devices, as well as work aimed at improving SPM tips. Experimental work that shows greater flexibility in arranging individual atoms and molecules should be supported, as the potential consequences of this work are very great.

This process of working backwards from our desired goal to near-term research objectives was called backward chaining by Drexler.[2] As can be seen, it is a method of analyzing a long-term objective (e.g. using respirocytes to treat medical conditions) and breaking down the steps needed to achieve that objective into nearer-term objectives (e.g. improving PEFs, experimental work in SPMs). While the outline of the process given here is necessarily very short, it should give the reader a feeling for the basic idea.

The procedure of targeting near-term research goals based on their utility in achieving long-term objectives not only provides a focus for research, it also produces a wealth of results which further bolster the underlying arguments supporting the feasibility of the objectives and the desirability of such research. This creates a recursive spiral of knowledge. A little research shows there are no fundamental barriers that prevent us from achieving the objectives of molecular nanotechnology. Further research gives a better understanding of which molecular machine systems should be feasible and provides initial targets for additional research. Ongoing work is providing a clearer picture of the routes that can move us from our present technology base to the proposed molecular machines of the future, and produces yet more targets for near-term efforts.

The Recursive Spiral of Knowledge

Every time we pursue further research in nanotechnology we find that our original assessment of its basic feasibility is strengthened, our understanding of the specific near-term research targets that we must pursue is broadened, our conviction that further research can speed the development of this fundamentally new and revolutionary technology grows stronger, and our awareness of the astonishingly pervasive benefits this technology can bring is widened. In this recursive spiral of knowledge, research emboldens our interest and increasing interest produces yet more research. The rate-limiting process is the speed with which people take the first step, for having taken the first step the second step comes a little faster, and the third step faster still.

This should come as no real surprise, for either the ability to arrange and rearrange molecular structures in most of the ways permitted by physical law is feasible, or, alternatively, it is not. But since Feynman's famous 1959 talk *There's Plenty of Room at the Bottom,*[4] every informed observer who has studied the issue has drawn the same conclusion: it's feasible. The only way to break the recursive spiral would be to discover a fundamental objection that makes molecular machine systems impossible. As we are surrounded by biological molecular machines, this possibility seems remote. If thermal noise was a fundamental obstacle to molecular machine design, then biological systems could not copy DNA and molecular rotary motors could not rotate. If quantum uncertainty was a fundamental obstacle, then ribosomes could not synthesize proteins and sodium channels could not distinguish between sodium and potassium.

A New Medical Technology And A New Era Of Medicine

We are left, then, with a fairly clear set of conclusions. Living systems exist. Living systems can usually heal and cure their own injuries, unless those injuries are severe enough to prevent the living system from functioning. Too often, we suffer injuries that are indeed this severe. Molecular nanotechnology is feasible. As we master the ability to design molecular machines that can continue to function when the living system around them has failed, those molecular machines can restore the function of the living system. They can support and sustain the processes of the living system until that living system can once again function on its own. Whether this is done by a temporary assist from respirocytes[3] or by any of the myriad other techniques discussed in *Nanomedicine*, the underlying message is clear: life and health can be restored and sustained in the face of greater injury, greater damage, greater trauma, and greater dysfunction than has ever before been realized. This will usher in a new era of medicine—an era in which health and long life will be the usual state of affairs while sickness, debility and death will be the mercifully rare exceptions.

The future capabilities of nanomedicine give hope and inspiration to those of us who still have decades of life to look forward to, but some are not so fortunate. Many others who rightfully should live several decades more might find that chance cuts short their expected time. Heart attacks and cancer can strike us down even in the prime of our lives. They do not always wait their turn and politely arrive only when expected. How can today's dying patient take advantage of a future medical technology that is as yet only described in a handful of theoretical publications? How can we preserve the physical structure of our bodies well enough to permit that future medical technology to restore our health?

The extraordinary medical prospects ahead of us have renewed interest in a proposal made long ago: that the dying patient could be frozen, then stored at the temperature of liquid nitrogen for decades or even centuries until the necessary medical technology to restore health is developed. Called cryonics, this service is now available from several companies. Because final proof that this will work must wait until after we have developed a medical technology based on the foundation of a mature nanotechnology, the procedure is experimental. We cannot prove today that medical technology will (or will not) be able to reverse freezing injury 100 years from now. But the patient dying today must choose whether to join the experimental group or the control group. The luxury of waiting for a definitive answer before choosing is simply not available. So the decision must be made today, on the basis of incomplete information. We already know what happens to the control group. The outcome for the experimental group has not yet been confirmed. But given the wonderful advances that we see coming, it seems likely that we should be able to reverse freezing injury—especially when that injury is minimized by the rapid introduction through the vascular system of cryoprotectants and other chemicals to cushion the tissues against further injury.

Conclusion

The development of nanomedicine depends on us: what we do and how rapidly we do it. Research is not done by a faceless "them," nor is it something that happens spontaneously and without any human intervention. It is done by and supported by people. Unless we decide to support and pursue this research, it won't happen. How long it takes to develop depends on us. We are not idle bystanders watching the world go by. We are a part of it. If we sit and wait for someone else to develop this technology, it will happen much more slowly. If we jump in and work to make it happen, it will happen sooner. And developing a life saving medical technology within our lifetimes seems like a very good idea—certainly better than the alternative.

References

1. For more examples of this kind and references for the above quotations, see http://www.foresight.org/News/negativeComments.html#loc026).
2. K. Eric Drexler, Nanosystems: Molecular Machinery, Manufacturing, and Computation, John Wiley & Sons, NY, 1992.
3. Robert A. Freitas Jr., "Exploratory Design in Medical Nanotechnology: A Mechanical Artificial Red Cell," Artificial Cells, Blood Substitutes, and Immobil. Biotech. 26(1998):411-430. See also: http://www.foresight.org/Nanomedicine/Respirocytes.html.
4. Richard P. Feynman, "There's Plenty of Room at the Bottom," Engineering and Science (California Institute of Technology), February 1960, pp. 22-36. Reprinted in B.C. Crandall, James Lewis, eds, Nanotechnology: Research and Perspectives, MIT Press, 1992. pp. 347–63, and in D.H. Gilbert, ed, Miniaturization, Reinhold, New York, 1961, pp. 282-296. See also: http://nano.xerox.com/nanotech/feynman.html.

APPENDIX A

APPENDIX A. Useful Data in Medical Nanodevice Design

Compiled from various sources, including (but not limited to) the following References: 10, 460, 536-537, 567, 763, 1164, 1597, 1662, 2036, 2153, 2154, 2223-2224, 3229-3232, 3429-3431, 3469.

I. Systeme International (SI) Metric Prefixes

10^{24}	Y-	yotta-
10^{21}	Z-	zetta-
10^{18}	E-	exa-
10^{15}	P-	peta-
10^{12}	T-	tera-
10^{9}	G-	giga-
10^{6}	M-	mega-
10^{3}	k-,K-	kilo-
10^{2}	h-	hecto-
10^{1}	da-, dk-	deka-
10^{-1}	d-	deci-
10^{-2}	c-	centi-
10^{-3}	m-	milli-
10^{-6}	µ-	micro-
10^{-9}	n-	nano-
10^{-12}	p-	pico-
10^{-15}	f-	femto-
10^{-18}	a-	atto-
10^{-21}	z-	zepto-
10^{-24}	y-	yocto-

II. Units of Measurement and Useful Conversions

Angles and Rotations:

180 degrees = π radians
1 radian = 57.29578 deg = 0.1591549 cycle (revolution)
1 cycle (revolution) = 6.2831853 radians = 360 deg
1 deg = 0.01745329 radian = 0.0027777 cycle
= 60 arcmin = 3600 arcsec
1 arcsec = 4.848136 microradians
1 hertz (Hz) = 1 cycle/sec = 6.2831853 radians/sec
1 radian/sec = 9.5492966 revolutions per minute (rpm)

Areas and Surfaces:

1 m^2 = 10^4 cm^2 = 10^6 mm^2 = 10^{12} $micron^2$ = 10^{18} nm^2
= 1.1959900 yd^2 = 10.763910 ft^2 = 1550.0031 $inch^2$
1 acre = 43,560 ft^2 = 4046.8564 m^2 = 0.0015625 $mile^2$
1 steradian = 0.079577472 spheres = 3282.8063 deg^2
1 sphere = 12.566371 steradians

Concentration:

1 molar (M) = 1 mole/liter = 0.602257 molecules/nm^3
1 molecule/nm^3 = 1.66042 moles/liter
1 molal = 1 mole/kg
milliequivalent:
mEq/liter = (mg/liter) x valence / molecular weight
mEq/kg = (mg/kg) x valence / molecular weight

Density:

1 gm/cm^3 = 1000 kg/m^3 = 8.3454044 lbs/gallon (U.S. liq.)
= 1 gm/ml = 1000 gm/liter = 62.42621 lbs/ft^3
1 gallon water at 4°C (U.S. liq.) = 8.34517 lbs = 3.785305 kg

Electrical:

1 coulomb (C) = 1 ampere-sec = 6.24196 x 10^{18} electron charges
1 ampere (A) = 1 coulomb/sec
1 volt (V) (electric potential, emf) = 1 joule/coulomb
= 1 watt/ampere
1 ohm (Ω) = 1 volt/ampere
1 siemen (S) (conductance) = 1 ampere/volt = 1 mho
1 farad (F) (capacitance) = 1 coulomb/volt

Energy:

1 joule (J) (work, heat) = 1 N-m = 1 W-sec = 1 kg-m^2/sec^2
= 0.000239006 Kcal
= 10^7 ergs = 0.000948451 Btu
= 2.7777 x 10^{-7} kilowatt-hours
= 0.00986895 liter-atm
= 6.241506 x 10^{18} eV
1 nanojoule (nJ) = 1000 picojoules (pJ) = 10^{-9} joules
1 zeptojoule (zJ) = 10^{-21} J = 6.241506 x 10^{-3} eV
= 0.1439325 Kcal
1 electron-volt (eV) = 160.217733 zJ
1 MeV = 10^6 eV = 1000 KeV = 0.001 GeV = 10^{-6} TeV
1 kilocalorie (Kcal) (dietary Calories) = 1000 calories = 4184 J
1 kT at 310 K = 4.28004 zJ = 0.026714 eV
1 Hartree = 627.5095 Kcal/mole = 27.2116 eV = 4359.7482 zJ
1 foot-pound = 1.355818 J
1 megaton (of TNT explosive) ~ 5 x 10^{15} J

Energy (molar):

1 Kcal/mole = 6.947700141 zJ/molecule
1 KJ/mole = 29.069177 zJ/molecule
1 zJ/molecule = 0.1439325 Kcal/mole = 0.0344007 KJ/mole
1 eV/atom = 23.0622 Kcal/mole = 160.217733 zJ/atom

Force:

1 newton (N) (force) = 1 kg-m/sec^2
= 10^5 dynes = 0.22480894 pounds
1 nanonewton (nN) = 1000 piconewtons (pN) = 10^{-9} newtons

Illumination:

1 candela (cd) (luminous intensity) = 1 lumen/m^2
1 lumen (luminous flux) (at 550 nm wavelength) = 0.0014705882 watt
1 candle = 1 lumen/steradian
1 candle/m^2 (at 550 nm wavelength) = 0.00462 watt/m^2

Length and Distance:

1 Angstrom (A) = 0.1 nm = 10^{-10} meters
1 nanometer (nm) = 1000 picometers = 10^{-9} meters
1 micron = 1000 nm = 0.001 mm = 10^{-6} m
1 mile = 5280 ft = 63,360 inches = 1609.344 m
1 light-year = 9.46055 x 10^{15} m

Magnetism:

1 weber (Wb) (magnetic flux) = 1 volt-sec
1 henry (H) (inductance) = 1 weber/ampere
1 tesla (T) (magnetic flux density) = 1 weber/m^2
= 1 N/ampere-m

Mass:

1 kilogram (kg) = 1000 grams (gm) = 2.2046226 pounds (lbs)
= 771.61792 scruples (apoth) = 15,432.358 grains
1 nanogram (ng) = 1000 picograms (pg) = 10^{-9} grams
1 pound = 16 ounces (avdp oz) = 453.59237 gm
1 troy ounce = 31.103486 gm = 1.0971429 (avdp) oz
1 gram (gm) = 0.25720597 drams (apoth/troy)
= 0.56438339 drams (avdp)
= 15.432358 grains = 0.77161792 scruples (apoth)
1 ton (metric) = 1000 kg
1 ton (long) = 2240 lbs = 1016.0469 kg
1 ton (short) = 2000 lbs = 907.18474 kg
1 carat (metric) = 0.200 grams = 3.08647 grains
1 dalton = 1 amu = 931.752 MeV (mass energy)
= 1.661 x 10^{-27} kg/molecule = 1 gm/mole

Power:

1 watt (W) = 1 joule/sec = 0.00134102 horsepower
= 10^7 erg/sec
= 3.41443 Btu/hour = 20.650 Kcal/day
1 nanowatt (nW) = 1000 picowatts (pW) = 10^{-9} watts
1 horsepower (hp) = 746 W
2000 Kcal/day = 96.85 W

Pressure or Stress:

1 Pascal (Pa) = 1 N/m^2
1 dyne/cm^2 = 0.1 N/m^2 (Pa) = 10^{-6} bars = 0.986923 x 10^{-6} atm
1 atm = 101,325 N/m^2 (Pa) = 1.01325 bars
= 760 mmHg = 760 torr = 14.6960 lbs/inch^2 (PSI)
1 mmHg = 0.00131579 atm = 133.32 N/m^2 (Pa)
= 0.00133322 bar
= 0.0193368 lbs/inch^2 = 1.35953 cmH_2O
1 kg/mm^2 = 96.784 atm = 9.80665 x 10^6 N/m^2 (Pa)
= 1422.33 lbs/inch^2 = 98.0665 bars
= 10^6 kg/m^2 = 100 kg/cm^2

Radioactivity:

1 curie (Ci) = 3.70 x 10^{10} nuclear disintegrations/sec
1 bequerel (Bq) = 1 nuclear disintegration/sec
= 3.70 x 10^{10} curies

Temperature:

Kelvin (K) degrees = Celsius (C) degrees + 273.15
1 deg K = 1 deg C (Celsius or Centigrade)
Fahrenheit (F) degrees = 32 + (9 x Celsius degrees / 5)
Celsius (C) degrees = 5 x (Fahrenheit degrees - 32) / 9
310 K = 37°C = 98.6°F

Time:

1 second = (1 / 31,556,925.9747) of a tropical year
1 day = 24 hours = 1440 minutes = 86,400 sec
1 year (tropical) = 365.24219 mean solar days ~ π x 10^7 sec

Velocity:

1 m/sec = 3.2808399 ft/sec = 3.6 km/hr = 2.2369363 mph
= 1.94385 knots (nautical miles per hour)
1 mph = 1.609344 km/hr

Viscosity (absolute or dynamic):

1 Poise = 0.1 kg/m-sec = 100 centipoise (cp) = 0.1 Pascal-sec

Volume:

1 cm^3 (cc) = 1 milliliter (ml)
1 m^3 = 10^3 liters = 10^6 cm^3 = 10^{18} micron^3 = 10^{27} nm^3
1 cm^3 = 10^{12} micron^3= 10^{21} nm^3 = 10^{-6} m^3 = 10^{-3} liters
1 micron^3 = 10^9 nm^3 = 10^{-18} m^3 = 10^{-15} liters = 10^{-12} cm^3
1 nm^3 = 10^{-27} m^3 = 10^{-24} liters = 10^{-21} cm^3 = 10^{-9} micron^3
1 liter = 0.001 m^3 = 1000 cm^3 = 10^{15} micron^3 = 10^{24} nm^3
1 dram (U.S. fluid) = 3.696588 cm^3 = 1.040843 drachms (Brit.)
= 60 minims = 0.125 U.S. fluid ounces
1 teaspoon ~ 60 drops ~ 5 cm^3
1 cup = 1 glass = 8 fl. oz. = 16 tablespoons = 48 teaspoons
1 ft^3 = 1728 inch^3 = 28,316.847 cm^3 = 0.037037037 yd^3
1 gallon (U.S. liq.) = 3785.4118 cm^3 = 0.133680555 ft^3
= 4 quarts = 8 pints = 16 cups = 128 fl. oz. (U.S.)
1 barrel (U.S. petroleum) = 158.9873 liters
1 acre-foot = 1233.4818 m^3

III. Mathematical and Physical Constants

Absolute viscosity:

Water, 310 K: 0.6915 x 10^{-3} kg/m-sec
Blood plasma, 310 K: 1.1 x 10^{-3} kg/m-sec

Acceleration of gravity:

g = 9.780 39 m/sec^2 (sea level at equator)
g = 9.806 21 m/sec^2 (sea level at 45° latitude)
g = 9.832 17 m/sec^2 (sea level at 90° latitude)

Acoustic impedance:

Water: 1.5 x 10^6 kg/m^2-sec
Nylon: 2.9 x 10^6 kg/m^2-sec
Diamond: 6.3 x 10^7 kg/m^2-sec

Albedo

Earth, mean: 31%

Angular momentum:
proton (quantized spin): 5.28×10^{-35} J-sec

Areal number density:
C atoms, monoatomic graphite sheet: ~38.2 /nm^2

Atmosphere, Earth:

N_2	78.084% (by volume)
O_2	20.946%
H_2O	0.01% (arctic) - 3% (tropical)
Ar	0.00934%
CO_2	0.00031%

Atom and ion diameters (approx.):

H	0.060 nm
F	0.128 nm
O	0.132 nm
N	0.140 nm
C	0.154 nm
He	0.186 nm
Na^+	0.190 nm
S	0.208 nm
P	0.220 nm
Ne	0.224 nm
F^-	0.272 nm
O^{--}	0.280 nm
S^{--}	0.368 nm
Na	0.372 nm
K	0.462 nm
Fr	0.544 nm

Atomic mass unit (amu):
1.661×10^{-27} kg (1/12th of C^{12} nuclide mass)

Avogadro's number:
$N_A = 6.02257 \times 10^{23}$ molecules/mole

Bandgap:

Silicon:	1.12 eV
Diamond:	5.47 eV

Bohr radius: $5.291\ 772\ 49 \times 10^{-11}$ m

Boltzmann's constant:
k = $1.380\ 658 \times 10^{-23}$ J/molecule-K
= 8.625×10^{-5} eV/molecule-K

Bond energy (covalent, dissociation): 556 zJ (C-C)

Bond length:

C-C in graphite:	0.141 5 nm
C-C in diamond:	0.154 448 nm

Breakdown voltage, electrical:

Air:	$1\text{-}3 \times 10^6$	volts/m
Porcelain:	4×10^6	volts/m
Titanium dioxide:	$3.9\text{-}8.3 \times 10^6$	volts/m
Paraffin, 25°C:	9.8×10^6	volts/m
Pyrex glass:	1.3×10^7	volts/m
Paper:	1.4×10^7	volts/m
Nylon, 20°C:	1.9×10^7	volts/m
Rubber, hard, 25°C:	1.9×10^7	volts/m
Polystyrene:	$2.0\text{-}2.8 \times 10^7$	volts/m
Teflon:	6×10^7	volts/m
Ruby mica:	1.6×10^8	volts/m
SiC:	4×10^8	volts/m
Diamond:	2×10^9	volts/m

Bulk modulus, diamond: K = $(4.4\text{-}5.9) \times 10^{11}$ N/m^2

Cleavage energy:

Diamond {111} crystal plane:	10.6	J/m^2
Diamond {110} crystal plane:	13.0	J/m^2
Diamond {100} crystal plane:	18.4	J/m^2

Compressibility, diamond: 1.7×10^{-11} m^2/kg

Crack velocity:

Soda-lime glass (maximum):	1580 m/sec
Sapphire (maximum):	4500 m/sec
Diamond (maximum):	7200 m/sec

Density:

H_2, STP:	0.0899 kg/m^3
He, STP:	0.1785 kg/m^3
Air, 1 atm, 20°C:	1.205 kg/m^3
Air, STP:	1.2929 kg/m^3
N_2 at 1000 atm, 37°C:	493 kg/m^3
O_2 at 1000 atm, 37°C:	672 kg/m^3
CO_2 at 1000 atm, 37°C:	816 kg/m^3
Crude oil:	862 kg/m^3
CO_2 at 1000 atm, 37°C:	816 kg/m^3 (137 kg/barrel)
Water-ice, STP:	917 kg/m^3
Water, 100°C:	958.384 kg/m^3
Water, 37°C:	993.360 kg/m^3
Water, 0°C:	999.868 kg/m^3
Water, 4°C:	1000.000 kg/m^3
Blood plasma, 37°C:	1025 kg/m^3
Glucose:	1562 kg/m^3
Silicon, 25°C:	2330 kg/m^3
Boron:	2340 kg/m^3
Quartz:	2650 kg/m^3
Diamond:	3510 kg/m^3
Sapphire:	3970 kg/m^3
Germanium, 25°C:	5323 kg/m^3
Earth (mean):	5522 kg/m^3
Gadolinium:	7895 kg/m^3
Polonium:	9320 kg/m^3
Silver, 20°C:	10,500 kg/m^3
Lead, 20°C:	11,350 kg/m^3
Gold, 20°C:	19,320 kg/m^3
Platinum, 20°C:	21,450 kg/m^3

Dielectric constant:

Vacuum:	1.00000
Air:	1.00059
Paraffin, 25°C:	2.0-2.5
Teflon:	2.1
Polystyrene:	2.4-2.65
Rubber, hard, 25°C:	2.8

Nylon, 25°C:	3.5
Paper:	3.5
Pyrex glass:	4.5
Diamond, 300 K:	5.7
Porcelain:	6.5
Sapphire:	9.0
SiC:	9.0
Ruby, parallel to optical axis:	11.28
Silicon:	12.0
Ruby, normal to optical axis:	13.27
Ethanol, 25°C:	24.3
Glycerol, 25°C:	42.5
Water, pure, 37°C K:	74.31
Water-ice, 0°C:	88.0
Titanium dioxide:	100.0

Distance between adjacent graphite sheets: 0.335 nm

e: 2.718 281 828 459

Electron mobility:

Diamond (holes):	0.12 m^2/volt-sec
Silicon:	0.15 m^2/volt-sec
Diamond:	0.18-0.19 m^2/volt-sec

Electron-volt: $1.602\ 177\ 33 \times 10^{-19}$ J

Elementary charge: $1.602\ 177\ 33 \times 10^{-19}$ coulomb

Energy content:

Glucose (burned in pure oxygen at 100% efficiency): 4.765×10^{-18} J/molecule

Sugar: ~26 Kcal (~10^5 J) per "lump"

Faraday constant: 96,487.0 coulomb/mole

Gravitational constant: $G = 6.67259 \times 10^{-11}$ N-m^2/kg^2

Gyromagnetic ratio, protons: 4.26×10^7 Hz/tesla

Heat capacity (C_V):

Air, room temp.:	1.19×10^3 J/m^3-K
Water-ice, 77 K:	0.63×10^6 J/m^3-K
Water-ice, 249 K:	1.76×10^6 J/m^3-K
Diamond:	1.82×10^6 J/m^3-K
Water-ice, 271 K:	1.93×10^6 J/m^3-K
Platinum, 298 K:	2.84×10^6 J/m^3-K
Sapphire:	2.89×10^6 J/m^3-K
Water, 310 K:	4.19×10^6 J/m^3-K

Heat of fusion:

Water, 1 atm, 0°C: 3.34×10^8 J/m^3 (79.7 cal/gm)

Heat of vaporization:

Water, 1 atm, 100°C: 2.17×10^9 J/m^3 (539 cal/gm)

Hemoglobin:

Atom count, per molecule:	~10,000	atoms/molecule
Free Hb, phagocytic half-life:	10-30	minutes
Molecular weight:	~67,000	daltons
Molecule count, per red cell:	~2.7×10^8	molecules/RBC

Lattice spacing at 300 K:

Diamond:	0.356 683 nm
Silicon:	0.543 095 nm
Germanium:	0.564 613 nm
Tin, grey:	0.648 920 nm

Magnetic moment:

Electron:	9.2732×10^{-24} J/tesla (Bohr magneton)
Proton:	1.41049×10^{-26} J/tesla

Mass, particle:

Electron rest mass:	$m_e = 9.109\ 389\ 7 \times 10^{-31}$ kg
Proton rest mass:	$m_p = 1.672\ 623\ 1 \times 10^{-27}$ kg
Neutron rest mass:	$m_n = 1.674\ 928\ 6 \times 10^{-27}$ kg

Mass, planetary:

Atmosphere (Earth):	5.27×10^{18} kg
Oceans (Earth):	1.36×10^{21} kg
Moon:	7.34×10^{22} kg
Earth:	5.98×10^{24} kg
Jupiter:	1.90×10^{27} kg
Sun:	1.97×10^{30} kg

Molar volume of ideal gas at STP:

0.022 414 10 m^3/mole
37.22 nm^3/molecule
0.02687 molecule/nm^3

Molecular mass:

Diamond:	1.99×10^{-26} kg/atom
Water:	2.99×10^{-26} kg/molecule
N_2:	4.65×10^{-26} kg/molecule
O_2:	5.32×10^{-26} kg/molecule
CO_2:	7.31×10^{-26} kg/molecule
Glucose:	2.99×10^{-25} kg/molecule

Molecular number density:

Glucose, solid:	5.24 molecules/nm^3
N_2 at 1000 atm:	10.6 molecules/nm^3
CO_2 at 1000 atm:	11.1 molecules/nm^3
O_2 at 1000 atm:	12.6 molecules/nm^3
Water-ice at 273 K:	~30 molecules/nm^3
Water, liquid:	33.4 molecules/nm^3
Diamond:	~176 carbons/nm^3

Molecular volume:

Diamond:	0.00567 nm^3/atom
Water, liquid:	0.0299 nm^3/molecule
O_2 at 1000 atm:	0.0791 nm^3/molecule
CO_2 at 1000 atm:	0.0897 nm^3/molecule
N_2 at 1000 atm:	0.0943 nm^3/molecule
Glucose, solid:	0.1910 nm^3/molecule

Permeability (magnetic) constant:

$\mu_0 = 1.256\ 637\ 061\ 4 \times 10^{-6}$ henry/m

Permittivity (electric) constant:

$\varepsilon_0 = 8.854\ 187\ 817 \times 10^{-12}$ farad/m

π: 3.141 592 653 589

Planck's constant:

$h = 6.626\ 075\ 5 \times 10^{-34}$ J-sec

$\hbar = h / 2\pi = 1.054\ 572\ 7 \times 10^{-34}$ J-sec

Power dissipation, global:

Human physiological worldwide:	5.3×10^{11} W (in 1998)
Human technological worldwide:	1.2×10^{13} W (in 1998)
Earth vegetation worldwide:	1.4×10^{14} W

Radius, particle:

Proton (Compton wavelength):	1.3214×10^{-15} m
Electron (classical):	2.81777×10^{-15} m

Radius, mean planetary:

Moon:	1.738×10^{6} m
Earth:	6.371×10^{6} m
Jupiter:	6.988×10^{7} m
Sun:	6.938×10^{8} m
Earth-Moon orbit:	3.80×10^{8} m
Earth-Sun orbit:	1.496×10^{11} m

Refractive index at λ = 589.29 nm (Na):

Air, STP, rel. to vacuum:	1.0002926
Water-Ice:	1.3104
Water, pure, 37°C:	1.33093
Water, pure, 20°C:	1.33299
Ethanol, 99.8%, 37°C:	1.35348
Sucrose, 25% aq. solution, 20°C:	1.3723
Sucrose, 50% aq. solution, 20°C:	1.4200
Quartz, fused, 18°C:	1.45845
Sucrose, 75% aq. solution, 20°C:	1.4774
Sucrose, 75% aq. solution, 30°C:	1.4793
Rock salt:	1.544
Glass:	1.52-1.89
Diamond:	2.41726

Resistivity:

Diamond, synthesized:	10^{7}-10^{8} ohm-m
Diamondoid materials:	up to 10^{10} ohm-m
Diamond, natural, dark:	up to 10^{18} ohm-m

Rest mass energy:

$(mc^2/m) = 8.99 \times 10^{16}$ J/kg

Saturation velocity (electronic), diamond: 2.7×10^{5} m/sec

Shear modulus, diamond: $G = (4.8\text{-}5.5) \times 10^{11}$ N/m²

Solar constant (at Earth): 1370 W/m²

Solar luminosity (mean, total): 3.92×10^{26} W

Speed of light in vacuo:

$c = 2.99\ 792\ 458 \times 10^{8}$ m/sec

Speed of sound:

Air, dry, STP:	331.36 m/sec
Water, 15°C:	1450 m/sec
Water, 37°C:	1500 m/sec
Sapphire:	10,000 m/sec
Diamond:	17,300 m/sec

Standard atmosphere: 1.01325×10^{5} N/m² (760 mmHg)

Standard molar gas volume at STP: 22.4141 liter-atm/mole

Standard temperature and pressure (STP): 273.15 K and 1 atm

Stefan-Boltzmann constant: $\sigma = 5.6697 \times 10^{-8}$ W/m²-K⁴

Surface area, Earth: 5.10×10^{14} m²

Surface energy of graphite: 0.234 J/m²

Thermal conductivity (K_t):

Air, 1 atm, 290 K:	0.02524 W/m-K
Glass wool, 293 K:	0.038 W/m-K
Cork, 293 K:	0.042 W/m-K
Wood, 293 K:	0.10 W/m-K
Water, 273 K:	0.561 W/m-K
Water, 310 K:	0.623 W/m-K
Water, 373 K:	0.681 W/m-K
Brick, 293 K:	0.71 W/m-K
Water-ice, 270 K:	1.56 W/m-K
Water-ice, 249 K:	2.21 W/m-K
Sapphire:	
normal to c-axis, 310 K:	2-20 W/m-K
parallel to c-axis, 310 K:	20-40 W/m-K
Lead, 293 K:	35 W/m-K
Platinum, 300 K:	73 W/m-K
Iron, 300 K:	80.3 W/m-K
Aluminum, 300 K:	237 W/m-K
Gold, 300 K:	315 W/m-K
Silver, 300 K:	427 W/m-K
Diamond, natural, 293 K:	2000 W/m-K
Diamond, pure C^{12}, 293 K:	3500 W/m-K
Diamond, natural, 65 K:	17,500 W/m-K

Thermal emissivity (e_r):

Silver, polished:	0.02
Aluminum:	0.022-0.08
Platinum:	0.037-0.05
Porcelain:	0.25-0.50
Brass:	0.60
Water:	0.67
Earth's surface, mean:	0.69
Glass:	0.76-0.94
Cotton cloth:	0.77
Wood:	0.80-0.90
Corundum, emory, 80°C:	0.86
Snow:	0.89
Paper:	0.93
Asphalt pavement:	0.93
Concrete, rough:	0.94
Water-ice:	0.97
Human skin:	0.97-0.99
Carbon black:	0.97-0.99

Thermal expansion coefficient, linear:

Diamond, 293 K:	0.8×10^{-6}/K
Glass, pyrex, 273-373 K:	3.6×10^{-6}/K
Sapphire, normal to c-axis, 293 K:	4.5×10^{-6}/K
Sapphire, parallel to c-axis, 293 K:	5.5×10^{-6}/K
Glass, ordinary, 273-373 K:	8.9×10^{-6}/K
Platinum, 273-373 K:	9.0×10^{-6}/K
Steel, 273-373 K:	12.0×10^{-6}/K
Marble, 273-373 K:	11.7×10^{-6}/K
Copper, 273-373 K:	14.1×10^{-6}/K
Brass, 273-373 K:	19.3×10^{-6}/K
Aluminum, 273-373 K:	23.8×10^{-6}/K
Lead, 273-373 K:	29×10^{-6}/K
Water-ice, 363-373 K:	51×10^{-6}/K
Hard rubber, 273-373 K:	80×10^{-6}/K

Thermal expansion coefficient, volumetric:

Vitreous silica, 298 K:	1.2×10^{-6}/K
Diamond, 298 K:	3.5×10^{-6}/K
Silicon, 298 K:	7.5×10^{-6}/K
Silicon carbide, 298 K:	11.1×10^{-6}/K
Sapphire, 298 K:	15.6×10^{-6}/K
Crystalline silica or quartz, 298 K:	36×10^{-6}/K

Universal gas constant:

$R_{gas} = 8.206 \times 10^{-5}$ m^3-atm/mole-K
= 8.314 510 J/mole-K
= 1.99 cal/mole-K

Year, tropical, in ephemeris (mean solar) seconds:

$3.155\ 692\ 6 \times 10^7$ sec

Young's modulus:

Sapphire:	$E = 4.0 \times 10^{11}$ N/m^2
Diamond:	$E = 1.05 \times 10^{12}$ N/m^2

APPENDIX B

Appendix B. Concentrations of Human Blood Components
(compiled and adapted from References 749, 753–757, 825, 1019, 1604, 1712, 2223).

Component	In Whole Blood (gm/cm^3)	In Plasma or Serum (gm/cm^3)
Water	0.81-0.86	0.93-0.95
Acetoacetate	8-40 x 10^{-7}	4-43 x 10^{-7}
Acetone		3-20 x 10^{-6}
Acetylcholine		6.6-8.2 x 10^{-8}
Adenosine triphosphate		
- total	3.1-5.7 x 10^{-4}	
- phosphorus	5-10 x 10^{-5}	
Adrenocorticotrophic hormone		2.5-12 x 10^{-11}
- @ 6AM, mean		5.5 x 10^{-11}
- @ 6AM, maximum		<12 x 10^{-11}
- @ 6PM, mean		3.5 x 10^{-11}
- @ 6PM, maximum		<7.5 x 10^{-11}
Alanine	2.7-5.5 x 10^{-5}	2.4-7.6 x 10^{-5}
Albumin		3.5-5.2 x 10^{-2}
Aluminum	1-40 x 10^{-8}	1-88 x 10^{-8}
Aldosterone		
- supine		3-10 x 10^{-11}
- standing, male		6-22 x 10^{-11}
- standing, female		5-30 x 10^{-11}
Amino acids		
- total	3.8-5.3 x 10^{-4}	
- nitrogen	4.6-6.8 x 10^{-5}	3.0-5.5 x 10^{-5}
α-Aminobutyric acid	1-2 x 10^{-6}	1-2 x 10^{-6}
δ-Aminolevulinic acid		1.5-2.3 x 10^{-7}
Ammonia nitrogen	1-2 x 10^{-6}	1.0-4.9 x 10^{-7}
AMP, cyclic		
- male		5.6-10.9 x 10^{-9}
- female		3.6-8.9 x 10^{-9}
Androstenedione		
- male >18 yrs		2-30 x 10^{-10}
- female >18 yrs		8-30 x 10^{-10}
Androsterone		1.5 x 10^{-7}
Angiotensin I		1.1-8.8 x 10^{-11}
Angiotensin II (Renin)		1.2-3.6 x 10^{-11}
α-Antitrypsin		7.8-20 x 10^{-4}
Arginine	6-17 x 10^{-6}	1.3-3.6 x 10^{-5}
Arsenic		
- normal range	2-62 x 10^{-9}	
- chronic poisoning	100-500 x 10^{-9}	
- acute poisoning	600-9300 x 10^{-9}	

Component	In Whole Blood (gm/cm^3)	In Plasma or Serum (gm/cm^3)
Ascorbic acid (Vitamin C)	1-15 x 10^{-6}	6-20 x 10^{-6}
Aspartic acid		0-3 x 10^{-6}
Aspartic acid (in WBCs)	2.5-4.0 x 10^{-4}	9-12 x 10^{-6}
Bicarbonate		5-5.7 x 10^{-4}
Bile acids	2-30 x 10^{-6}	3-30 x 10^{-6}
Bilirubin	2-14 x 10^{-6}	1-10 x 10^{-6}
Biotin (Vitamin H)	7-17 x 10^{-9}	9-16 x 10^{-9}
Blood Urea Nitrogen (BUN)		8-23 x 10^{-5}
Bradykinin		7 x 10^{-11}
Bromide		7-10 x 10^{-9}
Cadmium		
- normal	1-5 x 10^{-9}	
- toxic	0.1-3 x 10^{-6}	
Calciferol (Vitamin D_2)		1.7-4.1 x 10^{-8}
Calcitonin (CT)		<1.0 x 10^{-10}
Calcium		
- ionized	4.48-4.92 x 10^{-5}	4.25-5.25 x 10^{-5}
- total		8.4-11.5 x 10^{-5}
Carbon dioxide (respiratory gas)		
-arterial	8.8-10.8 x 10^{-4}	3.0-7.9 x 10^{-5}
-venous	9.8-11.8 x 10^{-4}	3.3-8.3 x 10^{-5}
Carbon monoxide (as HbCO)		
- nonsmokers	0.5-1.5% total Hb	
- smokers, 1-2 packs/day	4-5% total Hb	
- smokers, 2 packs/day	8-9% total Hb	
- toxic	>20% total Hb	
- lethal	>50% total Hb	
Carcinoembryonic antigen		<2.5 x 10^{-9}
β-Carotene		3-25 x 10^{-7}
Carotenoids	2.4-23.1 x 10^{-7}	
Cephalin	3-11.5 x 10^{-4}	0-1 x 10^{-4}
Ceruloplasmin		1.5-6 x 10^{-4}
Chloride, as NaCl	4.5-5 x 10^{-3}	3.5-3.8 x 10^{-3}

Component	In Whole Blood (gm/cm³)	In Plasma or Serum (gm/cm³)
Cholecalciferol (Vitamin D3)		
- 1, 25-dihydroxy		$2.5\text{-}4.5 \times 10^{-11}$
- 24,25-dihydroxy		1.5×10^{-9}
- 25-hydroxy		$1.4\text{-}8 \times 10^{-8}$
Cholecystokinin (pancreozymin)		6.04×10^{-11}
Cholesterol		
-LDLC		$0.5\text{-}2.0 \times 10^{-3}$
-HDLC		$2.9\text{-}9.0 \times 10^{-4}$
-total	$1.15\text{-}2.25 \times 10^{-3}$	$1.2\text{-}2 \times 10^{-3}$
Choline, total	$1.1\text{-}3.1 \times 10^{-4}$	$3.6\text{-}3.5 \times 10^{-4}$
Chorionic gonadotropin		
- Menstrual		$0\text{-}3 \times 10^{-11}$
- Pregnancy, 1st trimester		$5\text{-}3300 \times 10^{-10}$
- Pregnancy, 2nd trimester		$20\text{-}1000 \times 10^{-10}$
- Pregnancy, 3rd trimester		$20\text{-}50 \times 10^{-10}$
- Menopausal		$3\text{-}30 \times 10^{-11}$
Citric acid	$1.3\text{-}2.5 \times 10^{-5}$	$1.6\text{-}3.2 \times 10^{-5}$
Citrulline		$2\text{-}10 \times 10^{-6}$
Clotting Factors		
- I Fibrinogen	$1.2\text{-}1.6 \times 10^{-3}$	$2\text{-}4 \times 10^{-3}$
- II Prothrombin		1×10^{-4}
- III Tissue thromboplastin		1×10^{-6}
- V Proaccelerin		$5\text{-}12 \times 10^{-6}$
- VII Proconvertin		1×10^{-6}
- VIII Antihemophilic factor		1×10^{-7}
- IX Christmas factor		4×10^{-6}
- X Stuart factor		5×10^{-6}
- XI Plasma thrmb. anteced.		4×10^{-6}
- XII Hageman factor		2.9×10^{-5}
- XIII Fibrin stabiliz. factor		1×10^{-5}
- Fibrin split products		$<1 \times 10^{-5}$
- Fletcher factor		5×10^{-5}
- Fitzgerald factor		7×10^{-5}
- von Willebrand factor		7×10^{-6}
Cobalamin (Vitamin B_{12})	$6\text{-}14 \times 10^{-10}$	$1\text{-}10 \times 10^{-10}$
Cocarboxylase		$7\text{-}9 \times 10^{-8}$
Complement		
- C1q		$5.8\text{-}7.2 \times 10^{-5}$
- C1r		$2.5\text{-}3.8 \times 10^{-5}$
- C1s (C1 esterase)		$2.5\text{-}3.8 \times 10^{-5}$
- C2		$2.2\text{-}3.4 \times 10^{-5}$
- C3 (β_1C-globulin)		$8\text{-}15.5 \times 10^{-4}$
- Factor B (C3 proactivator)		$2\text{-}4.5 \times 10^{-4}$
- C4 (β_1E-globulin)		$1.3\text{-}3.7 \times 10^{-4}$
- C4 binding protein		$1.8\text{-}3.2 \times 10^{-4}$
- C5 (β_1F-globulin)		$5.1\text{-}7.7 \times 10^{-5}$
- C6		$4.8\text{-}6.4 \times 10^{-5}$
- C7		$4.9\text{-}7 \times 10^{-5}$
- C8		$4.3\text{-}6.3 \times 10^{-5}$
- C9		$4.7\text{-}6.9 \times 10^{-5}$
- Properdin		$2.4\text{-}3.2 \times 10^{-5}$
Compound S		$1\text{-}3 \times 10^{-9}$

Component	In Whole Blood (gm/cm³)	In Plasma or Serum (gm/cm³)
Copper	$9\text{-}15 \times 10^{-7}$	
- male		$7\text{-}14 \times 10^{-7}$
- female		$8\text{-}15.5 \times 10^{-7}$
Corticosteroids (male & female)		$1\text{-}4 \times 10^{-6}$
Corticosterone		$4\text{-}20 \times 10^{-9}$
Cortisol		$3\text{-}23 \times 10^{-8}$
- 8 AM		$6\text{-}23 \times 10^{-8}$
- 4 PM		$3\text{-}15 \times 10^{-8}$
- 10 PM		~50% of 8 AM value
C-peptide		
- fasting		$0.5\text{-}2.0 \times 10^{-9}$
- maximum		4×10^{-9}
C-reactive protein		$6.8\text{-}820 \times 10^{-8}$
Creatine		
- male		$1.7\text{-}5.0 \times 10^{-6}$
- female		$3.5\text{-}9.3 \times 10^{-6}$
Creatinine	$1\text{-}2 \times 10^{-5}$	$5\text{-}15 \times 10^{-6}$
- male		$0.8\text{-}1.5 \times 10^{-5}$
- female		$0.7\text{-}1.2 \times 10^{-5}$
Cyanide		
- nonsmokers		4×10^{-9}
- smokers		6×10^{-9}
- nitroprusside therapy		$10\text{-}60 \times 10^{-9}$
- toxic		$>100 \times 10^{-9}$
- lethal		$>1000 \times 10^{-9}$
Cystine	$6\text{-}12 \times 10^{-6}$	$1.8\text{-}5 \times 10^{-5}$
Dehydroepiandrosterone DHEA		
- aged 1-4 yrs		$0.2\text{-}0.4 \times 10^{-9}$
- aged 4-8 yrs		$0.1\text{-}1.9 \times 10^{-9}$
- aged 8-10 yrs		$0.2\text{-}2.9 \times 10^{-9}$
- aged 10-12 yrs		$0.5\text{-}9.2 \times 10^{-9}$
- aged 12-14 yrs		$0.9\text{-}20 \times 10^{-9}$
- aged 14-16 yrs		$2.5\text{-}20 \times 10^{-9}$
- male		$0.8\text{-}10 \times 10^{-9}$
- female, premenopausal		$2.0\text{-}15 \times 10^{-9}$
DHEA sulfate (male)		$1.99\text{-}3.34 \times 10^{-6}$
DHEA sulfate (female)		
- newborn		$1.67\text{-}3.64 \times 10^{-6}$
- pre-pubertal children		$1.0\text{-}6.0 \times 10^{-7}$
- premenopausal		$8.2\text{-}33.8 \times 10^{-7}$
- pregnancy		$2.3\text{-}11.7 \times 10^{-7}$
- postmenopausal		$1.1\text{-}6.1 \times 10^{-7}$
11-Deoxycortisol		$1\text{-}7 \times 10^{-8}$
Dihydrotestosterone (DHT)		
- male		$3\text{-}8 \times 10^{-9}$
- female		$1\text{-}10 \times 10^{-10}$
Diphosphoglycerate (phosphate)	$8\text{-}16 \times 10^{-5}$	
DNA		$0\text{-}1.6 \times 10^{-5}$
Dopamine		$<1.36 \times 10^{-10}$
Enzymes, total		$<6 \times 10^{-5}$
Epidermal growth factor (EGF)		$<1 \times 10^{-11}$
Epinephrine		
- after 15 min rest		$3.1\text{-}9.5 \times 10^{-11}$
- when emitted	3.8×10^{-9}	$2\text{-}2.5 \times 10^{-9}$
Ergothioneine	$1\text{-}20 \times 10^{-5}$	

Component	In Whole Blood (gm/cm^3)	In Plasma or Serum (gm/cm^3)
Erythrocytes ($\#/cm^3$)		
- adult male, avg. (range)	5.2 (4.6-6.2) x 10^9	
- adult female, avg. (range)	4.6 (4.2-5.4) x 10^9	
- children, varies with age	4.5-5.1 x 10^9	
- reticulocytes	25-75 x 10^6	
Erythropoietin		
- adult, normal		0.5-2.5 x 10^{-10}
- pregnant		2.7-6.2 x 10^{-10}
- hypoxia or anemia		0.8-8.0 x 10^{-8}
Estradiol (E_2) (male)		8-36 x 10^{-12}
Estradiol (E_2) (female)		
- follicular (days 1-10)		1-9 x 10^{-11}
- mean		5 x 10^{-11}
- pre-fertile (days 10-12)		10-15 x 10^{-11}
- fertile (days 12-14)		35-60 x 10^{-11}
- luteal (days 15-28)		20-40 x 10^{-11}
- pregnancy		3-70 x 10^{-7}
- postmenopausal		1-3 x 10^{-11}
Estriol (E_3)		
- nonpregnant		<2 x 10^{-9}
- pregnancy, weeks 22-30		3-5 x 10^{-9}
- pregnancy, weeks 32-37		6-11 x 10^{-9}
- pregnancy, weeks 38-41		25-170 x 10^{-9}
Estrogen (male)		4-11.5 x 10^{-11}
Estrogen (female)		
- prepubertal		<4 x 10^{-11}
- 1-10 days		6.1-39.4 x 10^{-11}
- 11-20 days		12.2-43.7 x 10^{-11}
- 21-30 days		15.6-35 x 10^{-11}
- postmenopausal		<4 x 10^{-11}
Estrone (E_1)		
- male		2.9-17 x 10^{-11}
- female, follicular		2-15 x 10^{-11}
- female, 1-10 days of cycle		4.3-18 x 10^{-11}
- female, 11-20 days of cycle		7.5-19.6 x 10^{-11}
- female, 20-29 days of cycle		13.1-20.1 x 10^{-11}
- pregnancy, weeks 22-30		3-5 x 10^{-9}
- pregnancy, weeks 32-37		5-6 x 10^{-9}
- pregnancy, weeks 38-41		7-10 x 10^{-9}
Ethanol		
- social high		0.5 x 10^{-3}
- reduced coordination		0.8 x 10^{-3}
- depression of CNS		>1 x 10^{-3}
- confusion, falling down		2.0 x 10^{-3}
- loss of consciousness		3.0 x 10^{-3}
- coma, death		>4 x 10^{-3}
Fat, neutral (see Triglycerides)		
Fatty acids, nonesterified (free)		8-25 x 10^{-5}
Fatty acids, esterified	2.5-3.9 x 10^{-3}	7-20 x 10^{-5}
Fatty acids, total		1.9-4.5 x 10^{-3}
Ferritin		
- male		1.5-30 x 10^{-8}
- female		0.9-18 x 10^{-8}

Component	In Whole Blood (gm/cm^3)	In Plasma or Serum (gm/cm^3)
α_1-Fetoprotein		0-2 x 10^{-8}
Flavine adenine dinucleotide		8-12 x 10^{-8}
Fluoride	1-4.5 x 10^{-7}	1-4.5 x 10^{-7}
Folate		2.2-17.3 x 10^{-9}
- in erythrocyte		1.67-7.07 x 10^{-7}
Folic acid (Vitamin M)	2.3-5.2 x 10^{-8}	1.6-2 x 10^{-8}
Fructose	0-5 x 10^{-5}	7-8 x 10^{-5}
Furosemide glucuronide		1-400 x 10^{-6}
Galactose (children)		<2 x 10^{-4}
Gastric inhibitory peptide (GIP)		<1.25-4.0 x 10^{-10}
Gastrin		
- mean		7 x 10^{-11}
- maximum		<20 x 10^{-11}
Globulin, total		2.2-4 x 10^{-2}
α_1-Globulin		1-4 x 10^{-3}
α_2-Globulin		4-10 x 10^{-3}
β-Globulin		5-12 x 10^{-3}
γ-Globulin		6-17 x 10^{-3}
Glucagon		
- range		5-15 x 10^{-11}
- mean		7.1-7.9 x 10^{-11}
Glucosamine		
- fetus	4-6 x 10^{-4}	4.2-5.5 x10^{-4}
- child	5-7 x 10^{-4}	5.2-6.9 x 10^{-4}
- adult	6-8 x 10^{-4}	6.1-8.2 x 10^{-4}
- aged	7-9 x 10^{-4}	7.0-8.9 x 10^{-4}
Glucose		
- newborn	2-3 x 10^{-4}	
- adult	6.5-9.5 x 10^{-4}	7-10.5 x 10^{-4}
- diabetic	14-120 x 10^{-4}	
Glucuronic acid	4.1-9.3 x 10^{-5}	8-11 x 10^{-6}
Glutamic acid		2-28 x 10^{-6}
Glutamine		4.6-10.6 x 10^{-5}
Glutathione, reduced	2.5-4.1 x 10^{-4}	0
Glycerol, free		2.9-17.2 x 10^{-6}
Glycine	1.7-2.3 x 10^{-5}	8-54 x 10^{-6}
Glycogen	1.2-16.2 x 10^{-5}	0
Glycoprotein, acid		4-15 x 10^{-4}
GMP, cyclic		0.6-4.4 x 10^{-9}
Gonadotropic releasing hormone		1-80 x 10^{-12}
Guanidine	1.8-2.3 x 10^{-6}	
Haptoglobin		3-22 x 10^{-4}
Hemoglobin	1.2-1.75 x 10^{-1}	1-4 x 10^{-5}
- newborn	1.65-1.95 x 10^{-1}	
- children, varies with age	1.12-1.65 x 10^{-1}	
- adult, male	1.4-1.8 x 10^{-1}	
- adult, female	1.2-1.6 x 10^{-1}	
- inside erythrocyte	~3.3 x 10^{-1}	
- per red blood cell	27-32 picograms	
Hexosephosphate P	1.4-5 x 10^{-5}	0-2 x 10^{-6}
Histamine	6.7-8.6 x 10^{-8}	
Histidine	9-17 x 10^{-6}	1.1-3.8 x 10^{-5}
Hydrogen ion (pH 7.4)	4 x 10^{-11}	
β-Hydroxybutyric acid	1-6 x 10^{-6}	1-9 x 10^{-6}
17-Hydroxycorticosteroids	4-10 x 10^{-8}	

Component	In Whole Blood (gm/cm^3)	In Plasma or Serum (gm/cm^3)
17-Hydroxyprogesterone, - male		20-250 x 10^{-11}
17-Hydroxyprogesterone		
- female:		
- follicular		20-80 x 10^{-11}
- luteal		80-300 x 10^{-11}
- postmenopausal		4-50 x 10^{-11}
17-Hydroxyprogesterone		
- child		20-140 x 10^{-11}
Immunoglobin A (IgA)		5-39 x 10^{-4}
Immunoglobin D (IgD)		0.5-8.0 x 10^{-5}
Immunoglobin G (IgG)		5.0-19 x 10^{-3}
Immunoglobin M (IgM)		3.0-30 x 10^{-4}
Immunoglobin E (IgE)		<5 x 10^{-7}
Indican		8-50 x 10^{-7}
Inositol		3-7 x 10^{-6}
Insulin		2.0-8.4 x 10^{-10}
Insulin-like growth factor I		9.9-50 x 10^{-8}
Iodine, total	2.4-3.2 x 10^{-8}	4.5-14.5 x 10^{-8}
Iron, adult	4-6 x 10^{-4}	6-18 x 10^{-7}
Isoleucine	9-15 x 10^{-6}	1.2-4.2 x 10^{-5}
Ketone bodies	2.3-10 x 10^{-6}	1.5-30 x 10^{-6}
α-Ketonic acids, adult	1-30 x 10^{-6}	
L-Lactate		
- arterial	<11.3 x 10^{-5}	4.5-14.4 x 10^{-5}
- venous	8.1-15.3 x 10^{-5}	4.5-19.8 x 10^{-5}
Lead		
- normal	1-5 x 10^{-7}	1-7.8 x 10^{-8}
- toxic	>6-10 x 10^{-7}	
Lecithin	1.1-1.2 x 10^{-3}	1-2.25 x 10^{-3}
Leptin	1.2 x 10^{-8}	
Leucine	1.4-2 x 10^{-5}	1.2-5.2 x 10^{-5}
Leukocytes (#/cm^3)		
Total:		
- birth	9.0-30.0 x 10^{6}	
- pediatric	4.5-15.5 x 10^{6}	
- adult, range	4.3-11.0 x 10^{6}	
- adult, median	7.0 x 10^{6}	
Neutrophils: birth	6.0-26.0 x 10^{6}	
- pediatric	1.5-8.5 x 10^{6}	
- adult, range	1.83-7.25 x 10^{6}	
- adult, median	3.65 x 10^{6}	
Eosinophils: birth	0.4 x 10^{6}	
- pediatric	0.2-0.3 x 10^{6}	
- adult, range	0.05-0.7 x 10^{6}	
- adult, median	0.15 x 10^{6}	
Basophils: adult, range	0.015-0.15 x 10^{6}	
- adult, median	0.03 x 10^{6}	
Lymphocytes: birth	2-11 x 10^{6}	
- pediatric	1.5-8.0 x 10^{6}	
- adult, range	1.5-4.0 x 10^{6}	
- adult, median	2.5 x 10^{6}	
Monocytes: birth, range	0.4-3.1 x 10^{6}	
- birth, median	1.05 x 10^{6}	
- pediatric	0.4 x 10^{6}	
- adult, range	0.21-1.05 x 10^{6}	
- adult, median	0.43 x 10^{6}	

Component	In Whole Blood (gm/cm^3)	In Plasma or Serum (gm/cm^3)
Phagocytes: birth, range	6-26 x 10^{6}	
- birth, median	11 x 10^{6}	
- pediatric, range	1.5-8.5 x 10^{6}	
- pediatric, median	4.1 x 10^{6}	
- adult, range	3.5-9.2 x 10^{6}	
- CD4 cell count	0.5-1.5 x 10^{6}	
Lipase P	1.2-1.4 x 10^{-4}	
Lipids, total	4.45-6.1 x 10^{-3}	4-8.5 x 10^{-3}
Lipoprotein (S_f 12-20)		1-10 x 10^{-4}
Lithium	1.5-2.5 x 10^{-8}	
Lysine	1.3-3 x 10^{-5}	2-5.8 x 10^{-5}
Lysozyme (muramidase)		1-15 x 10^{-6}
α_2-Macroglobulin		
- pediatric		2-7 x 10^{-3}
- male, adult		0.9-4.0 x 10^{-3}
- female, adult		1.2-5.4 x 10^{-3}
Magnesium	3.2-5.5 x 10^{-5}	1.8-3.6 x 10^{-5}
Malic acid	4.6 x 10^{-6}	1-9 x 10^{-6}
Manganese	0-2.5 x 10^{-7}	0-1.9 x 10^{-7}
Melatonin		
- Day		1.35-1.45 x 10^{-11}
- Night		6.07-7.13 x 10^{-11}
Mercury		
- normal	<1 x 10^{-8}	
- chronic	>20 x 10^{-8}	
Methemoglobin	4-6 x 10^{-4}	
Methionine	4-6 x10^{-6}	1-15 x 10^{-6}
Methyl guanidine	2-3 x 10^{-6}	
β-2-microglobulin		8-24 x 10^{-7}
MIP-1α		2.3 x 10^{-11}
MIP-1β		9 x 10^{-11}
Mucopolysaccharides		1.75-2.25 x 10^{-3}
Mucoproteins		8.65-9.6 x 10^{-4}
Nerve growth factor (NGF)		6-10 x 10^{-9}
Nicotinic acid	5-8 x 10^{-6}	2-15 x 10^{-7}
Nitrogen		
- respiratory gas	8.2 x 10^{-6}	9.7 x 10^{-6}
- total, nonrespiratory	3-3.7 x 10^{-2}	
Norepinephrine		
- after 15 min rest		2.15-4.75 x 10^{-10}
- when emitted	8.1 x 10^{-9}	8.5 x 10^{-9}
Nucleotide, total	3.1-5.2 x 10^{-4}	
Ornithine		4-14 x 10^{-6}
Oxalate		1-2.4 x 10^{-6}
Oxygen (respiratory gas)		
- arterial	2.4-3.2 x 10^{-4}	3.9 x 10^{-6}
- venous	1.6-2.3 x 10^{-4}	1.6 x 10^{-6}
Oxytocin		
- male		2 x 10^{-12}
- female, nonlactating		2 x 10^{-12}
- female, pregnant 33-40 wks		32-48 x 10^{-12}
Pancreatic polypeptide		5-20 x 10^{-11}
Pantothenic acid (Vitamin B_5)	1.5-4.5 x 10^{-7}	6-35 x 10^{-8}
Para-aminobenzoic acid	3-4 x 10^{-8}	
Parathyroid hormone (PTH)		2-4 x 10^{-10}

Component	In Whole Blood (gm/cm^3)	In Plasma or Serum (gm/cm^3)
Pentose, phosphorated		2-2.3 x 10^{-5}
Phenol, free	7-10 x 10^{-7}	
Phenylalanine	8-12 x 10^{-6}	1.1-4 x 10^{-5}
Phospholipid	2.25-2.85 x 10^{-3}	5-12 x 10^{-5}
Phosphatase, acid, prostatic		<3 x 10^{-9}
Phosphorus		
- inorganic, adult	2-3.9 x 10^{-5}	2.3-4.5 x 10^{-5}
- inorganic, children		4.0-7.0 x 10^{-5}
- total	3.5-4.3 x 10^{-4}	1-1.5 x 10^{-4}
Phytanic acid		<3 x 10^{-6}
Platelets (#/cm^3)		
- range	1.4-4.4 x 10^{8}	
- median	2.5 x 10^{8}	
Platelet Derived Growth Factor		5.0 x 10^{-8}
Polysaccharides, total		7.3-13.1 x 10^{-4}
Potassium	1.6-2.4 x 10^{-3}	1.4-2.2 x 10^{-4}
Pregnenolone		3-20 x 10^{-10}
Progesterone (male)		12-20 x 10^{-11}
Progesterone (female)		
- follicular		0.4-0.9 x 10^{-9}
- midluteal		7.7-12.1 x 10^{-9}
- pregnancy, weeks 16-18		30-66 x 10^{-9}
- pregnancy, weeks 28-30		70-126 x 10^{-9}
- pregnancy, weeks 38-40		131-227 x 10^{-9}
Proinsulin		
- fasting		0.5-5 x 10^{-10}
- mean		1.42-1.70 x 10^{-10}
Prolactin (male)		<20 x 10^{-9}
- while awake		1-7 x 10^{-9}
- during sleep		9-20 x 10^{-9}
Prolactin (female)		
- follicular		<23 x 10^{-9}
- luteal		5-40 x 10^{-9}
Proline		1.2-5.7 x 10^{-5}
Prostaglandins		
- PGE		3.55-4.15 x 10^{-10}
- PGF		1.26-1.56 x 10^{-10}
- 15-keto-$PGF_{2\alpha}$		5 x 10^{-10}
- 15-keto-PGE_2		<5 x 10^{-11}
Protein, total	1.9-2.1 x 10^{-1}	6.0-8.3 x 10^{-2}
Protoporphyrin	2.7-6.1 x 10^{-7}	
PSA (prostate-specific antigen)	0-5 x 10^{-9}	
Pseudoglobulin I		8-19 x 10^{-3}
Pseudoglobulin II		2-8 x 10^{-3}
Purine, total	9.5-11.5 x 10^{-5}	
Pyrimidine nucleotide	2.6-4.6 x 10^{-5}	2-12 x 10^{-7}
Pyridoxine (Vitamin B_6)		3.6-90 x 10^{-9}
Pyruvic acid	3-10 x 10^{-6}	3-12 x 10^{-6}
RANTES		7 x 10^{-11}
Relaxin		
- day <100 preparturition		<2 x 10^{-9}
- day 100 to 2 days preceding		5-40 x 10^{-9}
- day preceding parturition		100-200 x 10^{-9}
- day following parturition		<2 x 10^{-9}
Retinol (Vitamin A)		1-8 x 10^{-7}
Riboflavin (Vitamin B_2)	1.5-6 x 10^{-7}	2.6-3.7 x 10^{-8}
RNA	5-8 x 10^{-4}	4-6 x 10^{-5}
Secretin		2.9-4.5 x 10^{-11}
Serine		3-20 x 10^{-6}
Serotonin (5-hydroxytryptamine)	1.55-1.81 x 10^{-7}	0.8-2.1 x 10^{-7}
Silicon	1.4-2.95 x 10^{-6}	2.2-5.7 x 10^{-6}
Sodium		3.1-3.4 x 10^{-3}
Solids, total	2-2.5 x 10^{-1}	8-9 x 10^{-2}
Somatotropin (growth hormone)		4-140 x 10^{-10}
Sphingomyelin	1.5-1.85 x 10^{-3}	1-4 x 10^{-4}
Succinic acid		5 x 10^{-6}
Sugar, total	7-11 x 10^{-4}	
Sulfates, inorganic		8-12 x 10^{-6}
Sulfur, total	3.8-5 x 10^{-2}	3.1-3.8 x 10^{-2}
Taurine		3-21 x 10^{-6}
Testosterone (male)		
- free		5.6-10.2 x 10^{-11}
- total		275-875 x 10^{-11}
Testosterone (female)		
- free		0.24-0.38 x 10^{-11}
- total		23-75 x 10^{-11}
- pregnant		38-190 x 10^{-11}
Thiamine (Vitamin B_1)	3-10 x 10^{-8}	1-9 x 10^{-8}
Thiocyanate	5-14 x 10^{-6}	
- nonsmoker		1-4 x 10^{-6}
- smoker		3-12 x 10^{-6}
Threonine	1.3-2 x 10^{-5}	0.9-3.2 x 10^{-5}
Thyroglobulin (Tg)		<5 x 10^{-8}
Thyroid hormone		4-8 x 10^{-8}
Thyrotropin-releasing hormone		5-60 x 10^{-12}
Thyroxine (FT_4)		
- free		8-24 x 10^{-12}
- total		4-12 x 10^{-8}
Thyroxine-binding prealbumin		2.8-3.5 x 10^{-4}
Thyroxine-binding globulin		1.0-3.4 x 10^{-7}
Tin	0-4 x 10^{-7}	0-1 x 10^{-7}
α-Tocopherol (Vitamin E)		5-20 x 10^{-6}
Transcortin		
- male		1.5-2 x 10^{-5}
- female		1.6-2.5 x 10^{-5}
Transferrin		
- newborn		1.3-2.75 x 10^{-3}
- adult		2.2-4 x 10^{-3}
- age >60 yrs		1.8-3.8 x 10^{-3}
Triglycerides	8.5-23.5 x 10^{-4}	2.5-30 x 10^{-4}
Tri-iodothyronine		
- free		2.3-6.6 x 10^{-12}
- total (T_3)		0.75-2.50 x 10^{-9}
Tryptophan	5-10 x 10^{-6}	9-30 x 10^{-6}
Tyrosine	8-14 x 10^{-6}	4-25 x 10^{-6}
Urea	2-4 x 10^{-4}	2.8-4 x10^{-4}

Component	In Whole Blood (gm/cm^3)	In Plasma or Serum (gm/cm^3)	Component	In Whole Blood (gm/cm^3)	In Plasma or Serum (gm/cm^3)
Uric acid	$6-49 \times 10^{-6}$	$2-7 \times 10^{-5}$	Vasointestinal peptide (VIP)		$6-16 \times 10^{-12}$
- child		$3.5-7.2 \times 10^{-5}$	Vasopressin		
- adult, male		$2.6-6.0 \times 10^{-5}$	- hydrated		4.5×10^{-13}
- adult, female		$2.0-5.5 \times 10^{-5}$	- dehydrated		3.7×10^{-12}
Valine	$2-2.9 \times 10^{-5}$	$1.7-4.2 \times 10^{-5}$	Zinc	$5-13 \times 10^{-6}$	$7-15 \times 10^{-7}$

APPENDIX C

Appendix C. Catalog of Distinct Cell Types in the Adult Human Body[531]

I. Keratinizing Epithelial Cells

1. Epidermal keratinocyte (differentiating epidermal cell)
2. Epidermal basal cell (stem cell)
3. Keratinocyte of fingernails and toenails
4. Nail bed basal cell (stem cell)
5. Medullary hair shaft cell
6. Cortical hair shaft cell
7. Cuticular hair shaft cell
8. Cuticular hair root sheath cell
9. Hair root sheath cell of Huxley's layer
10. Hair root sheath cell of Henle's layer
11. External hair root sheath cell
12. Hair matrix cell (stem cell)

II. Wet Stratified Barrier Epithelial Cells

13. Surface epithelial cell of stratified squamous epithelium of cornea, tongue, oral cavity, esophagus, anal canal, distal urethra and vagina
14. Basal cell (stem cell) of epithelia of cornea, tongue, oral cavity, esophagus, anal canal, distal urethra and vagina
15. Urinary epithelium cell (lining bladder and urinary ducts)

III. Exocrine Secretory Epithelial Cells

16. Salivary gland mucous cell (polysaccharide-rich secretion)
17. Salivary gland serous cell (glycoprotein enzyme-rich secretion)
18. Von Ebner's gland cell in tongue (washes taste buds)
19. Mammary gland cell (milk secretion)
20. Lacrimal gland cell (tear secretion)
21. Ceruminous gland cell in ear (wax secretion)
22. Eccrine sweat gland dark cell (glycoprotein secretion)
23. Eccrine sweat gland clear cell (small molecule secretion)
24. Apocrine sweat gland cell (odoriferous secretion, sex-hormone sensitive)
25. Gland of Moll cell in eyelid (specialized sweat gland)
26. Sebaceous gland cell (lipid-rich sebum secretion)
27. Bowman's gland cell in nose (washes olfactory epithelium)
28. Brunner's gland cell in duodenum (enzymes and alkaline mucus)
29. Seminal vesicle cell (secretes seminal fluid components, including fructose for swimming sperm)
30. Prostate gland cell (secretes seminal fluid components)
31. Bulbourethral gland cell (mucus secretion)
32. Bartholin's gland cell (vaginal lubricant secretion)
33. Gland of Littre cell (mucus secretion)
34. Uterus endometrium cell (carbohydrate secretion)
35. Isolated goblet cell of respiratory and digestive tracts (mucus secretion)
36. Stomach lining mucous cell (mucus secretion)
37. Gastric gland zymogenic cell (pepsinogen secretion)
38. Gastric gland oxyntic cell (HCl secretion)
39. Pancreatic acinar cell (bicarbonate and digestive enzyme secretion)
40. Paneth cell of small intestine (lysozyme secretion)
41. Type II pneumocyte of lung (surfactant secretion)
42. Clara cell of lung

IV. Hormone Secreting Cells

43. Anterior pituitary cell secreting growth hormone
44. Anterior pituitary cell secreting follicle-stimulating hormone
45. Anterior pituitary cell secreting luteinizing hormone
46. Anterior pituitary cell secreting prolactin
47. Anterior pituitary cell secreting adrenocorticotropic hormone
48. Anterior pituitary cell secreting thyroid-stimulating hormone
49. Intermediate pituitary cell secreting melanocyte-stimulating hormone
50. Posterior pituitary cell secreting oxytocin
51. Posterior pituitary cell secreting vasopressin
52. Gut and respiratory tract cell secreting serotonin
53. Gut and respiratory tract cell secreting endorphin
54. Gut and respiratory tract cell secreting somatostatin
55. Gut and respiratory tract cell secreting gastrin
56. Gut and respiratory tract cell secreting secretin
57. Gut and respiratory tract cell secreting cholecystokinin
58. Gut and respiratory tract cell secreting insulin
59. Gut and respiratory tract cell secreting glucagon
60. Gut and respiratory tract cell secreting bombesin
61. Thyroid gland cell secreting thyroid hormone
62. Thyroid gland cell secreting calcitonin
63. Parathyroid gland cell secreting parathyroid hormone
64. Parathyroid gland oxyphil cell
65. Adrenal gland cell secreting epinephrine
66. Adrenal gland cell secreting norepinephrine
67. Adrenal gland cell secreting steroid hormones (mineralcorticoids and gluco corticoids)

68. Leydig cell of testes secreting testosterone
69. Theca interna cell of ovarian follicle secreting estrogen
70. Corpus luteum cell of ruptured ovarian follicle secreting progesterone
71. Kidney juxtaglomerular apparatus cell (renin secretion)
72. Macula densa cell of kidney
73. Peripolar cell of kidney
74. Mesangial cell of kidney

V. Epithelial Absorptive Cells (Gut, Exocrine Glands and Urogenital Tract)

75. Intestinal brush border cell (with microvilli)
76. Exocrine gland striated duct cell
77. Gall bladder epithelial cell
78. Kidney proximal tubule brush border cell
79. Kidney distal tubule cell
80. Ductulus efferens nonciliated cell
81. Epididymal principal cell
82. Epididymal basal cell

VI. Metabolism and Storage Cells

83. Hepatocyte (liver cell)
84. White adipocyte (fat cell)
85. Brown adipocyte (fat cell)
86. Liver lipocyte

VII. Barrier Function Cells (Lung, Gut, Exocrine Glands and Urogenital Tract)

87. Type I pneumocyte (lining air space of lung)
88. Pancreatic duct cell (centroacinar cell)
89. Nonstriated duct cell (of sweat gland, salivary gland, mammary gland, etc.)
90. Kidney glomerulus parietal cell
91. Kidney glomerulus podocyte
92. Loop of Henle thin segment cell (in kidney)
93. Kidney collecting duct cell
94. Duct cell (of seminal vesicle, prostate gland, etc.)

VIII. Epithelial Cells Lining Closed Internal Body Cavities

95. Blood vessel and lymphatic vascular endothelial fenestrated cell
96. Blood vessel and lymphatic vascular endothelial continuous cell
97. Blood vessel and lymphatic vascular endothelial splenic cell
98. Synovial cell (lining joint cavities, hyaluronic acid secretion)
99. Serosal cell (lining peritoneal, pleural, and pericardial cavities)
100. Squamous cell (lining perilymphatic space of ear)
101. Squamous cell (lining endolymphatic space of ear)
102. Columnar cell of endolymphatic sac with microvilli (lining endolymphatic space of ear)
103. Columnar cell of endolymphatic sac without microvilli (lining endolymphatic space of ear)
104. Dark cell (lining endolymphatic space of ear)
105. Vestibular membrane cell (lining endolymphatic space of ear)
106. Stria vascularis basal cell (lining endolymphatic space of ear)
107. Stria vascularis marginal cell (lining endolymphatic space of ear)
108. Cell of Claudius (lining endolymphatic space of ear)
109. Cell of Boettcher (lining endolymphatic space of ear)
110. Choroid plexus cell (cerebrospinal fluid secretion)
111. Pia-arachnoid squamous cell
112. Pigmented ciliary epithelium cell of eye
113. Nonpigmented ciliary epithelium cell of eye
114. Corneal endothelial cell

IX. Ciliated Cells with Propulsive Function

115. Respiratory tract ciliated cell
116. Oviduct ciliated cell (in female)
117. Uterine endometrial ciliated cell (in female)
118. Rete testis cilated cell (in male)
119. Ductulus efferens ciliated cell (in male)
120. Ciliated ependymal cell of central nervous system (lining brain cavities)

X. Extracellular Matrix Secretion Cells

121. Ameloblast epithelial cell (tooth enamel secretion)
122. Planum semilunatum epithelial cell of vestibular apparatus of ear (proteoglycan secretion)
123. Organ of Corti interdental epithelial cell (secreting tectorial membrane covering hair cells)
124. Loose connective tissue fibroblasts
125. Corneal fibroblasts
126. Tendon fibroblasts
127. Bone marrow reticular tissue fibroblasts
128. Other (nonepithelial) fibroblasts
129. Blood capillary pericyte
130. Nucleus pulposus cell of intervertebral disc
131. Cementoblast/cementocyte (tooth root bonelike cementum secretion)
132. Odontoblast/odontocyte (tooth dentin secretion)
133. Hyaline cartilage chondrocyte
134. Fibrocartilage chondrocyte
135. Elastic cartilage chondrocyte
136. Osteoblast/osteocyte
137. Osteoprogenitor cell (stem cell of osteoblasts)
138. Hyalocyte of vitreous body of eye
139. Stellate cell of perilymphatic space of ear

XI. Contractile Cells

140. Red skeletal muscle cell (slow)
141. White skeletal muscle cell (fast)
142. Intermediate skeletal muscle cell
143. Muscle spindle — nuclear bag cell
144. Muscle spindle — nuclear chain cell
145. Satellite cell (stem cell)
146. Ordinary heart muscle cell
147. Nodal heart muscle cell
148. Purkinje fiber cell
149. Smooth muscle cell (various types)
150. Myoepithelial cell of iris
151. Myoepithelial cell of exocrine glands

XII. Blood and Immune System Cells

152. Erythrocyte (red blood cell)
153. Megakaryocyte
154. Monocyte
155. Connective tissue macrophage (various types)
156. Epidermal Langerhans cell
157. Osteoclast (in bone)
158. Dendritic cell (in lymphoid tissues)
159. Microglial cell (in central nervous system)
160. Neutrophil
161. Eosinophil
162. Basophil
163. Mast cell
164. Helper T lymphocyte cell
165. Suppressor T lymphocyte cell
166. Killer T lymphocyte cell
167. IgM B lymphocyte cell
168. IgG B lymphocyte cell
169. IgA B lymphocyte cell
170. IgE B lymphocyte cell
171. Killer cell
172. Stem cells and committed progenitors for the blood and immune system (various types)

XIII. Sensory Transducer Cells

173. Photoreceptor rod cell of eye
174. Photoreceptor blue-sensitive cone cell of eye
175. Photoreceptor green-sensitive cone cell of eye
176. Photoreceptor red-sensitive cone cell of eye
177. Auditory inner hair cell of organ of Corti
178. Auditory outer hair cell of organ of Corti
179. Type I hair cell of vestibular apparatus of ear (acceleration and gravity)
180. Type II hair cell of vestibular apparatus of ear (acceleration and gravity)
181. Type I taste bud cell
182. Olfactory neuron
183. Basal cell of olfactory epithelium (stem cell for olfactory neurons)
184. Type I carotid body cell (blood pH sensor)
185. Type II carotid body cell (blood pH sensor)
186. Merkel cell of epidermis (touch sensor)
187. Touch-sensitive primary sensory neurons (various types)
188. Cold-sensitive primary sensory neurons
189. Heat-sensitive primary sensory neurons
190. Pain-sensitive primary sensory neurons (various types)
191. Proprioceptive primary sensory neurons (various types)

XIV. Autonomic Neuron Cells

192. Cholinergic neural cell (various types)
193. Adrenergic neural cell (various types)
194. Peptidergic neural cell (various types)

XV. Sense Organ and Peripheral Neuron Supporting Cells

195. Inner pillar cell of organ of Corti
196. Outer pillar cell of organ of Corti
197. Inner phalangeal cell of organ of Corti
198. Outer phalangeal cell of organ of Corti
199. Border cell of organ of Corti
200. Hensen cell of organ of Corti
201. Vestibular apparatus supporting cell
202. Type I taste bud supporting cell
203. Olfactory epithelium supporting cell
204. Schwann cell
205. Satellite cell (encapsulating peripheral nerve cell bodies)
206. Enteric glial cell

XVI. Central Nervous System Neurons and Glial Cells

207. Neuron cell (large variety of types, still poorly classified)
208. Astrocyte glial cell (various types)
209. Oligodendrocyte glial cell

XVII. Lens Cells

210. Anterior lens epithelial cell
211. Crystallin-containing lens fiber cell

XVIII. Pigment Cells

212. Melanocyte
213. Retinal pigmented epithelial cell

XIX. Germ Cells

214. Oogonium/oocyte
215. Spermatocyte
216. Spermatogonium cell (stem cell for spermatocyte)

XX. Nurse Cells

217. Ovarian follicle cell
218. Sertoli cell (in testis)
219. Thymus epithelial cell

GLOSSARY

This glossary includes words useful in the study of nanomedicine, mostly from the fields of physics, engineering, chemistry, biochemistry, biology, anatomy and medicine. Specialists are cautioned that terms may be described, but not rigorously defined, in order to encourage the quickest possible cross-disciplinary understanding by the nonspecialist reader. A very small number of the entries identify new terms introduced for the first time in this text. Much of the material was compiled or modified from pre-existing sources including the following References: 9, 10, 750, 763, 869, 996, 997, 1095, 1259, 1736, 2219-2221, 2223, 2224.

Ab initio — from the beginning; from first principles.

Abscess — a circumscribed collection of pus appearing in acute or chronic localized infection, and associated with tissue destruction and frequently with swelling; a cavity formed by liquefaction necrosis within solid tissue.

Abstraction — specific removal of bonded atom from a structure. A reaction that removes an atom from a structure.

AC — alternating current.

Accommodation — voluntarily thickening the lens of the eye to focus diverging rays of light from nearby objects on the fovea of the retina; visual focusing on nearby objects.

Acellular — cell-free.

Acetylcholine — a chemical neurotransmitter.

Acetylcholinesterase — enzyme that rapidly degrades acetylcholine.

Acidophilic — acid-loving.

Acoustomechanical conversion — conversion of acoustic energy into mechanical energy.

Action potential — complete sequence of electrical events accompanying and following the nerve impulse.

Active site — the restricted part of a protein to which a substrate binds.

Adduct — in chemistry, an addition product or complex; in biomechanics, to draw together physically separated components.

Adiabatic — change in pressure or volume without loss or gain of heat.

Adipocyte — fat cell.

Adipose — fatty; pertaining to fat.

ADP — adenosine diphosphate; has one energy-rich phosphate bond.

Adrenergic — activated or energized by adrenalin (epinephrine).

Adsorption — attachment of a substance to the surface of another material.

Aerobic — needing oxygen to live or function.

Aerobots (aerobotics) — aerial (flying) robots.

Afferent — in relation to nerves or blood vessels, conducting toward structure or organ; carrying impulses toward a center, as when sensory nerves carry sensory information toward the brain or spinal cord.

Affinity (constant) — the strength of the binding of a ligand to a receptor, or the reciprocal of the dissociation rate constant; a measure of the binding energy of a ligand in a receptor; the greater the affinity, the more securely the receptor binds the ligand.

AFM — see Atomic Force Microscope.

Aft — toward the rear.

Agglutinin — an antibody present in the blood that attaches to antigens, such as those found on the surfaces of red blood cells, causing them to clump together; agglutinins cause transfusion reactions when blood from a different group is given.

Agonist — in pharmacology, a drug which binds to a receptor and thus stimulates the receptor's function, possibly mimicking the body's own regulatory function. Compare antagonist.

Albumin — one of a group of simple proteins widely distributed in plant and animal tissues.

ALC — airborne lethal concentration.

Algorithm — in general, a formula or set of rules for solving a particular problem; in medicine, a set of steps used in diagnosing and treating a disease.

Alimentary — pertaining to the digestive tract.

Alimentography — a physical description (and mapping) of the human alimentary canal.

Aliquot — a portion obtained by dividing the whole into equal parts without a remainder; loosely, any one of two or more samples of something, of the same volume or weight.

Alkali — strongly basic substance, especially the metal hydroxides, usually associated with the alkali metals (e.g. sodium and potassium).

Allele — one of several alternative forms of a gene occupying a given locus on paired chromosomes.

Alloantigen — a substance present in certain individuals that stimulates antibody production in other members of the same species, but not in the original donor. See also antiserum.

Allometric scaling laws — in biology, scaling laws that involve a biological variable that is an exponential function of the mass of the organism.

Allosteric control — the ability of an interaction at one site of a protein to influence the activity of another site.

Allotropic — pertains to the existence of a chemical element or compound in two or more distinct forms with different physical and chemical properties (e.g. diamond and graphite are allotropes of C).

Alphanumeric — able to contain both alphabetic and numeric characters.

Alveolus (alveolar) — in anatomy, a small cell or cavity; a saclike dilation. Most commonly, a small air sac found at the lowest levels of the branching tube system comprising the lungs.

AM — amplitude modulation.

Amide — a molecule containing an amine bonded to a carboxyl group (e.g. $CONH_2$). Amide bonds link amino acids in peptides and proteins.

Amine — a molecule containing N with a single bond to C and two other single bonds to H or C (but not an amide); the amine group or moiety (e.g. $-NH_2$).

Amino acid — a molecule containing both an amine and a carboxylic acid group; there are 20 genetically encoded amino acids in biology.

Amniotic — pertaining to the amnion (the innermost of the fetal membranes).

Amphipathic — molecular structures which have two surfaces or ends, one of which is hydrophilic and the other of which is hydrophobic. Lipids are amphipathic, and some protein regions may form amphipathic helices with one charged face and one neutral face.

Anabolism — the constructive phase of metabolism and the opposite of catabolism; in anabolism, a cell takes from the blood the substances required for repair and growth, building them into a cytoplasm, thus converting nonliving material into the living cytoplasm of the cell.

Anaerobic — able to live or function without oxygen.

Analgesia — absence of normal sense of pain.

Analog — pertaining to data measurable and representable through continuously variable physical quantities. Compare digital.

Anaphase — the phase of mitosis (cell division) beginning with centromere division and the movement of chromosomes away from the metaphase plate toward opposite spindle poles.

Anaphylactoid-type reaction — a physiological response similar to anaphylaxis.

Anaphylaxis — the immediate transient kind of immunologic (allergic) reaction characterized by contraction of smooth muscle and dilation of capillaries due to release of pharmacologically active substances (e.g. histamine, bradykinin, serotonin, etc.); a powerful allergic response. Anaphylaxis is classically initiated by the combination of antigen (allergen) with mast cell-fixed, cytophilic antibody (chiefly IgE immunoglobulin), but can also be initiated by relatively large quantities of serum aggregates (antibody-antigen complexes, and other) that seemingly activate complement leading to production of anaphylatoxin.

Anastomose — to open one structure into another directly or by connecting channels, usually said of blood vessels, lymphatics, and hollow viscera; to unite by means of an anastomosis, or a connection between formerly separate structures.

AND gate — a logical gate that returns a high (1) output if and only if both input signals are high (1). See bit.

Anergic — unresponsive.

Aneutronic — without neutrons.

Angioedema — a condition characterized by development of urticaria (hives) and edematous (swollen with excessive fluid) areas of skin, mucous membranes, or viscera.

Angiogenesis — growth of new blood vessels, especially capillaries.

Anion — a negatively charged ion.

Anisotropic — not isotropic.

Anode — the positive pole of an electrical source.

ANS — see autonomic nervous system.

Antagonist — in pharmacology, a drug that prevents receptor function. Compare agonist.

Anterior — the front of the human body, on or nearest the abdominal surface; the front of something.

Anteroinferior — in front and below.

Anteroposterior — passing from front to rear.

Anthropogenic — caused by human activity.

Antibody — a protein (immunoglobulin) produced by B-lymphocyte cells that recognizes a particular foreign antigen, thus triggering the immune response.

Antigen — any molecule or foreign substance that, when introduced into the body, provokes synthesis of an antibody, thus stimulating an immune response.

Antiserum — serum that contains demonstrable antibody or antibodies specific for one (monovalent) or more (polyvalent) antigens.

Aorta — the largest artery in the human body, leading away from the heart.

Apheresis — removal of blood from an individual patient, separating certain elements (e.g. red cells, platelets, white cells) for use elsewhere, and reintroducing the remaining components into the patients; also known as cytapheresis, hemapheresis, leukapheresis, pheresis, and plasmapheresis, depending on the type of cells being harvested.

Apical — pertaining to the apex (e.g. the point of a cone) of a structure.

Apoptosis — an orderly disintegration of eukaryotic cells into membrane-bound particles that may then be phagocytosed by other cells.

Aqueous humor — transparent liquid contained in the anterior chamber of the eyeball in front of the lens.

Aromatic compounds — in chemistry, ring or cyclic compounds related to benzene, many having a fragrant odor.

Arrhythmia — irregularity or loss of rhythm, especially of the heartbeat.

Arteriovenous — relating to both arteries and veins.

Artery — in anatomy, a blood vessel that sends blood to the tissues from the heart.

Aseptic — characterized by the absence of living pathogenic organisms; a state of sterility.

Asperities — protruding elements of roughness on a surface, e.g., burrs or spurs.

Asphyxia — condition of hypoxia caused by insufficient oxygen intake.

Assembler — see molecular assembler.

Asymptotic — in geometry and mathematics, a curve that approaches closer and closer, but never quite reaches, another curve or line.

Asynchronous —not synchronized in time.

atm — atmosphere, a unit of pressure; mean air pressure at Earth's surface is 1 atmosphere ($\sim 1.01 \times 10^5$ N/m^2).

Atomic Force Microscope (AFM) — an instrument that uses atomic forces between a sample and a sharp scanning needle tip to image surfaces to molecular accuracy by mechanically probing their surface contours; the AFM measures the tiny upward and downward motions of the tip as the tip is dragged over the surface, producing an atomic-resolution topographic map of the surface. The AFM has also been used to physically manipulate individual molecules.

Atom laser — a laserlike device that uses beams of coherent atoms rather than photons.

ATP — adenosine triphosphate; has two energy-rich phosphate bonds.

Auscultation — the process of listening for sounds within the body, usually to the sounds of thoracic or abdominal viscera, in order to detect some abnormal condition, or to detect fetal heart sounds, or to diagnose vascular abnormalities such as arteriovenous fistulas.

Autogenous control — in medical nanorobotics, the conscious control of in vivo nanorobotic systems by the human user or patient; in biochemistry, the action of a gene product that either inhibits (negative autogenous control) or activates (positive autogenous control) expression of the gene coding for it.

Autonomic (nervous system) — the part of the nervous system that is concerned with the control of involuntary bodily functions.

Automated engineering — Engineering design done by a computer system, with detailed designs generated from broad specifications with little or no human help, a specialized form of artificial intelligence.

Automated manufacturing — molecular manufacturing that requires little human labor.

Autosomes — all the chromosomes except the sex chromosomes; a diploid cell has two copies of each autosome.

Avascular — having no blood vessels.

Avulsion — a tearing away forcibly of a part or structure.

Axisymmetric — symmetric relative to a geometric axis.

Axon — the (usually long and straight) protoplasmic process of a neuron that conducts impulses away from the cell body. There is usually one to a neuron cell.

Axoplasm — the cytoplasm (neuroplasm) of an axon that encloses the neurofibrils.

Bacterium — a single-celled prokaryotic microorganism, typically ~1-10 micron (~1000 nm) in diameter or length.

Bacteriophages — viruses that infect selected bacteria; often abbreviated as phages.

Barographics — pressure mapping of the human body.

Baronatation — in medical nanorobotics, locomotion through a frozen fluid by applying mechanical pressure along the path travelled to induce melting ahead, followed by regelation (refreezing) behind.

Basal lamina — basement lamina, e.g. basement membrane.

Basal Metabolic Rate (BMR) — a measure of the metabolic rate taken with the patient fasting and at rest. The oxygen consumed in breathing under these conditions indicates the minimum rate of chemical reactions in the body.

Basement membrane (basement lamina) — a thin layer of delicate noncellular material of a fine filamentous texture underlying the epithelium; its principal component is collagen.

Base pair (bp) — a complementary purine-pyrimidine hydrogen-bonded residue pair, one from each strand of DNA double helix, designating one unit (bp) of sequence. A partnership of adenine (A) with thymine (T) or of cytosine (C) with guanine (G) in a DNA double helix; other pairs can be formed in RNA under certain circumstances.

Basophil — a type of granulocytic white blood cell comprising less than 1% of all leukocytes, that is essential to the nonspecific immune response to inflammation because of its important role in releasing histamine and other chemicals that act on blood vessels.

Bearing — A mechanical device that permits the motion of a component (ideally, with minimal resistance) in one or more degrees of freedom while resisting motion (ideally, with a stiff restoring force) in all other degrees of freedom.

Beriberi — a thiamine deficiency disease, characterized by peripheral neurologic, cerebral, and cardiovascular abnormalities; early deficiency produces fatigue, irritation, poor memory, sleep disturbances, precordial pain, anorexia, abdominal discomfort, and constipation.

Biaxial — pertaining to two distinct geometric or spatial axes.

Bicuspid — having two cusps.

Bifurcate — to separate into two separate branches.

Bilobate — having two lobes.

Billion — this book follows the American convention in which a billion is 10^9.

Bimorph — a simple mechanical actuator capable of flexing in a single plane.

Binding — the process by which a molecule (or ligand) becomes bound, that is, confined in position (and often orientation) with respect to a receptor. Confinement occurs because structural features of the receptor create a potential well for the ligand; van der Waals and electrostatic interactions commonly contribute.

Binding energy — in chemistry, the reduction in the free energy of a system that occurs when a ligand binds to a receptor. In nuclear physics, the energy which binds neutrons and protons together in an atomic nucleus, which may be calculated from the decrease in mass that would occur if the appropriate numbers of neutrons and protons were brought together to form the nucleus in question; Fe^{56} has the maximum binding energy of any nucleus. Generally used to describe the total energy required to remove something, or to take a system apart into its constituent particles.

Binding site — the active region of a receptor; any site at which a chemical species of interest tends to bind.

Biocompatibility — the ability of the body to tolerate the presence or implantation of foreign objects.

Bioinformatics — most generally, the study and compilation of the information content of biological materials, especially genetic materials.

Biomimetic — mimicking biology.

Biosensor — A device that senses and analyzes biological information (e.g. temperature, pressure, chemical content, etc.), commonly using a biological recognition mechanism combined with a physical transduction technique.

Biotechnology — The application of biological systems and organisms to technical and industrial processes, with production carried out using intact organisms (e.g. yeasts and bacteria) or natural substances from organisms (e.g. enzymes), or by modifying the genetic structure of organisms (genetic engineering); most generally, the engineering of all biological systems, even completely artificial organic living systems, using biological instrumentalities.

Birefringence — in optics, a crystal having a different index of refraction for different polarizations of incident light (e.g. calcite).

Bit — a binary digit. In a binary code, one of the two possible characters, usually 0 (e.g. low voltage) and 1 (e.g. high voltage); in information theory, the fundamental unit of information.

Blackbody radiator — an absorber which ideally absorbs all electromagnetic energy incident upon it; such an ideal absorber is also an ideal emitter of such radiant energy.

Blepharitis — inflammation of the edges of the eyelids involving hair follicles and glands that open onto the surface.

Blockade — prevention of the action of something, such as the effect of a drug or of a body function (e.g. halting immune system blood cleansing, by overloading the RES).

B-lymphocytes (B cells) — thymus-independent white blood cells responsible for synthesizing antibodies.

Boolean functions — see logic gate.

Bose-Einstein condensate — low-temperature collection of bosons (particles with integral spin, e.g. deuterium nuclei and alpha particles) in their ground state.

Bottom-up — an approach to nanotechnology that aims to construct nanodevices molecule by molecule, making larger and larger objects with atomic precision.

Boutons terminaux — bulblike expansions at the tips of axons that come into synaptic contact with the cell bodies of other neurons.

bp — see base pair.

Brachiation — locomotion by alternately swinging the arms (e.g. swinging hand-over-hand).

Bradycardia — slowness of heartbeat or heart action.

Bronchial — pertaining to the lungs.

Bronchiography — a physical description (and mapping) of the human bronchial system.

Brownian assembly — Brownian motion in a fluid brings molecules together in various positions and orientations; if molecules have suitable complementary surfaces, they can bind, assembling to form a specific structure. The term also may apply to the self-assembly of nanoscale parts having complementary surfaces.

Brownian motion — random motion of small particles in a fluid owing to thermal agitation, first observed in 1827 by Robert Brown; originally attributed to a vital force, Brownian motion plays a vital role in the assembly and activity of the molecular structures of life.

Bruit — an adventitious (arising sporadically) sound of venous or arterial origin, heard upon auscultation, such as murmurs at the carotid (a major artery) bifurcation.

Bubonic plague — the usual form of plague; primarily a disease of rodents that is transmitted to humans by fleas that have bitten infected animals.

Buccal — pertaining to the cheeks (mouth).

Buckyballs — ball-like molecules of fullerene carbon, C_{60}.

Bulimia — excessive and insatiable appetite for food.

Bulk technology — technology in which atoms and molecules are manipulated in bulk, rather than individually.

Bumpers — in medical nanorobotics, expansible surfaces placed at interfaces between adjacent nanorobots to achieve a tight seal between nanodevices.

Byte — a sequence of N adjacent bits operated on as a unit for the sake of convenience and frequently used as a measure of memory or information, with one byte corresponding to a single alphabetic character or some other symbol; N may equal 8, 16, 32, 64, or 128, in different 20th century computers.

c (velocity) — the speed of light, in vacuo.

CAD — Computer-Aided Design.

Caliber — inside diameter of a tube or cylinder.

Calmodulin — a 17,000-dalton protein that binds calcium ions in eukaryotic cells, thereby becoming the agent for many or most of the cellular effects ascribed to calcium ions.

CAM — Computer-Aided Manufacturing.

Cam — in mechanical engineering, a mechanical component that translates or rotates to move a contoured surface past a follower; the contours impose a sequence of motions (potentially complex) on the follower. See follower.

cAMP — cyclic AMP (adenosine monophosphate), an intracellular messenger molecule.

Capillary — in anatomy, a thin-walled tiny blood vessel, averaging 8 microns in diameter.

Capsid — the external protein coat of a virus particle.

Carbohydrates — a group of chemical substances, including sugars, glycogen, starches, dextrins, and celluloses, that contain only C, H, and O; usually the ratio of H:O is 2:1. Glucose and its polymers (including starch and cellulose) represent the most abundant organic chemical compounds on Earth.

Carbonyl — a chemical moiety consisting of O with a double bond to C (e.g. -CO-). If the C is bonded to N, the resulting structure is termed an "amide"; if it is bonded to O, it is termed a carboxylic acid or an ester linkage.

Carboxylic acid — a molecule that includes a C having a double bond to O and a single bond to OH (e.g. -COOH).

Carbyne — a chain of carbon atoms with alternating single and triple bonds.

Cardiac — pertaining to the heart.

Cardiostasis — pertaining to a heart that has stopped beating.

Carnot efficiency — in thermodynamics, the energy efficiency of a heat engine (a device that converts thermal energy into mechanical energy).

Cartotaxis — in medical nanorobotics, in vivo nanorobotic navigation by following a series of landmarks recorded on a previously drawn map.

Cartilage — specialized type of dense connective tissue consisting of cells embedded in a firm, compact fibrous collagenous matrix.

Catabolism — the destructive phase of metabolism, the opposite of anabolism. Catabolism includes all processes in which complex substances are converted into simpler substances (the end products commonly being excreted), usually with the release of energy.

Catalysis — increase in the speed of a chemical reaction or process produced by the presence of a catalyst (a substance that is not consumed in the net chemical reaction or process).

Catalyst — a chemical species or other structure that facilitates a chemical reaction without itself undergoing a permanent change.

Catacholamines — biologically active amines (e.g. epinephrine, norepinephrine) derived from the amino acid tyrosine, that have marked effects on the nervous and cardiovascular systems, on metabolic rate and temperature, and on smooth muscle.

Cathode — the negative pole of an electrical source.

Cation — a positively charged ion.

Caudal (caudad, inferior) — away from the head or the lower part of a structure (literally means "toward the tail").

Cauterize — to apply a cautery (an agent or device used for scarring, burring, or cutting the skin or tissues by means of heat, electric current, or caustic chemicals).

Cavitation — in physics, the formation of bubbles in a fluid during high-power sonication of that fluid; in medicine, formation of a cavity by either normal or pathological biological processes.

Cell — a small biological structural unit, surrounded by a plasma membrane, making up living things.

Cell engineering — deliberate artificial modifications to biological cellular systems on a cell-by-cell basis.

Cell surgery — in medical nanorobotics, modifying cellular structures using medical nanomachines.

Cell typing — a method of identifying a cell's type by comparing it to a typology of cell characteristics.

Cellular immunity — immunity resulting from activation of sensitized T-lymphocytes.

Cellular topographics — description of the cell and its parts.

Central Processing Unit (CPU) — the main computational engine of a computer, responsible for interpreting and executing instructions to process information.

Centrioles — small hollow cylinders consisting of microtubules, residing within the centrosomes, that become located near the poles during mitosis (cell division).

Centromere — a constricted region of a chromosome that divides the chromosome into two arms; the attachment point for the spindle fiber concerned with chromosome movement during mitosis (cell division).

Centrosomes — the regions from which microtubules are organized at the poles of a mitotic (dividing) cell; see also MTOC.

Centrum — middle part.

Cephalic (cephalad, superior) — nearest or toward the head or the upper part of a structure; also, pertaining to the head or top.

Cervical — usually pertaining to, or in the region of, the neck (i.e. below the skull); more generally, pertaining to the neck of an organ, such as the uterine cervix.

C fiber — an unmyelinated nerve fiber, 0.4-1.2 microns in diameter, conducting nerve impulses at 0.7-2.3 m/sec.

Chalcogenide — a glassy material containing arsenic and selenium.

Chaperone — a molecular chaperone is a protein needed for the assembly or proper folding of some other target protein, but which is not itself a component of the target protein complex.

Chemical force microscopy — an AFM with a functionalized tip, used to probe the chemical characteristics (especially adhesiveness) of surface-bound molecules.

Chemoelectric conversion — conversion of chemical energy into electrical energy.

Chemoergic — pertaining to the conversion of chemical energy into forms of energy of various other kinds.

Chemographics — chemical mapping of the human body.

Chemomechanical conversion — conversion of chemical energy into mechanical energy.

Chemotactic — pertaining to chemotaxis.

Chemotactic nanosensor — in medical nanorobotics, a nanosensor used to determine the chemical characteristics of surfaces, possibly configured as a pad coated with an array of reversible, perhaps reconfigurable, artificial molecular receptors.

Chemotaxis — the movement of additional white blood cells to an area of inflammation in response to the release of chemical mediators by neutrophils, monocytes, or injured tissue.

Chiral — a chiral molecule is an asymmetric molecule that cannot be superimposed on its mirror image. The molecule has two forms, or isomers, called enantiomorphs, that are mirror images of each other, the solutions of which rotate the plane of polarized light in different directions, left (levo) or right (dextro), making the enantiomers levorotatory or dextrorotatory. Only levorotatory amino acids are present in biological systems.

Chirurgeon — surgeon (obsolete).

Cholinergic — activated or energized by acetylcholine.

CHON — Carbon (C), Hydrogen (H), Oxygen (O), and Nitrogen (N).

Choroideremia — congenital absence of the choroid of the eye; progressive degeneration of the choroid, leading to complete blindness, due to X-linked chromosome inheritance.

Chromatin — the complex of DNA and protein in the nucleus of the interphase eukaryotic cell; individual chromosomes cannot be distinguished in it.

Chromomorphic — in medical nanorobotics, a nanorobot capable of altering its external surface color or other external surface optical characteristics.

Chromophore — a color-producing chemical substance.

Chromosome — a discrete unit of the genome carrying many genes; a structure in the nucleus of a eukaryotic cell containing a long linear molecule of duplex DNA (and an approximately equal mass of proteins) which conveys genetic information.

Chronobiology — that aspect of biology concerned with the timing of biological events, especially repetitive or cyclic phenomena in individual organisms; the study of biological clocks.

Chronocyte — in medical nanorobotics, a theorized mobile, mass-storage (nanorobotic) device, similar to a communicyte, that may be used as a mobile source of precisely synchronized universal time inside the human body.

Chronometer — a clock or other timekeeping device.

Cilium — in anatomy, hairlike processes projecting from epithelial cells, as in the bronchi, for propelling mucus, pus, and dust particles, or in the inner ear, for sensing fluid motion to allow hearing; in microbiology, a means of manipulation and propulsion for motile microorganisms.

Circadian — pertaining to physiological events that occur at approximately 24-hour intervals.

Circumcorporeal — around or surrounding the human body.

Circumvascular — around or surrounding a blood vessel.

Cisterna — a reservoir or cavity.

Clinical — founded on actual observation and treatment of patients, as distinguished from data or facts obtained by experimentation or pathology; pertaining to a clinic.

Clinicopathological correlation — correlating (1) the signs and symptoms manifested by a patient, plus the results of any laboratory studies, with (2) the findings of the gross and histological examination of the patient's tissue, to arrive at a correct diagnosis.

Clyster — an enema (obsolete).

Cochlea — the coiled, fluid-filled structure of the inner ear that transduces sound, allowing hearing.

Codon — in DNA and RNA, a sequence of three nucleotidyl residues designating an amino acid to be placed in polypeptide sequence during translation.

Coenzyme — a substance that enhances or is necessary for the action of enzymes; coenzymes are of smaller molecular size than the enzymes themselves, are dialyzable and relatively heat-stable, and are usually easily dissociable from the protein portion of the enzyme. See also vitamins.

Collagen — the major protein of the white fibers of connective tissue, cartilage, and bone, rich in glycine, alanine, proline, and hydroxyproline (amino acids), low in sulfur, and completely lacking in tryptophan (another amino acid); the collagen family comprises ~25% of all mammalian protein.

Colloid — see macromolecule.

Comminution — breaking into fragments.

Communicyte — in medical nanorobotics, a theorized mobile, mass-storage (nanorobotic) device that can be used for information transport throughout the human body.

Complement — a group of proteins in the blood that influences the inflammatory process and serves as the primary mediator in the antigen-antibody reactions of the B-cell mediated immune response. Components of complement are labeled C1-C9; C3 and C5 are most commonly involved in promoting vasodilation, chemotaxis, opsonization of antigens, lysis of cells, and blood clotting.

Complementary — supplying something that is lacking in another object, system, or entity; (shapes) fitting together tightly without any gaps.

Compliance — the reciprocal of stiffness; in a linear elastic system, displacement equals force times compliance.

Computerized Axial Tomography (CAT) — see Computerized Tomography.

Computerized Tomography (CT) — tomography in which transverse planes of tissue are swept by a pinpoint radiographic beam (e.g. X-rays) and a computerized analysis of the variance in absorption produces a precise reconstructed image of that area.

Conformation — molecular folding; a molecular geometry that differs from other geometries chiefly by rotation about single or triple bonds; distinct conformations (termed conformers) are associated with distinct potential wells. Typical biomolecules and products of organic synthesis can interconvert among many conformations. Typical diamondoid structures are locked into a single potential well, and thus lack conformational flexibility.

Congeries — a collection of things or parts in a single mass or aggregate.

Conjugated — in chemistry, a conjugated π system is one in which π bonds alternate with single bonds; the resulting electron distribution gives the intervening single bonds partial double-bond character, the π electrons become delocalized (useful in molecular wires), and the energy of the system is reduced. More generally, joined or paired.

Conjugation — in medical nanorobotics, the docking of two or more nanorobots for the purpose of exchanging information, energy or materials, or to establish a larger multirobotic structure; in biology, the union of two unicellular organisms accompanied by an interchange of nuclear material, as in *Paramecium*.

Conjunctiva — a mucous membrane that lines the eyelid and is reflected onto the eyeball.

Conserved — in genomics, a portion of genetic code that remains almost unchanged among many different species.

Convection — conveyance of heat in liquids or gases by movement or currents of the heated fluids.

Coordinated Universal Time (UTC) — in observational astronomy and chronometry, the local time at the meridian of Greenwich near

London, England; a precision time stamp that is broadcast continuously by radio (e.g. NIST's station WWV).[3302]

Corium — the layer of the skin lying immediately under the epidermis.

Corneal — pertaining to the cornea (the clear, transparent anterior portion of the fibrous coat of the eye comprising about one-sixth of its surface).

Coronal — vertical, but at right angles to sagittal sections, dividing the body into anterior (front) and posterior (back) portions.

Cortex (cortical) — the outer layer of an organ or of the body. Compare medulla.

Covalent bond — in chemistry, a bond formed by sharing a pair of electrons between two atoms.

CPU — see Central Processing Unit.

Cranial — nearest or toward the head.

Crepitation — a crackling sound heard in certain diseases, such as the rale heard in pneumonia; a grating sound heard on movement of ends of a broken bone; a clicking or crackling sound often heard in movements of joints, such as the temporomandibular (jaw), elbow, or patellofemoral (knee) joints, due to roughness and irregularities in the articulating surfaces.

Crinal — pertaining to hair.

Crista — in cell biology, a projection, sometimes branched, of the inner wall of a mitochondrion into its fluid-filled cavity; in anatomy, a ridge of sensory cells inside the ampulla, thrusting hair endings into the cupula (the cells respond to rotary acceleration and deceleration of the head).

Critical pressure — the highest pressure at which gas and liquid may exist as separate phases at any temperature.

Critical temperature — the highest temperature at which gas and liquid may exist as separate phases at any pressure.

Cross-links — in biochemistry, additional bonds formed between normally separate parts of a polymer, typically increasing the tensile strength and stiffness of the chain.

Cryobiology — the study of the effects of cold on biological systems.

Cryogenic — producing, of pertaining to, low temperatures, typically the temperature of liquid nitrogen (77 K) or below.

Cryonic suspension — a currently non-standard medical technique that attempts to prevent the permanent cessation of life, usually by promptly immersing the body of a post-pronouncement patient in a storage fluid maintained at cryogenic temperatures. A person who is cryonically suspended cannot be revived by 20th century medical technology because the freezing process does too much damage, but once frozen the patient's biological condition does not further deteriorate. The procedure is attempted in the belief that future medical technology may allow reversal of tissue damage and the successful revival of the patient.

Crystallescence — in medical nanorobotics, the crystallization of solid solute that is offloaded by nanorobot sorting rotors at a concentration that exceeds the solvation capacity of the surrounding solvent.

Cutaneous — pertaining to the skin.

Cyclic — a structure is termed cyclic if its covalent bonds form one or more rings.

Cycloaddition — a chemical synthesis reaction in which two unsaturated molecules (or moieties within a molecule) bond to form a ring.

Cystic — (usually) pertaining to the gallbladder or urinary bladder.

Cytapheresis — see apheresis.

Cytoambulation — in medical nanorobotics, cell surface walking.

Cytocarriage — in medical nanorobotics, the commandeering of a natural motile cell, by a medical nanorobot, for the purposes of in vivo transport (of the nanorobot), or to perform a herding function (of the affected cell), or for other purposes.

Cytocide — the killing of living cells.

Cytography — a physical description (and mapping) of the living cell.

Cytoidentification — identification of cell type.

Cytokine — a group of extracellular biochemical substances that may be produced by a variety of cells, for the purposes of chemical messaging, regulation, and control; proteins that exert changes in the function or activity of a cell, such as differentiation, proliferation, secretion, or motility.

Cytology (cytological) — the study of biological cells.

Cytometrics — the quantitative measurement of cell sizes, shapes, structures, and numbers.

Cytonatation — in medical nanorobotics, swimming around inside a living cell.

Cytonavigation — in medical nanorobotics, navigation inside the cell; cellular navigation.

Cytopenetration — in medical nanorobotics, entry into cells by penetrating the plasma membrane.

Cytoplasm — the filling substance between the plasma membrane and the nucleus of a cell.

Cytoskeletolysis — in medical nanorobotics, purposeful destruction of the cellular cytoskeleton by a nanorobot, for cytocidal purposes.

Cytoskeleton — the internal structural framework of a cell consisting of at least three types of filaments (microfilaments, microtubules, and intermediate filaments), forming a dynamic framework for maintaining cell shape and motion and allowing rapid changes in the three-dimensional structure of the cell.

Cytosol — the liquid that fills all of the cytoplasmic region, except for fluids filling the interior of the cell organelles.

Cytotomography — tomographic imaging of an individual cell.

Cytotoxic — tending to kill cells.

Cytovehicle — in medical nanorobotics, a living cell that has been commandeered by a medical nanorobot for use during cytocarriage.

Dalton — unit of molecular weight (1 dalton ~ 1 proton).

DC — direct current.

Decoction — liquor extract, from vegetable matter boiled in water.

Deglutition — swallowing.

Degrees of Freedom (DOF) — distinct axes of allowed mechanical motion; the number of directions that a mechanism is free to translate or rotate.

Demarcation — in medical nanorobotics, a crude form of functional navigation in which artificial conditions detectable by in vivo medical nanorobots are created at or near the target treatment site, such as warm or cold spots, pressure spots, or injected chemical plumes.

Denaturation — conversion of a protein from the physiological conformation to some other (possibly inactive) conformation.

Dendrimers — large, regularly-branching molecules.

Dendrite — a branched protoplasmic process of a neuron that conducts impulses toward the cell body. There are usually many to a cell, forming synaptic connections with other neurons.

De novo — created anew.

Deoxyribonucleic acid (DNA) — a complex molecule of very high molecular weight encoding genetic information. DNA consists of deoxyribose (a sugar), phosphoric acid, and four bases (purines or pyrimidines), arranged as two long chains that twist around each other to form a double helix joined by bonds between the complementary purine and pyrimidine components (analogous to rungs on a twisted ladder). DNA is present in the chromosomes of all cells and is the chemical basis of heredity and the carrier of genetic information for almost all organisms (e.g. except the RNA virus, etc.).

Dermatoglyphics — the study of dermal ridge patterns of fingers, toes, palms and soles.

Dermis — inner layer of the skin that lies below the epidermis.

Desiccate — removal of water; dehydration.

Desquamation — shedding epidermis in scales or shreds.

Diagnosis — the determination of the cause and nature of a disease, in order to provide a logical basis for treatment and prognosis.

Dialysis — the passage of a solute through a membrane; process of diffusing blood across a semipermeable membrane to remove toxic materials and to maintain fluid, electrolyte, and acid-base balance in cases of impaired kidney function.

Diametral — pertaining to a diameter.

Diamondoid — structures that resemble diamond in a broad sense; strong, stiff structures containing dense, three-dimensional networks of covalent bonds, formed chiefly from first and second row atoms with a valence of three or more. Many of the most useful diamondoid structures will be rich in tetrahedrally coordinated carbon.

Diamondophagy — eating diamond.

Diapedesis — transendothelial migration (passing through blood vessel endothelial coated walls) to exit the bloodstream and enter the surrounding tissues.

Diaphragm — in human anatomy, the musculomembranous partition between the abdominal and thoracic cavities, whose motions induce lung movements, enabling respiration.

Diaphysis — the shaft or middle part of a long cylindrical bone.

Diastereomeric — having two stereoisomers.

Diastole — the normal period in the heart cycle during which the muscle fibers loosen and lengthen, the heart dilates, and the cavities fill with blood; roughly, the period of relaxation alternating with systole or contraction.

Diathermy — local elevation of temperature within the tissues, produced by high-frequency (~MHz) current, ultrasonic waves, or microwave radiation.

Dielectric — a material capable of storing electrical energy; the interior of a capacitor.

Diels-Alder cycloaddition — in chemical synthesis, the cycloaddition of a conjugated diolefin (an olefin or alkene is a hydrocarbon possessing one or more double bonds in the carbon chain). Diels-Alder reactions are highly stereospecific.

Differentiation — acquisition of character or functions that are different from those of the original type; specialization of cell type within a cell line of increasingly specialized types, by a change in physical form of a cell.

Diffusion — a process by which populations of molecules intermingle and become mixed as a result of their incessant thermal motions.

Digital — pertaining to the use of combinations of bits to represent all quantities that arise during a problem or computation. Compare analog.

Dimer — in chemistry, a combination of two similar or identical molecules, usually by elimination of H_2O or a similar small molecule between the two, or by simple noncovalent association.

Diode — an electronic device that allows current to flow in only one direction.

Diploe — in anatomy, spongy tissue that lies between two layers of the compact bone of the skull.

Diploid — a set of chromosomes that contains two copies of each autosome plus two sex chromosomes; generally found in the somatic body cells.

Dipole — two equal and opposite charges separated by a distance. See also electric dipole moment.

Disassembler — in molecular nanotechnology, a nanomachine or system of nanomachines able to take an object apart while at each step recording the structure and composition of that object at the molecular level.

Disassimilation — in biology, changing assimilated material into less complex compounds for the production of energy.

Disease — see volitional normative model of disease.

Disequilibration — in medical nanorobotics, maintenance or inducement of a state of perpetual ionic, chemical, or energetic disequilibrium in a living cell by a medical nanorobot, usually for the purpose of inducing cytocide.

Dispersion force (London dispersion force) — see van der Waals forces.

Dissociation — in chemistry, the separation of a molecular complex into simpler molecules due to lytic reaction, heat, or ionization.

Dissociation constant — For systems in which ligands of a particular kind bind to a receptor in a solvent, there will be a characteristic frequency with which existing ligand-receptor complexes dissociate as a result of thermal excitation, and a characteristic frequency with which empty receptors bind ligands as a result of Brownian encounters, forming new complexes. The frequency of binding is proportional to the concentration of the ligand in solution. The dissociation constant is the magnitude of the ligand concentration at which the probability that the receptor will be found occupied is 0.5.

Distal — away from a source or a point of attachment or origin; in the extremities, farthest from the trunk.

Diurnal — daily.

DNA — see deoxyribonucleic acid.

DNase — an enzyme that attacks bonds in DNA.

DNA polymerase — an enzyme that synthesizes a daughter strand of DNA under direction from a DNA template; may be involved in repair or replication.

DOF — see Degrees of Freedom.

Domain — in protein chemistry, a discrete continuous part of the amino acid sequence that can be equated with a particular function; proteins such as immunoglobulins may possess several active domains.

Dorsal — the backside of the human body, nearest the spine; the backside of something.

Ductility — see plasticity.

Duodenum — the first ~12 inches of the small intestine.

Dysopsonic — tending to remove opsonization molecules that have become adhered to an exposed in vivo surface.

ECG (EKG) — electrocardiogram.

ECM — see extracellular matrix.

Edema — swollen with excessive fluid.

EEG — electroencephalogram.

Efferent — in relation to nerves or blood vessels, conducting away from a structure or organ; carrying impulses away from a center, as when motor nerves carry impulses from the brain and spinal cord to an effector (e.g. a muscle).

Effervescence — in medical nanorobotics, bubble formation by a gaseous solute that is offloaded by nanorobot sorting rotors at a concentration that exceeds the solvation capacity of the surrounding solvent.

Eigenmode — in linear matrix algebra, a nonzero solution of the characteristic equation of a vector or tensor system.

Elasticity — a property of an object or material, wherein the object or material returns to its original shape after a force is applied and then removed.

Electret — a material that retains a permanent charge.

Electric dipole moment — a measure of the strength of an electric dipole (in units of coulomb-meters). See also dipole.

Electrodynamics — in physics, the study of the motions of charged particles.

Electrolyte — a substance that, in solution, conducts an electric current and is decomposed by the passage of an electric current; a solution that is a conductor of electricity.

Electrometer — an instrument for detecting or measuring differences of electrical potential (e.g. volts) by the effects of electrostatic forces.

Electron Beam Lithography (EBL) — lithography using electron beams rather than light beams.

Electronegativity — a measure of the tendency of an atom (or moiety) to withdraw electrons from structures to which it is bonded. In most circumstances, sodium (Na) tends to donate electron density (low electronegativity) whereas fluorine (F) tends to withdraw electron density (high electronegativity); nitrogen (N) and oxygen (O) are also electronegative atoms.

Electrophoresis — the movement of charged colloidal particles through the medium in which they are dispersed as a result of changes in electrical potential; used in the analysis of protein mixtures because protein particles move with different characteristic velocities dependent principally on the number of charges carried by each particle.

Electroporation — insertion of macromolecules (e.g. DNA) into cells by employing a brief intense pulse of electricity to open cellular pores.

Electrostatic Force Microscope (EFM) — a kind of SPM that images electrostatic forces.

Electrostatic force — a force arising between charged bodies produced by electrostatic fields.

Embolus — a mass of undissolved matter (solid, liquid, or gaseous) present in a blood or lymphatic vessel, brought there by the blood or lymph current.

Emesis — vomiting; may be chemically induced using an emetic.

emf — in physics, "electromotive force" (typically, the electrical potential established across the terminals of a battery), measured in volts.

Emissivity — relative intensity of emission of electromagnetic radiation by a heated body, as compared to a blackbody radiator whose emissivity is defined as 1.

EMP — electromagnetic pulse (e.g. as typically generated during a nuclear explosion).

Enantiomer — in chemistry, a special class of stereoisomers whose structure is not superimposable on its mirror image; a chiral molecule. Two enantiomers of a compound have identical chemical properties, but differ in a characteristic physical property, the ability to rotate the plane of plane-polarized light.

Endocrine gland — a gland that secretes biochemical substances (especially hormones) directly into the bloodstream.

Endocytosis — a process by which proteins arriving at the surface of a cell are internalized, being transported inside the cell within membranous vesicles.

Endoergic — a transformation that absorbs energy; such a reaction increases molecular potential energy. Opposite of exoergic.

Endogenous — originating inside an organ, part, or system.

Endohedral — lying entirely within a (fullerene) cage molecule.

Endometrial — pertaining to the lining of the uterus.

Endoplasmic reticulum — in cell biology, a highly convoluted sheet of membranes, extending from the outer layer of the nuclear envelope into the cytoplasm.

Endosome — the vacuole formed when material is absorbed into a cell by the process of endocytosis; the vacuole fuses with lysosomes.

Endothelium — a form of squamous epithelium consisting of flat cells that line the blood and lymphatic vessels, the heart, and various other body cavities.

Endotheliocyte — in medical nanorobotics, a theorized (nanorobotic) device capable of performing repairs of an injured vascular luminal surface.

Endothermic — a transformation that absorbs energy in the form of heat. A typical endothermic reaction increases both entropy and molecular potential energy, and thus is analogous to a gas expanding while absorbing heat and compressing a spring. Opposite of exothermic.

Energy — in physics, a conserved quantity that can be interconverted among many forms, including kinetic energy, potential energy, and electromagnetic energy.

Engulf formation — in medical nanorobotics, a configuration that may be adopted by a metamorphic nanorobot, in which the nanorobot reshapes itself to create an interior cavity capable of trapping a living cell, virion, or other biological particle.

Enthalpy — in thermodynamics, the internal energy of a system plus the product of its volume and the external pressure.

Entropy — in the physical sciences, a measure of uncertainty regarding the state of a system; free energy can be extracted by converting a low-entropy state to a high-entropy state. In other contexts, the term is often used by analogy to describe the extent of randomness and disorder in a system and the consequent lack of knowledge or information about it.

Enucleated cell — a cell from which the nucleus has been removed.

Enzyme - a protein molecule that often acts as a specific catalyst, facilitating specific chemical or metabolic reactions necessary for cell growth and reproduction; a biological chemosynthetic molecular machine.

Eosinophil — a type of granulocytic white blood cell comprising 1%-4% of all leukocytes, that is known to destroy parasitic organisms and to play a major role in allergic reactions (some of the major chemical mediators that cause bronchoconstriction in asthma are released by eosinophils).

Epidermis — the outer epithelial portion of the skin.

Epitaxial methods — a class of methods for inducing crystal growth.

Epithelium — the avascular layer of cells forming the epidermis of the skin and the surface layer of mucous (secreting mucus) and serous (secreting serum or serumlike fluid) membranes, including the glands. The cells rest on a basement membrane and lie closely approximated to each other with little intercellular material between them.

Epitope — any component of an antigen molecule that functions as an antigenic determinant by permitting the attachment of certain antibodies.

Equilibrium — a system is said to be at equilibrium (with respect to some set of feasible transformations) if that system has minimal free energy. A system containing objects at different temperatures is in disequilibrium, because heat flow can reduce the free energy (causing the different temperatures to converge). Springs have equilibrium lengths, reactants and products in solution have equilibrium concentrations, thermally excited systems have equilibrium probabilities of occupying various states, and so forth.

Ergoacoustic — pertaining to the conversion of energy of various kinds into acoustic energy.

Ergooptical (ergophotonic) — pertaining to the conversion of energy of various kinds into optical (photonic) energy.

Eructations — producing gas from the stomach, usually with a characteristic sound; belching.

Erysipelas — acute febrile disease with localized inflammation, eruption and redness of skin and subcutaneous tissue, accompanied by systemic signs and symptoms, caused by a hemolytic streptococcus.

Erythrocyte — red blood cell.

Erythropoietin — a hormone that controls the production rate of red blood cells in the human body.

Euchromatin — all of the genome in the interphase nucleus, except for the heterochromatin.

Eukaryote — an organism or cell that contains its genome within a nucleus.

Eutactic — characterized by precise molecular order.

Excimer laser — a kind of high-energy ultraviolet (UV) laser based on excited state transitions.

Excision — an act of cutting away or taking out.

Excluded volume — the presence of one molecule or moiety reduces the physical volume available for other molecules or moieties to occupy, thus partially crowding them out.

Excoriation — abrasion of the epidermis or of the coating of any organ of the body by trauma, chemicals, burns, or other causes.

Exfusion — generally, to remove from the body; distinguished from infusion.

Exocrine — external secretion of a gland.

Exocytosis — the process of secreting proteins from a cell into the surrounding medium, by transport in membranous vesicles from the endoplasmic reticulum, through the Golgi, to storage vesicles, and finally (upon a regulatory signal) through the plasma membrane.

Exodermal — lying outside of the skin surface.

Exoergic — a transformation that releases energy; such a reaction decreases molecular potential energy. Opposite of endoergic.

Exogenous — originating outside an organ, part, or system.

Exohedral — lying entirely outside a (fullerene) cage molecule.

Exons — portions of genes represented in mRNA.

Exothermic — a transformation that releases energy in the form of heat. Exoergic reactions in solution are commonly exothermic. Opposite of endothermic.

Exploratory engineering — design and analysis of systems that are theoretically possible but cannot be built yet, owing to the limitations of currently available tools.

Exponential — refers to a mathematical function (e.g. $y = 10^x$) which has an exponented quantity as its independent variable (e.g. x); more informally, may denote a very steeply rising (or falling) quantity, function or variable.

Extracellular — outside of the cell.

Extracellular matrix (ECM) — an extracellular fibrous scaffolding that helps organize cells into tissues.

Extrasomatic — originating or existing outside of the human body.

Extravasation — exiting the bloodstream.

Exudate — accumulation of a fluid in a cavity; matter that penetrates through vessel walls into adjoining tissue; the production of pus or serum.

Ex vivo — outside of the living human body.

Facultative — having the ability to do something which is not mandatory.

Fascia — a fibrous membrane covering, supporting, and separating muscles; also, unites the skin with underlying (e.g. muscular) tissue.

Fatty acid — a hydrocarbon in which one of the H atoms has been replaced by a carboxyl group.

Febrile — pertaining to fever.

Fenestrated — having openings.

Fibroblast — a stellate or spindle-shaped motile cell with cytoplasmic processes present in connective tissue, capable of forming collagen fibers.

Fission (fissile) — in physics, the release of energy when an atomic nucleus more massive than Fe^{56} (see binding energy) is split into two or more less massive fragments; the fission of nuclei lighter than Fe^{56} is typically endoergic. In microbiology, a method of asexual reproduction in bacteria, protozoa, and other lower forms of life; in cell biology, the partition of one organelle into two, as for example the fissioning mitochondrion.

Fistula — in anatomy, an abnormal tubelike passage from a normal cavity or tube to a free surface or to another cavity; may be due to congenital incomplete closure of parts, or may result from abscesses, injuries, or inflammatory processes.

Flagellum — in cell biology, a whiplike locomotory organelle consisting of nine double peripheral microtubules and two single central microtubules.

Flatus — gas in the digestive tract; expelling of gas from a body orifice, especially the anus (e.g. to fart).

FLOP — in computer science, a floating point operation, an individual computational step as software executes in a computer. A floating point number is a number expressed as a product of a bounded number and an exponential scale factor, as in scientific notation.

Fluidity — in cellular biomechanics, a property of cell membranes, indicating the ability of lipids to move laterally within their particular monolayer.

Flux (fluence) — generally, a rate of flow.

FM — frequency modulation.

Follower — in mechanical engineering, a mechanical component in a cam system that is driven through a pattern of displacements as it rests against a moving contoured surface. See cam.

Foramen magnum — in anatomy, an opening in the occipital bone through which passes the spinal cord from the brain.

Formed elements — the cellular components of the blood, usually including red cells, white cells, and platelets.

Fourier transform — in mathematical physics, the expression of a complex waveform as a weighted sum of an infinite series of monofrequency waves.

Fovea — the clearest point of vision in the retina of the eye.

Fractionation — to separate components of a mixture into distinct molecular submixtures or pure components.

Free energy — a measure of the ability of a system to do work, such that a reduction in free energy could in principle yield an equivalent quantity of work. The Helmholtz free energy describes the free energy within a system; the Gibbs free energy does not.

Fresnel lens — a glass lens cast in a series of adjacent annular rings of various heights and shapes, commonly employed in lighthouses to produce powerful directed beams of light.

Friction Force Microscopy (FFM) — a kind of SPM that measures the frictional force between a sample and a sharp tip.

FTP — file transfer protocol (used for large-block data transfers on the Internet).

Fullerene — a closed-cage molecule consisting of linked pentagons, hexagons, heptagons, or other polygonal elements; originally referred to carbon-only structures but has since been broadened to represent the entire class of molecules having this geometry, regardless of atomic constituency.

Functionalized — in chemistry, an otherwise chemically inert structure is functionalized when a chemically active ligand or moiety is covalently bonded to it.

Functional navigation — in medical nanorobotics, a form of nanorobotic navigation in which nanodevices seek to detect subtle variations in their environment, comparing sensor readings with target tissue/cell profiles and then congregating wherever a precisely defined set of preconditions exists.

Fundamental mode — the lowest natural frequency of vibration of an object or system.

Fusion — in physics, the release of energy when atomic particles of total atomic mass less than the atomic mass of Fe^{56} (see binding energy) join together to form a more massive single particle; the fusion of nuclei heavier than Fe^{56} is typically endoergic. In cell biology, fusion is the merging of vesicles budded from the ER into the Golgi complex, or of endosomes with lysosomes, or of the contents of two cells by artificial means without the destruction of either, resulting in a heterokaryon that, for at least a few generations, will reproduce its kind (this was once an important method in assigning loci to chromosomes). In sensory physiology, the sensation that results when two different sensory qualities merge to give a third quality, such as the fusion of red and yellow into orange. Most generally, to combine together.

g — unit of gravitational acceleration (9.81 m/sec^2); describes the mean gravitation force experienced by a mass at rest on Earth's surface.

Galvanic — pertaining to electrical direct current, usually chemically generated.

Gamete — either type of reproductive or germ cell (e.g. sperm or egg) with haploid chromosome content. Compare somatic cell.

Ganglion — a mass of nervous tissue composed principally of nerve-cell bodies and lying outside the brain or spinal cord (e.g. the chains of ganglia that form the main sympathetic trunks, or the dorsal root ganglion of a spinal nerve).

Gangrene — a necrosis (death) of tissue, usually due to deficient, obstructed, or lost blood supply; it may be localized to a small area or it may involve an entire organ or extremity.

Gastro — pertaining to the stomach.

Gate — see logic gate.

GDP — guanosine diphosphate.

Gene — a segment of a chromosome; an hereditary unit comprised of DNA occupying a locus in the genome which bears base sequential information for regulation, for transcription into RNA, or for transcription into mRNA destined for translation into protein.

Genome — the total hereditary material of a cell, containing the entire chromosomal set found in each nucleus of a given species.

Genomics — concerning the genome, the study of genes and how they affect the human body.

Genotype — the basic combination of genes of an organism. The genetic constitution of an organism.

Geodesic — pertaining to the mapping of the surface of the Earth.

Germ line — the cell line from which gametes derive.

GHz — gigahertz; billions of cycles per second.

Gibbs free energy — equals the Helmholtz free energy plus the product of the system volume and the external pressure. Changes in the Gibbs free energy at a constant pressure thus include work done against external pressure as a system undergoes volumetric changes.

Gimbal — in mechanical engineering, a device consisting of a pair of rings pivoted on axes at right angles to each other so that one is free to swing within the other.

Glioblastoma — a neuroglial (brain) cell tumor.

Global Positioning System (GPS) — a system of Earth-orbiting satellites that broadcasts navigational radio signals, allowing a ground receiver to precisely fix its position on the Earth's surface.

Glottis — the sound-producing apparatus of the larynx, consisting of two vocal cords and the intervening space.

Glucose — simple blood sugar ($C_6H_{12}O_6$).

Glycocalyx — a thin layer of glycoprotein and polysaccharide that covers the surface of some cells, such as muscle cells, fibroblasts, pericytes, and epithelial cells, and contributes to the basal lamina.

Glycogen — a polysaccharide commonly called animal starch, with chemical formula $(C_6H_{10}O_5)_n$; glycogen is the form in which carbohydrate is stored in the animal body (mostly in the liver and muscles) for future conversion into sugar. The formation of glycogen from carbohydrate sources is called glycogenesis, while the reverse process is called glycogenolysis.

Glycolysis — enzyme-mediated energy-yielding anaerobic hydrolysis of glucose to lactic acid in various cells and tissues, notably muscle.

Glycoprotein — a protein molecule with carbohydrate moieties attached.

Glycosylation — the covalent bonding of carbohydrate moieties to another molecule.

Golgi complex/apparatus — in cell biology, individual stacks of membranes near the endoplasmic reticulum involved in glycosylating proteins and sorting them for transport to different intracellular locations.

Gorget — in surgery, an instrument grooved to protect soft tissues from injury as a pointed instrument is inserted into a body cavity.

G-proteins — guanine nucleotide-binding trimeric proteins that reside in the plasma membrane. When bound by GDP, the trimer remains intact and is inert; when GDP is replaced by GTP, the trimer separates into a monomer and a dimer, one of which may then activate or repress a target protein.

GPS — see Global Positioning System.

Gradient — a slope or grade; an increase or decrease of varying degrees or the curve that represents such; rate of change of temperature, pressure, chemical concentration, or other physical variable, as a function of time, distance, frequency, etc.

Granules — a small, grainlike body. Small granules may be found in cells, containing stores of nutrients; large granules may be formed in tissues following a granulomatous reaction.

Granulocyte — a granular leukocyte; a polymorphonuclear (nucleus composed of two or more lobes or parts) leukocyte, including basophils, eosinophils, and neutrophils.

Granuloma — a nodular inflammatory lesion, usually small or granular, that is firm, persistent, and contains compactly grouped mononuclear phagocytes.

Granulomatous reaction — producing a granuloma, a granular tumor or growth, usually of lymphoid and epithelioid cells; an encapsulation reaction to the presence of a foreign object in the body that cannot be readily phagocytosed.

Gravimeter — a device for measuring gravitational acceleration.

Ground state — the lowest-energy state of a system. A system in its electronic ground state cannot further reduce its energy by an electronic transition, but may still contain vibrational energy.

GTP — guanosine triphosphate.

Gustatory — pertaining to the sense of taste.

Halogen — pertaining to fluorine, chlorine, bromine, iodine, or astatine.

Haploid — a set of chromosomes that contains one copy of each autosome and one sex chromosome.

Haploid number — the number of chromosomes in sperm or ova (23 in humans), half the number found in somatic (e.g. diploid) cells; characteristic of the gametes of diploid organisms.

Haptic — operated by, or pertaining to, the sense of touch.

Harmonic oscillator — in physics, any system of particles that displays harmonic (periodic oscillating) motion, such as a pendulum or spring with an attached mass; a system in which a mass is subject to a linear restoring force. A harmonic oscillator vibrates at a fixed frequency, independent of amplitude.

Haustra — in anatomy, the sacculated pouches of the colon.

Hawk — to make an audible effort to force up phlegm from the throat.

Hct — see hematocrit.

Heat — as defined in thermodynamics, heat is the energy that flows between two systems as a result of temperature differences, as distinguished from thermal energy. (A system contains neither heat nor work, but can produce heat or do work.)

Heat capacity — the ratio of the heat input to the temperature increase in a system.

Hectomicron — 100 microns.

Helmholtz free energy — the internal energy of a system minus the product of its entropy and temperature.

Hemapheresis — see apheresis.

Hemato — pertaining to blood.

Hematocrit (Hct) — volume-fraction or bloodstream concentration of erythrocytes (red blood cells), expressed as a percentage.

Hematoma — a swelling or mass of blood (usually clotted), confined to an organ, tissue, or other space, caused by a break in a blood vessel.

Hemobaric — pertaining to blood pressure.

Hemolytic — tending to destroy red blood cells, liberating hemoglobin.

Hemorrhagic — pertaining to bleeding.

Hemostasis — arrest of bleeding.

Hepatic — pertaining to the liver.

Hepatocyte — the most common tissue cell found in the liver.

Heterochromatin — regions of the genome that remain permanently in a highly condensed state and are not genetically expressed.

Histamine — a chemical substance, produced from the amino acid histidine, normally present in the body; exerts a pharmacological action when released from injured cells.

Histaminergic — activated or energized by histamine.

Histology — the study of tissues.

Histonatation — in medical nanorobotics, locomotion (swimming) through tissues by a nanorobot.

Histonavigation — in medical nanorobotics, navigation through tissues by a nanorobot.

Histones — conserved DNA-binding proteins of eukaryotes that form the nucleosome, the basic subunit of chromatin; histones are rich in arginine and lysine residues.

HLA complex — Histocompatibility Locus Antigens, formerly known as Human Leukocyte Antigen (or Associated) complex.

Holliday junction — a connection between two DNA duplex molecules (as during recombination), wherein one duplex rotates relative to the other, creating a junction with 3-D topology.[3154]

Homeodomain — a DNA-binding motif in a transcriptional regulator that identifies, or at least is common in, the genes concerned with early embryonic developmental regulation.

Homeostasis — in physiology, a state of equilibrium of the internal environment of the body that is maintained by dynamic processes of feedback and regulation; homeostasis is a dynamic equilibrium (changing balance), keeping cells within the physical and chemical limits that can support life.

Homeothermic — tending to maintain a constant temperature, despite temperature variations in the surrounding environment.

Homochirality — chirality is a property of certain asymmetric molecules, the property being that the mirror images of the molecules cannot be superimposed one on the other while facing in the same direction. Homochirality is the preference of a process or system for a single optical isomer in a pair of isomers.

Homologous — similar in form (e.g. fundamental structure and origin), but not necessarily in function.

Hormone — a chemical substance that originates in an organ, gland, or part and is conveyed through the blood to another part of the body, stimulating that other part by chemical action to increase functional activity or to increase secretion of another hormone.

Hyaline cartilage — true cartilage; a smooth and pearly layer that covers the articular (place of union between two or more bones) surfaces of bones.

Hydrocarbon — a molecule consisting only of H and C.

Hydrodynamics — in physics, the study of the action of and motion of (and in) water and other liquids.

Hydrogen bond — the weak bond between a positively charged hydrogen atom that is covalently bound to one electronegative atom, and another electronegative atom.

Hydrolysis — a (hydrolytic) reaction in which a covalent bond is broken with the incorporation of a water molecule.

Hydrophilicity — tending to mix with water; wettable. Hydrophilic groups interact with water, so that hydrophilic regions of protein or the faces of a lipid bilayer reside in an aqueous environment.

Hydrophobic force — water molecules are linked by a network of hydrogen bonds; a nonpolar nonwetting surface such as wax cannot form hydrogen bonds, hence repels water.

Hydrophobicity — tending not to mix with water; nonwetting. Hydrophobic groups repel water, so that they interact with one another to generate a nonaqueous environment.

Hydrostatic — pertaining to the pressure of fluids or to fluid properties when in equilibrium.

Hygroscopic — readily absorbing and retaining moisture.

Hypercholesterolemia — presence of an abnormal amount of cholesterol in the cells and plasma of the circulating blood.

Hypergolic — refers to two substances which, although stable when stored separately, spontaneously combust or react when mixed.

Hypogravity — conditions of below-normal gravity (e.g. microgravity in Earth orbit).

Hypotension — low blood pressure.

Hypoxia — a condition in which the tissues are not receiving enough oxygen to sustain their metabolic activity.

Hypsithermal limit — the maximum amount of energy that may be released at Earth's surface, as a result of human technological activities, without significantly altering the natural global energy balance; estimated as 10^{13}-10^{15} watts.

Hz — hertz (MKS unit of frequency); cycles per second of an oscillation.

Iatrogenic disorder — an adverse condition induced in a patient by the actions of a physician.

Icosahedral — a solid figure with 20 planar faces.

Iliac crest — in anatomy, pertaining to the top of the ilium (the uppermost of the three sections of the hipbone).

Immunoglobulin — see antibody.

Impedance — opposition to flow (e.g. fluid, electrical, etc.) when flow is steady, or the driving pressure per unit flow when flow is changing; the resistance of an acoustic system to being set in motion.

Incision — a cut made with a knife.

In cyto — within a biological cell.

Inertia — in physics, the tendency of a body to remain in its kinematic state (e.g. at rest or in motion) until acted upon by an outside force; in biology, sluggishness or lack of activity.

Infarct — an area of tissue in an organ or part that undergoes necrosis following cessation of blood supply.

Inferior — beneath or lower; often refers to the undersurface of an organ or indicates a structure below another structure. See also caudal.

Infrasonic — inaudible (to human ears); sounds with acoustic frequencies less than ~16 Hz.

Infusion — the introduction of a fluid, other than blood, into a vein.

Inmessaging — in medical nanorobotics, conveyance of information from a source external to the human body, or external to working nanodevices, to a receiver located inside the human body.

Inner ear — the portion of the ear consisting of the cochlea, containing the sensory receptors for hearing, and the vestibule and semicircular canals, which include the receptors for balance and the sense of position.

Innervated — having nerves.

In nucleo — within the nucleus of a cell.

In sanguo — within the bloodstream.

Integral membrane protein — in cell biology, an amphipathic protein embedded in the lipid bilayer of the cell which cannot be extracted from the membrane without disrupting the lipid bilayer; most integral proteins are transmembrane proteins.

Intercalated — inserted between two others, as something interposed.

Intercostal — between the ribs.

Interferometry — measurement of very small spatial or frequency displacements using wave interference patterns.

Intermolecular — an interaction (e.g. a chemical reaction) between different molecules.

Internal energy — the sum of the kinetic and potential energies (including electromagnetic field energies) of the particles that make up a system.

Interphase — in cell biology, the quiescent period of time between mitotic cell divisions.

Interstitial — pertaining to extracellular interstices or spaces within an organ or tissue.

Intracellular fluid — all of the fluid inside a cell; the cytosol plus the fluid inside each organelle, including the nucleus.

Intracorporeal — inside the human body.

Intramolecular — an interaction (e.g. chemical reaction) within a single molecule. Intramolecular interactions between widely separated parts of a molecule resemble intermolecular interactions in most respects.

Intraperitoneal — within the peritoneal (abdominal) cavity.

Intravascular — inside a blood vessel.

In vacuo — in a vacuum (viz. the ablative case of the 2nd-declension Latin adjective "vacuus").

Invaginate — to place or receive into a sheath; to receive within itself or into another part.

In vivo — inside the living human body.

Ion — an atom or molecule with a net charge.

Ion Beam Lithography (IBL) — lithography using ions rather than light beams.

Ion channels — a large heterogeneous family of voltage-activated proteins that control the permeability of cells to specific ions by opening or closing in response to differences in potentials across the plasma membrane. Ion channels participate in the generation and transmission of electrical activity in the nervous system and in the hormonal regulation of cellular physiology.

Ionic bond — a chemical bond resulting chiefly from the electrostatic attraction between positive and negative ions.

Ionosphere — an upper region of Earth's atmosphere.

IR — infrared.

Ischemia — local and temporary deficiency of blood supply due to obstruction of the circulation into a body part.

Isoareal — occurring without any change in surface area.

Isobaric — held, or existing, at a constant pressure.

Isomer — one of two more chemical substances that have the same molecular formula but different chemical and physical properties due to a different arrangement of the atoms in the molecule; for example, dextrose is an isomer of levulose. Isomers may be geometric, optical, or structural. See also chiral, enantiomer, stereochemistry, and stereoisomer.

Isomagnetic — having the same magnetic field strength.

Isometric — in general, having equal dimensions; in physiology (or biomechanics), denoting a condition wherein the ends of a contracting muscle (or motor protein) are held fixed so that contraction produces increased tension at constant overall length.

Isoporous — having pores of the same size.

Isostatic — denoting a condition in which there is equal pressure on every side; in hydrostatic equilibrium.

Isotherm — region, section, or surface of constant temperature.

Isothermal — held, or existing, at a constant temperature.

Isotonic — animal cells containing a solution which exerts an osmotic pressure approximately equal to that of the surrounding fluid are isotonic or isoosmotic to that fluid. Stronger solutions that cause cells to shrink are hypertonic; weaker solutions that cause cells to swell are hypotonic.

Isotope — any of two or more forms of the same chemical element that have nearly identical chemical properties but which differ in the number of neutrons contained in each atomic nucleus; many isotopes are radioactive.

Isotropic — the same in all directions.

Isovolemic — occurring without any change in volume.

IV — intravenous (inserted into a vein).

J — joule (MKS unit of energy).

Kelvins (K) — kelvin degrees (MKS unit of temperature).

Keratin — a sulfur-rich scleroprotein or albuminoid present largely in cuticular (pertaining to cuticles) structures.

Keratinocyte — a cell of the epidermis, and parts of the mouth, that produces keratin.

kg — kilogram (MKS unit of mass).

KHz — kilohertz; thousands of cycles per second.

Kinematic — pertaining to motion.

Kinesthesis — sensations of position, movement, direction and extent from the limbs, neck and body trunk.

Kinetic energy — energy resulting from the motion of masses.

Kupffer cells — macrophages lining the sinusoids of the liver.

Labial — pertaining to the lips.

Lacrimal — pertaining to the tears (eye fluid).

Lamellipodium — a cytoplasmic veil produced on all sides of a migrating polymorphonuclear leukocyte (granulocyte).

Laminar (Poiseuille) flow — fluid flow that moves exclusively along separate and independent parallel flow planes (i.e. streamlines), generally with an axisymmetric parabolic profile if in a tube. Laminar flow minimizes the impedance (resistance) and energy dissipation of fluid flow.

Langmuir-Blodgett (LB) film — a technique for producing highly regular stacks of monomolecular films.

Lateral — on the side, or farthest from, the midsagittal plane; away from the midline of the body (to the side).

Lathe — in mechanical engineering, a machine for shaping an object, by holding and turning the object rapidly against the edge of a cutting tool.

LD50 — a dose of or exposure to a toxic influence that produces death in 50% of organisms exposed to it.

LED — light emitting diode.

Leukapheresis — see apheresis.

Leukocytes (white blood cells) — the primary effector cells that respond to infection and tissue damage in the human body. There are two types: granulocytes (including basophils, eosinophils, and neutrophils) and agranulocytes (including monocytes and lymphocytes). Leukocytes are formed from two stem cell populations in the bone marrow. The myeloid stem cell line produces granulocytes and monocytes, while the lymphoid stem cell line produces lymphocytes. Lymphoid cells travel to the thymus, spleen and lymph nodes, where they mature and differentiate into active, antigen-specific lymphocytes.

Leukokine — a cytokine secreted by a leukocyte.

Leukotaxis — active amoeboid movement of leukocytes, especially neutrophils, either toward (positive leukotaxis) or away from (negative leukotaxis) certain microorganisms or substances that frequently are formed in inflamed tissue; the property of attracting or repelling leukocytes.

Ligand — in protein chemistry, a small molecule that is (or can be) bound by a larger molecule; in organometallic chemistry, a moiety bonded to a central metal atom (this latter definition is more common in general chemistry).

Ligation — the formation of a phosphodiester bond to link two adjacent bases separated by a nick in one strand of a double helix of DNA; the term can also be applied to blunt-end ligation and to the joining of RNA.

Linear — in control theory, describes systems in which an output is directly proportional to an input.

Lingual — pertaining to the tongue.

Lipid bilayer — in cell biology, the form taken by a concentration of lipids in which the hydrophobic fatty acids occupy the interior and the hydrophilic polar heads face the exterior; primary constituent of the plasma membranes of cells.

Lipids — molecules having hydrophilic polar heads, containing phosphate (phospholipid), sterol (such as cholesterol), or saccharide (glycolipid) connected to a hydrophobic tail consisting of fatty acid.

Lipofuscin — brown pigment granules representing lipid-containing nondegradable residues of lysosomal digestion.

Lipophilic — having an affinity for lipids (fats).

Lipophobic — repulsed by lipids (fats).

Liposomes — the sealed concentric microscopic shells formed when certain lipid substances are in an aqueous solution. See also micelles.

Lithography — a technique for surface patterning commonly used to make semiconductor devices.

Lithotomy — in surgery, incision of a duct or organ, especially of the bladder, to remove a calculus (any abnormal concretion within the animal body, usually composed of mineral salts, commonly called stone).

Lithotripsy — crushing of a stone in the bladder or urethra.

Load error — in control theory, minimum range of variation in a control variable that is necessary to provoke a response from a control system.

Logic gate — in digital logic, a component that can switch the state of an output depending on the states of one or more inputs; a device implementing any of the elementary logic (or Boolean) functions (e.g. AND, NAND, NOR, NOT, OR, XOR). A logic gate is characterized by the relationship between its inputs and outputs, and not by its internal mechanisms.

Loin (lumbar) — lower part of the back and sides, between the thorax (ribs) and the pelvis (hips).

LPS — lipopolysaccharide, the lipid used to construct the outer leaflet of the outer bilayer membrane of Gram-negative bacteria.

LR oscillator — an electrical oscillator circuit comprised of resistors and inductors (solenoids).

Lumbar — see loin.

Lumen — the interior, especially of a compartment bounded by membranes, as for instance the endoplasmic reticulum or the mitochondrion.

Luminal — pertaining to the interior of a cavity, tube, or vessel.

Lymph — an alkaline fluid found in the lymphatic system.

Lymphatic system — includes all structures involved in the conveyance of lymph from the tissues to the bloodstream, including lymph capillaries, lacteals, lymph nodes, lymph vessels, main lymph ducts, and cisterna chyli.

Lymphocyte — a morphologically distinct variety of leukocytes, comprising 20%-44% of all white blood cells. But only ~2% of all lymphocytes present in the human body are in the bloodstream; most reside elsewhere, particularly in the lymph and the lymph nodes. B-lymphocytes differentiate into antibody-secreting plasma cells, whereas T-lymphocytes play diverse regulatory roles in the immune response.

Lysis (lytic) — in microbiology, the death of a bacterium at the end of a bacteriophage infective cycle when the bacterium bursts open to release the progeny of an infecting phage; also applies to eukaryotic cells, as for example infected cells that are attacked by the immune system. More generally, dissolution or decomposition.

Lysosomes — small bodies inside cells, enclosed by membranes, that contain hydrolytic enzymes that are part of the cell's digestive apparatus.

Lysozyme (muramidase) — an enzyme that is destructive to cell walls of certain bacteria, found in white blood cells of the granulocytic and monocytic series.

m — meter (MKS unit of length)

M — see molarity.

Macromolecule — a molecule of colloidal size, typically 1-100 nm in diameter or length, consisting most notably of proteins, nucleic acids, and polysaccharides.

Macrophage — a monocyte that has left the circulation and settled and matured in a tissue; found in large numbers in the spleen, lymph nodes, alveoli, and tonsils, with ~50% found in the liver as Kupffer cells. Along with neutrophils, macrophages are the major phagocytic cells of the immune system, able to recognize (and then ingest) foreign antigens via chemical receptors on the surface of their cell membranes. Macrophages also serve a vital role by processing antigens and presenting them to T cells, activating the specific immune response.

Macroscopic — easily visible to the human naked eye; typically ~1 mm^3 or larger.

Macrosensing — in medical nanorobotics, the detection of global somatic states (inside the human body) and extrasomatic states (sensory data originating outside of the human body) by in vivo nanorobots.

Magnetic Force Microscope (MFM) — a kind of SPM that images surfaces using magnetic forces.

Maillard reaction — in food science, the "browning" reaction that occurs between proteins and reducing sugars as they are heated.

Major histocompatibility complex (MHC) — the complex of HLA genes on the short arm of human chromosome 6.

Manometer (manometry) — a device for measuring liquid or gaseous pressure such as blood, spinal fluid, or atmosphere (air).

Manustupration — masturbation.

Margination — adhesion of leukocytes to endothelial cells lining the walls of a blood vessel, during the relatively early stages of inflammation; more generally, the process of differential radial migration among suspended particles of different sizes during fluid flow through a tube.

Massometer — in medical nanorobotics, a nanosensor device for measuring the mass of individual molecules or small physical objects to single-proton resolution.

Mast cells — cells resident in connective tissue just below epithelial surfaces, serous cavities, and around blood vessels, that synthesize, store, and release (upon stimulation) histamine and other local chemical mediators of inflammation (e.g. leukotrienes).

Mastication — chewing.

Mechanical nanocomputers — nano-sized computers that use mechanical rather than chemical or electronic logic switches.

Mechanomechanical conversion — conversion of one form of mechanical energy into another form of mechanical energy.

Mechanochemistry — the chemistry of processes in which mechanical systems operating with atomic-scale precision guide, drive, or are driven by chemical transformations; in more general usage, the chemistry of processes in which energy is converted from mechanical to chemical form, or vice versa (aka. piezochemistry).

Mechanosynthesis — chemical synthesis controlled by mechanical systems operating with atomic-scale precision, enabling direct positional selection of reaction sites; synthetic applications of mechanochemistry.

Medial — middle or nearest to the midsagittal plane; toward the midline of a body or vessel.

Medulla (medullary) — the inner or central portion of an organ. Compare cortex.

Medulla oblongata — enlarged portion of the spinal cord in the cranium, after the cord enters the foramen magnum of the occipital bone; the lower portion of the brain stem.

Melanoma — a malignant, darkly pigmented mole or tumor of the skin.

Membrane — in cell biology, an asymmetrical lipid bilayer that has lateral fluidity and contains proteins; in anatomy, a thin, soft, pliable layer of tissue that lines a tube or cavity, covers an organ or structure, or separates one part from another.

Membrane proteins — in cell biology, plasma membrane proteins that have hydrophobic regions that allow part or all of the protein structure to reside within the membrane; the bonds involved in this association are usually noncovalent.

Membranolytic — causing the physical failure of a membrane.

MEMS — see microelectromechanical systems.

Meniscus — the curved upper surface of a liquid in contact with a container.

-mer — see oligomer.

Mesenchyme — a diffuse network of cells forming the embryonic mesoderm and giving rise to connective tissues, blood, and blood vessels, the lymphatic system, and cells of the RES.

Mesentery — a peritoneal fold encircling the greater part of the small intestines and connecting the intestine to the posterior abdominal wall.

Mesoderm — a tissue layer in the embryo from which arises all connective tissues, including the muscular, skeletal, circulatory, lymphatic, and urogenital systems, and the linings of the body cavities.

Mesoscopic — lying midway in size between the nanoscale (~nanometers) and the microscale (~microns).

Mesothelium — the layer of cells derived from the mesoderm that lines the primitive body cavity; in the adult, it becomes the epithelium covering the serous membranes.

Messenger molecule — a chemically recognizable molecule which can convey information after it is received and decoded by an appropriate chemical sensor.

Messenger RNA (mRNA) — the RNA whose sequence corresponds to that of exons in the transcribed gene, which embodies the codons and is translated into the protein gene product.

Metabolism — the sum of all physical and chemical changes that take place within an organism; all energy and material transformations that occur within living cells, including anabolism and catabolism.

Metamorphic — in medical nanorobotics, capable of adopting multiple physical configurations via smooth changes from one configuration to another.

Metaphase — stage of mitosis (cell division) in which all chromosomes are aligned equidistant between the spindle poles.

Metastable state — a high energy state that requires an input of energy to relax to the ground state.

Metastasize — usually refers to the manifestation of a malignancy (e.g. of cancerous body cells) as a secondary growth arising from the primary growth, but in a new location.

Metazoa — all multicellular life.

Metrology — the science of weights and measures.

MeV — million electron volts (unit of energy).

MHC — see major histocompatibility complex.

MHz — megahertz; millions of cycles per second.

Micelle — a self-assembling hollow spheroidal aggregate of amphipathic lipids in a polar liquid (e.g. aqueous) medium.

Michaelis-Menten enzyme — an enzyme whose saturation kinetics obey the Michaelis-Menten equation, which describes the half-maximal reaction velocity as a function of substrate concentration; certain enzymes and other ligand-binding proteins such as hemoglobin may obey sigmoid (e.g., Hill equation) substrate saturation kinetics instead.

Microbarom — a low-amplitude, slowly-varying atmospheric pressure wave.

Microbiotagraphics — mapping the microbiotic populations present in the human body.

Microelectromechanical systems (MEMS) — micron-scale devices combining electronic and mechanical elements.

Micron — one-millionth of a meter; a micrometer.

Micro-opto-mechanical systems (MOMS) — micron-scale devices combining electronic, optical and mechanical elements.

Microsensors — micron-scale chemical and physical sensors.

Microtubules — filaments consisting of dimers of tubulin; interphase microtubules are reorganized into spindle fibers during mitosis (cell division), when they are responsible for chromosome movement.

Microvasculature — pertaining to the very fine blood vessels of the body.

Midsagittal — vertical at midline, dividing the body into right and left halves.

Mince — progressive reduction in size of biological tissue samples by mechanical means; more generally, to cut or chop into very small pieces, or to subdivide minutely.

MIPS — a conventional measure of computing speed, defined as millions of instructions per second.

Mitochondrion — a self-reproducing organelle that provides energy for eukaryotic cells via oxidative phosphorylation.

Mitosis — in cell biology, the division of a eukaryotic somatic cell. The four (or five) sequential stages are prophase, (prometaphase), metaphase, anaphase, and telophase; the absence of mitosis is the interphase.

MKS — meter-kilogram-second; standard system of units adopted by the international physics community.

Moiety — a portion of a molecular structure having some property of interest.

Molality — in chemistry, moles of solute per kilogram of solvent.

Molar — in anatomy, pertaining to a grinding (back) tooth.

Molarity (M) — in chemistry, moles of solute per liter of solvent.

Mole — a number of instances of something (e.g. molecular objects) equal to ~6.023×10^{23} objects.

Molecular assembler — a general-purpose device for molecular manufacturing, able to guide chemical reactions by positioning individual molecules to atomic accuracy (e.g. mechanosynthesis) and to construct a wide range of useful and stable molecular structures according to precise specifications.

Molecular Beam Epitaxy (MBE) — a technique for producing single-layer crystals.

Molecular electronics — any system of atomically precise electronic devices of nanometer dimensions, especially if made of discrete molecular parts rather than the continuous bulk materials found in 20th century semiconductor devices.

Molecular machine — a mechanical device that performs a useful function using components of nanometer scale and a well-defined molecular structure; may include both artificial nanomachines and naturally occurring devices found in biological systems.

Molecular machine system — a system of molecular machines.

Molecular manipulator — a manipulator device able to position molecular tools with high precision, for example to direct varying sequences of mechanosynthetic steps; a major component of a molecular assembler.

Molecular manufacturing — manufacturing using molecular machinery, giving molecule-by-molecule control of products via positional chemical synthesis, to produce complex molecular structures manufactured to precise specifications.

Molecular medicine — a variety of pharmaceutical techniques and gene therapies that address specific molecular diseases or molecular defects in biological systems.

Molecular mill — a mechanochemical molecular transport and processing system characterized by limited motions and repetitive operations without programmable flexibility.

Molecular nanotechnology — thorough, inexpensive control of the structure of matter based on molecule-by-molecule control of products and byproducts; the products and processes of molecular manufacturing, including molecular machinery; a technology based on the ability to build structures to complex, atomic specifications by mechanosynthesis or other means; most broadly, the engineering of all complex mechanical systems constructed from the molecular level.

Molecular recognition — a chemical term referring to processes in which molecules adhere in a highly specific way, forming a larger structure; a possible enabling technology for nanotechnology.

Molecular sorting rotor — a class of nanomechanical device capable of selectively binding (or releasing) molecules from (or to) solution, and of transporting these bound molecules against significant concentration gradients.

Molecular surgery (molecular repair) — in medical nanorobotics, the analysis and physical correction of molecular structures in the body using medical nanomachines.

Molecular systems engineering — design, analysis, and construction of systems of molecular parts working together to carry out a useful purpose.

Molecule — group of atoms held together by chemical bonds; the typical unit manipulated by molecular nanotechnology.

Monkeywrenching — in medical nanorobotics, the mechanical or chemical jamming of cellular equilibrium processes, with a cytocidal objective. See also disequilibration.

Monocyte — a mononuclear phagocytic white blood cell derived from the myeloid stem cells, that is short-lived (~1 day half-life) and circulates in the bloodstream from which it moves into tissues, at which point it matures into a macrophage (which is long-lived). Monocytes represent 3%-8% of all white blood cells.

Monomer — any molecule that can be bound to similar molecules to form a polymer.

Morcellation — fragmentation of biological materials as they are excised from the body.

Morphogen — a (biochemical) factor that induces development of particular cell types in a manner that depends on its concentration.

Morphology — the science of structure and form, without regard to function.

Motif — main element, theme, or design feature that may occur in slightly different forms.

Motile — capable of voluntary movement. Opposite of sessile.

MRI — magnetic resonance imaging.

MRFM — magnetic resonance force microscope.

mRNA — see messenger RNA.

MTOC — microtubule organizing center; a cellular structure from which microtubules may be extended. The major MTOCs in a mitotic (dividing) cell are the centrosomes.

Mucosa — a mucous membrane; the moist tissue layer that lines a hollow organ or body cavity.

Muller cells — neuroglial cells with fine fibers that form supporting elements of the retina.

Multivalent — in chemistry, able to form more than one covalent or ionic bond; in biomedicine, efficacious in more than one direction, or active against several strains of an organism.

Mutagenesis, site-directed — a biotechnological technique whereby a gene encoding an enzyme is mutated, then overexpressed in a unicellular host, then characterized. By altering the base sequence of a single codon, site-directed mutagenesis can replace a given amino acid with any other protein amino acid, and can also generate multiple point mutants.

Mycelium — the mass of hyphae (branching tubular cells characteristic of the growth of filamentous fungi) making up a colony of fungi.

Myelin — a fatlike substance forming a sheath around the axons of certain nerves; composed of lipids and protein.

Myocardium — heart muscle.

Myoepithelium — tissue containing contractile epithelial cells (e.g. contractile spindle-shaped cells arranged longitudinally or obliquely around sweat glands and around the secretory alveoli of the mammary and salivary glands).

Myopotential — pertaining to an action potential in an axon innervating a muscle cell.

N — in physics, newton (MKS unit of force); in solution chemistry, see Normal.

Naked DNA — DNA that is not surrounded by an outer protein envelope.

Nanapheresis — in medical nanorobotics, the removal of bloodborne medical nanorobots from the body using aphersis-like processes.

NAND gate — a logical gate equivalent to a negated (NOT-) AND gate.

nano — a prefix meaning one billionth (1/1,000,000,000); more specifically, may refer to sizes of ~10^{-9} meters or to physical objects constructed or processes performed at the atomic or molecular scale.

Nanocentrifuge — in medical nanorobotics, a proposed nanodevice that can spin materials at very high speed, imparting rotational accelerations of up to one trillion gravities (g's), thus permitting rapid sortation.

Nanochronometer — in medical nanorobotics, a proposed clock or timing mechanism constructed of nanoscale components.

Nanoclusters — nanoscale aggregates of atoms or molecules.

Nanocomputer — a proposed computer with parts built on a molecular scale, possibly employing molecular electronics, mechanical rod logic, or biological molecules.

Nanocrit (Nct) — in medical nanorobotics, volume-fraction or bloodstream concentration of medical nanorobots, expressed as a percentage.

Nanolithography — the process of transferring nanometer-sized surface patterns.

Nanomachine — functional machine systems on the scale of nanometers; an artificial mechanical device constructed with precise molecular order using nanometer-scale components; any molecular structure large and complex enough to function as a machine.

Nanomanipulator — a nanorobotic manipulator device.

Nanomanufacturing — see molecular manufacturing.

Nanomechanical — pertaining to nanomachines.

Nanomedicine — (1) the comprehensive monitoring, control, construction, repair, defense, and improvement of all human biological systems, working from the molecular level, using engineered nanodevices and nanostructures; (2) the science and technology of diagnosing, treating, and preventing disease and traumatic injury, of relieving pain, and of preserving and improving human health, using molecular tools and molecular knowledge of the human body; (3) the employment of molecular machine systems to address medical problems, using molecular knowledge to maintain and improve human health at the molecular scale.

Nanometer — a billionth of a meter, roughly the diameter of 3-7 atoms.

Nanorobot — a computer-controlled robotic device constructed of nanometer-scale components to molecular precision, usually microscopic in size (often abbreviated as "nanobot").

Nanosensor — a chemical or physical sensor constructed using nanoscale components, usually microscopic or submicroscopic in size.

Nanosieving — in medical nanorobotics, a nanodevice that can sort molecules or other nanoscale objects by physical sieving.

Nanosystem — a set of nanoscale components, characterized by precise molecular order, working together to serve a set of purposes; complex nanosystems can be of macroscopic size.

Nanotechnology — engineering and manufacturing at nanometer scales; any technology related to features of nanometer scale, including thin films, fine particles, chemical synthesis, advanced microlithography, and so forth, as well as complex mechanical systems constructed from the molecular level.

Nanotubes — hollow fullerene tubes, including but not limited to single- and multi-walled carbon nanotubes, with submicroscopic, often nanoscale, diameters and a wide range of continuous lengths.

NASA — National Aeronautics and Space Administration.

Nasal septum — in anatomy, the cartilage, covered with mucous membrane, that divides the two nostrils and nasal passages.

Nasopharynx — in anatomy, the nasal passages, mouth, and upper throat.

Natation — swimming.

Naturophilia — an exclusive love of Nature, disdaining everything that is artificial or technological.

Nauseogenic — tending to produce nausea.

Navicyte — in medical nanorobotics, a mobile, mass-storage (nanorobotic) device, similar to a communicyte, that may be used to establish a navigational network inside the human body.

N/C — numeric control machining (e.g. computer-aided manufacturing).

Nct — see nanocrit.

Necrosis (necrotic) — the death of areas of tissue or bone, surrounded by healthy parts.

Neoplastic — pertaining to, or of the nature of, new and abnormal tissue (i.e. neoplasm) formation and growth.

Neurofibrils — a filamentous aggregation of microfilaments and microtubules found in the main cell body, dendrites, and axon of the nerve cell, and sometimes in its synaptic endings.

Neuron — a nerve cell, the principal structural and functional unit of the nervous system.

Neuropeptide — any of a variety of neurotransmitter peptides found in neural tissue (e.g. endorphins, enkephalins).

Neurotransmitter — a biochemical substance released when the axon terminal of a presynaptic neuron is excited. The substance travels across the synapse to act on the target cell to either inhibit or excite it.

Neutrophil — the most common type of granulocytic white blood cell. Neutrophils are responsible for much of the body's protection against infection. Comprising ~60% of all white blood cells, neutrophils play the primary role in inflammation, easily recognizing foreign antigens and destroying them through phagocytosis. Neutrophils also may overreact to stimuli and become involved in tissue destruction, as in rheumatoid arthritis, myocardial reperfusion injury, respiratory distress syndrome, and ulcerative colitis.

NMR — see Nuclear Magnetic Resonance.

NIST — National Institute of Standards and Technology.

Nociceptors — pain receptors.

Nodes of Ranvier — constrictions of the myelin sheath of a myelinated nerve fiber.

Nonpolar liquid — a liquid consisting of molecules that have zero electric dipole moment (e.g. ethane, benzene, liquefied carbon dioxide). Compare polar liquid.

NOR gate — a logical gate equivalent to a negated (NOT) OR gate.

Normal (N) — in solution chemistry, 1 liter of solution which contains 1 gram-equivalent of solute.

Nosogenic — tending to cause disease.

NOT gate — a logical gate that inverts or negates the input signal, as its output.

NSOM — Near-field Scanning Optical Microscope.

Nuclear cortex — a proteinaceous layer on the inside of the cellular nuclear envelope, consisting of up to three kinds of laminin proteins.

Nuclear envelope — a layer consisting of two membranes surrounding the cellular nucleus, penetrated by nuclear pores and bounded on the interior by the nuclear cortex.

Nuclear lamina — see nuclear cortex.

Nuclear Magnetic Resonance (NMR) — in physics and radiology, an analytical technique that relies on the absorption of certain electromagnetic frequencies by atomic nuclei.

Nuclear matrix — a network of fibers surrounding and penetrating the cell nucleus.

Nuclear pores — holes in the cellular nuclear envelope used for transport of macromolecules.

Nucleic acids — polymers of nucleotidyl residues.

Nucleoelectric conversion — conversion of nuclear energy into electrical energy.

Nucleography — a physical description (and mapping) of the nucleus of a human cell.

Nucleolus — an RNA-rich spherical body made up of dense fibers and granules within the cell nucleus, associated with chromosomal loci for rRNA genes, created by the transcription of rRNA genes.

Nucleoplasm — the protoplasm of a cell nucleus.

Nucleosides — compounds consisting of a purine or pyrimidine attached to ribose or deoxyribose at the 1' carbon.

Nucleosome — the basic structural subunit of chromatin, consisting of 146 base pairs of DNA wrapped around a core of eight histone protein molecules.

Nucleotide (nucleotidyl) — phosphorylated nucleosides; nucleotidyl residues are the monomeric units of RNA and DNA. The building blocks of nucleic acids. Each nucleotide is composed of sugar (ribose or deoxyribose), phosphate, and one of four nitrogen bases (purine or pyrimidine). The sequence of the bases within the nucleic acid determines what proteins will be made.

Nucleus — in physics, the positively-charged core of an atom, an object of ~0.00001 atomic diameters containing >99.9% of the atomic mass; in cell biology, a cellular organelle containing the genome, separated from the cytoplasm by a membrane.

Nyctalopia — a vitamin A deficiency disease, characterized by decreased ability to see in reduced illumination or at night.

Obligate — to make necessary or require, without alternative.

Occipital — pertaining to the back part of the head.

Occlusal surface — in dental medicine, the masticating surface of the premolar and molar teeth.

Olfaction (olfactory) — pertaining to the sense of smell.

Oligomer — any short polymeric molecular chain consisting of well-defined subunits; N-mer refers to an oligomer that has exactly N subunits.

Oligonucleotide — a polymeric chain that consists of a small number of (possibly different) nucleotides.

Opsonin — a biochemical substance that coats foreign antigens, making them more susceptible to macrophages and other leukocytes, thus increasing phagocytosis of the organism. Complement and antibodies are the two main opsonins in human blood.

Opsonization — the coating action of opsonins, thus facilitating phagocytosis.

Organelle — most commonly described subcellular compartment, located in the cytoplasm, that is surrounded by a membrane (e.g. lysosome, mitochondrion).

Organography — a physical description (and mapping) of the body organs.

OR gate — a logical gate that returns a high (1) output if either input signal is high (1). See bit.

Orthogonal — at right angles; mutually perpendicular.

Orthotropic — capable of alternating between bent and straight configurations.

Osmosis — the passage of solvent through a semipermeable membrane that separates solutions of different concentrations.

Osmotic pressure — the pressure that would develop if a solution is enclosed in a solvent-permeable membrane that is impermeable to all solutes present, and is then surrounded by pure solvent.

Osseous — pertaining to bone.

Ossicle — any small bone, especially one of the three bones of the ear.

Osteoblast — a bone-forming cell derived from mesenchyme to form the osseous matrix in which it becomes enclosed as an osteocyte.

Osteoclast — a giant multinuclear cell with abundant acidophilic cytoplasm, formed in the bone marrow of growing bones, which functions to absorb and remove unwanted osseous tissue.

Osteocyte — a mesodermal bone-forming cell that has become entrapped within the bone matrix, helping to maintain bone as living tissue.

Osteography — a physical description (and mapping) of the human skeletal system.

Osteomalacia — a vitamin D deficiency disease, characterized by a gradual and painful softening and bending of the bones.

Ostium — small opening, especially one into a tubular organ.

Otolith — a crystalline particle of calcium carbonate and protein, adhering to the gelatinous membrane of the maculae (thickened areas in the utricle and saccule) of the inner ear.

Ouabain — a glycoside ($C_{29}H_{44}O_{12}$•H_2O) obtained from the wood of *Acocanthera ouabaio* or from the seeds of *Strophanthus gratus*; its action is qualitatively identical to that of the digitalis glycosides (e.g. increasing the contractility of cardiac muscle).

Outmessaging — in medical nanorobotics, conveyance of information from a transmitter located inside the human body, especially from working nanodevices, to the patient or to a recipient external to the human body.

Ovariotomy — incision into an ovary.

Oxidation — in chemistry, a combination with oxygen, or an increase in positive valence of an ion, atom, or molecule, either by the loss from it of hydrogen or by the loss of one or more electrons. In bacteriology, the aerobic disassimilation of substrates with the production of energy and water; in contrast to fermentation, the transfer of electrons is accomplished via the respiratory chain, which utilizes oxygen as the final electron acceptor.

Oxidation-reduction reaction (redox) — chemical interaction in which one substance is oxidized and loses electrons, thus is increased in positive valence, while another substance gains an equal number of electrons by being reduced, thus is decreased in positive valence.

Oxyglucose — pertaining to a chemoergic energy conversion system involving the glucose/oxygen reaction; a glucose (fuel) and oxygen (oxidant) supply or mixture.

Palatine — pertaining to the palate (roof of the mouth).

Papilla — in anatomy, a small nipple-like protuberance or elevation.

Paracrine control — a general form of bioregulation in which one cell type in a tissue selectively influences the activity of an adjacent cell type by secreting chemicals that diffuse into the tissue and act specifically on cells in that area.

Paradigm — a conceptual model, pattern, or system.

Parenchyma — the essential parts of an organ that are concerned with its function as opposed to its framework; opposite of stroma. The distinguishing or specific cells of a gland or organ, contained within and supported by the connective tissue framework.

Parenteral — denoting any medication route other than the alimentary canal, such as intravenous, subcutaneous, intramuscular, or mucosal.

Parietal — pertaining to, or forming, the walls of a cavity; often specifically refers to the parietal bone, one of two bones that together form the roof and sides of the skull.

Partition — in medical nanorobotics, a cessation of the process of conjugation.

Parturition — the act of giving birth to young; childbirth.

Passivation — the covalent bonding of a layer of atoms to a surface, in order to neutralize (occupy) any dangling surface bonds, thus chemically stabilizing the surface.

Patency — the state of being freely open.

Pathogen — a microorganism or agent capable of producing disease.

Pathognomonic — characteristic or indicative of a disease; relating to one or more of the typical symptoms of a disease.

Pathological — diseased or due to a disease; more informally, pertaining to an adverse condition.

PEG — polyethylene glycol.

Pellagra — a niacin deficiency disease, characterized by gastrointestinal disturbances, erythema (inflammatory skin redness) followed by desquamation (shedding epidermis in scales or shreds), and nervous and mental disorders.

Peptide — a short chain of amino acids joined by amide bonds, up to 100 residues in length.

Peptidergic — activated or energized by neuropeptides.

Peptidoglycan layer — the dense material consisting of cross-linked polysaccharide chains present in the cell wall of most bacteria.

Periaxonal — near or around the neural axon.

Perineum — in anatomy, the area between the thighs extending from the coccyx to the pubis and lying below the pelvic diaphragm; the structures forming the pelvic floor.

Perinuclear space — in cell biology, the space that lies between the inner and outer membranes of the nuclear envelope.

Periportal — near the portal end.

Periosteum — in anatomy, the fibrous membrane forming the investing covering of bones except at their articular (joint) surfaces.

Peripheral — pertaining to a part of a body or object that is away from the center.

Peripheral protein — a non-amphipathic protein bound to the hydrophilic region of an integral membrane protein, or bound to the hydrophilic heads of plasma membrane lipids, of a cell; most peripheral proteins are located near the cytoplasmic side of the plasma membrane.

Peristalsis — a progressive wavelike movement that occurs involuntarily in hollow tubes of the body, especially the alimentary canal; it is characteristic of tubes possessing longitudinal and circular layers of smooth muscle fibers.

Peritoneum — in anatomy, the serous membrane reflected over the viscera and lining the abdominal cavity.

Periurethral — in anatomy, located near or around the urethra (which discharges urine).

Permittivity (relative) — in physics, the dielectric constant, a measure of the ability of a material to store electrical energy.

Peroxisome — in cell biology, an organelle found in vertebrate animal cells that contains a great number and variety of enzymes important in cell metabolism.

PET — Positron Emission Tomography; see Computerized Tomography.

Phage — see bacteriophage.

Phagocyte — a cell with the ability to ingest and destroy particulate substances such as bacteria, protozoa, cells and cell debris, dust particles, and colloids.

Phagocytosis — ingestion and digestion of bacteria and particles by phagocytes.

Pharmacodynamics — the study of the action of drugs on living organisms, and the physiological and clinical changes produced in organisms by those drugs.

Pharmacogenetics — the study of the influence of hereditary factors on the response of individual organisms to drugs; a branch of genetics dealing with hereditary aspects of drug metabolism.

Pharmacokinetics — study of the metabolism of drugs with particular emphasis on the time required for absorption, duration of action, distribution in the body, and method of excretion.

Pharmacyte — in medical nanorobotics, a theorized (nanorobotic) device capable of delivering precise doses of biologically active chemicals to individually-addressed human body tissue cells (e.g. cell-by-cell drug delivery).

Pharynx — the passageway for air from the nasal cavity to the larynx (also acting as a resonating cavity), and for food from the mouth to the esophagus; more specifically, a musculomembranous tube extending from the base of the skull to the level of the 6th cervical vertebra, where the tube becomes continuous with the esophagus.

Phase — fraction of a periodic cycle, often expressed as an angle.

Phasic (muscular) — refers to muscles with origins and insertions on skeleton or skin, that have rapid, brief contraction cycles. Compare tonic.

Phenotype — the appearance or other characteristics of an organism, resulting from the interaction of its genetic constitution with the environment; any observable characteristic that expresses the genotype of an individual.

Pheresis — see apheresis.

Pheromone — a substance permitting chemical communication between animals, and between certain insects, of the same species; may affect development, reproduction, or behavior of like individuals.

Phonons — in physics, a quantum of acoustic energy, analogous to the quantum of electromagnetic energy, the photon. Thermal excitations in a crystal (lattice vibrations) or in an elastic continuum can be described as a population of phonons (analogous to black-body electromagnetic radiation).

Photolithography — a surface patterning technique that employs light, used to make semiconductor devices.

Physiognomy — the countenance (physical features) of the face.

Phytotoxic — pertaining to a poisonous plant.

Piezoelectric — the property of some materials to generate a voltage when mechanical stress is applied, and vice versa.

Pinocytosis — the process by which cells absorb or ingest nutrients and fluid, in which minute incuppings or invaginations are first formed in the surface of the plasma membrane and then close to form fluid-filled vesicles; resembles phagocytosis.

Pixel — abbreviation for picture element; a single square cell within a two-dimensional geometric grid or array.

Plague — see bubonic plague, pneumonic plague.

Planetary gear — in machinery, an epicyclic train of gears as found in an automobile transmission, for the purpose of transforming the rotational speeds of rotating shafts.

Plasma — in anatomy, the fluid (noncellular) part of the lymph and of the blood, usually distinguished from the serum obtained after coagulation; in cell biology, the part of the protoplasm (cell substance) outside of the nucleus.

Plasma membrane — the outermost membrane of a cell, with cell contents on one side and the extracellular environment on the other side; the continuous membrane defining the boundary of every cell.

Plasmapheresis — see apheresis.

Plasmid — an autonomous self-replicating extrachromosomal circular DNA molecule present intracellularly and symbiotically in most bacteria, encoding a protein product that confers drug resistance or some other advantageous phenotype. Plasmids reproduce inside the bacterial cell but are not essential to its viability, and can influence a great number of bacterial functions.

Plasticity — a property of an object or material, wherein the object or material suffers a permanent deformation in its original shape after a force is applied and then removed.

Platelet — a round or ovoid 2-4 micron disk found in the blood of vertebrates; platelets play an important role in blood coagulation and hemostasis.

Plateletocrit — volume-fraction or bloodstream concentration of platelets, expressed as a percentage.

Pleura — serous membranes that enfold both lungs and are reflected on the walls of the thorax and diaphragm, and are moistened with a serous secretion that reduces friction during the respiratory movements of the lungs.

Pluripotent — concerning an embryonic stem cell that can differentiate into many different kinds of cells.

Plexus — an extensive two-dimensional meshwork.

Pneumatic — driven to motion or extension by pressurized gas or fluid.

Pneumonic plague — highly virulent and frequently fatal form of plague, having an extensive involvement of the lungs.

Poiseuille flow — laminar (nonturbulent) fluid flow.

Polarization — in optical physics, a change effected in a ray of light passing through certain media, whereby the transverse vibrations of the emerging ray occur in one plane only, instead of in all planes as in the ordinary incident light; in biology and electrical physics, the development of differences in electrical potential between two points on an object, such as between the inside and outside of a cell wall or along the length of a piezoelectric bone subjected to shear stress.

Polar liquid — a liquid consisting of molecules that have an electric dipole moment (e.g. water, ethanol, liquefied ammonia). Compare nonpolar liquid.

Polymer — a long molecular chain of well-defined linked subunits.

Polymorphonuclear leukocyte — see granulocyte.

Polynucleotides — polymers of nucleotidyl residues, as in RNA and DNA.

Polysaccharide — complex carbohydrates of high molecular weight; one of a group of carbohydrates that upon hydrolysis yields more than two molecules of simple sugars.

Polysome (polyribosome) — an mRNA associated with a series of ribosomes engaged in translation.

Polyyne — see carbyne.

Portal — in anatomy, pertaining to any porta or entrance to an organ, but especially to the portal vein through which nutrient-laden blood is carried from the gastrointestinal tract to the liver for filtration.

Positional navigation — in medical nanorobotics, a form of nanorobotic navigation in which nanodevices know their exact location inside the human body to ~micron accuracy continuously at all times.

Positional synthesis — in molecular nanotechnology, control of chemical reactions by precisely positioning specific moieties; possibly a basic component of molecular assemblers.

Positron Emission Tomography (PET) — see Computerized Tomography.

Posterior — the backside of the human body; the backside of something.

Postpartum — after childbirth.

Potential energy — the energy associated with a configuration of particles, as distinct from their motions.

Power — the rate at which energy is produced or consumed.

Precession — movement of the axis of rotation of a fixed-pivot gyroscope under the influence of gravity, describing a conical surface.

(to) Present — used as verb in medicine, meaning "to exhibit" a symptom or a condition (a medical idiom).

Presentation semaphore — in medical nanorobotics, a mechanical device used to display specific antigens, chemical ligands, or other molecular objects to the external environment, with the purpose of selectively modifying the chemical or other surface characteristics of a nanorobot exterior.

Process — used as a noun in cell biology and medicine; a projection or outgrowth of bone or tissue.

Prognosis — a judgement or forecast, based upon a correct diagnosis, of the future course of a disease or injury, and the patient's prospects for partial or full recovery.

Prokaryote — in microbiology, an organism or cell that lacks a nucleus.

Prometaphase — stage of mitosis (cell division) beginning with a fragmentation of the nuclear membrane and marked by kinetochore formation on the centromeres of the condensed chromosomes.

Promoter — a region of DNA involved in the binding of RNA polymerase to initiate transcription.

Pronouncement — a legally sufficient assertion of the biological death of a patient, usually attested by a physician.

Prophase — stage of mitosis (cell division) during which the chromosomes begin to condense within the still-intact nucleus, the nucleolus disperses, and the mitotic spindle begins to develop.

Prophylaxis — that which helps to prevent disease.

Proprioception — sensations of position and movement, including kinesthesis and the vestibular senses.

Protease — a class of enzymes that break down, or hydrolyze, the peptide bonds that join the amino acids in a protein.

Proteasomes — an extra-lysosomal ATP-driven system for selectively degrading endogenous ubiquinated proteins in virtually all human cells.

Protein — a long chain of amino acids joined by amide bonds, exceeding 100 residues in length; shorter chains are peptides. More generally, living cells contain many molecules that consist of amino acid polymers folded to form more-or-less definite three-dimensional structures, termed proteins. Short polymers lacking definite three-dimensional structures are termed peptides. Many proteins incorporate structures other than amino acids, either as covalently attached side chains or as bound ligands. Molecular objects made of protein form much of the molecular machinery of living cells.

Protein engineering (protein design) — design and construction of new artificial proteins with desired functions; a possible enabling technology for molecular manufacturing.

Proteolytic — hastening the hydrolysis (breakdown) of proteins, usually by enzyme action, into simpler substances.

Proteomics — the study of proteins and how they affect the human body.

Protoplasm — a thick, viscous colloidal substance that constitutes the physical basis of all living activities; the entire contents of a living cell.

Protozoa — the simplest animals, mostly unicellular although some are colonial.

Proximal — near the source or point of attachment or origin; in the extremities, closer to the trunk.

Proximal probes — a generic name for devices that exploit interactions between a sample and a sharp probe tip; a family of devices capable of fine positional control and sensing, including scanning tunneling microscopes and atomic force microscopes; a possible enabling technology for molecular manufacturing.

Pseudopod — in microbiology, a temporary protruding protoplasmic process in protozoa for the purpose of taking up food and aiding in locomotion.

Pseudostratified — apparently composed of layers.

Psychosomatic — pertaining to the influence of the mind or of higher functions of the brain upon the functions of the body, especially in relation to bodily disorders or disease.

Puerperal — relating to the period after childbirth.

Pulmonary — pertaining to the lungs.

Purgative — an agent used for purging the bowels.

Purine — parent molecule of a group of heterocyclic compounds (e.g. adenine, caffeine, guanine, uric acid, xanthine), which have fused five- and six-member carbon-nitrogen rings. Purines are the end products of nucleoprotein digestion; they may be synthesized in the body, and break down to form uric acid.

Pyemia — septicemia due to pyogenic (pus-forming) organisms causing multiple abscesses.

Pylorus — the lower orifice of the stomach, opening into the duodenum.

Pyrimidine — parent molecule of a group of heterocyclic compounds (e.g. cytosine, thymine, uracil), which have a six-member carbon-nitrogen ring.

Pyroelectric — producing electrical energy directly from heat.

Q (resonator or circuit) — in engineering, a measure of the sharpness of a resonance peak.

Quantum computer — a computer that relies upon quantum effects such as superposition and interference.

Quantum confinement — restriction of particle to small physical regions so that quantum effects are exhibited. See also tunneling.

Quantum dot — a zero-dimensional quantum system.

Quantum dot lasers — lasers that exploit the energy levels of quantum dots.

Quantum Hall effect — phenomenon in which certain semiconductors at low temperatures display quantized resistance.

Quantum mechanics — theory of matter and radiation in which certain physical properties are quantized.

Quantum uncertainty — a measurement indeterminacy associated with the dual wave/particle nature of matter; e.g. the Heisenberg uncertainty principle.

Qubits — quantum bits; the equivalent of bits, for quantum computers.

Racemic (mixture) — a mixture of two optical isomers in equal amounts; a racemic mixture does not show optical activity.

Radiolarian — an order of single-celled sea animals with long slender pseudopodia and a perforated outer skeleton of silica.

Radionuclide — a radioactive isotope.

Rale — an abnormal sound heard upon auscultation of the chest. Rales are produced by the passage of air through bronchi that contain secretion or exudate, or that are constricted by spasm or a thickening of bronchial walls.

RAM — random access memory (a data storage device for computers).

Raoult's law — in an ideal solution, molar weights of non-volatile non-electrolytes, when dissolved in a definite weight of a given solvent under the same conditions, lower the solvent's freezing point, elevate its boiling point, and reduce its vapor pressure equally for all such solutes.

Ratchet — a hinged catch (pawl) arranged so as to engage with a toothed wheel or bar whose teeth slope in one direction, thus imparting forward movement and preventing backward movement.

RBC — red blood cell (erythrocyte).

RC time — the characteristic exponential decay time of an RC (resistor-capacitor) circuit; the capacitive time constant of a circuit.

Reaction — in chemistry, a process that transforms one or more chemical species into others; typical reactions make or break bonds, while others change the state of ionization or other properties taken to distinguish chemical species. In medicine, a response of a living organism to a chemical, mechanical, or other stimulus.

Reagent — a chemical species that undergoes change as a result of a chemical reaction.

Receptor — most generally, a structure that can capture a molecule (often of a specific type in a specific orientation) owing to complementary surface shapes, charge distributions, and so forth, without forming a covalent bond. In biology, a receptor is a transmembrane protein, located in the plasma membrane, that binds a ligand in a domain on the extracellular side, and as a result has a change in activity of the cytoplasmic domain of the protein.

Recombination — in genetics, the inclusion of a chromosomal part or extrachromosomal element of one microbial strain in the chromosome of another; the interchange of chromosomal parts between different microbial strains. Most generally, the joining together of gene combinations in the offspring that were not present in the parents.

Red blood cell (RBC) — see erythrocyte.

Redox — see oxidation-reduction reaction.

Reduced mass — many dynamical properties of a system consisting of two interacting masses m_1 and m_2 are equivalent to those of a system in which one mass is fixed in space and the other has a mass (the reduced mass) with the value $m_1 m_2 / (m_1 + m_2)$. The reduced mass description has fewer dynamical variables.

Reference man — a man 22 years of age, weight 70 kg, engaged in light physical activity in a 20°C environment, consuming ~2800 Kcal/day.

Reference woman — a woman 22 years of age, weight 58 kg, engaged in light physical activity in a 20°C environment, consuming ~2000 Kcal/day.

Refractive index — in optics, the ratio of the sine of the angle of incidence to the sine of the angle of refraction when light is transmitted through a refracting substance (that bends the light beam).

Regioselectivity — selection of the precise position of a ligand group addition to a molecule, e.g. ortho-, meta-, and para- positions in substituted benzenes.

Register — a temporary storage location for an array of bits of data within a digital logic system.

Relaxation time — the measure of the rate at which a disequilibrium distribution decays toward an equilibrium distribution.

Renal — pertaining to the kidney.

Replicator — any system that can build copies of itself when provided with the appropriate raw materials and energy.

Repression — the ability of bacteria to prevent synthesis of certain enzymes when the products of those enzymes are present; more generally, the inhibition of transcription (or translation) by the binding of repressor protein to a specific site on DNA or mRNA.

Repressor protein — a protein molecule that binds to an operator on DNA or RNA to prevent transcription or translation, respectively.

RES — see reticuloendothelial system.

Resection — the partial excision of a bone or other structure.

Residue — in biochemistry, a portion of a single amino acid or nucleotide, linked as part of a peptide/protein or polynucleotide polymer chain, respectively.

Resistor — in electrical engineering, an electronic device that resists the flow of current.

Resonance — in engineering and in control theory, the tendency of an object or system to vibrate or oscillate at a characteristic frequency.

Resonant tunneling — increased probability of quantum tunneling under favorable resonance conditions.

Respirocrit — in medical nanorobotics, the volume-fraction or bloodstream concentration of respirocyte[1400] nanorobots, expressed as a percentage.

Respirocyte — in medical nanorobotics, a theorized bloodborne spherical 1-micron (nanorobotic) device having a 1000-atm pressure vessel with active pumping powered by endogenous serum glucose, that serves as a mechanical artificial red blood cell.[1400]

Reticular — relating to a reticulum.

Reticulum — a fine network formed by cells, or formed of certain structures within cells, or formed of connective tissue between cells.

Reticuloendothelial system (RES) — in anatomy, the network of fixed and mobile phagocytes that engulf (and dispose of) foreign antigens and cell debris found inside the human body.

Reticuloendothelium — tissue of the reticuloendothelial system (RES); the system of mononuclear phagocytes located in the reticular connective tissue of the body that is responsible for the phagocytosis of damaged or old cells, cellular debris, foreign substances, and pathogens, removing them from the circulation.

Reticuloplasm — the fluid that fills the lumen of the endoplasmic reticulum.

Retinitis — inflammation of the retina of the eye.

Reversible computer — a computer capable of reversing its computational steps (after storing the final answer), thus recovering most of the energy that was employed during the computation.

Reynolds number — the ratio of inertial to viscous forces in fluid flow. Macroscopic objects and flows typically experience Reynolds numbers >> 1, where mass and inertia dominate object motions; microscopic and especially nanoscale objects and flows typically experience Reynolds numbers << 1, where the viscosity of the environment dominates object motions.

rf — radio frequency.

Rheology — study of the deformation and flow properties of materials, especially fluids, such as blood.

Ribonucleic acid (RNA) - the ribonucleotide polymer into which DNA is transcribed.

Ribosomal RNA (rRNA) — the RNA components of ribosomes.

Ribosome — a naturally occurring molecular machine that manufactures proteins according to instructions derived from the cell's genes; a cytoplasmic ribonucleoprotein complex that serves as the site of translation in the cell. Each ribosome has a large and a small subunit, 60S and 40S in eukaryotes. These subunits dissociate and reassociate in a cycle related to their functions, during translation.

Rickets — a vitamin D deficiency disease characterized by overproduction and deficient calcification of osteoid (bony) tissue, with associated skeletal deformities, enlargement of the liver and spleen, profuse sweating, and general tenderness of the body when touched.

Rigidity — see stiffness.

RMS — root mean square. Refers to a kind of average molecular speed; the speeds of individual molecules vary over a wide range of magnitude, with a characteristic temperature-dependent distribution of molecular speeds.

RNA — see ribonucleic acid.

RNase — an enzyme that attacks bonds in RNA.

RNA polymerase — an enzyme that synthesizes RNA under direction from a DNA template (formally described as DNA-dependent RNA polymerase).

Robot — a programmable device usually consisting of mechanisms for sensing and mechanical manipulation, often connected to (or including) a computer that provides control.

Rough ER — regions of endoplasmic reticulum that are associated with ribosomes.

Rouleaux — stack-of-coins configuration of a cluster of red blood cells.

rRNA — see ribosomal RNA.

Rugosity — condition of being folded or wrinkled; surface roughness.

Sacculation — formation into a sac or sacs; group of sacs, collectively.

Saccule — the smaller of the two membranous sacs in the vestibule (central cavity) of the osseous labyrinth (the inner ear).

Sagittal — in anatomy, a vertical plane or section that divides the body into right and left portions.

Salt bridge — in biochemistry, an ionic bond between charged groups that are part of larger covalent structures; salt bridges occur in many proteins.

SAM — in microscopy, a Scanning Acoustic Microscope; in polymer chemistry, a self-assembled monolayer or a spontaneously assembled monolayer.

Sanguinatation — in medical nanorobotics, locomotion (especially swimming by a nanorobot) through the bloodstream.

Sapphirophagy — eating sapphire (corundum).

Sarcoplasmic reticulum — specialized, elaborate smooth ER, found in muscle cells.

Saturated — a molecule which is a closed-shell species lacking double or triple bonds; forming a new bond to a saturated molecule requires the cleavage of an existing bond.

Scanning Electron Microscope (SEM) — a kind of microscope that uses electrons rather than light.

Scanning Force Microscope — see Atomic Force Microscope.

Scanning Probe Microscope (SPM) — a class of microscope (including AFMs and STMs) that exploits physical interactions that are sensitive to the separation of a sample and a sharp tip.

Scanning Tunneling Microscope (STM) — an instrument able to image conducting surfaces to atomic accuracy. A sharp conductive tip is moved across a conductive surface close enough (typically a nanometer or less) to permit a substantial tunneling current. In a common mode of operation, a constant voltage is established and the current is monitored and kept constant by controlling the height of the tip above the surface using a feedback circuit, ultimately producing an atomic-resolution map of the surface reflecting a combination of topography and electronic properties. Increasing the voltage enables a researcher to move atoms around, pile them up, or trigger chemical reactions.

Schistosomiasis — a parasitic disease due to infestation with blood flukes; endemic throughout Asia, Africa, and tropical America.

Sclerosis (sclerotic) — hardening of a tissue or organ, especially due to excessive growth of fibrous tissue; also, thickening and hardening of the tissue layers comprising the walls of an artery.

Scurvy — a vitamin C deficiency disease characterized by hemorrhagic manifestations and abnormal formation of bones and teeth, including spongy condition of the gums, sometimes with ulceration.

Self-assembly — see Brownian assembly.

Semaphores — see presentation semaphores.

Semicircular canals — superior, posterior, and inferior passages forming part of the inner ear.

Semilunar — shaped like a crescent.

Sepsis — the presence of various pus-forming and other pathogenic organisms, or their toxins, in the blood or tissues.

Septic — pertaining to or caused by sepsis.

Septicemia — septic fever; systemic disease caused by the multiplication of microorganisms in the circulating blood.

Septum — a wall dividing two cavities (e.g. the interalveolar septa between the alveoli).

Serotonin — a biochemical substance, 5-hydroxytryptamine (5-HT), that is present in platelets, gastrointestinal mucosa, mast cells, and in carcinoid tumors. Serotonin is a potent vasoconstrictor involved in neural mechanisms important in sleep and sensory perception.

Serous membrane — a membrane lining a serous cavity, specifically the pleural (lung), peritoneal (abdominal), and pericardial (heart) cavities.

Serum — the watery portion of the blood after coagulation; a fluid found when clotted blood is left standing long enough for the clot to shrink. More generally, any serous fluid, especially the fluid that moistens the surfaces of serous membranes.

Sessile — incapable of voluntary movement. Opposite of motile.

Shear — a shear deformation is one that displaces successive layers of a material transversely with respect to one another, like a crooked stack of cards. Shear is a dimensionless quantity measured by the ratio of the transverse displacement to the thickness over which it occurs.

Shear modulus — shear stress divided by shear strain (units of force per unit area).

Shirr — a series of parallel rows of short, running stitches with gatherings between rows.

Sinoatrial node — a node at the junction of the superior vena cava with the right cardiac atrium (one of the upper chambers of the heart), regarded as the starting point of the heartbeat.

Sinusoid — resembling a sinus (a cavity having a relatively narrow opening); a minute blood vessel found in such organs as the liver, spleen, adrenal glands, and bone marrow, that is slightly larger than a capillary and has a lining of reticuloendothelium.

Site-directed mutagenesis — see mutagenesis.

Smooth ER — in cell biology, regions of endoplasmic reticulum that are devoid of ribosomes.

SNR — signal-to-noise (power) ratio.

Solenoid — in physics and electrical engineering, a coil of wire carrying an electric current; an electromagnet.

Solute — the dissolved substance in a solution.

Solvation — the process of dissolving a solute in a solvent, making a solution.

Solvent — a substance, usually a liquid, that can hold another substance in solution.

Somatic — in general, relating to the body, as opposed to the mind or soul; corporeal.

Somatic cell — in cell biology, all the cells of an organism except those of the germ line (gametes).

Somatography — a physical description (and mapping) of the human body.

Somesthesis — sensations from the skin and viscera, including pressure, warmth, cold, and pain.

Sonication — to bombard with high-energy acoustic waves, often for the purpose of fragmenting or destroying the sonicated object.

Sonolucent — in ultrasonography, the condition of not reflecting the ultrasound waves back to their source.

Sonoluminescence — generation of visible light during high-powered sonication of a fluid, usually water.

Sortation — the act of separating or sorting, especially of molecular species.

Sorting rotor — see molecular sorting rotor.

Species — in chemistry, a distinct kind of molecule, ion, or other structure.

Specific gravity — relative density, as a ratio to the density of pure water.

Specificity — in biochemistry, defines the degree to which a receptor can distinguish between similar ligands.

Specular reflection — in physics, reflection as from a mirror, requiring that the wavelength of the reflected wave is smaller than the characteristic dimension of the reflector.

Sphincter — in anatomy, circular muscle constricting an orifice. In normal tonic (i.e. under tension or in contraction) condition, it closes the orifice; the muscle must relax in order to allow the orifice to open.

Spindle — in cell biology, the reorganized structure of a eukaryotic cell that is passing through mitosis (cell division); the nucleus has been dissolved and chromosomes are attached to the spindle by microtubules.

Splenic — pertaining to the spleen.

SPM — see Scanning Probe Microscope.

Sputum — substance expelled by coughing or clearing the throat.

Squamous cell — a flat, scaly epithelial cell.

SQUID — superconducting quantum interference device.

Stable — in the physical sciences, a system is termed stable if no rearrangement of its parts can produce a system having lower free energy; in biology, a living system is stable so long as homeostasis can be maintained.

Stationkeeping — active maintenance of location in a specific physical place, area, or volume.

Stellate — star-shaped.

Steric — pertaining to the spatial relationships among atoms in a molecular structure; in particular, pertaining to the space-filling properties of a molecule.

Steric hindrance — in chemistry, slowing of the rate of a chemical reaction owing to the presence of molecular structures possessed by the reagents that mechanically interfere with the motions associated with the reaction, typically by obstructing the reaction site; in hematodynamics, the reduction in hematocrit near small blood vessel bifurcations due to the elongation and orientation of red cells along the direction of shear flow.

Stereochemistry — the branch of chemistry concerned with the three-dimensional spatial relationships among atoms in molecules and the effects of such relationships on the properties (especially optical rotation) of molecules.

Stereoisomers — isomeric forms that have different configurations in space; may be geometric (non-enantiomeric, achiral) or enantiomeric (chiral).

Steroids — a large family of chemical substances, comprising many hormones, vitamins, body constituents, and drugs, each containing the tetracyclic cyclopentophenanthrene skeleton.

Stewart platform — in engineering, a manipulator employing a 6-DOF mobile platform.

Sticky ends — in biochemistry, complementary single strands of DNA that protrude from opposite ends of a duplex or from ends of different duplex (two-stranded) molecules; can be generated by staggered cuts in duplex DNA.

Stiffness — in mechanical engineering, the stiffness of a system with respect to a deformation (e.g. the stiffness of a spring with respect to stretching) is the second derivative of the energy with respect to the corresponding displacement. Positive stiffness is associated with stability, and a large stiffness can result in a small positional uncertainty in the presence of thermal excitation. Negative stiffnesses correspond to unstable locations on the potential energy surface.

Stirling engine — invented by Robert Stirling in 1816; generates power not by burning fuels explosively in an otherwise empty cylinder, but by heating and cooling working gas from the outside of a cylinder which always contains a pressurized working gas.

STM — see Scanning Tunneling Microscope.

Stoichiometric — in chemistry, pertaining to the precise quantities of reagents required to complete a chemical reaction; in particular, to the exact amounts needed to balance the chemical reaction equation.

Strain — in mechanical engineering, strain (a dimensionless quantity) is a measure of the deformation resulting from stress (an applied force per unit area); the displacement of one point with respect to another, divided by their equilibrium separation in the absence of stress. In chemistry, a molecular fragment generally has some equilibrium geometry (e.g. bond lengths, interbond angles) when the rest of the molecular structure does not impose special constraints (e.g. bending bonds to form a small ring); deviations from this molecular equilibrium geometry are described as strain, and increase the energy of the molecule. Strain in the mechanical engineering sense also causes strain in the chemical sense.

Stratum corneum — in anatomy, the outermost (horny) layer of the epidermis, consisting of many layers of flat, keratinized, enucleated cells.

Streamline — the movement or flow of a small portion of fluid, especially in relation to a solid body which lies in the path of this flow. Compare turbulence.

Stress — in mechanical engineering, the force per unit area applied by one part of an object to another. Pressure is an isotropic compressive stress. Suspending a mass from a fiber places the fiber in tensile stress. Gluing a layer of rubber between two plates and then sliding one plate over the other (while holding their separation constant) places the rubber in shear stress. Twisting one end of a rod while holding fixed the other end places the rod in torsional stress.

Striated — striped; marked by streaks or striae (lines or bands elevated above or depressed below surrounding tissue, or differing in color or texture).

Stroma — foundation-supporting tissues of an organ, defining the framework of an organ; opposite of parenchyma.

Sublimation — in chemistry, passing directly from solid to vapor state.

Submaxillary — below the maxilla (upper jaw).

Substrate — in biology, the substance acted upon and changed by an enzyme; in replicator theory, the set of all material inputs to the replication process.

Superconductivity — in physics, a physical phenomenon in which the electrical resistance of certain materials drops to zero at moderate or low temperatures.

Superficial — near the surface of the skin, as opposed to keep inside the body.

Superior — upper or higher than; situated above something else. See also cephalic.

Supine — lying on the back, with the face up.

Suppuration — producing or associated with the generation of pus, often involving an infection with pyogenic (pus-forming) bacteria.

Supraglottal — located above the glottis.

Supramolecular chemistry — the study of interactions between molecules; chemistry beyond the molecule; the chemistry of the noncovalent bond.

Surfactant — in physical chemistry, a chemical agent that lowers surface tension.

Sympathetic (nervous system) — a major component of the autonomic nervous system, consisting of ganglia, nerves (mostly motor, some sensory), and plexuses that supply the involuntary muscles.

Synapse — the point of junction between two neurons in a neural pathway, where the termination of the axon of one neuron comes into close proximity with the cell body or dendrites of another neuron.

Synovial membrane — a membrane lining the capsule of a joint.

Synthesis — in chemistry, the production of a specific molecular structure by a series of chemical reactions.

System — in engineering usage, a set of components working together to serve a common set of purposes.

Systems theory — in clinical medicine, an approach that considers the human being as a whole as opposed to his parts; human beings are considered as open systems constantly exchanging information, matter, and energy with the environment.

Systole — the normal period in the heart cycle during which the muscle fibers tighten and shorten, the heart constricts, and the cavities empty of blood; roughly, the period of contraction alternating with diastole or relaxation. Occurs in the interval between the first and second heart sounds during which blood is surged through the aorta and pulmonary artery.

Tachometer — a device for measuring the speed of rotation.

Tachyiatria — the art of curing quickly.

Teleoperation — remote control.

Telepresence — in control engineering, teleoperation with full sensor feedback (see virtual reality system).

Telomerase — in biochemistry, the ribonucleoprotein enzyme that creates repeating units of one strand at the telomere, by adding individual bases.

Telomere — the natural end of a chromosome; the telomeric DNA sequence consists of a simple repeating unit (in humans, TTAGGG) with a protruding single-stranded end that may fold into a hairpin.

Telophase — the final stage of mitosis (cell division), in which chromosomes at opposite spindle poles begin to decondense as spindle fibers disappear and the nuclear membrane reforms.

Temperature — a system in which internal vibrational modes have equilibrated with one another can be said to have a particular temperature; two systems are at different temperatures if heat flows between them when they are brought into physical contact. The most common measurement units of temperature are Centigrade or Celsius (°C), Fahrenheit (°F), and Kelvin (K).

Temporal — pertaining to time.

Tensile — pertaining to extension or stretching.

Teragravity — one trillion times normal terrestrial gravity.

Tessellation — in physical geometry, laid out or paved in a mosaic pattern of small squares or blocks, usually with the objective of completely covering a surface or completely filling a volume.

Tetanic — in medicine, tending to produce spasms characteristic of tetanus.

Tether — a cable, tube, or other physical linkage that allows information, matter, or energy to flow between two or more objects.

Thermal conductivity — transport of thermal energy due to a temperature gradient; the energy flux (W/m^2) per unit of spatial temperature gradient (K/m) equals the coefficient of thermal conductivity (W/m-K).

Thermal energy — the internal energy present in a system as a result of the energy of thermally equilibrated vibrational modes and other motions (including both kinetic energy and molecular potential energy); the mean thermal energy of a classical harmonic oscillator is kT.

Thermal expansion coefficient — the rate of change of length with respect to temperature for a particular material.

Thermogenesis — the production of heat, especially in the body (e.g. by shivering).

Thermogenic limit — in medical nanorobotics, the maximum amount of waste heat that may safely be released by a population of in vivo medical nanorobots that are operating within a given tissue volume.

Thermography — temperature mapping of the human body.

Thiol — in chemistry, an -SH group, or a molecule containing such a group; also known as a sulfhydryl or mercapto group.

Thoracic — in anatomy, pertaining to the chest or thorax.

Thorax — that part of the body between the base of the neck superiorly and the diaphragm inferiorly.

Thrombus — blood clot.

THz — terahertz; trillions of cycles per second.

Tight-receptor structure — in molecular nanotechnology, a molecular receptor structure in which a bound ligand of a particular kind is confined on all sides by repulsive interactions. A tight-receptor structure discriminates strongly against all molecules larger than the target.

Tinnitis — a subjective ringing or tinkling sound in the ear.

Titer — in analytical chemistry, the standard of strength of a volumetric test solution; assay value of an unknown measure by volumetric means.

T-lymphocytes (T cells) — White blood cells that are produced in the bone marrow but later mature in the thymus. T cells are important in the body's defense against certain bacteria and fungi, help B cells make antibodies, and assist in the recognition and rejection of foreign tissues.

Tomography — a noninvasive imaging technique designed to show detailed images of structures in a selected plane of tissue by blurring images of structures in all other planes.

Tonic (osmotic) — see isotonic.

Tonic (muscular) — refers to muscles arranged around hollow structures that contract slowly and can hold for a long period of time. Compare phasic.

Tonic (physiological) — pertaining to or characterized by tension or contraction; in a state of continuous action, denoting especially a muscular contraction.

Top-down — an approach to nanotechnology that aims to construct nanodevices by progressive miniaturization of existing bulk components.

Torque — in physics, a force that produces torsion.

Torsional — relating to, producing, or resulting from twisting.

Toxic shock — a disease caused by the release of toxins produced by certain strains of various bacteria.

Trabecular — inner part of organ or body.

Transcription — synthesis of RNA on a DNA template.

Transcutaneous (percutaneous) — effected through the skin.

Transdermal — through the skin.

Transducer — any mechanism or device that can convert energy or signals from one physical form to another.

Transduction — in physics and engineering, the conversion of energy or signals from one form to another; in biology and biotechnology, a phenomenon causing genetic recombination in bacteria in which DNA is carried from one bacterium to another, usually by a bacteriophage.

Transendothelial migration — see diapedesis.

Transfer RNA (tRNA) — the adaptor RNA that carries amino acid residues into polypeptide linkage during translation, as the codon sequence in mRNA is read.

Transgenic organism — in biotechnology, an organism modified by the insertion of foreign genetic material into its germ line cells. Recombinant DNA techniques are commonly used to produce transgenic organisms.

Translation — in biochemistry, the synthesis of protein on the mRNA template; the process of reading the codon sequence in mRNA to synthesize the corresponding polypeptide with the involvement of ribosomes, tRNA, and many enzymes.

Transmembrane — crossing the plasma membrane of a living cell.

Transmembrane protein — in cell biology, a membrane component, wherein a hydrophobic region or regions of the protein resides within the membrane, and hydrophilic regions are exposed on one or both sides of the membrane. See integral membrane protein.

Transtegumental — crossing or passing through the skin or covering of a body.

Transvenue outmessaging — in medical nanorobotics, outmessaging from the nanorobots present within the body of one patient to the nanorobots present in another (physically separated) human body.

Transverse — horizontal, hence at right angles to both sagittal and coronal sections, dividing the body into upper and lower portions; more generally, extending crossways or from side to side.

Triage — in emergency medicine, the screening of sick and wounded patients during war, disasters, or other emergencies. During triage, patients are classified into one of three groups: (1) those who will not survive even if given treatment, (2) those who will recover without treatment, and (3) those who need treatment in order to survive (the priority treatment group).

Tribology — the study of friction.

Trichinosis — a pathogenic disease caused by ingestion of *Trichinella spiralis* in raw or insufficiently cooked infected pork.

Trillion — this book follows the American convention in which a trillion is 10^{12}.

Trimer — in chemistry, a compound of three similar or identical molecules.

Triple point — a single condition of temperature and pressure in which three distinct phases of a substance (e.g. solid, liquid, and gas) can exist simultaneously and in equilibrium.

tRNA — see transfer RNA.

Trypanosomiasis — any disease caused by trypanosomes (asexual protozoan flagellates parasitic in the blood plasma of many vertebrates).

Tubulin — a protein present in the microtubules of cells, which are polymers of α-tubulin (~53,000 dalton) and β-tubulin (~55,000 dalton) dimers.

Tunneling — in quantum physics, a probabilistic effect in classically-forbidden transitions that is a consequence of the wave nature of matter. In classical physics, a particle or system cannot penetrate regions of negative energy (e.g. barrier regions in which the potential energy is greater than the system energy). In quantum physics, a wave function of significant amplitude may extend into and beyond such regions; if the wave function extends into another region of positive energy, the barrier is crossed with some nonzero probability, a process called tunneling (since the barrier is penetrated rather than climbed).

Turbulence — in hydrodynamics, fluid flow which does not follow parallel streamlines, which has a blunt (nonparabolic) profile in tube flow, and often involves eddies, vortices, and significant variations in fluid velocities, accelerations and shear stress between adjacent fluid elements. Turbulence dissipates more energy, and presents more resistance to flow, than laminar flow.

Turgid — swollen.

Turing machine — a programmable computing device.

Tympanic — pertaining to the tympanum (the middle ear or tympanic cavity; eardrum).

Ubiquitin — a small protein present in eukaryotic cells that combines with other proteins and makes those other proteins susceptible to destruction; this protein is also important in promoting the functions of proteins that make up the ribosomes.

Ullage — the amount by which a fluid container falls short of being full.

Ultrasonic — inaudible (to human ears) sounds with frequencies greater than ~20,000 Hz.

Unsaturated — possessing double or triple bonds; capable of making additional covalent bonds.

Urethra — a canal for the discharge of urine extending from the bladder to the outside of the body.

Urticaria — vascular reaction of the skin characterized by the eruption of pale evanescent wheals (round elevations of the skin, white in the center with a pale red periphery), which are associated with severe itching; hives.

UTC — see coordinated universal time.

Utricle — the larger of the two membranous sacs in the vestibule (central cavity) of the osseous labyrinth (the inner ear).

UV — ultraviolet.

Uveitis — a nonspecific term for any intraocular inflammatory disorder, usually of the uveal tract structures (iris, ciliary body, and choroid, forming the pigmented layer) although nonuveal parts such as the retina and cornea may also be involved.

Valence — in chemistry, regarding covalent compounds, the valence of an atom is the number of bonds that the atom forms to other atoms. In immunology, antiserum contains antibodies that may have specificity for one (monovalent) or more (polyvalent) antigens.

Vallate papilla — one of a group of papillae (small nipple-like protuberances or elevations) forming a V-shaped row on the posterior dorsal surface of the tongue.

Van der Waals forces — weak electrostatic forces between atoms and molecules; any of several intermolecular attractive forces not resulting from ionic charges; also known as the London dispersion force.

Vascular — containing, or pertaining to, blood or lymph vessels.

Vasculography — a physical description (and mapping) of the human vascular system.

Vasoconstriction — in physiology, a decrease in the diameter of blood vessels.

Vasodilation — in physiology, an increase in the diameter of blood vessels.

Vaults — in cell biology, barrel-shaped protein particles found in the cytoplasm, that are of the right size size and shape to be able to dock at the nuclear pore complex.

Vein — in anatomy, generally, a blood vessel that returns blood from the tissues to the heart.

Velum palatinum — the soft palate.

Vena cava — the largest vein in the human body, leading toward the heart.

Venesection — blood-letting (phlebotomy, venotomy).

Ventral — the front of the human body, hence on or nearest the abdominal surface; pertaining to the belly.

Ventricle — either of two lower chambers of the heart.

Ventricular fibrillation — the primary mechanism and arrhythmia seen in sudden cardiac arrest (cessation of blood circulation).

Vernier — a short, graduated scale, permitting accurate measurement of the relative movement of mechanical parts.

Vertigo — the sensation of moving around in space; sometimes used as a synonym for dizziness, lightheadedness, or giddiness.

Vesicles — small bodies bounded by membrane, derived by budding from one membrane and often able to fuse with another membrane.

Vesicles (endocytotic) — membranous particles that transport proteins through endocytosis; also known as clathrin-coated vesicles, having on their surfaces a layer of the protein clathrin.

Vesicles (exocytic) — membranous particles that transport and store proteins during exocytosis.

Vestibular senses — sensory receptors in the labyrinth of the human inner ear that respond to human head position and movement, imparting a sense of balance.

Virion — a physical virus particle.

Virtual reality system — a combination of computer and interface devices (goggles, gloves, etc.) that presents a user with the illusion of being in a three dimensional world of computer-generated objects. These three dimensional environments and force-feedback systems can aid in the visualization of complex molecules, and in telepresence systems.

Virucide — the destruction of active or dormant virus particles.

Virus — A parasite (consisting primarily of genetic material enclosed in a protein capsid shell) that invades cells and takes over their molecular machinery in order to copy itself.

Viscera — internal organs enclosed within a cavity, especially the abdominal organs.

Viscosity — resistance of a fluid to shearing, when the fluid is in motion.

Vitamins (biology) — a group of organic substances, present in minute amounts in natural foodstuffs, that are essential to normal metabolism, growth, and development of the body. Vitamins serve principally to regulate metabolic processes and to play a role in energy transformations, usually acting as coenzymes in enzymatic systems. See also coenzyme.

Vitamins (engineering) — in machine replication theory, vitamin parts are components of a self-replicating machine which the machine is incapable of producing itself, therefore these vital parts must be supplied from an external source.

Vitreous humor — in anatomy, a delicate network enclosing in its meshes a clear watery fluid filling the interior of the eyeball behind the lens.

Volitional normative model of disease — in medical nanorobotics, disease is said to be present in a human being upon either: (1) the failure of optimal physical (e.g. biological) functioning, or (2) the failure of desired (by the patient) functioning.

Vomeronasal organ — in anatomy, a small tubular epithelial sac lying on the anteroinferior surface of the nasal septum.

Voxel (volume pixel) — abbreviation for volume element; a single cubic cell within a three-dimensional geometric solid grid or array.

W — watt (MKS unit of power).

Watt governor — in control engineering, a governor is a mechanism by which the speed of an engine, turbine, wheel, or motor may be regulated. The Watt governor employs rotating weights attached to a pivoted lever arm; the weights extend as the pair rotates faster, depressing the attached lever arm and throttling the motor down, thus slowing the rotation, and vice versa.

Wave function — in quantum mechanics, a complex mathematical function extending over the configuration space of a material system.

WBC — white blood cell (see leukocyte).

White blood cell (WBC) — see leukocyte.

Whitlow — in medicine, a suppurative inflammation at the end of a finger or toe.

Work — in physics, the energy transferred by applying a force across a distance; for example, lifting a mass does work against gravity and stores gravitational potential energy.

WWV — a radio station that continuously broadcasts the exact Coordinated Universal Time.

Xenotransplantation — transplantation of cells or organs from an organism of a different species.

Xerophthalmia — a vitamin A deficiency disease, characterized by extreme dryness of the conjunctiva with keratinization of epithelium.

Young's modulus — in mechanical engineering, a modulus relating tensile (or compressive) stress to strain in a rod that is free to contract or expand transversely. The relevant measure of strain is the elongation divided by the initial length (see also strain and stress).

Zippocytes — in medical nanorobotics, a theorized medical nanorobot that can rapidly perform incision-wound repairs to the dermis and epidermis; dermal zippers.

Zwitterions — dipolar ions that contain positive and negative charges of equal strength, and are therefore not attracted to either anode or cathode; in a neutral solution, some amino acids function as zwitterions.

Zymogenic — pertaining to a substance (a zymogen or proenzyme) that develops into an enzyme capable of producing or causing fermentation or digestion (e.g. pepsinogen, trypsinogen); a cell that produces zymogens (proenzymes).

REFERENCES

1. Hans Moravec, Mind Children: The Future of Robot and Human Intelligence, Harvard University Press, Cambridge, MA, 1988.
6. Seth Lloyd, "A Potentially Realizable Quantum Computer," Science 261(17 September 1993):1569-1571 and 263(4 February 1994):695. See also: "Quantum-Mechanical Computers," Scientific American 273(October 1995):140-145.
8. K. Eric Drexler, Engines of Creation: The Coming Era of Nanotechnology, Anchor Press/Doubleday, New York, 1986.
9. K. Eric Drexler, Chris Peterson, Gayle Pergamit, Unbounding the Future: The Nanotechnology Revolution, William Morrow/Quill Books, NY, 1991.
10. K. Eric Drexler, Nanosystems: Molecular Machinery, Manufacturing, and Computation, John Wiley & Sons, NY, 1992.
16. Yun Kim, Charles M. Lieber, "Machining Oxide Thin Films with an Atomic Force Microscope: Pattern and Object Formation on the Nanometer Scale," Science 257(17 July 1992):375-7.
17. T. Ross Kelly, Michael C. Bowyer, K. Vijaya Bhaskar, David Bebbington, Alberto Garcia, Fengrui Lang, Min H. Kim, Michael P. Jette, "A Molecular Brake," J. Am. Chem. Soc. 116(1994):3657-3658. See also: Stu Borman, "Molecular Brake: Side Chain Reversibly Slows Rotating Wheel," Chemical & Engineering News 72(25 April 1994):6-7.
18. A. K. Dewdney, "Nanotechnology—Wherein Molecular Computers Control Tiny Circulatory Submarines," Scientific American 258(January 1988):100-103.
19. Robert A. Freitas Jr., "The Future of Computers," Analog 116(March 1996):57-73.
20. Brian Wowk, Michael Darwin, eds., Cryonics: Reaching for Tomorrow, Alcor Life Extension Foundation, Tucson, AZ, December 1993.
21. Robert R. Birge, "Introduction to Molecular and Biomolecular Electronics," in Robert R. Birge, editor, Molecular and Biomolecular Electronics, Advances in Chemistry Series 240 (American Chemical Society, Washington, DC, 1994), Chapter 1, pp. 1-14.
27. Gregory Fahy, "Appendix B: A 'Realistic' Scenario for Nanotechnological Repair of the Frozen Human Brain," in Brian Wowk, Michael Darwin, eds., Cryonics: Reaching for Tomorrow, Alcor Life Extension Foundation, Tucson, AZ, December 1993.
70. Frederick A. Fiedler, Glenn H. Reynolds, "Legal Problems of Nanotechnology: An Overview," Southern California Interdisciplinary Law Journal 3(1994):593-629.
71. Arthur C. Guyton, Textbook of Medical Physiology, Seventh Edition, W.B. Saunders Company, Philadelphia PA, 1986.
72. K. Eric Drexler, "Machines of Inner Space," 1990 Yearbook of Science and the Future, Encyclopedia Britannica, Chicago, 1989, pp. 160-167. Reprinted as "Appendix A" in B.C. Crandall, James Lewis, eds., Nanotechnology: Research and Perspectives, MIT Press, 1992. pp. 325-346.
73. New Technologies for a Sustainable World: Hearing before the Subcommittee on Science, Technology, and Space of the Senate Committee on Commerce, Science, and Transportation, 102nd Congress, 2nd Session, 1992, S. HRG. 102-967. Statements of K. Eric Drexler.
96. Kris Sperry, "Tattoos & Tattooing: Part I: History and Methodology," Am. J. Forensic Med. & Pathology 12(1991):313-319.
115. Robert A. Freitas Jr., William P. Gilbreath, eds., Advanced Automation for Space Missions, Proceedings of the 1980 NASA/ASEE Summer Study held at the University of Santa Clara, Santa Clara, CA, June 23-August 29, 1980; NASA Conference Publication CP-2255, November 1982. See also at: http://www.islandone.org/MMSG/aasm/.
116. Ralph C. Merkle, "Replicating Systems and Molecular Manufacturing," Journal of the British Interplanetary Society 45(1992):407-413. See at: http://nano.xerox.com/nanotech/selfRepJBIS.html.
121. Allen J. Bard, Integrated Chemical Systems: A Chemical Approach to Nanotechnology, John Wiley & Sons, New York, 1994.
122. T.M. Beardsley, "Nanofuture: How much Fun Would It Be To Live Forever?" Scientific American 262 (January 1990):15-16.
123. Wiley P. Kirk, Mark A. Reed, eds., Nanostructures and Mesoscopic Systems, Academic Press, 1992.
125. Roald Hoffmann, "How Should Chemists Think?" Scientific American 268(February 1993):66-73.
129. Robert W. Keyes, "The Future of the Transistor," Scientific American 268(June 1993):70-78.
131. Julius Rebek, Jr., "Synthetic Self-Replicating Molecules," Scientific American 271(July 1994):48-55.
132. Marvin Minsky, "Will Robots Inherit the Earth?" Scientific American 271(October 1994):109-113.
153. Conrad Schneiker, "NanoTechnology with Feynman Machines: Scanning Tunneling Engineering and Artificial Life," in Christopher G. Langton, ed., Artificial Life, Santa Fe Institute, Studies in the Sciences of Complexity, Volume VI, Addison-Wesley, NY, 1989, pp.443-500.
154. A. Franks, "Nanotechnology," J. Phys. E:Sci. Instrum. 20(December 1987):1442-1451.
155. R.A. Heinlein, Waldo and Magic, Inc., Doubleday & Co., NY, 1950. First story in series ("Waldo"), published August 1942 in Astounding Science Fiction.
156. R.P. Feynman, "There's Plenty of Room at the Bottom," Engineering and Science (California Institute of Technology), February 1960, pp. 22-36. Reprinted in B.C. Crandall, James Lewis, eds., Nanotechnology: Research and Perspectives, MIT Press, 1992. pp. 347-363, and in D.H. Gilbert, ed., Miniaturization, Reinhold, New York, 1961, pp. 282-296. See also: http://nano.xerox.com/nanotech/feynman.html.
157. Robert C.W. Ettinger, The Prospect of Immortality, Doubleday, NY, 1964.
158. K.W. Jeon, I.J. Lorch, J.F. Danielli, "Reassembly of Living Cells from Dissociated Components," Science 167(1970):1626-1627.
159. H.J. Morowitz, "Manufacturing a Living Organism," Hospital Practice 9(November 1974):210-215.
160. Robert C.W. Ettinger, Man Into Superman, St. Martin's Press, NY, 1972.
161. T. Donaldson, "How Will They Bring Us Back, 200 Years From Now?" The Immortalist 12(March 1981):5-10.
162. J.P. Changeux, "The Control of Biochemical Reactions," Scientific American 212 (April 1965):36-45.
163. H. Iwamura, "Molecular Design of Correlated Internal Rotation," J. Molecular Struct. 126(1985):401-412.
164. G. Yamamoto, "Molecular Gears with Two-Toothed and Three-Toothed Wheels," J. Molecular Struct. 126(1985):413-420.
165. Chris Peterson, K. Eric Drexler, "Nanotechnology," Analog 107(Mid-December 1987):48-60.
168. Christopher Lampton, "Nanotechnology Promises to Revolutionize the Diagnosis and Treatment of Diseases," Genetic Engineering News 15(1 April 1995):4, 23.
172. T.E. Creighton, Proteins, W.H. Freeman & Co., NY, 1984.
182. K. Eric Drexler, "Molecular Engineering: An Approach to the Development of General Capabilities for Molecular Manipulation," Proc. National Academy of Sciences (USA) 78(September 1981):5275-5278.
202. Marvin Minsky, "Our Robotized Future," in Marvin Minsky, ed., Robotics, Omni Publications International, NY, 1985, pp. 286-307.
204. Robert A. Freitas Jr., "The Birth of the Cyborg," in Marvin Minsky, ed., Robotics, Omni Publications International, NY, 1985, pp. 146-183.
215. Gregory M. Fahy, "Possible Medical Applications of Nanotechnology," in B.C. Crandall, James Lewis, eds., Nanotechnology: Research and Perspectives, MIT Press, 1992, pp. 251-267.
216. Robert M. Macnab, "Genetics and Biogenesis of Bacterial Flagella," Annual Review of Genetics 26(1992):131-158.
217. K. Eric Drexler, John S. Foster, "Synthetic Tips," Nature 343(15 February 1990):600.
222. T.W. Bell, Z. Hou, Y. Luo, M.G.B. Drew, E. Chapoteau, B.P. Czech, A. Kumar, "Detection of Creatinine by a Designed Receptor," Science 269(4 August 1995):671-674.
223. Harley H. McAdams, Lucy Shapiro, "Circuit Simulation of Genetic Networks," Science 269(4 August 1995):650-656.
224. Gregory M. Fahy, "Short-Term and Long-Term Possibilities for Interventive Gerontology," Mount Sinai Journal of Medicine 58(4 September 1991):328-340.

258. Ralph Merkle, "Algorithmic Feasibility of Molecular Repair of the Brain," Cryonics 16(1995QI):15-16.
259. Eric Drexler, "Molecular Technology and Cell Repair Machines," paper presented at the 1985 Lake Tahoe Life Extension Festival, 25 May 1985; reprinted and published in Claustrophobia Magazine (August-October 1985) and Cryonics (Dec 1985 - January 1986).
261. Brian Wowk, "Cell Repair Technology," Cryonics (July 1988) reprint.
262. Ralph C. Merkle, "The Molecular Repair of the Brain," Cryonics (January 1994):16-31 (Part I); Cryonics (April, 1994):20-32 (Part II).
278. D.M. Eigler, E.K. Schweizer, "Positioning Single Atoms with a Scanning Tunnelling Microscope," Nature 344(1990):524-526.
279. K. Eric Drexler, "Introduction to Nanotechnology," in Markus Krummenacker, James Lewis, eds., Prospects in Nanotechnology: Toward Molecular Manufacturing, John Wiley & Sons, New York, 1995, pp. 1-22.
280. Ralph C. Merkle, "Design-Ahead for Nanotechnology," in Markus Krummenacker, James Lewis, eds., Prospects in Nanotechnology: Toward Molecular Manufacturing, John Wiley & Sons, New York, 1995, pp. 23-52.
282. N. Taniguchi, "Current Status in, and Future Trends of, Ultraprecision Machining and Ultrafine Materials Processing," Annals of the CIRP 32(1983, No.2):573-582.
289. Marvin Minsky, "Virtual Molecular Reality," in Markus Krummenacker, James Lewis, eds., Prospects in Nanotechnology: Toward Molecular Manufacturing, John Wiley & Sons, New York, 1995, pp. 187-195.
292. Thomas Kuhn, The Structure of Scientific Revolutions, Second Edition, University of Chicago Press, Chicago, 1970.
296. C. Bennett, "The Thermodynamics of Computation -- A Review," Intl. J. Theoret. Phys. 21(1981):905-940.
300. Ed Regis, Nano: The Emerging Science of Nanotechnology, Little, Brown and Company, New York, 1995.
306. R.C. Merkle, "The Technical Feasibility of Cryonics," Medical Hypotheses 39(1992):6-16.
308. Klaus Weber, Mary Osborn, "The Molecules of the Cell Matrix," Scientific American 253(October 1985):110-120.
310. Fred Hapgood, "Tinytech," Omni 9(November 1986):56-62, 102.
311. Eric Drexler, "Mightier Machines from Tiny Atoms May Someday Grow," Smithsonian 13(November 1982):145-155.
312. David S. Goodsell, The Machinery of Life, Springer-Verlag, New York, 1993.
313. Wayne M. Becker, The World of the Cell, The Benjamin/Cummings Publishing Company, Menlo Park, CA, 1986.
317. Richard J. Lagow et al., "Synthesis of Linear Acetylenic Carbon: The 'sp' Carbon Allotrope," Science 267(20 January 1995):362-367.
322. Gregory M. Fahy, "Molecular Nanotechnology," Clinical Chemistry 39(September 1993):2011-2016.
328. Richard Preston, The Hot Zone, Anchor Books Doubleday, NY, 1994.
330. Christopher Lampton, Nanotechnology Playhouse: Building Machines from Atoms, Waite Group Press, Corte Madera, CA, 1993.
336. Robert Dillon, Lisa Fauci, Donald Gaver III, "A Microscale Model of Bacterial Swimming, Chemotaxis and Substrate Transport," J. Theoret. Biology 177(December 1995):325-340.
337. Howard C. Berg, Edward M. Purcell, "Physics of Chemoreception," Biophysical Journal 20(1977):193-219.
338. George T. Yates, "How Microorganisms Move through Water," American Scientist 74(July-August 1986):358-365.
339. Isaac Asimov, Fantastic Voyage, Houghton Mifflin Company, Boston, 1966.
340. Isaac Asimov, Fantastic Voyage II: Destination Brain, Doubleday, NY, 1987.
341. Jonathan Murphy, Bob Carr, Tony Atkinson, "Nanotechnology in Medicine and the Biosciences," Trends in Biotechnology 12(August 1994):289-290.
343. Elton Elliott, ed., Nanodreams, Baen Books, Riverdale NY, 1995.
346. B. Magnussen, S. Fatikow, U. Rembold, "Actuation in Microsystems: Problem Field Overview and Practical Example of the Piezoelectric Robot for Handling of Microobjects," in Proceedings of the 1995 INRIA/IEEE Symposium on Emerging Technologies and Factory Automation, IEEE Computer Society Press, Vol. 3, 1995, pp. 21-27.
347. Y. Kubo, Isao Shimoyama, T. Kaneda, Hirofumi Miura, "Study on Wings of Flying Microrobots," in Proceedings IEEE International Conference on Robotics and Automation, IEEE Computer Society Press, Vol. 1, 1994, pp. 834-9.
348. Y. Kubo, Isao Shimoyama, Hirofumi Miura, "Study of Insect-Based Flying Microrobots," in Proceedings IEEE International Conference on Robotics and Automation, IEEE Computer Society Press, Vol. 2, 1994, pp. 386-391.
352. Takashi Yasuda, Isao Shimoyama, Hirofumi Miura, "Microrobot Actuated by a Vibration Energy Field," Sensors and Actuators 43A(1994):366-370.
355. Richard Feynman, "Infinitesimal Machinery," Journal of Microelectromechanical Systems 2(March 1991):4-14.
357. Cyberlife, Sams Publishing, Indianapolis, IN, 1994.
358. Wesley M. DuCharme, Becoming Immortal: Nanotechnology, You, and the Demise of Death, Blue Creek Ventures, Evergreen CO, 1995.
359. Erle E. Peacock, Jr., Wound Repair, W.B. Saunders Company, Philadelphia, 1984.
360. Thomas K. Hunt, J. Englebert Dunphy, Fundamentals of Wound Management, Appleton-Century-Crofts, New York, 1979.
361. Y.C. Fung, Biodynamics: Circulation, Springer-Verlag, New York, 1984.
362. Y.C. Fung, Biomechanics: Mechanical Properties of Living Tissues, Second Edition, Springer-Verlag, New York, 1993.
363. Y.C. Fung, Biomechanics: Motion, Flow, Stress, and Growth, Springer-Verlag, New York, 1990.
364. S.A. Wainwright, W.D. Biggs, J.D. Currey, J.M. Gosline, Mechanical Design in Organisms. John Wiley & Sons, New York, 1976.
365. D.L. Fry, "Acute vascular endothelial changes associated with increased blood velocity gradients," Circulation Res. 22(1968):165-197.
366. G.W. Schmid-Schonbein, Y.C. Fung, B.W. Zweifach, "Vascular endothelium-leukocyte interaction," Circulation Res. 36(1975):173-184.
368. E.A. Evans, W. Rawicz, "Entropy-driven tension and bending elasticity in condensed-fluid membranes," Phys. Rev. Lett. 64(1990):2094-2097.
371. Robert M. Hochmuth, "Chapter 12: Properties of red blood cells." In Richard Skalak, Shu Chien, eds., Handbook of Bioengineering, McGraw-Hill, New York, 1987.
374. M.I. Gregersen, C.A. Bryant, W.E. Hammerle, S. Usami, S. Chien, "Flow characteristics of human erythrocytes through polycarbonate sieves," Science 157(1967):825-827.
381. Kevin Kelly, Out of Control: The New Biology of Machines, Social Systems, and the Economic World, Addison-Wesley Publishing Company, New York, 1994.
382. Philip Ball, Designing the Molecular World: Chemistry at the Frontier, Princeton University Press, Princeton NJ, 1994.
383. Michael Fossel, Reversing Human Aging, William Morrow and Company, NY, 1996.
384. Laurie Garrett, The Coming Plague, Penguin Books USA, New York, 1994.
385. Albert Einstein, "Investigations on the Theory of Brownian Movement," with notes by R. Furth, translated into English from German by A.D. Cowper, Methuen, London (1926), Dover Publications (1956); original paper in Ann. Phys. 17(1905):549.
386. H.L. Goldsmith, V.T. Turitto, "Rheological aspects of thrombosis and haemostasis: basic principles and applications," Thromb. Haemostasis 55(1986):415-435.
388. Kenneth H. Keller, "Effect of fluid shear on mass transport in flowing blood," Proc. Fed. Am. Soc. Exp. Biol. 30 (September-October 1971):1591-1599.
389. E.M. Purcell, "Life at low Reynolds number," Am. J. Physics 45(January 1977):3-11.
390. Farrington Daniels, Robert A. Alberty, Physical Chemistry, Third Edition, John Wiley & Sons, New York, NY, 1966.
391. Gary L. Westbrook, "Ligand-Gated Ion Channels," in Nicholas Sperelakis, ed., Cell Physiology Source Book, Academic Press, New York, 1995, Chapter 31, pp. 431-441.
392. William A. Catterall, "Structure and function of voltage-gated ion channels," Annual Rev. Biochemistry 64(1995):493-531.
393. Paul Burgmayer, Royce W. Murray, "An ion gate membrane: Electrochemical control of ion permeability through a membrane with an embedded electrode," J. Amer. Chem. Soc. 104(1982):6139-6140.
394. Matsuhiko Nishizawa, Vinod P. Menon, Charles R. Martin, "Metal nanotubule membranes with electrochemically switchable ion-transport selectivity," Science 268(5 May 1995):700-702.
395. David A. Langs, David J. Triggle, "Structural motifs for ion channels in membranes," in Philip Yeagle, ed., The Structure of Biological Membranes, CRC Press, Boca Raton, 1992, Chapter 16, pp. 721-772.
396. Lubert Stryer, Biochemistry, 4th Edition, W.H. Freeman and Company, New York, 1995.
397. Nicholas Sperelakis, "Diffusion and Permeability," in Nicholas Sperelakis, ed., Cell Physiology Source Book, Academic Press, New York, 1995, Chapter 5, pp. 61-66.
398. Thomas M. Devlin, ed., Textbook of Biochemistry with Clinical Correlations, Third Edition, Wiley-Liss, New York, 1992.
399. Michael M. Gottesman, Ira Pastan, "Biochemistry of multidrug resistance mediated by the multidrug transporter," Ann. Rev. Biochemistry 62(1993):385-427.
400. Hiroshi Nikaido, "Prevention of Drug Access to Bacterial Targets: Permeability Barriers and Active Efflux," Science 264(15 April 1994):382-388.
401. Michel Delaage, "Physico-Chemical Aspects of Molecular Recognition," in Michel Delaage, ed., Molecular Recognition Mechanisms, VCH Publishers, Inc., 1991, Chapter 1, pp. 1-13.
402. Cyrus Chothia, Joel Janin, "Principles of protein-protein recognition," Nature 256(28Aug 1975):705-708.
403. George Scatchard, Alan C. Batchelder, Alexander Brown, "Preparation and Properties of Serum and Plasma Proteins. VI. Osmotic Equilibria in Solutions of Serum Albumin and Sodium Chloride," J. Amer. Chem. Soc. 68(November 1946):2320-2329.
404. F. Harold, The Vital Force: A Study of Bioenergetics, W.H. Freeman & Co., New York, 1986.
405. M. Fehlman, A. le Cam, P. Kitabgi, J.F. Ray, P. Freychet, "Regulation of amino acid transport in the liver," J. Biol. Chem. 254(1978):401-407.
406. J.P. Vincent, M. Lazdunski, "Trypsin-pancreatic trypsin inhibitor association: Dynamics of the interaction and role of disulfide bridges," Biochemistry 11(1972):2967-2977.
407. M. Green, in C.B. Anfisen, J.T. Edsall, F.M. Richards, eds., Advances in Protein Chemistry, Volume 29, Academic Press, New York, 1975, pp. 85-133.
408. M.A. Delaage, J.J. Puizillout, "Radioimmunoassays for serotonine and 5-hydroxyindole acetic acid," J. Physiol. 77(1981):339-347.
409. M. Karplus, J.A. McCammon, "Dynamics of Proteins: Elements and Function," Annual Rev. Biochem. 53(1983):263-300.

410. Donald J. Cram, "Molecular container compounds," Nature 356(5 March 1992):29-36.
411. C.D. Gutsche, Calixarenes, Royal Society of Chemistry, London, 1993.
412. Arthur M. Lesk, Cyrus Chothia, "Evolution of Proteins Formed by β-Sheets: II. The Core of the Immunoglobulin Domains," J. Mol. Biol. 160(1982):325-342.
413. Cyrus Chothra, "Principles that Determine the Structure of Proteins," Ann. Rev. Biochem. 53(1984):537-572.
414. Russell F. Doolittle, "The Multiplicity of Domains in Proteins," Ann. Rev. Biochem. 64(1995):287-314.
415. Nathan Sharon, Halina Lis, "Carbohydrates in Cell Recognition," Scientific American 268(January 1993):82-89.
416. T.N. Bhat, G.A. Bentley, T.O. Fischmann, G. Boulot, R.J. Poljak, "Small rearrangements in structures of Fv and Fab fragments of antibody D1.3 on antigen binding," Nature 347(4 October 1990):483-485.
417. K.N. Houk, Kensuke Nakamura, Chimin Sheu, Amy E. Keating, "Gating as a Control Element in Constrictive Binding and Guest Release by Hemicarcerands," Science 273(2 August 1996):627-629.
418. Lei Jin, James A. Wells, "Dissecting the energetics of an antibody-antigen interface by alanine shaving and molecular grafting," Protein Science 3(1994):2351-2357.
419. A. Bertazzon, B.M. Conti-Tronconi, M.A. Raftery, "Scanning tunneling microscopy imaging of *Torpedo* acetylcholine receptor," Proc. Natl. Acad. Sci. USA 89(October 1992):9632-9636.
421. Klaus Mosbach, "Molecular Imprinting," Trends in Biochemical Sciences 19(1994):9-14.
422. Richard J. Ansell, Olof Ramstrom, Klaus Mosbach, "Towards artificial antibodies prepared by molecular imprinting," Clinical Chemistry 42(1996):1506-1512.
423. S. Roper, "Olfactory/Taste Receptor Transduction," in Nicholas Sperelakis, ed., Cell Physiology Source Book, Academic Press, New York, 1995, Chapter 38, pp. 514-522.
424. Suzanne B. Shuker, Philip J. Hajduk, Robert P. Meadows, Stephen W. Fesik, "Discovering High-Affinity Ligands for Proteins: SAR by NMR," Science 274(29 November 1996):1531-1534.
425. Markus Krummenacker, "Cavity Stuffer," 1993; see at: http://www.ai.sri.com/-kr/nano/cavstuf/cavstuf.html.
426. Monty Krieger, Joachim Herz, "Structures and Functions of Multiligand Lipoprotein Receptors: Macrophage Scavenger Receptors and LDL Receptor-Related Protein (LRP)," Ann. Rev. Biochem. 63(1994):601-637.
427. Joel Janin, Cyrus Chothia, "Role of Hydrophobicity in the Binding of Coenzymes. Appendix: Translational and Rotational Contribution to the Free Energy of Dissociation," Biochemistry 17(25 July 1978):2943-2948.
430. Mark E. Davis, "Design for Sieving," Nature 382(15 August 1996):583-584.
431. D.W. Lewis, C.M. Freeman, C.R.A. Catlow, "Predicting the Templating Ability of Organic Additives for the Synthesis of Microporous Materials," J. Phys. Chem. 99(1995):11194-11202.
432. Dewi W. Lewis, David J. Willock, C. Richard A. Catlow, John Meurig Thomas, Graham J. Hutchings, "De novo design of structure-directing agents for the synthesis of microporous solids," Nature 382 (15 August 1996):604-606.
433. R. Wiesendanger, Scanning Probe Microscopy and Spectroscopy: Methods and Applications. Cambridge University Press, Cambridge, MA, 1994.
434. W.C. Gardiner Jr., Rates and Mechanisms of Chemical Reactions, Benjamin, New York, 1969.
435. R. Macnab, D.E. Koshland Jr., "The gradient-sensing mechanism in bacterial chemotaxis," Proc. Natl. Acad. Sci. USA 69(1972):2509-2512.
436. D.E. Koshland Jr., "A Response Regulator Model in a Simple Sensory System," Science 196(3 June 1977):1055-1063.
437. John S. Parkinson, David F. Blair, "Does *E. coli* Have a Nose?" Science 259 (19 March 1993):1701-1702.
438. H. Meixner, R. Jones, eds., Volume 8: Micro- and Nanosensor Technology / Trends in Sensor Markets. In W. Gopel, J. Hesse, J.N. Zemel, eds., Sensors: A Comprehensive Survey, VCH Verlagsgesellschaft mbH, Weinheim Germany, 1995.
439. Robert G. Urban, Roman M. Chicz, eds., MHC Molecules: Expression, Assembly and Function, Chapman & Hall, New York, 1996.
440. C. Daniel Frisbie, Lawrence F. Rozsnyai, Aleksandr Noy, Mark S. Wrighton, Charles M. Lieber, "Functional Group Imaging by Chemical Force Microscopy", Science 265(30 September 1994):2071-2074.
441. Ross C. Thomas, J.E. Houston, Richard M. Crooks, Taisun Kim, Terry A. Michalske, "Probing Adhesion Forces at the Molecular Scale," J. Amer. Chem. Soc. 117(1995):3830-3834.
442. V. Gass, B.H. van der Schoot, N.F. de Rooij, "Nanofluid Handling by Micro-Flow-Sensor Based on Drag Force Measurements," Proceedings 6th IEEE Micro Electro Mechanical Systems, IEEE Robotics and Automation Society, 1993, pp. 167-172.
443. S.D. Rapoport, M.L. Reed, L.E. Weiss, "Fabrication and Testing of a Microdynamic Rotor for Blood Flow Measurements," J. Micromech. Microeng. 1(1991):60-65.
444. C.S.F. Lee, L. Talbot, "A fluid mechanical study on the closure of heart valves," J. Fluid Mechanics 91(1979):41-63.
445. G. Binnig, C.F. Quate, Ch. Gerber, "Atomic Force Microscopy," Phys. Rev. Lett. 56(3 March 1986):930-933.
446. A.J. Hudspeth, "The Hair Cells of the Inner Ear," Scientific American 248(January 1983):54-64.
447. J. Bernstein, S. Cho, A.T. King, A. Kourepenis, P. Maciel, M. Weinberg, "A Micromachined Comb-Drive Tuning Fork Rate Gyroscope," Proceedings 6th IEEE Micro Electro Mechanical Systems, IEEE Robotics and Automation Society, 1993, pp. 413-418.
448. Keith R. Symon, Mechanics, 3rd edition, Addison-Wesley Publishing Co., Reading MA, 1971.
449. William C. Van Buskirk, J. Wallace Grant, "Chapter 31: Vestibular Mechanics," in Richard Skalak, Shu Chien, eds., Handbook of Bioengineering, McGraw-Hill Book Company, New York, 1987.
450. R. Wiesendanger, "Chapter 11. Future Nanosensors." In H. Meixner, R. Jones, eds., Volume 8: Micro- and Nanosensor Technology / Trends in Sensor Markets. In W. Gopel, J. Hesse, J.N. Zemel, eds., Sensors: A Comprehensive Survey, VCH Verlagsgesellschaft mbH, Weinheim Germany, 1995; pp. 337-356.
451. D. Rugar, C.S. Yannoni, J.A. Sidles, "Mechanical detection of magnetic resonance," Nature 360(1992):563-566.
452. Shinji Kamimura, Keiichi Takahashi, "Direct measurement of the force of microtubule sliding in flagella," Nature 293(15 October 1981):566-568.
453. A. Ashkin, Karin Schutze, J.M. Dziedzic, Ursula Euteneuer, Manfred Schliwa, "Force generation of organelle transport measured in vivo by infrared laser trap," Nature 348(22 November 1990):346-348.
454. Steven M. Block, Lawrence S.B. Goldstein, Bruce J. Schnapp, "Bead movement by single kinesin molecules studied with optical tweezers," Nature 348(22 November 1990):348-352.
455. Akihiko Ishijima, Takashi Doi, Katsuhiko Sakurada, Toshio Yanagida, "Sub-piconewton force fluctuations of actomyosin in vitro," Nature 352(25 July 1991):301-306.
456. M. Kandler, Y. Manoli, W. Mokwa, E. Spiegel, H. Vogt, "A miniature single-chip pressure and temperature sensor," J. Micromech. Microeng. 2(1992):199-201.
457. Lars Rosengren, Ylva Backlund, Tom Sjostrom, Bertil Hok, Bjorn Svedbergh, "A system for wireless intra-ocular pressure measurements using a silicon micromachined sensor," J. Micromech. Microeng. 2(1992):202-204.
458. R.C. Hughes, A.J. Ricco, M.A. Butler, S.J. Martin, "Chemical Microsensors," Science 254(4 October 1991):74-80.
459. John R. Vig, Raymond L. Filler, Yoonkee Kim, "Chemical Sensor Based on Quartz Microresonators," J. Microelectromechanical Systems 5(June 1996):138-140.
460. Max N. Yoder, "Diamond Properties and Applications," in Robert F. Davis, ed., Diamond Films and Coatings: Development, Properties, and Applications, Noyes Publications, Park Ridge NJ, 1993, pp. 1-30.
461. J.K. Gimzewski, Ch. Gerber, E. Meyer, R.R. Schlittler, "Observation of a chemical reaction using a micromechanical sensor," Chem. Phys. Lett. 217(28 January 1994):589-594.
462. W.L. Smith, W.J. Spencer, "Quartz crystal thermometer for measuring temperature deviations in the 10^{-3} to 10^{-6}°C range," Rev. Sci. Instr. 34(1963):268-270.
463. C.C. Williams, H.K. Wickramasinghe, "Scanning thermal profiler," Appl. Phys. Lett. 49(8 December 1986):1587-1589.
464. C.C. Williams, H.K. Wickramasinghe, "Microscopy of chemical-potential variations on an atomic scale," Nature 344(22 March 1990):317-319.
465. Richard I. Morimoto, "Cells in Stress: Transcriptional Activation of Heat Shock Genes," Science 259(5 March 1993):1409-1410.
466. Joseph P. Hendrick, Franz-Ulrich Hartl, "Molecular Chaperone Functions of Heat-Shock Proteins," Ann. Rev. Biochem. 62(1993):349-384.
467. Robert F. Service, "Folding Proteins Caught in the Act," Science 273(5 July 1996):29-30.
468. Jason W. Armstrong, Richard A. Gerren, Stephen K. Chapes, "The Effect of Space and Parabolic Flight on Macrophage Hematopoiesis and Function," Experimental Cell Research 216 (1995):160-168.
469. Augusto Cogoli, "The effect of hypogravity and hypergravity on cells of the immune system," J. Leukocyte Biol. 54(September 1993):259-268.
470. Augusto Cogoli, Birgitt Bechler, Marianne Cogoli-Greuter, Sue B. Criswell, Helen Joller, Peter Joller, Elisabeth Hunzinger, Ottfried Muller, "Mitogenic signal transduction in T lymphocytes in microgravity," J. Leukocyte Biol. 53(May 1993):569-575.
471. D.K. Kondepudi, I. Prigogine, "Sensitivity in nonequilibrium chemical systems to gravitation field," Adv. Space Res. 3(1983):171-176.
472. M. Limouse, S. Manie, I. Konstantinova, B. Ferrua, L. Schaffar, "Inhibition of phorbol ester-induced cell activation in microgravity," Exp. Cell Res. 197(1991):82-86.
473. R.P. deGroot, P.J. Rijken, J. den Hertog, J. Boonstra, A.J. Verkleij, S.W. deLaat, W. Kruijer, "Nuclear responses to protein kinase C signal transduction are sensitive to gravity changes," Exp. Cell Res. 197(1991):87-90.
475. T.R. Anthony, W.F. Banholzer, J.F. Fleischer, Lanhua Wei, P.K. Kuo, R.L. Thomas, R.W. Pryor, "Thermal diffusivity of isotopically enriched C^{12} diamond," Phys. Rev. B 42(15 July 1990):1104-1111.
476. Eliot Marshall, "GE's Cool Diamonds Prompt Warm Words," Science 250(5 October 1990):25-26; and "Letters: Cool Diamonds," Science 250(30 November 1990):1194-1195.
477. B. Reipert, "Alterations in gene expression induced by low-frequency, low-intensity electromagnetic fields," in F. Lyall, A.J. El Haj, eds., Biomechanics and Cells, Cambridge University Press, 1994, pp. 131-143.

478. A.M. Chang, H.D. Hallen, L. Harriott, H.F. Hess, H.L. Kao, J. Kwo, R.E. Miller, R. Wolfe, J. van der Ziel, T.Y. Chang, "Scanning Hall probe microscopy," Appl. Phys. Lett. 61(19 October 1992):1974-1976.

479. S.J. Swithenby, "SQUID Magnetometer: Uses in Medicine," Phys. Technol. 18(January 1987):17-24.

480. Robert R. Birge, "Molecular Electronics," in B.C. Crandall, James Lewis, eds., Nanotechnology: Research and Perspectives, MIT Press, 1992, pp. 149-170.

481. Caridad Rosette, Michael Karin, "Ultraviolet Light and Osmotic Stress: Activation of the JNK Cascade Through Multiple Growth Factor and Cytokine Receptors," Science 274(15 November 1996):1194-1197.

482. B. Hadimioglu, J.S. Foster, "Advances in superfluid helium acoustic microscopy," J. Appl. Phys. 56 (1 October 1984):1976-1980.

483. Jurgen Bereiter-Hahn, "Probing Biological Cells and Tissues with Acoustic Microscopy," in Andrew Briggs, ed., Advances in Acoustic Microscopy, Volume 1, Plenum Press, New York, 1995, pp. 79-115.

484. H.J. Butt, E.K. Wolff, S.A. Gould, B.D. Northern, C.M. Peterson, P.K. Hansma, "Imaging cells with the atomic force microscope," J. Struct. Biol. 105(1990):54-61.

485. E. Henderson, P.G. Haydon, D.S. Sakaguchi, "Actin filament dynamics in living glial cells imaged by atomic force microscopy," Science 257(1992):1944-1946.

486. J.K.H. Horber, W. Haberle, F. Ohnesorge, G. Binnig, H.G. Liebich, C.P. Czerny, H. Mahnel, A. Mayr, "Investigation of living cells in the nanometer regime with the scanning force microscope," Scanning Microsc. 6(1992):919-930.

488. H. Luers, J. Bereiter-Hahn, J. Litniewski, in H. Ermert, H.P. Harjes, eds., Acoustical Imaging, Volume 19, Plenum Press, New York, 1992, pp. 511-516.

489. D. Rugar, O. Zuger, S. Hoen, C.S. Yannoni, H.M. Vieth, R.D. Kendrick, "Force Detection of Nuclear Magnetic Resonance," Science 264(10 June 1994):1560-1563.

490. Michael K. Stehling, Robert Turner, Peter Mansfield, "Echo-Planar Imaging: Magnetic Resonance Imaging in a Fraction of a Second," Science 254(4 October 1991):43-50.

491. Kevin Strange, ed., Cellular and Molecular Physiology of Cell Volume Regulation, CRC Press, Boca Raton FL, 1994.

492. E. Betzig, J.K. Trautman, T.D. Harris, J.S. Weiner, R.L. Kostelak, "Breaking the Diffraction Barrier: Optical Microscopy on a Nanometric Scale," Science 251(22 March 1991):1468-1470.

493. Eric Betzig, Robert J. Chichester, "Single Molecules Observed by Near-Field Scanning Optical Microscopy," Science 262(26 November 1993):1422-1425.

494. R. Berndt, R. Gaisch, J.K. Gimzewski, B. Reihl, R.R. Schlittler, W.D. Schneider, M. Tschudy, "Photon Emission at Molecular Resolution Induced by a Scanning Tunneling Microscope," Science 262(26 November 1993):1425-1427.

495. F. Zenhausern, Y. Martin, H.K. Wickramasinghe,"Scanning Interferometric Apertureless Microscopy: Optical Imaging at 10 Angstrom Resolution," Science 269(25 August 1995):1083-1085.

496. C. Thomas, P. DeVries, J. Hardin, J. White, "Four-Dimensional Imaging: Computer Visualization of 3D Movements in Living Specimens," Science 273 (2 August 1996):603-607.

497. Jack L. Jewell, James P. Harbison, Axel Scherer, "Microlasers," Scientific American 265(November 1991):86-94.

498. Chaya Nanavati, Julio M. Fernandez, "The Secretory Granule Matrix: A Fast-Acting Smart Polymer," Science 259(12 February 1993):963-965.

499. Masuo Aizawa, Hiroaki Shinohara, "Designing Artificial Structures from Biological Models," in Paolo Dario, Giulio Sandini, Patrick Aebischer, eds., Robots and Biological Systems: Towards a New Bionics? Springer-Verlag, New York, 1993, pp. 571-578.

500. T. Gualtierotti, V. Capraro, "The Action of Magnetic Field on the Sodium Transport Across the Cell Membrane," in M. Florkin, A. Dollfus, eds., Life Sciences and Space Research III, North-Holland Publishing Company, Amsterdam, 1964, pp. 311-316.

501. R.P. Blakemore, "Magnetotactic Bacteria," Science 190(1975):377-379.

502. Ellen D. Yorke, "A Possible Magnetic Transducer in Birds," J. Theoret. Biol. 77(1979):101-105.

503. Moshe Kisliuk, Jacob S. Ishay, "Hornet Building Orientation in Additional Magnetic Fields," in Richard Holmquist, ed., Life Sciences and Space Research XVI, Pergamon Press, New York, 1978, pp. 57-62.

504. T.F. Budinger, C.A. Tobias, R.H. Huesman, F.T. Upham, T.F. Wieskamp, R.A. Hoffman, "Apollo-Soyuz Light-Flash Observations," in Richard Holmquist, ed., Life Sciences and Space Research XV, Pergamon Press, New York, 1977, pp. 141-146.

505. Wesley L. Nyborg, Marvin C. Ziskin, eds., Biological Effects of Ultrasound, Churchill Livingstone, New York, 1985.

506. Sandra L. Hagen-Ansert, Textbook of Diagnostic Ultrasonography, Third Edition, C.V. Mosby Company, St. Louis MO, 1989.

507. Rudolph L. Leibel, "A Biologic Radar System for the Assessment of Body Mass: The Model of a Geometry Sensitive Endocrine System is Presented," J. Theoret. Biol. 66(1977):297-306.

508. R. Rox Anderson, John A. Parrish, "The Optics of Human Skin," J. Investigative Dermatology 77(1981):13-19.

509. M.J.C. Van Gemert, Steven L. Jacques, H.J.C.M. Sterenborg, W.M. Star, "Skin Optics," IEEE Trans. Biomed. Eng. 36(December 1989):1146-1154.

510. Wai-Fung Cheong, Scott A. Prahl, Ashley J. Welch, "A Review of the Optical Properties of Biological Tissues," IEEE J. Quantum Electronics 26(December 1990):2166-2185.

512. H. Rada, A. Dittmar, G. Delhomme, C. Collet, R. Roure, E. Vernet-Maury, A. Priez, "Bioelectric and microcirculation cutaneous sensors for the study of vigilance and emotional response during tasks and tests," Biosensors and Bioelectronics 10(1995):7-15.

513. Peter Fromherz, Alfred Stett, "Silicon-Neuron Junction: Capacitive Stimulation of an Individual Neuron on a Silicon Chip," Phys. Rev. Lett. 75(21 August 1995):1670-1673.

514. Sergey M. Bezrukov, Igor Vodyanoy, "Noise-induced enhancement of signal transduction across voltage-dependent ion channels," Nature 378(23 November 1995):362-364.

517. Eugene M. Renkin, "Chapter 42. Microcirculation and Exchange," in Harry D. Patton, Albert F. Fuchs, Bertil Hille, Alan M. Scher, Robert Steiner, eds., Textbook of Physiology, 21st Edition, W.B. Saunders, Philadelphia, 1989, pp. 860-878.

518. Peter Pearce, Susan Pearce, Polyhedra Primer, Van Nostrand Reinhold Company, New Yrok, 1978.

519. Peter C. Gasson, Geometry of Spatial Forms, John Wiley & Sons, New York, 1983.

520. D'Arcy Wentworth Thompson, On Growth and Form, Second Edition, Cambridge University Press, Cambridge, UK, 1942. (First Edition, 1917)

521. Frederick H. Silver, Biological Materials: Structure, Mechanical Properties, and Modeling of Soft Tissues, New York University Press, New York, 1987.

522. Robert F. Curl, Richard E. Smalley, "Fullerenes," Scientific American 265(October 1991):54-63.

523. H.W. Kroto, J.E. Fischer, D.E. Cox, eds., The Fullerenes, Pergamon Press, New York, 1993.

524. H. Weyl, Symmetry, Princeton University Press, Princeton, NJ, 1952.

525. Uwe B. Sleytr, Margit Sara, Paul Messner, Dietmar Pum, "Two-Dimensional Protein Crystals (S-Layers): Fundamentals and Applications," J. Cellular Biochemistry 56(1994):171-176.

526. James A. Wilson, Principles of Animal Physiology, Macmillan Publishing Company, New York, 1972.

527. H.J. Morowitz, M.E. Tourtellotte, "The Smallest Living Cells," Scientific American 206(March 1962):117-126.

528. Yong Li, Toyoichi Tanaka, "Phase Transitions of Gels," Ann. Rev. Materials Sci. 22(1992):243-277. See also: E.S. Matsuo, T. Tanaka, "Patterns in shrinking gels," Nature 358(6 August 1992):482-485; and A.H. Mitwalli et al., "Closed-loop feedback control of magnetically-activated gels," J. Intell. Mater. Syst. Struct. 8(July 1997):596-604.

529. R.B. Clark, J.B. Cowey, "Factors controlling the change of shape of certain Nemertean and Turbellarian worms," J. Experimental Biology 35(1958):731-748.

530. Tadayoshi Okumura, G.A. Jamieson, "Platelet Glycocalicin. I. Orientation of Glycoproteins of the Human Platelet Surface," J. Biol. Chem. 251(10 October 1976):5944-5949.

531. Bruce Alberts, Dennis Bray, Julian Lewis, Martin Raff, Keith Roberts, James D. Watson, The Molecular Biology of the Cell, Second Edition, Garland Publishing, Inc., New York, 1989.

532. Hongtao Han, Lee E. Weiss, Michael L. Reed, "Micromechanical Velcro," J. Microelectromechanical Systems 1(March 1992):37-43.

533. W. Nachtigall, Biological Mechanisms of Attachment: The Comparative Morphology and Bioengineering of Organs for Linkage, Suction, and Adhesion, Springer-Verlag, New York, 1974.

534. K.S.J. Pister, M.W. Judy, S.R. Burgett, R.S. Fearing, "Microfabricated hinges," Sensors and Actuators A 33(1992):249-256.

535. Joyce Y. Wong, Tonya L. Kuhl, Jacob N. Israelachvili, Nasreen Mullah, Samuel Zalipsky, "Direct Measurement of a Tethered Ligand-Receptor Interaction Potential," Science 275(7 February 1997):820-822.

536. J.E. Field, "Chapter 9. Strength and Fracture Properties of Diamond," in J.E. Field, ed., The Properties of Diamond, Academic Press, New York, 1979, pp. 281-324.

537. National Materials Advisory Board; Status and Applications of Diamond and Diamond-Like Materials: An Emerging Technology, Report of the Committee on Superhard Materials, NMAB-445, National Academy Press, 1990.

538. Richard P. Feynman, Robert B. Leighton, Matthew Sands, The Feynman Lectures on Physics, Addison-Wesley Publishing Company, Reading, MA, 1963.

539. R. Buckminster Fuller, E.J. Applewhite, Synergetics: Explorations in the Geometry of Thinking, Macmillan Publishing Company, New York, 1975.

540. Harry Chesley, "Early Applications," in B.C. Crandall, ed., Nanotechnology: Molecular Speculations on Global Abundance, MIT Press, Cambridge MA, 1996, pp. 89-105.

541. Naomasa Nakajima, Kazuhiro Ogawa, Iwao Fujimasa, "Study on Microengines: Miniaturizing Stirling Engines for Actuators," Sensors and Actuators 20(1989):75-82.

543. Seth J. Putterman, "Sonoluminescence: Sound into Light," Scientific American 272(February 1995):46-51.

544. K.F. Hale, C. Clarke, R.F. Duggan, B.E. Jones, "Incremental Control of a Valve Actuator Employing Optopneumatic Conversion," Sensors and Actuators A21-A23(1990):207-210.

545. Paul L. Bergstrom, Jin Ji, Yu-Ning Liu, Massoud Kaviany, Kensall D. Wise, "Thermally Driven Phase-Change Microactuation," J. Microelectromechanical Systems 4(March1995):10-17.

546. V.P. Jaecklin, C. Linder, N.F. de Rooij, J.-M. Moret, R. Vuilleumier, "Optical Microshutters and Torsional Micromirrors for Light Modulator Arrays," Proceedings 6th IEEE Micro Electro Mechanical Systems, IEEE Robotics and Automation Society, 1993, pp. 124-127.

547. W. Riethmuller, W. Benecke, U. Schnakenberg, A. Heuberger, "Micromechanical silicon actuators based on thermal expansion effects," Dig. Int. Conf. Solid-State Sensors and Actuators, Tokyo, Japan, June 1987, pp. 834-837.

548. K. Ikuta, M. Tsukamoto, S. Hirose, "Mathematical model and experimental verification of shape memory alloy for designing microactuators," in Proc. IEEE Micro Electro Mechanical Systems Workshop, February 1991, pp. 103-108.

549. Richard I. Epstein, Melvin I. Buchwald, Bradley C. Edwards, Timothy R. Gosnell, Carl E. Mungan, "Observation of laser-induced fluorescent cooling of a solid," Nature 377(12 October 1995):500-503.

550. P.C.W. Chu, "High-Temperature Superconductors," Scientific American 273(September 1995):162-165.

551. P.H. Egli, ed., Thermoelectricity, John Wiley & Sons, New York, 1960.

552. B. Wagner, G. Fuhr, T. Muller, Th. Schnelle, W. Benecke, "Fluid-Filled Dielectric Induction Micromotor with Al-SiO_2 Rotor," Proceedings 6th IEEE Micro Electro Mechanical Systems, IEEE Robotics and Automation Society, 1993.

553. Bernard Jaffe, William R. Cook Jr., Hans Jaffe, Piezoelectric Ceramics, Academic Press, New York, 1971.

554. J.R. Vig, J.W. LeBus, R.L. Filler, "Chemically polished quartz," in Proc. 31st Annual Symposium on Frequency Control, 1977, pp. 131-143.

555. J.R. Hunt, R.C. Smythe, "Chemically milled VHF and UHF AT-cut resonators," in Proc. 39st Annual Symposium on Frequency Control, 1985, pp. 292-300.

556. Mehran Mehregany, Yu-Chong Tai, "Surface micromachined mechanisms and micromotors," J. Micromech. Microeng. 1(1991):73-85.

557. U. Beerschwinger, N.G. Milne, S.J. Yang, R.L. Reuben, A.J. Sangster, H. Ziad, "Coupled Electrostatic and Mechanical FEA of a Micromotor," J. Microelectromechanical Systems 3(December 1994):162-171.

558. Yogesh Gianchandani, Khalil Najafi, "Batch fabrication and assembly of micromotor-driven mechanisms with multi-level linkages," Proceedings 5th IEEE Micro Electro Mechanical Systems, IEEE Robotics and Automation Society, 1992, pp. 141-146.

559. Takashi Yasuda, Isao Shimoyama, Hirofumi Miura, "Microrobot locomotion in a mechanical vibration field," Advanced Robotics 9(1995):165-176.

560. E.P. Muntz, G.R. Shiflett, D.A. Erwin, J.A. Kunc, "Transient Energy-Release Pressure-Driven Microdevices," J. Microelectromechanical Systems 1(September 1992):155-163.

561. Alexander Hellemans, "Trapped Buckyball Turns Up the Amp," Science 275 (21 February 1997):1069.

562. H.M. Hubbard, "Photovoltaics Today and Tomorrow," Science 244(1989):297-304.

563. "Microsensors Move Into Biomedical Applications", Electronic Design (28 May 1996):75.

564. Toshio Fukuda, Hidemi Hosokai, Hiroaki Ohyama, Hideki Hashimoto, Fumihito Arai, "Giant Magnetostrictive Alloy (GMA): Applications to Micro Mobile Robot as a Micro Actuator without Power Supply Cables," Proceedings 4th IEEE Micro Electro Mechanical Systems, IEEE Robotics and Automation Society, 1991, pp. 210-215.

565. Peter G.O. Freund, Christopher T. Hill, "A possible practical application of heavy quark physics," Nature 276(16 November 1978):250.

566. Bruce J. Gluckman, Theoden I. Netoff, Emily J. Neel, William L. Ditto, Mark L. Spano, Steven J. Schiff, "Stochastic Resonance in a Neuronal Network from Mammalian Brain," Phys. Rev. Lett. 77(4 November 1996):4098-4101. See also: B.J. Gluckman et al., "Stochastic resonance in mammalian neuronal networks," Chaos 8(September 1998):588-598.

567. Dwight E. Gray, ed., American Institute of Physics Handbook, Third Edition, McGraw-Hill Book Company, New York, 1972.

568. H.K. Mao, P.M. Bell, "Observations of Hydrogen at Room Temperature (25°C) and High Pressure (to 500 Kilobars)," Science 203(9 March 1979):1004-1006.

570. Richard R.H. Coombs, Dennis W. Robinson, eds., Nanotechnology in Medicine and the Biosciences, Gordon & Breach Publishers, Netherlands, 1996.

572. J.A.T. Dow, P. Clark, P. Connolly, A.S.G. Curtis, "Novel methods for the guidance and monitoring of single cells and simple networks in culture," J. Cell. Science Suppl. 8(1987):55-79.

573. D.J. Edell, "A peripheral information transducer for amputees: long term multichannel recordings from rabbit peripheral nerves," IEEE Trans. Biomed. Eng. 33(1986):204-214.

574. P. Connolly, P. Clark, A.S.G. Curtis, J.A.T. Dow, C.D.W. Wilkinson, "An extracellular microelectrode array for monitoring electrogenic cells in culture," Biosens. Bioelectron. 5(1989):223-234.

575. R. Wilson, L. Breckenridge, S.E. Blackshaw, P. Connolly, J.A.T. Dow, A.S.G. Curtis, "Simultaneous multi site recordings and stimulation of single isolated leech neurons using planar extracellular electrode arrays," J. Neurosci. Methods 53(1994):101-110.

576. D.W. Pohl, W. Denk, M. Lanz, "Optical stethoscopy: image recording with resolution λ/20," Appl. Phys. Lett. 44(1984):651-654.

577. W. Tan, Z-Y. Shi, S. Smith, D. Birnbaum, R. Kopelman, "Submicrometer Intracellular Chemical Optical Fiber Sensors," Science 258(1992):778-781.

578. James A. Spudich, "How molecular motors work," Nature 372(8 December 1994):515-518.

579. M. Meister, S.R. Caplan, H.C. Berg, "Dynamics of a tightly coupled mechanism for flagellar rotation. Bacterial motility, chemiosmotic coupling, protonmotive force," Biophys. J. 55(1989):905-914.

580. L.L McCarter, "MotY, a component of the sodium-type flagellar motor," J. Bacteriol. 176(1994):4219-4225; and "MotX, the channel component of the sodium-type flagellar motor," J. Bacteriol. 176(1994):5988-5998.

581. Christopher J. Jones, Shin-Ichi Aizawa, "The Bacterial Flagellum and Flagellar Motor: Structure, Assembly and Function," Adv. Microbial Physiol. 32(1991):109-172.

582. Paul Loubeyre, Rene LeToullec, "Stability of O_2/H_2 mixtures at high pressure," Nature 378(2 November 1995):44-46.

583. Charles W. Shilling, Margaret F. Werts, Nancy R. Shandelmeier, The Underwater Handbook: A Guide to Physiology and Performance for the Engineer, Plenum Press, NY, 1976.

584. J.U. Steinle, E.U. Franck, "High Pressure Combustion—Ignition Temperatures to 1000 bar," Berichte der Bunsen. fur Phys. 99(January 1995):66-73.

585. William S. Spector, ed., Handbook of Biological Data, W.B. Saunders Company, Philadelphia PA, 1956.

587. Yoichi Tatara, "Mechanochemical Actuators," Advanced Robotics 2(1987):69-85.

588. J.B. Bates, G.R. Gruzalski, C.F. Luck, "Rechargeable solid state lithium microbatteries," Proceedings 6th IEEE Micro Electro Mechanical Systems, IEEE Robotics and Automation Society, 1993, pp. 82-86.

589. Wenjie Li, Jorma A. Virtanen, Reginald M. Penner, "A Nanometer-Scale Galvanic Cell," J. Phys. Chem. 96(August 1992):6529-6532.

590. O.Z. Roy, "Biological Energy Sources: A Review," Bio-Medical Engineering 6(June 1971):250-256.

592. W. Roth, "Bioenergy electrical power sources," Digest of the 7th International Conference on Medical and Biological Engineering, August 1967, p. 518.

593. G. Lewin, G.H. Myers, V. Parsonnet, K.V. Raman, "An improved biological power source for cardiac pacemakers," Trans. Amer. Soc. Artif. Intern. Organs 14(1968):215-219.

594. B.Y.C. Wan, A.C.C. Tseung, "Some studies related to electricity generation from biological fuel cells and galvanic cells, in vitro and in vivo," Medical and Biological Engineering 12(January 1974):14-28.

595. L.R. Pinneo, M.L. Kesselman, "Tapping the Electric Power of the Nervous System for Biological Telemetering," ASTIA Document AD-209-607, May 1959.

596. L.W. Reynolds, "Utilization of Bioelectricity as Power Supply for Implanted Electronic Devices," Aerospace Medicine 35(February 1964):115-117.

597. M.V. Sussmann, A. Katchalsky, "Mechanochemical Turbine: A New Power Cycle," Science 167(2 January 1970):45-47.

598. A.N. Oksendal, "Biodistribution and toxicity of MR imaging contrast media," J. Magn. Reson. Imaging 3(1993):157-165.

599. P. Galle, J.P. Berry, C. Galle, "Role of alveolar macrophages in precipitation of mineral elements inhaled as soluble aerosols," Environ. Health Perspect. 97(1992):145-147.

600. Y. Berthezene, A. Muhler, P. Lang, D.M. Shames, O. Clement, W. Rosenau, R. Kuwatsuru, R.C. Brasch, "Safety aspects and pharmacokinetics of inhaled aerosolized gadolinium," J. Magn. Reson. Imaging 3(1993):125-130.

601. Seishiro Hirano, Kazuo T. Suzuki, "Exposure, Metabolism, and Toxicity of Rare Earths and Related Compounds," Environ. Health Perspect. 104 (March 1996):85-95.

602. Anthony R. Martin, Alan Bond, "Project Daedalus: The Propulsion System. Part I. Theoretical considerations and calculations," in Anthony R. Martin, ed. Project Daedalus, J. Brit. Interplanet. Soc. Suppl., 1978, pp. S44-S62.

603. Wen H. Ko, Jaroslav Hynecek, "Implant Evaluation of a Nuclear Power Source—Betacel Battery," IEEE Trans. Biomed. Eng. 21(May 1974):238-241.

604. L.W. Alvarez et al., "Catalysis of Nuclear Reactions by Mu Mesons," Phys. Rev. 105(1957):1127-1128.

605. George Zweig, "Quark Catalysis of Exothermal Nuclear Reactions," Science 201(15 September 1978):973-979.

606. F.C. Frank, "Hypothetical Alternative Energy Sources for the Second Meson Events," Nature 160(1947):525.

607. S.E. Jones et al., "Observation of cold nuclear fusion in condensed matter," Nature 338(27 April 1989):737-740.

608. J. Rafelski, S.E. Jones, "Cold Nuclear Fusion," Scientific American 257(July 1987):84-89.

609. C. DeW. Van Siclen, S.E. Jones, "Piezonuclear fusion in isotopic hydrogen molecules," J. Phys. G 12(March 1986):213-221.

610. S.E. Jones et al., "Experimental Investigation of Muon-Catalyzed d-t Fusion," Phys. Rev. Lett. 51(7 November 1983):1757-1760.

611. Steven Earl Jones, "Muon-catalysed fusion revisited," Nature 321(8 May 1986):127-133.

612. W.K. Hensley, W.A. Bassett, J.R. Huizenga, "Pressure Dependence of the Radioactive Decay Constant of Beryllium-7," Science 181(21 September 1973):1164-1165.

613. Gustave K. Kohn, "Letters," Science 274(25 October 1996):481. See also: T.N. Claytor, D.D. Jackson, D.G. Tuggle, "Tritium Production from a Low Voltage Deuterium Discharge on Palladium and Other Metals," LAUR#95-2687, 1995, at: http://nde.lanl.gov/cf/tritweb.htm.

614. V.A. Klyuev, A.G. Lipson, Yu.P. Toporov, B.V. Deryagin, V.J. Lushchikov, A.V. Streikov, E.P. Shabalin, "High-energy processes accompanying the fracture of solids," Sov. Tech. Phys. Lett. 12(1986):551-552.
615. M. Fleischmann, S. Pons, M. Hawkins, "Electrochemically Induced Nuclear Fusion of Deuterium," J. Electroanalytical Chem. 261(1989):301-308.
616. M. Fleischmann, S. Pons, "Calorimetry of the Pd-D_2O system: From simplicity via complications to simplicity," Phys. Lett. A 176(1993):118-129.
617. Edmund Storms, "Warming up to Cold Fusion," Technology Review (MIT) (May/June 1994):19-29.
618. J.T. Dickinson, L.C. Jensen, S.C. Langford, R.R. Ryan, E. Garcia, "Fracto-emission from deuterated titanium: Supporting evidence for a fracto-fusion mechanism," J. Materials Res. 5(January 1990):109-122.
619. B.V. Derjaguin, A.G. Lipson, V.A. Kluev, D.M. Sakov, Yu.P. Toporov, "Titanium fracture yields neutrons?" Nature 341(1989):492.
620. P.I. Golubnichii, V.A. Kurakin, A.D. Filonenko, V.A. Tsarev, A.A. Tsarik, "A possible mechanism for cold nuclear fusion," Sov. Phys. Dokl. 34(July 1989):628-629.
621. Tatsuoki Tekeda, Tomonori Takizuka, "Fractofusion Mechanism," J. Phys. Soc. Japan 58(September 1989):3073-3076.
622. W. Lochte-Holtgreven, Z. Naturf. 42A(1987):538 et seq.
624. Melvin H. Miles, Benjamin F. Bush, David E. Stilwell, "Calorimetric Principles and Problems in Measurements of Excess Power during Pd-D_2O Electrolysis," J. Phys. Chem. 98(1994):1948-1952.
625. Kenneth S. Suslick, "The Chemical Effects of Ultrasound," Scientific American 260(February 1989):80-86.
626. "Statement of mammalian in vivo ultrasonic biological effects," Reflections 4(1978):311. (See also W. Nyborg, HEW Publ. No. FDA 788062, 1978.)
627. American Institute of Ultrasound in Medicine, "Bioeffects considerations for the safety of diagnostic ultrasound," J. Ultrasound Med. 7(September 1988):suppl. See also: "American Institute of Ultrasound in Medicine Guidelines," J. Ultrasound Med. 11(April 1992):171-172.
628. W.N. McDicken, Diagnostic Ultrasonics: Principles and Use of Instruments, Third Edition, Churchill Livingstone, New York, 1991.
629. Stewart C. Bushong, Benjamin R. Archer, Diagnostic Ultrasound: Physics, Biology, and Instrumentation, Mosby Year Book, St. Louis, MO, 1991.
630. William J. Heetderks, "RF Powering of Millimeter- and Submillimeter-Sized Neural Prosthetic Implants," IEEE Trans. Biomed. Eng. 35(May 1988):323-327.
631. W. Greatbatch, T.S. Bustard, "A $^{238}PuO_2$ nuclear power source for implantable cardiac pacemakers," IEEE Trans. Biomed. Eng. 20(1973):336-345.
633. W.H. Ko, "Power Sources for Implant Telemetry and Stimulation Systems, in Charles J. Amlaner Jr., David W. MacDonald, eds., A Handbook of Biotelemetry and Radio Tracking, Pergamon Press, New York, 1979, pp. 225-245.
634. R. Stuart Mackay, Bio-Medical Telemetry, Second Edition, John Wiley & Sons, Inc., New York, 1970.
635. Cesar A. Caceres, ed., Biomedical Telemetry, Academic Press, New York, 1965.
636. Philip R. Troyk, Martin A.K. Schwan, "Closed-Loop Class E Transcutaneous Power and Data Link for MicroImplants," IEEE Trans. Biomed. Eng. 39(June 1992):589-599.
637. Charles J. Amlaner Jr., David W. MacDonald, eds., A Handbook of Biotelemetry and Radio Tracking, Pergamon Press, New York, 1979.
638. R. Stuart Mackay, Bertil Jacobson, "Endoradiosonde," Nature 179(15 June 1957):1239-1240. See also: "A Radio Pill," Nature 179(4 May 1957):898.
639. J. Lange, B.P. Brockway, "Telemetric monitoring of laboratory animals: An advanced technique that has come of age," Lab. Animal 20(1991):28-33.
640. Hideo Mizoguchi, Mitsuhiro Ando, Tomokimi Mizuno, Tarou Takagi, Naomasa Nakajima, "Design and Fabrication of Light Driven Micropump," Proceedings 5th IEEE Micro Electro Mechanical Systems, IEEE Robotics and Automation Society, 1992, pp. 31-36.
641. Marc Bockrath, David H. Cobden, Paul L. McEuen, Nasreen G. Chopra, A. Zettl, Andreas Thess, R.E. Smalley, "Single-Electron Transport in Ropes of Carbon Nanotubes," Science 275(28 March 1997):1922-1925.
642. L.D. Landau, E.M. Lifshitz, Theory of Elasticity, Pergamon Press, New York, 1986.
643. A.G. Rinzler, J.H. Hafner, P. Nikolaev, L. Lou, S.G. Kim, D. Tomanek, P. Nordlander, D.T. Colbert, R.E. Smalley, "Unraveling Nanotubes: Field Emission from an Atomic Wire," Science 269(15 September 1995):1550-1553.
644. Arthur F. Hebard, "Superconductivity in Doped Fullerenes," Physics Today 45(November 1992):26-32.
645. Malcolm Gower, "Chapter 12. Excimer Lasers for Surgery and Biomedical Fabrication," in Richard R.H. Coombs, Dennis W. Robinson, eds., Nanotechnology in Medicine and the Biosciences, Gordon & Breach Publishers, Netherlands, 1996, pp. 169-193.
646. Gavin Pearson, "Precision Milling of Teeth for Dental Caries," in Richard R.H. Coombs, Dennis W. Robinson, eds., Nanotechnology in Medicine and the Biosciences, Gordon & Breach Publishers, Netherlands, 1996, pp. 195-208.
647. M. Minnaert, "On musical air-bubbles and the sounds of running water," Phil. Mag. 16(1933):235-248.
649. George Walter Stewart, Robert Bruce Linday, Acoustics: A Text on Theory and Applications, D. Van Nostrand Company, New York, 1930.
650. A.B. Wood, A Textbook of Sound, G. Bell and Sons Ltd., London, 1960.
651. Henrik W. Anthonsen, Antonio Baptista, Finn Drablos, Paulo Martel, Steffen B. Petersen, "The blind watchmaker and rational protein engineering," J. Biotechnology 36(1994):185-220.
652. C.M. Hargreaves, "Anomalous radiative transfer between closely-spaced bodies," Phys. Lett. 30A(29 December 1969):491-492.
653. D. Polder, M. Van Hove, "Theory of Radiative Heat Transfer between Closely Spaced Bodies," Phys. Rev. B 4(15 November 1971):3303-3314.
654. R.F. Wuerker, H. Shelton, R.V. Langmuir, "Electrodynamic Containment of Charged Particles," J. Appl. Phys. 30(March 1959):342-349.
655. S. Arnold, L.M. Folan, "Spherical void electrodynamic levitator," Rev. Sci. Instrum. 58(September 1987):1732-1735.
656. Suresh Kumar, Dan Cho, William N. Carr, "A Proposal for Electrically Levitating Micromotors," Sensors and Actuators 24A(1990):141-149.
657. Suresh Kumar, Dan Cho, William N. Carr, "Experimental Study of Electric Suspension for Microbearings," J. Microelectromech. Syst. 1(March 1992):23-30.
658. D. Hu, B. Makin, "Design and operation of a multi-electrode quadrupole levitation system—theoretical and experimental aspects," in B.C. O'Neill, ed., Electrostatics 1991, Institute of Physics Conference Series Number 118, Institute Of Physics, New York, 1991, pp. 177-184.
659. D.R.G. Rodley, S.J. Belmont, B. Makin, K. Dastoori, "Observation and Computer Modeling of Particle Trajectories in a Seven-Electrode Levitation System," in Samia Cunningham, ed., Electrostatics 1995, Institute of Physics Conference Series Number 143, Institute Of Physics, New York, 1995, pp. 315-318.
660. T.B. Jones, "Electrical forces and torques on bioparticles," in Samia Cunningham, ed., Electrostatics 1995, Institute of Physics Conference Series Number 143, Institute of Physics, New York, 1995, pp. 135-144.
661. J.S. Zmuidzinas, "Electronically Excited Solid Helium," in D.D. Papailiou, ed., Frontiers in Propulsion Research: Lasers, Matter-Antimatter, Excited Helium, Energy Exchange Thermonuclear Fusion, NASA/JPL Technical Memorandum 33-722 (N75-22373), March 1975, pp. 120-123.
662. W.E. Sweeney Jr., J.B. Marion, "Gamma-Ray Transitions Involving Isobaric-Spin Mixed States in Be^8," Physical Review 182(20 June 1969):1007-1021.
663. P. Froelich, "Muon catalysed fusion," Advances in Physics 41(1992):405-508.
664. Shalom Eliezer, Zohar Henis, "Muon-Catalyzed Fusion—An Energy Production Perspective," Fusion Technology 26(August 1994):46-73.
665. A.J. McCevoy, C.T.D. O'Sullivan, "Cold fusion: what's going on?" Nature 338(27 April 1989):711-712.
666. "Fusion in 1926: plus ca change," Nature 338(27 April 1989):706.
667. Yuk Fukai, Nobuyuki Okuma, "Formation of Superabundant Vacancies in Pd Hydride under High Hydrogen Pressures," Phys. Rev. Lett. 12(19 September 1994):1640-1643.
668. C.T. White, D.W. Brenner, R.C. Mowrey, J.W. Mintmire, P.P. Schmidt, B.I. Dunlap, "D-D (H-H) Interactions within Interstices of Pd," Jap. J. Appl. Phys. 30(January 1991):182-189. See also: C.T. White, B.I. Dunlap, D.W. Brenner, R.C. Mowrey, J.W. Mintmire, "Limits of Chemical Effects on Cold Fusion," J. Fusion Energy 9(1990):363-366; B.I. Dunlap, D.W. Brenner, R.C. Mowrey, J.W. Mintmire, C.T. White, "Linear combination of Gaussian-type orbitals—local-density-functional cluster studies of D-D interactions in titanium and palladium," Phys. Rev. B. 41(13 May 1990):9683-9687; J.W. Mintmire, B.I. Dunlap, D.W. Brenner, R.C. Mowrey, H.D. Ladouceur, P.P. Schmidt, C.T. White, W.E. O'Grady, "Chemical Forces Associated with Deuterium Confinement in Palladium," Phys. Lett. A. 138(12 June 1989):51-54.
676. M.C.H. McKubre et al., "Development of Advanced Concepts for Nuclear Processes in Deuterated Metals," EPRI TR-104195, Research Project 3170-01, Final Report, August 1994.
677. M.C.H. McKubre et al., "Isothermal flow calorimetric investigations of the D/Pd and H/Pd systems," J. Electroanalytical Chem. 386(1994):55-66.
678. Pontus Eriksson, Jan Y. Andersson, Goran Stemme, "Thermal Characterization of Surface Micromachined Silicon Nitride Membranes for Thermal Infrared Detectors," J. Microelectromech. Syst. 6(March 1997):55-61.
679. C.C. Chancey, S.A. George, P.J. Marshall, "Calculations of Quantum Tunnelling Between Closed and Open States of Sodium Channels," J. Biol. Phys. 18(1992):307-321.
680. H. Frohlich, "Evidence for Bose condensation-like excitation of coherent modes in biological systems," Phys. Lett. 51A(27 January 1975):21-22. See also: "Long-range coherence and energy storage in biological systems," Intl. J. Quantum Chem. 2(1968):641-649; "Long range coherence and the actions of enzymes," Nature 228(1970):1093; "The extraordinary dielectric properties of biological materials and the action of enzymes," Proc. Natl. Acad. Sci. 72(1975):4211-4215; and Adv. Electron. Electron. Phys. 53(1980):85.
681. H. Frohlich, F. Kremer, eds., Coherent Excitations in Biological Systems, Springer-Verlag, Berlin, 1983.
682. W. Grundler, F. Keilmann, H. Frohlich, "Resonant growth rate response of yeast cells irradiated by weak microwaves," Phys. Lett. 62A(19 September 1977):463-466. See also: W. Grundler, F. Keilmann, "Sharp resonances in yeast growth prove nonthermal sensitivity to microwaves," Phys. Rev. Lett. 51(1983):1214-1216.
683. Herbert A. Pohl, J. Kent Pollock, "Biological Dielectrophoresis. The Behavior of Biologically Significant Materials in Nonuniform Electric Fields." In F. Gutmann, H. Keyzer, eds., Modern Bio-Electrochemistry, Plenum Press, New York, 1986, pp.329-376.
684. E. Del Giudice, S. Doglia, M. Milani, "Self-focusing of Frohlich waves and cytoskeleton dynamics," Phys. Lett. 90A(21 June 1982):104-106.
685. S. Rowlands, "Some Physics Aspects for 21st Century Biologists," J. Biol. Phys. 11(1983):117-122.

686. Felix Gutmann, "A proposed source of electromagnetic radiation from biological systems," Appl. Phys. Commun. 11(1992):205-222.
687. J. Pokorny, K. Vacek, J. Fiala, "Frohlich Electromagnetic Field Generated by Living Cells: Computer Results," J. Biol. Phys. 12(1984):79-84.
688. J.A. Tuszynski, E. Kimberly Strong, "Application of the Frohlich Theory to the Modelling of Rouleau Formation in Human Erythrocytes," J. Biol. Phys. 17(1989):19-40.
689. Bjorn E.W. Nordenstrom, Biologically Closed Electric Circuits: Clinical, Experimental and Theoretical Evidence for an Additional Circulatory System, Nordic Medical Publications, Stockholm, Sweden, 1983.
690. Bjorn E.W. Nordenstrom, "An Additional Circulatory System: Vascular-Interstitial Closed Electric Circuits (VICC)," J. Biol. Phys. 15(1987):43-55.
691. F. Albert Cotton, Geoffrey Wilkinson, Advanced Inorganic Chemistry: A Comprehensive Text, Second Edition, John Wiley & Sons, New York, 1966.
692. A.E. Nixon, M.S. Warren, Steven J. Benkovic, "Assembly of an active enzyme by the linkage of two protein molecules," Proc. Nat. Acad. Sci. 94(18 February 1997):1069-1073.
693. X. Feng, G.E. Fryxell, L.-Q. Wang, A.Y. Kim, J. Liu, K.M. Kemner, "Functionalized Monolayers of Ordered Mesoporous Supports," Science 276(9 May 1997):923-926.
695. Victoria A. Russell, Cara C. Evans, Wenjie Li, Michael D. Ward, "Nanoporous Molecular Sandwiches: Pillared Two-Dimensional Hydrogen-Bonded Networks with Adjustable Porosity," Science 276(25 April 1997):575-579. See also: Steven C. Zimmerman, "Putting Molecules Behind Bars," Science 276(25 April 1997):543-544.
696. R. Dean Astumian, "Thermodynamics and Kinetics of a Brownian Motor," Science 276(9 May 1997):917-922.
697. Constance Holden, "Berkeley Cooks Up Powerful Magnet," Science 276(16 May 1997):1035-1037.
698. Geoffrey B. West, James H. Brown, Brian J. Enquist, "A General Model for the Origin of Allometric Scaling Laws in Biology," Science 276(4 April 1997):122-126.
699. C.E. Shannon, W. Weaver, The Mathematical Theory of Communication, University of Illinois Press, Urbana IL, 1949.
700. Rolf Landauer, "Minimal Energy Requirements in Communication," Science 272 (28 June 1996):1914-1918.
701. Lucien Gerardin, Bionics, McGraw-Hill, New York, 1968.
702. M. Ruderfer, "Are Solar Neutrinos Detected by Living Things?" Phys. Lett. 54A (6 October 1975):363-364.
703. William H. Bossert, Edward O. Wilson, "The Analysis of Olfactory Communication Among Animals," J. Theoret. Biol. 5(1963):443-469.
704. Thomas F. Zuck, Jean G. Riess, "Current Status of Injectable Oxygen Carriers," Crit. Rev. Clin. Lab. Sci. 31(1994):295-324.
705. J.A. Jones, "Red blood cell substitutes: current status," Brit. J. Anaesthes. 74(1995):697-703.
706. Y. Ohnishi, M. Kitazawa, "Application of perfluorocarbons in human beings," Acta Pathologica Japonica 30(1980):489-504.
707. S.F. Flaim, "Pharmacokinetics and side effects of perfluorocarbon-based blood substitutes," Blood Subst. Art. Cells Immob. Biotech. 22(1994):1043-1054.
708. G.M. Vercellotti, D.E. Hammerschmidt, P.R. Craddock, H.S. Jacob, "Activation of plasma complement by perfluorocarbon artificial blood: probably mechanism of adverse pulmonary reactions in treated patients and rationale for corticosteroid prophylaxis," Blood 59(1982):1299-1304.
709. K. Yokoyama, R. Naito, Y. Tsuda, et al., "Selection of 53 PFC substances for better stability of emulsion and improved artificial blood substitutes," Prog. Clin. Biol. Res. 122(1983):189-196.
710. J. Lutz, "Effects of perfluorochemicals on host defense, especially on the reticuloendothelial system," Int. Anesthes. Clin. 23(1985):63-93.
711. R. Naito, K. Yokoyama, Perfluorochemical Blood Substitutes. Technical Information Series n°5 and n°7, Gress Cross Corp., Osaka, Japan, 1978, 1981; see also Fluosol 20% Intravascular Perfluorochemical Emulsion, Product Monograph, Alpha Therapeutic Corporation, 1990.
712. J.G. Riess, C. Cornelus, R. Follana, M.P. Krafft, A.M. Mahe, M. Postel, L. Zarif, "Novel fluorocarbon-based injectable oxygen-carrying formulations with long-term room-temperature storage stability." In Peter Vaupel, Rolf Zander, Duane F. Bruley, eds., Oxygen Transport to Tissue XV, Plenum Press, New York, 1994, pp. 227-234.
713. R.C. Merkle, "Reversible electronic logic using switches," Nanotechnology 4(1993):21-40.
714. Alexander Hellemans, "Optoelectronics: Storing Light by Surfing on Silicon," Science 276(30 May 1997):1339.
715. Yoshio Idota, Tadahiko Kubota, Akihiro Matsufuji, Yukio Maekawa, Tsutomu, "Tin-Based Amorphous Oxide: A High-Capacity Lithium-Ion-Storage Material," Science 276(30 May 1997):1395-1397.
716. William C. Moss, Douglas B. Clarke, David A. Young, "Calculated Pulse Widths and Spectra of a Single Sonoluminescing Bubble," Science 276(30 May 1997):1398-1401; 1348-1349.
718. Christopher S. Chen, Milan Mrksich, Sui Huang, George M. Whitesides, Donald E. Ingber, "Geometric Control of Cell Life and Death," Science 276(30 May 1997):1425-1428; and see pp. 1345-1346.
721. D. Vasilescu, H. Kranck, "Noise in Biomolecular Systems." In Felix Gutmann, Hendrik Keyzer, eds., Modern Bioelectrochemistry, Plenum Press, NY, 1986, pp. 397-430.
722. G.H. Myers, V. Parsonnet, I.R. Zucker, H.A. Lotman, M.M. Asa, "Biologically energized cardiac pacemaker," IEEE Trans. Biomed. Electronics 10(1963):83.
723. J.H. Kennedy, C.C. Enger, A.G. Michel, "Implantable pacemaker powered by ventricular contractions," JAMA 195(Suppl., 21 February 1966):48; "Tiny pacemaker is powered by heart itself," World Medicine 1(1966):11.
724. Thomas F. Hursen, Steve A. Kolenik, "Nuclear Energy Sources," Annals N.Y. Acad. Sci. 162(October 1969):661-673 and panel discussion pp. 674-678.
725. William H. Bossert, "Temporal Patterning in Olfactory Communication," J. Theoret. Biol. 18(1968):157-170.
727. Paul Lorrain, Dale R. Corson, Electromagnetic Fields and Waves, Second Edition, W.H. Freeman and Company, San Francisco, CA, 1970.
728. Ronald Pethig, "A.C. Electrokinetic Manipulation of Bioparticles," in Richard R.H. Coombs, Dennis W. Robinson, eds., Nanotechnology in Medicine and the Biosciences, Gordon & Breach Publishers, Netherlands, 1996, Chapter 11, pp. 153-168.
729. Steven L. Jacques, "Time-Resolved Reflectance Spectroscopy in Turbid Tissues," IEEE Trans. Biomed. Eng. 36(December 1989):1155-1161.
730. Matthew Hussey, Basic Physics and Technology of Medical Diagnostic Ultrasound, Elsevier, New York, 1985.
731. William Tomkins, Indian Sign Language, Dover Publications, New York, 1969.
732. Zilan Shen, Paul E. Burrows, Vladimir Bulovic, Stephen R. Forrest, Mark E. Thompson, "Three Color, Tunable, Organic Light-Emitting Devices," Science 276(27 June 1997):2009-2011.
733. Robert F. Service, "Tripping the Light at Fantastic Speeds," Science 276(27 June 1997):1970.
735. Rainer H. Kohler, Jun Cao, Warren R. Zipfel, Watt W. Webb, Maureen R. Hanson, "Exchange of Protein Molecules Through Connections Between Higher Plant Plastids," Science 276(27 June 1997):2039-2042.
736. Guillermo J. Tearney, Mark E. Brezinski, Brett E. Bouma, Stephen A. Boppart, Costas Pitris, James F. Southern, James G. Fujimoto, "In Vivo Endoscopic Optical Biopsy with Optical Coherence Tomography," Science 276(27 June 1997):2037-2039.
737. Gary Taubes, "Firefly Gene Lights Up Lab Animals From Inside Out," Science 276(27 June 1997):1993.
738. David A. Benaron, Wai-Fung Cheong, David K. Stevenson, "Tissue Optics," Science 276(27 June 1997):2002-2003.
739. Norris McWhirter, Ross McWhirter, Guiness Book of World Records, 12th Bantam Edition, Sterling Publishing Co., NY, 1974.
740. Yoshiaki Arata, Yue-Chang Zhang, "Solid-State Plasma Fusion," J. Japan. High-Temp. Society 23(January 1997), entire issue. See also: "Deuterium Nuclear Reaction Process within Solid," Proc. Japan Acad. 72B(November 1996):179-184.
742. D.H. Hubel, T.N. Wiesel, "Receptive fields and functional architecture of monkey striate cortex," J. Physiol. (London) 195(1968):215-243.
743. G.R. Lee, T.C. Bithell, J. Foerster, J.W. Athens, J.N. Lukens, eds., Wintrobe's Clinical Hematology, Ninth Edition, Lea & Febiger, Philadelphia PA, 1993.
744. Knut Schmidt-Nielsen, Scaling: Why is Animal Size So Important? Cambridge University Press, Cambridge, 1984.
745. Martin Davies, "On Body Size and Tissue Respiration," J. Cellular Comp. Physiol. 57(1961):135-147.
746. Michel A. Hofman, "Energy Metabolism, Brain Size and Longevity in Mammals," Quart. Rev. Biology 58(December 1983):495-512.
747. R. Duara et al., "Human Brain Glucose Utilization and Cognitive Function in Relation to Age," Annals of Neurology 16(1984):702-713.
749. Philip B. Hawk, Bernard L. Oser, William H. Summerson, Practical Physiological Chemistry, 12th Edition, The Blakiston Company, New York NY, 1951.
750. Nellie D. Millard, Barry G. King, Maryjane Showers, Human Anatomy and Physiology, 4th Edition, W.B. Saunders Company, Philadelphia PA, 1956.
751. Benjamin Harrow, Abraham Mazur, Textbook of Biochemistry, 7th Edition, W.B. Saunders Company, Philadelphia PA, 1958.
752. Mary Dan Eades, The Doctor's Complete Guide to Vitamins and Minerals, Dell Publishing, New York, 1994.
753. I. Newton Kugelmass, Biochemistry of Blood in Health and Disease, Charles C. Thomas, Springfield IL, 1959, pp. 502-506.
754. Herbert A. Sober, ed., Handbook of Biochemistry: Selected Data for Molecular Biology, 2nd Edition, CRC Press, Cleveland OH, 1970.
755. Anthony W. Norman, Gerald Litwack, "Appendix A. Human Blood Concentrations of Major Hormones," in Hormones, Academic Press, New York, 1987, pp. 758-760.
756. Ronald J. Elin, "Part XXVI: Laboratory Reference Range Values of Clinical Importance." In James Wyngaarden, Lloyd H. Smith, Jr., eds., Cecil Textbook of Medicine, 18th Edition, W.B. Saunders Company, Harcourt Brace Jovanovich, Philadelphia PA, 1988, pp. 2394-2404.
757. "Normal Blood Values", in Robert I. Handin, Samuel E. Lux, Thomas P. Stossel, eds., Blood: Principles and Practice of Hematology, J.B. Lippincott Company, Philadelphia PA, 1995, pp. 2133-2165.
758. Arthur C. Giese, Cell Physiology, 5th Edition, W.B. Saunders Company, Philadelphia PA, 1979.
759. Geoffrey Zubay, Biochemistry, 3rd Edition, William C. Brown Publishers, Dubuque IA, 1993.
760. Philip L. Altman, Dorothy S. Dittmer, eds., Biology Data Book, Federation of American Societies for Experimental Biology, Washington DC, 1964.

761. H.S. Harned, B.B. Owen, The Physical Chemistry of Electrolytic Solutions, 3rd Edition, Reinhold Publishing, New York NY, 1958.
762. C. Tanford, Physical Chemistry of Macromolecules, John Wiley & Sons, New York NY, 1961.
763. Robert C. Weast, Handbook of Chemistry and Physics, 49th Edition, CRC, Cleveland OH, 1968.
764. Edgardo Browne, Richard B. Firestone, Table of Radioactive Isotopes, John Wiley & Sons, New York NY, 1986.
765. Jean-Marie Lehn, Supramolecular Chemistry: Concepts and Perspectives, VCH, New York NY, 1995.
766. Stuart A. Kauffman, The Origins of Order: Self-Organization and Selection in Evolution, Oxford University Press, New York, 1993.
767. Robin E. Callard, Andy J.H. Gearing, The Cytokine FactsBook, Academic Press, New York, 1994.
768. T.K. Hughes Jr., R. Chin, "Interactions of Neuropeptides and Cytokines," in B. Scharrer, E.M. Smith, G.B. Stefano, eds., Neuropeptides and Immunoregulation, Springer-Verlag, Berlin, 1994, pp. 101-119.
769. A.J. Turner, ed., Neuropeptides and Their Peptidases, VCH, New York NY, 1987.
770. Andrzej W. Lipkowski, Daniel B. Carr, "Neuropeptides: Peptide and Nonpeptide Analogs," in Bernd Gutte, ed., Peptides: Synthesis, Structures, and Applications, Academic Press, New York, 1995, pp. 287-320.
771. L.C. Katz, C.J. Shatz, "Synaptic Activity and the Construction of Cortical Circuits," Science 274(15 November 1996):1133-1138.
772. I.J. Russell, P.M. Sellick, "Intracellular studies of hair cells in the mammalian cochlea," J. Physiol. (London) 284(1978):261-290.
773. R.S. Woodworth, H. Schlosberg, Experimental Psychology, Revised Edition, Holt, Rinehart & Winston, New York, 1954.
775. Gerard J. Milburn, Schrodinger's Machines: The Quantum Technology Reshaping Everyday Life, W.H. Freeman and Company, NY, 1997.
776. Nigel Williams, "Biologists Cut Reductionist Approach Down to Size," Science 277(25 July 1997):476-477.
777. Dennis A. Carson, "Chapter 94. Composition and biochemistry of lymphocytes and plasma cells," in Ernest Beutler, Marshall A. Lichtman, Barry S. Coller, Thomas J. Kipps, eds., William's Hematology, Fifth Edition, McGraw-Hill, New York, 1995, pp. 916-921.
779. Louis Sokoloff, "Localization of Functional Activity in the Central Nervous System by Measurement of Glucose Utilization with Radioactive Deoxyglucose," J. Cerebral Blood Flow and Metabolism 1(1981):7-36.
780. J.F. Nunn, Nunn's Applied Respiratory Physiology, 4th Edition, Butterworth-Heinemann Ltd., London, 1993.
781. Robert E. Smith, "Quantitative Relations Between Liver Mitochondria Metabolism and Total Body Weight in Mammals," Ann. N.Y. Acad. Sci. 62.17(31 January 1956):403-422.
782. M.A. Holliday, D. Potter, A. Jarrah, S. Bearg, "The Relation of Metabolic Rate to Body Weight and Organ Size," Pediatric Res. 1(1967):185-195.
783. Roland A. Coulson, Thomas Hernandez, Jack D. Herbert, "Metabolic Rate, Enzyme Kinetics In Vivo," Comp. Biochem. Physiol. 56A(1977):251-262.
784. Jonathan W. Mink, Robert J. Blumenschine, David B. Adams, "Ratio of central nervous system to body metabolism in vertebrates: its constancy and functional basis," Amer. J. Physiol. 241(1981):R203-R212.
785. Graeme F. Mason et al., "Simultaneous Determination of the Rates of the TCA Cycle, Glucose Utilization, α-Ketoglutarate/Glutamate Exchange, and Glutamine Synthesis in Human Brain by NMR," J. Cerebral Blood Flow and Metabolism 15(1995):12-25.
786. Jan Nedergaard, Barbara Cannon, "Chapter 10. Thermogenic mitochondria," in L. Ernster, ed., Bioenergetics, Elsevier, New York, 1984, pp. 291-314.
787. Richard J. Kones, Glucose, Insulin, Potassium and the Heart: Selected Aspects of Cardiac Energy Metabolism, Futura Publishing Company, 1975.
788. C.L. Gibbs, W.F.H.M. Mommaerts, N.V. Ricchiuti, "Energetics of cardiac contractions," J. Physiol. (London) 191(1967):25-46.
789. M. Trumpa, B. Wendt, "Microcalorimetric Measurements of Heat Production in Human Erythrocytes with a Batch Calorimeter," in I. Lamprecht, B. Schaarschmidt, eds., Application of Calorimetry in Life Sciences, Walter de Gruyter, New York, 1977, pp. 241-249.
790. J. Anthony Ware, Barry S. Coller, "Chapter 119. Platelet morphology, biochemistry, and function." In Ernest Beutler, Marshall A. Lichtman, Barry S. Coller, Thomas J. Kipps, eds., William's Hematology, Fifth Edition, McGraw-Hill, New York, 1995, pp. 1161-1201.
791. Philip D. Ross, A.P. Fletcher, G.A. Jamieson, "Microcalorimetric Study of Isolated Blood Platelets in the Presence of Thrombin and Other Aggregating Agents," Biochimica Biophysica Acta 313(1973):106-118.
792. K. Levin, "Heat Production by Leucocytes and Thrombocytes Measured with a Flow Microcalorimeter in Normal Man and During Thyroid Dysfunction," Clinica Chimica Acta 32(1971):87-94.
793. E. Gylfe, B. Hellman, "The heat production of pancreatic β-cells stimulated by glucose," Acta Physiol. Scand. 93(1975):179-183.
794. A. Anders, G. Welge, B. Schaarschmidt, I. Lamprecht, H. Schaefer, "Calorimetric Investigations of Metabolic Regulation in Human Skin," in I. Lamprecht, B. Schaarschmidt, eds., Application of Calorimetry in Life Sciences, Walter de Gruyter, New York, 1977, pp. 199-208.
795. Beatrice A. Wittenberg, "Intracellular Oxygen Delivery in Heart Cells," in Arie Pinson, ed., The Heart Cell in Culture, Vol. III, CRC Press, Boca Raton, Florida, 1987, pp. 83-89.
796. K. Levin, "A Modified Flow Microcalorimeter Adapted for the Study of Human Leucocyte Phagocytosis," Scand. J. Clin. Lab. Investig. 32(1973):67-73.
797. E.A. Dawes, D.W. Ribbons, "The Endogenous Metabolism of Microorganisms," Ann. Rev. Microbiol. 16(1962):241-263.
798. W.W. Forrest, D.J. Walker, "Calorimetric Measurements of Energy of Maintenance of *Streptococcus faecalis*," Biochem. Biophys. Res. Commun. 13(1963):217-222.
799. John G. Nicholls, A. Robert Martin, Bruce G. Wallace, From Neuron to Brain, Third Edition, Sinauer Associates, Inc., Sunderland, MA, 1992.
800. D. Landowne, J.M. Ritchie, "The binding of tritiated ouabain to mammalian non-myelinated nerve fibers," J. Physiol. (London) 207(1970):529-537.
801. J.V. Howarth, R.D. Keynes, J.M. Ritchie, "The origin of the initial heat associated with a single impulse in mammalian non-myelinated nerve fibers," J. Physiol. (London) 194(1968):745-793.
802. M.M. Salpeter, ed., The Vertebrate Neuromuscular Junction, Alan R. Liss, NY, 1987.
803. Stephen W. Kuffler, Doju Yoshikami, "The distribution of acetylcholine sensitivity at the post-synaptic membrane of vertebrate skeletal twitch muscles: iontophoretic mapping in the micron range," J. Physiol. (London) 244(1975):703-730.
804. Bertil Hille, "Ionic Channels in Nerve Membranes," Prog. Biophys. Mol. Biol. 21(1970):1-32.
805. L.B. Cohen, P. De Weer, "Structural and metabolic processes directly related to action potential propagation," in Handbook of Physiology, Section 1, Volume I, Part 1, Chapter 5, American Physiological Society, Bethesda MD, 1977, pp. 137-159.
807. Randall R. Reed, "How Does the Nose Know?" Cell 60(12 January 1990):1-2.
808. L. Buck, R. Axel, "A novel multigene family may encode odorant receptors: a molecular basis for odor recognition," Cell 65(1991):175-187.
809. Linda B. Buck, "A Novel Multigene Family May Encode Odorant Receptors," in David P. Corey, Stephen D. Roper, eds., Sensory Transduction, The Rockefeller University Press, NY, 1992, pp. 39-51.
810. Steven M. Block, "Biophysical Principles of Sensory Transduction," in David P. Corey, Stephen D. Roper, eds., Sensory Transduction, The Rockefeller University Press, NY, 1992, pp. 1-17.
811. W. Bialek, "Physical limits to sensation and perception," Ann. Rev. Biophysics and Biophysical Chemistry 16(1987):455-478.
812. G. Corbiere-Tichane, R. Loftus, "Antennal thermal receptors of the cave beetle, *Speophyes lucidulus*," J. Compar. Physiol. 153(1983):343-351.
813. A.D. Kalmijn, "Electric and magnetic field detection in elasmobranch fishes," Science 218(1982):916-918.
814. J. Weaver, R.D. Astumian, "The Response of Living Cells to Very Weak Electric Fields: The Thermal Noise Limit," Science 247(1990):459-462.
815. J.L. Gould, "Magnetic field sensitivity in animals," Ann. Rev. Physiol. 46(1984):585-598.
816. J.L. Kirschvink, "Magnetite biomineralization and geomagnetic sensitivity in higher animals," Bioelectromagnetics 10(1989):239-259.
817. Gilbert B. Forbes, Human Body Composition: Growth, Aging, Nutrition, and Activity, Springer-Verlag, New York, 1987.
818. K. Michael Sekins, Ashley F. Emery, "Chapter 2. Thermal Science for Physical Medicine," in Justus F. Lehmann, ed., Therapeutic Heat and Cold, Fourth Edition, Williams & Wilkins, Baltimore MD, 1990, pp. 62-112.
819. Arthur W. Guy, "Chapter 5. Biophysics of High-Frequency Currents and Electromagnetic Radiation," in Justus F. Lehmann, ed., Therapeutic Heat and Cold, Fourth Edition, Williams & Wilkins, Baltimore MD, 1990, pp. 179-236.
821. E.F. DuBois, Fever and the Regulation of Body Temperature, Charles C. Thomas, Springfield IL, 1948.
822. H.P. Schwan, "Biophysics of Diathermy," in S. Licht, ed., Therapeutic Heat and Cold, Second Edition, Waverly Press, Baltimore MD, 1965, pp. 63-125.
823. S.M. Michaelson, "Human exposure to nonionizing radiant energy -- potential hazards and safety standards," Proc. IEEE 60(1972):389-421.
824. P. Czerski, "The development of biomedical approaches and concepts in radiofrequency radiation protection," Microwave Power 21(1986):9-23.
825. Robert P. Lanza, Robert Langer, William L. Chick, eds., Principles of Tissue Engineering, R.G. Landes Company, Georgetown TX, 1997.
826. R. Igor Gamow, John F. Harris, "The Infrared Receptors of Snakes," Scientific American 228(May 1973):94-100.
827. David Y. Chung, Keith Mason, R. Patrick Gannon, Glenn N. Willson, "The ear effect as a function of age and hearing loss," J. Acoust. Soc. Amer. 73(April 1983):1277-1282.
828. S. Singhal, R. Henderson, K. Horsfield, K. Harding, G. Cumming, "Morphometry of the human pulmonary arterial tree," Circ. Res. 33(1973):190-197.
829. A. Maseri, P. Caldini, S. Permutt, K.L. Zierler, "Frequency function of transit times through dog pulmonary circulation," Circ. Res. 26(1970):527-543.
830. Alan C. Burton, "Physical principles of circulatory phenomena: The physical equilibria of the heart and blood vessels," Handbook of Physiology, Section 2: Circulation, Volume I, American Physiological Society, Bethesda MD, 1962, pp. 85-106.
831. Alan C. Burton, Physiology and Biophysics of the Circulation, Second Edition, Year Book Medical Publishers, Chicago IL, 1972.

832. R.F. Schmidt, G. Thews, eds., Human Physiology, Second Edition, Springer-Verlag, New York, 1989.
833. Robert C. Little, William C. Little, Physiology of the Heart and Circulation, Fourth Edition, Year Book Medical Publishers, Chicago IL, 1989.
834. John Ross, Jr., "Section 2: Cardiovascular System," in Best and Taylor's Physiological Basis of Medical Practice, Twelfth Edition, Williams & Wilkins, Baltimore MD, 1991.
835. Solomon N. Albert, Blood Volume and Extracellular Fluid Volume, Second Edition, Charles C. Thomas, Springfield IL, 1971.
836. Arthur C. Guyton, John E. Hall, Human Physiology and Mechanisms of Disease, Sixth Edition, W.B. Saunders Company, Philadelphia PA, 1997.
837. B. Folkow, E. Neil, Circulation, Oxford University Press, New York, 1971.
838. Don W. Fawcett, A Textbook of Histology, Twelfth Edition, Chapman & Hall, New York, 1994.
839. Herbert H. Lipowsky, Colin B. McKay, Junji Seki, "Trans Time Distributions of Blood Flow in the Microcirculation," in Jen-Shih Lee, Thomas C. Skalak, eds., Microvascular Mechanics: Hemodynamics of Systems and Pulmonary Microcirculation, Springer-Verlag, NY, 1989, pp. 13-27.
840. R.L. Whitmore, Rheology of the Circulation, Pergamon Press, Oxford, 1968.
841. P. Gaehtgens, "Flow of blood through narrow capillaries: Rheological mechanisms determining capillary hematocrit and apparent viscosity," Biorheology 17(1980):183-189.
842. M.S. Roy, K.S. Harrison, E. Harvey, T. Mitchell, "Ocular Blood Flow in Dogs Using Radiolabelled Microspheres," Nucl. Med. Biol. 16(1989):81-84.
843. R.E. Records, ed., Ocular Circulation in Physiology of the Human Eye and Visual System, Harper & Row, NY, 1979.
844. S. Chien, "Chapter 26. Biophysical Behavior of Red Cells in Suspensions," in D.M. Surgenor, ed., The Red Blood Cell, 2nd Edition, Volume II, Academic Press, NY, 1975, pp. 1031-1133.
845. P.S. Lingard, "Capillary pore rheology of erythrocytes," Microvasc. Res. 8(1974):53-63, 181-191; 13(1977):29-77; 17(1979):272-289.
846. Geert W. Schmid-Schonbein, "Chapter 13: Rheology of Leukocytes," in Richard Skalak, Shu Chien, eds., Handbook of Bioengineering, McGraw-Hill, New York, 1987.
847. Mario Battezzati, Ippolito Donini, The Lymphatic System, Revised Edition, John Wiley & Sons, New York, 1972. Translation by Vilfrido Cameron-Curry.
848. Joseph Mendel Yoffey, Frederick Colin Courtice, Lymphatics, Lymph and the Lymphomyeloid Complex, Academic Press, New York, 1970.
849. G. Hauck, "Chapter 12: Vital microscopic results of the substance transport in the extravascular space and quantitative aspects of the video analysis," in M. Foldi, ed., Ergebnisse der Angiologie, Schattauer, Stuttgart, 1976, pp. 51-60.
850. John R. Casley-Smith, "Chapter 19: Lymph and Lymphatics," in Gabor Kaley, Burton M. Altura, eds., Microcirculation, Volume I, University Park Press, Baltimore MD, 1977, pp. 423-502.
851. L. Allen, "On the penetrability of the lymphatics of the diaphragm," Anat. Record 124(1956):639-652.
852. Istvan Rusznyak, Mihaly Foldi, Gyorgy Szabo, Lymphatics and Lymph Circulation: Physiology and Pathology, Pergamon Press, New York, 1967.
853. Gerard J. Tortora, Principles of Human Anatomy, Fifth Edition, Harper & Row Publishers, New York, 1989.
854. Peter L. Williams, Roger Warwick, Mary Dyson, Lawrence H. Bannister, eds., Gray's Anatomy, Thirty-Seventh Edition, Churchill Livingstone, New York, 1989.
855. Mary P. Wiedeman, "Chapter 2. Architecture," Handbook of Physiology, Section 2: The Cardiovascular System, Volume IV, Microcirculation, Part I, American Physiological Society, Bethesda MD, 1984, pp. 11-40.
856. P. Kinnaert, "Anatomical variations of the cervical portion of the thoracic duct in man," J. Anat. 115(1973):45-52.
857. C.D. Haagensen, "Chapter 3. General Anatomy of the Lymphatic System," in The Lymphatics in Cancer, W.B. Saunders Company, Philadelphia PA, 1972, pp. 22-40.
858. Jack W. Shields, J.M. Yoffey, The Trophic Function of Lymphoid Elements, Charles C. Thomas, Springfield IL, 1972.
859. S. Kubik, M. Manestar, "Anatomy of the lymph capillaries and pre-collectors of the skin," in A. Bollinger, H. Partsch, J.H.N. Wolfe, eds., The Initial Lymphatics, Thieme-Stratton Inc., New York, 1985, pp. 66-74.
860. David I. Abramson, Blood Vessels and Lymphatics, Academic Press, New York, 1962.
861. J.R. Casley-Smith, "Prelymphatics," in Prokop Malek, Vladimir Bartos, Horst Weissleder, Marlys H. Witte, eds., Lymphology, Georg Thieme Publishers, Stuttgart, 1979, pp. 17-21.
862. Michael Foldi, Diseases of Lymphatics and Lymph Circulation, Charles C. Thomas, Springfield IL, 1969.
863. Arthur C. Guyton, Anatomy and Physiology, Saunders College Publishing, New York, 1985.
864. E.R. Weibel, Morphometry of the Human Lung, Academic Press, New York, 1963.
865. C. Bruce Wenger, James D. Hardy, "Chapter 4. Temperature Regulation and Exposure to Heat and Cold," in Justus F. Lehmann, ed., Therapeutic Heat and Cold, Fourth Edition, Williams & Wilkins, Baltimore, MD, 1990, pp. 150-178.
866. Arthur J. Vander, James H. Sherman, Dorothy S. Luciano, Human Physiology: The Mechanisms of Body Function, Fifth Edition, McGraw-Hill Publishing Company, New York, 1990.
867. R.O. Greep, L. Weiss, Histology, Third Edition, McGraw-Hill Book Company, New York, 1973.
868. H. Davis, S.R. Silverman, eds., Hearing and Deafness, Revised Edition, Holt, Rinehart & Winston, New York, 1960.
869. Francis Leukel, Introduction to Physiological Psychology, Second Edition, C.V. Mosby Company, St. Louis, MO, 1972.
870. Isaac Asimov, The Human Body: Its Structure and Operation, Houghton Mifflin Company, New York, 1963.
871. Henry D. Janowitz, Your Gut Feelings, Consumers Union, New York, 1987.
872. Peter Chalmers Mitchell, Leslie Brainerd Arey, "Gastrointestinal Tract," Encyclopedia Britannica 10(1963):54B-54F.
873. Paul Spinrad, Guide to Bodily Fluids, RE/Search Publications, San Francisco CA, 1994.
874. Frank H. Netter, The Ciba Collection of Medical Illustrations, Ciba Pharmaceutical Products, Inc., Summit, NJ, 1948.
875. Samuel Glasstone, Sourcebook on Atomic Energy, D. Van Nostrand Company, New York NY, 1950.
877. P. Krecmer, A.M. Moulin, R.J. Stephenson, T. Rayment, M.E. Welland, S.R. Elliott, "Reversible Nanocontraction and Dilatation in a Solid Induced by Polarized Light," Science 277(19September 1997):1799-1802; see also pp. 1786-1787.
878. Fu-Ren F. Fan, Allen J. Bard, "An Electrochemical Coulomb Staircase: Detection of Single Electron-Transfer Events at Nanometer Electrodes," Science 277 (19 September 1997):1791-1793.
879. Gary Stix, "Beam It Up," Scientific American 277(September 1997):40-41.
880. Hagan Bayley, "Building Doors into Cells," Scientific American 277(September 1997):62-67.
881. International Commission on Radiation Protection, Committee II, 1959, "Permissible Dose for Internal Radiation," Health Phys. 3(1960):1.
882. Irving L. Weissman, Max D. Cooper, "How the Immune System Develops," Scientific American 269(September 1993):65-71.
883. Hans Elias, "Liver," Encyclopedia Britannica 14(1963):227-231.
884. Robert G. Meeks, Steadman D. Harrison, Richard J. Bull, eds., Hepatotoxicology, CRC Press, Boca Raton, 1991.
885. E. Wisse, "Ultrastructure and Function of Kupffer Cells and Other Sinusoidal Cells in the Liver, " in E. Wisse, D.L. Knook, eds., Kupffer Cells and Other Liver Sinusoidal Cells, Elsevier/North-Holland Biomedical Press, New York, 1977, pp. 33-60.
886. E. Anthony Jones, John A. Summerfield, "Chapter 37. Kupffer Cells," in Irwin M. Arias, William B. Jakoby, Hans Popper, David Schachter, David A. Shafritz, eds., The Liver: Biology and Pathobiology, Second Edition, Raven Press, New York, 1988, pp. 683-704.
887. Richard C. Willson, "Total Solar Irradiance Trend During Solar Cycles 21 and 22," Science 277(26 September 1997):1963-1965.
888. R.C. Merkle, "Nanotechnology and Medicine," in R.M. Klatz, Frances A. Kovarik, eds., Advances in Anti-Aging Medicine, Volume 1, Mary Ann Liebert Press, 1996, pp. 277-286. (See also http://nano.xerox.com/nanotech/nanotechAndMedicine.html)
889. Frank Massa, "Chapter 3i. Radiation of Sound," in Dwight E. Gray, ed., American Institute of Physics Handbook, Third Edition, McGraw-Hill Book Company, New York, 1972, pp. 3.139-3.153.
890. H. Precht, J. Christophersen, H. Hensel, W. Larcher, Temperature and Life, Springer-Verlag, New York, 1973.
891. Von Jurgen Aschoff, Rutger Wever, "Kern und Schale im Warmehaushalt des Menschen," Naturwissenschaften 45 (1958):477-485.
892. H.A. Krebs, H.L. Kornberg, Energy Transformations in Living Matter, Springer-Verlag, Berlin, 1957.
893. Duncan Mitchell, C.H. Wyndham, A.R. Atkins, A.J. Vermeulen, H.S. Hofmeyr, N.B. Strydom, T. Hodgson, "Direct Measurement of the Thermal Responses of Nude Resting Men in Dry Environment," Pflugers Arch. Ges. Physiol. 303(1968):324-343.
894. Eugene F. Du Bois, "The Many Different Temperatures of the Human Body and Its Parts," Western J. Surg. 59(1951):476-490.
895. Alan C. Burton, "Human Calorimetry II: The Average Temperature of the Tissues of the Body," J. Nutr. 9(March 1935):261-280.
896. K. Wezler, G. Neuroth, Z. Exp. Med. 115(1949):127 et seq.
897. Merrill Edwards, Alan C. Burton, "Temperature distribution over the human head, especially in the cold," J. Appl. Physiol. 15(1960):209-211.
898. James D. Hardy, Eugene F. Du Bois, "Basal Metabolism, Radiation, Convection and Vaporization at Temperatures of 22 to 35°C," J. Nutr. 15(1938):477-497.
899. E. Francis J. Ring, Barbara Phillips, eds., Recent Advances in Medical Thermology, Plenum Press, New York, 1984.
900. James N. Hayward, "Cerebral Cooling During Increased Cerebral Blood Flow in the Monkey," Proc. Soc. Exp. Biol. (NY) 124(1967):555-557.
901. Jose M.R. Delgado, Taiji Hanai, "Intracerebral temperatures in free-moving cats," Am. J. Physiol. 211(1966):755-769.
902. J. Grayson, T. Kinnear, "Temperature of human liver," Proc. Federation Amer. Soc. Exp. Biol. 22(1963):775-776.
903. H.C. Bazett, "Blood Temperature and its Control," Am. J. Med. Sci. 218(November 1949):483-492.
904. J. Aschoff, B. Gunther, K. Kramer, Energiehaushalt und Temperaturregulation, Urban & Schwarzenberg, Munchen-Berlin-Wein, Germany, 1971.

905. Edward Rubenstein, Daniel W. Meub, Frederic Eldridge, "Common carotid blood temperature," J. Appl. Physiol. 15(1960):603-604.
906. Skoda Afonso, George G. Rowe, Cesar A. Castillo, Charles W. Crumpton, "Intravascular and intracardiac blood temperatures in man," J. Appl. Physiol. 17(1962):706-708.
907. J.S. Hepburn, H.M. Eberhard, R. Ricketts, C.L. Rieger, "Temperature of the Gastrointestinal Tract," Arch. Intern. Med. 52(1933):603-615.
908. Henry C. Mellette, B.K. Hutt, S.I. Askovitz, Steven M. Horvath, "Diurnal Variations in Body Temperature," J. Appl. Physiol. 3(1951):665-675.
909. R. Von Wurster, "Influence of Head Skin Temperature on Tympanic Membrane and Oral Temperatures," Pflugers Arch. Ges. Physiol. 300(1968):R47.
910. Steven M. Horvath, H. Menduke, George Morris Piersol, "Oral and Rectal Temperatures of Man," J. Amer. Med. Assoc. 144(1950):1562-1565.
912. Ashley F. Emery, K. Michael Sekins, "Computer Modeling of Thermotherapy," in Justus F. Lehmann, ed., Therapeutic Heat and Cold, Fourth Edition, Williams & Wilkins, Baltimore MD, 1990, pp. 113-149.
913. Theodor Hellbrugge, "The Development of Circadian Rhythms in Infants," Cold Spring. Harb. Symp. Quant. Biol. 25(1960):311-323.
915. Sutherland Simpson, J.J. Galbraith, "An Investigation into the Diurnal Variation of the Body Temperature of Nocturnal and Other Birds, and a Few Mammals," J. Physiol. (London) 33(1905):225-238.
916. R.P. Clark, "Human skin temperature and its relevance in physiology and clinical assessment," in E. Francis J. Ring, Barbara Phillips, eds., Recent Advances in Medical Thermology, Plenum Press, New York, 1984, pp. 5-15.
917. R.P. Clark, J.K. Stothers, "Neonatal skin temperature distribution using infrared color thermography," J. Physiol. 302(1980):323-333.
918. R.P. Clark, M.R. Goff, "Human skin temperature during rest and sleep visualized with color infrared thermography," J. Physiol. 300(1979):14-15.
919. L.B. Rowell, "Chapter 27. Cardiovascular Adjustments to Thermal Stress," Handbook of Physiology, Section 2: The Cardiovascular System, Volume III, American Physiological Society, Bethesda MD, 1983.
920. M.A. Vince, "Rapid response sequences and the psychological refractory period," Brit. J. Psychol. 40(1949):23-40.
921. H. Quastler, V.J. Wulff, "Human performance in information transmission," Technical Report R-62, Control Systems Laboratory, University of Illinois, Urbana IL, 1955.
922. A.F. Clift, F.A. Glover, G.W. Scott Blair, "Rheology of Human Cervical Secretions: Effects of Menstrual Cycle and Pregnancy," Lancet 258(1950):1154-1155.
923. R.M. Olson, "Aortic blood pressure and velocity as a function of time and position," J. Appl. Physiol. 24(1968):563-569.
924. C.J. Mills, I.T. Gabe, J.H. Gault, D.T. Mason, J. Ross Jr., E. Braunwald, J.P. Shillingford, "Pressure-flow relationships and vascular impedance in man," Cardiovascular Res. 4(October 1970):405-417.
925. B.W. Zweifach, H.H. Lipowsky, "Quantitative studies of microcirculatory structure and function. III. Microvascular hemodynamics of cat mesentery and rabbit omentum," Circulation Res. 41(1977):380-390.
926. K. Fronek, B.W. Zweifach, "The effect of vasodilator agents on microvascular pressures in skeletal muscle," Angiologia 3(1974):35-39 (Unione Intern. di Angiologia).
927. H.H. Lipowsky, S. Usami, S. Chien, "In vivo measurements of `apparent viscosity' and microvessel hematocrit in the mesentery of the cat," Microvascular Res. 19(1980):297-319.
928. R. Muthupillai, D.J. Lomas, P.J. Rossman, J.F. Greenleaf, A. Manduca, R.L. Ehman, "Magnetic Resonance Elastography by Direct Visualization of Propagating Acoustic Strain Waves," Science 269(29 September 1995):1854-1857.
929. B.W. Zweifach, "Quantitative studies of microcirculatory structure and function," Circulation Res. 34(1974):843-857, 858-868.
930. Weiguo Xi, Maria A. Stuchly, Om P. Gandhi, "Induced Electric Currents in Models of Man and Rodents from 60 Hz Magnetic Fields," IEEE Trans. Biomed. Eng. 41(November 1994):1018-1023.
931. Gordon H. Sato, "Chapter 8. Animal Cell Culture," in Robert P. Lanza, Robert Langer, William L. Chick, eds., Principles of Tissue Engineering, R.G. Landes Company, Georgetown TX, 1997, pp. 101-109.
932. Albert L. Lehninger, David L. Nelson, Michael M. Cox, Principles of Biochemistry, Second Edition, Worth Publishers, NY, 1993.
933. William C. Moss, Douglas B. Clarke, John W. White, David A. Young, "Sonoluminescence and the prospects for table-top micro-thermonuclear fusion," Physics Letters A 211(5 February 1996):69-74.
934. Kenton D. Hammonds, Hui Deng, Volker Heine, Martin T. Dove, "How Floppy Modes Give Rise to Adsorption Sites in Zeolites," Physical Review Letters 78(12 May 1997):3701-3704.
935. Michael H. Ross, Edward J. Reith, Lynn J. Romrell, Histology: A Text and Atlas, Second Edition, Williams & Wilkins, Baltimore MD, 1989.
936. David H. Cormack, Ham's Histology, J.B. Lippincott Company, Philadelphia PA, 1987.
937. Ted A. Yednock, Steven D. Rosen, "Lymphocyte Homing," Advances in Immunology 44(1989):313-378.
938. Ariel G. Loewy, Philip Siekevitz, John R. Menninger, Jonathan A.N. Gallant, Cell Structure and Function: An Integrated Approach, Third Edition, Saunders College Publishing, Philadelphia PA, 1991.
939. Wayne M. Becker, David W. Deamer, The World of the Cell, Second Edition, Benjamin/Cummings Publishing Company, Redwood City CA, 1991.
940. Elaine N. Marieb, Human Anatomy and Physiology, Benjamin/Cummings Publishing Company, Redwood City CA, 1989.
941. Alice B. Fulton, "How Crowded is the Cytoplasm?" Cell 30(September 1982):345-347.
942. Andrew J. Maniotis, Christopher S. Chen, Donald E. Ingber, "Demonstration of mechanical connections between integrins, cytoskeletal filaments, and nucleoplasm that stabilize nuclear structure," Proc. Natl. Acad. Sci. USA 94(February 1997):849-854.
943. G.N. Jenkins, The Physiology and Biochemistry of the Mouth, Fourth Edition, Blackwell Scientific Publications, Oxford, 1978.
944. Victor A. Politano, "Periurethral Polytetrafluoroethylene Injection for Urinary Incontinence," J. Urology 127(March 1982):439-442.
945. Anthony A. Malizia, Jr., Herbert M. Reiman, Robert P. Myers, Jonathan R. Sande, Steven S. Barham, Ralph C. Benson, Jr., Mrinal K. Dewanjee, William J. Utz, "Migration and Granulomatous Reaction After Periurethral Injection of Polytef (Teflon)," J. Amer. Med. Assn. 251(1984):3277-3281.
946. H. Claes, D. Stroobants, J. Van Meerbeek, E. Verbeken, D. Knockaert, L. Baert, "Pulmonary Migration Following Periurethral Polytetrafluoroethylene Injection for Urinary Incontinence," J. Urology 142(September 1989):821-822.
947. Carlos Lois, Jose-Manuel Garcia-Verdugo, Arturo Alvarez-Buylla, "Chain Migration of Neuronal Precursors," Science 271(16 February 1996):978-981.
948. Gautam R. Desiraju, "Crystal Gazing: Structure Prediction and Polymorphism," Science 278(17 October 1997):404-405.
949. Marcia Barinaga, "Researchers Find Signals That Guide Young Brain Neurons," Science 278(17 October 1997):385-386.
950. S.A. Anderson, D.D. Eisenstat, L. Shi, J.L.R. Rubenstein, "Interneuron Migration from Basal Forebrain to Neocortex: Dependence on Dlx Genes," Science 278(17 October 1997):474-476.
951. John Travis, "Axon Guidance: Wiring the Nervous System," Science 266(28 October 1994):568-570.
952. Bassil I. Dahiyat, Stephen L. Mayo, "De Novo Protein Design: Fully Automated Sequence Selection," Science 278(3 October 1997):82-87.
953. Stewart Sell, Immunology, Immunopathology and Immunity, Fourth Edition, Elsevier, New York, 1987.
954. John W. Kimball, Introduction to Immunology, Third Edition, Macmillan Publishing Company, New York, 1990.
955. Ivan M. Roitt, Jonathan Brostoff, David K. Male, Immunology, Gower Medical Publishing, New York, 1989.
956. Emily G. Reisner, "Chapter 149. Human leukocyte and platelet antigens," in Ernest Beutler, Marshall A. Lichtman, Barry S. Coller, Thomas J. Kipps, eds., William's Hematology, Fifth Edition, McGraw-Hill, New York, 1995, pp. 1611-1617.
957. Loni Calhoun, Lawrence D. Petz, "Chapter 148. Erythrocyte antigens and antibodies," in Ernest Beutler, Marshall A. Lichtman, Barry S. Coller, Thomas J. Kipps, eds., William's Hematology, Fifth Edition, McGraw-Hill, New York, 1995, pp. 1595-1610.
958. Avrion Mitchison, "Will We Survive?" Scientific American 269(September 1993):136-144.
959. Roger K. Cunningham, "Chapter 14. Immunochemistry of Polysaccharide and Blood Group Antigens," in Carel J. van Oss, Marc H. van Regenmortel, eds., Immunochemistry, Marcel Dekker, New York, 1994, pp. 319-335.
960. P.L. Mollison, C.P. Engelfriet, M. Contreras, Blood Transfusions in Clinical Medicine, Ninth Edition, Blackwell Scientific, Oxford, 1993.
961. P. Hawkins, S.E. Anderson, J.L. McKenzie, K. McLoughlin, M.E.J. Beard, D.N.J. Hart, "Localization of MN Blood Group Antigens in Kidney," Transplant. Proc. 17(1985):1697-1700.
962. D.J. Anstee, G. Mallinson, J.E. Yendle, et al., "Evidence for the occurrence of Lu^b-active glycoproteins in human erythrocytes, kidney, and liver," International Congress ISBT-BBTS Book of Abstracts, 1988, p. 263.
963. Aron E. Szulman, "The ABH antigens in human tissues and secretions during embryonal development," J. Histochem. Cytochem. 13(1965):752-754.
964. Thomas J. Kunicki, Peter J. Newman, "The molecular immunology of human platelet proteins," Blood 80(1992):1386-1404.
965. Una Chen, "Chapter 33. Lymphocyte Engineering, Its Status of Art and Its Future," in Robert P. Lanza, Robert Langer, William L. Chick, eds., Principles of Tissue Engineering, R.G. Landes Company, Georgetown TX, 1997, pp. 527-561.
966. Lola M. Reid, "Chapter 31. Stem Cell/Lineage Biology and Lineage-Dependent Extracellular Matrix Chemistry: Keys to Tissue Engineering of Quiescent Tissues such as Liver," in Robert P. Lanza, Robert Langer, William L. Chick, eds., Principles of Tissue Engineering, R.G. Landes Company, Georgetown TX, 1997, pp. 481-514.
967. Janet Hardin Young, Jeffrey Teumer, Paul D. Kemp, Nancy L. Parenteau, "Chapter 20. Approaches to Transplanting Engineered Cells and Tissues," in Robert P. Lanza, Robert Langer, William L. Chick, eds., Principles of Tissue Engineering, R.G. Landes Company, Georgetown TX, 1997, pp. 297-307.
968. Norio Haneji, Takanori Nakamura, Koji Takio, et al., "Identification of α-Fodrin as a Candidate Autoantigen in Primary Sjogren's Syndrome," Science 276(25 April 1997):604-607.
970. Mark J. Poznansky, Rudolph L. Juliano, "Biological Approaches to the Controlled Delivery of Drugs: A Critical Review," Pharmacological Reviews 36(1984):277-336.

971. E.D. Hay, ed., Cell Biology of Extracellular Matrix, Second Edition, Plenum Press, New York, 1991.
972. Jayne Lesley, Robert Hyman, Paul W. Kincade, "CD44 and Its Interaction with Extracellular Matrix," Advances in Immunology 54(1993):271-335.
973. Tod A. Brown, Todd Bouchard, Tom St. John, Elizabeth Wayner, William G. Carter, "Human Keratinocytes Express a New CD44 Core Protein (CD44E) as a Heparin-Sulfate Intrinsic Membrane Proteoglycan with Additional Exons," J. Cell Biology 113(April 1991):207-221.
974. Lloyd M. Stoolman, "Adhesion Molecules Controlling Lymphocyte Migration," Cell 56(24 March 1989):907-910.
975. Richard O. Hynes, "Integrins: Versatility, Modulation, and Signaling in Cell Adhesion," Cell 69(3 April 1992):11-25.
976. Ajit Varki, "Selectin ligands," Proc. Natl. Acad. Sci. USA 91(August 1994):7390-7397.
977. Masatoshi Takeichi, "Cadherins: A molecular family important in selective cell-cell adhesion," Ann. Rev. Biochem. 59(1990):237-252.
978. Laurence A. Lasky, "Selectins: Interpreters of Cell-Specific Carbohydrate Information During Inflammation," Science 258(6 November 1992):964-969.
980. Elizabeth J. Luna, Anne L. Hitt, "Cytoskeleton-Plasma Membrane Interactions," Science 258(6 November 1992):955-964.
981. Karl-Anders Karlsson, "Glycobiology: A Growing Field for Drug Design," Trends in Pharmacological Sciences 12(July 1991):265-272.
982. Carlo Laudanna, James J. Campbell, Eugene C. Butcher, "Role of Rho in Chemoattractant-Activated Leukocyte Adhesion Through Integrins," Science 271 (16 February 1996):981-983.
983. Mark Halper, "Putting Mount Everest into an Anthill," Forbes 160(7 July 1997):208-213.
984. Bjorn Reino Olsen, "Chapter 4. Matrix Molecules and Their Ligands," in Robert P. Lanza, Robert Langer, William L. Chick, eds., Principles of Tissue Engineering, R.G. Landes Company, Georgetown TX, 1997, pp. 47-65.
985. Donald E. Ingber, "Chapter 7. Mechanochemical Switching Between Growth and Differentiation by Extracellular Matrix," in Robert P. Lanza, Robert Langer, William L. Chick, eds., Principles of Tissue Engineering, R.G. Landes Company, Georgetown TX, 1997, pp. 89-100.
986. Patricia Parsons-Wingerter, E. Helene Sage, "Chapter 9. Regulation of Cell Behavior by Extracellular Proteins," in Robert P. Lanza, Robert Langer, William L. Chick, eds., Principles of Tissue Engineering, R.G. Landes Company, Georgetown TX, 1997, pp. 111-131.
987. Kshama B. Jirage, John C. Hulteen, Charles R. Martin, "Nanotubule-Based Molecular-Filtration Membranes," Science 278(24 October 1997):655-658.
988. Ch. Spielmann, N.H. Burnett, S. Sartania, R. Koppitsch, M. Schnurer, C. Kan, M. Lenzner, P. Wobrauschek, F. Krausz, "Generation of Coherent X-rays in the Water Window Using 5-Femtosecond Laser Pulses," Science 278(24 October 1997):661-664.
989. See journal: Biosensors and Bioelectronics 1(1985)-present.
990. V.G. Kozlov, V. Bulovic, P.E. Burrows, S.R. Forrest, "Laser action in organic semiconductor waveguide and double-heterostructure devices," Nature 389(25 September 1997):362-364.
991. James H. Jett, Richard A. Keller, John C. Martin, Babetta L. Marrone, Robert K. Moyzis, Robert L. Ratliff, Newton K. Seitzinger, E. Brooks Shera, Carleton C. Stewart, "High-Speed DNA Sequencing: An Approach Based Upon Fluorescence Detection of Single Molecules," J. Biomol. Struct. Dynam. 7(1989):301-309.
992. E. Brooks Shera, Newton K. Seitzinger, Lloyd M. Davis, Richard A. Keller, Steven A. Soper, "Detection of single fluorescent molecules," Chem. Phys. Lett. 174(1990):553-557.
993. J. Fraden, AIP Handbook of Modern Sensors, American Institute of Physics, New York, 1993.
996. Robert K. Murray, Daryl K. Granner, Peter A. Mayes, Victor W. Rodwell, Harper's Biochemistry, 23rd Edition, Appleton & Lange, Norwalk CT, 1993.
997. Benjamin Lewin, Genes V, Oxford University Press, New York NY, 1995.
998. E.D.P. de Robertis, E.M.F. de Robertis, Cell and Molecular Biology, Eighth Edition, Lea & Febiger, Philadelphia PA, 1987.
999. Gordon L.E. Koch, "Chapter 8. The Endoplasmic Reticulum," in E. Edward Bittar, Neville Bittar, eds., Cellular Organelles, JAI Press, Greenwich CT, 1995, pp. 189-214.
1000. Colin Masters, Denis Crane, The Peroxisome: A Vital Organelle, Cambridge University Press, New York, 1995.
1001. John Travis, "What's in the Vault?" Science News 150(27 July 1996):56-57.
1003. Laura I. Davis, "The Nuclear Pore Complex," Ann. Rev. Biochem. 64(1995):865-896.
1004. N. Pokrywka, D. Goldfarb, M. Zillmann, A. DeSilva, "The Transport of Macromolecules Across the Nuclear Envelope," in E. Edward Bittar, Neville Bittar, eds., Cellular Organelles, JAI Press, Greenwich CT, 1995, pp. 19-54.
1005. James M. Cork, Radioactivity and Nuclear Physics, Second Edition, D. Van Nostrand Company, New York, 1950.
1006. F.K. Richtmyer, E.H. Kennard, Introduction to Modern Physics, Third Edition, McGraw-Hill Book Company, New York, 1942.
1007. Rutherford and Chadwick, Phil. Mag. 42(1921):809; 44(1922):417; Proc. Phys. Soc. 36(1924):417.
1008. F.A. Paneth, E. Gluckauf, H. Loleit, "Spectroscopic Identification and Manometric Measurement of Artificially Produced Helium," Proc. Roy. Soc. 147(2 December 1936):412-422.
1009. G. Preparata, "A New Look at Solid-State Fractures, Particle Emission and Cold Nuclear Fusion," Il Nuovo Cimento 104A(August 1991):1259-1263.
1010. Allen P. Minton, "Excluded Volume as a Determinant of Macromolecular Structure and Reactivity," Biopolymers 20(October 1981):2093-2120.
1011. Edwin H. McConkey, "Molecular evolution, intracellular organization, and the quinary structure of proteins," Proc. Natl. Acad. Sci. USA 79(1982):3236-3240.
1012. B. Brett Finlay, Pascale Cossart, "Exploitation of Mammalian Host Cell Functions by Bacterial Pathogens," Science 276(2 May 1997):718-725.
1013. Tobias A. Knoch, Christian Munkel, Jorg Langowski, "New Three-Dimensional Organization of Chromosome Territories and the Human Cell Nucleus: About the Structure of a Self-Replicating Nano Fabrication Site," poster presentation at the Sixth Foresight Conference on Molecular Nanotechnology, November 1998. See also: http://www.DKFZ-Heidelberg.de/Macromol/Welcome.html.
1014. J.S. O'Brien, "Stability of the Myelin Membrane," Science 147(1965):1099-1107.
1015. S.J. Yao, A.J. Appleby, A. Geisel, H.R. Cash, S.K. Wolfson Jr., "Anodic Oxidation of Carbohydrates and their Derivatives in Neutral Saline Solution," Nature 224(29 November 1969):921-922.
1016. Edwin B. Newman, "Chapter 3k. Speech and Hearing," in Dwight E. Gray, ed., American Institute of Physics Handbook, Third Edition, McGraw-Hill Book Company, New York, 1972, pp. 3.154-3.165.
1017. Steven H. Bergens, Christopher B. Gorman, G. Tayhas, R. Palmore, George M. Whitesides, "A Redox Fuel Cell That Operates with Methane as Fuel at 120°C," Science 265(2 September 1994):1418-1420.
1018. Arthur E. Johnson, "Protein translocation at the ER membrane: a complex process becomes more so," Trends Cell. Biol. 7(March 1997):90-95.
1019. Eric S. Rosenberg et al., "Vigorous HIV-1-Specific $CD4^+$ T Cell Responses Associated with Control of Viremia," Science 278(21 November 1997):1447-1450.
1020. Donald E. Ingber, "Tensegrity: The Architectural Basis of Cellular Mechanotransduction," Ann. Rev. Physiol. 59(1997):575-599.
1021. Donald E. Ingber, "The Architecture of Life," Scientific American 278(January 1998):48-57.
1022. Humphrey Maris, "Picosecond Ultrasonics," Scientific American 278(January 1998):86-89.
1023. Norman Rostoker, Michl W. Binderbauer, Hendrik J. Monkhorst, "Colliding Beam Fusion Reactor," Science 278(21 November 1997):1419-1422.
1024. Roland Beckmann, Doryen Bubeck, Robert Grassucci, Pawel Penczek, Adriana Verschoor, Gunter Blobel, Joachim Frank, "Alignment of Conduits for the Nascent Polypeptide Chain in the Ribosome-Sec61 Complex," Science 278(19 December 1997):2123-2126.
1025. T.A. Mary, J.S.O. Evans, T. Vogt, A.W. Sleight, "Negative Thermal Expansion from 0.3 to 1050 Kelvin in ZrW_2O_8," Science 272(5 April 1996):90-92.
1026. P.L. Kuhns, A. Kleinhammes, W.G. Moulton, N.S. Sullivan, "NMR in Resistive Magnets at Fields up to 30 T," J. Magnetic Reson. A 115(August 1995):270-272.
1027. Eugene C. Butcher, Louis J. Picker, "Lymphocyte Homing and Homeostasis," Science 272(5 April 1996):60-66.
1028. Peter Parham, Tomoko Ohta, "Population Biology of Antigen Presentation by MHC Class I Molecules," Science 272(5 April 1996):67-74.
1029. Tyrone L. Daulton, Minoru Ozima, "Radiation-Induced Diamond Formation in Uranium-Rich Carbonaceous Materials," Science 271(1 March 1996):1260-1263.
1030. Herman J.C. Berendsen, "Bio-Molecular Dynamics Comes of Age," Science 271(16 February 1996):954-955.
1031. F. Reif, Fundamentals of Statistical and Thermal Physics, McGraw-Hill Book Company, New York, 1965.
1032. Richard C. Kurten, Deborah L. Cadena, Gordon N. Gill, "Enhanced Degradation of EGF Receptors by a Sorting Nexin, SNX1," Science 272(17 May 1996):1008-1010.
1033. V. Nathan Subramaniam, Frank Peter, Robin Philp, Siew Heng Wong, Wanjin Hong, "GS28, a 28-Kilodalton Golgi SNARE That Participates in ER-Golgi Transport," Science 272(24 May 1996):1161-1163.
1034. D.M. Rowe, ed., CRC Handbook of Thermoelectrics, CRC Press, Boca Raton, FL, 1995.
1035. H.J. Goldsmid, Electronic Refrigeration, Pion Limited, London UK, 1986.
1036. V.B. Mountcastle, The Mindful Brain, MIT Press, Cambridge MA, 1978.
1037. Gang Wang, Keiji Tanaka, Manabu Tanifuji, "Optical Imaging of Functional Organization in the Monkey Inferotemporal Cortex," Science 272(14 June 1996):1665-1668.
1038. Susan Acton, Attilio Rigotti, Katherine T. Landschulz, Shangzhe Xu, Helen H. Hobbs, Monty Krieger, "Identification of Scavenger Receptor SR-BI as a High Density Lipoprotein Receptor," Science 271(26 January 1996):518-520.
1039. D.H. Hubel, T.N. Wiesel, "Receptive Fields, Binocular Interaction and Functional Architecture in the Cat's Visual Cortex," J. Physiol. 160(1962):106-154.
1040. M.-L. Mittelstaedt, H. Mittelstaedt, "Homing by Path Integration in a Mammal," Naturwissenschaften 67(1980):566-567.
1041. Hideki Masuda, Kenji Fukuda, "Ordered Metal Nanohole Arrays Made by a Two-Step Replication of Honeycomb Structures of Anodic Alumina," Science 268(9 June 1995):1466-1468.

1043. L.P. Faucheux, L.S. Bourdieu, P.D. Kaplan, Albert J. Libchaber, "Optical Thermal Ratchet," Phys. Rev. Lett. 74(27 February 1995):1504-1507.
1044. Wade Roush, "Envisioning an Artificial Retina," Science 268(5 May 1995):637-638.
1045. Frank A. Schabert, Christian Henn, Andreas Engel, "Native *Escherichia coli* OmpF Porin Surfaces Probed by Atomic Force Microscopy," Science 268(7 April 1995):92-94.
1046. Olaf Schneewind, Audree Fowler, Kym F. Faull, "Structure of the Cell Wall Anchor of Surface Proteins in *Staphylococcus aureus*," Science 268(7 April 1995):103-106.
1047. James A. Ernst, Robert T. Clubb, Huan-Xiang Zhou, Angela M. Gronenborn, G. Marius Clore, "Demonstration of Positionally Disordered Water Within a Protein Hydrophobic Cavity by NMR," Science 267(24 March 1995):1813-1817. See also: "Use of NMR to Detect Water Within Nonpolar Protein Cavities," Science 270 (15 December 1995):1847-1849.
1048. Junji Kido, Masato Kimura, Katsutoshi Nagai, "Multilayer White Light-Emitting Organic Electroluminescent Device," Science 267(3 March 1995):1332-1334.
1049. Magnus Granstrom, Magnus Berggren, Olle Inganas, "Micrometer- and Nanometer-Sized Polymeric Light-Emitting Diodes," Science 267(10 March 1995):1479-1481.
1050. Camillo Peracchia, ed., Handbook of Membrane Channels: Molecular and Cellular Physiology, Academic Press, San Diego, CA, 1994.
1051. Michael Seul, David Andelman, "Domain Shapes and Patterns: The Phenomenology of Modulated Phases," Science 267(27 January 1995):476-483.
1052. Jeff Hall, Doreen Kimura, "Dermatoglyphic Asymmetry and Sexual Orientation in Man," Behavioral Neuroscience 108 (December 1994):1203-1206.
1053. Tilman Schirmer, Thomas A. Keller, Yan-Fei Wang, Jurg P. Rosenbusch, "Structural Basis for Sugar Translocation Through Maltoporin Channels at 3.1 Angstrom Resolution," Science 267(27 January 1995):512-514.
1054. H. Morkoc, S.N. Mohammad, "High-Luminosity Blue and Blue-Green Gallium Nitride Light-Emitting Diodes," Science 267(6 January 1995):51-55.
1055. Jean Marx, "Helping Neurons Find Their Way," Science 268(19 May 1995):971-973.
1056. Huxiong Chen, Gerald Diebold, "Chemical Generation of Acoustic Waves: A Giant Photoacoustic Effect," Science 270(10 November 1995):963-966.
1057. Robert S. Meissner, Julius Rebek Jr., Javier de Mendoza, "Autoencapsulation Through Intermolecular Forces: A Synthetic Self-Assembling Spherical Complex," Science 270(1 December 1995):1485-1488.
1058. Hong Yin, Michelle D. Wang, Karel Svoboda, Robert Landick, Steven M. Block, Jeff Gelles, "Transcription Against an Applied Force," Science 270(8 December 1995):1653-1657.
1059. G. Yu, J. Gao, J.C. Hummelen, F. Wudl, A.J. Heeger, "Polymer Photovoltaic Cells: Enhanced Efficiencies via a Network of Internal Donor-Acceptor Heterojunctions," Science 270(15 December 1995):1789-1791.
1060. Robert Nagele, Theresa Freeman, Lydia McMorrow, Hsin-yi Lee, "Precise Spatial Positioning of Chromosomes During Prometaphase: Evidence for Chromosomal Order," Science 270(15 December 1995):1831-1835.
1061. Dean L. Olson, Timothy L. Peck, Andrew G. Webb, Richard L. Magin, Jonathan V. Sweedler, "High-Resolution Microcoil ^{1}H-NMR for Mass-Limited, Nanoliter-Volume Samples," Science 270(22 December 1995):1967-1970.
1062. Jon Cohen, "Interdisciplinary Talkfest Prompts Flurry of Questions," Science 270(24 November 1995):1294.
1063. Kouichi Itoh, Beth Stevens, Melitta Schachner, R. Douglas Fields, "Regulated Expression of the Neural Cell Adhesion Molecule L1 by Specific Patterns of Neural Impulses," Science 270(24 November 1995):1369-1372.
1065. Robert F. Service, "Capturing Sound, Light, and Strength With New Materials," Science 266(16 December 1994):1807-1808.
1066. Gil U. Lee, Linda A. Chrisey, Richard J. Colton, "Direct Measurement of the Forces Between Complementary Strands of DNA," Science 266(4 November 1994):771-773.
1068. Ruth S. Spolar, M. Thomas Record Jr., "Coupling of Local Folding to Site-Specific Binding of Proteins to DNA," Science 263(11 February 1994):777-784.
1069. Benno Hess, Alexander Mikhailov, "Self-Organization in Living Cells," Science 264(8 April 1994):223-224.
1070. Kenneth A. Johnson, Gary G. Borisy, "Kinetic Analysis of Microtubule Self-assembly in Vitro," J. Mol. Biol. 117(1977):1-31.
1071. Eckhard Mandelkow, Eva-Maria Mandelkow, Hirokazu Hotani, Benno Hess, Stefan C. Muller, "Spatial Patterns from Oscillating Microtubules," Science 246(1989):1291-1293.
1073. James Tabony, "Morphological Bifurcations Involving Reaction-Diffusion Processes During Microtubule Formation," Science 264(8 April 1994):245-248.
1074. Patrizia Fabrizio, Sybille Esser, Berthold Kastner, Reinhard Luhrmann, "Isolation of *S. cerevisiae* snRNPs: Comparison of U1 and U4/U6.U5 to Their Human Counterparts," Science 264(8 April 1994):261-265.
1075. Ernst-Ludwig Florin, Vincent T. Moy, Hermann E. Gaub, "Adhesion Forces Between Individual Ligand-Receptor Pairs," Science 264(15 April 1994):415-417.
1076. Lionel F. Jaffe, Kenneth R. Robinson, Richard Nuccitelli, "Local Cation Entry and Self-Electrophoresis as an Intracellular Localization Mechanism," Ann. N.Y. Acad. Sci. 238(1974):372-389.
1077. Bryan C. Gibbon, Darryl L. Kropf, "Cytosolic pH Gradients Associated with Tip Growth," Science 263(11 March 1994):1419-1421.
1078. Robert D. Jenison, Stanley C. Gill, Arthur Pardi, Barry Polisky, "High-Resolution Molecular Discrimination by RNA," Science 263(11 March 1994):1425-1429.
1079. Nicole Calakos, Mark K. Bennett, Karen E. Peterson, Richard H. Scheller, "Protein-Protein Interactions Contributing to the Specificity of Intracellular Vesicular Trafficking," Science 263(25 February 1994):1146-1149.
1080. Craig Hammond, Ari Helenius, "Folding of VSV G Protein: Sequential Interaction with BiP and Calnexin," Science 266(21 October 1994):456-458.
1081. Carol A. Vasconcellos, Philip G. Allen, Mary Ellen Wohl, Jeffrey M. Drazen, Paul A. Janmey, Thomas P. Stossel, "Reduction in Viscosity of Cystic Fibrosis Sputum in Vitro by Gelsolin," Science 263(18 February 1994):969-971.
1082. Carl P. Blobel, Tyra G. Wolfsberg, Christoph W. Turck, Diana G. Myles, Paul Primakoff, Judith M. White, "A potential fusion peptide and an integrin ligand domain in a protein active in sperm-egg fusion," Nature 356(19 March 1992):248-252.
1083. Nobuyuki Shiina, Yukiko Gotoh, Nobuko Kubomura, Akihiro Iwamatsu, Eisuke Nishida, "Microtubule Severing by Elongation Factor 1α," Science 266(14 October 1994):282-285.
1084. Kenneth S. Suslick, "Sonochemistry," Science 247(1990):1439-1445.
1085. Kenneth S. Suslick, Edward B. Flint, Mark W. Grinstaff, Kathleen A. Kemper, "Sonoluminescence from Metal Carbonyls," J. Phys. Chem. 97(1 April 1993):3098-3099.
1087. A. Jennifer Rivett, "Proteasomes: multicatalytic proteinase complexes," Biochem. J. 291(1993):1-10.
1088. Alfred L. Goldberg, Kenneth L. Rock, "Proteolysis, proteasomes and antigen presentation," Nature 357(1992):375-379.
1089. Chin-Yuan Hsu, Chia-Wei Li, "Magnetoreception in Honeybees," Science 265 (1 July 1994):95-97.
1090. Marcia Barinaga, "Watching the Brain Remake Itself," Science 266(2 December 1994):1475-1476.
1091. Olga O. Blumenfeld, Anthony M. Adamany, "Structural polymorphism within the amino-terminal region of MM, NN, and MN glycoproteins (glycophorins) of the human erythrocyte membrane," Proc. Natl. Acad. Sci. (USA) 75(1978):2727-2731.
1092. P. Dustin, Microtubules, Second Edition, Springer-Verlag, Berlin, 1987.
1093. Rebecca Howland, Lisa Benatar, A Practical Guide to Scanning Probe Microscopy, Park Scientific Instruments, Sunnyvale CA, 1996.
1094. Thure E. Cerling, John M. Harris, Bruce J. MacFadden, Meave G. Leakey, Jay Quade, Vera Eisenmann, James R. Ehleringer, "Global vegetation change through the Miocene/Pliocene boundary," Nature 389(11 September 1997):153-158.
1095. Robert Olson, Focused Study on Biotechnology and Nanotechnology, Military Health Service System (MHSS)-2020, U.S. Department of Defense, Health Affairs, September 1997. See also: http://keydet.sra.com/hs2020/homepage/hs2020.htm.
1097. Ralph C. Merkle, K. Eric Drexler, "Helical Logic," Nanotechnology 7(1996):325-339. See also: http://nano.xerox.com/nanotech/helical/helical.html.
1098. H. Sakaki, "Scattering Suppression and High-Mobility Effect of Size-Quantized Electrons in Ultrafine Semiconductor Wire Structures," Japanese Journal of Applied Physics 19(December 1980):L735-L738.
1099. Janet Raloff, "EMFs' Biological Influences," Science News 153(10 January 1998):29-31.
1100. Martin Jenkner, Peter Fromherz, "Bistability of Membrane Conductance in Cell Adhesion Observed in a Neuron Transistor," Phys. Rev. Lett. 79(8 December 1997):4705-4708.
1101. Robert Williams, The Geometrical Foundation of Natural Structure: A Sourcebook of Design, Dover Publications, New York, 1979.
1102. James M. Sakoda, Modern Origami, Simon and Schuster, New York, 1969.
1103. H. Lulli, "Nested tetrahedrons," School Science and Mathematics 78(May-June 1978):408-409; "Nested hexahedrons," School Science and Mathematics 76(March 1976):246-247; "The icosahedron and tangled tetrahedron," J. Recreational Mathematics 12(1979-1980):170-176; "The truncated tetrahedron," Mathematics in School 5(March 1976):33.
1104. Eric Kenneway, Complete Origami, Ebury Press, London, 1987. (ISBN 0-85223-617-4)
1105. J.J. Vittal, "A simple paper model for buckminsterfullerene," J. Chemical Education 66(1989):282.
1106. T. Sundra Rao, Geometric Exercises in Paper Folding, Dover Publications, New York, 1966.
1107. Michel Mendes France, "Folding paper and thermodynamics," Physics Reports (review section of Physics Letters) 103(1984):161-172.
1108. Patrick Morton, W. Mourant, "Paper folding, digit patterns, and groups in arithmetic fractals," Proc. London Math. Soc. 59(March 1989):253-293.
1109. Thomas Hull, "On the mathematics of flat origamis," Congressus Numerantium 100(1994):215-224.
1110. Robert J. Lang, "Mathematical algorithms for origami design," Symmetry: Culture and Science 5(1994):115-152.
1111. Koryo Miura, ed. in chief, Origami Science and Art: Proceedings of the Second International Meeting of Origami Science and Scientific Origami, 29 November - 2 December 1994, Otsu, Japan; published by organizing committee with support of Seian University of Art and Design, 1997. (560 pp Proceedings available by mail order from Toshikazu Kawasaki; see Origami Detectives web page.)
1112. Paul A. Schulte, Frederica P. Perera, eds., Molecular Epidemiology: Principles and Practices, Academic Press, San Diego, CA, 1993.
1113. Mark S. Bretscher, Sean Munro, "Cholesterol and the Golgi Apparatus," Science 261(3 September 1993):1280-1281.

1114. Y.K. Levine, M.H.F. Wilkins, "Structure of Oriented Lipid Bilayers," Nature New Biology 230(17 March 1971):69-72.
1115. Frank A. Nezil, Myer Bloom, "Combined influence of cholesterol and synthetic amphiphillic peptides upon bilayer thickness in model membranes," Biophys. J. 61(May 1992):1176-1183.
1116. James E. Rothman, "The Golgi Apparatus: Two Organelles in Tandem," Science 213(1981):1212-1219.
1117. L. Orci, R. Montesano, P. Meda, F. Malaisse-Lagae, D. Brown, A. Perrelet, P. Vassalli, "Heterogeneous distribution of filipin-cholesterol complexes across the cisternae of the Golgi apparatus," Proc. Natl. Acad. Sci. USA 78(1981):293-297.
1118. Jurgen Roth, "Subcellular organization of glycosylation in mammalian cells," Biochim. Biophys. Acta 906(1987):405-436.
1119. Tommy Nilsson, Marc Pypaert, Mee. H. Hoe, Paul Slusarewicz, Eric G. Berger, Graham Warren, "Overlapping Distribution of Two Glycosyltransferases in the Golgi Apparatus of HeLa Cells," J. Cell Biol. 120(1993):5-13.
1120. Haiqing Zhao, Lidija Ivic, Joji M. Otaki, Mitsuhiro Hashimoto, Katsuhiro Mikoshiba, Stuart Firestein, "Functional Expression of a Mammalian Odorant Receptor," Science 279(9 January 1998):237-242.
1121. Paul De Koninck, Howard Schulman, "Sensitivity of CaM Kinase II to the Frequency of Ca^{2+} Oscillations," Science 279(9 January 1998):227-230. See also: James W. Putney, Jr., "Calcium Signaling: Up, Down, Up, Down....What's the Point?" Science 279(9 January 1998):191-192.
1122. R.C. Dunbar, T.B. McMahon, "Activation of Unimolecular Reactions by Ambient Blackbody Radiation," Science 279(9 January 1998):194-197.
1123. John M. Bekkers, "Enhancement by Histamine of NMDA-Mediated Synaptic Transmission in the Hippocampus," Science 261(2 July 1993):104-106.
1124. T.J. Mitchison, "Localization of an Exchangeable GTP Binding Site at the Plus End of Microtubules," Science 261(20 August 1993):1044-1047.
1125. Ajay Verma, David J. Hirsch, Charles E. Glatt, Gabriele V. Ronnett, Solomon H. Snyder, "Carbon Monoxide: A Putative Neural Messenger," Science 259(15 January 1993):381-384.
1126. Christoph F. Schmidt, Karel Svoboda, Ning Lei, Irena B. Petsche, Lonny E. Berman, Cyrus R. Safinya, Gary S. Grest, "Existence of a Flat Phase in Red Cell Membrane Skeletons," Science 259(12 February 1993):952-955.
1127. Tania Ewing, "Genetic 'Master Switch' for Left-Right Symmetry Found," Science 260(30 April 1993):624-625.
1128. Gary Taubes, "Physicists Explore the Driplines," Science 260(25 June 1993):1874-1876.
1129. Min Zhuo, Scott A. Small, Eric R. Kandel, Robert D. Hawkins, "Nitric Oxide and Carbon Monoxide Produce Activity-Dependent Long-Term Synaptic Enhancement in Hippocampus," Science 260(25 June 1993):1946-1950.
1130. Richard A. Kerr, "Magnetism Triggers a Brain Response," Science 260(11 June 1993):1590.
1131. M.W. Chase, Jr., et al., J. Phys. Chem. Ref. Data 14(1985, Suppl. 1):1.
1132. Michelle Hoffman, "The Cell's Nucleus Shapes Up," Science 259(26 February 1993):1257-1259.
1133. Yigong Xing, Carol V. Johnson, Paul R. Dobner, Jeanne Bentley Lawrence, "Higher Level Organization of Individual Gene Transcription and RNA Splicing," Science 259(26 February 1993):1326-1330.
1134. Ronald Berezney, Donald S. Coffey, "Identification of a Nuclear Protein Matrix," Biochem. Biophys. Res. Commun. 60(1974):1410-1417.
1135. Kenneth C. Carter, Douglas Bowman, Walter Carrington, Kevin Fogarty, John A. McNeil, Fredric S. Fay, Jeanne Bentley Lawrence, "A Three-Dimensional View of Precursor Messenger RNA Metabolism Within the Mammalian Nucleus," Science 259(26 February 1993):1330-1335.
1136. C.W.M. Haest, "Interactions Between Membrane Skeleton Proteins and the Intrinsic Domain of the Erythrocyte Membrane," Biochim. Biophys. Acta 694(1982):331-352.
1137. John Travis, "Cell Biologists Explore Tiny Caves," Science 262(19 November 1993):1208-1209.
1138. James O. Deshler, Martin I. Highett, Bruce J. Schnapp, "Localization of Xenopus Vg1 mRNA by Vera Protein and the Endoplasmic Reticulum," Science 276 (16 May 1997):1128-1131.
1139. Michael J. Pazin, Purnima Bhargava, E. Peter Geiduschek, James T. Kadonaga, "Nucleosome Mobility and the Maintenance of Nucleosome Positioning," Science 276(2 May 1997):809-812.
1140. Colin Dingwall, Ronald Laskey, "The Nuclear Membrane," Science 258(6 November 1992):942-947.
1141. Danielle Hernandez-Verdun, Henriette R. Junera, "Chapter 4. The Nucleolus," in E. Edward Bittar, Neville Bittar, eds., Cellular Organelles, JAI Press, Greenwich CT, 1995, pp. 73-92.
1142. Carla M. Koehler, Ernst Jarosch, Kostas Tokatlidis, Karl Schmid, Rudolf J. Schweyen, Gottfried Schatz, "Import of Mitochondrial Carriers Mediated by Essential Proteins of the Intermembrane Space," Science 279(16 January 1998):369-373.
1143. Wadih Arap, Renata Pasqualini, Erkki Ruoslahti, "Cancer Treatment by Targeted Drug Delivery to Tumor Vasculature in a Mouse Model," Science 279(16 January 1998):377-380.
1144. For current tabulation and online access to Protein Data Bank data, see at: http://pdb.pdb.bnl.gov/ or at: http://www.rcsb.org. See also the "Image Library of Biological Macromolecules" at: http://www.imb-jena.de/IMAGE.html.
1145. T. Koritsanszky, R. Flaig, D. Zobel, H.-G. Krane, W. Morgenroth, P. Luger, "Accurate Experimental Electronic Properties of DL-Proline Monohydrate Obtained Within 1 Day," Science 279(16 January 1998):356-258.
1146. R. Allen Bowling, "A Theoretical Review of Particle Adhesion," in K.L. Mittal, ed., Particles on Surfaces I: Detection, Adhesion, and Removal, Plenum Press, NY, 1988, pp.129-142.
1147. Ronald S. Fearing, "Survey of Sticking Effects for Micro Parts Handling," in Proceedings of the 1995 IEEE/RSJ International Conference on Intelligent Robots and Systems, Volume 2, IEEE Computer Society Press, Los Alamitos CA, 1995.
1148. Fumihito Arai, Daisuke Ando, Toshio Fukuda, Yukio Nonoda, Tomoya Oota, "Micro Manipulation Based on Micro Physics Strategy Based on Attractive Force Reduction and Stress Measurement," in Proceedings of the 1995 IEEE/RSJ International Conference on Intelligent Robots and Systems, Volume 2, IEEE Computer Society Press, Los Alamitos CA, 1995.
1149. Jacob N. Israelachvili, Intermolecular and Surface Forces, Second Edition, Academic Press, NY, 1992.
1150. H. Yeh, J.S. Smith, "Fluidic self-assembly for the integration of GaAs light-emitting diodes on Si substrates," IEEE Photonics Technology Letters 6(June 1994):706-708.
1151. J. Lowell, A.C. Rose-Innes, "Contact electrification," Adv. Phys. 29(1980):947-1023.
1152. Kevin Kendall, "Adhesion: Molecules and Mechanics," Science 263(25 March 1994):1720-1725.
1153. W.R. Harper, Contact and Frictional Electrification, Clarendon Press, Oxford, 1967.
1154. R.G. Horn, D.T. Smith, "Contact Electrification and Adhesion Between Dissimilar Materials," Science 256(17 April 1992):362-364.
1155. K.L. Johnson, K. Kendall, A.D. Roberts, "Surface energy and the contact of elastic solids," Proc. Royal Soc. London Series A 324(1971):301-313.
1160. Manoj K. Chaudhury, George M. Whitesides, "Direct Measurement of Interfacial Interactions between Semispherical Lenses and Flat Sheets of Poly(dimethyl siloxane) and Their Chemical Derivatives," Langmuir 7(1991):1013-1025.
1162. Geoffrey V. F. Seaman, "Chapter 27. Electrokinetic Behavior of Red Cells," in Douglas MacN. Surgenor, ed., The Red Blood Cell, Second Edition, Volume II, Academic Press, NY, 1975, pp. 1135-1224.
1163. J.S. Rowlinson, B. Widom, Molecular Theory of Capillarity, Clarendon Press, Oxford, 1982.
1164. Joseph Morgan, Introduction to University Physics, Allyn and Bacon, Inc., Boston MA, 1963.
1165. Roger G. Horn, Jacob N. Israelachvili, "Direct measurement of structural forces between two surfaces in a nonpolar liquid," J. Chem. Phys. 75(1 August 1981):1400-1411.
1166. Jacob Israelachvili, Richard Pashley, "The hydrophobic interaction is long range, decaying exponentially with distance," Nature 300(1982):341-342.
1167. Mark R. Pederson, Jeremy Q. Broughton, "Nanocapillarity in Fullerene Tubules," Phys. Rev. Lett. 69(2 November 1992):2689-2692.
1168. E. Dujardin, T.W. Ebbesen, H. Hiura, K. Tanigaki, "Capillarity and Wetting of Carbon Nanotubes," Science 265(23 September 1994):1850-1852.
1169. D. Ugarte, A. Chatelain, W.A. de Heer, "Nanocapillarity and Chemistry in Carbon Nanotubes," Science 274(13 December 1996):1897-1899.
1170. Thomas W. Ebbesen, "Wetting, Filling and Decorating Carbon Nanotubes," J. Phys. Chem. Solids 57(1996):951-955.
1171. P.G. de Gennes, "Wetting: statics and dynamics," Rev. Mod. Physics 57(1985):827-863.
1172. Jianping Gao, W.D. Luedtke, Uzi Landman, "Nano-Elastohydrodynamics: Structure, Dynamics, and Flow in Nanouniform Lubricated Junctions," Science 270 (27 October 1995):605-608.
1173. Robert E. Tuzun, Donald W. Noid, Bobby G. Sumpter, Ralph C. Merkle, "Dynamics of fluid flow inside carbon nanotubes," Nanotechnology 7(1996):241-246.
1174. Robert E. Tuzun, Donald W. Noid, Bobby G. Sumpter, Ralph C. Merkle, "Dynamics of He/C_{60} flow inside carbon nanotubes," Nanotechnology 8(1997):112-118.
1175. Newton E. Harvey, W.D. McElroy, A.H. Whiteley, "On Cavity Formation in Water," J. Appl. Phys. 18(February 1947):162-172.
1176. Richard M. Holman, Wilfred W. Robbins, A Textbook of General Botany, Second Edition, John Wiley & Sons, NY, 1928.
1177. M. Reza Ghadiri, Juan R. Granja, Lukas K. Buehler, "Artificial transmembrane ion channels from self-assembling peptide nanotubes," Nature 369(26 May 1994):301-304; 276-277.
1178. V. Zarybnicky, "Mechanism of T-Even DNA Ejection," J. Theoret. Biol. 22(1969):33-42.
1179. B.F. Poglazov, Morphogenesis of T-Even Bacteriophages, S. Karger, NY, 1973.
1180. Christopher K. Mathews, Elizabeth M. Kutter, Gisela Mosig, Peter B. Berget, Bacteriophage T4, American Society for Microbiology, Washington DC, 1983.
1181. D.L.D. Caspar, "Movement and self-control in protein assemblies. Quasi-equivalence revisited," Biophys. J. 32(1980):103-135.
1182. R. Kilkson, M.F. Maestre, "Structure of T-2 Bacteriophage," Nature 195(1962):494-495.
1183. Sabine A. Lauer, Pradipsinh K. Rathod, Nafisa Ghori, Kasturi Haldar, "A Membrane Network for Nutrient Import in Red Cells Infected with the Malaria Parasite," Science 276(16 May 1997):1122-1125.
1185. C.R. Thomas, M. Al-Rubeai, Z. Zhang, "Prediction of mechanical damage to animal cells in turbulence," Cytotechnology 15(1994):329-335.

1186. J.T. Davies, Turbulence Phenomena, Academic Press, NY, 1972.
1187. O. Reynolds, "An experimental investigation of the circumstances which determine whether the motion of water shall be direct or sinuous, and of the law of resistance in parallel channels," Phil. Trans. Roy. Soc. 174(1883):935-982.
1188. M.A. Tenan, S. Hackwood, G. Beni, "Friction in Capillary Systems," J. Appl. Phys. 53(1982):6687-6692.
1189. S.J. Singer, Garth L. Nicolson, "The Fluid Mosaic Model of the Structure of Cell Membranes," Science 175(18 February 1972):720-731.
1190. R.T. Yen, L. Foppiano, "Elasticity of small pulmonary veins in the cat," J. Biomech. Eng. Trans. ASME 103(1981):38-42.
1191. Martin Schnorf, Ingo Potrykus, Gunther Neuhaus, "Microinjection Technique: Routine System for Characterization of Microcapillaries by Bubble Pressure Measurement," Experimental Cell Research 210(1994):260-267.
1192. Julio E. Celis, "Microinjection of somatic cells with micropipettes: comparison with other transfer techniques," Biochem. J. 223(1984):281-291.
1193. Steven M. Jones, Kathryn E. Howell, John R. Henley, Hong Cao, Mark A. McNiven, "Role of Dynamin in the Formation of Transport Vesicles from the Trans-Golgi Network," Science 279(23 January 1998):573-577.
1194. Tatyana M. Svitkina, Alexander B. Verkhovsky, Gary G. Borisy, "Plectin Sidearms Mediate Interaction of Intermediate Filaments with Microtubules and Other Components of the Cytoskeleton," J. Cell Biol. 135(1996):991-1007.
1195. V. Kislov, V. Kolesov, I. Taranov, A. Saskovets, "Mechanical features of the SPM microprobe and nanoscale mass detector," Nanotechnology 8(1997):126-131.
1196. John A. Rogers, Rebecca J. Jackman, George M. Whitesides, "Constructing Single- and Multiple-Helical Microcoils and Characterizing Their Performance as Components of Microinductors and Microelectromagnets," J. Microelectromech. Syst. 6(September 1997):184-192.
1197. Paul B. Koeneman, Ilene J. Busch-Vishniac, Kristin L. Wood, "Feasibility of Micro Power Supplies for MEMS," J. Microelectromech. Syst. 6(September 1997):355-362.
1198. Florian Lang, Siegfried Waldegger, "Regulating Cell Volume," American Scientist 85(September-October 1997):456-463.
1199. Ralph C. Merkle, "Binding sites for use in a simple assembler," Nanotechnology 8(1997):23-28.
1200. Charles W. Bauschlicher Jr., Alessandra Ricca, Ralph Merkle, "Chemical storage of data," Nanotechnology 8(1997):1-5.
1201. K.J. Pienta, D.S. Coffey, "Cellular Harmonic Information Transfer Through A Tissue Tensegrity-Matrix System," Medical Hypotheses 34(1991):88-95.
1202. G. Forgacs, "On the possible role of cytoskeletal filamentous networks in intracellular signaling: an approach based on percolation," J. Cell Sci. 108(1995):2131-2143.
1203. Charles S. Peskin, Garrett M. Odell, George F. Oster, "Cellular Motions and Thermal Fluctuations: The Brownian Ratchet," Biophys. J. 65(July 1993):316-324.
1204. J.G. Chu, Z.Y. Hua, "The statistical theory of turbomolecular pumps," J. Vac. Sci. Tech. 20(1982):1101-1104.
1205. A. Richter, A. Plettner, K.A. Hofmann, H. Sandmaier, "A micromachined electrohydrodynamic (EHD) pump," Sensors and Actuators 29A(1991):159-168.
1206. A. Richter, A. Plettner, K.A. Hofmann, H. Sandmaier, "Electrohydrodynamic Pumping and Flow Measurement," MEMS-4 IEEE, New York, 1991, pp. 271-276.
1207. Axel Richter, Hermann Sandmaier, "An Electrohydrodynamic Micropump," in MEMS-3 (1990):99-104.
1208. Otmar M. Stuetzer, "Ion Drag Pumps," J. Appl. Phys. 31(January 1960):136-146.
1209. William F. Pickard, "Ion Drag Pumping. I. Theory," J. Appl. Phys. 34(1963):246-250; "Ion Drag Pumping. II. Experiment," J. Appl. Phys. 34(1963):251-258.
1210. J.R. Melcher, U.S. Firebaugh, "Traveling wave bulk electroconvection induced across a temperature gradient," Physics of Fluids 10(1967):1178-1185.
1211. S.F. Bart, L.S. Tavrow, M. Mehregany, J.H. Lang, "Microfabricated electrohydrodynamic pumps," Sensors and Actuators 21-23A(1990):193-197.
1212. Gunter Fuhr, Rolf Hagedorn, Torsten Muller, Wolfgang Benecke, Bernd Wagner, "Microfabricated Electrohydrodynamic (EHD) Pumps for Liquids of Higher Conductivity," J. Microelectromech. Syst. 1(September 1992):141-146.
1213. D.J. Harrison, K. Seiler, A. Manz, Z. Fan, "Chemical analysis and electrophoresis systems integrated on glass and silicon chips," Digest of IEEE Solid State Sensor and Actuator Workshop, 1993, pp. 110-113. See also: D. Jed Harrison, Karl Fluri, Kurt Seiler, Zhonghui Fan, Carlo S. Effenhauser, Andreas Manz, "Micromachining a Miniaturized Capillary Electrophoresis-Based Chemical Analysis System on a Chip," Science 261(13 August 1993):895-897; H. Salimi-Moosavi, Thompson Tang, D. Jed Harrison, "Electroosmotic Pumping of Organic Solvents and Reagents in Microfabricated Reactor Chips," J. Am. Chem. Soc. 119(1997):8716-8717.
1214. R.M. Moroney, R.M. White, R.T. Howe, "Ultrasonically Induced Microtransport," MEMS-4 (1991):277-282.
1215. Shun-ichi Miyazaki, Takashi Kawai, Muneki Araragi, "A Piezo-Electric Pump Driven by a Flexural Progressive Wave," MEMS-4 (1991):283-288.
1216. Jan G. Smits, "Piezoelectric Micropump with Three Valves Working Peristaltically," Sensors and Actuators 21-23A(1990):203-206.
1217. A. Manz, J.C. Fettinger, E. Verpoorte, D.J. Harrison, H. Ludi, H.M. Widmer, "Design of integrated electroosmotic pumps and flow manifolds for total chemical analysis systems," Tech. Digest MME 1990 (Berlin), pp. 127-132; see also Tech. Digest IEEE Transducers 1991 (San Francisco), IEEE, New York, 1991, pp. 939-941.
1218. M. Himmelhaus, P. Bley, J. Mohr, U. Wallrabe, "Integrated measuring system for the detection of the revolutions of LIGA microturbines in view of a volumetric flow sensor," J. Micromech. Microeng. 2(1992):196-198.
1219. M. Elwenspoek, T.S.J. Lammerink, R. Miyake, J.H.J. Fluitman, "Towards integrated microliquid handling systems," J. Micromech. Microeng. 4(1994):227-245.
1220. Cecil D. Murray, "The Physiological Principle of Minimum Work. I. The Vascular System and the Cost of Blood Volume," Proc. Natl. Acad. Sci. (USA) 12(1926):207-214; see also: "The Physiological Principle of Minimum Work Applied to the Angle of Branching of Arteries," J. Gen. Physiol. 9(1926):835-841.
1221. Hirofumi Matsumoto, James E. Colgate, "Preliminary Investigations of Micropumping based on Electrical Control of Interfacial Tension," MEMS-3 (1990):107-110.
1222. Sheila H. DeWitt (Orchid Biocomputer, 201 Washington Road, Princeton, NJ 08543-2197), "Massively Parallel, Microfabricated Systems for High-Throughput Drug Discovery," Laboratory Robotics Interest Group (http://lab-robotics.org), February 1998 Meeting on Drug Discovery, Somerset Marriott Hotel, 25 February 1998. See also: http://www.orchidbio.com/.
1223. Jan H. Hoh, Ratneshwar Lal, Scott A. John, Jean-Paul Revel, Morton F. Arnsdorf, "Atomic Force Microscopy and Dissection of Gap Junctions," Science 253 (20 September 1991):1405-1408.
1225. Don E. Meyer, Robert Buchanan, eds., Biological Science, Second Edition, Harcourt, Brace & World, Inc., NY, 1968.
1226. Chao-Tsen Chen, Holger Wagner, W. Clark Still, "Fluorescent, Sequence-Selective Peptide Detection by Synthetic Small Molecules," Science 279(6 February 1998):851-853.
1227. See, for example, the NOR logic elements available from Air Logic Pneumatic Components and Systems; website at: http://www.air-logic.com/LogicControls.html.
1228. Emmanuel Delamarche, Andre Bernard, Heinz Schmid, Bruno Michel, Hans Biebuyck, "Patterned Delivery of Immunoglobulins to Surfaces Using Microfluidic Networks," Science 276(2 May 1997):779-781.
1229. Laura Capelli, Sergey V. Ermakov, Pier Giorgio Righetti, "Tunable positive and negative surface charges on a capillary wall: exploiting the Immobiline chemistry," J. Biochem. Biophys. Methods 32(1996):109-124.
1230. George F. Oster, Alan S. Perelson, "The Physics of Cell Motility," J. Cell Sci. Suppl. 8(1987):35-54.
1231. J.F. Wilson, D. Li, Z. Chen, R.T. George Jr., "Flexible Robot Manipulators and Grippers: Relatives of Elephant Trunks and Squid Tentacles," in Paolo Dario, Giulio Sandini, Patrick Aebischer, eds., Robots and Biological Systems: Towards a New Bionics, Springer-Verlag, New York, 1993, pp. 475-494.
1232. Koichi Suzumori, Shoichi Iikura, Hirohisa Tanaka, "Flexible Microactuator for Miniature Robots," MEMS-4 (1991), pp. 204-209.
1233. Shugen Ma, Shigeo Hirose, Hiroshi Yoshinada, "Development of a hyper-redundant multijoint manipulator for maintenance of nuclear reactors," Advanced Robotics 9(1995):281-300.
1234. Hiroyuki Noji, Ryohei Yasuda, Masasuke Yoshida, Kazuhiko Kinosita Jr., "Direct observation of the rotation of F_1-ATPase," Nature 386(20 March 1997):299-302.
1235. Jie Han, Al Globus, Richard Jaffe, Glenn Deardorff, "Molecular Dynamics Simulation of Carbon Nanotube Based Gears," Nanotechnology 8(September 1997):95-102.
1236. Deepak Srivastava, "A phenomenological model of the rotation dynamics of carbon nanotube gears with laser electric fields," Nanotechnology 8(1997):186-192.
1237. D. Stewart, "A Platform with Six Degrees of Freedom," The Institution of Mechanical Engineers, Proceedings 1965-66, 180 Part 1, No. 15, pp. 371-386.
1238. R.S. Stoughton, T. Arai, T., "A Modified Stewart Platform Manipulator with Improved Dexterity, IEEE Transactions on Robotics and Automation 9 (1993):166-173.
1239. Ralph C. Merkle, "A New Family of Six Degree Of Freedom Positional Devices," Nanotechnology 8(June 1997):47-52.
1240. Robert F. Valentini, Patrick Aebischer, "Chapter 42. Strategies for the Engineering of Peripheral Nervous Tissue Regeneration," in Robert P. Lanza, Robert Langer, William L. Chick, eds., Principles of Tissue Engineering, R.G. Landes Company, Georgetown TX, 1997, pp. 671-684.
1241. R.E. Rosensweig, Ferrohydrodynamics, Cambridge University Press, New York, 1985.
1242. Thomas C. Halsey, "Electrorheological Fluids," Science 258(30 October 1992):761-766.
1243. W.M. Winslow, "Induced fibration of suspensions," J. Appl. Phys. 20(1949):1137-1140.
1244. W.A. Bullough, "Electro-rheological fluids: an introduction for biomedical applications," J. Biomed. Eng. 13(May 1991):234-238.
1245. Lawrence C. Rome, Douglas A. Syme, Stephen Hollingworth, Stan L. Lindstedt, Stephen M. Baylor, "The whistle and the rattle: The design of sound producing muscles," Proc. Natl. Acad. Sci. USA 93(23 July 1996):8095-8100.
1246. Ivan Rayment et al., "Three-Dimensional Structure of Myosin Subfragment-1: A Molecular Motor," Science 261(2 July 1993):50-58; and "Structure of the Actin-Myosin Complex and Its Implications for Muscle Contraction," Science 261(2 July 1993):58-65.
1247. Scot C. Kuo, Michael P. Sheetz, "Force of Single Kinesin Molecules Measured with Optical Tweezers," Science 260(9 April 1993):232-234.

1248. Ulrich Dammer, Octavian Popescu, Peter Wagner, Dario Anselmetti, Hans-Joachim Guntherodt, Gradimir N. Misevic, "Binding Strength Between Cell Adhesion Proteoglycans Measured by Atomic Force Microscopy," Science 267(24 February 1995):1173-1175.
1249. Michael P. Koonce, Manfred Schliwa, "Bidirectional Organelle Transport Can Occur in Cell Processes That Contain Single Microtubules," J. Cell Biol. 100(1985):322-326.
1250. A.M. Flynn, "Gnat robots (and how they will change robotics)," Proc. IEEE Microrobotics and Teleoperators Workshop, Hyannis, MA, USA, 9-11 November 1987.
1251. Elisabeth Smela, Olle Inganas, Ingemar Lundstrom, "Controlled Folding of Micrometer-Size Structures," Science 268(23 June 1995):1735-1738.
1252. N. Tinbergen, Animal Behavior, Time Inc., NY, 1965.
1253. Richard Yeh, Ezekiel J.J. Kruglick, Kristofer S.J. Pister, "Surface-Micromachined Components for Articulated Microrobots," J. Microelectromech. Syst. 5(March 1996):10-17.
1254. J.-M. Breguet, Ph. Renaud, "A 4-degrees-of-freedom microrobot with nanometer resolution," Robotica 14(March/April 1996):199-203.
1255. Yutaka Tanaka, "Study of Artificial Rubber Muscle," Mechatronics 3(1993):59-75.
1256. Robert G. McNeil, Rogers C. Ritter, Bert Wang, Michael A. Lawson, George T. Gillies, Kevin G. Wika, Elizabeth G. Quate, Matthew A. Howard III, M. Sean Grady, "Functional Design Features and Initial Performance Characteristics of a Magnetic-Implant Guidance System for Stereotactic Neurosurgery," IEEE Trans. Biomed. Eng. 42(August 1995):793-801; and "Characteristics of an Improved Magnetic-Implant Guidance System," IEEE Trans. Biomed. Eng. 42(August 1995):802-808.
1257. J.A. Molloy et al., "Experimental determination of the force required for insertion of a thermoseed into deep brain tissues," Ann. Biomed. Eng. 18(May/June 1990):299-313.
1258. Thomas Hans Keller, Trevor Rayment, David Klenerman, Robert J. Stephenson, "Scanning near-field optical microscopy in reflection mode imaging in liquid," Rev. Sci. Instrum 68(March 1997):1448-1454.
1259. David Howie, Nanotechnology: Progress and Prospects, Oxford Nanotechnology PLC, August 1997; see at: http://www.oxfordnano.com.
1260. T.P. Flanagan, "Nanotechnology, bioscience and medicine: New scientific and industrial opportunities for the UK," Meas. Sci. Tech. 4(1993):1299-1300.
1261. D. Urry, "Elastic Biomolecular Machines," Scientific American 272(January 1995):44-49.
1262. Jose M. Rivera, Tomas Martin, Julius Rebek, Jr., "Chiral Spaces: Dissymmetric Capsules Through Self-Assembly," Science 279(13 February 1998):1021-1023.
1263. Daniel T. Chiu, Sheri J. Lillard, Richard H. Scheller, Richard N. Zare, Sandra E. Rodriguez-Cruz, Evan R. Williams, Owe Orwar, Mats Sandberg, J. Anders Lundqvist, "Probing Single Secretory Vesicles with Capillary Electrophoresis," Science 279(20 February 1998):1190-1193.
1264. Elizabeth Pennisi, "The Nucleus's Revolving Door," Science 279(20 February 1998):1129-1131.
1265. H. Quastler, "Studies of human channel capacity," in E.C. Cherry, ed., Information Theory -- Third London Symposium, Academic Press, New York, 1955, pp. 361-371.
1266. S.A. Kauffman, "Metabolic Stability and Epigenesis in Randomly Constructed Genetic Nets," J. Theoret. Biol. 22(1969):437-467.
1267. Chang-Jin Kim, Albert P. Pisano, Richard S. Muller, Martin G. Lim, "Polysilicon microgripper," Sensors and Actuators A 33(1992):221-227. See also: "Silicon-Processed Overhanding Microgripper," J. Microelectromech. Syst. 1(March 1992):31-36 and "Design, Fabrication and Testing of a Polysilicon Microgripper," Microstructures, Sensors, and Actuators, ASME, New York, DSC-19(1990):99-109.
1268. Diann E. Brei, James Blechschmidt, "Design and Static Modeling of a Semicircular Polymeric Piezoelectric Microactuator," J. Microelectromech. Syst. 1(September 1992):106-115.
1269. M. Elwenspoek, L. Smith, B. Hok, "Active joints for microrobot limbs," J. Micromech. Microeng. 2(1992):221-223.
1270. Shannon C. Ridgeway, Phillip D. Adsit, Carl D. Crane, "Development of an articulated transporter/manipulator system," Advanced Robotics 9(1995):301-316.
1271. W.K. Taylor, D. Lavie, I.I. Esat, "A curvilinear snake arm robot with gripper-axis fiber-optic image processor feedback," Intl. J. Robotics 1(1983):33-39.
1272. S. Hirose, Biologically Inspired Robots, Oxford University Press, Oxford, 1993.
1273. J.W. Burdick, J. Radford, G.S. Chirikjian, "A 'sidewinding' locomotion gait for hyper-redundant robots," Advanced Robotics 9(1995):195-216.
1274. Manabu Ataka, Akito Omodaka, Naohiro Takeshima, Hiroyuki Fujita, "Fabrication and Operation of Polyimide Bimorph Actuators for a Ciliary Motion System," J. Microelectromech. Syst. 2(December 1993):146-150.
1275. Melvin H. Miles, Benjamin F. Bush, Kendall B. Johnson, "Anomalous Effects in Deuterated Systems," Research amd Technology Division, U.S. Naval Air Warfare Center Weapons Division (China Lake, CA 93555-6100), Report NAWCWPNS TP 8302, September 1996, 98 pp.
1276. K.S. Shea, V. Samper, A.J. Sangster, R.L. Reuben, S.J. Yang, "An electrostatic harmonic microactuator for arterial plaque removal," J. Micromech. Microeng. 5(1995):297-304.
1277. T. Evans, "Chapter 13. Changes Produced by High Temperature Treatment of Diamond," in J.E. Field, ed., The Properties of Diamond, Academic Press, New York, 1979, pp. 403-424.
1278. M.M.J. Treacy, T.W. Ebbesen, J.M. Gibson, "Exceptionally high Young's modulus observed for individual carbon nanotubes," Nature 381(20 June 1996):678-680.
1279. Eric W. Wong, Paul E. Sheehan, Charles M. Lieber, "Nanobeam Mechanics: Elasticity, Strength, and Toughness of Nanorods and Nanotubes," Science 277(26 September 1997):1971-1975.
1280. Harry Bateman, "Elasticity," Encyclopedia Britannica 8(1963):107-114.
1281. A. Kelly, N.H. Macmillan, Strong Solids, Clarendon Press, Oxford U.K., 1986.
1282. W.B. Hillig, Modern Aspects of the Vitreous State, Butterworths, Washington DC, 1962.
1283. David A. Tirrell, "Putting a New Spin on Spider Silk," Science 271(5 January 1996):39-40.
1284. Antonio Regalado, "Another Step Toward a Diamond-Beater," Science 267(24 February 1995):1089.
1285. David M. Teter, Russell J. Hemley, "Low-Compressibility Carbon Nitrides," Science 271(5 January 1996):53-55.
1286. Michael Parkin, "Glass," Encyclopedia Britannica 10(1963):398-407.
1287. Albert John Phillips, "Lead," Encyclopedia Britannica 13(1963):820-824.
1288. Robert S. Williams, Victor O. Homerberg, Principles of Metallography, McGraw-Hill Book Company, NY, 1939.
1289. R. Stringham, R. George, "Cavitation Induced Solid State Production of Heat, He^3, and He^4," 209th American Chemical Society (ACS) National Meeting, 2-6 April 1995, Anaheim CA, Book of Abstracts, No. NUCL-044.
1290. T. Evans, P.F. James, "A study of the transformation of diamond to graphite," Proc. R. Soc. London A 277(1964):260-269.
1291. A.V. Hamza, G.D. Kubiak, R.H. Stulen, "The role of hydrogen on the diamond C(111)-(2x1) reconstruction," Surface Sci. 206(1988):L833-L844.
1292. C.A. Brookes, V.R. Howes, A.R. Parry, "Multiple slip in diamond due to a nominal contact pressure of 10 GPa at 1,000°C," Nature 332(1988):139-141.
1293. Michael Frenklach, Sergei Skokov, "Surface Migration in Diamond Growth," J. Phys. Chem. B 101(1997):3025-3036.
1294. J. Raloff, "EMFs Attract Controversy," Science News 153(28 February 1998):131, 141.
1295. Joan Zimmermann, ed., BMDO Technologies for Biomedical Applications, report prepared by the National Technology Transfer Center, Washington Operations for the Ballistic Missile Defense Organization, The Pentagon, Washington DC 20301-7100, 1997.
1296. David Kennedy, How To Save Your Teeth: Toxic-Free Preventive Dentistry, Health Action Press, Delaware OH, 1993.
1297. Ray H. Baughman, Sven Stafstrom, Changxing Cui, Socrates O. Dantas, "Materials with Negative Compressibilities in One or More Dimensions," Science 279(6 March 1998):1522-1524.
1298. Stephen H. Koslow, Michael F. Huerta, eds., Neuroinformatics: An Overview of the Human Brain Project, Erlbaum, Mahwah, NJ, 1997.
1301. Yoseph Bar-Cohen, "Artificial Muscles from Electrostrictive Polymers," in NASA-JPL Telerobotics Program Plan, 1996; see at: http://ranier.oact.hq.nasa.gov/telerobotics_page/FY96Plan/Chap2i.html.
1302. J.R. Bulgrin, B.J. Rubal, C.R. Thompson, J.M. Moody, "Comparison of short-time Fourier, wavelet and time domain analyses of intracardiac sounds," Biomedical Sciences Instrumentation 29(1993):465-472; J.R. Bulgrin, B.J. Rubal, "Time-Frequency Analysis of Heart Sounds," Scientific Computing and Automation (August 1994):15 et seq.
1303. Ralph Merkle, "Re Bacterial Motors and Nanotech," http://crit.org/critmail/sci_nano/1729.html.
1304. National Library of Medicine, Visible Human Project, http://www.nlm.nih.gov/research/visible/visible_human.html. See also the "Digital Anatomist Project," University of Washington, Seattle, WA, at: http://sig.biostr.washington.edu/projects/da.
1306. H. Hisakuni, K. Tanaka, "Optical Microfabrication of Chalcogenide Glasses," Science 270(10 November 1995):974-975.
1307. Michael Curry, Jeffrey Hobbs, Ronald Toub, "Will Using a Head Mounted Display Affect Pointing on Wearable Computers?" 2nd ACM International Conference on Mobile Computing and Networking (MobiCom 96), White Plains, NY, 11-12 November 1996. See also: http://www.cs.uoregon.edu/research/wearables/Papers/.
1308. Boris I. Yakobson, Richard E. Smalley, "Fullerene Nanotubes: $C_{1,000,000}$ and Beyond," American Scientist 85(July-August 1997):324-337.
1309. Slava Grebenev, J. Peter Toennies, Andrei F. Vilesov, "Superfluidity Within a Small Helium-4 Cluster: The Microscopic Andronikashvili Experiment," Science 279(27 March 1998):2083-2086.
1310. Thomas A. Herring, "The Global Positioning System," Scientific American 274(February 1996):44-50.
1311. Declan A. Doyle et al., "The Structure of the Potassium Channel: Molecular Basis of K^+ Conduction and Selectivity," Science 280(3 April 1998):69-76.
1312. H.L. Goldsmith, S.G. Mason, "Chapter 4. The Microrheology of Dispersions," in F.R. Eirich, ed., Rheology: Theory and Applications, Volume IV, Academic Press, NY, 1967, pp. 87-205.
1313. R. Fahraeus, "The suspension stability of blood," Physiol. Rev. 9(1929):241-274.
1314. S. Chien, "Shear dependence of effective cell volume as a determinant of blood viscosity," Science 168(1970):977-979.
1315. R.L. Whitmore, "A theory of blood flow in small vessels," J. Appl. Physiol. 22(1967):767-771.

1316. P.C. Hiemenz, Principles of Colloid and Surface Chemistry, Second Edition, Marcel Dekker, NY, 1986.
1317. H.L. Goldsmith, S.G. Mason, "The Flow of Suspensions Through Tubes. I. Single Spheres, Rods, and Discs," J. Colloid Sci. 17(1962):448-476.
1318. G.R. Cokelet, E.W. Merrill, E.R. Gilliland, H. Shin, A. Britten, R.E. Wells, "The rheology of human blood measurement near and at zero shear rate," Trans. Soc. Rheol. 7(1963):303-317.
1319. S.G. Mason, H.L. Goldsmith, "The Flow Behavior of Particulate Suspensions," in G.E.W. Wolstenholme, Julie Knight, eds., Circulatory and Respiratory Mass Transport, Little, Brown & Co., Boston, 1969, pp. 105-129.
1320. A. Karnis, H.L. Goldsmith, S.G. Mason, "The Flow of Suspensions Through Tubes. V. Inertial Effects," Can. J. Chem. Eng. 44(August 1966):181-193.
1321. G. Segre, A. Silberberg, "Behavior of macroscopic rigid spheres in Poiseuille flow. Part 2. Experimental results and interpretation," J. Fluid Mech. 14(1962):136-157.
1322. A. Karnis, H.L. Goldsmith, S.G. Mason, "The Kinetics of Flowing Dispersions. I. Concentrated Suspensions of Rigid Particles," J. Colloid Interface Sci. 22(1966):531-553.
1323. R. Fahraeus, T. Lindqvist, "The viscosity of the blood in narrow capillary tubes," Am. J. Physiol. 96(1931):562-568.
1324. J.H. Barbee, G.R. Cokelet, "The Fahraeus effect," Microvasc. Res. 3(1971):6-16; "Prediction of blood flow in tubes with diameters as small as 29 microns," Microvasc. Res. 3(1971):17-21.
1325. Shu Chien, "Chapter 26. Biophysical Behavior of Red Cells in Suspensions," in Douglas MacN. Surgenor, ed., The Red Blood Cell, Second Edition, Volume II, Academic Press, NY, 1975, pp. 1031-1133.
1326. A. Krogh, The Anatomy and Physiology of Capillaries, Yale University Press, New Haven, CT, 1922.
1327. G.R. Cokelet, "Blood rheology interpreted through the flow properties of the red cell," in J. Grayson, W. Zingg, eds., Microcirculation, Volume I, Plenum Press, New York, 1976, pp. 9-32.
1328. Shu Chien, Shunichi Usami, Richard Skalak, "Chapter 6. Blood flow in small tubes," Handbook of Physiology, Section 2: The Cardiovascular System, Volume IV, Microcirculation, Part I, American Physiological Society, Bethesda MD, 1984, pp. 217-249.
1329. P. Gaehtgens, "In vitro studies of blood rheology in microscopic tubes," in D.R. Gross, N.H.C. Hwang, eds., The Rheology of Blood, Blood Vessels, and Associated Tissues, Sijthoff & Noordhoff, Amsterdam, 1981, pp. 257-275.
1330. P. Gaehtgens, "Flow of blood through narrow capillaries: Rheological mechanisms determining capillary hematocrit and apparent viscosity," Biorheology 17(1980):183-189.
1331. S.M. Targ, Basic Problems of the Theory of Laminar Flow, Moskva, 1951. (in Russian)
1332. Giles R. Cokelet, "Chapter 14: The Rheology and Tube Flow of Blood," in Richard Skalak, Shu Chien, eds., Handbook of Bioengineering, McGraw-Hill, New York, 1987.
1333. G. Vejlens, "The distribution of leukocytes in the vascular system," Acta Pathol. Microbiol. Scand. Suppl. 33(1938):11-239.
1334. U. Nobis, A.R. Pries, P. Gaehtgens, "Rheological mechanisms contributing to WBC-margination," in U. Bagge, G.V.R. Born, P. Gaehtgens, eds., White Blood Cells: Morphology and Rheology as Related to Function, Martinus Nijhoff, The Hague, 1982, pp. 57-65.
1335. H.L. Goldsmith, S. Spain, "Margination of leukocytes in blood flow through small tubes," Microvasc. Res. 27(1984):204-222.
1336. U. Nobis, A.R. Pries, G.R. Cokelet, P. Gaehtgens, "Radial distribution of white cells during blood flow in small tubes," Microvasc. Res. 29(1985):295-304.
1337. A.A. Palmer, "Platelet and leukocyte skimming," Bibl. Anat. 9(1967):300-393.
1338. M.R. Beck, E.C. Eckstein, "Preliminary reports on platelet concentration in capillary tube flows of whole blood," Biorheology 17(1980):455-464.
1339. J.R. Casley-Smith, A.H. Vincent, "Variations in the numbers and dimensions of tissue channels after injury," Tissue Cell 12(1980):761-771.
1340. G.J. Tangelder, D.W. Slaaf, T. Arts, R.S. Reneman, "Wall shear rate in arterioles in vivo: Least estimates from platelet velocity profiles," Am. J. Physiol. 254(1988):H1059-H1064.
1341. H.C. Teirlinck, G.J. Tangelder, D.W. Slaaf, A.M.M. Muijtjens, T. Arts, R.S. Reneman, "Orientation and diameter distributions of rabbit blood platelets flowing in small arterioles," Biorheology 21(1984):317-331.
1342. G.J. Tangelder, D.W. Slaaf, H.C. Teirlinck, R.S. Reneman, "Distribution of blood platelets flowing in arterioles," Am. J. Physiol. 248(1985):H318-H323.
1343. E. Anczurowski, S.G. Mason, "Kinetics of Flowing Dispersions. III. Equilibrium Orientation of Rods and Disks (Experimental)," J. Colloid Interface Sci. 23(1967):533-546.
1344. Harry L. Goldsmith, "The Microrheology of Red Blood Cell Suspensions," J. Gen. Physiol. 52(1968):5S-27S.
1345. H.L. Goldsmith, S.G. Mason, "The flow of suspensions through tubes. III. Collisions of small uniform spheres," Proc. R. Soc. A 282(1964):569-591.
1346. Z.M. Ruggeri, "Mechanisms of shear-induced platelet adhesion and aggregation," Thromb. Haemostasis 70(1993):119-123.
1347. J.L. Moake, N.A. Turner, N.A. Stathopoulos, L. Nolasco, J.D. Hellums, "Shear-induced platelet aggregation can be mediated by vWF released from platelets, as well as by exogenous large or unusually large vWF multimers, requires adenosine diphosphate, and is resistant to aspirin," Blood 71(1988):1366-1374.
1348. J.L. Moake, N.A. Turner, N.A. Stathopoulos, L. Nolasco, J.D. Hellums, "Involvement of large plasma von Willebrand factor (vWF) multimers and unusually large vWF forms derived from endothelial cells in shear stress-induced platelet aggregation," J. Clin. Invest. 78(1986):1456-1461.
1349. Y. Ikeda, M. Murata, Y. Araki, K. Watanabe, Y. Ando, I. Itagaki, Y. Mori, M. Ichitani, K. Sakai, "Importance of fibrinogen and platelet membrane glycoprotein IIb/IIIa in shear-induced platelet aggregation," Thromb. Res. 51(1988):157-163.
1350. M.H. Kroll, J.D. Hellums, Z. Guo, W. Durante, K. Razdan, J.K. Hrbolich, A.I. Schafer, "Protein kinase C is activated in platelets subjected to pathological shear stress," J. Biol. Chem. 268(1993):3520-3524.
1351. Y. Ikeda, M. Handa, K. Kawano, T. Kamata, M. Murata, Y. Araki, H. Anbo, Y. Kawai, K. Watanabe, K. Sakai, Z.M. Ruggeri, "The role of von Willebrand factor and fibrinogen in platelet aggregation under varying shear stress," J. Clin. Invest. 87(1991):1234-1240.
1352. D.P. Giddens, C.K. Zarins, S. Glagov, "Response of arteries to near-wall fluid dynamic behavior," Appl. Mech. Rev. 43(1990):S98-S102.
1353. H.N. Mayrovitz, "The relationship between leukocytes and erythrocytes velocity in arterioles," in U. Bagge, G.V.R. Born, P. Gaehtgens, eds., White Blood Cells: Morphology and Rheology as Related to Function, Martinus Nijhoff, The Hague, 1982.
1354. P-I. Branemark, Intravascular Anatomy of Blood Cells in Man, Karger, Basel, 1971.
1355. U. Bagge, P-I. Branemark, "White blood cell rheology: An intravital study in man," Adv. Microcirc. 7(1977):1-17.
1356. G.W. Schmid-Schonbein, S. Usami, R. Skalak, S. Chien, "The interaction of leukocytes and erythrocytes in capillary and postcapillary vessels," Microvasc. Res. 19(1980):45-70.
1357. U. Bagge, A. Blixt, K-G. Strid, "The initiation of post-capillary margination of leukocytes: Studies in vitro on the influence of erythrocyte concentration and flow velocity," Int. J. Microcirc. Clin. Exp. 2(1983):215-222.
1358. Harry L. Goldsmith, Takeshi Karino, "Chapter 21. Flow-Induced Interactions of Blood Cells with the Vessel Wall," in Una S. Ryan, Endothelial Cells, Volume I, CRC Press, Boca Raton FL, 1988, pp. 139-171.
1359. Takeshi Karino, Harry L. Goldsmith, Mineo Motomiya, Shoji Mabuchi, Yasunori Sohara, "Flow Patterns in Vessels of Simple and Complex Geometries," in Edward F. Leonard, Vincent T. Turitto, Leo Vroman, eds., Blood in Contact with Natural and Artificial Surfaces, Annals N.Y. Acad. Sci. 516(1987):422-441.
1360. T. Karino, H.M. Kwong, H.L. Goldsmith, "Particle flow behavior in models of branching vessels. I. Vortices in 90° T-junctions," Biorheology 16(1979):231-248.
1361. T. Karino, H.L. Goldsmith, "Flow behavior of blood cells and rigid spheres in an annular vortex," Phil. Trans. Roy. Soc. London Ser. B 279(10 June 1977):413-445.
1362. T. Karino, H.L. Goldsmith, "Aggregation of human platelets in an annular vortex distal to a tubular expansion," Microvasc. Res. 17(1979):217-237.
1363. Takeshi Karino, Mineo Motomiya, "Flow visualization in isolated transparent natural blood vessels," Biorheology 20(1983):119-127.
1364. Mineo Motomiya, Takeshi Karino, "Flow patterns in the human carotid artery bifurcation," Stroke 15(1984):50-56.
1365. Takeshi Karino, Mineo Motomiya, "Flow through a venous valve and its implication in thrombogenesis," Thromb. Res. 36(1984):245-257.
1366. Takeshi Karino, Harry L. Goldsmith, "Particle flow behavior in models of branching vessels. II. Effects of branching angle and diameter ratio on flow patterns," Biorheology 22(1985):87-104.
1367. J. Lighthill, "Flagellar hydrodynamics," SIAM Review 18(1976):161-230.
1368. J.J.L. Higdon, "The hydrodynamics of flagellar propulsion: Helical waves," J. Fluid Mech. 94(1979):331-351.
1369. D.C. Guell, H. Brenner, R.B. Frankel, H. Hartman, "Hydrodynamic forces and band formation in swimming magnetotactic bacteria," J. Theoret. Biol. 135(1988):525-542.
1370. M. Ramia, D.L. Tullock, N. Phan-Thien, "The role of hydrodynamic interaction in the locomotion of microorganisms," Biophys. J. 65(1993):755-778.
1371. Z. Liu, K.D. Papadopoulos, "Unidirectional motility of *Escherischia coli* in restrictive capillaries," Appl. Environ. Microbiol. 61(1995):3567-3572.
1372. Martin L. Lenhardt, Ruth Skellett, Peter Wang, Alex M. Clarke, "Human Ultrasonic Speech Perception," Science 253(5 July 1991):82-85. See also: http://www.flantech.com/neuropho.htm.
1373. G.G. Stokes, "On the effect of the internal friction of fluids on the motion of pendulums," Trans. Cambridge Philosophical Soc. 9(1851):8; Mathematical and Physical Papers, Vol. 3, pp. 1-141.
1374. C.S. Yih, Fluid Mechanics: A Concise Introduction to the Theory, corrected edition, West River Press, Ann Arbor MI, 1977.
1375. E. Cunningham, "On the Velocity of Steady Fall of Spherical Particles through Fluid Medium," Proc. Royal Soc. London A 83(1910):357-365.
1376. J. Lighthill, Mathematical Biofluiddynamics, Soc. Indus. Appl. Math., Philadelphia PA, 1975.
1377. A.T. Chwang, T.Y. Wu, "A note on the helical movement of micro-organisms," Proc. Roy. Soc. Ser. B 178(1971):327-346.
1378. C.M. White, "The drag of cylinders in fluids at slow speeds," Proc. Roy. Soc. Ser. B 186(1946):472-479.
1379. J.R. Blake, "A spherical envelope approach to ciliary propulsion," J. Fluid Mech. 46(1971):199-208; "Infinite models for ciliary propulsion," J. Fluid Mech. 49(1971):209-222; "Self-propulsion due to oscillations on the surface of a cylinder at low Reynolds number," Bull. Aust. Math. Soc. 5(1971):255-264.

1380. D.V. Holberton, "Chapter 11. Locomotion of Protozoa and Single Cells," in R. McN. Alexander, G. Goldspink, eds., Mechanics and Energetics of Animal Locomotion, Chapman and Hall, London, 1977, pp. 279-332.
1381. Howard C. Berg, Robert A. Anderson, "Bacteria Swim by Rotating their Flagellar Filaments," Nature 245(1973):380-382.
1382. R.S. Fearing, "Micro Structures and Micro Actuators for Implementing Sub-millimeter Robots," in H.S. Tzou, T. Fukuda, eds., Precision Sensors, Actuators and Systems, Kluwer Academic Publishers, Boston MA, 1992, pp. 39-72.
1383. P. Greiff, B. Boxenhorn, T. King, L. Niles, "Silicon Monolithic Micromechanical Gyroscope," 1991 Intl. Conf. on Solid-State Sensors and Actuators (Transducers '91), San Francisco, CA, June 1991, pp. 966-968.
1385. Toshio Fukuda, Atsushi Kawamoto, Fumihito Arai, Hideo Matsuura, "Mechanism and Swimming Experiment of Micro Mobile Robot in Water," MEMS-7, 1994, pp. 273-278.
1386. S. Childress, Mechanics of Swimming and Flying, Cambridge University Press, Cambridge, UK, 1981.
1387. J. Happel, H. Brenner, Low Reynolds Number Hydrodynamics, Prentice-Hall, Englewood Cliffs, NJ, 1965.
1388. Howard A. Stone, Aravinthan D.T. Samuel, "Propulsion of Microorganisms by Surface Distortions," Phys. Rev. Lett. 77(4 November 1996):4102-4104.
1389. A. Shapere, F. Wilczek, Phys. Rev. Lett. 58(1987):2051-2054; J. Fluid Mech. 198(1989):557-585.
1390. R.P. Benedict, Fundamentals of Pipe Flow, John Wiley and Sons, New York, 1980.
1391. S.H. Lee, L.G. Leal, "Motion of a sphere in the presence of a plane interface. Part 2: An exact solution in bipolar coordinates," J. Fluid Mech. 98(1980):193-24.
1392. D.F. Katz, T.D. Bloom, R.H. BonDurant, "Movement of bull spermatozoa in cervical mucus," Bio. Reproduction 25(1981):931-937.
1393. H. Winet, "Wall drag on free-moving ciliated micro-organisms," J. Exp. Biol. 59(1973):753-766.
1394. Michael A. Sleigh, "Chapter 16. Cell Motility," in Bittar, ed., Cell Biology in Medicine, 1973, pp. 525-567.
1395. Howard C. Berg, "Dynamic properties of bacterial flagellar motors," Nature 249 (3 May 1974):77-79.
1396. L.D. Landau, E.M. Lifshitz, Fluid Mechanics, Pergamon Press, London, 1959.
1397. David F. Blair, "How Bacteria Sense and Swim," Annual Rev. Microbiol. 49(1995):489-522.
1398. V.T. Turitto, H.J. Weiss, "Red Cells: Their Dual Role in Thrombus Formation," Science 207(1 February 1980):541-543.
1399. R.M. Hochmuth, R.N. Marple, S.P. Sutera, "Capillary blood flow. 1. Erythrocyte deformation in glass capillaries," Microvasc. Res. 2(1970):409-419.
1400. Robert A. Freitas Jr., "Exploratory Design in Medical Nanotechnology: A Mechanical Artificial Red Cell," Artificial Cells, Blood Substitutes, and Immobil. Biotech. 26(1998):411-430. See also: http://www.foresight.org/Nanomedicine/Respirocytes.html.
1401. J. Gray, G.J. Hancock, "The propulsion of sea-urchin spermatozoa," J. Exp. Biol. 32(1955):802-814.
1402. G.R. Cokelet, M.A. Lichtman, "Rheology of leukocyte suspensions," in U. Bagge, G.V.R. Born, P. Gaehtgens, eds., White Blood Cells: Morphology and Rheology as Related to Function, Martinus Nijhoff, The Hague, 1982.
1403. Vicki Glaser, "Carbohydrate-Based Drugs Move CLoser to Market," Genetic Engineering News, 15 April 1998, pp. 1, 12, 32, 34.
1404. T. Karino, M. Motomiya, H.L. Goldsmith, "Flow patterns in model and natural vessels," in J.C. Stanley, ed., Biologic and Synthetic Vascular Prostheses, Grune & Stratton, New York, 1982.
1405. E.W. Knight-Jones, "Relations between metachronism and the direction of ciliary beat in Metazoa," Q. J. Micros. Sci. 95(1954):503-521.
1406. H. Machemer, "Ciliary activity and the origin of metachrony in *Paramecium*: Effects of increased viscosity," J. Exp. Biol. 57(1972):239-259.
1407. Jurgen Bereiter-Hahn, "I.1 Mechanical Principles of Architecture of Eukaryotic Cells," in J. Bereiter-Hahn, O.R. Anderson, W.-E. Reif, eds., Cytomechanics: The Mechanical Basis of Cell Form and Structure, Springer-Verlag, Berlin, 1987, pp. 3-30.
1408. M. Dembo, M. Maltrud, F. Harlow, "Numerical studies of unreactive contractile networks," Biophys. J. 50(1986):123-137.
1409. Christopher W. Akey, "Visualization of transport-related configurations of the nuclear pore transporter," Biophys. J. 58(August 1990):341-355.
1410. Carmen Perez-Terzic, Jason Pyle, Marisa Jaconi, Lisa Stehno-Bittel, David E. Clapham, "Conformational States of the Nuclear Pore Complex Induced by Depletion of Nuclear Ca^{2+} Stores," Science 273(27 September 1996):1875-1877.
1411. Evan Evans, Howard Bowman, Andrew Leung, David Needham, David Tirrell, "Biomembrane Templates for Nanoscale Conduits and Networks," Science 273 (16 August 1996):933-935.
1412. R. Waugh, E.A. Evans, "Thermoelasticity of red blood cell membrane," Biophys. J. 26(1979):115-132.
1413. E.A. Evans, R. Waugh, "Osmotic correction to elastic area compressibility measurements on red cell membrane," Biophys. J. 20(1977):307-313.
1414. D. Needham, R.S. Nunn, "Elastic deformation and failure of lipid bilayer membranes containing cholesterol," Biophys. J. 58(1990):997-1009.
1415. E.A. Evans, R. Waugh, L. Melnik, "Elastic area compressibility modulus of red cell membrane," Biophys. J. 16(1976):585-595.
1416. S.G. Shultz, "Volume Preservation: Then and Now," News in Physiol. Sci. 4(1989):169-172.
1417. L.E. Lanyon, A.E. Goodship, C.J. Pye, J.H. MacFie, "Mechanically adaptive bone remodeling," J. Biomechanics 15(1982):141-154.
1418. L.E. Lanyon, "Functional strain as a determinant for bone remodeling," Calcif. Tiss. Res. 36(1984):556-561.
1419. C.T. Rubin, L.E. Lanyon, "Regulation of bone mass by mechanical strain magnitude," Calcif. Tiss. Res. 37(1985):411-417.
1420. D.B. Jones, H. Nolte, J.-G. Scholubbers, E. Turner, D. Veltel, "Biochemical signal transduction of mechanical strain in osteoblastlike cells," Biomaterials 12(1991):101-110.
1421. R.P. Rand, "Mechanical properties of the red cell membrane. II. Viscoelastic breakdown of the membrane," Biophys. J. 4(1964):303-316.
1422. R. Skalak, A. Tozeren, R.P. Zarda, S. Chien, "Strain energy function of red blood cell membranes," Biophys. J. 13(1973):245-264.
1423. E. Schulze, M. Kirschner, "Microtubule dynamics in interphase cells," J. Cell Biol. 102(1986):1020-1031.
1424. R.B. Nicklas, "A quantitative comparison of cellular motile systems," Cell Motil. 4(1984):1-5.
1425. A. Ben-Ze'ev, "Cell shape, the complex cellular networks, and gene expression," J. Muscle Res. Cell Motil. 6(1985):23-53.
1426. A.S.G. Curtis, G.M. Seehar, "The control of cell division by tension or diffusion," Nature 274(1978):52-53.
1427. C. Yeh, G.A. Rodan, "Tensile forces enhance prostaglandin E synthesis in osteoblastic cells grown on collagen ribbons," Calcif. Tissue Int. 36(1984):S67-S71.
1428. C. Masters, "Interactions between glycolytic enzymes and components of the cytomatrix," J. Cell Biol. 99(1984):222s-225s.
1429. U. Tillmann, J. Bereiter-Hahn, "Relation of actin fibrils to energy metabolism of endothelial cells," Cell Tissue Res. 243(1986):579-585.
1430. Konrad Beck, "II.1 Mechanical Concepts of Membrane Dynamics: Diffusion and Phase Separation in Two Dimensions," in J. Bereiter-Hahn, O.R. Anderson, W.-E. Reif, eds., Cytomechanics: The Mechanical Basis of Cell Form and Structure, Springer-Verlag, Berlin, 1987, pp. 79-99.
1431. K. Jacobson, Y. Hou, Z. Derzko, J. Wojcieszyn, D. Organisciak, "Lipid lateral diffusion in the surface membranes of cells and in multibilayers formed from plasma membrane lipids," Biochemistry 20(1981):5268-5275.
1432. D.E. Koppel, M.P. Sheetz, M. Schindler, "Matrix control of protein diffusion in biological membranes," Proc. Natl. Acad. Sci. USA 78(1981):3576-3580.
1433. J.A. Bloom, W.W. Webb, "Lipid diffusibility in the intact erythrocyte membrane," Biophys. J. 42(1983):295-305.
1434. D.E. Golan, W. Veatch, "Lateral mobility of band 3 in the human erythrocyte membrane studied by fluorescence photobleaching recovery: evidence for control by cytoskeletal interactions," Proc. Natl. Acad. Sci. USA 77(1980):2537-2541.
1435. M. McCloskey, M. Poo, "Protein diffusion in cell membranes: some biological implications," Intern. Rev. Cytol. 87(1984):19-81.
1436. D.A. Pink, "Protein lateral movement in bilipid layers. Simulation studies of its dependence upon protein concentration," Biochim. Biophys. Acta 818(1985):200-204.
1437. R.D. Allen, D.G. Weiss, J.H. Hayden, D.T. Brown, H. Fujiwake, M. SImpson, "Gliding movement of and bidirectional transport along single native microtubules from squid axoplasm: evidence for an active role of microtubules in cytoplasmic transport," J. Cell Biol. 100(1985):1736-1752.
1439. R.H. Miller, R.J. Lasek, "Crossbridges mediate anterograde and retrograde vesicle transport along microtubules in squid axoplasm," J. Cell Biol. 101(1985):2181-2193.
1440. M. Schliwa, K.B. Pryzwansky, J. van Blerkom, "Implications of cytoskeletal interactions for cellular architecture and behavior," Philos. Trans. Roy. Soc. London B Biol. Sci. 299(1982):199-205.
1441. S. Sasaki, J.K. Stevens, N. Bodick, "Serial reconstruction of microtubule arrays within dendrites of the cat retinal ganglion cell: the cytoskeleton of a vertebrate dendrite," Brain Res. 259(1982):193-206.
1442. H. Stebbings, C. Hunt, "The nature of the clear zone around microtubules," Cell Tissue Res. 227(1982):609-617.
1443. H.C. MacGregor, H. Stebbings, "A massive system of microtubules associated with cytoplasmic movement in telotrophic ovarioles," J. Cell Sci. 6(March 1970):431-449.
1444. D.G. Weiss, G.W. Gross, "Intracellular transport in axonal microtubular domains. I. Theoretical considerations on the essential properties of a force generating mechanism," Protoplasma 114(1983):179-197.
1445. W.A. Voter, H.P. Erickson, "Electron microscopy of MAP 2 (microtubule associated protein 2)," J. Ultrastruct. Res. 80(1982):374-382.
1446. L. Cassimeris, P. Wadsworth, E.D. Salmon, "Dynamic instability and differential stability of cytoplasmic microtubules in human monocytes," in M. De Brabander, J. de Mey, eds., Microtubules and Microtubule Inhibitors, Elsevier, Amsterdam, 1985, pp. 119-125.
1447. T. Mitchison, M. Kirschner, "Dynamic instability of microtubule growth," Nature 312(1984):237-242.
1448. Dieter G. Weiss, George M. Langford, Robert D. Allen, "II.2 Implications of Microtubules in Cytomechanics: Static and Motile Aspects," in J. Bereiter-Hahn, O.R. Anderson, W.-E. Reif, eds., Cytomechanics: The Mechanical Basis of Cell Form and Structure, Springer-Verlag, Berlin, 1987, pp. 100-113.

1449. Michael E.J. Holwill, Peter Satir, "II.4 Generation of Propulsive Forces by Cilia and Flagella," in J. Bereiter-Hahn, O.R. Anderson, W.-E. Reif, eds., Cytomechanics: The Mechanical Basis of Cell Form and Structure, Springer-Verlag, Berlin, 1987, pp. 120-130.
1450. Y. Yano, T. Miki-Noumura, "Sliding velocity between outer doublet microtubules of sea-urchin sperm axonemes," J. Cell Sci. 44(1980):169-186.
1451. C.B. Lindemann, W.G. Rudd, R. Rikmenspoel, "The stiffness of the flagella of impaled bull sperm," Biophys. J. 13(1973):437-448.
1452. R.P. Rand, A.C. Burtun, "Mechanical Properties of the Red Cell Membrane. I. Membrane Stiffness and Intracellular Pressure," Biophys. J. 4(1964):115-135.
1453. D.B. Lairand, N.B. Matveeva, V.A. Teplov, S.I. Beylina, "The role of elastoosmotic parameters in locomotion of myxomycete plasmodia," Acta Protozool. 11(1972):339-354.
1454. Michal Opas, "V.3 The Transmission of Forces Between Cells and Their Environment," in J. Bereiter-Hahn, O.R. Anderson, W.-E. Reif, eds., Cytomechanics: The Mechanical Basis of Cell Form and Structure, Springer-Verlag, Berlin, 1987, pp. 273-285.
1455. M.A. Hubbe, "Adhesion and detachment of biological cells in vitro," Prog. Surf. Sci. 11(1981):65-138.
1456. M. Opas, L. Kalinina, "Comparison of locomotion and adhesion in four strains of *Amoeba proteus*," Acta Protozool. 19(1980):339-344.
1457. C.S. Izzard, L.R. Lochner, "Formation of cell-to-substrate contacts during fibroblast motility: an interference-reflexion study," J. Cell Sci. 42(1980):81-116.
1458. K.-L.P. Sung, L.A. Sung, M. Crimmins, S.J. Burakoff, S. Chien, "Determination of Junction Avidity of Cytolytic T Cell and Target Cell," Science 234(1986):1405-1408.
1459. K.-L.P. Sung, L.A. Sung, M. Crimmins, S.J. Burakoff, S. Chien, "Biophysical basis of cell killing by cytotoxic T lymphocytes," J. Cell Sci. 91(1988):179-189.
1460. J.R. Blake, M.A. Sleigh, "Mechanics of ciliary locomotion," Biol. Rev. 49(1974):85-125.
1461. D.W. James, J.F. Taylor, "The stress developed by sheets of chick fibroblasts in vitro," Exp. Cell Res. 54(1969):107-110.
1462. R.J. Goldacre, "The role of the cell membrane in the locomotion of *Amoebae* and the source of the motive force and its control by feedback," Exp. Cell Res. 8(1961):1-16.
1463. Arthur Forer, "Chapter 23. Chromosome movements during cell-division," in A. Lima-de-Faria, ed., Handbook of Molecular Cytology, Volume 15, North Holland Publ. Co., Amsterdam, 1969, pp. 553-601.
1464. M. Haberey, "Cinematography of cell membrane behavior and flow phenomena in *Amoeba proteus*," Acta Protozoologica 11(1972):95-102.
1465. L. Wolpert, C.M. Thompson, C.H. O'Neill; in R.D. Allen, N. Kamiya, eds., Primitive Motile Systems in Cell Biology, Academic Press, New York, 1964, pp. 143-172.
1466. H. Komnick, W. Stockem, K.E. Wohlfarth-Bottermann, "Cell Motility: Mechanisms in Protoplasmic Streaming and Amoeboid Movement," Int. Rev. Cytol. 34(1973):169-252.
1467. E.J. Ambrose, J.A. Forrester, "Electrical phenomena associated with cell movements," Symposia of the Society for Experimental Biology 22(1968):237-248.
1468. Marileen Dogterom, Bernard Yurke, "Measurement of the Force-Velocity Relation for Growing Microtubules," Science 278(31 October 1997):856-860.
1469. R.D. Allen, "The consistency of amoeba cytoplasm and its bearing on the mechanism of amoeboid movement. II. The effects of centrifugal acceleration observed in the centrifuge microscope," J. Biophys. Biochem. Cytol. 8(1960):379-397.
1470. K. Yagi, "The mechanical and colloidal properties of *Amoeba* protoplasm and their relations to the mechanism of amoeboid movement," Comp. Biochem. Physiol. 3(1961):73-91.
1471. N. Kamiya; in R.D. Allen, N. Kamiya, eds., Primitive Motile Systems in Cell Biology, Academic Press, New York, 1964, pp. 257-278.
1472. D. Nichols, (tube feet papers), Quart. J. Microsc. Sci. 100(1959):73-87, 100(1959):539-555, 101(1960):105-117, and 102(1961):157-180.
1473. J.B. Buchanan, J.D. Woodley, "Extrusion and retraction of the tube-feet of Ophiuroids," Nature 197(1963):616-617.
1474. J.D. Woodley, (Ophiuroid water-vascular system); in N. Millott, ed., Echinoderm Biology, Academic Press, London, 1967, pp. 75-104.
1475. J.E. Smith, (tube feet of starfish), Phil. Trans. Roy. Soc. B 232(1946):279-310.
1476. A. Kusumi, Y. Sako, M. Yamamoto, "Confined lateral diffusion of membrane receptors as studied by single particle tracking (nanovid microscopy). Effects of calcium-induced differentiation in cultured epithelial cells," Biophys. J. 65(1993):2021-2040.
1477. Yasushi Sako, Akihiro Kusumi, "Barriers for Lateral Diffusion of Transferrin Receptor in the Plasma Membrane as Characterized by Receptor Dragging by Laser Tweezers: Fence vs. Tether," J. Cell Biol. 129(June 1995):1559-1574.
1478. Y. Sako, A. Kusumi, "Compartmentalized structure of the plasma membrane for lateral diffusion of receptors as revealed by nanometer-level motion analysis," J. Cell Biol. 125(1994):1251-1264.
1479. Michael Edidin, Scot C. Kuo, Michael P. Sheetz, "Lateral Movements of Membrane Glycoproteins Restricted by Dynamic Cytoplasmic Barriers," Science 254(1991):1379-1382.
1480. R. Simpson, B. Yang, P. Doherty, S. Moore, F. Walsh, K. Jacobson, "The Mosaic Structure of Cell Membranes Revealed by Transient Confinement of GPI-Linked NCAM-125," Biophys. J. 68(February 1995):A436.
1481. Philip L. Yeagle, "Chapter 3. The Dynamics of Membrane Lipids," in Philip Yeagle, ed., The Structure of Biological Membranes, CRC Press, Boca Raton, 1992, pp. 157-174.
1482. Michael Edidin, "Chapter 12. Translational Diffusion of Membrane Proteins," in Philip Yeagle, ed., The Structure of Biological Membranes, CRC Press, Boca Raton, 1992, pp. 539-567.
1483. Richard J. Cherry, "Chapter 11. Membrane Protein Dynamics: Rotational Dynamics," in Philip Yeagle, ed., The Structure of Biological Membranes, CRC Press, Boca Raton, 1992, pp. 507-537.
1484. James J. Campbell, Joseph Hedrick, Albert Zlotnik, Michael A. Siani, Darren A. Thompson, Eugene C. Butcher, "Chemokines and the Arrest of Lymphocytes Rolling Under Flow Conditions," Science 279(16 January 1998):381-384.
1485. Paul T. Englund,"The Structure and Biosynthesis of Glycosyl Phosphatidylinositol Protein Anchors," Annu. Rev. Biochem. 62(1993):121-138.
1486. Jeff Koechling, Marc H. Raibert, "How Fast Can a Legged Robot Run?" in Paolo Dario, Giulio Sandini, Patrick Aebischer, eds., Robots and Biological Systems: Towards a New Bionics, Springer-Verlag, New York, 1993, pp. 239-269.
1488. Eliot R. Clarke, Eleanor Linton Clarke, "Observations on Changes in Blood Vascular Endothelium in the Living Animal," Amer. J. Anat. 57(1935):385-438.
1489. J.V. Hurley, "An Electron Microscopic Study of Leucocytic Emigration and Vascular Permeability in Rat Skin," Austral. J. Exp. Biol. 41(1963):171-186.
1490. M.E. Smith, W.L. Ford, "The recirculating lymphocyte pool of the rat: a systematic description of the migratory behavior of recirculating lymphocytes," Immunology 49(1983):83-94.
1491. Una S. Ryan, "Chapter 30. Endothelial Cells," in John H. Barker, Gary L. Anderson, eds., Clinically Applied Microcirculation Research, CRC Press, Boca Raton FL, 1995, pp. 407-418.
1492. Stanley Davis, "Chapter 16. Biomedical Applications of Particle Engineering," in Richard R.H. Coombs, Dennis W. Robinson, eds., Nanotechnology in Medicine and the Biosciences, Gordon & Breach Publishers, Netherlands, 1996, pp. 243-262.
1493. Werner W. Franke, Pamela Cowin, Christine Grund, Caecilia Kuhn, Hans-Peter Kapprell, "The Endothelial Junction: The Plaque and Its Components," in Nicolae Simionescu, Maya Simionescu, eds., Endothelial Cell Biology in Health and Disease, Plenum Press, New York, 1988, pp. 147-166.
1494. Stephen M. Schwartz, Ronald L. Heimark, Mark W. Majesky, "Developmental Mechanisms Underlying Pathology of Arteries," Physiol. Rev. 70(October 1990):1177-1209.
1495. Timothy A. Springer, "Traffic Signals on Endothelium for Lymphocyte Recirculation and Leukocyte Emigration," Annu. Rev. Physiol. 57(1995):827-872.
1496. Joseph A. Madri, Bruce M. Pratt, Judith Yannariello-Brown, "Endothelial Cell-Extracellular Matrix Interactions: Matrix as a Modulator of Cell Function," in Nicolae Simionescu, Maya Simionescu, eds., Endothelial Cell Biology in Health and Disease, Plenum Press, New York, 1988, pp. 167-188.
1497. M. van der Rest, P. Bruckner, "Collagens: Diversity at the Molecular and Supramolecular Levels," Curr. Opin. Cell. Biol. 3(1993):430-436.
1498. D.J. Prockop, K.I. Kivirikko, "Collagens: Molecular Biology, Diseases, and Potentials for Therapy," Ann. Rev. Biochem. 64(1995):403-434.
1499. R.B. Vernon, J.C. Angello, M.L. Iruela-Arispe, et al., "Reorganization of basement membrane matrices by cellular traction promotes the formation of cellular networks in vitro," Lab. Invest. 66(1992):536-547.
1501. D. Mooney, L. Hansen, J. Vacanti, et al., "Switching from differentiation to growth in hepatocytes: control by extracellular matrix," J. Cell Physiol. 151(1992):497-505.
1502. B.J. Spargo, M.A. Testoff, T.B. Nielsen, et al., "Spatially controlled adhesion, spreading, and differentiation of endothelial cells on self-assembled molecular monolayers," Proc. Natl. Acad. Sci. USA 91(1994):11070-11074.
1503. G. Bauriedel, U. Windstetter, S.J. DeMaio, R. Kandolf, B. Hofling, "Migratory activity of human smooth muscle cells cultivated from coronary and peripheral primary and restenotic lesions removed by percutaneous atherectomy," Circulation 85(1992):554-564.
1505. Herbert H. Lipowsky, Dorethea Riedel, Guo Shan Shi, "In Vivo Mechanical Properties of Leukocytes During Adhesion to Venular Endothelium," Biorheology 28(1991):53-64.
1506. Jingdong Liu, Bertold Schrank, Robert H. Waterston, "Interaction Between a Putative Mechanosensory Membrane Channel and a Collagen," Science 273 (19 July 1996):361-364.
1507. David A. Jones, C. Wayne Smith, Larry V. McIntire, "Leucocyte adhesion under flow conditions: principles important in tissue engineering," Biomaterials 17(1996):337-347.
1508. K.-L.P. Sung, M.M. Frojmovic, T.E. O'Toole, Zhu Cheng, M.H. Ginsberg, "Determination of adhesion force between single cell pairs generated by activated GpIIb-IIIa receptors," Blood 81(1993):419-423.
1509. M.B. Lawrence, T.A. Springer, "Leukocytes roll on a selectin at physiologic flow rates: distinction from and prerequisite for adhesion through integrins," Cell 65(1991):859-873.

1510. B.J. Hughes, J.C. Hollers, E. Crockett-Torabi, C.W. Smith, "Recruitment of CD11b/CD18 to the neutrophil surface and adherence-dependent cell locomotion," J. Clin. Invest. 90(1992):1687-1696.
1511. Alan F. Horwitz, "Integrins and Health," Scientific American 276(May 1997):68-75.
1512. W. Heagy, M. Laurance, E. Cohen, R. Finberg, "Neurohormones regulate T-cell function," J. Exp. Med. 171(1990):1625-1633.
1513. G.B. Stefano, M.A. Shipp, B. Scharrer, "A possible immunoregulatory function for Met-enkephalin-Arg^6-Phe^7 involving human and invertebrate granulocytes," J. Neuroimmunology 31(February 1991):97-103.
1515. P. Sacerdote, M.R. Ruff, C.B. Pert, "Cholecystokinin and the immune system: receptor-mediated chemotaxis of human and rat monocytes," Peptides 9(1988, Suppl. 1):29-34.
1516. H.U. Keller, A. Zimmermann, H. Cottier, "Cell Shape, Movement, and Chemokinesis," Advances in the Biosciences 66(1987):21-27.
1517. A. Maureen Rouhi, "Nanotechnology -- from the ACS meeting," C&EN (20 April 1998):57-62.
1518. "Star Wars Technology Targets Tumors," BMDO Update (Spring 1998):10.
1519. Oscar Khaselev, John A. Turner, "A Monolithic Photovoltaic-Photoelectrochemical Device for Hydrogen Production via Water Splitting," Science 280(17 April 1998):425-427.
1520. Alan R. Fersht, "Sieves in Sequence," Science 280(24April 1998):541.
1522. Wuzong Zhou et al., "Ordering of Ruthenium Cluster Carbonyls in Mesoporous Silica," Science 280(1 May 1998):705-708.
1523. T.J. Mason, J.P. Lorimer, Sonochemistry: Theory, Applications and Uses of Ultrasound in Chemistry, Halsted Press, New York, 1988.
1524. Samuel F. McKay, "Expansion of Annealed Pyrolytic Graphite," J. Appl. Phys. 35(1964):1992-1993.
1525. Jie Liu et al., "Fullerene Pipes," Science 280(22 May 1998):1253-1256.
1526. Philip Morrison, "Double Bass Redoubled," Scientific American 278(May 1998):109, 111.
1527. Robin E. Bell, "Gravity Gradiometry," Scientific American 278(June 1998):74-79.
1528. S. Milius, "Red-flashing fish have chlorophyll eyes," Science News 153(6 June 1998):359.
1529. Angus I. Lamond, William C. Earnshaw, "Structure and Function in the Nucleus," Science 280(24 April 1998):547-553.
1530. Chavela M. Carr, Peter S. Kim, "Flu Virus Invasion: Halfway There," Science 266(14 October 1994):234-236.
1531. Y.N. Vaishnav, F. Wong-Staal, "The biochemistry of AIDS," Annu. Rev. Biochem. 60(1991):577-630.
1532. Yeon Gyu Yu, David S. King, Yeon-Kyun Shin, "Insertion of a Coiled-Coil Peptide from Influenza Virus Hemagglutinin into Membranes," Science 266(14 October 1994):274-276.
1533. Robert J. Geraghty, Claude Krummenacher, Gary H. Cohen, Roselyn J. Eisenberg, Patricia G. Spear, "Entry of Alphaherpesviruses Mediated by Poliovirus Receptor-Related Protein 1 and Poliovirus Receptor," Science 280(5 June 1998):1618-1620.
1534. Richard A. Steinhardt, Guoqiang Bi, Janet M. Alderton, "Cell Membrane Resealing by a Vesicular Mechanism Similar to Neurotransmitter Release," Science 263(21 January 1994):390-393.
1535. John Travis, "Stepping Out With Kinesin," Science 261(27 August 1993):1112-1113.
1536. Nobutaka Hirokawa, "Kinesin and Dynein Superfamily Proteins and the Mechanism of Organelle Transport," Science 279(23 January 1998):519-526.
1537. Richard A.F. Clark, "Chapter 46. Wound Repair: Lessons for Tissue Engineering," in Robert P. Lanza, Robert Langer, William L. Chick, eds., Principles of Tissue Engineering, R.G. Landes Company, Georgetown TX, 1997, pp. 737-768.
1538. Anne J. Ridley, Alan Hall, "The Small GTP-Binding Protein Rho Regulates the Assembly of Focal Adhesions and Actin Stress Fibers in Response to Growth Factors," Cell 70(1992):389-399.
1539. Alan Hall, "Rho GTPases and the Actin Cytoskeleton," Science 279(23 January 1998):509-514.
1540. A.J. Ridley, H.F. Paterson, C.L. Johnston, D. Diekmann, A. Hall, "The small GTP-binding protein rac regulates growth factor-induced membrane ruffling," Cell 70(7 August 1992):401-410.
1541. C.D. Nobes, A. Hall, "Rho, race, and cdc42 GTPases regulate the assembly of multimolecular focal complexes associated with actin stress fibers, lamellipodia, and filopodia," Cell 81(7 April 1995):53-62.
1542. R. Kozma, S. Ahmed, A. Best, L. Lim, "The Ras-related protein Cdc42Hs and bradykinin promote formation of peripheral actin microspikes and filopodia in Swiss 3T3 fibroblasts," Mol. Cell. Biol. 15(April 1995):1942-1952.
1543. Elaine Fuchs, Don W. Cleveland, "A Structural Scaffolding of Intermediate Filaments in Health and Disease," Science 279(23 January 1998):514-519.
1544. Janine R. Maddock, Lucille Shapiro, "Polar Location of the Chemoreceptor Complex in the *Escherichia coli* Cell," Science 259(1993):1717-1723.
1545. Julie A. Gegner, Daniel R. Graham, Amy F. Roth, Frederick W. Dahlquist, "Assembly of an MCP Receptor, CheW, and Kinase CheA Complex in the Bacterial Chemotaxis Signal Transduction Pathway," Cell 70(1992):975-982.
1546. J.E. Segall, A. Ishihara, H.C. Berg, "Chemotactic signaling in filamentous cells of *Escherichia coli*," J. Bacteriol. 161(January 1985):51-59.
1547. Carol A. Erikson, "Chapter 2. Organization of Cells Into Higher Ordered Structures: The Role of the Epithelial-Mesenchymal Transformation in the Generation and Stabilization of Embryonic Tissues," in Robert P. Lanza, Robert Langer, William L. Chick, eds., Principles of Tissue Engineering, R.G. Landes Company, Georgetown TX, 1997, pp. 9-22.
1548. L.A. Liotta, R. Mandler, G. Murano et al., "Tumor cell autocrine motility factor," Proc. Natl. Acad. Sci. (USA) 83(1986):3302-3306.
1549. A.-M. Grey, A.M. Schor, G. Rushton et al., "Purification of the migration stimulating factor produced by fetal and breast cancer patient fibroblasts," Proc. Natl. Acad. Sci. (USA) 86(1989):2438-2442.
1550. C.D. Roskelly, P.Y. Desprez, M.J. Bissell, "Extracellular matrix-dependent tissue-specific gene expression in mammary epithelial cells requires both physical and biochemical signal transduction," Proc. Natl. Acad. Sci. (USA) 91(1994):12378-12382.
1551. S. Cheng, W.S. Craig, D. Mullen et al., "Design and synthesis of novel cyclic RGD-containing peptides as highly potent and selective integrin $\alpha_{IIb}\beta_3$ antagonists," J. Med. Chem. 37(1994):1-8.
1552. W.E. Pullman, W.F. Bodmer, "Cloning and characterization of a gene that regulates cell adhesion," Nature 356(1992):529-532.
1553. Manuela Martins-Green, "Chapter 3. The Dynamics of Cell-ECM Interactions with Implications for Tissue Engineering," in Robert P. Lanza, Robert Langer, William L. Chick, eds., Principles of Tissue Engineering, R.G. Landes Company, Georgetown TX, 1997, pp. 23-46.
1554. Thomas F. Deuel, "Chapter 10. Growth Factors," in Robert P. Lanza, Robert Langer, William L. Chick, eds., Principles of Tissue Engineering, R.G. Landes Company, Georgetown TX, 1997, pp. 133-149.
1555. R. Singhvi, A. Kumar, G. Lopez, et al., "Engineering Cell Shape and Function," Science 264(1994):696-698.
1556. William E. Paul, "Infectious Diseases and the Immune System," Scientific American 269(September 1993):90-97.
1557. N. Pender, C.A.G. McCulloch, "Effects of mechanical stretch on actin polymerisation in fibroblasts of the periodontium," in F. Lyall, A.J. El Haj, eds., Biomechanics and Cells, Cambridge University Press, 1994, pp. 228-243.
1558. Sergio Arruda, Gloria Bomfim, Ronald Knights, Tellervo Huima-Byron, Lee W. Riley, "Cloning of an *M. tuberculosis* DNA Fragment Associated with Entry and Survival Inside Cells," Science 261(10 September 1993):1454-1457.
1559. Pamela L.C. Small, Lalita Ramakrishnan, Stanley Falkow, "Remodeling Schemes of Intracellular Pathogens," Science 263(4 February 1994):637-639.
1560. Vladimir I. Rodionov, Gary G. Borisy, "Microtubule Treadmilling in Vivo," Science 275(10 January 1997):215-218.
1561. Li-Mei Chen, Silke Hobbie, Jorge E. Galan, "Requirement of CDC42 for Salmonella-Induced Cytoskeletal and Nuclear Responses," Science 274(20 December 1996):2115-2118.
1562. Vassiliki A. Boussiotis, Gordon J. Freeman, Alla Berezovskaya, Dwayne L. Barber, Lee M. Nadler, "Maintenance of Human T Cell Anergy: Blocking of IL-2 Gene Transcription by Activated Rap1," Science 278(3 October 1997):124-128.
1563. Roman Sakowicz, Michael S. Berdelis, Krishanu Ray, Christine L. Blackburn, Cordula Hopmann, D. John Faulkner, Lawrence S.B. Goldstein, "A Marine Natural Product Inhibitor of Kinesin Motors," Science 280(10 April 1998):292-295.
1564. Thomas P. Stossel, "On the Crawling of Animal Cells," Science 260(21 May 1993):1086-1094.
1565. Christopher Haslett, Peter J. Jose, Patricia C. Giclas, Timothy J. Williams, Peter M. Henson, "Cessation of Neutrophil Influx in C5a-Induced Acute Experimental Arthritis is Associated with Loss of Chemoattractant Activity from the Joint Space," J. Immunology 142(15 May 1989):3510-3517.
1566. C.A. Nacy, S.J. Green, D.L. Leiby, B.A. Nelson, R.M. Crawford, A.H. Fortier, D.L. Hoover, M.S. Meltzer, "Intercellular Communication: Macrophages and Cytokines," in H. Kiyono, E. Jirillo, C. DeSimone, Molecular Aspects of Immune Response and Infectious Diseases, Raven Press, NY, 1990, pp. 47-53.
1567. Jo Van Damme, "Chapter 10. Interleukin-8 and Related Chemotactic Cytokines," in Angus W. Thomson, ed., The Cytokine Handbook, Second Edition, Academic Press, NY, 1994, pp. 185-208.
1568. Thomas J. Schall, "Chapter 22. The Chemokines," in Angus W. Thomson, ed., The Cytokine Handbook, Second Edition, Academic Press, NY, 1994, pp. 419-460.
1569. Marco Baggiolini, Beatrice DeWald, Bernhard Moser, "Interleukin-8 and Related Chemotactic Cytokines -- CXC and CC Chemokines," Adv. Immunology 55(1994):97-179.
1570. Donald Metcalf, "The molecular control of granulocytes and macrophages," in The Molecular Basis of Cellular Defense Mechanisms, Ciba Foundation Symposium 204, John Wiley & Sons, 1997, NY, pp. 40-56.
1571. Howard Tomb, Dennis Kunkel, MicroAliens: Dazzling Journeys with an Electron Microscope, Farrar, Straus and Giroux, NY, 1993.
1572. Helmut E. Landsberg, "Dust," Encyclopedia Britannica 7(1963):787-791.
1573. Gregory Getzan, Masahito Shimada, Isao Shimoyama, Yoichiro Matsumoto, Hirofumi Miura, "Aerodynamic Behavior of Microstructures," in Proceedings of the 1995 IEEE/RSJ International Conference on Intelligent Robots and Systems, Volume 2, IEEE Computer Society Press, Los Alamitos CA, 1995.

1574. Isao Shimoyama, Yayoi Kubo Fujisawa, Gregory Getzan, Hirofumi Miura, Masahito Shimada, Yoichiro Matsumoto, "Fluid Dynamics of Micro Wing," MEMS-8(1995):380-385.
1575. Isao Shimoyama, Yayoi Kubo, Tomoyuki Kaneda, Hirofumi Miura, "Simple Microflight Mechanism on Silicon Wafer," MEMS-7(1994):148-152.
1576. K.I. Arai, W. Sugawara, K. Ishiyama, T. Honda, M. Yamaguchi, "Fabrication of Small Flying Machines Using Magnetic Thin Films," IEEE Transactions on Magnetics 31(November 1995):3758-3760.
1577. Torkel Weis-Fogh, "Unusual Mechanisms for the Generation of Lift in Flying Animals," Scientific American 233(November 1975):81-87.
1578. Torkel Weis-Fogh, "Quick Estimates of Flight Fitness in Hovering Animals, Including Novel Mechanisms for Lift Production," J. Exp. Biol. 59(1973):169-230.
1579. G.A. Horridge, "The flight of very small insects," Nature 178(1956):1334-1335.
1580. Jon F. Harrison, Jennifer H. Fewell, Stephen P. Roberts, H. Glenn Hall, "Achievement of Thermal Stability by Varying Metabolic Heat Production in Flying Honeybees," Science 274(4 October 1996):88-90. See also: "Honeybee Thermoregulation," Science 276(16 May 1996):1015-1017.
1581. Wai Pang Chan, Frederick Prete, Michael H. Dickinson, "Visual Input to the Efferent Control System of a Fly's 'Gyroscope'," Science 280(10 April 1996):289-291.
1582. Michael H. Dickinson, John R.B. Lighton, "Muscle Efficiency and Elastic Storage in the Flight Motor of Drosophila," Science 268(7 April 1995):87-90.
1583. Torkel Weis-Fogh, "Energetics of Hovering Flight in Hummingbirds and Drosophila," J. Exp. Biol. 56(1972):79-104.
1584. L. Prandtl, Essentials of Fluid Dynamics, Blackie, London, 1952.
1585. M.J. Lighthill, "On the Weis-Fogh Mechanism of Lift Generation," J. Fluid Mech. 60(21 August 1973):1-17.
1586. J. Brainard, "Ultrasound prevents blood loss in surgery," Science News 153(27 June 1998):407.
1587. Richard Wyatt, Joseph Sodroski, "The HIV-1 Envelope Glycoproteins: Fusogens, Antigens, and Immunogens," Science 280(19 June 1998):1884-1888.
1588. David Bieber, Sandra W. Ramer, Cheng-Yen Wu, William J. Murray, Toru Tobe, Rosemary Fernandez, Gary K. Schoolnik, "Type IV Pili, Transient Bacterial Aggregates, and Virulence of Enteropathogenic *Escherichia coli*," Science 280(26 June 1998):2114-2118. See also: Kristin Weidenbach, "A Tangled Tale of *E. coli* Virulence," Science 280(26 June 1998):2048.
1590. K.L. Lu, R.M. Lago, Y.K. Chen, M.L.H. Green, P.J.F. Harris, S.C. Tsang, "Mechanical Damage of Carbon Nanotubes by Ultrasound," Carbon 34(1996):814-816.
1591. Michael T. Madigan, Barry L. Marrs, "Extremophiles," Scientific American 276(April 1997):82-87.
1592. Richard Monastersky, "Deep Dwellers: Microbes Thrive Far Below Ground," Science News 151(29 March 1997):192-193.
1593. D.E. Koshland, T.J. Mitchison, M.W. Kirschner, "Polewards chromosome movement driven by microtubule depolymerization in vitro," Nature 331(1988):255-318.
1594. Q.M. Zhang, Vivek Bharti, X. Zhao, "Giant Electrostriction and Relaxor Ferroelectric Behavior in Electron-Irradiated Poly(vinylidene fluoride-trifluoroethylene) Copolymer," Science 280(26 June 1998):2101-2104.
1595. HandyKey Corporation website: "http://www.handykey.com"
1596. Stephen Evans, "Chapter 4. Surface Properties of Diamond," in J.E. Field, ed., The Properties of Natural and Synthetic Diamond, Academic Press, NY, 1992, pp. 181-214.
1597. J.E. Field, "Appendix: Tables of Properties," in J.E. Field, ed., The Properties of Natural and Synthetic Diamond, Academic Press, NY, 1992, pp. 667-699.
1598. J.L. Margrave, R.B. Badachhape, Proc. Electrochem. Soc. 84(1984):525-535.
1599. S. Evans, "Some effects of heteroatom size and reactivity on low-energy ion implantation in diamond, revealed by X-ray induced electron spectroscopy and oxidative depth profiling," Proc. R. Soc. London A 370(1980):107-129; "Depth profiles of ion-induced structural changes in diamond from X-ray photoelectron spectroscopy," Proc. R. Soc. London A 360(1978):427-443.
1600. R. Sappok, H.P. Boehm, Carbon 6(1968):283-295, 573-588. In German.
1601. Handbook of Aluminum, Aluminum Company of Canada, Ltd., Toronto, 1957.
1602. Richard W. Hughes, Ruby & Sapphire, RWH Publishing, Boulder CO, 1997.
1603. K. Wefers, "Nomenclature, Preparation, and Properties of Aluminum Oxides, Oxide Hydroxides, and Trihydroxides," in L.D. Hart, ed., Alumina Chemicals Science and Technology Handbook, The American Ceramic Society, Inc., Westerville OH, 1990, pp.13-22.
1604. Robert Berkow, Mark H. Beers, Andrew J. Fletcher, eds., The Merck Manual of Medical Information, Merck Research Laboratories, Whitehouse Station NJ, 1997.
1605. Richard C. Bradt, "Mechanical Properties of Alumina," in L.D. Hart, ed., Alumina Chemicals Science and Technology Handbook, The American Ceramic Society, Inc., Westerville OH, 1990, pp.23-48.
1606. Joseph C. Yater, "Power conversion of energy fluctuations," Phys. Rev. A 10(October 1974):1361-1369. See also: Phys. Rev. A 18(August 1978):767-772, Phys. Rev. A 20(August 1979):623-627, and Phys. Rev. A 20(October 1979):1614-1618.
1607. Joseph C. Yater, "Physical basis of power conversion of energy fluctuations," Phys. Rev. A 26(July 1982):522-538.
1608. N.A. Tsytovich, The Mechanics of Frozen Ground, Scripta Book Company, Washington DC, 1975.
1609. N.K. Sinha, G.W. Timco, R. Frederking, "Recent advances in ice mechanics in Canada," in Jin S. Chung, S.D. Hallam, M. Maatanen, N.K. Sinha, D.S. Sodhi, eds., Advances in Ice Mechanics—1987, The American Society of Mechanical Engineers, New York, 1987, pp. 15-35.
1610. A. De Ninno, A. La Barbera, V. Violante, "Deformations induced by high loading ratios in palladium-deuterium compounds," J. Alloys and Compounds 253-254(1997):181-184.
1611. Naoto Asami, Toshio Senjuh, Hiroshi Kamimura, Masao Sumi, Elliot Kennel, Takeshi Sakai, Kenya Mori, Hisashi Watanabe, Kazuaki Matsui, "Material characteristics and behavior of highly deuterium loaded palladium by electrolysis," J. Alloys and Compounds 253-254(1997):185-190.
1612. T. Senjuh, H. Kamimura, T. Uehara, M. Sumi, S. Miyasita, T. Sigemitsu, N. Asami, "Experimental Study of Electrochemical Deuterium Loading of Pd Cathodes in the LiOD/D_2O System," J. Alloys and Compounds 253-254(1997):617-620.
1613. Jay T. Groves, Steven G. Boxer, Harden M. McConnell, "Electric field-induced critical demixing in lipid bilayer membranes," Proc. Natl. Acad. Sci. USA 95(February 1998):935-938.
1614. See Reference #2811.
1615. Michael LaBarbera, "Principles of Design of Fluid Transport Systems in Zoology," Science 249(31 August 1990):992-1000.
1616. W.F. Ganong, Review of Medical Physiology, Lange Medical, Los Altos CA, 1975.
1617. Elizabeth H. Gladfelter, "Circulation of Fluids in the Gastrovascular System of the Reef Coral *Acropora cervicornis*," Biol. Bull. Woods Hole 165(December 1983):619-636.
1618. J.C. Grimmer, N.D. Holland, Zoomorphology Berl. 94(1979):93 et seq; N.D. Holland, J.C. Grimmer, "Fine structure of the cirri and a possible mechanism for their motility in stalkless crinoids (Echinodermata)," Cell and Tissue Res. 214(1981):207-217.
1619. Wolfgang Zesch, Markus Brunner, Ariel Weber, "Vacuum Tool for Handling Microobjects with a Nanorobot," Proc. 1997 IEEE International Conference on Robotics and Automation, 20-25 April 1997, IEEE Robotics and Automation Society, pp. 1761-1766.
1620. N. Masuyaki, I. Kazuhisha et al., "Prototypes of non-tweezing handling tools with releasing mechanisms," Trans. of Japan Soc. of Mech. Engineers C 61/583(1995):1021-1026.
1621. Jun Nakanishi, Toshio Fukuda, Daniel E. Koditschek, "Preliminary Studies of a Second Generation Brachiation Robot Controller," Proc. 1997 IEEE International Conference on Robotics and Automation, 20-25 April 1997, IEEE Robotics and Automation Society, pp. 2050-2056.
1622. A.M. Okamura, M.L. Turner, M.R. Cutkosky, "Haptic Exploration of Objects with Rolling and Sliding," Proc. 1997 IEEE International Conference on Robotics and Automation, 20-25 April 1997, IEEE Robotics and Automation Society, pp. 2485-2490.
1623. M. Khatib, B. Bouilly, T. Simeon, R. Chatila, "Indoor Navigation with Uncertainty using Sensor-Based Motions," Proc. 1997 IEEE International Conference on Robotics and Automation, 20-25 April 1997, IEEE Robotics and Automation Society, pp. 3379-3384.
1624. Nitin Juneja, A.A. Goldenberg, "Kinematic Calibration of A Re-configurable Robot (RoboTwin)," Proc. 1997 IEEE International Conference on Robotics and Automation, 20-25 April 1997, IEEE Robotics and Automation Society, pp. 3178-3183.
1625. Martin Nilsson, "Snake Robot Free Climbing," Proc. 1997 IEEE International Conference on Robotics and Automation, 20-25 April 1997, IEEE Robotics and Automation Society, pp. 3415-3420.
1627. E. Benes, "Trapping of Suspended Biological Particles by Use of Ultrasonic Resonance Fields," 1993 Ultrasonics International Abstract, p. 39.
1628. H.A. Pohl, Dielectrophoresis, Cambridge University Press, Cambridge, 1978.
1629. X.-B. Wang, "Selective Dielectrophoretic Confinement of Bioparticles in Potential Energy Wells," J. Phys. D: Appl. Phys. 26(1993):1278-1285.
1630. Steven Chu, "Laser Trapping of Neutral Particles," Scientific American 266(February 1992):70-76.
1631. Steven Chu, "Laser Manipulation of Atoms and Particles," Science 253(23 August 1991):861-866.
1632. P. Dario, M.C. Carrozza, L. Lencioni, B. Magnani, S. D'Attanasio, "A Micro Robotic System for Colonoscopy," Proc. 1997 IEEE International Conference on Robotics and Automation, 20-25 April 1997, IEEE Robotics and Automation Society, pp. 1567-1572.
1633. R.F. Schmidt, Fundamentals of Sensory Physiology, Springer-Verlag, Berlin, 1985.
1634. F.A. Geldard, The Human Senses, Second Edition, John Wiley & Sons, New York, 1972.
1635. I. Darian-Smith, "The Nervous System," Handbook of Physiology, American Physiological Society, 1984.
1636. S.J. Bolanowski Jr., G.A. Gescheider, R.T. Verrillo, C.M. Chechosky, "Four channels mediate the mechanical aspects of touch," J. Acoust. Soc. Amer. 84(1988):1680-1694.

1637. Darwin G. Caldwell, N. Tsagarakis, A. Wardle, "Mechano Thermo and Proprioceptor Feedback for Integrated Haptic Feedback," Proc. 1997 IEEE International Conference on Robotics and Automation, 20-25 April 1997, IEEE Robotics and Automation Society, pp. 2491-2496.
1638. Barmeshwar Vikramaditya, Bradley J. Nelson, "Visually Guided Microassembly Using Optical Microscopes and Active Vision Techniques," Proc. 1997 IEEE International Conference on Robotics and Automation, 20-25 April 1997, IEEE Robotics and Automation Society, pp. 3172-3177.
1639. Karl-Fredrich Bohringer, John W. Suh, Bruce Randall Donald, Gregory T.A. Kovacs, "Vector Fields for Task-level Distributed Manipulation: Experiments with Organic Micro Actuator Arrays," Proc. 1997 IEEE International Conference on Robotics and Automation, 20-25 April 1997, IEEE Robotics and Automation Society, pp. 1779-1786.
1640. Murilo G. Coutinho, Peter M. Will, P. Selvan Viswanathan, "The Intelligent Motion Surface: A hardware/software tool for the assembly of meso-scale devices," Proc. 1997 IEEE International Conference on Robotics and Automation, 20-25 April 1997, IEEE Robotics and Automation Society, pp. 1755-1760.
1641. P. Will, W. Liu, "Parts Manipulation on a MEMS Intelligent Motion Surface," ISI Research Report -- ISI/RR-94-391, Marina del Rey, CA, May 1994.
1642. W. Liu, P. Will, "Parts Manipulation on an Intelligent Motion Surface," Human Robot Interaction and Cooperative Robots, Proc. IEEE/RSJ Intl. Conf. on Intell. Robots and Systems (IROS), August 1995, pp. 399-404.
1643. K.-F. Bohringer, B.R. Donald, R. Mihailovich, N.C. Macdonald, "A theory of manipulation and control for microfabricated actuator arrays," Proc. IEEE Workshop on Micro Electro Mechanical Systems (MEMS), January 1994, pp. 102-107.
1644. K.-F. Bohringer, B.R. Donald, N.C. Macdonald, "Upper and lower bounds for programmable vector fields with applications to MEMS and vibratory plate parts feeders," Intl. Workshop on Algorithmic Foundations of Robotics (WAFR), Toulouse, France, July 1996.
1645. K. Bohringer, B. Donald, N. MacDonald, "Single-crystal silicon actuator arrays for micro manipulation tasks," IEEE Workshop on Micro Electro Mechanical Systems (MEMS), San Diego CA, February 1996.
1646. Dan Reznik, Stan Brown, John Camy, "Dynamic Simulation as a Design Tool for a Microactuator Array," Proc. 1997 IEEE International Conference on Robotics and Automation, 20-25 April 1997, IEEE Robotics and Automation Society, pp. 1675-1680.
1647. Ian Rivens, Ian Rowland, Gail ter Haar, Mark Denbow, Nicholas Fisk, "Occlusion of blood flow by high-intensity focused ultrasound," Paper 2pBV4, presented Tuesday afternoon, 23 June 1998, at the International Congress on Acoustics and the Acoustical Society of America (ICA/ASA) Conference, Seattle, WA, 1998.
1648. J.F. Holzrichter, G.C. Burnett, L.C. Ng, W.A. Lea, "Speech articulator measurements using low power EM-wave sensors," J. Acoustic Soc. Amer. 103(January 1998):622-625. See also: http://speech.llnl.gov.
1649. Philip Morrison, Phylis Morrison, "The Sum of Human Knowledge?" Scientific American 279(July 1998):115, 117.
1650. T.S. Rappaport, Wireless Communications, Principles and Practice, Prentice Hall, NJ, 1996.
1651. C. Smith, C. Gervelis, Cellular System Design and Optimization, McGraw-Hill, NY, 1996.
1652. Andrew S. Tanenbaum, Computer Networks, Third Edition, Prentice Hall, NJ, 1996.
1653. Jan P.H. Van Santen, Richard W. Sproat, Joseph P. Olive, eds., Progress in Speech Synthesis, Springer-Verlag, Berlin, 1996.
1654. Eric Keller, ed., Fundamentals of Speech Synthesis and Speech Recognition: Basic Concepts, State of the Art and Future Challenges, John Wiley & Sons, NY, 1994.
1655. Lawrence Rabiner, Biing-Hwang Juang, Fundamentals of Speech Recognition, Prentice Hall, NJ, 1993.
1656. A. Kindoz, A.M. Kondoz, Digital Speech: Coding for Low Bit Rate Communication Systems, John Wiley & Sons, NY, 1995.
1657. Richard L. Klevans, Robert D. Rodman, Voice Recognition, Artech House, 1997.
1658. Renato De Mori, ed., Spoken Dialogues With Computers, Academic Press, NY, 1998.
1659. Esther Schindler, The Computer Speech Book, Ap Professional, 1996.
1660. Michael Koerner, Lori Hawkins, Joseph Polimeni, eds., Speech Recognition: The Future Now!, Prentice-Hall, NJ, 1997.
1661. Mark S. Schwartz, Biofeedback: A Practitioner's Guide, Second Edition, Guilford Press, 1995.
1662. Robert Resnick, David Halliday, Physics, John Wiley & Sons, New York, 1966.
1663. Elias Towe, "MicroOptoElectroMechanical Systems (MOEMS) at DARPA: Overview Briefing," DARPA Electronics Technology Office, Summer 1997; see at: http://www.darpa.mil/ETO/MOEMS/Briefing/index.html.
1664. Virginia Morell, "A 24-Hour Circadian Clock Is Found in the Mammalian Retina," Science 272(19 April 1995):349.
1665. L.N. Edwards, Cellular and Molecular Bases of Biological Clocks, Springer-Verlag, Berlin, 1988.
1666. Albert Goldbeter, Biochemical Oscillations and Cellular Rhythms: The Molecular Bases of Periodic and Chaotic Behavior, Cambridge University Press, New York, 1996.
1667. Marcia Barinaga, "New Clock Gene Cloned," Science 270(3 November 1995):732-733.
1668. Susan K. Crosthwaite, Jay C. Dunlap, Jennifer J. Loros, "Neurospora wc-1 and wc-2: Transcription, Photoresponses, and the Origins of Circadian Rhythmicity," Science 276(2 May 1997):763-769.
1669. Z.S. Sun, U. Albrecht, O. Zhuchenko, J. Bailey, Gregor Eichele, Cheng Chi Lee, "RIGUI, a putative mammalian ortholog of the Drosophila period gene," Cell 90(19 September 1997):1003-1011.
1670. Mary E. Morris, N. Viswanathan, Sandra Kuhlman, Fred C. Davis, Charles J. Weitz, "A Screen for Genes Induced in the Suprachiasmatic Nucleus by Light," Science 279(6 March 1998):1544-1547.
1671. Nicholas Gekakis, David Staknis, Hubert B. Nguyen, Fred C. Davis, Lisa D. Wilsbacher, David P. King, Joseph S. Takahashi, Charles J. Weitz, "Role of the CLOCK Protein in the Mammalian Circadian Mechanism," Science 280(5 June 1998):1564-1569.
1672. Thomas K. Darlington, Karen Wager-Smith, M. Fernanda Ceriani, David Staknis, Nicholas Gekakis, Thomas D.L. Steeves, Charles J. Weitz, Joseph S. Takahashi, Charles J. Weitz, "Closing the Circadian Loop: CLOCK-Induced Transcription of Its Own Inhibitors per and tim," Science 280(5 June 1998):1599-1603.
1673. L. Wetterberg, ed., Light and Biological Rhythms in Man, Pergamon Press, Oxford, 1993.
1674. Jeffrey D. Plautz, Maki Kaneko, Jeffrey C. Hall, Steve A. Kay, "Independent Photoreceptive Circadian Clocks Throughout Drosophila," Science 278(28 November 1997):1632-1635.
1675. Scott S. Campbell, Patricia J. Murphy, "Extraocular Circadian Phototransduction in Humans," Science 279(16 January 1998):396-399.
1676. Gianluca Tosini, Michael Menaker, "Circadian Rhythms in Cultured Mammalian Retina," Science 272(19 April 1996):419-421.
1677. Charles A. Czeisler, Richard E. Kronauer, James S. Allan, Jeanne F. Duffy, Megan E. Jewett, Emery N. Brown, Joseph M. Ronda, "Bright Light Induction of Strong (Type O) Resetting of the Human Circadian Pacemaker," Science 244(16 June 1989):1328-1333.
1678. D.C. Klein, R.Y. Moore, S.M. Reppert, eds., Suprachiasmatic Nucleus: The Mind's Clock, Oxford University Press, NY, 1991.
1679. R.Y. Moore, D.C. Klein, "Visual pathways and the central neural control of a circadian rhythm in pineal serotonin N-acetyltransferase activity," Brain Res. 71(10 May 1974):17-33. See also D.C. Klein, R.Y. Moore, "Pineal N-acetyltransferase and hydroxyindole-O-methyltransferase: Control by the retinohypothalamic tract and the suprachiasmatic nucleus," Brain Res. 174(5 October 1979):245-262.
1680. R.F. Johnson, R.Y. Moore, L.P. Morin, "Loss of entrainment and anatomical plasticity after lesions of the hamster retinohypothalamic tract," Brain Res. 460(20 September 1988):297-313.
1681. Jay Dunlap, "An End in the Beginning," Science 280(5 June 1998):1548-1549.
1682. Zuoshi J. Huang, Kathryn D. Curtin, Michael Rosbash, "PER Protein Interactions and Temperature Compensation of a Circadian Clock in Drosophila," Science 267(24 February 1995):1169-1172.
1683. Lesley A. Sawyer, J. Michael Hennessy, Alexandre A. Peixoto, Ezio Rosato, Helen Parkinson, Rodolfo Costa, Charalambos P. Kyriacou, "Natural Variation in a Drosophila Clock Gene and Temperature Compensation," Science 278(19 December 1997):2117-2120.
1684. Michael P. Myers, Karen Wager-Smith, Adrian Rothenfluh-Hilfiker, Michael W. Young, "Light-Induced Degradation of TIMELESS and Entrainment of the Drosophila Circadian Clock," Science 271(22 March 1996):1736-1740.
1685. Choogon Lee, Vaishali Parikh, Tomoko Itsukaichi, Kiho Bae, Isaac Edery, "Resetting the Drosophila Clock by Photic Regulation of PER and a PER-TIM Complex," Science 271(22 March 1996):1740-1744.
1686. Ernst Knobil, "The circhoral hypothalmic clock that governs the 28-day menstrual cycle," in A. Goldbetter, ed., Cell to Cell Signalling: From Experiments to Theoretical Models, Academic Press, NY, 1989, pp. 353-358.
1687. R.C. Wilson, J.S. Kesner, J.-M. Kaufman, T. Uemura, T. Akema, E. Knobil, "Central electrophysiologic correlates of pulsatile luteinizing hormone secretion in the rhesus monkey," Neuroendocrinology 39(1984):256-260.
1688. Elizabeth Pennisi, "New Developmental Clock Discovered," Science 278(28 November 1997):1563.
1689. Esther M. Chipps, Norma J. Clanin, Victor G. Campbell, Neurologic Disorders, Mosby Year Book, St. Louis, MO, 1992.
1690. Brian O'Rourke, Brian M. Ramza, Eduardo Marban, "Oscillations of Membrane Current and Excitability Driven by Metabolic Oscillations in Heart Cells," Science 265(12 August 1994):962-966.
1691. Virginia Morell, "Setting a Biological Stopwatch," Science 271(16 February 1996):905-906.
1692. R.W. Schoenlein, L.A. Peteanu, R.A. Mathies, C.V. Shank, "The First Step in Vision: Femtosecond Isomerization of Rhodopsin," Science 254(18 October 1991):412-415.
1693. Peter J. Steinbach, Bernard R. Brooks, "Protein hydration elucidated by molecular dynamics simulation," Proc. Natl. Acad. Sci. USA 90(1 October 1993):9135-9139.

1694. H. Eyring, "The activated complex and the absolute rate of chemical reactions," Chem. Rev. 17(1935):65-77. See also: H. Eyring, D.W. Urry, "Thermodynamics and chemical kinetics," in T.H. Waterman, H.J. Morowitz, eds., Theoretical and Mathematical Biology, Blaisdell Publishing Company, Waltham, MA, 1965, pp. 57-96.
1695. J. Gray, "The mechanism of ciliary movement. III. The effect of temperature," Proc. Roy. Soc. B 95(1923):6-15. See also: J. Gray, Ciliary Movement, Cambridge University Press, NY, 1928.
1696. Thomas Rufer Barnard Robinson, Francis Alan Burnett Ward, "Clock," Encyclopedia Britannica 5(1963):933-936.
1697. Louis Bevier Spinney, A Textbook of Physics, The Macmillan Company, NY, 1941.
1698. Robert W. Young, "3h. Frequencies of Simple Vibrators. Musical Scales," in Dwight E. Gray, ed., American Institute of Physics Handbook, Third Edition, McGraw-Hill Book Company, New York, 1972, pp. 3-130 - 3-138.
1699. John R. Vig, Raymond L. Filler, Yoonkee Kim, "Uncooled IR Imaging Array Based on Quartz Microresonators," J. Microelectromechanical Systems 5(June 1996):131-137.
1700. F.L. Walls, J.R. Vig, "Fundamental limits on the frequency stabilities of crystal oscillators," IEEE Trans. Ultrason. Ferroelect. Freq. Contr. 42(1995):576-589.
1701. V.E. Bottom, Introduction to Quartz Crystal Unit Design, Van Nostrand-Reinhold, NY, 1982.
1702. E.A. Gerber, A. Ballato, eds., Precision Frequency Control, Academic Press, NY, 1985.
1703. Natarajan D. Bhaskar, Joseph White, Leo A. Mallette, Thomas A. McClelland, James Hardy, "A Historical Review of Atomic Frequency Standards Used in Space Systems," 1997; see at: http://bul.eecs.umich.edu/uffc/fc_history/bhaskar.html.
1704. T.A McClelland, I. Pascaru, I. Shaterman, C. Stone, C. Szekely, J. Zacharski, N.D. Bhaskar, "Subminiature Rubidium Frequency Standard: Performance Improvements," Proc. 1996 IEEE Freq. Contr. Symposium, 1996.
1705. R. Frueholz, "The Effects of Ambient Temperature Fluctuations on the Long-Term Frequency Stability on the Miniature Rubidium Atomic Frequency Standard," Proc. 1996 IEEE Freq. Contr. Symposium, 1996.
1706. K. Hisadome, M. Kihara, "Prototype of an Optically Pumped Frequency Standard," Proc. 45th Ann. Freq. Contr. Symposium, 1991, pp. 513-520.
1707. N.D. Bhaskar, "Potential for Improving the Rubidium Frequency Standard with a Novel Optical Pumping Scheme Using Diode Lasers," IEEE Trans. Ultrason. Ferroelect. Freq. Contr. 42(1995):15-22.
1708. J.C. Camparo, "Reducing the Light-Shift in the Diode Laser Pumped Atomic Clock," Proc. 1996 IEEE Freq. Contr. Symposium, 1996.
1709. J.D. Prestage, R.L. Tjoelker, G.J. Dick, L. Maleki, "Space Flyable Hg^+ Frequency Standard," Proc. 48th Ann. Freq. Contr. Symposium, 1994, p. 747. See also: "Mercury Trapped Ion Frequency Standards" at: http://tycho.usno.navy.mil/CD/ion.html.
1710. X.D. Huang, Y. Ariki, M.A. Jack, Hidden Markov Models for Speech Recognition, Edinburgh University Press, 1990.
1711. Philip Morrison, "The Timekeeping ELF," Scientific American 278(April 1998):105, 107.
1712. Thomas R. Koch, Show-Hong Duh, "Laboratory Reference Range Values," in James T. McDonough, Jr., ed., Stedman's Concise Medical Dictionary, Second Edition, Williams & Wilkins, Baltimore MD, 1994, pp. 1147-1168.
1713. G.S. Brindley, W.S. Lewin, "The Sensations Produced by Electrical Stimulation of the Visual Cortex," J. Physiol. 196(1968):479-493.
1714. J.P. Stapp, "Human tolerance to deceleration," Am. J. of Surgery 93(1957):734-740. See also: "Human tolerance to severe, abrupt deceleration," in O.H. Gauer, G.D. Zuidema, eds., Gravitational Stress in Aerospace Medicine, Little, Brown, Boston MA, 1961, pp. 165-188; and "Voluntary human tolerance levels," in E.S. Gurdjian, W.A. Lange, L.M. Partrick, L.M. Thomas, eds., Impact Injury and Crash Protection, Charles C. Thomas, Springfield IL, 1970.
1715. E.M. Roth, W.G. Teichner, R.L. Craig, Compendium of Human Response to the Aerospace Environment, Vol. II, Sec. 7, Acceleration, NASA Contractor Report No. CR-1205 (II), 1968.
1716. A.M. Eiband, "Human tolerance to rapidly applied accelerations: A summary of the literature," NASA Memorandum No. 5-19-59E, 1959.
1717. Jacob Kulowski, Crash Injuries: The Integrated Medical Aspects of Automobile Injuries and Deaths, Charles C. Thomas, Springfield IL, 1960.
1718. H.J. Rogers, in Aspects of Microbiology, Volume 7, Van Nostrand Reinhold, Wokingham, UK, 1983, pp. 6-25.
1719. J.-M. Ghuysen, G.D. Shockman, in L. Leive, ed., Bacterial Membranes and Walls, Volume 1, Marcel Dekker, New York, 1973.
1720. Christopher B. Field, Michael J. Behrenfeld, James T. Randerson, Paul Falkowski, "Primary Production of the Biosphere: Integrating Terrestrial and Oceanic Components," Science 281(10 July 1998):237-240.
1721. Philip L. Felgner, "Nonviral Strategies for Gene Therapy," Scientific American 276(June 1997):102-106.
1722. Ilya Koltover, Tim Salditt, Joachim O. Radler, Cyrus R. Safinya, "An Inverted Hexagonal Phase of Cationic Liposome-DNA Complexes Related to DNA Release and Delivery," Science 281(3 July 1998):78-81.
1723. Peixuan Guo, C. Zhang, C. Chen, K. Garver, M. Trottier, "Inter-RNA interaction of phage φ29 pRNA to form a hexameric complex for viral DNA transportation," Mol. Cell 2(July 1998):149-155. See also: F. Zhang, S. Lemieux, X. Wu, D. St.-Arnaud, C.T. McMurray, F. Major, D. Anderson, "Function of hexameric RNA in packaging of bacteriophage φ29 DNA in vitro," Mol. Cell 2(July 1998):141-147, 405.
1724. Thomas Donaldson, "24th Century Medicine," Analog 108(September 1988):64-80.
1725. L. Thomsen, T.L. Robinson, J.C. Lee, L.A. Farraway, M.J. Hughes, D.W. Andrews, Jan D. Huizinga, "Interstitial cells of Cajal generate a rhythmic pacemaker current," Nature Medicine 4(July 1998):848-851.
1726. J.M. Pullan, The History of the Abacus, Hutchinson, London, 1968.
1727. Parry H. Moon, The Abacus: Its History, Its Design, Its Possibilities in the Modern World, Gordon and Breach, New York, 1971.
1728. Stan Augarten, Bit by Bit: An Illustrated History of Computers, Ticknor and Fields, New York, 1984.
1729. Henry Prevost Babbage, Babbage's Calculating Engines, Charles Babbage Institute Reprint Series for the History of Computing, Volume 2, Tomash Publishers, Los Angeles, CA, 1982. Originally published in 1889.
1730. Anthony Hyman, Charles Babbage: Pioneer of the Computer, Oxford University Press, Oxford, 1982.
1731. H.W. Buxton, Memoirs of the Life and Labours of the Late Charles Babbage, Esq., F.R.S., Anthoy Hyman, ed., Tomash Publishers, Los Angeles, 1988.
1732. Doron D. Swade, "Redeeming Charles Babbage's Mechanical Computer," Scientific American 268(February 1993):86-91.
1733. Doron D. Swade, "It Will Not Slice A Pineapple: Babbage, Miracles and Machines," F. Spufford, J. Uglow, eds., Cultural Babbage: Technology, Time and Invention, Faber and Faber, London, 1996.
1734. P.L. Bergstrom, T. Tamagawa, D.L. Polla, "Design and Fabrication of Micromechanical Logic Elements," MEMS-3, 1990, pp. 15-20.
1735. M.T. Cuberes, R.B. Schlittler, James K. Gimzewski, "Room-temperature repositioning of individual C_{60} molecules at Cu steps: Operation of a molecular counting device," Appl. Phys. Lett. 69(11 November 1996):3016-3018.
1736. Raymond Kurzweil, The Age of Intelligent Machines, MIT Press, Cambridge MA, 1990.
1737. Paul E. Sheehan, Charles M. Lieber, "Nanotribology and Nanofabrication of MoO_3 Structures by Atomic Force Microscopy," Science 272(24 May 1996):1158-1161.
1738. A.K. Dewdney, "A Tinkertoy computer that plays tic-tac-toe," Scientific American (October 1989):120-123. See also: A.K. Dewdney, The Tinkertoy Computer and Other Machinations, W.H. Freeman & Co., San Francisco, CA, 1993.
1739. S. Hosaka, A. Kikukawa, H. Koyanagi, T. Shintani, M. Miyamoto, K. Nakamura, K. Etoh, "SPM-based data storage for ultrahigh density recording," Nanotechnology 8(1997):A58-A62.
1740. J.I. Pascual, J. Mendez, J. Gomez-Herrero, A.M. Baro, N. Garcia, Uzi Landman, W.D. Luedtke, E.N. Bogachek, H.-P. Cheng, "Properties of Metallic Nanowires: From Conductance Quantization to Localization," Science 267(24 March 1995):1793-1795.
1741. Y.W. Mo, "Reversible Rotation of Antimony Dimers on the Silicon (001) Surface with a Scanning Tunneling Microscope," Science 261(13 August 1993):886-888.
1742. B. Halg, "On a nonvolatile memory cell based on micro-electro-mechanics," MEMS-3, 1990, pp. 172-176.
1743. J. Storrs Hall, "Nanocomputers and reversible logic," Nanotechnology 5(1994):157-167.
1744. Doron Swade, Charles Babbage and his Calculating Engines, Science Museum, London, 1991.
1745. Charles W. Bauschlicher Jr., Marzio Rosi, "Differentiating between hydrogen and fluorine on a diamond surface," Theor. Chem. Accounts 96(1997):213-216.
1746. C.J. Brabec et al., "Growth of Carbon Nanotubes: A Molecular Dynamics Study," Chem. Phys. Lett. 236(1995):150-155.
1747. David Goldhaber-Gordon, Michael S. Montemerlo, J. Christopher Love, Gregory J. Opiteck, James C. Ellenbogen, "Overview of Nanoelectronic Devices," Proc. IEEE 85(April 1997):(31pp). See also: MITRE Nanosystems Group, "The Nanoelectronics and Nanocomputing Home Page," http://www.mitre.org/research/nanotech.
1749. Y. Xu, N.C. MacDonald, S.A. Miller, "Integrated micro-scanning tunneling microscope," Appl. Phys. Lett. 67(16 October 1995):2305-2307.
1750. J.J. Hopfield, Jose Nelson Onuchic, David N. Beratan, "A Molecular Shift Register Based on Electron Transfer," Science 241(12 August 1988):817-820.
1751. M. Ono et al., "A 40 nm Gate Length n-MOSFET," IEEE Trans. Electron Devices 42(October 1995):1822-1830.
1752. J. Han, D. Ferry, P. Newman, "Ultra-Submicrometer-Gate AlGaAs/GaAs HEMT's," IEEE Electron Device Letters 11(May 1990):209-21.
1753. M. Nagata, "Limitations, Innovations, and Challenges of Circuits and Devices into a Half Micrometer and Beyond," J. Solid State Circuits 27(April 1992):465-472.
1754. Robert W. Keyes, "The Future of the Transistor," Scientific American 268(June 1993):70-78.
1755. C. Mead, "Scaling of MOS Technology to Submicrometer Feature Size," J. VLSI Signal Process. (1994):9-25.

1756. S. Asai, Y. Wada, "Technology Challenges for Integration Below 0.1 Microns," Proc. IEEE 85(April 1997):505-520.
1757. Y. Taur, D.A. Buchanan, "CMOS Scaling into the Nanometer Regime," Proc. IEEE 85(April 1997):486-504.
1758. C. Joachim, J.F. Vinuesa, "Length Dependence of the Electronic Transparence (Conductance) of a Molecular Wire," Europhys. Lett. 33(1996):635-640.
1759. V. Mujica, M. Kemp, M.A. Ratner, "Electron Conduction in Molecular Wires. I. A Scattering Formalism," J. Chem. Phys. 101(1994):6849-6855; "Electron Conduction in Molecular Wires. II. Application to Scanning Tunneling Microscopy," J. Chem. Phys. 101(1994):6856-6864.
1760. V. Mujica et al., "Current-Voltage Characteristics of Molecular Wires: Eigenvalue Staircase, Coulomb Blockade, and Rectification," J. Chem. Phys. 104(1996):7296-7305.
1761. M. Samanta, W. Tian, S. Datta, "Electronic Conduction Through Organic Molecules," Phys. Rev. B 53(1996):5-9.
1762. J.M. Tour, R. Wu, J.S. Schumm, "Extended Orthogonally Fused Conducting Oligomers for Molecular Electronic Devices," J. Am. Chem. Soc. 113(1991):7064-7066.
1763. R.A. English, S.G. Davison, "Transmission properties of molecular switches in semiconducting polymers," Phys. Rev. B 49(1994):8718-8731.
1764. J.M. Tour, et al., "Self-Assembled Monolayers and Multilayers of Conjugated Thiols, α,ω-Dithiols, and Thioacetyl-Containing Adsorbates. Understanding Attachments between Potential Molecular Wires and Gold Surfaces," J. Am. Chem. Soc. 117(1995):9529-9534.
1765. C. Joachim, J.K. Gimzewski, "Analysis of Low-Voltage I(V) Characteristics of a Single C_{60} Molecule," Europhys. Lett. 30(1995):409-414.
1766. J.S. Schumm, D.L. Pearson, J.M. Tour, "Iterative Divergent/Convergent Approach to Linear Conjugated Oligomers by Successive Doubling of the Molecular Length: A Rapid Route to a 128 Angstrom-Long Potential Molecular Wire," Angew. Chem. Int. Ed. Engl. 33(1994):1360-1363.
1767. L.A. Bumm, J.J. Arnold, M.T. Cygan, T.D. Dunbar, T.P. Burgin, L. Jones II, D.L. Allara, J.M. Tour, P.S. Weiss, "Are Single Molecular Wires Conducting?" Science 271(22 March 1996):1705-1707.
1768. C. Joachim, J.K. Gimzewski, "An Electromechanical Amplifier Using A Single Molecule," Chem. Phys. Lett. 265(1997):353-357.
1769. A. Aviram, "Molecules for Memory, Logic, and Amplification," J. Am. Chem. Soc. 110(1988):5687-5692.
1770. A. Aviram, M.A. Ratner, "Molecular Rectifiers," Chem. Phys. Lett. 29(1974):277-283.
1771. Y.G. Krieger, "Molecular Electronics: Current State and Future Trends," J. Structural Chem. 34(1993):896-904.
1772. S.V. Subramanyam, "Molecular Electronics," Current Science 67(1994):844-852.
1773. F.L. Carter, ed., Molecular Electronic Devices, Marcel Dekker, New York, 1982. See also: F.L. Carter et al., eds., 2nd International Workship on Molecular Electronic Devices, 13-15 April 1983, Naval Research Laboratory, Chemistry Division, Washington DC; and F.L. Carter, "The Molecular Device Computer: Point of Departure for Large Scale Cellular Automata," Physica D 10(1984):175-194.
1774. F.L. Carter, ed., Molecular Electronic Devices II, Marcel Dekker, New York, 1987. See also: F.L. Carter, R.E. Siatkowski, H. Wohltjen, eds., Molecular Electronic Devices, North-Holland, Amsterdam, 1988.
1775. A. Aviram, ed., Molecular Electronics: Science and Technology, AIP Conf. Proc. No. 262, AIP Press, New York, 1992.
1776. F.T. Hong, "Molecular Electronics: Science and Technology for the Future," IEEE Engineering in Medicine and Biology 13(1994):25-32.
1777. Robert R. Birge, ed., Molecular and Biomolecular Electronics, Advances in Chemistry Series, Volume 240, American Chemical Society, Washington, DC, 1994.
1778. S. Nespurek, J. Sworakowski, "Electroactive and Photochromic Molecular Materials for Wires, Switches, and Memories," IEEE Engineering in Medicine and Biology 13(1994):45-57.
1779. A. Prasanna de Silva, H.Q. Guaratne, Colin McCoy, "A molecular photoionic AND gate based on fluorescent signalling," Nature 364(1 July 1993):42-44.
1780. Robert R. Birge, "Protein-Based Three-Dimensional Memory," American Scientist 82(July-August 1994):348-355.
1781. D. Gust et al., "Photosynthesis Mimics as Molecular Electronics Devices," IEEE Engineering in Medicine and Biology 13(1994):58-66.
1782. M. Hampp, D. Ziesel, "Mutated Bacteriorhodopsins," IEEE Engineering in Medicine and Biology 13(1994):67-74.
1783. F.T. Hong, "Photovoltaic Effects in Biomembranes," IEEE Engineering in Medicine and Biology 13(1994):75-93.
1784. Mark A. Reed, "Quantum Dots," Scientific American 268(January 1993):118-123.
1785. C.S. Lent, P.D. Tougaw, "A Device Architecture for Computing with Quantum Dots," Proc. IEEE 85(April 1997):541-557.
1786. Simon C. Benjamin, Neil F. Johnson, "A possible nanometer-scale computing device based on an adding cellular automaton," Appl. Phys. Lett. 70(28 April 1997):2321-2323.
1787. R. Turton, The Quantum Dot: A Journey into the Future of Microelectronics, Oxford University Press, Oxford UK, 1995.
1788. A.C. Seabaugh, et al., "Pseudomorphic Bipolar Quantum Resonant Tunneling Transistor," IEEE Trans. Electron Devices 36(1989):2328-2334.
1789. Frederico Capasso, "Quantum Transistors and Integrated Circuits," in B.C. Crandall, James Lewis, eds., Nanotechnology: Research and Perspectives, MIT Press, 1992, pp. 171-197.
1790. J.N. Randall, "A Lateral-Resonant-Tunneling Universal Quantum-Dot Cell," Nanotechnology 4(1993):41-48.
1791. A.C. Seabaugh, J.H. Luscombe, J.N. Randall, "Quantum Functional Devices: Present Status and Future Prospects," Future Electron Devices (FED) Journal 3(1993):9-20.
1792. R. Landauer, in M.A. Reed, W.R. Kirk, eds., Nanostructure Physics and Fabrication, Academic Press, New York, 1989, pp. 17-30.
1793. Y. Nakajima, et al., "Fabrication of a Silicon Quantum Wire Surrounded by Silicon Dioxide and its Transport Properties," Appl. Phys. Lett. 65(1994):2833-2835.
1794. Y. Takahashi, et al., "Fabrication Techniques for Si Single-Electron Transistor Operating at Room Temperature," Electronics Letters 31(1995):136-137.
1795. T.A. Fulton, G.J. Dolan, "Observation of Single-Electron Charging Effects in Small Tunnel Junctions," Phys. Rev. Lett. 59(1987):109-112.
1796. Konstantin K. Likarev, Tord Claeson, "Single Electronics," Scientific American 266(June 1992):80-85.
1797. S.Y. Chou, Y. Wang, "Single-Electron Coulomb Blockade in a Nanometer Field-Effect Transistor with a Single Barrier," Appl. Phys. Lett. 61(1992):1591-1593.
1798. M.A. Kastner, "The Single-Electron Transistor," Rev. Mod. Phys. 64(1992):849-858.
1799. H. Ahmed, K. Nakazoto, "Single-Electron Devices," Microelectronic Engineering 32(1996):297-315.
1800. A. Aviram, C. Joachim, M. Pomerantz, "Evidence of Switching and Rectification by a Single Molecule Effected with a Scanning Tunneling Microscope," Chem. Phys. Lett. 146(1988):490-495. Errata, Chem. Phys. Lett. 162(1989):416.
1801. Z. Cai, et al., "Molecular and Supramolecular Origins of Enhanced Electronic Conductivity in Template-Synthesized Polyheterocyclic Fibrils," Supramolecular Effects Chem. Mater. 3(1992):960.
1802. Chun-Guey Wu, Thomas Bein, "Conducting Polyaniline Filaments in a Mesoporous Channel Host," Science 264(17 June 1994):1757-1759; "Conducting Carbon Wires in Ordered, Nanometer-Sized Channels," Science 266(11 November 1994):1013-1015.
1803. M. Aizawa, "Molecular Interfacing for Protein Molecular Devices and Neurodevices," IEEE Engineering in Medicine and Biology 13(1994):94-102.
1804. M. Todd, et al., "Electron Transfer Rates From Time-Dependent Correlation Functions. Wavepacket Dynamics, Solvent Effects, and Applications," J. Photochem. Photobiol. A:Chem 82(1994):87-101.
1805. R.A. Bissell, E. Cordova, A.E. Kaifer, J.F. Stoddart, "A Chemically and Electrochemically Switchable Molecular Shuttle," Nature 369(1994):133-137.
1806. Y. Wada, et al., "A Proposal of Nanoscale Devices Based on Atom/Molecule Switching," J. Appl. Phys. (15 December 1993):7321-7328.
1807. D.M. Eigler, C.P. Lutz, W.E. Rudge, "An atomic switch realized with the scanning tunnelling microscope," Nature 352(15 August 1991):600-603.
1808. J.J. Saenz, N. Garcia, "Quantum Atom Switch: Tunneling of Xe Atoms," Phys. Rev. B 47(1993):7537-7541.
1809. H.J. Schneider, R. Price, T. Keller, "Conformational Studies by Low Temperature Carbon-13 NMR Spectroscopy," Angew. Chem. Int. Ed. Engl. 10(1971):730-731.
1810. W. Kitching, D. Doddrell, J.B. Grutzner, "Conformational Equilibria in Cyclohexyltrimethylstannane and Cyclohexyltrimethylplumbane by Low Temperature Carbon-13 NMR Spectroscopy," J. Organomet. Chem. 107(1976):C5-C10.
1811. R.P. Andres, Thomas Bein, Matt Dorogi, Sue Feng, Jason I. Henderson, Clifford P. Kubiak, William Mahoney, Richard G. Osifchin, R. Reifenberger, "Coulomb Staircase at Room Temperature in a Self-Assembled Molecular Nanostructure," Science 272(31 May 1996):1323-1325.
1812. R.P. Andres, J. Bielefeld, J. Henderson, D. Janes, V. Kolagunta, C. Kubiak, W. Mahoney, R. Osifchin, "Self-Assembly of a Two-Dimensional Superlattice of Molecularly Linked Metal Clusters," Science 273(20 September 1996):1690-1693.
1813. D.K. Ferry, Quantum Mechanics: An Introduction for Device Physicists and Electrical Engineers, IOP Publishing Ltd, London, 1995.
1814. K. Matsumoto, M. Ishii, K. Segawa, Y. Oka, "Room temperature operation of a single electron transitor made by the scanning tunneling microscope nanooxidation process for the TiO_x/Ti system," Appl. Phys. Lett. 68(1 January 1996):34-36.
1815. Lingjie Guo, Effendi Leobandung, Stephen Y. Chou, "A Silicon Single-Electron Transistor Memory Operating at Room Temperature," Science 275(31 January 1997):649-651.
1816. Wei Chen, Haroon Ahmed, "Fabrication and physics of ~2 nm islands for single electron devices," J. Vac. Sci. Technol. B 13(November/December 1995):2883-2887.
1817. M. Derogi, et al., "Room-Temperature Coulomb Blockade from a Self-Assembled Molecular Nanostructure," Phys. Rev. B 52(1995):9071-9077.
1818. P.W. Atkins, Quanta: A Handbook of Concepts, Second Edition, Oxford University Press, Oxford UK, 1992.

1819. C.D. Bain, G.M. Whitesides, "Formation of Monolayers by the Coadsorption of Thiols on Gold: Variation in the Length of the Alkyl Chain," J. Am. Chem. Soc. 111(1989):7164-7175.
1820. M.D. Ward, "Current developments in molecular wires," Chemistry and Industry (5 August 1996):568-573.
1821. M.S. Dresselhaus, G. Dresselhaus, P.C. Eklund, Science of Fullerenes and Carbon Nanotubes, Academic Press, San Diego, 1996.
1822. G.M. Whitesides, C.S. Weisbecker, "Measurements of the Conductivity of Individual 10 nm Carbon Nanotubes," Materials Research Soc. Symp. Proc. 349(1994):263-268.
1823. Y. Wada, et al., "A Proposal for Nanoscale Devices Based on Atom/Molecule Switching," J. Appl. Phys. (15 December 1993):7321-7328.
1824. S. Takeda, G. Soda, H. Chihara, "Solid Neopentane $C(CH_3)_4$ as Studied by Nuclear Magnetic Resonance: A Detailed Examination of Methyl and Molecular Reorientation in the Low Temperature Phase," Mol. Phys. 47(1982):501-517.
1825. J.M. Tour, "Organic Molecules for Application as Nanometer-Scale Electronic Devices," unpublished briefing, University of South Carolina, Columbia, SC, 1996; presented at the DARPA ULTRA Program Review, Estes Park, CO, 6-10 October 1996.
1826. R.C. Haddon et al., "Conducting films of C_{60} and C_{70} by alkali-metal doping," Nature 350(28 March 1991):320-322.
1827. R.C. Haddon, A.S. Perel, R.C. Morris, T.T.M. Palstra, A.F. Hebard, R.M. Fleming, "C_{60} thin film transistors," Appl. Phys. Lett. 67(3 July 1995):121-123.
1828. Y. Miyamoto, S.G. Louie, M.L. Cohen, "Chiral conductivities of nanotubes," Phys. Rev. Lett. 76(1996):2121-2124. See also: Science 271(1 March 1996):1232.
1829. S.N. Song, X.K. Wang, R.P.H. Chang, J.B. Ketterson, "Electronic Properties of Graphite Nanotubules from Galvanomagnetic Effects," Phys. Rev. Lett. 72(31 January 1994):697-700.
1830. D.P.E. Smith, "Quantum Point Contact Switches," Science 269(21 July 1995):371-373.
1831. Donal D.C. Bradley, "Molecular electronics—aspects of the physics," Chemistry in Britain 27(August 1991):719-723.
1832. John Barker, "Building molecular electronic systems," Chemistry in Britain 27(August 1991):718, 728-731.
1833. Richard B. Kaner, Alan G. MacDiarmid, "Plastics That Conduct Electricity," Scientific American 258(February 1988):106-111.
1835. Martin P. Debreczeny, Walter A. Svec, Michael R. Wasielewski, "Optical Control of Photogenerated Ion Pair Lifetimes: An Approach to a Molecular Switch," Science 274(25 October 1996):584-587.
1836. Michael P. O'Neil, Mark P. Niemczyk, Walter A. Svec, David Gosztola, George L. Gaines III, Michael R. Wasielewski, "Picosecond Optical Switching Based on Biphotonic Excitation of an Electron Donor-Acceptor-Donor Molecule," Science 257(3 July 1992):63-65.
1837. M.A. Reed, C. Zhou, C.J. Muller, T.P. Burgin, J.M. Tour, "Conductance of a Molecular Junction," Science 278(10 October 1997):252-254.
1838. Philip G. Collins, Alex Zettl, Hiroshi Bando, Andreas Thess, R.E. Smalley, "Nanotube Nanodevice," Science 278(3 October 1997):100-103.
1839. Corrine L. Curtis, Jason E. Ritchie, Michael J. Sailor, "Fabrication of Conducting Polymer Interconnects," Science 262(24 December 1993):2014-2016.
1840. O. Kahn, C. Jay Martinez, "Spin-Transition Polymers: From Molecular Materials Toward Memory Devices," Science 279(2 January 1998):44-48.
1841. Craig Halvorson, Andrew Hays, Brett Krabel, Rulian Wu, Fred Wudl, Alan J. Heeger, "A 160-Femtosecond Optical Image Processor Based on a Conjugated Polymer," Science 265(26 August 1994):1215-1216.
1842. A. Dodabalapur, L. Torsi, H.E. Katz, "Organic Transistors: Two-Dimensional Transport and Improved Electrical Characteristics," Science 268(14 April 1995):270-271.
1843. Alfredo M. Morales, Charles M. Lieber, "A Laser Ablation Method for the Synthesis of Crystalline Semiconductor Nanowires," Science 279(9 January 1998):208-211.
1844. Hongjie Dai, Eric W. Wong, Charles M. Lieber, "Probing Electrical Transport in Nanomaterials: Conductivity of Individual Carbon Nanotubes," Science 272(26 April 1996):523-526.
1845. Alexander S. Lane, David A. Leigh, Aden Murphy, "Peptide-Based Molecular Shuttles," J. Am. Chem. Soc. 119(12 November 1997):11092-11093.
1846. Myriam Linke, Jean-Claude Chambron, Valerie Heitz, Jean-Pierre Sauvage, "Electron Transfer Between Mechanically Linked Porphyrins in a [2]Rotaxane," J. Am. Chem Soc. 119(19 November 1997):11329-11330.
1847. Jeroen W.G. Wildoer, Liesbeth C. Venema, Andrew G. Rinzler, Richard E. Smalley, Cees Dekker, "Electronic structure of atomically resolved carbon nanotubes," Nature 391(1 January 1998):59-61.
1848. Teri Wang Odom, Jin-Lin Huang, Philip Kim, Charles M. Lieber, "Atomic structure and electronic properties of single-walled carbon nanotubes," Nature 391(1 January 1998):62-64.
1849. Philippe Lambin, A. Fonseca, J.P. Vigneron, J.B. Nagy, A.A. Lucas, "Structural and electronic properties of bent carbon nanotubes," Chem. Phys. Lett. 245(20 October 1995):85-89.
1850. S.J. Tans, M.H. Devoret, H. Dai, A. Thess, R.E. Smalley, L.J. Geerligs, C. Dekker, "Individual single-wall carbon nanotubes as quantum wires," Nature 386(1997):474-476.
1852. J.W. Mintmire, B.I. Dunlap, C.T. White, "Are fullerene tubules metallic?" Phys. Rev. Lett. 68(1992):631-634.
1853. Noriaki Hamada, Shin-ichi Sawada, Atsushi Oshiyama, "New One-Dimensional Conductors: Graphitic Microtubules," Phys. Rev. Lett. 68(9 March 1992):1579-1581.
1854. R. Saito, M. Fujita, G. Dresselhaus, M.S. Dresselhaus, "Electronic structure of chiral graphene tubules," Appl. Phys. Lett. 60(1992):2204-2206.
1855. R.J. Schoelkopf, P. Wahlgren, A.A. Kozhevnikov, P. Delsing, D.E. Prober, "The Radio-Frequency Single-Electron Transistor (RF-SET): A Fast and Ultrasensitive Electrometer," Science 280(22 May 1998):1238-1242.
1857. Stefan Frank, Philippe Poncharal, Z.L. Wang, Walt A. de Heer, "Carbon Nanotube Quantum Resistors," Science 280(12 June 1998):1744-1746.
1858. L. Chico, Vincent H. Crespi, Lorin X. Benedict, Steven G. Louie, Marvin L. Cohen, "Pure carbon nanoscale devices: nanotube heterojunctions," Phys. Rev. Lett. 76(5 February 1996):971-974.
1859. R. Saito, G. Dresselhaus, M.S. Dresselhaus, "Tunneling conductance of connected carbon nanotubes," Phys. Rev. B 53(15 January 1996):2044-2050.
1860. J.-C. Charlier, T.W. Ebbesen, Ph. Lambin, "Structural and electronic properties of pentagon-heptagon pair defects in carbon nanotubes," Phys. Rev. B 53(15 April 1996):11108-11113.
1861. Leonor Chico, Lorin X. Benedict, Stephen G. Louie, Marvin L. Cohen, "Quantum conductance of carbon nanotubes with defects," Phys. Rev. B 54(15 July 1996):2600-2606.
1862. C. Guerret-Piecourt, Y. Le Bouar, A. Loiseau, H. Pascard, "Relation between metal electronic structure and morphology of metal compounds inside carbon nanotubes," Nature 372(22/29 December 1994):761-765.
1863. T.M. Whitney, J.S. Jiang, P.C. Searson, C.L. Chien, "Fabrication and Magnetic Properties of Arrays of Metallic Nanowires," Science 261(3 September 1993):1316-1319.
1864. Josh H. Golden, Francis J. DiSalvo, Jean M.J. Frechet, John Silcox, Malcolm Thomas, Jim Elman, "Subnanometer-Diameter Wires Isolated in a Polymer Matrix by Fast Polymerization," Science 273(9 August 1996):782-784.
1865. J.R. Olson, K.A. Topp, R.O. Pohl, "Specific Heat and Thermal Conductivity of Solid Fullerenes," Science 259(19 February 1993):1145-1148.
1866. R.C. Haddon, "Chemistry of the Fullerenes: The Manifestation of Strain in a Class of Continuous Aromatic Molecules," Science 261(17 September 1993):1545-1550.
1867. Ruilan Wu, Jeffry S. Schumm, Darren L. Pearson, James M. Tour, "Convergent Synthetic Routes to Orthogonally Fused Conjugated Oligomers Directed Toward Molecular Scale Electronic Device Applications," J. Org. Chem. 61(1996):6906-6921.
1868. J.M. Tour, "Conjugated Macromolecules of Precise Length and Constitution. Organic Synthesis for the Construction of Nanoarchitectures," Chem. Rev. 96(January-February 1996):537-553.
1869. D.L. Pearson, J.M. Tour, "Rapid Syntheses of Oligo(2,5-thiophene-ethynylene)s with Thioester Termini: Potential Molecular Scale Wires With Alligator Clips," J. Org. Chem. 62(1997):1376-1387.
1870. L. Jones II, J.S. Schumm, J.M. Tour, "Rapid Solution and Solid Phase Syntheses of Oligo(1,4-phenylene-ethynylene)s With Thioester Termini: Molecular Scale Wires With Alligator Clips. Derivation of Iterative Reaction Efficiencies on a Polymer Support," J. Org. Chem. 62(1997):1388-1410.
1871. Abbas Farazdel, Michel Dupuis, Enrico Clementi, Ari Aviram, "Electric Field Induced Intramolecular Electron Transfer in Spiro π-Electron Systems and Their Suitability as Molecular Electronic Devices. A Theoretical Study," J. Am. Chem. Soc. 112(1990):4206-4214.
1872. Deepak Srivastava, Steve T. Barnard, S. Saini, M. Menon, "Carbon Nanotubes: Nanoscale Electromechanical Sensors", 2nd NASA Semiconductor Device Modeling Workshop, NASA Ames Research Center, August 1997.
1873. Philip G. Collins, Hiroshi Bando, Alex Zettl, "Nanoscale Electronic Devices on Carbon Nanotubes," Nanotechnology 9(September 1998):153-157; paper presented at the 5th Foresight Conference on Molecular Nanotechnology, November 1997.
1874. Barry C. Stipe, Mohammad A. Rezaei, Wilson Ho, "Inducing and Viewing the Rotational Motion of a Single Molecule," Science 279(20 March 1998):1907-1909.
1875. S.J. Tans, A.R.M. Verschueren, C. Dekker, "Room-temperature transistor based on a single carbon nanotube," Nature 393(7 May 1998):49-52.
1876. Jie Han, M.P. Anantram, Richard Jaffe, "Design and Study of Carbon Nanotube Electronic Devices," paper presented at the Fifth Foresight Conference on Molecular Nanotechnology, 5-8 November 1997, Palo Alto, CA.
1877. M. Menon, D. Srivastava, S. Saini, "Carbon Nanotube Junctions as Building Blocks for Nanoscale Electronic Devices," Semiconductor Device Modeling Workshop at NASA Ames Research Center, August 1997.
1878. Madhu Menon, Deepak Srivastava, "Carbon Nanotube T-Junctions: Nanoscale Metal-Semiconductor-Metal Contact Devices," Phys. Rev. Lett. 79(1 December 1997):4453-4456.
1879. James M. Tour, Masatoshi Kozaki, Jorge M. Seminario, "Molecular Scale Electronics: A Synthetic/Computational Approach to Digital Computing," J. Am. Chem. Soc. 120(1998):8486-8493.
1880. Stephen H. Unger, Asynchronous Sequential Switching Circuits, Wiley-Interscience, New York, 1969.

1881. C. L. Seitz, "System Timing," in Carver Mead, Lynn Conway, eds., Introduction to VLSI Systems, Addison-Wesley, Reading, MA, 1980, pp. 242-262.

1882. Ivan E. Sutherland, "Micropipelines," Commun. CM 32(June 1989):720-738.

1883. Ilana David, Ran Ginosar, Michael Yoeli, "An Efficient Implementation of Boolean Functions as Self-Timed Circuits," IEEE Trans. Comp. 41(January 1992):2-10.

1884. J. A. Brzozowski, C-J. H. Seger, "Advances in Asynchronous Circuit Theory. Part I: Gate and Unbounded Inertial Delay Models," Bulletin of the European Association for Computer Science 42(October 1990):198-248.

1885. Karl M. Fant, Scott A. Brandt, "NULL Convention Logic: A Complete and Consistent Logic for Asynchronous Digital Design," at http://www.theseus.com/NCLPaper/index.html; NULL Convention Logic System, US Patent 5,305,463; 19 April 1994.

1886. Paul Wilhelm Karl Rothemund, "A DNA and restriction enzyme implementation of Turing Machines," in Richard J. Lipton, Eric B. Baum, eds., DNA Based Computers, American Mathematical Society, Providence RI, 1996, pp. 75-120.

1887. T. Yagi, N. Ito, M. Watanabe, T. Matsushima, Y. Uchikawa, "A Study on Hybrid Artificial Retina with Cultured Neural Cells and Semiconductor Microdevice," Proc. 1998 IEEE Intl. Joint Conf. Neural Networks (IJCNN'98), 1998.

1888. N. Ito, A. Shirahata, T. Yagi, T. Matsushima, K. Kawase, M. Watanabe, Y. Uchikawa, "Development of Artificial Retina using Cultured Neural Cells and Photoelectric Device: A Study on Electric Current with Membrane Model," Proc. 4th Intl. Conf. Neural Information Proc. (ICONIP'97), 1997.

1889. T. Yagi, N. Ito, T. Matsushima, Y. Ishikawa, K. Kawase, A. Shirahata, Y. Uchikawa, "Artificial Retina using Cultured Neural Cells and Photoelectric Device," Proc. 7th Intl. Conf. Human-Computer Interaction (HCI'97), 1997, p. 109.

1890. N. Ito, T. Yagi, T. Matsushima, Y. Uchikawa, "Development of an Artificial Retina for Light Sense Restoration," Neuroscience Res. 21(1997):S302.

1891. A. van Schaik, R. Meddis, "The Electronic Ear: Towards a Blueprint," in Vincent Torre, Franco Conti, eds., Neurobiology: Ionic Channels, Neurons, and the Brain, Plenum Press, New York, 1997, pp. 233-250.

1892. I. Honjo, H. Takahashi, eds., Cochlear Implant and Related Sciences Update, 1st Asia Pacific Symposium on Cochlear Implant and Related Sciences, Kyoto, 3-5 April 1996, S. Karger Publishing, 1997.

1893. Graeme M. Clark, Robert S.C. Cowan, Richard C. Dowell, eds., Cochlear Implantation for Infants and Children, Singular Publishing Group, 1997.

1894. Charles H. Bennett, Rolf Landauer, "The Fundamental Physical Limits of Computation," Scientific American 253(July 1985):48-56.

1895. Leonard M. Adleman, "Molecular Computation of Solutions to Combinatorial Problems," Science 266(11 November 1994):1021-1024.

1896. Leonard M. Adleman, "Computing with DNA," Scientific American 279(August 1998):54-61.

1897. "On the Potential of Molecular Computing," Science 268(28 April 1995):481-484.

1898. Richard J. Lipton, "DNA Solution of Hard Computational Problems," Science 268(28 April 1995):542-545.

1899. Willem P.C. Stemmer, "The Evolution of Molecular Computation," Science 270(1 December 1995):1510.

1900. Frank Guarnieri, Makiko Fliss, Carter Bancroft, "Making DNA Add," Science 273(12 July 1996):220-223.

1901. E. Csuhaj-Varju, R. Freund, L. Kari, G. Paun, "DNA computing based on splicing: universality results," Pacific Symposium on Biocomputing, 1996, pp. 179-190; G. Paun, J. Autom. Lang. Comb. 1(1996):27 et seq.

1902. Qi Ouyang, Peter D. Kaplan, Shumao Liu, Albert Libchaber, "DNA Solution of the Maximal Clique Problem," Science 278(17 October 1997):446-449.

1903. Eric B. Baum, "Building an Associative Memory Vastly Larger Than the Brain," Science 268(28 April 1995):583-585.

1904. C.A. Mirkin, R.L. Letsinger, R.C. Mucic, J.J. Storhoff, "A DNA-based method for rationally assembling nanoparticles into macroscopic materials," Nature 382(15 August 1996):607-609.

1905. C.M. Niemeyer, T. Sano, C.L. Smith, C.R. Cantor, "Oligonucleotide-directed self-assembly of proteins," Nucl. Acids Res. 22(1994):5530-5539.

1906. A.J. Epstein, J.S. Miller, "Linear Chain Conductors," Scientific American (October 1979):52-61.

1907. M. Kanatzidis, "Conductive Polymers," Chem. Eng. News (3 December 1990):36-54.

1908. S. Roth, W. Graupner, P. McNellis, "Survey of Industrial Applications of Conducting Polymers," Acta Physica Polonica A 87(1995):699-711.

1909. T.A. Skotheim, ed., Handbook of Conducting Polymers, Marcel Dekker, New York, 1986.

1910. Hava T. Siegelmann, "Computation Beyond the Turing Limit," Science 268(28 April 1995):545-548.

1911. A. Hjelmfelt, F.W. Schneider, J. Ross, "Pattern Recognition in Coupled Chemical Kinetic Systems," Science 260(16 April 1993):335-337.

1912. Jean-Pierre Laplante, Thomas Erneux, "Propagation Failure in Arrays of Coupled Bistable Chemical Reactors," J. Phys. Chem. 96(1992):4931-4934.

1913. B.H. Robinson, N.C. Seeman, "Design of a Biochip," Protein Eng. 1(1987):295-300.

1914. Junghuei Chen, Nadrian C. Seeman, "Synthesis from DNA of a molecule with the connectivity of a cube," Nature 350(1991):631-633.

1915. Yuwen Zhang, Nadrian C. Seeman, "Construction of a DNA-Truncated Octahedron, "J. Am. Chem. Soc. 116(1994):1661-1669.

1916. Nadrian C. Seeman et al., "New Motifs in DNA Nanotechnology," Nanotechnology 9(September 1998):257-273.

1917. C. Mao, W. Sun, N.C. Seeman, "Assembly of Borromean rings from DNA," Nature 386(1997):137-138.

1918. C. Liang, K. Mislow, "On Borromean links," J. Math. Chem. 16(1994):27-35.

1919. Eric Winfree, "On the computational power of DNA annealing and ligation," in Richard J. Lipton, Eric B. Baum, eds., DNA Based Computers, American Mathematical Society, Providence RI, 1996, pp. 199-219. See also: "Erik's Molecular Computation Page," http://dope.caltech.edu/winfree/DNA.html.

1920. T.J. Fu, N.C. Seeman, "DNA double crossover structures," Biochemistry 32(1993):3211-3220.

1921. M. Gellert, K. Mizuuchi, M.H. O'Dea, H. Ohmori, J. Tomizawa, "DNA gyrase and DNA supercoiling," Cold Spring Harbor Symp. Quant. Biol. 43(1978):35-40.

1922. X. Yang, A.V. Vologodskii, B. Liu, B. Kemper, N.C. Seeman, "Torsional control of double-stranded DNA branch migration," Biopolymers 45(1997):69-83.

1923. A.R. Brown, A. Pomp, C.M. Hart, D.M. de Leeuw, "Logic Gates Made from Polymer Transistors and Their Use in Ring Oscillators," Science 270(10 November 1995):972-974.

1924. M.C. Petty, M.R. Bryce, D. Bloor, eds., Introduction to Molecular Electronics, Oxford University Press, New York, 1995.

1925. Robert R. Birge, "Protein-Based Computers," Scientific American 272(March 1995):90-95.

1926. R. Shashidhar, J.M. Schnur, "Self-Assembling Tubules from Phospholipids," in Robert R. Birge, ed., Molecular and Biomolecular Electronics, American Chemical Society, Washington, DC, 1994, pp. 455-474.

1927. Elisabeth Smela, Olle Inganas, Ingemar Lundstrom, "New Devices Made from Combining Silicon Microfabrication and Conducting Polymers," in C. Nicolini, ed., Molecular Manufacturing, Plenum Press, New York, 1996, pp. 189-213.

1928. Michael D. Toney, Erhard Hohenester, Sandra W. Cowan, Johan N. Jansonius, "Dialkylglycine Decarboxylase Structure: Bifunctional Active Site and Alkali Metal Sites," Science 261(6 August 1993):756-759.

1929. M. Matsumura, B.W. Matthews, "Control of Enzyme Activity by an Engineered Disulfide Bond," Science 243(10 February 1989):792-794.

1930. H.J. Sices, T.M. Kristie, "A genetic screen for the isolation and characterization of site-specific proteases," Proc. Natl. Acad. Sci. 95(17 March 1998):2828-2833.

1931. Janos H. Fendler, "Colloid Chemical Approach to Band-Gap Engineering and Quantum-Tailored Devices," in Robert R. Birge, ed., Molecular and Biomolecular Electronics, American Chemical Society, Washington, DC, 1994, pp. 413-438.

1932. A. Ottova-Leitmannova, T. Martynski, A. Wardak, H.T. Tien, "Self-Assembling Bilayer Lipid Membranes on Solid Support: Building Blocks of Future Biosensors and Molecular Devices," in Robert R. Birge, ed., Molecular and Biomolecular Electronics, American Chemical Society, Washington, DC, 1994, pp. 439-454.

1933. Patrick S. Stayton, Jill M. Olinger, Susan T. Wollman, Paul W. Bohn, Stephen G. Sligar, "Engineering Proteins for Electrooptical Biomaterials," in Robert R. Birge, ed., Molecular and Biomolecular Electronics, American Chemical Society, Washington, DC, 1994, pp. 475-490.

1934. M.R. Arkin, E.D.A. Stemp, R.E. Holmlin, J.K. Barton, A. Hormann, E.J.C. Olson, P.F. Barbara, "Rates of DNA-Mediated Electron Transfer Between Metallointercalators," Science 273(26 July 1996):475-480.

1935. F. Garnier et al., "All-Polymer Field-Effect Transistor Realized by Printing Techniques," Science 265(1994):1684-1686.

1936. J.S. Clegg, "Properties and metabolism of the aqueous cytoplasm," Am. J. Physiol. 246(1984):R133-R151.

1937. S. Pauser, A. Zschunke, A. Khuen, K. Keller, "Estimation of water content and water mobility in the nucleus and cytoplasm of *Xenopus laevis* oocytes by NMR microscopy," Magnetic Resonance Imaging 13(1995):269-276.

1938. C. Neubauer, A.M. Phelan, H. Keus, D.G. Lange, "Microwave irradiation of rats at 2.45 GHz activates pinocytotic-like uptake of tracer by capillary endothelial cells of cerebral cortex," Bioelectromagnetics 11(1990):261-268.

1939. C.A.L. Bassett, "Electrical Effects in Bone," Scientific American 213(October 1965):18-25.

1940. A. Gjelsvik, "Bone remodelling and piezoelectricity," J. Biomech. 6(1973):69-77, 187-193.

1941. Sergio Mascarenhas, "The electret effect in bone and biopolymers and the bound water problem," Ann. N.Y. Acad. Sci. 238(11 October 1974):36-52. See also: "The electret state: A new property of bone," in M.M. Perlman, ed., Electrets, The Electrochemical Society, Princeton, NJ, 1973, pp. 650 et seq.

1942. H. Athenstaedt, "Pyroelectric and piezoelectric properties of vertebrates," Ann. N.Y. Acad. Sci. 238(1974):68-93.

1943. David H. Freedman, "Exploiting the Nanotechnology of Life," Science 254(29 November 1991):1308-1310.

1956. T.T. Puck, A. Krystosek, "Role of the cytoskeleton in genome regulation and cancer," Intl. Rev. Cytology 132(1992):75-108.

1960. G. Albrecht-Buehler, "Cellular infrared detector appears to be contained in the centrosome," Cell Motility and the Cytoskeleton 27(1994):262-271.

1961. E. Braun, Y. Eichen, U. Silvan, G. Ben-Yoseph, "DNA-templated assembly and electrode attachment of a conducting silver wire," Nature 391(19 February 1998):775-778.

1962. Thomas F. Knight Jr., Gerald Jay Sussman, "Cellular Gate Technology," paper presented at Proc. UMC98, First International Conference on Unconventional Models of Computation, Auckland, NZ, January 1998; see also: http://www-swiss.ai.mit.edu/~switz/amorphous/papers/cellgates.ps.gz (postscript version) or http://www-swiss.ai.mit.edu/~switz/amorphous/papers/cellgates (html version).
1963. Yi Liu, Martha Merrow, Jennifer J. Loros, Jay C. Dunlap, "How Temperature Changes Reset a Circadian Oscillator," Science 281(7 August 1998):825-829.
1964. E. Rios, M.D. Stern, "Calcium in close quarters: Microdomain feedback in excitation-contraction coupling and other cell biological phenomena," Annu. Rev. Biophys. Biomol. Struct. 26(1997):47-82.
1965. Steven O. Marx, Karol Ondrias, Andrew R. Marks, "Coupled Gating Between Individual Skeletal Muscle Ca^{2+} Release Channels (Ryanodine Receptors," Science 281(7 August 1998):818-821. See also: Donald M. Bers, Michael Fill, "Coordinated Feet and the Dance of Ryanodine Receptors," Science 281(7 August 1998):790-791.
1966. J.J. Hickman, S.K. Bhatia, J.N. Quong, P. Sheen, et al., "Rational pattern design for in vitro cellular networks using surface photochemistry," J. Vac. Sci. Technol. A 12(May-June 1994):607-616.
1967. D.R. Jung, D.S. Cuttino, J.J. Pancrazio, P. Manos, et al., "Cell-based sensor microelectrode array characterized by imaging X-ray photoelectron spectroscopy scanning electron microscopy, impedance measurements, and extracellular recordings," J. Vac. Sci. Technol. A 16(May-June 1998):1183-1188.
1968. Philip Yeagle, ed., The Structure of Biological Membranes, CRC Press, Boca Raton, FL 1992.
1969. Dick Hoekstra, Shlomo Nir, "Chapter 21. Cell Biology of Entry and Exit of Enveloped Virus," in Philip Yeagle, ed., The Structure of Biological Membranes, CRC Press, Boca Raton, FL, 1992, pp. 949-996.
1970. Erik Winfree, Furong Liu, Lisa A. Wenzler, Nadrian C. Seeman, "Design and self-assembly of two-dimensional DNA crystals," Nature 394(6 August 1998):539-544.
1971. L. Monti-Bloch, C. Jennings-White, D.S. Dolberg, D.L. Berliner, "The Human Vomeronasal System," Psychoneuroendocrinology 19(1994):673-686.
1972. Kathleen Stern, Martha K. McClintock, "Regulation of ovulation by human pheromones," Nature 392(12 March 1998):177-179. See also: Aron Weller, "Communication through body odour," Nature 392(12 March 1998):126-127.
1973. Ivan Damjanov, James Linder, Anderson's Pathology, Tenth Edition, Mosby, St. Louis MO, 1996.
1974. Kaigham J. Gabriel, "Engineering Microscopic Machines," Scientific American 273(September 1995):150-153.
1975. Richard Ravel, Clinical Laboratory Medicine: Clinical Application of Laboratory Data, Sixth Edition, Mosby, St. Louis MO, 1995.
1976. Mark Ptashne, A Genetic Switch: Phage Lambda and Higher Organisms, Second Edition, Cell Press and Blackwell Scientific Publications, Cambridge, 1992.
1980. James R. Heath, Philip J. Kuekes, Gregory S. Snider, R. Stanley Williams, "A Defect-Tolerant Computer Architecture: Opportunities for Nanotechnology," Science 280(12 June 1998):1716-1721.
1981. Jorge M. Seminario, James M. Tour, "Ab Initio Methods for the Study of Molecular Systems for Nanometer Technology: Toward the First-Principles Design of Molecular Computers," in A. Aviram, M. Ratner, eds., Molecular Electronics: Science and Technology, Ann. N.Y. Acad. Sci. 852(1998):68-94.
1982. Johndale C. Solem, "The Motility of Microrobots," in Christopher G.Langton, ed., Artificial Life III, Addison-Wesley Publishing Company, Reading, MA, 1994, pp. 359-380.
1983. Timothy J. Coutts, Mark C. Fitzgerald, "Thermophotovoltaics," Scientific American 279(September 1998):90-95.
1984. L. Brillouin, Science and Information Theory, Second Edition, Academic Press, London, 1962.
1985. John von Neumann, Theory of Self-Reproducing Automata, A.W. Burks, ed., University of Illinois Press, Urbana IL, 1966.
1986. R. Landauer, "Irreversibility and Heat Generation in the Computing Process," IBM J. Res. Develop. 3(1961):183-191.
1987. Edward Fredkin, Tommaso Toffoli, "Conservative logic," Intl. J. Theor. Phys. 21(1982):219-253.
1988. R. Landauer, "Energy Requirements in Computation," Appl. Phys. Lett. 51(1987):2056-2058.
1989. R. Landauer, "Dissipation and noise immunity in computation and communication," Nature 335(1988):779-784.
1990. Jacob D. Bekenstein, "Energy Cost of Information Transfer," Phys. Rev. Lett. 46(9 March 1981):623-626. See also: "Entropy content and information flow in systems with limited energy," Phys. Rev. D 30(1984):1669-1679.
1991. Marcelo Schiffer, Jacob D. Bekenstein, "Proof of the quantum bound on specific entropy for free fields," Phys. Rev. D 39(15 February 1989):1109-1115; and "Do zero-frequency modes contribute to the entropy?" Phys. Rev. D 42(15 November 1989):3598-3599.
1992. Konstantin K. Likharev, "Classical and Quantum Limitations on Energy Consumption in Computation," Intl. J. Theor. Phys. 21(1982):311-325.
1993. Konstantin K. Likharev, Alexander N. Korotkov, "Single-Electron Parametron: Reversible Computation in a Discrete-State System," Science 273(9 August 1996):763-765.
1994. Michael P. Frank, Thomas F. Knight, Jr., "Ultimate Theoretical Models of Nanocomputers," Nanotechnology 9(September 1998):162-176; or see: http://www.ai.mit.edu/~mpf/Nano97/paper.html.
1995. Jean-Marc Bonard, Thomas Stockli, Frederic Maier, Walt A. de Heer, Andre Chatelain, "Field-Emission-Induced Luminescence from Carbon Nanotubes," Phys. Rev. Lett. 81(17 August 1998):1441-1444.
1996. Richard P. Feynman, "Quantum Mechanical Computers," Optics News 11(February 1985):11-20; and "Simulating Physics with Computers," Intl. J. Theor. Phys. 21(1982):467-488. See also: http://feynman.stanford.edu/qcomp/.
1997. Paul Benioff, "Quantum Mechanical Models of Turing Machines That Dissipate No Energy," Phys. Rev. Lett. 48(7 June 1982):1581-1585.
1998. D. Deutsch, "Quantum theory, the Church-Turing principle and the universal quantum computer," Proc. Roy. Soc. London A 400(8 July 1985):97-117. See also: The Fabric of Reality, Penguin, New York, 1997, pp. 194-222.
1999. David P. DiVincenzo, "Quantum Computation," Science 270(13 October 1995):255-261.
2000. I.L. Chang, R. Laflamme, P.W. Shor, W.H. Zurek, "Quantum Computers, Factoring, and Decoherence," Science 270(8 December 1995):1633-1635.
2001. Seth Lloyd, "Universal Quantum Simulators," Science 273(23 August 1996):1073-1078; see also Science 279(20 February 1998):1117.
2002. Neil A. Gershenfeld, Isaac L. Chuang, "Bulk Spin-Resonance Quantum Computation," Science 275(17 January 1997):350-356. See also: "Quantum Computing with Molecules," Scientific American 278(June 1998):66-71; Isaac L. Chuang, Lievon M.K. Vandersypen, Xinlan Zhou, Debbie W. Leung, Seth Lloyd, "Experimental realization of a quantum algorithm," Nature 393(14 May 1998):143-146.
2003. Emanuel Knill, Raymond Laflamme, Wojciech H. Zurek, "Resilient Quantum Computation," Science 279(16 January 1998):342-345.
2004. Lov K. Grover, "The Advantages of Superposition," Science 280(10 April 1998):228; see also "Beyond Factorization and Search," Science 281(7 August 1998):792-794.
2005. C. Monroe, D.M. Meekhof, B.E. King, W.M. Itano, D.J. Wineland, "Demonstration of a Fundamental Quantum Logic Gate," Phys. Rev. Lett. 75(18 December 1995):4714-4717.
2006. Q.A. Turchette, C.J. Hood, W. Lange, H. Mabuchi, H.J. Kimble, "Measurement of Conditional Phase Shifts for Quantum Logic," Phys. Rev. Lett. 75(18 December 1995):4710-4713.
2007. Warren S. Warren, "The Usefulness of NMR Quantum Computing," Science 277(12 September 1997):1688-1689.
2008. Jonathan A. Jones, "Fast Searches with Nuclear Magnetic Resonance Computers," Science 280(10 April 1998):229; see also Science 281(25 September 1998):1963-1964.
2009. P.W. Shor, in Proceedings of the 35th Annual IEEE Symposium on Foundations of Computer Science, IEEE Computer Society Press, Los Alamitos, CA, 1994, pp. 124-134.
2010. J.I. Cirac, T. Pellizzari, P. Zoller, "Enforcing Coherent Evolution in Dissipative Quantum Dynamics," Science 273(30 August 1996):1207-1210.
2013. C.P. Williams, Explorations in Quantum Computing, Springer-Verlag, New York, 1998.
2014. B.E. Kane, "A silicon-based nuclear spin quantum computer," Nature 393(14 May 1998):133-137.
2015. A. Balsalobre, F. Damiola, Ueli Schibler, "A serum shock induces circadian gene expression in mammalian tissue culture cells," Cell 93(12 June 1998):929-937.
2016. Y. Zhang, K. Suenaga, C. Colliex, S. Iijima, "Coaxial Nanocable: Silicon Carbide and Silicon Oxide Sheathed with Boron Nitride and Carbon," Science 281(14 August 1998):973-975.
2017. E.D. Getzoff, D.E. Cabelli, C.L. Fisher, H.E. Parge, M.S. Viezzoli, L. Banci, R.A. Hallewell, "Faster Superoxide Dismutase Mutants Designed by Enhancing Electrostatic Guidance," Nature 358(1992):347-351.
2018. C. Grillot-Courvalin, S. Goussard, F. Hoetz, D.M. Ojcius, P. Courvalin, "Functional gene transfer from intracellular bacteria to mammalian cells," Nature Biotechnology 16(September 1998):862-866.
2019. Hal K. Hawkins, Jan L.E. Ericsson, Peter Biberfeld, Benjamin F. Trump, "Lysosome and Phagosome Stability in Lethal Cell Injury," Am. J. Physiol. 68(1972):255-288
2020. Hannu Kalimo, Julio H. Garcia, Yoshinari Kamijyo, Junichi Tanaka, Benjamin F. Trump, "The Ultrastructure of Brain Death. II. Electron Microscopy of Feline Cortex after Complete Ischemia," Virchows Archiv. B. Cell Path. 25(1977):207-220.
2021. Xiangyun Wei, Jagath Samarabandu, Rakendu S. Devdhar, Alan J. Siegel, Raj Acharya, Ronald Berezney, "Segregation of Transcription and Replication Sites Into Higher Order Domains," Science 281(4 September 1998):1502-1505.
2022. Steven Vogel, Cats' Paws and Catapults: Mechanical Worlds of Nature and People, W.W. Norton and Company, New York, 1998.
2023. Richard D. Johnson, Charles Holbrow, Space Settlements: A Design Study, NASA SP-413, 1977.
2024. A.C. Dillon, K.M. Jones, T.A. Bekkedahl, C.-H. Kiang, D.S. Bethune, M.J. Heben, "Storage of hydrogen in single-walled carbon nanotubes," Nature 386(27 March 1997):377-379.
2025. L.R. Cleveland, A.V. Grimstone, "The fine structure of the flagellate Mixotricha and its associated microorganisms," Proc. Roy. Soc. London B 159(1964):668-686.

2026. S.L. Tamm, "Flagellated ectosymbiotic bacteria propel a eukaryotic cell," J. Cell Biol. 94(1982):697-709.
2027. B.D. Dyer, R.A. Obar, Tracing the History of Eukaryotic Cells, Columbia University Press, New York, 1994.
2028. A.E. Walsby, "A square bacterium," Nature 283(1980):69-71.
2029. P.R. Grant, "Polyhedral territories of animals," Amer. Nat. 102(1968):75-80.
2030. G.W. Barlow, "Hexagonal territories," Anim. Behav. 22(1974):876-878.
2031. M.H. Zimmermann, Xylem Structure and the Ascent of Sap, Springer-Verlag, Berlin, 1983.
2032. W.H. Schlesinger, J.T. Gray, D.S. Gill, B.E. Mahall, "*Ceanothus megacarpus* chaparral: a synthesis of ecosystem processes during development and annual growth," Bot. Rev. 48(1982):71-117.
2033. O. Sotavalta, "Recordings of high wing-stroke and thoracic vibration frequency in some midges," Biol. Bull. Woods Hole 104(1953):439-444. See also: "The flight-tone (wing stroke frequency) of insects," Acta Entomol. Fenn. 4(1947):1-117.
2034. G.E. Gadd, M. Blackford, S. Moricca, N. Webb, P.J. Evans, A.M. Smith, G. Jacobsen, S. Leung, A. Day, Q. Hua, "The World's Smallest Gas Cylinders?" Science 277(15 August 1997):933-936.
2035. D.H. Liebenberg, R.L. Mills, J.C. Bronson, L.C. Schmidt, "High-Pressure Gases in Diamond Cells," Phys. Lett. 67A(24 July 1978):162-164.
2036. Linus Pauling, College Chemistry, Third Edition, W.H. Freeman and Company, San Francisco, 1964.
2037. J.M. Besson, J.P. Pinceaux, "Melting of Helium at Room Temperature and High Pressure," Science 206(30 November 1979):1073-1075.
2038. P. Loubeyre, R. LeToullec, D. Hausermann, M. Hanfland, R.J. Hemley, H.K. Mao, L.W. Finger, "X-ray diffraction and equation of state of hydrogen at megabar pressures," Nature 383(24 October 1996):702-704.
2039. P.V. Hobbs, Ice Physics, Clarendon Press, Oxford, 1974.
2040. I-Ming Chou, Jennifer G. Blank, Alexander F. Goncharov, Ho-kwang Mao, Russell J. Hemley, "In Situ Observations of a High-Pressure Phase of H_2O Ice," Science 281(7 August 1998):809-812.
2041. Donald J. Weidner, Yanbin Wang, Michael T. Vaughan, "Strength of Diamond," Science 266(21 October 1994):419-422.
2042. Robert M. Hazen, The New Alchemists: Breaking Through the Barriers of High Pressure, Times Books, NY, 1993.
2043. H.K. Mao, P.M. Bell, "High Pressure Physics: Sustained Static Generation of 1.36 to 1.72 Megabars," Science 200(9 June 1978):1145-1147.
2044. Manuel Nunez-Regueiro, Pierre Monceau, Jean-Louis Hodeau, "Crushing C_{60} to diamond at room temperature," Nature 355(16 January 1992):237-239.
2045. Y. Iwasa et al., "New Phases of C_{60} Synthesized at High Pressure," Science 264(10 June 1994):1570-1572. See also: M. Nunez-Regueiro, L. Marques, J.-L. Hodeau, O. Bethoux, M. Perroux, "Polymerized Fullerite Structures," Phys. Rev. Lett. 74(9 January 1995):278-281; L. Marques et al., "Debye-Scherrer Ellipses from 3D Fullerene Polymers: An Anisotropic Pressure Memory Signature," Science 283(12 March 1999):1720-1723.
2046. A.P. Jephcoat, R.J. Hemley, H.K. Mao, "X-ray Diffraction of Ruby (Al_2O_3:Cr^{3+}) to 175 GPa," Physica B 150(1988):115-121.
2047. Nobumasa Funamori, Raymond Jeanloz, "High-Pressure Transformation of Al_2O_3," Science 278(7 November 1997):1109-1111.
2048. Michell J. Sienko, Robert A. Plane, Chemistry, Second Edition, McGraw-Hill Book Company, New York, 1961.
2049. K.P. Johnston, K.L. Harrison, M.J. Clarke, S.M. Howdle, M.P. Heitz, F.V. Bright, C. Carlier, T.W. Randolph, "Water-in-Carbon Dioxide Microemulsions: An Environment for Hydrophiles Including Proteins," Science 271(2 February 1996):624-626.
2050. William L. Masterton, Emil J. Slowinski, Chemical Principles, Second Edition, W.B. Saunders Company, Philadelphia, 1969.
2051. Stanley Block, Gasper Piermarini, "The diamond cell stimulates high-pressure research," Physics Today 29(September 1976):44-55.
2052. M.I. Eremets, K. Shimizu, T.C. Kobayashi, K. Amaya, "Metallic CsI at Pressures of up to 220 Gigapascals," Science 281(28 August 1998):1333-1335.
2053. Henri Bader, Joseph K. Landauer, "Ice," Encyclopedia Britannica 12(1963):40-41.
2054. H.T. Haselton Jr., I.M. Chou, A.H. Shen, W.A. Bassett, Am. Mineral. 80(1995):1302 et seq.
2055. C.H. Chu, S.K. Estreicher, "Similarities, differences, and trends in the properties of interstitial H in cubic C, Si, BN, BP, AlP, and SiC," Phys. Rev. B 42(1990):9486-9495.
2056. J.H. Austin, T.S. Elleman, "Tritium diffusion in 304- and 316-stainless steels in the temperature range 25 to 222°C," J. Nucl. Materials 43(1972):119-125.
2057. J.J. Kearns, "Diffusion coefficient of hydrogen in α-zirconium, zircaloy-2 and zircaloy-4," J. Nucl. Materials 43(1972):330-338.
2058. Grazia Ambrosini, C. Adida, D.C. Altieri, "A novel anti-apoptosis gene, survivin, expressed in cancer and lymphoma," Nature Medicine 3(August 1997):917-921.
2059. Vicki Brower, "Biotech and Pharmaceutical Companies Target Apoptosis for the Potential Treatment of Disease," Gen. Eng. News (1 October 1996):1, 29, 34.
2060. Thomas G. Cotter, Mohamed Al-Rubeai, "Cell death (apoptosis) in cell culture systems," TIBTECH 13(April 1995):150-155.
2061. R.P. Singh, M. Al-Rubeai, C.D. Gregory, A.N. Emery, "Cell Death in Bioreactors: A Role for Apoptosis?" Biotechnol. Bioeng. 44(5 September 1994):720-726.
2062. J. John Cohen, Mohamed Al-Rubeai, "Apoptosis-targeted therapies: the next big thing in biotechnology?" TIBTECH 13(August 1995):281-283.
2063. Franziska A. Oberhammer et al., "Apoptotic death in epithelial cells: cleavage of DNA to 300 and/or 50 kb fragments prior to or in the absence of internucleosomal fragmentation," EMBO J. 12(1993):3679-3684.
2064. Daniel R. Catchpoole, Bernard W. Stewart, "Formation of Apoptotic Bodies Is Associated with Internucleosomal DNA Fragmentation during Drug-Induced Apoptosis," Exp. Cell. Res. 216(1995):169-177.
2065. Pierre Golstein, "Cell Death in Us and Others," Science 281(28 August 1998):1283.
2066. Shigekazu Nagata, Pierre Golstein, "The Fas Death Factor," Science 267(10 March 1995):1449-1456.
2067. Michael Hengartner, "Death by Crowd Control," Science 281(28 August 1998):1298-1299.
2068. Nancy A. Thornberry, Yuri Lazebnik, "Caspases: Enemies Within," Science 281(28 August 1998):1312-1316.
2069. Avi Ashkenazi, Vishva M. Dixit, "Death Receptors: Signaling and Modulation," Science 281(28 August 1998):1305-1308.
2070. Guohua Pan, Karen O'Rourke, Arul M. Chinnaiyan, Reiner Gentz, Reinhard Ebner, Jian Ni, Vishva M. Dixit, "The Receptor for the Cytotoxic Ligand TRAIL," Science 276(4 April 1997):111-113.
2071. E. Beltrami, J. Jesty, "Mathematical analysis of activation thresholds in enzyme-catalyzed positive feedbacks: application to the feedbacks of blood coagulation," Proc. Natl. Acad. Sci. USA 92(12 September 1995):8744-8748.
2072. Kornelia Polyak, Y. Xia, J.L. Zweier, K.W. Kinzler, B. Vogelstein, "A model for p53-induced apoptosis," Nature 389(18 September 1997):300-305.
2073. Douglas R. Green, John C. Reed, "Mitochondria and Apoptosis," Science 281(28 August 1998):1309-1312.
2074. Gerard Evan, Trevor Littlewood, "A Matter of Life and Cell Death," Science 281(28 August 1998):1317-1322.
2075. J.F. Kerr, A.H. Wyllie, A.R. Currie, "Apoptosis: A basic biological phenomenon with wide-ranging implications in tissue kinetics," Brit. J. Cancer 26(August 1972):239-257.
2076. L.H. Boise, C.B. Thompson, "Hierarchical Control of Lymphocyte Survival," Science 274(4 October 1996):67-68.
2077. B.A. Osborne, "Apoptosis and the maintenance of homeostasis in the immune system," Curr. Opin. Immunol. 8(April 1996):245-254.
2078. A. Winoto, "Cell death in the regulation of immune responses," Curr. Opin. Immunol. 9(June 1997):365-370.
2079. L.A. Tartaglia, D.V. Goeddel, "Two TNF receptors," Immunol. Today 13(May 1992):151-153.
2080. L.A. Tartaglia, T.M. Ayres, G.H.W. Wong, D.V. Goeddel, "A novel domain within the 55 kd TNF receptor signals cell death," Cell 74(10 September 1993):845-853.
2081. S. Nagata, "Apoptosis by death factor," Cell 88(7 February 1997):355-365.
2082. K. Orth, A.M. Chinnaiyan, M. Garg, C.J. Froelich, V.M. Dixit, "The CED-3/ICE-like protease Mch2 is activated during apoptosis and cleaves the death substrate lamin A," J. Biol. Chem. 271(12 July 1996):16443-16446.
2083. A. Takahashi et al., "Cleavage of lamin A by Mch2 alpha but not CPP32:...," Proc. Natl. Acad. Sci. USA 93(6 August 1996):8395-8400.
2084. Srinivas Kothakota et al., "Caspase-3-Generated Fragment of Gelsolin: Effector of Morphological Change in Apoptosis," Science 278(10 October 1997):294-298.
2085. L.P. Wen, J.A. Fahrni, S. Troie, J.L. Guan, K. Orth, G.D. Rosen, "Cleavage of focal adhesion kinase by caspases during apoptosis," J. Biol. Chem. 272(10 October 1997):26056-26061.
2086. T. Rudel, G.M. Bokoch, "Membrane and morphological changes in apoptotic cells regulated by caspase-mediated activation of PAK2," Science 276(6 June 1997):1571-1574.
2087. E. Rheaume et al., "The large subunit of replication factor C is a substrate for caspase-3 in vitro and is cleaved by a caspase-3-like protease during Fas-mediated apoptosis," EMBO J. 16(3 November 1997):6346-6354.
2088. V. Cryns, J. Yuan, "Proteases to die for," Genes Dev. 12(1 June 1998):1551-1570.
2089. N.A. Thornberry et al., "A combinatorial approach defines specificities of members of the caspase family and granzyme B. Functional relationships established for key mediators of apoptosis," J. Biol. Chem. 272(18 July 1997):17907-17911.
2090. Andrew Wyllie, "An endonuclease at last," Nature 391(1 January 1998):20-21.
2091. Masato Enari, Hideki Sakahira, Hideki Yokoyama, Katsuya Okawa, Akihiro Iwamatsu, Shigekazu Nagata, "A caspase-activated DNase that degrades DNA during apoptosis, and its inhibitor ICAD," Nature 391(1 January 1998):43-50.
2092. Hideki Sakahira, Masato Enari, Shigekazu Nagata, "Cleavage of CAD inhibitor in CAD activation and DNA degradation during apoptosis," Nature 391 (1 January 1998):96-99.
2093. A.H. Wyllie, J.F.R. Kerr, A.R. Currie, "Cell death: the significance of apoptosis," Int. Rev. Cytol. 68(1980):251-306.
2094. A.H. Wyllie, "Glucocorticoid-induced thymocyte apoptosis is associated with endogenous endonuclease activation," Nature 284(10 April 1980):555-556.
2095. J.S. Savill, I. Dransfield, N. Hogg, C. Haslett, "Vitronectin receptor-mediated phagocytosis of cells undergoing apoptosis," Nature 343(11 January 1990):170-173.
2096. Craig B. Thompson, "Apoptosis in the Pathogenesis and Treatment of Disease," Science 267(10 March 1995):1456-1462.

2097. Jerry M. Adams, Suzanne Cory, "The Bcl-2 Protein Family: Arbiters of Cell Survival," Science 281(28 August 1998):1322-1326.
2098. Adil A. Khan et al., "Lymphocyte Apoptosis: Mediation by Increased Type 3 Inositol 1,4,5-Trisphosphate Receptor," Science 273(26 July 1996):503-507.
2099. Hannes C.A. Drexler, "Activation of the cell death program by inhibition of proteasome function," Proc. Natl. Acad. Sci. USA 94(February 1997):855-860.
2100. Wen-Chen Yeh et al., "FADD: Essential for Embryo Development and Signaling from Some, But Not All, Inducers of Apoptosis," Science 279(20 March 1998):1954-1958.
2101. S.M. Srinivasula, M. Ahmad, T. Fernandes-Alnemri, E.S. Alnemri, "Autoactivation of procaspase-9 by Apaf-1-mediated oligomerization," Mol. Cell 1(June 1998):949-957.
2102. A.G. Uren, E.J. Coulson, D.L. Vaux, "Conservation of baculovirus inhibitor of apoptosis repeat proteins (BIRPs) in viruses, nematodes, vertebrates and yeasts," Trends Biochem. Sci. 23(May 1998):159-162.
2103. Luis del Peso, Maribel Gonzalez-Garcia, Carmen Page, Roman Herrera, Gabriel Nunez, "Interleukin-3-Induced Phosphorylation of BAD Through the Protein Kinase Akt," Science 278(24 October 1997):687-689.
2104. Pierre Golstein, "Cell death: TRAIL and its receptors," Curr. Biol. 7(1 December 1997):R750-R753.
2105. Guohua Pan, Jian Ni, Ying-Fei Wei, Guo-liang Yu, Reiner Gentz, Vishva M. Dixit, "An Antagonist Decoy Receptor and a Death Domain-Containing Receptor for TRAIL," Science 277(8 August 1997):815-818.
2106. James P. Sheridan et al., "Control of TRAIL-Induced Apoptosis by a Family of Signaling and Decoy Receptors," Science 277(8 August 1997):818-821.
2107. A. Desmouliere, M. Redard, I. Darby, G. Gabbiani, "Apoptosis mediates the decrease in cellularity during the transition between granulation tissue and scar," Am. J. Path. 146(1995):56-66.
2108. Vitaly A. Polunovsky, Baruch Chen, Craig Henke, Dale Snover, Christine Wendt, David H. Ingbar, Peter B. Bitterman, "Role of Mesenchymal Cell Death in Lung Remodeling after Injury," J. Clin. Invest. 92(1993):388-397.
2109. N.J. McCarthy, M.K.B. Whyte, C.S. Gilbert, G.I. Evan, "Inhibition of Ced-3/ICE-related proteases does not prevent cell death induced by oncogenes, DNA damage, or the Bcl-2 homologue Bak," J. Cell Biol. 136(13 January 1997):215-227.
2110. T. Hirsch et al., "The apoptosis-necrosis paradox. Apoptogenic proteases activated after mitochondrial permeability transition determine the mode of cell death," Oncogene 15(25 September 1997):1573-1581.
2111. Clare L. Brunet, Rosalind H. Gunby, Roderick S.P. Benson, John A. Hickman, Alastair J.M. Watson, Gerard Brady, "Commitment to cell death measured by loss of clonogenicity is separable from the appearance of apoptotic markers," Cell Death Differ. 5(January 1998):107-115.
2112. Gustavo P. Amarante-Mendes, Deborah M. Finucane, Seamus J. Martin, Thomas G. Cotter, Guys. Salvesen, Douglas R. Green, "Anti-apoptotic oncogenes prevent caspase-dependent and independent commitment for cell death," Cell Death Differ. 5(April 1998):298-306.
2113. Michael B. Yarmolinsky, "Programmed Cell Death in Bacterial Populations," Science 267(10 February 1995):836-837.
2114. Taku Naito, Kohji Kusano, Ichizo Kobayashi, "Selfish Behavior of Restriction-Modification Systems," Science 267(10 February 1995):897-899.
2115. Jean Claude Ameisen, "The Origin of Programmed Cell Death," Science 272(31 May 1996):1278-1279.
2116. Maria Mercedes Zambrano, Deborah A. Siegele, Marta Almiron, Antonio Tormo, Roberto Kolter, "Microbial Competition: *Escherichia coli* Mutants That Take Over Stationary Phase Cultures," Science 259(19 March 1993):1757-1760.
2117. V.A. Fadok, D.R. Voelker, P.A. Campbell, J.J. Cohen, D.L. Bratton, P.M. Henson, "Exposure of phosphatidylserine on the surface of apoptotic lymphocytes triggers specific recognition and removal by macrophages," J. Immunol. 148(1 April 1992):2207-2216.
2118. J.G. Teodoro, P.E. Branton, "Regulation of apoptosis by viral gene products," J. Virol. 71(March 1997):1739-1746.
2119. Physicians' Desk Reference, 48th Edition, Medical Economics Data Production Company, Montvale, NJ, 1994.
2120. Paul McEuen, "Carbon-based electronics," Nature 393(7 May 1998):15-17.
2121. Janet Raloff, "Staging Germ Warfare in Foods," Science News 153(7 February 1998):89-90.
2122. J. Willis Hurst, Medicine for the Practicing Physician, Third Edition, Butterworth-Heinemann, Boston MA, 1992.
2123. C.A. Lawrence, S.S. Block, Disinfection, Sterilization, and Preservation, Lee and Febiger, Philadelphia, PA, 1968.
2124. A.G. Goodman, L.S. Goodman, A. Gilman, Goodman and Gilman's Pharmacological Basis of Therapeutics, Sixth Edition, Macmillan Publishing Company, NY, 1980.
2125. Andrew A. Marino, Edwin A. Deitch, Visit Malakanok, James A. Albright, Robert D. Specian, "Electrical Augmentation of the Antimicrobial Activity of Silver-Nylon Fabrics," J. Biol. Phys. 12(1984):93-98.
2126. "Germ-Killing Silver Showing Up in Hundreds of Everyday Products," Silver News (April/May 1997):1-2.
2127. Lara K. Mahal, Kevin J. Yarema, Carolyn R. Bertozzi, "Engineering Chemical Reactivity on Cell Surfaces Through Oligosaccharide Biosynthesis," Science 276(16 May 1997):1125-1128.
2128. J. Travis, "Gene pushes cells into forced retirement," Science News 153(3 January 1998):7.
2129. Barry S. Schonwetter, Ethan D. Stolzenberg, Michael A. Zasloff, "Epithelial Antibiotics Induced at Sites of Inflammation," Science 267(17 March 1995):1645-1648.
2130. Mauro S. Malnati, Marta Peruzzi, Kenneth C. Parker, William E. Biddison, Ermanno Ciccone, Alessandro Moretta, Eric O. Long, "Peptide Specificity in the Recognition of MHC Class I by Natural Killer Cell Clones," Science 267(17 February 1995):1016-1018.
2131. Nafsika H. Georgopapadakou, Thomas J. Walsh, "Human Mycoses: Drugs and Targets for Emerging Pathogens," Science 264(15 April 1994):371-373.
2132. Joelle E. Gabay, "Ubiquitous Natural Antibiotics," Science 264(15 April 1994):373-374.
2133. Hiroshi Nikaido, "Porins and specific channels of bacterial outer membranes," Mol. Microbiol. 6(February 1992):435-442; see also "Porins and specific diffusion channels in bacterial outer membranes," J. Biol. Chem. 269(11 February 1994):3905-3908.
2134. Hiroshi Nikaido, "Prevention of Drug Access to Bacterial Targets: Permeability Barriers and Active Efflux," Science 264(15 April 1994):382-388.
2135. Brian G. Spratt, "Resistance to Antibiotics Mediated by Target Alterations," Science 264(15 April 1994):388-393.
2136. Wesley I. Sundquist, Stephen J. Lippard, "The Coordination Chemistry of Platinum Anticancer Drugs and Related Compounds with DNA," Coord. Chem. Rev. 100(1990):293-322.
2137. Michael J. Abrams, Barry A. Murrer, "Metal Compounds in Therapy and Diagnosis," Science 261(6 August 1993):725-730.
2138. E.R. Stadtman, "Protein oxidation and aging," Science 257(28 August 1992):1220-1224.
2139. M.F. Bachmann et al., "The Role of Antibody Concentration and Avidity in Antiviral Protection," Science 276(27 June 1997):2024-2027.
2140. A. Flamand, H. Raux, Y. Gaudin, R.W. Ruigrok, "Mechanisms of rabies virus neutralization," Virology 194(May 1993):302-313.
2141. David G. Cory, Raymond Laflamme, et al., "Experimental Quantum Error Correction," Phys. Rev. Lett. 81(7 September 1998):2152-2155.
2142. Cun-Yu Wang, Marty W. Mayo, Robert G. Korneluk, David V. Goeddel, Albert S. Baldwin Jr., "NF-κB Antiapoptosis: Induction of TRAF1 and TRAF2 and c-IAP1 and c-IAP2 to Suppress Caspase-8 Activation," Science 281(11 September 1998):1680-1683.
2143. Tomas Martin, Ulrike Obst, Julius Rebek Jr., "Molecular Assembly and Encapsulation Directed by Hydrogen-Bonding Preferences and the Filling of Space," Science 281(18 September 1998):1842-1845.
2144. Xiao-Hong Nancy Xu, Edward S. Yeung, "Long-Range Electrostatic Trapping of Single-Protein Molecules at a Liquid-Solid Interface," Science 281(11 September 1998):1650-1653.
2145. Robert Pool, "Trapping with Optical Tweezers, Science 241(26 August 1988):1042.
2146. Ronald Lawes, "Chapter 4. Microstructures and Microengineering," in Richard R.H. Coombs, Dennis W. Robinson, eds., Nanotechnology in Medicine and the Biosciences, Gordon & Breach Publishers, Netherlands, 1996, pp. 57-73.
2147. T. Burns, M. Wilson, G.J. Pearson, "Sensitization of cariogenic bacteria to killing by light from a helium-neon laser," J. Med. Microbiol. 38(1993):401-405; see also: "The effects of dentine and collagen on the lethal photosensitization of *Streptococcus mutans*," Caries Research 29(1995):192-197.
2148. W.M. Stanley, E.G. Valens, Viruses and the Nature of Life, Dutton, NY, 1961.
2149. E. Olavi Kajander, Neva Ciftcioglu, "Nanobacteria: An alternative mechanism for pathogenic intra- and extracellular calcification and stone formation," Proc. Natl. Acad. Sci. 95(7 July 1998):8274-8279. See also: John Travis, "Nanobacteria strike the kidney again," Science News 155(19 June 1999):395.
2150. Yeon-Kyun Shin, Cyrus Levinthal, Francoise Levinthal, Wayne L. Hubbell, "Colicin E1 Binding to Membranes: Time-Resolved Studies of Spin-Labeled Mutants," Science 259(12 February 1993):960-963.
2151. Virginia Morell, "Bacteria Diversify Through Warfare," Science 278(24 October 1997):575.
2152. Peter A. Fields, George N. Somero, "Hot spots in cold adaptation: Localized increases in conformational flexibility in lactate dehydrogenase A4 orthologs of Antarctic notothenoid fishes," Proc. Natl. Acad. Sci. 95(15 September 1998):11476-11481.
2153. Y.S. Touloukian, ed., Thermophysical Properties of High Temperature Solid Materials, Volume 4, The Macmillan Company, NY, 1967.
2154. Y.S. Touloukian, R.W. Powell, C.Y. Ho, P.G. Klemens, eds., Thermal Conductivity: Nonmetallic Solids, Thermophysical Properties of Matter, Volume 2, IFO/Plenum, NY, 1970.
2155. G.W. Willard, "Temperature Coefficient of Ultrasonic Velocity in Solutions," J. Acoust. Soc. Amer. 19(January 1947):235-241.
2156. Robert Bruce Lindsay, "Sound," Encyclopedia Britannica 21(1963):5-35.
2157. Archer E. Knowlton, ed., Standard Handbook for Electrical Engineers, Seventh Edition, McGraw-Hill Book Company, NY, 1941.
2158. W.J. Bishop, The Early History of Surgery, Robert Hale Ltd., 1960.

2159. James Glanz, "Making a Bigger Chill With Magnets," Science 279(27 March 1998):2045; see also: Mark Alpert, "A Cool Idea: Will Magnetic Refrigerators Come to Your Kitchen?" Scientific American 278(May 1998):44.
2160. B.C. Sales, D. Mandrus, R.K. Williams, "Filled Skutterudite Antimonides: A New Class of Thermoelectric Materials," Science 272(31 May 1996):1325-1328; see also: Terry M. Tritt, "Thermoelectrics Run Hot and Cold," Science 272(31 May 1996):1276-1277.
2161. Bruce H. Mahan, University Chemistry, Second Edition, Addison-Wesley Publishing Co., Reading MA, 1969.
2162. Isabel Marzo, Catherine Brenner, et al., "Bax and Adenine Nucleotide Translocator Cooperate in the Mitochondrial Control of Apoptosis," Science 281(25 September 1998):2027-2031.
2163. Y. Kuwana, I. Shimoyama, "A pheromone-guided mobile robot that behaves like a silkworm moth with living antennae as pheromone sensors," Intl. J. Robotics Res. 17(September 1998):924-933.
2164. Jian Chen, Mark A. Hamon, Hui Hu, Yongsheng Chen, Apparao M. Rao, Peter C. Eklund, Robert C. Haddon, "Solution Properties of Single-Walled Carbon Nanotubes," Science 282(2 October 1998):95-98.
2165. Steffen Stenger et al., "An Antimicrobial Activity of Cytolytic T Cells Mediated by Granulysin," Science 282(2 October 1998):121-125.
2166. G. Berke, "The binding and lysis of target cells by cytotoxic lymphocytes: Molecular and cellular aspects," Annu. Rev. Immunol. 12(1994):735-773.
2167. M. Leippe, "Ancient weapons: NK-lysin is a mammalian homolog to pore-forming peptides of a protozoan parasite," Cell 83(6 October 1995):17-18.
2168. Peter Weiss, "Another Face of Entropy," Science News 154(15 August 1998):108-109.
2169. Marie Adams, Zvonimir Dogic, Sarah L. Keller, Seth Fraden, "Entropically driven microphase transitions in mixtures of colloidal rods and spheres," Nature 393(28 May 1998):349-352.
2170. A.D. Dinsmore, D.J. Wang, Philip Nelson, Arjun G. Yodh, "Hard Spheres in Vesicles: Curvature-Induced Forces and Particle-Induced Curvature," Phys. Rev. Lett. 80(12 January 1998):409-412.
2171. D.B. Lacy, W. Tepp, A.C. Cohen, Bibhuti R. DasGupta, R.C. Stevens, "Crystal structure of botulinum neurotoxin type A and implications for toxicity," Nature Struct. Biol. 5(October 1998):898-902.
2172. W. Earnshaw, "On the nature of the molecular forces which regulate the constitution of the luminiferous ether," Trans. Camb. Phil. Soc. 7(1842):97-112.
2173. W. Braunbeck, "Free suspension of bodies in electric and magnetic fields," Zeitschrift fur Physik 112(1939):753-763.
2174. E.H. Brandt, "Levitation in Physics," Science 243(20 January 1989):349-355.
2175. M.V. Berry, "The Levitron^{TM}: an adiabatic trap for spins," Proc. Roy. Soc. London 452(8 May 1996):1207-1220.
2176. B.V. Jayawant, Electromagnetic Levitation and Suspension Systems, Edward Arnold, London, 1981.
2177. Joseph M. Crowley, Fundamentals of Applied Electrostatics, John Wiley & Sons, New York, 1986.
2178. B.H. Ketelle, G.E. Boyd, "The Exchange Adsorption of Ions from Aqueous Solutions by Organic Zeolites. IV. The Separation of the Yttrium Group Rare Earths," J. Am. Chem. Soc. 69(1947):2800-2812.
2179. J.A. Clements, D.F. Tierney, "Alveolar stability associated with altered surface tension," in W.O. Fenn, H. Rahn, eds., Handbook of Physiology, Section 3, Volume 2, American Physiological Society, Washington, DC, 1965, pp. 1565-1583.
2180. Lawrence M. Tierney, Jr., Stephen J. McPhee, Maxine A. Papadakis, eds., Current Medical Diagnosis and Treatment, 35th Edition, Appleton and Lange, Stamford, CT, 1996.
2181. P.J. Hore, Nuclear Magnetic Resonance, Oxford University Press, Cambridge, 1995.
2182. Frank H. Stillinger, Zelda Wasserman, "Molecular Recognition and Self-Organization in Fluorinated Hydrocarbons," J. Phys. Chem. 82(1978):929-940.
2183. J.C. Clark Jr., F. Gollan, "Survival of Mammals Breathing Organic Liquids Equilibrated with Oxygen at Atmospheric Pressure," Science 152(1966):1755-1757.
2184. R.P. Geyer, "Bloodless rats through the use of artificial blood substitutes," Fed. Proc. 34(May 1975):1499-1505.
2185. Randolph M. Nesse, George C. Williams, "Evolution and the Origins of Disease," Scientific American 279(November 1998):86-93.
2186. John E. Pfeiffer, The Emergence of Man, Second Edition, Harper & Row, New York, 1972.
2187. L.S.B. Leakey, "Exploring 1,750,000 Years into Man's Past," National Geographic 120(October 1961):564-589.
2188. Mary D. Leakey, "A Review of the Oldowan Culture from Olduvai Gorge, Tanzania," Nature 210(30 April 1966):462-466.
2189. L.J. Bruce-Chwatt, "Paleogenesis and Paleoepidemiology of Primate Malaria," W.H.O. Bulletin 32(1965):363-387.
2190. T. Aidan Cockburn, The Evolution and Eradication of Infectious Diseases, Johns Hopkins Press, Baltimore MD, 1963.
2191. Richard Fiennes, Zoonoses of Primates: The Epidemiology and Ecology of Simian Diseases in Relation to Man, Cornell University Press, Ithaca, New York, 1967.
2192. Thomas W.M. Cameron, Parasites and Parasitism, Wiley, New York, 1956.
2193. T. Aidan Cockburn, "Infectious Diseases in Ancient Populations," Curr. Anthropology 12(1971):51-56.
2194. Macfarlane Burnet, David O. White, Natural History of Infectious Disease, 4th Edition, Cambridge University Press, London, 1972.
2195. Francis L. Black, "Infectious Diseases in Primitive Societies," Science 187(1975):515-518.
2196. Francis L. Black, "Measles Endemicity in Insular Populations: Critical Community Size and Its Evolutionary Implications," J. Theoret. Biol. 11(1966):207-211.
2197. M.S. Bartlett, "Measles Periodicity and Community Size," J. Royal Statistical Soc. 120(1957):48-70.
2198. Theodor Rosebury, Microorganisms Indigenous to Man, McGraw-Hill, NY, 1962.
2199. T.D. Stewart, Alexander Spoehr, "Evidence on the Paleopathology of Yaws," Bull. History Med. 26(1952):538-553.
2200. Celsus, De Medicina, with an English Translation by W.G. Spencer, 3 Volumes, Loeb Classical Library, 1935-1938.
2201. J. Szilagyi, "Beitrage zur Statistik der Sterblichkeit in der Westeuropaischen Provinzen des Romischen Imperium," Acta Archaeologica Academica Scientiarum Hungaricae 13(1961):126-156.
2202. Michael Balter, "19th Century Rules of Causation Outdated?" Science 282(9 October 1998):220.
2203. N. Jewson, "The disappearance of the sick-man from medical cosmology, 1770-1870," Sociology 10(1976):225-244.
2204. Roy Porter, The Greatest Benefit to Mankind: A Medical History of Humanity, W.W. Norton & Company, New York, 1997.
2205. Roy Porter, ed., Medicine: A History of Healing, Ancient Traditions to Modern Practices, Barnes & Noble Books, New York, 1997.
2206. William H. McNeill, Plagues and Peoples, Anchor Press/Doubleday, Garden City NY, 1976.
2207. James B. Wyngaarden, Lloyd H. Smith, Jr., J. Claude Bennett, eds., Cecil Textbook of Medicine, 19th Edition, W.B. Saunders Company, Philadelphia PA, 1992.
2208. Henry W. Ruoff, ed., The Standard Dictionary of Facts, The Frontier Press Company, Buffalo NY, 1914.
2209. Statistical Abstract of the United States: 1996, 116th Edition, U.S. Bureau of the Census, Washington DC, 1996.
2210. A.R Bridbury, "The Black Death," Economic History Review 26(1973):577-592.
2211. Roger Mols, Introduction a la demographie historique des villes d'Europe du XIVe au XVIIIe siecle, 3 volumes, Louvain, 1954-56.
2212. Daniele Beltrami, Storia della popolazione di Venezia dalla fine del secolo XVI alla caduta della Repubblica, CEDAM, Padova, 1954.
2213. J.F.D. Shrewsbury, A History of Bubonic Plague in the British Isles, Cambridge University Press, London, 1970.
2214. R. Pollitzer, Plague, WHO Monograph Series, No. 22, World Health Organization (WHO), Geneva, 1954.
2215. Marvin Harris, Cows, Pigs, Wars and Witches: The Riddles of Culture, Random House, New York, 1974.
2216. Richard Gordon, The Alarming History of Medicine, St. Martin's Press, London, 1994.
2217. Lily E. Kay, The Molecular Vision of Life: Caltech, the Rockefeller Foundation, and the Rise of the New Biology, Oxford University Press, Cambridge, 1992.
2218. Theodore Friedmann, ed., Molecular Genetic Medicine, Academic Press, New York, 1994.
2219. Karl H. Muench, Genetic Medicine, Elsevier, New York, 1988.
2220. C.V. Brownlow, ed., Gould's Medical Dictionary, 5th Revised Edition, The Blakiston Company, Philadelphia PA, 1945.
2221. Jean L. McKechnie, ed., Webster's New Twentieth Century Dictionary of the English Language, Unabridged, 2nd Edition, The World Publishing Company, New York, 1961.
2222. Jonathan Campbell Meakins, "Medicine," Encyclopedia Britannica 15(1963):195-198.
2223. Clayton L. Thomas, ed., Taber's Cyclopedic Medical Dictionary, 17th Edition, F.A. Davis Company, Philadelphia PA, 1989.
2224. James T. McDonough, Jr., ed., Stedman's Concise Medical Dictionary, Second Edition, Williams & Wilkins, Baltimore MD, 1994.
2225. Knud Faber, Nosography: The Evolution of Clinical Medicine in Modern Times, Second Edition, Paul Hoeber, New York, 1930.
2226. Daniel A. Albert, Ronald Munson, Michael D. Resnik, Reasoning in Medicine: An Introduction to Clinical Inference, The Johns Hopkins University Press, Baltimore MD, 1988.
2227. Graham W. Bradley, Disease, Diagnosis and Decisions, John Wiley & Sons, New York, 1993.
2228. Edmond A. Murphy, The Logic of Medicine, 2nd Edition, The Johns Hopkins University Press, Balitmore MD, 1997.
2229. Huntington Sheldon, ed., Boyd's Introduction to the Study of Disease, 11th Edition, Lea & Febiger, Philadelphia PA, 1992.
2230. Eric J. Cassell, Mark Siegler, eds., Changing Values in Medicine, University Publications of America, Inc., 1979.
2231. T. McKeown, The Role of Medicine: Dream, Mirage, or Nemesis?, Princeton University Press, Princeton NJ, 1979.
2232. E.J.M. Campbell, J.G. Scadding, R.S. Roberts, "The concept of disease," Brit. Med. J. 2(29 September 1979):757-762.

2233. Dennis W. Ross, Introduction to Molecular Medicine, Second Edition, Springer-Verlag, New York, 1996.
2234. Otto E. Guttentag, "The Attending Physician as a Central Figure," in Eric J. Cassell, Mark Siegler, eds., Changing Values in Medicine, University Publications of America, Inc., 1979, pp. 107-126.
2235. Mack Lipkin, Jr., "Chapter 1. Generalist's Approach to the Medical Interview," in John Noble, ed., Textbook of Primary Care Medicine, Second Edition, Mosby, St. Louis, 1996, pp. 2-8.
2236. K. Jaspers, General Psychopathology, 7th Edition, translated by J. Hoenig, M.W. Hamilton, Manchester University Press, Manchester England, 1963.
2237. Thomas Addis, Glomerular Nephritis: Diagnosis and Treatment, Macmillan, New York, 1948.
2238. J. Claude Bennett, "Internal Medicine and Today's Internist," in James B. Wyngaarden, Lloyd H. Smith, Jr., J. Claude Bennett, eds., Cecil Textbook of Medicine, 19th Edition, W.B. Saunders Company, Philadelphia PA, 1992, pp. 2-6.
2239. Eric J. Cassell, The Nature of Suffering and the Goals of Medicine, Oxford University Press, New York, 1991.
2240. The Genuine Works of Hippocrates: The Book of Prognostics, translated by Francis Adams, Williams and Wilkins, Baltimore MD, 1939.
2241. N. Taniguchi, "On the Basic Concept of 'Nano-Technology'," Proc. Intl. Conf. Prod. Eng. Tokyo, Part II, Japan Society of Precision Engineering, 1974.
2242. Norio Taniguchi, ed., Nanotechnology: Integrated Processing Systems for Ultra-Precision and Ultra-Fine Products, Oxford University Press, Cambridge, 1996.
2243. K. Eric Drexler, "Molecular Machinery and Molecular Electronic Devices," 2nd International Workshop on Molecular Electronic Devices, 13-15 April 1983, Naval Research Laboratory, Chemistry Division, Washington DC.
2244. K. Eric Drexler, "Biological and Nanomechanical Systems: Contrasts in Evolutionary Capacity," in Christopher G. Langton, ed., Artificial Life, Santa Fe Institute, Studies in the Science of Complexity, Volume VI, Addison-Wesley, New York, 1989, pp. 501-519.
2245. A.R. von Hippel, "Molecular Designing of Materials," Science 138(1962):91-108.
2246. H. von Foester, "Molecular Bionics," Third Bionics Symposium, Defense Documentation Center, Alexandria VA, 1964, pp. 161-190.
2247. H.P. Zingsheim, "Molecular Engineering Using Nanometer Surface Microstructures," Proc. NSF Workshop on Opportunities for Microstructure Science, Engineering and Technology in Cooperation with the NRC Panel on Thin Film Microstructure Science and Technology, 19-22 November 1978, National Science Foundation, Washington DC, 1978, pp. 44-48. See also: Ber. d. Bunsengesellsch. Phys. Chem. 80(1976):1185.
2248. W.F. McClaire, "Chemical Machines, Maxwell's Demon and Living Organisms," J. Theoret. Biol. 30(1971):1-34.
2249. R. Laing, "Some Forms of Replication in Artificial Molecular Machines," Proc. 1974 Conf. on Biologically Motivated Automata Theory, McLean VA, 1974, pp. 6-8.
2250. R. Laing, "Some Alternative Reproductive Strategies in Artificial Molecular Machines," J. Theoret. Biol. 54(1975):63-84.
2251. R. Laing, "Machines as Organisms: An Exploration of the Relevance of Recent Results," BioSystems 11(1979):201-215.
2252. P. Mitchell, "Osmoenzymology: The Study of Molecular Machines," Cell Function and Differentiation, Alan R. Liss, New York, F.E.B.S. 65B(1982):399-408.
2253. Eric Drexler, "Cell Repair Machines and Tissue Reconstruction: Some Notes on Computational Complexity and Physical Constraints," unpublished privately circulated draft paper, February 1983 and January 1984.
2254. Christine L. Peterson, "Nanotechnology: Evolution of the Concept," J. Brit. Interplanet. Soc. 45(1992):395-400.
2255. Michael Kassler, "Robotics for health care: a review of the literature," Robotica 11(1993):495-516.
2256. Time-Life Editors, Alternative Computers, Time-Life Books, Richmond VA, 1989.
2257. Isaac Asimov, Is Anyone There? Ace Books, New York, 1967.
2258. G.R. Taylor, The Biological Time Bomb, World Publishing Company, New York, 1968.
2259. J. White, "Viral Induced Repair of Damaged Neurons with Preservation of Long-Term Information Content," paper presented at the Second Annual Cryonics Conference, Ann Arbor, Michigan, 11 April 1969; reprints available from Cryonics Society of Michigan.
2260. J.F. Danielli, "Artificial Synthesis of New Life Forms," Bull. Atomic Scientists 28(October 1972):20-24.
2261. D.S. Halacy, Jr., Genetic Revolution: Shaping Life for Tomorrow, Harper and Row, New York, 1974.
2262. Thomas Donaldson, "Cryonics: A Brief Scientific Bibliography," unpublished privately circulated discursive bibliography, 1976; revised version reprinted by Alcor Life Extension Foundation, 1978.
2263. Michael G. Darwin, "The Anabolocyte: A Biological Approach to Repairing Cryoinjury," Life Extension Magazine (July-August 1977):80-83.
2264. Isaac Asimov, Change!, Houghton Mifflin, Boston MA, 1981.
2265. K.R. Shoulders, "Microelectronics Using Electron-Beam-Activated Machining Techniques," in Franz Alt, ed., Advances in Computers, Academic Press, New York, 1961, pp. 135-293.
2266. K.R. Shoulders, "Toward Complex Systems," Microelectronics and Large Systems, Spartan Books, Washington DC, 1965, pp. 97-128.
2267. Mikhail V. Volkenstein, Molecules and Life: An Introduction to Molecular Biology, Plenum Press, New York, 1970.
2268. T. Nemes, Cybernetic Machines, Gordon and Breach Science Publishers, New York, 1970.
2269. G. Feinberg, Solid Clues: Quantum Physics, Molecular Biology, and the Future of Science, Simon and Schuster, Touchstone Books, New York, 1985.
2270. Richard Crawford, "Cosmetic Nanosurgery," in B.C. Crandall, ed., Nanotechnology: Molecular Speculations on Global Abundance, MIT Press, Cambridge MA, 1996, pp. 61-80.
2271. Gregory M. Fahy, "Molecular Nanotechnology and its Possible Pharmaceutical Implications," in Clement Bezold, Jerome A. Halperin, Jacqueline L. Eng, eds., 2020 Visions: Health Care Information Standards and Technologies, U.S. Pharmacopeial Convention Inc., Rockville MD, 1993, pp. 152-159.
2272. Ted Kaehler, "In-Vivo Nanoscope and the Two-Week Revolution," in B.C. Crandall, ed., Nanotechnology: Molecular Speculations on Global Abundance, MIT Press, Cambridge MA, 1996, pp. 49-60.
2273. Edward M. Reifman, "Diamond Teeth," in B.C. Crandall, ed., Nanotechnology: Molecular Speculations on Global Abundance, MIT Press, Cambridge MA, 1996, pp. 81-86.
2274. I.T. Dorn, K.R. Neumaier, R. Tampe, "Molecular Recognition of Histidine-Tagged Molecules by Chelator Lipids Monitored by Fluorescence Energy Transfer and Correlation Spectroscopy," J. Am. Chem. Soc. 120(1998):2753-2763.
2275. James C. Ellenbogen, "Architectures for Molecular Electronic Computer Logic," paper presented at the Sixth Foresight Conference on Molecular Nanotechnology, November 1998.
2276. Cees Dekker, "Carbon Nanotubes as Molecular Quantum Wires," paper presented at the Sixth Foresight Conference on Molecular Nanotechnology, November 1998.
2277. Boris I. Yacobson, "Mechanical relaxation and intramolecular plasticity in carbon nanotubes," Appl. Phys. Lett. 72(23 February 1998):918-920.
2278. Carlo D. Montemagno, George Bachand, Scott Stelick, Marlene Bachand, "Constructing Biological Motor Powered Nanomechanical Devices," paper presented at the Sixth Foresight Conference on Molecular Nanotechnology, November 1998. See also: http:www/foresight.org/Conferences/MNT6/Papers/Montemagno/index.html.
2279. Steven Block, "Using Optical Tweezers to Study Biological Motors," paper presented at the Sixth Foresight Conference on Molecular Nanotechnology, November 1998.
2280. B.T. Kelly, Physics of Graphite, Applied Science Press, 1981.
2281. Ralph C. Merkle, "Casing an Assembler," paper presented at the Sixth Foresight Conference on Molecular Nanotechnology, November 1998; see also: http://www.foresight.org/Conferences/MNT6/Papers/Merkle/index.html.
2282. K. Eric Drexler, "Rod logic and thermal noise in the mechanical nanocomputer," in F.L. Carter, R.E. Siatkowski, H. Wohltjen, eds., Molecular Electronic Devices, North-Holland, Amsterdam, 1988, pp. 39 et seq.
2284. Charles Ostman, "Chapter 23. Nanotechnology -- The Next Revolution," in Cyberlife, Sams Publishing, Indianapolis, IN, 1994, pp. 521-562.
2285. Barry Robson, "Doppelganger Proteins as Drug Leads," Nature Biotechnology 14(1996):892-893.
2286. Barry Robson, "Pseudoproteins: Non-Protein Protein-like Machines," paper presented at the Sixth Foresight Conference on Molecular Nanotechnology, November 1998.
2287. Alan Duncan Ross, Harlan Gibbs, The Medicine of ER, Basic Books, New York, 1996.
2288. C.S. Henriquez, "Bioelectric Phenomena," in J.D. Bronzoni, ed., Biomedical Engineering Handbook, CRC Press, 1995, pp. 99-251.
2289. J.A. Mattar, "Application of total body bioimpedance to the critically ill patient," New Horiz. 4(November 1996):493-503.
2290. H.J. Zdolsek, O.A. Lindahl, K.A. Angquist, F. Sjoberg, "Non-invasive assessment of intercompartmental fluid shifts in burn victims," Burns 24(May 1998):233-240.
2291. G. Majno, I. Joris, "Apoptosis, oncosis, and necrosis: An overview of cell death," Am. J. Pathol. 146(January 1995):3-15.
2292. C. Charriaut, I. Margaill, A. Represa, T. Popovici, M. Plotkine, Y. Ben-Ari, "Apoptosis and necrosis after reversible focal ischemia: An in situ DNA fragmentation analysis," J. Cerebral Blood Flow Metab. 16(March 1996):186-194.
2293. R.A. Nixon, A.M. Cataldo, "The lysosomal system in neuronal cell death," Ann. N.Y. Acad. Sci. 679(28 May 1993):87-109.
2294. J.S. Haller Jr., "The Beginnings of Ambulance Service in the United States and England," J. Emergency Med. 8(November-December 1990):743-755.
2295. T.E. Thompson, I. Bennett, "*Physalia* nematocysts utilized by mollusks for defense," Science 166(1969):1532-1533.
2296. E.O. Wilson, Biophilia, Harvard University Press, Cambridge, MA, 1984.
2297. A.L. Mackay, A Dictionary of Scientific Quotations, Adam Hilger, New York, 1991.
2298. M.S. Schneider, A Beginner's Guide to Constructing the Universe, Harper Collins, New York, 1994.
2299. Virginia Postrel, The Future and Its Enemies, The Free Press, New York, 1999.
2300. Robert A. Freitas Jr., "Respirocytes: High Performance Artificial Nanotechnology Red Blood Cells," NanoTechnology Magazine 2(October 1996):1, 8-13.

2301. Herbert Simon, The Sciences of the Artificial, Second Edition, MIT Press, Cambridge, MA, 1981.
2302. Lewis Mumford, The Myth and the Machine: Technics and Human Development, Harcourt Brace Jovanovich, New York, 1967.
2303. Richard Taylor, Medicine Out Of Control: The Anatomy of a Malignant Technology, Sun Books, Melbourne, 1979.
2304. Jeremy Rifkin, Algeny, Viking Press, New York, 1983.
2305. Leon R. Kass, Toward a More Natural Science: Biology and Human Affairs, Free Press, New York, 1985.
2306. Diana B. Dutton, Worse Than The Disease: Pitfalls of Medical Progress, Cambridge University Press, New York, 1988.
2307. Bill McKibben, The End of Nature, Anchor Books, New York, 1989.
2308. Daniel Callahan, False Hopes: Why America's Quest for Perfect Health is a Recipe for Failure, Simon & Schuster, New York, 1998.
2309. Raymond Kurzweil, The Age of Spiritual Machines, Viking Press, New York, 1999.
2310. William B. Schwartz, Life Without Disease: The Pursuit of Medical Utopia, University of California Press, Berkeley, CA, 1998.
2311. Lee M. Silver, Remaking Eden: Cloning and Beyond in a Brave New World, Avon Books, New York, 1997.
2312. Kevin McFarland, Incredible But True, Bell Publishing Company, New York, 1978.
2313. David R. Baselt, Gil U. Lee, Richard J. Colton, "A Biosensor Based on Force Microscope Technology," J. Vac. Sci. Technol. B 14(1996):789-793.
2314. Gregory T. Baxter, Luc J. Bousse, Timothy D. Dawes, Jeffrey M. Libby, Douglas N. Modlin, John C. Owicki, J. Wallace Parce, "Microfabrication in Silicon Microphysiometry," Clin. Chem. 40(1994):1800-1804.
2315. U.S. Department of Energy, Isotope Production and Distribution Catalog, 1996-1997: "Gadolinium-148"; see http://www.ornl.gov/isotopes/r_gd148.htm.
2316. Charles Tanford, The Hydrophobic Effect: Formation of Micelles and Biological Membranes, Second Edition, John Wiley and Sons, New York, 1980.
2317. Stephen J. Dodd, Mangay Williams, Joseph P. Suhan, Donald S. Williams, Alan P. Koretsky, Chien Ho, "Detection of Single Mammalian Cells by High-Resolution Magnetic Resonance Imaging," Biophys. J. 76(January 1999):103-109.
2318. Lev B. Levitin, "Energy cost of information transmission," Physica D 120(1998):162-167.
2319. Norman Margolus, Lev B. Levitin, "The maximum speed of dynamical evolution," Physica D 120(1998):188-195.
2320. J.G. Linner, S.A. Livesey, "Low Temperature Molecular Distillation Drying of Cryofixed Biological Samples," in J.J. McGrath, K.R. Diller, eds., Low Temperature Biotechnology: Emerging Applications and Engineering Contributions, ASME, New York, 1988, pp. 147-157.
2321. Andreas D. Baxevanis, B.F. Francis Ouellette, eds., Bioinformatics: A Practical Guide to the Analysis of Genes and Proteins, Wiley-Interscience, New York, 1998.
2322. Francis S. Collins, Ari Patrinos, Elke Jordan, Aravinda Chakravarti, Raymond Gesteland, LeRoy Walters, et al., "New Goals for the U.S. Human Genome Project: 1998-2003," Science 282(23 October 1998):682-689.
2323. M. Guyer, "Statement on the rapid release of genomic DNA sequence," Genome Res. 8(May 1998):413.
2324. Yong Duan, Peter A. Kollman, "Pathways to a Protein Folding Intermediate Observed in a 1-Microsecond Simulation in Aqueous Solution," Science 282(23 October 1998):740-744.
2325. Alexander Kazimirov, Jorg Zegenhagen, Manuel Cardona, "Isotopic Mass and Lattice Constant: X-ray Standing Wave Measurements," Science 282(30 October 1998):930-932.
2326. Matthew C. Coffey, James E. Strong, Peter A. Forsyth, Patrick W.K. Lee, "Reovirus Therapy of Tumors with Activated Ras Pathway," Science 282(13 November 1998):1332-1334.
2327. Elizabeth Pennisi, "Training Viruses to Attack Cancers," Science 282(13 November 1998):1244-1246.
2328. Matthew A. Mulvey, Yolanda S. Lopez-Boado, Carole L. Wilson, Robyn Roth, William C. Parks, John Heuser, Scott J. Hultgren, "Induction and Evasion of Host Defenses by Type 1-Piliated Uropathogenic *Escherichia coli*," Science 282(20 November 1998):1494-1497.
2329. Constance Holden, "How Much Like Us Were the Neandertals?" Science 282(20 November 1998):1456.
2330. Rafal E. Dunin-Borkowski, Martha R. McCartney, Richard B. Frankel, Dennis A. Bazylinski, Mihaly Posfai, Peter R. Buseck, "Magnetic Microstructure of Magnetotactic Bacteria by Electron Holography," Science 282(4 December 1998):1868-1870.
2331. Anthony G. Frutos, Lloyd M. Smith, Robert M. Corn, "Enzymatic Ligation Reactions of DNA 'Words' on Surfaces for DNA Computing," J. Amer. Chem Soc. 120(14 October 1998):10277-10282. See also: Q. Liu, A.G. Frutos, A.J. Thiel, R.M. Corn, L.M. Smith, "DNA computing on surfaces: Encoding information at the single base level," J. Comput. Biol. 5(Summer 1998):269-278.
2332. Kristine Coleman, David Sloan Wilson, "Shyness and boldness in pumpkinseed sunfish: Individual differences are context-specific," Animal Behavior 56(October 1998):927-936.
2333. Adrienne Mayor, "What's new, honey?" Science News 154(31 October 1998):275.
2334. Robert Root-Bernstein, Michele Root-Bernstein, Honey, Mud, Maggots, and Other Medical Marvels: The Science Behind Folk Remedies and Old Wives' Tales, Mariner Books, 1998.
2335. Yoshihiro Ito, "Signal-responsive gating by a polyelectrolyte pelage on a nanoporous membrane," Nanotechnology 9(September 1998):205-207.
2336. Thomas Heinz, Dmitry M. Rudkevich, Julius Rebek Jr., "Pairwise selection of guests in a cylindrical molecular capsule of nanometre dimensions," Nature 394(20 August 1998):764-766.
2337. H. Lawrence Clever, "The Hydrated Hydronium Ion," J. Chem. Ed. 40(December 1963):637-641.
2338. J.O. Bockris, A.K.N. Reddy, Modern Electrochemistry, Plenum Press, New York, 1970.
2339. Myra Shackley, Neanderthal Man, Archon Books, Hamden, 1980.
2340. Shari Rudavsky, "The Secret Life of the Neanderthal," Omni 14(1991):42-44, 55-56.
2341. Ralph Solecki, Shanidar: The First Flower People, Knopf, New York, 1971.
2342. Erik Trinkhaus, The Shanidar Neandertals, Academic Press, New York, 1983.
2343. K.A. Dettwyler, "Can paleopathology provide evidence for compassion?" Amer. J. Physical Anthropology 84(1991):375-384.
2344. V.D.D. Jabon, G.V. Fedorovich, N.V. Samsonenko, "Catalytically induced D-D fusion in ferroelectrics," Brazillian J. Phys. 27(December 1997):515-521.
2345. "Microbial soup," Science 282(18 December 1998):2147. See also: http://www.tigr.org/tdb/mdb/mdb.html.
2346. I. Laffafian, M.B. Hallett, "Lipid-assisted microinjection: Introducing material into the cytosol and membranes of small cells," Biophys. J. 75(November 1998):2558-2563.
2347. Carol Featherstone, "Coming to Grips With The Golgi," Science 282(18 December 1998):2172-2174.
2348. Geoffrey Chang, Robert H. Spencer, Allen T. Lee, Margaret T. Barclay, Douglas C. Rees, "Structure of the MscL Homolog from *Mycobacterium tuberculosis*: A Gated Mechanosensitive Ion Channel," Science 282(18 December 1998):2220-2226.
2349. Leo Szilard, "On the Decrease of Entropy in a Thermodynamic System by the Intervention of Intelligent Beings," Zeitschrift fur Physik 53(1929):840-856 and Behav. Sci. 9(1964):301-310. See also: B.T. Feld, G.W. Szilard, The Collected Works of Leo Sziland: Scientific Papers, The MIT Press, London, 1972.
2350. L. Brillouin, "Maxwell's Demon Cannot Operate: Information and Entropy," J. Appl. Phys. 22(March 1951):334-337; "Physical entropy and information," J. Appl. Phys. 22(March 1951):338-343. See also: L. Brillouin, Science and Information Theory, Second Edition, Academic Press, New York, 1962.
2351. Akihiko Teshigahara, Masakane Watanabe, Nobuaki Kawahara, Yoshinori Ohtsuka, Tadashi Hattori, "Performance of a 7-mm Microfabricated Car," J. Microelectromech. Syst. 4(June 1995):76-80.
2352. Harumi Suzuki, Nobuyuki Ohya, Nobuaki Kawahara, Masao Yokoi, Sigeru Ohyanagi, Takashi Kurahashi, Tadashi Hattori, "Shell-body fabrication for micromachines," J. Micromech. Microeng. 5(1995):36-40.
2353. Kenji Suzuki, Isao Shimoyama, Hirofumi Miura, "Insect-Model Based Microrobot with Elastic Hinges," J. Microelectromech. Syst. 3(March 1994):4-9.
2354. Dustin W. Carr, Harold G. Craighead, "Fabrication of nanoelectromechanical systems in single crystal silicon using silicon on insulator substrates and electron beam lithography," J. Vac. Sci. Technol. B 15(November/December 1997):2760-2765. See also: Science News 152(30 August 1997):143.
2355. Vasant Natarajan, R.E. Behringer, D.M. Tennant, G. Timp, "Nanolithography using a laser focused neutral atom beam," J. Vac. Sci. Technol. B 13(November/December 1995):2823-2827.
2356. Paul McWhorter, "Sandia National Laboratories Intelligent Micromachine Initiative," see at: http://www.mdl.sandia.gov/Micromachine.
2357. Stephen Y. Chou, P.R. Krauss, P.J. Renstrom, "Imprint Lithography with 25-Nanometer Resolution," Science 272(5 April 1996):85-87.
2358. "Nanoimprint Lithography" and "Nanoscale Transistors Fabricated using Nanoimprint Lithography," DARPA-ETO Electronics, 24 July 1998, at http://www.darpa.mil/eto/ULTRA/Weeklies.htm; see also http://www.ee.princeton.edu/~chouweb.
2359. U. Rembold, R. Dillmann, Institute for Real-Time Computer Systems & Robotics, MicroRobot Project Group, 16 October 1997, http://wwwipr.ira.uka.de/~santa/microrob.html.
2360. Jean-Marc Breguet, P. Renaud, "A 4-Degrees-of-Freedom Microrobot with Nanometer Resolution," Robotics 14(1996):199-203. See also: http://dmtwww.epfl.ch/isr/hpr/jmbreguet.html.
2361. "Smoovy Motor Applications: A 1 cc mobile robot," LAMI Miniature Robots and Subsystems Group, June 1997, http://diwww.epfl.ch/w3lami/mirobots/smoovy.html.
2362. "Microrobots: Features of Jemmy, our tiny 1 cm^3 robot," LAMI Miniature Robots and Subsystems Group, 31 August 1998, http://lamiwww.epfl.ch/lami/mirobots/1cubes.html.
2363. V.R. Dhuler, M. Mehregany, S.M. Philips, J.H. Lang, "A comparative study of bearing design and operational environments for harmonic side-drive micromotors," Proc. IEEE Micro Electro Mechanical Systems, Travemunde, Germany, 1992, pp. 171-176.

2364. Rebecca J. Jackman, Scott T. Brittain, Allan Adams, Mara G. Prentiss, George M. Whitesides, "Design and Fabrication of Topologically Complex, Three-Dimensional Microstructures," Science 280(26 June 1998):2089-2091.
2365. R.J. Tonucci, B.L. Justus, A.J. Campillo, C.E. Ford, "Nanochannel Array Glass," Science 258(30 October 1992):783-787.
2366. Doug Stewart, "New Machines are Smaller than a Hair, and Do Real Work," Smithsonian 21(November 1990):85-96.
2367. Ivan Amato, "The Small Wonders of Microengineering," Science 253(26 July 1991):387-388.
2368. Frank Caruso, Rachel A. Caruso, Helmuth Mohwald, "Nanoengineering of Inorganic and Hybrid Hollow Spheres by Colloidal Templating," Science 282(6 November 1998):1111-1114.
2369. Anvar A. Zakhidov et al., "Carbon Structures with Three-Dimensional Periodicity at Optical Wavelengths," Science 282(30 October 1998):897-901.
2370. Robert Pool, "Lining up Atoms With Laser Light," Science 255(20 March 1992):1514.
2371. Roberto Dizon, Hongtao Han, Armistead G. Russell, Michael L. Reed, "An Ion Milling Pattern Transfer Technique for Fabrication of Three-Dimensional Micromechanical Structures," J. Microelectromech. Syst. 2(December 1993):151-159.
2372. Yogesh Gianchandani, Khalil Najafi, "Batch-assembled multi-level micromachined mechanisms from bulk silicon," J. Micromech. Microeng. 2(1992):80-85.
2373. Shuichi Shoji, Masayoshi Esashi, "Microfabrication and Microsensors," Appl. Biochem. Biotech. 41(1993):21-34.
2374. S.S. Lee, L.Y. Lin, K.S.J. Pister, M.C. Wu, H.C. Lee, P. Grodzinski, "Passively Aligned Hybrid Integration of 8 x 1 Micromachined Micro-Fresnel Lens Arrays and 8 x 1 Vertical-Cavity Surface-Emitting Laser Arrays for Free-Space Optical Interconnect," IEEE Photonics Technol. Lett. 7(September 1995):1031-1033.
2375. "Diamond—A Gear's Best Friend," Science 261(24 September 1993):1673.
2376. John D. Hunn, S.P. Withrow, C.W. White, R.E. Clausing, L. Heatherly, C. Paul Christensen, "Fabrication of single-crystal diamond microcomponents," Appl. Phys. Lett. 65(12 December 1994)3072-3074.
2377. I.A. Waitz, G. Gauba, Y.-S. Tzeng, paper presented at the A.S.M.E. International Engineering Congress and Exposition, Atlanta, November 1996.
2378. A.H. Epstein, S.D. Senturia, "Macro Power from Micro Machinery," Science 276(23 May 1997):1211.
2379. M. Mehregany, K.J. Gabriel, W.S. Trimmer, "Integrated fabrication of polysilicon mechanisms," IEEE Trans. Electron. Devices ED-35(1988):719-723.
2380. L.S. Fan, Y.C. Tai, R.S. Miller, "Integrated movable micromechanical structures for sensors and actuators," IEEE Trans. Electron. Devices ED-35(1988):724-730.
2381. M. Fleischer, H. Meixner, "Ultrasonic Motors," Mechatronics 1(1991):403-415.
2382. Christian Burrer, Jaume Esteve, Emilio Lora-Tamayo, "Resonant Silicon Accelerometers in Bulk Micromachining Technology -- An Approach," J. Microelectromech. Syst. 5(June 1996):122-129.
2383. Ezekiel J.J. Kruglick, Brett A. Warneke, Kristofer S.J. Pister, "CMOS 3-Axis Accelerometers with Integrated Amplifier," Proc. IEEE Micro Electro Mechanical Systems Workshop 1998 (MEMS '98).
2384. M. Kraft, C.P. Lewis, T.G. Hesketh, "Closed Loop Silicon Accelerometers," IEE Proc. Circuits Devices Syst. 145(1998):325-331.
2385. A.F. Vakakis, J.W. Burdick, T.K. Caughey, "An Interesting Attractor in the Dynamics of a Hopping Robot," International Journal of Robotics Research 10(December 1991):606-618.
2386. R.T. M'Closkey, J.W. Burdick, "On the Periodic Motions of a Hopping Robot with Vertical and Forward Motion," International Journal of Robotics Research 12(June 1993):197-218.
2387. G.S. Chirikjian, J.W. Burdick, "The Kinematics of Hyper-Redundant Robotic Locomotion," IEEE Trans. on Robotics and Automation 11(December 1995):781-793.
2388. John D. Madden, Tanya Kanigan, Peter Madden, Ian W. Hunter, "Nanofabrication of Conducting Polymer-Based Artificial Muscle," paper presented at the 1997 Albany Conference on Biomolecular Motors and Nanomachines; see abstract at: http://www.wadsworth.org/albcon97/abstract/madden.htm.
2389. R.E. Smalley, "Chemistry on the Nanometer Scale -- Introductory Remarks," 1996 Welch Conference in Chemistry, at: http://cnst.rice.edu/NanoWelch.html.
2390. R. Sakowicz, M.S. Berdelis, K. Ray, C.L. Blackburn, C. Hopmann, D.J. Faulkner, L.S. Goldstein, "A marine natural product inhibitor of kinesin motors," Science 280(10 April 1998):292-295.
2391. Trevor Douglas, Mark Young, "Host-guest encapsulation of materials by assembled virus protein cages," Nature 393(14 May 1998):152-155.
2392. K. Eric Drexler, "Building molecular machine systems," Trends in Biotechnology 17(January 1999):5-7. See also: http://www.imm.org/Reports/Rep008.html.
2393. J.W. Bryson et al., "Protein Design: A Hierarchic Approach," Science 270(1995):935-941.
2394. W.F. DeGrado, L. Regan, S.P. Ho, "The Design of a Four-Helix Bundle Protein," Cold Spring Harbor Symposia on Qualitative Biology 52(1987):521-526. See also: W.F. Degrado, "Design of Peptides and Proteins," Adv. Protein Chem. 39(1988):51-124 and L. Regan, W.F DeGrado, "Characterization of a helical protein designed from first principles," Science 241(19 August 1988):976-978.
2395. M. Mutter et al., "The Construction of New Proteins, Artificial Folding Units by Assembly of Amphiphilic Secondary Structures on a Template," Helv. Chim. Acta 71(1988):835-847.
2396. K.W. Hahn, W.A. Klis, J.M. Steward, "Design and Synthesis of a Peptide Having Chymotrypsin-Like Esterase Activity," Science 248(1990):1544-1547.
2397. K.E. Drexler, "Nanotechnology and Aging," Age 15(October 1992):143.
2398. Tanja Kortemme, Marina Ramirez-Alvarado, Luis Serrano, "Design of a 20-Amino Acid, Three-Stranded β-Sheet Protein," Science 281(10 July 1998):253-256.
2399. S. Borman, "Peptoids Eyed for Gene Therapy Applications," C&EN (4 May 1998):56-57.
2400. Pehr B. Harbury, Joseph J. Plecs, Bruce Tidor, Tom Alber, Peter S. Kim, "High-Resolution Protein Design with Backbone Freedom," Science 282(20 November 1998):1462-1467.
2401. Pierre Broun, John Shanklin, Ed Whittle, Chris Somerville, "Catalytic Plasticity of Fatty Acid Modification Enzymes Underlying Chemical Diversity of Plant Lipids," Science 282(13 November 1998):1315-1317.
2402. Christopher J. Noren, Spencer J. Anthony-Cahill, Michael C. Griffith, Peter G. Shultz, "A General Method for Site-Specific Incorporation of Unnatural Amino Acids into Proteins," Science 244(14 April 1989):182-188.
2403. David Mendel, Jonathan A. Ellman, Zhiyuh Chang, David L. Veenstra, Peter A. Kollman, Peter G. Schultz, "Probing Protein Stability with Unnatural Amino Acids," Science 256(26 June 1992):1798-1802.
2404. Joseph A. Piccirilli, Tilman Krauch, Simon E. Moroney, Steven A. Benner, "Enzymatic incorporation of a new base pair into DNA and RNA extends the genetic alphabet," Nature 343(4 January 1990):33-37.
2405. Herman J.C. Berendsen, "A Glimpse of the Holy Grail?" Science 282(23 October 1998):642-643.
2406. Themis Lazaridis, Martin Karplus, "New View of Protein Folding Reconciled with the Old Through Multiple Unfolding Simulations," Science 278(12 December 1997):1928-1931.
2407. X. Daura, B. Jaun, D. Seebach, W.F. Van Gunsteren, A.E. Mark, "Reversible peptide folding in solution by molecular dynamics simulation," J. Mol. Biol. 280(31 July 1998):925-932.
2408. Vukica Srajer et al., "Photolysis of the Carbon Monoxide Complex of Myoglobin: Nanosecond Time-Resolved Crystallography," Science 274(6 December 1996):1726-1729.
2409. Chengde Mao, Weiqiong Sun, Zhiyon Shen, Nadrian C. Seeman, "A Nanomechanical Device Based on the B-Z Transition of DNA," Nature 397(14 January 1999):144-146.
2410. M.H. Hecht, J.S. Richardson, D.C. Richardson, R.C. Ogden, "De Novo Design, Expression, and Characterization of Felix: A Four-Helix Bundle Protein of Native-like Sequence," Science 249(24 August 1990):884-891.
2411. S. Kamtekar, J.M. Schiffer, H. Xiong, J.M. Babik, M.H. Hecht, "Protein Design by Binary Patterning of Polar and Nonpolar Amino Acids," Science 262(10 December 1993):1680-1685.
2412. M.D. Struthers, R.P. Cheng, B. Imperiali, "Design of a Monomeric 23-residue Polypeptide with Defined Tertiary Structure," Science 271(19 January 1996):342-345.
2413. C.E. Schafmeister, S.L. LaPorte, L.J.W. Miercke, R.M. Stroud, "A designed four helix bundle protein with native-like structure," Nature Struct. Biol. 4(December 1997):1039-1046.
2414. N.C. Seeman, "Nucleic acid junctions: Building blocks for genetic engineering in three dimensions," in R.H. Sarma, ed., Biomolecular Stereodynamics, Adenine, New York, 1981, pp. 269-277.
2415. A. Paul Alivisatos, Kai P. Johnsson, Xiaogang Peng, Troy E. Wilson, Colin J. Loweth, Marcel P. Bruchez Jr., Peter G. Schultz, "Organization of `nanocrystal molecules' using DNA," Nature 382(15 August 1996):609-611.
2416. J. Shi, D.E. Bergstrom, "Assembly of novel DNA cycles with rigid tetrahedral linkers," Angew. Chem. Int. Ed. Engl. 36(1997):111-113.
2417. J.H. Chen, N.R. Kallenbach, N.C. Seeman, "A specific quadrilateral synthesized from DNA branched junctions," J. Am. Chem. Soc. 111(1989):6402-6407.
2418. Y. Zhang, N.C. Seeman, "A solid-support methodology for the construction of geometrical objects from DNA," J. Am. Chem. Soc. 114(1992):2656-2663.
2419. N.C. Seeman, "Nucleic acid junctions and lattices," J. Theor. Biol. 99(1982):237-247.
2420. X. Li, X. Yang, J. Qi, N.C. Seeman, "Antiparallel DNA double crossover molecules as components for nanoconstruction," J. Am. Chem. Soc. 118(1996):6131-6140.
2421. P.J. Hagerman, "Flexibility of DNA," Ann. Rev. Biophys. Biophys. Chem. 17(1988):265-286.
2422. N.C. Seeman, J.M. Rosenberg, A. Rich, "Sequence specific recognition of double helical nucleic acids by proteins," Proc. Natl. Acad. Sci. USA 73(1976):804-808.
2423. Bruce Smith, Markus Krummenacker, "DNA-Guided Assembly of Proteins as a Pathway to an Assembler," paper presented at the 1997 Albany Conference on Biomolecular Motors and Nanomachines; see abstract at: http://www.wadsworth.org/albcon97/abstract/krummena.htm.
2424. Custom DNA and peptide sequence Web ordering; see: http://www.perkin-elmer.com:80/ds/230000/dsww0002.html; http://www.cris.com/~biotech/oligoweb.html; http://mmr.bmb.colostate.edu/dna/forms/orderDNANet.html; http://www.genosys.com/text/prods/olg_onl.htm;

http://www.biosyn.com/order.htm; and http://mbcf.dfci.harvard.edu/docs/oligoform.html.

2425. J.R. Dennis, J. Howard, V. Vogel, "Molecular shuttles: directed motion of microtubules along nanoscale kinesin tracks," Nanotechnology 10(December 1999):In press. John R. Dennis, Jonathan Howard, Viola Vogel, "Guiding Molecular Shuttles by Nanoscale Surface Topologies," paper presented at the Sixth Foresight Conference on Molecular Nanotechnology, November 1998.

2426. Robert F. Service, "Borrowing From Biology to Power the Petite," Science 283(1 January 1999):27-28. See also: Jonathan Knight, "The engine of creation," New Scientist 162(19 June 1999); see at: http://www.newscientist.com/ns/19990619/theengineo.html.

2427. Peter Bennetto, "Microbial Fuel Cell," Materials from the NCBE; see http://134.225.167.114/ncbe/MATERIALS/fuelcell.html.

2428. See: "The Lion Fuel Cell," http://www.lion-breath.com/Fteclionfuelcell.html; and "Breath alcohol analysis technology," http://www.lion-breath.com/Fbreathtech.html.

2429. Intoximeters, Inc., "Fuel Cell Technology Applied to Alcohol Breath Testing," 1995-1997; see: http://www.intox.com/Products/Fuel_Cell_WP.html.

2430. Steven S. Smith, Luming Niu, David J. Baker, John A. Wendel, Susan E. Kane, Darrin S. Joy, "Nucleoprotein-based nanoscale assembly," Proc. Natl. Acad. Sci. 94(18 March 1997):2162-2167. See also: http://www.pnas.org/cgi/content/full/94/6/2162.

2431. Russell Mills, "Steps Toward Nanotechnology," Foresight Update No. 8, 15 March 1990, pp. 8-9.

2432. Wade Roush, "Counterfeit Chromosomes for Humans," Science 276(4 April 1997):38-39.

2433. G.M. Whitesides, J.P. Mathias, C. Seto, "Molecular self-assembly and nanochemistry: A chemical strategy for the synthesis of nanostructures," Science 254(1991):1312-1319. See also: G.M Whitesides, "Self-Assembling Materials," Scientific American 273(September 1995):114-117.

2434. William B. Wood, R.S. Edgar, "Building a Bacterial Virus," Scientific American 217(July 1967):61-66.

2435. R.S. Edgar, I. Lielausis, "Some Steps in the Morphogenesis of Bacteriophage T4," J. Mol. Biol. 32(March 1968):263-276.

2436. M.R. Ghadiri, J.R. Granja, R.A. Milligan, D.E. McRee, N. Khazanovich, "Self-Assembling Organic Nanotubes Based on a Cyclic Peptide Architecture," Nature 366(1993):324-327.

2437. T.D. Clark, M.R. Ghadiri, "Supramolecular Design by Covalent Capture: Design of a Peptide Cylinder via Hydrogen Bond-Promoted Intermolecular Olefin Metathesis," J. Am. Chem. Soc. 117(1995):12364-12365.

2438. J.M. Buriak, M.R. Ghadiri, "Self-Assembly of Peptide Based Nanotubes," Mater. Sci. Eng. C4(1997):207-212.

2439. H.S. Kim, J.D. Hartgerink, M. Reza Ghadiri, "Oriented Self-Assembly of Cyclic Peptide Nanotubes in Lipid Membranes," J. Am. Chem. Soc. 120(1998):4417-4424.

2440. Thomas D. Clark, Lukas K. Buehler, M. Reza Ghadiri, "Self-Assembling Cyclic β-3-Peptide Nanotubes as Artificial Transmembrane Ion Channels," J. Am. Chem. Soc. 120(1998):651-656.

2441. K. Kobayashi, J.R. Granja, M.R. Ghadiri, "β-Sheet Peptide Architecture: Measuring the Relative Stability of Parallel vs. Antiparallel β-Sheets," Angew. Chem. Int. Ed. Engl. 34(1995):95-98.

2442. N. Khazanovich, J.R. Granja, D.E. McRee, R.A. Milligan, M.R. Ghadiri, "Nanoscale Tubular Ensembles with Specified Internal Diameters: Design of a Self-Assembled Nanotube with a 13-Angstrom Pore," J. Am. Chem. Soc. 116(1994):6011-6012.

2443. J.R. Granja, M.R. Ghadiri, "Channel-Mediated Transport of Glucose Across Lipid Bilayers," J. Am. Chem. Soc. 116(1994):10785-10786.

2444. Christof M. Niemeyer, "DNA as a Material for Nanotechnology," Angew. Chem. Int. Ed. Engl. 36(1997):585-587.

2445. Jean-Marie Lehn, "Supramolecular Chemistry -- Scope and Perspectives: Molecules, Supermolecules, and Molecular Devices (Nobel Lecture)," Angew. Chem. Int. Ed. Engl. 27(January 1988):89-112.

2446. J.L. Atwood, J.E.D. Davies, D.D. MacNicol, F. Vogtle, eds., Comprehensive Supramolecular Chemistry, Pergamon Press, New York, 1996.

2447. N. Herron, "Catalytic aspects of inclusion in zeolites," in J.L. Atwood, J.E.D. Davies, D.D. MacNicol, Inclusion Compounds, Vol. 5, Oxford University Press, Cambridge, 1991.

2448. Robert Pool, "The Smallest Chemical Plants," Science 263(25 March 1994):1698-1699.

2449. Seong Su Kim, Wenzhong Zhang, Thomas J. Pinnavaia, "Ultrastable Mesostructured Silica Vesicles," Science 282(13 November 1998):1302-1305.

2450. J. Rebek, "Molecular recognition with model systems," Angew. Chem. Int. Ed. Engl. 29(1990):245-255.

2451. T. Tjivikua, P. Ballester, J. Rebek, Jr., "A Self-Replicating System," J. Am. Chem. Soc. 112(1990):1249-1250.

2452. James S. Nowick, Qing Feng, Tjama Tjivikua, Pablo Ballester, Julius Rebeck, Jr., "Kinetic Studies and Modeling of a Self-Replicating System," J. Am. Chem. Soc. 113(1991):8831-8839.

2453. D.D. MacNicol, J.J. McKendrick, D.R. Wilson, "Clathrates and Molecular Inclusion Phenomena," Chem. Soc. Rev. 7(1978):65-87.

2454. M. Simard, S. Dan, J.D. Wuest, "Use of Hydrogen Bonds to Control Molecular Aggregation. Self-Assembly of Three-Dimensional Networks with Large Chambers," J. Am. Chem. Soc. 113(1991):4696-4698.

2455. A. Ulman, An Introduction to Ultrathin Organic Films From Langmuir-Blodgett to Self-Assembly, Academic Press, Boston, 1991.

2456. G.R. Fleischaker, S. Colonna, P.L. Luisi, eds., Self-Production of Supramolecular Structures From Synthetic Structures to Models of Minimal Living Systems, NATO ASI Ser. C Vol. 446, Kluwer Academic Publishers, Dordrecht, 1994.

2457. D.H. Lee, J.R. Granja, J.A. Martinez, K. Severin, M.R. Ghadiri, "A Self-Replicating Peptide," Nature 382(1996):525-528.

2458. D.H. Lee, K. Severin, M.R. Ghadiri, "Autocatalytic Networks: The Transition from Molecular Self-Replication to Ecosystems," Curr. Opin. Chem. Biol. 1(1997):491-496.

2459. D.H. Lee, K. Severin, Y. Yokobayashi, M.R. Ghadiri, "Emergence of Symbiosis in Peptide Self-Replication Through A Hypercyclic Network," Nature 390(1997):591-594.

2460. D.H. Lee, K. Severin, M.R. Ghadiri, "Dynamic Error Correction in Autocatalytic Peptide Networks," Angew. Chem. Int. Ed. Engl. 37(1998):126-128.

2461. Samson Jenekhe, X. Linda Chen, "Self-Assembly of Ordered Microporous Materials from Rod-Coil Block Copolymers," Science 283(15 January 1999):372-375.

2462. T.W.R. Petrie, "A Review of Possible Fusion Fuels," in G.H. Miley, ed., Advanced Energy Conversion for Fusion Reactors, Univ. of Illinois Report COO-2218-18, 1974, pp. A1-A17.

2463. Robert B. Leighton, Principles of Modern Physics, McGraw-Hill Book Company, New York, 1959.

2464. Christian Munkel, Jorg Langowski, "Chromosome structure predicted by a polymer model," Phys. Rev. E 57(May 1998):5888-5896.

2465. Tobias A. Knoch, "Three-Dimensional Organization of Chromosome Territories in Simulation and Experiments," (German), Diploma-Thesis, German Cancer Research Center, Heidelberg, Faculty for Physics and Astronomy, University of Heidelberg, 1998.

2466. R.K. Sachs, G. van den Engh, B. Trask, H. Yokota, J.E. Hearst, "A random-walk/giant-loop model for interphase chromosomes," Proc. Natl. Acad. Sci. 92(1995):2710-2714.

2467. Kenneth J. Pienta, Donald S. Coffey, "A structural analysis of the role of the nuclear matrix and DNA loops in the organization of the nucleus and chromosome," in P.R. Cook, R.A. Laskey, eds., Higher Order Structure in the Nucleus, J. Cell Sci. Suppl. 1(1984):123-135.

2468. H. van Bekkum, E.M. Flanigen, J.C. Jansen, eds., Introduction to Zeolite Science and Practice, Elsevier, Amsterdam, 1991. See also: W.M. Meier, D.H. Olson, C. Baerlocher, Atlas of Zeolite Structure Types, Elsevier, Boston MA, 1996.

2469. George T. Kerr, "Synthetic Zeolites," Scientific American 261(July 1989):100-105. See also: John Meurig Thomas, "Solid Acid Catalysts," Scientific American 266(April 1992):112-118.

2470. Donald A. Tomalia, "Dendrimer Molecules," Scientific American 272(May 1995):62-66.

2471. George R. Newkome, Claus D. Weis, Charles N. Moorefield, Ingrid Weis, "Detection and Functionalization of Dendrimers Possessing Free Carboxylic Acid Moieties," Macromolecules 30(1997):2300-2304.

2472. K. Mislow, "Molecular Machinery in Organic Chemistry," Chemtracts-Org. Chem. 2(1989):151-174.

2473. Robert F. Service, "Not-So-Square Molecules," Science 271(12 January 1996):145-146.

2474. J.K. Gimzewski, C. Joachim, R.R. Schlittler, V. Langlais, H. Tang, I. Johannsen, "Rotation of a Single Molecule Within a Supramolecular Bearing," Science 281(24 July 1998):531-533.

2475. Matthias Wintermantel, Markus Gerle, Karl Fischer, Manfred Schmidt, Isao Wataoka, Hiroshi Urakawa, Kanji Kajiwara, Yasuhisa Tsukhara, "Molecular Bottlebrushes," Macromolecules 29(29 January 1996):978-983.

2476. Philippe Cluzel, Anne Lebrun, Christoph Heller, Richard Lavery, Jean-Louis Viovy, Didier Chatenay, Francois Caron, "DNA: An Extensible Molecule," Science 271(9 February 1996):792-794.

2477. Steven B. Smith, Yujia Cui, Carlos Bustamonte, "Overstretching B-DNA: The Elastic Response of Individual Double-Stranded and Single-Stranded DNA Molecules," Science 271(9 February 1996):795-799.

2478. T. Kajiyama, H. Kikuchi, M. Katayose, S. Shinkai, "Photo-driven active transport of metal cations through polymer/(liquid crystal)/(Azobenzene crown ether) ternary composite thin films," New Polymeric Materials 1(1987/1988):99-106.

2479. G.W. Gokel, Crown Ethers and Cryptands, Royal Society of Chemistry, London, 1991.

2480. P.L. Anelli et al., "Molecular Meccano. 1. [2]Rotaxanes and a [2]Catenane Made to Order," J. Am. Chem. Soc. 114(1992):193-218.

2481. G. Schill, Catenanes, Rotaxanes and Knots, Academic Press, New York, 1971. See also: D.B. Amabilino, J.F. Stoddart, Chem. Rev. 95(1995):2725-2828.

2482. Fraser Stoddart, "Making molecules to order," Chem. in Britain 27(August 1991):714-718.

2483. Peter R. Ashton, Richard A. Bissell, Neil Spencer, J. Fraser Stoddart, Malcolm S. Tolley, "Towards Controllable Molecular Shuttles," Synlett (November 1992):914-926.

2484. Marcos Gomez-Lopez, Jon A. Preece, J. Fraser Stoddart, "The art and science of self-assembling molecular machines," Nanotechnology 7(September 1996):183-192.
2485. D.B. Amabilino, P.R. Ashton, A.S. Reder, N. Spencer, J.F. Stoddart, "The two-step self-assembly of [4]- and [5]-catenanes," Angew. Chem. Int. Ed. Engl. 33(1994):433-437. See also: "Another Gain in Self-Assembly," Science 265(29 July 1994):608.
2486. Robert L. Duda, "Protein chainmail: Catenated protein in viral capsids," Cell 94(10 July 1998):55-60. See also: J. Travis, "Protein chain mail offers armor for viruses," Science News 154(18 July 1998):38.
2487. Gerhard Wenz, Bruno Keller, "Threading Cyclodextrin Rings on Polymer Chains," Angew. Chem. Int. Ed. Engl. 31(1992):197-199. See also: Ivan Amato, "The Molecular Bead Game," Science 260(16 April 1993):293-294.
2488. Guang Li, Linda B. McGown, "Molecular Nanotube Aggregates of β- and γ-Cyclodextrins Linked by Diphenylhexatrienes," Science 264(8 April 1994):249-251.
2489. Franz H. Kohnke, John P. Mathias, J. Fraser Stoddart, "Structure-Directed Synthesis of New Organic Materials," Angew. Chem. Int. Ed. Engl. 28(1989):1103-1110.
2490. P.R. Ashton, N.S. Isaacs, F.H. Kohnke, J.P. Mathias, J.F. Stoddart, "Stereoregular Oligomerization by Repetitive Diels-Alder Reactions," Angew. Chem. Int. Ed. Engl. 28(1989):1258-1261.
2491. J.S. Lindsey, "Self-Assembly in Synthetic Routes to Molecular Devices. Biological Principles and Chemical Perspectives: A Review," New J. Chem. 15(1991):153-180.
2492. D.J. Cram, "Preorganization -- From Solvents to Spherands," Angew. Chem. Int. Ed. Engl. 25(1986):1039-1134.
2493. F. Diederich, Cyclophanes, Royal Society of Chemistry, London, 1991. See also: "Complexation of Neutral Molecules by Cyclophane Hosts," Angew. Chem. Int. Ed. Engl. 27(1988):362-386.
2494. P.J. Fagan, M.D. Ward, J.C. Calabrese, "Molecular Engineering of Solid-State Materials: Organometallic Building Blocks," J. Am. Chem. Soc. 111(1989):1698-1719.
2495. X. Yang, W. Jiang, C.B. Knobler, M.F. Hawthorne, "Rigid-Rod Molecules: Carborods. Synthesis of Tetrameric p-Carboranes and the Crystal Structure of Bis(tri-n-butylsilyl)tetra-p-carborane" J. Am. Chem.Soc. 114(1992):9719-9721.
2496. Roland Pease, "Nanoworlds Are Made of This," New Scientist 146(10 June 1995):26-29.
2497. F.H. Walker, K.B. Wiberg, J. Michl, "[2.2.1]Propellane," J. Am. Chem. Soc. 104(1982):2056-2057.
2498. J. Michl, "Synthesis of Giant Modular Structures," in C. Chatgilialoglu, V. Snieckus, eds., Chemical Synthesis: Gnosis to Prognosis, Kluwer: Dordrecht, The Netherlands, 1996, pp. 429 et seq.
2499. J. Michl, ed., Modular Chemistry, NATO ASI Series, Vol. C499, Kluwer: Dordrecht, The Netherlands, 1997.
2500. A.C. Friedli, P. Kaszynski, J. Michl, "Towards a Molecular-size Construction Set: 3,3(n-1)- Bisacetylthio[n]staffanes," Tetrahedron Lett. 30(1989):455-458.
2501. G.S. Murthy, K. Hassenruck, V.M. Lynch, J. Michl, "[n]Staffanes: The Parent Hydrocarbons," J. Am. Chem. Soc. 111(1989):7262-7264.
2502. Andrienne C. Friedli, Vincent M. Lynch, Piotr Kaszynski, Josef Michl, "Structures of Six Terminally Substituted [n]Staffanes, n = 1-4," Acta Cryst. B 46(1990):377-389.
2503. M.S. Gudipati, S.J. Hamrock, V. Balaji, J. Michl, "Infrared Spectra of [n]Staffanes," J. Phys. Chem. 96(1992):10165-10176.
2504. Huey C. Yang, Thomas F. Magnera, Chongmuk Lee, Allen J. Bard, Josef Michl, "Rigid-Rod Langmuir-Blodgett Films from [n]Staffane-3-carboxylates," Langmuir 8(1992):2740-2746.
2505. Tomasz Janecki, Shu Shi, Piotr Kaszynski, Josef Michl, "[n]Staffanes with Terminal Nitrile and Isonitrile Functionalities and Their Metal Complexes," Collect. Czech. Chem. Commun. 58(1993):89-104.
2506. Piotr Kaszynski, Josef Michl, "[n]Staffanes," in B. Halton, ed., Advances in Strain in Organic Chemistry, IV, JAI Press Inc., Greenwich CT, 1995, pp. 283 et seq.
2507. Josef Michl, "[n]Staffanes: Inert Rods for a Molecular Construction Set," 1995 McGraw Hill Yearbook of Science and Technology, McGraw Hill, New York, pp. 391 et seq.
2508. Ctibor Mazal, Alex J. Paraskos, Josef Michl, "Symmetric Bridgehead-to-Bridgehead Coupling of Bicyclo[1.1.1]pentanes and [n]Staffanes," J. Org. Chem. 63(1998):2116-2119.
2509. Piotr Kaszynski, Josef Michl, "[n]Staffanes: A Molecular-Size 'Tinkertoy' Construction Set for Nanotechnology. Preparation of End-functionalized Telomers and a Polymer of [1.1.1]Propellane," J. Am. Chem. Soc. 110(1988):5225-5226.
2510. Karin Hassenruck, Gudipati S. Murthy, Vincent M. Lynch, Josef Michl, "'Mixed Staffanes' as Intermediate Length Staffs for Molecular-size Tinkertoys. Parent Hydrocarbons and Terminal Diiodides Combining Bicyclo[1.1.1]pentane with Cubane or Bicyclo[2.2.2]octane Units," J. Org. Chem. 55(1990):1013-1016.
2511. Josef Michl, Piotr Kaszynski, Andrienne C. Friedli, Gudipati S. Murthy, Huey-Chin Yang, Randall E. Robinson, Neil D. McMurdie, Taisun Kim, "Harnessing Strain: From [1.1.1]Propellanes to Tinkertoys," in A. de Meijere, S. Blechert, eds., Strain and Its Implications in Organic Chemistry, NATO ASI Series, Vol. 273, Kluwer Academic Publishers:Dordrecht, The Netherlands, 1989, pp. 463-482.
2512. Piotr Kaszynski, Andrienne C. Friedli, Joseph Michl, "Toward a Molecular-Size 'Tinkertoy' Construction Set. Preparation of Terminally Functionalized [n]Staffanes from [1.1.1]Propellane," J. Am. Chem. Soc. 114(1992):601-620.
2513. J. Muller, K. Base, T.F. Magnera, J. Michl, "Rigid-Rod Oligo-p-Carboranes for Molecular Tinkertoys," J. Am. Chem. Soc. 114(1992):9721-9722.
2514. Josef Michl, "The 'Molecular Tinkertoy' Approach to Materials," Proceedings of the NATO ARW Applications of Organometallic Chemistry in the Preparation and Processing of Advanced Materials, Cap d'Agde, France, September 1994, Kluwer:Dordrecht, The Netherlands, 1995, pp. 243 et seq.
2515. Thomas F. Magnera, Laurence M. Peslherbe, Eva Korblova, Josef Michl, "The Organometallic 'Molecular Tinkertoy' Approach to Planar Grid Polymers," J. Organomet. Chem. 548(1997):83-89.
2516. Jaroslav Vacek, Josef Michl, "A Molecular Tinkertoy Construction Kit: Computer Simulation of Molecular Propellers," New J. Chem. 21(1997):1259-1268.
2517. Thomas F. Magnera, Jaroslav Pecka, Jaroslav Vacek, Josef Michl, "Synthesis and Handling of Single Sheets of a Covalent Monolayer Square Grid Polymer," in M. Moskovits, V. Shalaev, eds., Nanostructural Materials: Clusters, Composites, and Thin Films, ACS Symposium Series 679, American Chemical Society, Washington DC, 1997, pp. 213-220.
2518. Robin M. Harrison, Thierry Brotin, Bruce C. Noll, Josef Michl, "Towards a Square Grid Polymer: Synthesis and Structure of Pedestal-Mounted Tetragonal Star Connectors, C_4R_4-Co-C_5Y_5," Organometallics 16(1997):3401-3412.
2519. T. Magnera, J. Pecka, J. Michl, "Synthesis of a Covalent Square Grid," in Science and Technology of Polymers & Advanced Materials, Plenum Press, New York, 1998.
2520. Lubomir Pospisil, Michael Heyrovsk, Jaroslav Pecka, Josef Michl, "Towards a Hexagonal Grid Polymer: Interaction of Tentacled 1,3,5-Tricarboranylbenzene Derivatives with Mercury Surface," Langmuir 13(1997):6294-6301.
2521. U. Schoberl, T.F. Magnera, R. Harrison, F Fleischer, J.L. Pflug, P.F.H. Schwab, X. Meng, D. Lipiak, B.C. Noll, V.S. Allured, T. Rudalevige, S. Lee, J. Michl, "Towards a Hexagonal Grid Polymer: Synthesis, Coupling, and Chemically Reversible Surface-Pinning of the Star Connectors, 1,3,5-$C_6H_3(CB_{10}H_{10}CX)_3$," J. Am. Chem. Soc. 119(1997):3907-3917.
2522. H.W. Gibson, H. Marand, "Polyrotaxanes: molecular composites derived by physical linkage of cyclic and linear species," Advanced Materials 5(1993):11 et seq.
2523. Jon Preece, Fraser Stoddart, "From Biology to Materials," in Richard R.H. Coombs, Dennis W. Robinson, eds., Nanotechnology in Medicine and the Biosciences, Gordon & Breach Publishers, Netherlands, 1996, pp. 211-230.
2524. M. Famulok, J.S. Nowick, J. Rebek, Jr., "Self-replicating systems," Acta Chem. Scand. 46(1992):315-324.
2525. L.E. Orgel, "Molecular replication," Nature 358(1992):203-209.
2526. T. Achilles, G. von Kiedrowski, "A self-replicating system from three starting materials," Angew. Chem. Int. Ed. Engl. 32(1993):1198-1201. See also: G. von Kiedrowski, "A Self-Replicating Hexadeoxynucleotide," Angew. Chem. Int. Ed. Engl. 25(1986):932-935.
2527. D. Philip, J.F. Stoddart, "Self-assembly in organic synthesis," Synlett 7(1991):445-458.
2528. A.G. Johnston, D.A. Leigh, R.J. Pritchard, M.D. Deegan, "Facile Synthesis and Solid State Structure of a Benzylic Amide [2]Catenane," Angew. Chem. Int. Ed. Engl. 34(1995):1209-1212.
2529. A.S. Lane, D.A. Leigh, A. Murphy, "Peptide-based Molecular Shuttles," J. Am. Chem. Soc. 119(1997):11092-11093.
2530. D.A. Leigh, A. Murphy, J.P. Smart, A.M.Z. Slawin, "Glycylglycine Rotaxanes -- The Hydrogen Bond-Directed Assembly of Synthetic Peptide Rotaxanes," Angew. Chem. Int. Ed. Engl. 36(1997):728-732.
2531. O.A. Matthews, A.N. Shipway, J.F. Stoddart, "Dendrimers -- branching out from curiosities into new technologies," Prog. Poly. Sci. 23(1998):1-56.
2532. D.B. Amabilino, et al., "Molecular meccano. 30. Oligocatenanes made to order," J. Am. Chem. Soc. 120(1998):4295-4307.
2533. P.R. Ashton, et al., "Supramolecular daisy chains," Angew. Chem 110(1998):1344-1347; Angew. Chem. Int. Ed. 37(1998):1294-1297.
2534. P.R. Ashton, et al., "Self-assembling supramolecular daisy chains," Angew. Chem. 110(1998):2016-2019; Angew. Chem. Int. Ed. 37(1998):1913-1916.
2535. D.B. Amabilino, P.R. Ashton, S.E. Boyd, J.Y. Lee, S. Menzer, J.F. Stoddart, D.J. WIlliams, "The five-stage self-assembly of a branched heptacatenane," Angew. Chem. 109(1997):2160-2162; Angew. Chem. Int. Ed. Engl. 36(1997):2070-2072.
2536. F. Diederich, M. Gomez-Lopez, J.-F. Nierengarten, J.A. Preece, F.M. Raymo, J.F. Stoddart, "The self-assembly of the first fullerene-containing [2]catenane," Angew. Chem. 109(1997):1611-1614; Angew. Chem. Int. Ed. Engl. 36(1997):1448-1451.
2537. P.R. Ashton, A.N. Collins, M.C.T. Fyfe, S. Menzer, J.F. Stoddart, D.J. Williams, "Supramolecular weaving," Angew. Chem. 109(1997):760-763; Angew. Chem. Int. Ed. Engl. 36(1997):735-739.
2538. F.M. Raymo, J.F. Stoddart, "Polyrotaxanes and pseudopolyrotaxanes," Trends Polym. Sci. 4(1996):208-211.
2539. F.M. Raymo, J.F. Stoddart, "Slippage -- a simple and efficient way to self-assemble [n]rotaxanes," Pure Appl. Chem. 69(1997):1987-1997.
2540. A. Credi, V. Balzani, S.J. Langford, J.F. Stoddart, "Molecular logic. An XOR gate based on a mechanical molecular machine," J. Am. Chem. Soc. 119(1997):2679-2681.

2541. P.R. Ashton, et al., "Molecular meccano. 24. Multiple stranded and multiply encircled pseudorotaxanes," J. Am. Chem. Soc. 119(1997):12514-12524.

2542. Roberto Ballardini, Vincenzo Balzani, Alberto Credi, Maria Teresa Gandolfi, Steven J. Langford, Stephan Menzer, Luca Prodi, J. Fraser Stoddart, Margherita Venturi, David J. Williams, "Simple Molecular Machines. Cyclical Chemically-driven Unthreading and Re-threading of a [2]Pseudorotaxane," Angew. Chem. Int. Ed. Engl. 35(1996):978-981.

2543. M. Asakawa, et al., "Molecular meccano. 8. Cyclobis(paraquat-4,4c-biphenylene)? An organic molecular square," Chem. Eur. J. 2(1996):877-893.

2544. John A. Wendel, Steven S. Smith, "Uracil as an alternative to 5-fluorocytosine in addressable protein targeting," Nanotechnology 9(September 1998):297-304.

2545. Keren Deng, Wen H. Ko, "Static friction of diamond-like carbon film in MEMS," Sensors and Actuators A 35(1992):45-50.

2546. T. Ross Kelly, Imanol Tellitu, Jose Perez Sestelo, "In Search of Molecular Ratchets," Angew. Chem. Int. Ed. Engl. 36(1997):1866-1868. See also: T. Ross Kelly, Jose Perez Sestelo, Imanol Tellitu, "New Molecular Devices: In Search of a Molecular Ratchet," J. Org. Chem. 63(1998):3655-3665; George Musser, "Taming Maxwell's Demon," Scientific American 280(February 1999):24.

2547. B.C. Hamann, K.D. Shimizu, J. Rebek, Jr., "Reversible Encapsulation of Guest Molecules in a Calixarene Dimer," Angew. Chem. Int. Ed. Engl. 35(1996):1326-1329. See also: "The Littlest Test-tube," Science 273(16 August 1996):877.

2548. Z. Wu, J.S. Moore, "A Freely-Hinged Macrotricycle with a Molecular Cavity," Angew. Chem. Int. Ed. Engl. 35(1996):297-299.

2549. R. Grotzfeld, N. Branda, J. Rebek, Jr., "Reversible Encapsulation of Disc-Shaped Guests by a Synthetic, Self-Assembled Host," Science 271(1996):487-489.

2550. M.M. Conn, J. Rebek, Jr., ""Self-Assembling Capsules," Chem. Rev. 97(1997):1647-1668.

2551. T. Szabo, G. Hilmersson, J. Rebek, Jr., "Dynamics of Assembly and Guest Exchange in the Tennis Ball," J. Am. Chem. Soc. 120(1998):6193-6194. See also: David Bradley, "A Game of Molecular Tennis, Anyone?" Science 263(4 March 1994):1222-1223.

2552. Kingsley L. Taft, Stephen J. Lippard, "Synthesis and Structure of $[Fe(OMe)_2(O_2CCH_2Cl)]_{10}$. A Molecular Ferric Wheel," J. Am. Chem. Soc. 112(19 December 1990):9629-9630.

2553. K.C. Nicolaou, Zhen Yang, Guo-qiang Shi, Janet L. Gunzner, Konstantinos A. Agrios, Peter Gartner, "Total Synthesis of Brevetoxin A," Nature 392(19 March 1998):264-269. See also: Kyriacos Costa Nicolaou, "Total Synthesis of Brevetoxin B. A Twelve-Year Synthetic Odyssey," Angew. Chem. Int. Ed. Engl. 35(1996):588-607; K.C. Nicolaou, F.B.J.T. Rutjes, J. Tiebes, M. Sato, E. Untersteller, X.-Y. Xiao, E. Theodorakis, "Total Synthesis of Brevetoxin B...," J. Am. Chem. Soc. 117(1995):1171-1172, 1173-1174.

2554. Edwin C. Constable, "Oligopyridines as Helicating Ligands," Tetrahedron 48(1992):10013-10059; E.C. Constable, D.R. Smith, "Metallosupramolecular helicates," in The Polymeric Materials Encyclopedia, CRC Press, Boca Raton FL, 1996, pp. 4237-4243; E.C. Constable, F.R. Heirtzler, M. Neuburger, M. Zehnder, "Selectivity in the self-assembly of directional helicates," Chem. Commun. (1996):933-934.

2555. James C. Nelson, Jeffery G. Saven, Jeffrey S. Moore, Peter G. Wolynes, "Solvophobically Driven Folding of Nonbiological Oligomers," Science 277(19 September 1997):1793-1796.

2556. M.C.T. Fyfe, J.F. Stoddart, A.J.P. White, D.J. Williams, "Novel clay-like and helical superstructures generated using arene-arene interactions," New J. Chem. 22(1998):155-157.

2557. J. Kang, J. Santamaria, G. Hilmersson, J. Rebek, Jr., "Diels-Alder Reactions Through Reversible Encapsulation," J. Am. Chem. Soc. 120(1998):3650-3656; "Self-Assembled Molecular Capsule Catalyzes a Diels-Alder Reaction," J. Am. Chem. Soc. 120(1998):7389-7390.

2558. R. Beerli, J. Rebek, Jr., "Barrelene Derivatives -- Potential Modules for Assembly," Tetrahedron Lett. 36(1995):1813-1816.

2559. E.C. Constable, E. Schofield, "Metal-directed assembly of box-like structures," Chem. Commun. (1998):403-404.

2560. James R. Sheats, et al., "Organic Electroluminescent Devices," Science 273(16 August 1996):884-888.

2561. Stuart R. Batten, Bernard F. Hoskins, Richard Robson, "Two Interpenetrating 3D Networks...," J. Am. Chem. Soc. 117(17 May 1995):5385-5386.

2562. Riccardo F. Carina, Christiane Dietrich-Buchecker, Jean-Pierre Sauvage, "Molecular Composite Knots," J. Am. Chem. Soc. 118(25 September 1996):9110-9116.

2563. S.I. Stupp, V. LeBonheur, K. Walker, L.S. Li, K.E. Huggins, M. Keser, A. Amstutz, "Supramolecular Materials: Self-Organized Nanostructures," Science 276(18 April 1997):384-389.

2564. I.A. Aksay, et al., "Biomimetic Pathways for Assembling Inorganic Thin Films," Science 273(16 August 1996):892-898.

2565. Rudiger Berger, Emmanuel Delamarche, Hans Peter Lang, Christoph Gerber, James K. Gimzewski, Ernst Meyer, Hans-Joachim Guntherodt, "Surface Stress in the Self-Assembly of Alkanethiols on Gold," Science 276(27 June 1997):2021-2024.

2566. Masad J. Damha, Kanjana Ganeshan, Robert H.E. Hudson, Steven V. Zabarylo, "Solid-phase synthesis of branched oligoribonucleotides related to messenger RNA splicing intermediates," Nucleic Acid Res. 20(December 1992):6565-6573.

2567. Paul A. Giannaris, Masad J. Damha, "Oligoribonucleotides containing 2'-5'-phosphodiester linkages exhibit binding selectivity for 3'-5'-RNA over 3'-5'-ssDNA," Nucleic Acid Res. 21(October 1993):4742-4749.

2568. R.H.E. Hudson, M.J. Damha, "Nucleic acid dendrimers -- novel biopolymer structures," J. Am. Chem. Soc. 115(24 March 1993):2119-2124.

2569. A.H. Uddin, M.A. Roman, J. Anderson, M.J. Damha, "A novel N3-functionalized thymidine linker for the stabilization of triple helical DNA," Chem. Commun. (1996):171-172.

2570. Philip E. Eaton, "Cubane: Starting Material for the 1990s and the New Century," Angew. Chem. Int. Ed. Engl. 31(1992):1421-1436.

2571. Philip E. Eaton, Kirill A. Lukin, "Through Space Amide-Activation of C-H Bonds in Triangulanes," J. Am. Chem. Soc 115(1993):11370-11375.

2572. J.S. Moore, "Hollow Organic Solids," Nature 374(1995):495-496.

2573. T.C. Bedard, J.S. Moore, "Design and Synthesis of a `Molecular Turnstile'" J. Am. Chem. Soc. 117(1995):10662-10671.

2574. J. Zhang, J.S. Moore, Z. Xu, R.A. Aguirre, "Nanoarchitectures. 1. Controlled-Synthesis of Phenylacetylene Sequences," J. Am. Chem. Soc. 114(1992):2273-2274.

2575. Jeffrey S. Moore, Jinshan Zhang, "Nanoarchitectures. 2. Efficient Preparation of Nanoscale Macrocyclic Hydrocarbons," Angew. Chem. Int. Ed. Engl. 31(1992):922 924

2576. J. Zhang, J.S. Moore, "Nanoarchitectures. 3. Aggregation of Hexa(Phenylacetylene) Macrocycles in Solution: A Model System for Studying _-_ Interactions," J. Am. Chem. Soc. 114(1992):9701-9702.

2577. Z. Wu, S. Lee, J.S. Moore, "Nanoarchitectures. 4. Synthesis of Three-Dimensional Nanoscaffolding," J. Am. Chem. Soc. 114(1992):8730-8732.

2578. Jeffrey S. Moore, "Carborod molecular scaffolding," Nature 361(1993):118-119.

2579. J.S. Moore, "Shape-Persistent Molecular Architectures of Nanoscale Dimension," Acc. Chem. Res. 30(1997):402-413.

2580. Z. Xu, J.S. Moore, "Synthesis and Characterization of a High Molecular Weight Stiff Dendrimer," Angew. Chem. 105(1993):261; Angew. Chem. Int. Ed. Engl. 32(1993):246-248.

2581. Z. Xu, J.S. Moore, "Rapid Construction of Large-Size Phenylacetylene Dendrimers up to 12.5 Nanometers in Molecular Diameter," Angew. Chem. 105(1993):1394; Angew. Chem. Int. Ed. Engl. 32(1993):1354-1357.

2582. Z. Xu, B. Kyan, J.S. Moore, "Stiff Dendritic Macromolecules Based on Phenylacetylenes," in G.R. Newkome, ed., Advances in Dendritic Macromolecules, Volume 1, JAI Press, Greenwich CT, 1994, pp. 69-104.

2583. Z. Xu, M. Kahr, K.L. Walker, C.L. Wilkins, J.S. Moore, "Phenylacetylene Dendrimers by the Divergent, Convergent and Double-Stage Convergent Methods," J. Am. Chem. Soc. 116(1994):4537-4550.

2584. T. Kawaguchi, K.L. Walker, C.L. Wilkins, J.S. Moore, "Double Exponential Dendrimer Growth," J. Am. Chem. Soc. 117(1995):2159-2165.

2585. D.J. Pesak, J.S. Moore, T.E. Wheat, "Synthesis and Characterization of Water-Soluble Dendritic Macromolecules with a Stiff Hydrocarbon Interior," Macromolecules 30(1997):6467-6482.

2586. Z. Xu, J.S. Moore, "Design and Synthesis of a Convergent and Directional Molecular Antenna," Acta Polymerica 45(1994):83-87.

2587. C. Devadoss, P. Bharathi, J.S. Moore, "Energy Transfer in Dendritic Macromolecules: Molecular Size Effects and the Role of an Energy Gradient," J. Am. Chem. Soc. 118(1996):9635-9644.

2588. M.R. Shortreed, S.F. Swallen, Z.-Y. Shi, W. Tan, Z. Xu, C. Devadoss, J.S. Moore, R. Kopelman, "Directed Energy Transfer Funnels in Dendrimeric Antenna Supermolecules," J. Phys. Chem. 101(1997):6318-6322.

2589. C. Devadoss, P. Bharathi, J.S. Moore, "Photoinduced Electron Transfer in Dendritic Macromolecules: I. Intermolecular Electron Transfer," Macromolecules 31(1998):8091-8099.

2590. S.F. Swallen, M.R. Shortreed, Z.-Y. Shi, W. Tan, Z. Xu, C. Devadoss, J.S. Moore, R. Kopelman, "Dendrimeric Antenna Supermolecules with Multistep Directed Energy Transfer," in P.N. Prasad et al., eds., Science and Technology Polymers and Advanced Materials, Plenum Press, NY, 1998.

2591. C. Devadoss, J.S. Moore, "Synthetic Light Harvesting Antennas," 1999 McGraw-Hill Yearbook of Science and Technology, Mcgraw-Hill, NY, 1999, pp. 284-287.

2592. G.C. Abeln, D.S. Thompson, S.Y. Lee, J.S. Moore, J.W. Lyding, "Nanopatterning Organic Monolayers on Si(100) by Selective Chemisorption of Norbornadiene," Appl. Phys. Lett. 70(1997):2747-2749.

2593. G.C. Abeln, M.C. Hersam, D.S. Thompson, S.-T. Hwang, H. Choi, J.S. Moore, J.W. Lyding, "Approaches to Nanofabrication on Si(100) Surfaces: Selective Area Chemical Vapor Deposition of Metals and Selective Chemisorption of Organic Molecules," J. Vac. Sci. Technol. B 16(1998):3874-3878.

2594. K.A. Hirsch, S.R. Wilson, J.S. Moore, "A Packing Model for Interpenetrated Diamondoid Structures -- An Interpretation Based on the Constructive Interference of Supramolecular Networks," Chem. Eur. J. 3(1997):765-71.

2595. Judith Konnert, Doyle Britton, "The Crystal Structure of $AgC(CN)_3$," Inorg. Chem. 5(1966):1193-1196.

2596. David J. Duchamp, Richard E. Marsh, "The Crystal Structure of Trimesic Acid (Benzene-1,3,5-tricarboxylic Acid)," Acta Crystallogr. Sect. B 25(1969):5-19.

2597. Robert W. Gable, Bernard F. Hoskins, Richard Robson, "A New Type of Interpenetration Involving Enmeshed Independent Square Grid Sheets. The Structure of Diaquabis-(4,4'-bipyridine)zinc Hexafluorosilicate," Chem. Commun. (1990):1677-1678.
2598. Humberto O. Stumpf, Lahcene Ouahab, Yu Pei, Daniel Grandjean, Olivier Kahn, "A Molecular-Based Magnet with a Fully Interlocked Three-Dimensional Structure," Science 261(23 July 1993):447-449. See also: Peter Day, "The Chemistry of Magnets," Science 261(23 July 1993):431-432.
2599. Jose Antonio Real, Enrique Andres, M. Carmen Munoz, Miguel Julve, Thierry Granier, Azzedine Bousseksou, Francois Varret, "Spin Crossover in a Catenane Supramolecular System," Science 268(14 April 1995):265-267.
2600. Olivier Kahn, Molecular Magnetism, VCH, New York, 1993.
2601. M. Reza Ghadiri, "Molecular Self-Assembly, Self-Organization, and Self-Replication," paper presented at the Sixth Foresight Conference on Molecular Nanotechnology, November 1998.
2602. Ralph C. Merkle, "A proposed 'metabolism' for a hydrocarbon assembler," Nanotechnology 8(1997):149-162.
2603. Russell Mills, "Chiral metal complexes as molecular catalysts," Foresight Update #10, 30 October 1990, pp. 8-9.
2604. Cyrus Chothia, "Proteins. One thousand families for the molecular biologist," Nature 357(18 June 1992):543-544.
2605. Brett Lovejoy, Seunghyon Choe, Duilio Cascio, Donald K. McRorie, William F. DeGrado, David Eisenberg, "Crystal Structure of a Synthetic Triple-Stranded α-Helical Bundle," Science 259(26 February 1993):1288-1293.
2606. T. Horn, M.S. Urdea, "Forks and combs and DNA: The synthesis of branched oligodeoxyribonucleotides," Nucleic Acid Res. 17(12 September 1989):6959-6967.
2607. J.D. Bain, C. Switzer, A. Chamberlin, S. Benner, "Ribosome-mediated incorporation of a non-standard amino acid into a peptide through expansion of the genetic code," Nature 356(9 April 1992):537-539.
2608. J.A. Zasadzinski, R. Viswanathan, L. Madsen, J. Garnaes, D.K. Schwartz, "Langmuir-Blodgett Films," Science 263(25 March 1994):1726-1733.
2609. W. Muller et al., "Attempts to Mimic Docking Processes of the Immune System: Recognition-Induced Formation of Protein Multilayers," Science 262(10 December 1993):1706-1708.
2610. Steven C. Zimmerman, Fanwen Zeng, "Dendrimers in Supramolecular Chemistry: From Molecular Recognition to Self-Assembly," Chem. Rev. 97(1997):1681-1712. See also: Steven C. Zimmerman, Fanwen Zeng, David E.C. Reichert, Sergei V. Kolotuchin, "Self-Assembling Dendrimers," Science 271(23 February 1996):1095-1098; Thomas W. Bell, "Molecular Trees: A New Branch of Chemistry," Science 271(23 February 1996):1077-1078.
2611. Richard P. Feynman, "Ratchet and pawl," Volume I, Chapter 46, The Feynman Lectures on Physics, Addison-Wesley Publishing Company, Reading, MA, 1963.
2612. H.W. Kroto, J.R. Heath, S.C. O'Brien, R.F. Curl, R.E. Smalley, "C_{60}: Buckminsterfullerene," Nature 318(14 November 1985):162-163.
2613. H.W. Kroto, "The stability of the fullerenes C_n with n = 24, 28, 32, 36, 50, 60, and 70," Nature 329(8 October1987):529-531.
2614. Gustavo E. Scuseria, "Ab Initio Calculations of Fullerenes," Science 271(16 February 1996):942-945.
2615. Gary B. Adams, Otto F. Sankey, John B. Page, Michael O'Keeffe, David A. Drabold, "Energetics of Large Fullerenes: Balls, Tubes, and Capsules," Science 256(26 June 1992):1792-1795.
2616. Craig C. Henderson, Paul A. Cahill, "$C_{60}H_2$: Synthesis of the Simplest C_{60} Hydrocarbon Derivative," Science 259(26 March 1993):1885-1887.
2617. Craig C. Henderson, Celeste McMichael Rohlfing, Kenneth T. Gillen, Paul A. Cahill, "Synthesis, Isolation, and Equilibration of 1,9- and 7,8-$C_{70}H_2$," Science 264(15 April 1994):397-399.
2618. M. Prato, T. Suzuki, H. Foroudian, Q. Li, K. Khemani, F. Wudl, "[3+2] and [4+2] Cycloadditions of C_{60}," J. Am. Chem. Soc. 115(1993):1594-1595.
2619. A. Hirsch, The Chemistry of the Fullerenes, Thieme, Stuttgart, 1994.
2620. K.L. Wooley, C.J. Hawker, J.M.J. Frechet, F. Wudl, G. Srdanov, S. Shi, C. Li, M. Kao, "Fullerene-Bound Dendrimers: Soluble, Isolated Carbon Clusters," J. Am. Chem. Soc. 115(1993):9836-9837.
2621. S. Shi, K.C. Khemani, Q. Li, F. Wudi, "A Polyester and Polyurethane of Diphenyl C_{61}: Retention of Fulleroid Properties in a Polymer," J. Am. Chem. Soc. 114(1992):10656-10657.
2622. F. Diederich, C. Dietrich-Buchecker, J.-F. Nierengarten, J.P. Sauvage, "A Copper(I)-complexed Rotaxane with Two Fullerene Stoppers," Chem. Commun. 1995(1995):781-782.
2623. Alexandre S. Boutorine, Hidetoshi Tokuyama, Masashi Takasugi, Hiroyuki Isobe, Eiichi Nakamura, Claude Helene, "Fullerene-Oligonucleotide Conjugates: Photoinduced Sequence-Specific DNA Cleavage," Angew. Chem. Int. Ed. Engl. 33(1994):2462-2465.
2624. Francois Diederich, Carlo Thilgen, "Covalent Fullerene Chemistry," Science 271(19 January 1996):317-323.
2625. Paul J. Fagan, Paul J. Krusic, C.N. McEwen, J. Lazar, Deborah Holmes Parker, N. Herron, E. Wasserman, "Production of Perfluoroalkylated Nanospheres from Buckminsterfullerene," Science 262(15 October 193):404-407.
2626. Sumio Iijima, "Helical microtubules of graphitic carbon," Nature 354(7 November 1991):56-58.
2627. W. Kratschmer, Lowell D. Lamb, K. Fostiropoulos, Donald R. Huffman, "Solid C_{60}: A new form of carbon," Nature 347(27 September 1990):354-358.
2628. Martin Saunders, R. James Cross, Hugo A. Jimenez-Vazquez, Rinat Shimshi, Anthony Khong, "Noble Gas Atoms Inside Fullerenes," Science 271(22 March 1996):1693-1697.
2629. Guanghua Gao, Tahir Cagin, William A. Goddard III, "Energetics, structure, mechanical and vibrational properties of single-walled carbon nanotubes," Nanotechnology 9(September 1998):184-191. See at: http://www.wag.caltech.edu/foresight/foresight_2.html.
2630. V.V. Kolesov, V.I. Panov, E.A. Fedorov, J. Commun. Technol. Electron. (Russia) 42(July 1997):818-821.
2631. Robert F. Service, "The Kitchen Chemistry of Nanoholes," Science 282(18 December 1998):2179.
2632. J. Liu, H. Dai, J.H. Hafner, D.T. Colbert, R.E. Smalley, S.J. Tans, C. Dekker, "Fullerene crop circles," Nature 385(27 February 1997):781-782.
2633. Simon H. Friedman, Dianne L. DeCamp, Rint P. Sijbesma, Gordana Srdanov, Fred Wudl, George L. Kenyon, "Inhibition of the HIV-1 Protease by Fullerene Derivatives: Model Building Studies and Experimental Verification," J. Am. Chem. Soc. 115(1993):6506-6509. See also: S.H. Friedman, P.S. Ganapathi, Y. Rubin, G.L. Kenyon, "Optimizing the binding of fullerene inhibitors of the HIV-1 protease through predicted increases in hydrophobic desolvation," J. Med. Chem. 41(18 June 1998):2424-2429.
2634. C. Toniolo et al., "A bioactive fullerene peptide," J. Med. Chem. 37(1994):4558-4562.
2635. H. Terrones, M. Terrones, W.K. Hsu, "Beyond C_{60}: Graphite Structures for the Future," Chem. Soc. Reviews 24(1995):341-350. See also: http://www.ch.ic.ac.uk/motm/spiral.html.
2636. T.W. Ebbesen, Carbon Nanotubes: Preparation and Properties, CRC Press, 1997.
2637. R. Saito, G. Dresselhaus, M.S. Dresselhaus, Physical Properties of Carbon, Imperial College Press, 1998.
2638. Francois Diederich, Robert L. Whetten, Carlo Thilgen, Roland Etti, Ita Chao, Marcos M. Alvarez, "Fullerene Isomerism: Isolation of C_{2v}-C_{78} and D_3-C_{78}," Science 254(20 December 1991):1768-1770.
2639. T. Jon Seiders, Kim K. Baldridge, Jay S. Siegel, "Synthesis and Characterization of the First Corannulene Cyclophane," J. Am. Chem. Soc. 118(1996):2754-2755.
2640. S. Wei, B.C. Guo, J. Purnell, S. Buzza, A.W. Castleman, Jr., "Metallo-Carbohedrenes: Formation of Multicage Structures," Science 256(8 May 1992):818-820.
2641. Yu. L. Orlov, The Mineralogy of the Diamond, John Wiley & Sons, NY, 1977.
2642. A.W. Jensen, S.R. Wilson, D.I. Schuster, "Biological Applications of Fullerenes—A Review," Bioorg. Med. Chem. 4(1996):767-779.
2643. Daniel T. Colbert, Richard E. Smalley, "Fullerene Tinkertoys," Proc. NATO Advanced Research Workshop on Modular Chemistry, Estes Park, CO, September 1995; see at: http://cnst.rice.edu/Modular.html.
2644. Steven H. Hoke, Jay Molstad, Dominique Dilettato, Mary Jennifer Jay, Dean Carlson, Bart Kahr, R. Graham Cooks, "Cooks Reaction of Fullerenes and Benzyne," J. Org. Chem. 57(11 September 1992):5069-5071.
2645. Richard Jaffe, Jie Han, Al Globus, "Formation of Carbon Nanotube Based Gears: Quantum Chemistry and Molecular Dynamics Simulations of the Electrophilic Addition of o-Benzyne to Fullerenes, Graphene, and Nanotubes," First Electronic Molecular Modelling & Graphics Society Conference, presented to the American Physical Society (MO Division of Materials Physics, Focused Session on Fullerenes, Carbon Nanotubes and Related Materials), Kansas City, 17-21 March 1997.
2646. Richard L. Jaffe, Grant D. Smith, "A Quantum Chemistry Study of Benzene Dimer," J. Chem. Phys. 105(15 August 1996):2780-2788.
2647. T.A. Jung, R.R. Schlittler, J.K. Gimzewski, H. Tang, C. Joachim, "Controlled Room-Temperature Positioning of Individual Molecules: Molecular Flexure and Motion," Science 271(12 January 1996):181-184.
2648. Jie Han, Al Globus, Richard Jaffe, Glenn Deardorff, "Molecular dynamics simulations of carbon nanotube-based gears," Nanotechnology 8(1997):95-102.
2649. Roger Taylor, David R.M. Walton, "The Chemistry of Fullerenes," Nature 363(24 June 1993):685-693.
2650. P.M. Ajayan, T. Ichihashi, S. Iijima, "Distribution of pentagons and shapes in carbon nano-tubes and nano-particles," Chem. Phys. Lett. 202(1993):384-388.
2651. S. Iijima, T. Ichihashi, Y. Ando, "Pentagons, heptagons and negative curvature in graphite microtubule growth," Nature 356(1992):756-778.
2652. S. Iijima, "Growth of carbon nanotubes," Mater. Sci. Eng. B 19(1993):172-180.
2653. Maohui Ge, Klaus Sattler, "Observation of fullerene cones," Chem. Phys. Lett. 220(1994):192-196. See also: K. Sattler, "Scanning tunneling microscopy of carbon nanotubes and nanocones," Carbon 33(1995):915-920.
2654. M. Endo, K. Takeuchi, K. Kobori, K. Takashi, H.W. Kroto, A. Sarkar, "Pyrolytic carbon nanotubes from vapor-grown carbon fibers," Carbon 33(1995):873-881.
2655. S. Amelinckx, X.B. Zhang, D. Bernaets, X.F. Zhang, V. Ivanov, J.B. Nagy, "A formation mechanism for catalytically grown helix-shaped graphite nanotubes," Science 265(1994):635-639.
2656. O.-Y. Zhong-can, Z.-B. Su, C.-L. Wang, "Coil formation in multishell carbon nanotubes: Competition between curvature elasticity and interlayer adhesion," Phys. Rev. Lett. 78(1997):4055-4058.

2657. S. Ihara, S. Itoh, "Helically coiled and toroidal cage forms of graphitic carbon," Carbon 33(1995):931-939. See also: http://shachi.cochem2.tutkie.tut.ac.jp/Fuller/fsl/torus.html.

2658. T.W. Ebbesen, T. Takada, "Topological and SP3 defect structures in nanotubes," Carbon 33(1995):973-978.

2659. B.I. Yacobson, C.J. Brabec, J. Bernholc, "Nanomechanics of carbon tubes—instabilities beyond linear response," Phys. Rev. Lett. 76(1996):2511-2514.

2660. Bobby G. Sumpter, Donald W. Noid, "The onset of instability in nanostructures: The role of nonlinear resonance," J. Chem. Phys. 102(22 April 1995):6619-6622.

2661. S. Iijima, C. Brabec, A. Maiti, J. Bernholc, "Structural flexibility of carbon nanotubes," J. Chem. Phys. 104(1996):2089-2092.

2662. Robert E. Tuzun, Donald W. Noid, Bobby G. Sumpter, "The dynamics of molecular bearings," Nanotechnology 6(April 1995):64-74.

2663. Karl Sohlberg, Robert E. Tuzun, Bobby G. Sumpter, Donald W. Noid, "Application of rigid-body dynamics and semiclassical mechanics to molecular bearings," Nanotechnology 8(1997):103-111.

2664. Donald W. Noid, Robert E. Tuzun, Bobby G. Sumpter, "On the importance of quantum mechanics for nanotechnology," Nanotechnology 8(1997):119-125. See also: R.E. Tuzun, D.W. Noid, B.G. Sumpter, "An internal coordinate quantum Monte Carlo method for calculating vibrational ground state energies and wave functions of large molecules: A quantum geometric statement function approach," J. Chem. Phys. 105(1 October 1996):5494-5502.

2665. B.I. Dunlap, "Connecting carbon tubules," Phys. Rev. B 46(1992):1933-1936; "Relating carbon tubules," Phys. Rev. B 49(1994):5643-5649; "Constraints on small graphitic helices," Phys. Rev. B 50(1994):8134-8137.

2666. X.F. Zhang, Z. Zhang, "Polygonal spiral of coil-shaped carbon nanotubes," Phys. Rev. B 52(1995):5313-5317.

2667. Al Globus, Charles W. Bauschlicher Jr., Jie Han, Richard L. Jaffe, Creon Levit, Deepack Srivastava, "Machine phase fullerene nanotechnology," Nanotechnology 9(1998):192-199.

2668. Robert E. Tuzun, Donald W. Noid, Bobby G. Sumpter, "Dynamics of a laser driven molecular motor," Nanotechnology 6(April 1995):52-63.

2669. Jeremy Q. Broughton, "Direct Atomistic Simulation of Next Generation Quartz Crystal Oscillators," NRL DoD HPCMP Annual Report, Computational Technology Areas, FY 1996; see also: http://ccs-www.nrl.navy.mil/hpc/annual-reports/fy96/broughton278.html.

2670. D.H. Robertson, B.I. Dunlap, D.W. Brenner, J.W. Mintmire, C.T. White, et al., "Molecular Dynamics Simulations of Fullerene-based Nanoscale Gears," in C.L. Renschler, D.M. Cox, J.J. Pouch, Y. Achiba, eds., Novel Forms of Carbon II, MRS Symposium Proceedings Series, Volume 349, 1994, pp. 283-288; see also: http://chem.iupui.edu/Chem/Research/Robertson/Robertson.html.

2671. Jean Haensler, Francis C. Szoka Jr., "Polyamidoamine Cascade Polymers Mediate Efficient Transfection of Cells in Culture," Bioconjugate Chemistry 4(September 1993):372-379.

2672. Weiquiang Han, Shoushan Fan, Qunqing Li, Yongdan Hu, "Synthesis of Gallium Nitride Nanorods Through a Carbon Nanotube-Confined Reaction," Science 277(29 August 1997):1287-1289.

2673. Y. Feldman, E. Wasserman, D.J. Srolovitz, R. Tenne, "High-Rate, Gas-Phase Growth of MoS_2 Nested Inorganic Fullerenes and Nanotubes," Science 267(13 January 1995):222-225.

2674. Nasreen G. Chopra, R.J. Luyken, K. Cherrey, Vincent H. Crespi, Marvin L. Cohen, Steven G. Louie, A. Zettl, "Boron Nitride Nanotubes," Science 269(18 August 1995):966-967.

2675. Slavi C. Sevov, John D. Corbett, "Carbon-Free Fullerenes: Condensed and Stuffed Anionic Examples in Indium Systems," Science 262(5 November 1993):880-883.

2676. Steven C. Zimmerman, Philippe Schmitt, "Model Studies Directed Toward a General Triplex DNA Recognition Scheme: A Novel DNA Base that Binds a CG Base-Pair in an Organic Solvent," J. Am. Chem. Soc. 117(1995):10769-10770.

2677. Steven C. Zimmerman, "Rigid Molecular Tweezers as Hosts for the Complexation of Neutral Guests," in E. Weber, ed., Topics in Current Chemistry, Springer-Verlag, Berlin, 1993, Vol. 165, Supramolecular Chemistry I, pp. 71-102 (Chapter 2).

2678. M.J. Zaworotko, "Crystal Engineering of Diamondoid Networks," Chem. Soc. Rev. 23(1994):283-288.

2679. "The Shape of Things to Come," Chemical and Engineering News, 8 June 1998.

2680. C.M. Drain, J.-M. Lehn, "Self-assembly of square multiporphyrin arrays by metal ion coordination," Chem. Commun. (1994):2313-2315.

2681. C.M. Drain, F. Nifiatis, A. Vasenko, J. Batteas, "Porphyrin Tessellation by Design: Metal Mediated Self-Assembly of Large Arrays and Tapes," Angew. Chem. Int. Ed. Engl. 37(1998):2344-2347.

2682. Werner Trabesinger, Gerhard J. Scetz, Herrmann J. Gruber, Hansgeorg Schindler, Thomas Schmidt, "Detection of Individual Oligonucleotide Pairing by Single-Molecule Microscopy," Anal. Chem. 71(1999):279-283.

2683. Vishwanath R. Iyer et al., "The Transcriptional Program in the Response of Human Fibroblasts to Serum," Science 283(1 January 1999):83-87.

2684. Barbie K. Ganser, Su Li, Victor Y. Klishko, John T. Finch, Wesley I. Sundquist, "Assembly and Analysis of Conical Models for the HIV-1 Core," Science 283(1 January 1999):80-83.

2685. Liesbeth C. Venema, J.W.G. Wildoer, H.L.J. Temminck Tuinstra, C. Dekker, "Length control of individual carbon nanotubes by nanostructuring with a scanning tunneling microscope," Appl. Phys. Lett. 71(3 November 1997):2629-2631.

2686. Atsushi Harada, Kazunori Kataoka, "Chain Length Recognition: Core-Shell Supramolecular Assembly from Oppositely Charged Block Copolymers," Science 283(1 January 1999):65-67.

2687. Rohini Kuner, Georg Kohr, Sylvia Grunewald, Gisela Eisenhardt, Alfred Bach, Hans-Christian Karnau, "Role of Heteromer Formation in $GABA_B$ Receptor Formation," Science 283(1 January 1999):74-77.

2688. A. Krishnan, E. Dujardin, M.M.J. Treacy, J. Hugdahl, S. Lynum, T.W. Ebbesen, "Graphitic cones and the nucleation of curved carbon surfaces," Nature 388(1997):451-454.

2689. Bernhard H. Weigl, Paul Yager, "Microfluidic Diffusion-Based Separation and Detection," Science 283(15 January 1999):346-347.

2690. K. Mauersberger, B. Erbacher, D. Krankowsky, J. Gunther, R. Nickel, "Ozone Isotope Enrichment: Isotopomer-Specific Rate Coefficients," Science 283(15 January 1999):370-372.

2691. Shoushan Fan, Michael G. Chapline, Nathan R. Franklin, Thomas W. Tombler, Alan M. Cassell, Hongjie Dai, "Self-Oriented Regular Arrays of Carbon Nanotubes and Their Field Emission Properties," Science 283(22 January 1999):512-514.

2692. Eugene R. Zubarev, Martin U. Pralle, Leiming Li, Samuel I. Stupp, "Conversion of Supramolecular Clusters to Macromolecular Objects," Science 283(22 January 1999):523-526.

2693. Jan Born, K. Hansen, L. Marshall, M. Molle, H.L. Fehm, "Timing the end of nocturnal sleep," Nature 397(7 January 1999):29-30.

2694. Hank Wittemore, Your Future Self: A Journey to the Frontiers of Molecular Medicine, Thames Hudson, 1998.

2695. Upinder S. Bhalla, Ravi Iyengar, "Emergent Properties of Networks of Biological Signaling Pathways," Science 283(15 January 1999):381-387.

2696. Gregory T.A. Kovacs, Micromachined Transducers Sourcebook, McGraw-Hill, Boston, 1998.

2697. Hartmut Gau, Stephan Herminghaus, Peter Lenz, Reinhard Lipowsky, "Liquid Morphologies on Structured Surfaces: From Microchannels to Microchips," Science 283(1 January 1999):46-49.

2698. Benedict S. Gallardo, Vinay K. Gupta, Franklin D. Eagerton, Lana I. Jong, Vincent S. Craig, Rahul R. Shah, Nicholas L. Abbott, "Electrochemical Principles for Active Control of Liquids on Submillimeter Scales," Science 283(1 January 1999):57-60.

2699. N. Materer, U. Starke, A. Barbieri, Michel A. Van Hove, Gabor A. Somorjai, G.-J. Kroes, C. Minot, "Molecular Surface Structure of a Low-Temperature Ice Ih(0001) Crystal," J. Phys. Chem. 99(1995):6267-6269.

2700. T.G. Zimmerman, "Personal Area Networks: Near-field intrabody communication," IBM Reprint No. G321-5627, 8 April 1996; see also: http://www.almaden.ibm.com/journal/sj/mit/sectione/zimmerman.html.

2701. Astrid Doppenschmidt, "The Surface of Ice," at http://wintermute.chemie.uni-mainz.de/astrid/eis/eis.html.

2702. Morinubo Endo, Sumio Iijima, Mildred S. Dresselhaus, eds., Carbon Nanotubes (Carbon, Vol. 33), Pergamon Press, New York, 1996.

2703. B.C. Stipe, M.A. Rezaei, W. Ho, "Single-Molecule Vibrational Spectroscopy and Microscopy," Science 280(12 June 1998):1732-1735.

2704. J. Vesekna, T. Marsh, R. Miller, E. Henderson, "Atomic force microscopy reconstruction of G-wire DNA," J. Vac. Sci. Technol. B 14(1996):1413-1417.

2705. G.I. Leach, R.E. Tuzun, D.W. Noid, B.G. Sumpter, "Positional stability of some diamondoid and graphitic nanomechanical structures: A molecular dynamics study," presentation at the Fifth Foresight Conference on Molecular Nanotechnology, November 1997; see also: http://goanna.cs.rmit.edu.au/~gl/research/nano/nano97/html/nano97.html.

2706. T.C. Marsh, E.R. Henderson, "G-wires: Self-assembly of a telomeric oligonucleotide, d(GGGGTTGGGG), into large superstructures," Biochemistry 33(1994):10718-10724.

2707. T.C. Marsh, J. Vesenka, E.R. Henderson, "A new DNA nanostructure, the G-wire, imaged by scanning probe microscopy," Nucl. Acids Res. 23(1995):696–700.

2708. Shuji Kiyohara, Iwao Miyamoto, "Reactive ion beam machining of diamond using an ECR-type oxygen source," Nanotechnology 7(September 1996):270-274.

2709. L.J. Geerligs et al., "Frequency-locked turnstile device for single electrons," Phys. Rev. Lett. 64(1990):2691-2694.

2710. Hongjie Dai, Eric Wong, Yuan Z. Lu, Shoushan Fan, Charles M. Lieber, "Synthesis and Characterization of Carbide Nanorods," Nature 375(29 June 1995):769-772.

2711. H. Dai, Franklin, Han, Applied Physics Letters, 14 September 1998. See also: T.-C. Shen, C. Wang, G.C. Abeln, J.R. Tucker, J.W. Lyding, Ph. Avouris, R.E. Walkup, "Atomic-Scale Desorption Through Electronic and Vibrational Excitation Mechanisms," Science 268(16 June 1995):1590-1592.

2712. R.A. Lewis, S.A. Gower, P. Groombridge, D.T.W. Cox, L.G. Adorni-Braccesi, "Student scanning tunneling microscope," Am. J. Phys. 59(January 1991):38-42.

2713. P.J. de Pablo, E. Graugnard, B. Walsh, R.P. Andres, S. Datta, R. Reifenberger, "A simple, reliable technique for making electrical contact to multiwalled carbon nanotubes," Appl. Phys. Lett. 74(15 January 1999):323-325.

2714. P. Bhyrappa, G. Vaijayanthimala, Kenneth S. Suslick, "Shape-Selective Ligation to Dendrimer-Metalloporphyrins," J. Am. Chem. Soc. 121(13 January 1999):262-263.
2715. D.H. Robertson, D.W. Brenner, J.W. Mintmire, "Energetics of nanoscale graphitic tubules," Phys. Rev. B. 45(1992):592-595. See also: D.W. Brenner, J.A. Harrison, C.T. White, R.J. Colton, "Molecular dynamics simulations of the nanometer-scale mechanical properties of compressed Buckminsterfullerene," Thin Solid Films 206(1991):220-223; and R.C. Mowrey, D.W. Brenner, B.I. Dunlap, J.W. Mintmire, C.T. White, "Simulations of C_{60} collisions with a hydrogen terminated diamond(111) surface," J. Phys. Chem. 95(19 September 1991):7138-7142.
2716. R. Luthi, E. Meyer, H. Haefke, L. Howard, W. Gutmannsbauer, H.-J. Guntherodt, "Sled-Type Motion on the Nanometer Scale: Determination of Dissipation and Cohesive Energies of C_{60}," Science 266(23 December 1994):1979-1981.
2717. Michael R. Falvo, Russell M. Taylor II, Aron Helser, Vren Chi, Frederich P. Brooks Jr., Sean Washburn, Richard Superfine, "Nanometer-scale rolling and sliding of carbon nanotubes," Nature 397(21 January 1999):236-238.
2718. Michael R. Falvo, G. Clary, Aron Helser, Scott Paulson, Russell M. Taylor II, Vern Chi, Frederick P. Brooks Jr., Sean Washburn, Richard Superfine, "Nanomanipulation experiments exploring frictional and mechanical properties of carbon nanotubes," Microscopy and Microanalysis 4(1998):In press.
2719. M.R. Falvo, G.J. Clary, R.M. Taylor II, V. Chi, F.P. Brooks Jr., S. Washburn, R. Superfine, "Bending and buckling of carbon nanotubes under large strain," Nature 389(9 October 1997):582-584.
2720. R.M. Taylor II, R. Superfine, "Advanced Interfaces to Scanning Probe Microscopes," in H.S. Nalwa, ed., Handbook of Nanostructured Materials and Nanotechnology, Academic Press, New York, 1998.
2721. M. Falvo, R. Superfine, S. Washburn, M. Finch, R.M. Taylor, V.L. Chi, F.P. Brooks Jr., "The Nanomanipulator: A Teleoperator for Manipulating Materials at the Nanometer Scale," Proceedings of the International Symposium on the Science and Technology of Atomically Engineered Materials, 30 October—4 November 1995, Richmond VA, World Scientific Publishing, 1996, pp. 579-586.
2722. R.M. Taylor, "The Nanomanipulator: A virtual-reality interface for a scanning tunneling microscope," Proc. 20th SIGGRAPH Conf. Comp. Graphics, 1993, pp. 127-134. See also: http://www.cs.unc.edu/Research/nano/.
2723. Martin Guthold, W. Garrett Matthews, Atsuko Negishi, Russell M. Taylor II, Dorothy A. Erie, Frederick P. Brooks Jr, Richard Superfine, "Quantitative Manipulation of DNA and Viruses with the Nano-Manipulator Scanning Force Microscope," Surf. Interf. Anal. 27(1999):In press.
2724. M.R. Falvo, S. Washburn, R. Superfine, M. Finch, F.P. Brooks, Jr., V. Chi, R.M. Taylor II, "Manipulation of Individual Viruses: Friction and Mechanical Properties," Biophys. J. 72(March 1997):1396-1403.
2725. M.D. Antonik, N.P. D'Costa, J.H. Hoh, "A biosensor based on micromechanical interrogation of living cells," IEEE Engin. Med. Biol. 16(1997):66-72.
2726. H.G. Hansma, J.H. Hoh, "Biomolecular imaging with the AFM," Ann. Rev. Biophys. Biomol. Struct. 23(1994):115-139.
2727. L.D. Martin, J.P. Vesenka, E.R. Henderson, D.L. Dobbs, "Visualization of nucleosomal structure in native chromatin by atomic force microscopy," Biochemistry 34(1995):4610-4616.
2728. H. Kumar Wickramasinghe, "Scanned-Probe Microscopes," Scientific American 260(October 1989):98-105.
2729. J.A. Stroscio, W.J. Kaiser, eds., Scanning Tunneling Microscopy, Academic Press, Boston MA, 1993. See also: Joseph A. Stroscio, D.M. Eigler, "Atomic and Molecular Manipulation with the Scanning Tunneling Microscope," Science 254(29 November 1991):1319-1326.
2730. R. Wiesendanger, Scanning Probe Microscopy Methods and Applications, Cambridge University Press, Cambridge, 1994.
2731. G. Binnig, H. Rohrer, "Scanning tunneling microscopy," Helv. Phys. Acta 55(1982):726-735.
2732. G. Binnig, H. Rohrer, C. Gerber, E. Weibel, "Surface studies by scanning tunneling microscopy," Phys. Rev. Lett. 49(1982):57-61; Phys. Rev. Lett. 50(1983):120-123.
2733. Gerd Binnig, Heinrich Rohrer, "The Scanning Tunneling Microscope," Scientific American 253(August 1985):50-56.
2734. G. Binnig, H. Rohrer, "Scanning tunneling microscopy," IBM J. Res. Develop. 30(1986):355-369.
2735. Gerd Binnig, Heinrich Rohrer, "Scanning tunneling microscopy from birth to adolescence," Rev. Modern. Phys. 59(July 1987):615-625.
2736. H.J. Mamin, D. Rugar, J.E. Stern, R.E. Fontana, Jr., P. Kasiraj, "Magnetic force microscopy of thin Permalloy films," Appl. Phys. Lett. 55(17 July 1989):318-320.
2737. Daniel Rugar, Paul Hansma, "Atomic Force Microscopy," Phys. Today 43(October 1990):23-30.
2738. H.J. Mamin et al., "Atomic Emission from a Gold Scanning-Tunneling-Microscope Tip," Phys. Rev. Lett. 65(1990):2418-2421.
2739. H.J. Mamin et al., "Gold deposition from a scanning tunneling microscope tip," J. Vac. Sci. Technol. B 9(1991):1398-1402.
2740. S.S. Wong, J.D. Harper, P.T. Lansbury, C.M. Lieber, "Carbon Nanotube Tips: High-Resolution Probes for Imaging Biological Systems," J. Am. Chem. Soc. 120(1998):603-604.
2741. S.S. Wong, A.T. Woolley, E. Joselevich, C.L. Cheung, C.M. Lieber, "Covalently-Functionalized Single-Walled Carbon Nanotube Probe Tips for Chemical Force Microscopy," J. Am. Chem. Soc. 120(1998):8557-8558.
2742. S.S. Wong, A.T. Woolley, T.W. Odom, K.-L. Huang, P. Kim, D.V. Vezenov, C.M. Lieber, "Single-walled carbon nanotube probes for high-resolution nanostructure imaging," Appl. Phys. Lett. 73(7 December 1998):3465-3467.
2743. R.P. Andres et al., "Room temperature Coulomb blockade and Coulomb staircase from self-assembled nanostructures," J. Vac. Sci. Technol. A 14(May/June 1996):1178-1183.
2744. F.K. Perkins, E.A. Dobisz, S.L. Brandow, J.M. Calvert, J.E. Kosakowski, C.R.K. Marrian, "Fabrication of 15 nm wide trenches in Si by vacuum scanning tunneling microscope lithography of an organosilane self-assembled film and reactive ion etching," Appl. Phys. Lett. 68(22 January 1996):550-552.
2745. Pamela C. Ohara, James R. Heath, William M. Gelbart, "Self-Assembly of Submicrometer Rings of Particles from Solutions of Nanoparticles," Angew. Chemie Int. Ed. Engl. 36(1997):1077-1080.
2746. In-Whan Lyo, Phaedon Avouris, "Field-Induced Nanometer- to Atomic-Scale Manipulation of Silicon Surfaces with the STM," Science 253(12 July 1991):173-176.
2747. M. Aono, A. Kobayashi, F. Grey, H. Uchida, D.H. Huang, "Tip-sample interactions in the scanning tunneling microscope for atomic-scale structure fabrication," J. Appl. Phys. 32(1993):1470-1477.
2748. C.T. Salling, M.G. Lagally, "Fabrication of Atomic-Scale Structures on Si(001) Surfaces," Science 265(22 July 1994):502-506.
2749. Dehuan Huang, Hironaga Uchida, Masakazu Aono, "Deposition and subsequent removal of single Si atoms on the Si(111)-7x7 surface by a scanning tunneling microscope," J. Vac. Sci. Technol. B 12(July/August 1994):2429-2433.
2750. P. Avouris, "Manipulation of matter at the atomic and molecular levels," Acc. Chem. Res. 28(1995):95-102.
2751. G. Meyer, K.H. Rieder, "Controlled manipulation of single atoms and small molecules with the scanning tunneling microscope," Surf. Sci. 377-9(1997):1087-1093.
2752. S. Li et al., "Submicrometer lithography of a silicon substrate by machining of a photoresist using atomic force microscopy followed by wet chemical etching," Nanotechnology 8(1997):76-81.
2753. E.S. Snow, P.M. Campbell, "AFM Fabrication of Sub-Nanometer Metal-Oxide Devices with In Situ Control of Electrical Properties," Science 270(8 December 1995):1639-1641.
2754. L.L. Sohn, R.L. Willett, "Fabrication of Nanostructures Using Atomic-Force-Microscope-Based Lithography," Appl. Phys. Lett. 67(11 September 1995):1552-1554.
2755. A. Noy, C.D. Frisbie, L.F. Rozsnyai, M.S. Wrighton, and C.M. Lieber, "Chemical Force Microscopy: Exploiting Chemically-Modified Tips to Quantify Adhesion, Friction, and Functional Group Distributions in Molecular Assemblies," J. Am. Chem. Soc. 117(1995):7943-7951.
2756. C.M. Lieber, D. Vezenov, A. Noy, C. Sanders, "Chemical Force Microscopy," Microscopy and Microanalysis 3(1997):1253-1254.
2757. A.L. Weisenhorn, P.K. Hansma, T.R. Albrecht, C.F. Quate, "Forces in atomic force microscopy in air and water," Appl. Phys. Lett. 54(1989):2651-2653.
2758. C. Julian Chen, Introduction to Scanning Tunneling Microscopy, Oxford University Press, Cambridge, 1993.
2760. R.C. Merkle, "Computational Nanotechnology," Nanotechnology 2(1991):134-141. See also: http://nano.xerox.com/nanotech/compNano.html.
2761. R.C. Merkle, "Molecular Manufacturing: Adding Positional Control to Chemical Synthesis," Chemical Design Automation News 8(September/October 1993):1 et seq. See also: http://nano.xerox.com/nanotech/CDAarticle.html.
2762. C.B. Musgrave, J.K. Perry, R.C. Merkle, W.A. Goddard III, "Theoretical studies of a hydrogen abstraction tool for nanotechnology," Nanotechnology 2(1991):187-195. See also: http://nano.xerox.com/nanotech/Habs/paper.html.
2763. Susan B. Sinnott, Richard J. Colton, Carter T. White, Donald W. Brenner, "Surface patterning by atomically-controlled chemical forces: Molecular dynamics simulations," Surf. Sci. 316(1994):L1055-L1060.
2764. D.W. Brenner, S.B. Sinnott, J.A. Harrison, O.A. Shenderova, "Simulated engineering of nanostructures," Nanotechnology 7(1996):161-167. See also: http://nano.xerox.com/nanotech/nano4/brennerPaper.pdf.
2765. Michael Frenklach, Karl E. Spear, "Growth mechanism of vapor-deposited diamond," J. Mater. Res. 3(January/February 1988):133-140. See also: M. Frenklach, H. Wang, "Detailed surface and gas-phase chemical kinetics of diamond deposition," Phys. Rev. B 43(1991):1520-1545.
2766. Stephen J. Harris, "Mechanism for diamond growth from methyl radicals," Appl. Phys. Lett. 56(4 June 1990):2298-2300.
2767. D.W. Brenner, D.H. Robertson, R.J. Carty, D. Srivastava, B.J. Garrison, "Combining Molecular Dynamics and Monte Carlo Simulations to Model Chemical Vapor Deposition: Application to Diamond," Mat. Res. Soc. Symp. Proc. 278(1992):255 et seq.
2768. J.E. Butler, R. Woodin, "Thin film diamond growth mechanisms," Phil. Trans. R. Soc. Lond. A 342(1993):209-224. See also: F.G. Celii, J.E. Butler, "Diamond Chemical Vapor Deposition," Ann. Rev. Phys. Chem. 42(1991):643-684.
2769. J.C. Angus, A. Argoitia, R. Gat, Z. Li, M. Sunkara, L. Wang, Y. Wang, "Chemical vapour deposition of diamond," Phil. Trans. R. Soc. Lond. A 342(1993):195-208.
2770. Stephen P. Walch, Ralph C. Merkle, "Theoretical studies of diamond mechanosynthesis reactions," Nanotechnology 9(September 1998):285-296.

2771. Tobias Hertel, Richard Martel, Phaedon Avouris, "Manipulation of Individual Carbon Nanotubes and Their Interaction with Surfaces," J. Phys. Chem. B 102(1998):910-915.

2772. Thomas R. Albrecht, Shinya Akamine, Mark J. Zdeblick, Calvin F. Quate, "Microfabrication of integrated scanning tunneling microscope," J. Vac. Sci. Technol. A 8(January/February 1990):317-318.

2773. M.I. Lutwyche, Y. Wada, "Observation of a vacuum tunnel gap in a transmission electron microscope using a micromechanical tunneling microscope," Appl. Phys. Lett. 66(22 May 1995):2807-2809.

2774. D.A. Walters, J.P. Cleveland, N.H. Thomson, P.K. Hansma, M.A. Wendman, G. Gurley, V. Elings, "Short cantilevers for atomic force microscopy," Rev. Sci. Instrum. 67(October 1996):3583-3590.

2775. T. Boland, B.D. Ratner, "Direct measurement of hydrogen bonding in DNA nucleotide bases by atomic force microscopy," Proc. Natl. Acad. Sci. USA 92(1995):5297-5301.

2776. K. Wago et al., "Magnetic resonance force detection and spectroscopy of electron spins in phosphorus-doped silicon," Rev. Sci. Instr. 68(1997):1823-1826.

2777. "1995 Scientist of the Year," R&D Magazine, July 1995, pp. 22-25.

2778. Peter Weiss, "Atom-viewing 101: Make STMs at home," Science News 154(24 October 1998):269.

2779. Paul E. Sheehan, Charles M. Lieber, "Nanomachining, manipulation and fabrication by force microscopy," Nanotechnology 7(September 1996):236-240.

2780. Richard D. Piner, Jin Zhu, Feng Xu, Seunghun Hong, Chad A. Mirkin, "Dip Pen Nanolithography," Science 283(29 January 1999):661-663.

2781. A. Kobayashi, F. Grey, R.S. Williams, M. Aono, "Formation of Nanometer-Scale Grooves in Silicon with a Scanning Tunneling Microscope," Science 259(19 March 1993):1724-1726.

2782. Kazuhiko Matsumoto, Shu Takahashi, Masami Ishii, Masakatsu Hoshi, Akira Kurokawa, Shingo Ichimura, Atsushi Ando, "First Application of STM Nano-Meter Size Oxidation Process to Planar-Type MIM Diode," Extended Abstracts Int. Conf. Solid State Devices and Materials, 23-26 August 1994, Yokohama, pp.46-48.

2783. R. Gomer, "Possible mechanisms of atom transfer in scanning tunneling microscopy," IBM J. Res. Dev. 30(July 1986):428-430.

2784. H.H. Farrell, M. Levinson, "Scanning tunneling microscope as a structure-modifying tool," Phys. Rev. B 31(1985):3593-3598.

2785. R.S. Becker, J.A. Golovchenko, B.S. Swartzentruber, "Atomic-scale surface modifications using a tunneling microscope," Nature 325(1987):419-421.

2786. J.S. Foster, J.E. Frommer, P.C. Arnett, "Molecular manipulation using a tunnelling microscope," Nature 331(28 January 1988):324-326.

2787. D.M. Kolb, R. Ullmann, T. Will, "Nanofabrication of Small Copper Clusters on Gold(111) Electrodes by a Scanning Tunneling Microscope," Science 275(21 February 1997):1097-1099.

2788. John Foster, "Atomic Imaging and Positioning," in B.C. Crandall, James Lewis, eds., Nanotechnology: Research and Perspectives, MIT Press, Cambridge MA, 1992, pp. 15-36.

2789. David L. Patrick, Victor J. Cee, Thomas P. Beebe Jr., "Molecular Corrals for Studies of Monolayer Organic Films," Science 265(8 July 1994):231-234.

2790. M.F. Crommie, C.P. Lutz, D.M. Eigler, "Confinement of Electrons to Quantum Corrals on a Metal Surface," Science 262(8 October 1993):218-220. See also: M.F. Crommie, C.P. Lutz, D.M. Eigler, E.J. Heller, "Waves on a metal surface and quantum corrals," Surface Review and Letters 2(1995):127-137.

2791. Malcolm Ritter, "World's smallest moving job shifts just one atom at a time," Sacramento Bee, Thursday, April 5, 1990, p. A8.

2792. J. Madeleine Nash, "Adventures in Lilliput," Time (30 December 1991):75, 78.

2793. C. Baur, B.C. Gazen, B. Koel, T.R. Ramachandran, A. Requicha, L. Zini, "Robotic nanomanipulation with a scanning probe microscope in a networked computing environment," J. Vac. Sci. Technol. B 15(July/August 1997):1577-1580.

2794. Zyvex corporate website is at: http://www.zyvex.com. See also: "Zyvex: Current Research Projects, 2 nm high gold dots" at: http://zyvex.com/Research/Research.html.

2795. Shigeyuki Hosoki, Sumio Hosaka, Tsuyoshi Hasegawa, "Surface modification of MoS_2 using an STM," Appl. Surf. Sci. 60/61(1992):643-647.

2796. R.S. Becker, G.S. Higashi, Y.J. Chabal, A.J. Becker, "Atomic Scale Conversion of Clean Si(111):H-1 x 1 to Si(111)-2 x 1 by Electron-Stimulated Desorption," Phys. Rev. Lett. 65(8 October 1990):1917-1920.

2797. Wolfgang T. Muller, David L. Klein, Thomas Lee, John Clarke, Paul L. McEuen, Peter G. Schultz, "A Strategy for the Chemical Synthesis of Nanostructures," Science 268(14 April 1995):272-273. See also: B.J. McIntyre, M. Salmeron, G.A. Somorjai, "Nanocatalysis by the Tip of a Scanning Tunneling Microscope Operating Inside a Reactor Cell," Science 265(2 September 1994):1415-1418.

2798. Peter Hinterdorfer, Werner Baumgartner, Hermann J. Gruber, Kurt Schilcher, Hansgeorg Schindler, "Detection and localization of individual antibody-antigen recognition events by atomic force microscopy," Proc. Natl. Acad. Sci. USA 93(16 April 1996):3477-3481.

2799. Hongjie Dai, Jason H. Hafner, Andrew G. Rinzler, Daniel T. Colbert, Richard E. Smalley, "Nanotubes as nanoprobes in scanning probe microscopy," Nature 384(14 November 1996):147-151. See at: http://cnst.rice.edu/TIPS_rev.htm.

2800. S.S. Wong, E. Joselvich, A.T. Woolley, C.L. Cheung, C.M. Lieber, "Covalently functionalized nanotubes as nanometer probes for chemistry and biology," Nature 394(2 July 1998):52-55.

2801. M.F. Shostakovskii, A.V. Bogdanova, The Chemistry of Diacetylenes, Wiley, New York, 1974.

2802. John M. Michelsen, Mark J. Dyer, Jim Von Ehr, "Assembler Construction by Proximal Probe", presentation at the Fifth Foresight Conference on Molecular Nanotechnology; see also: http://www.zyvex.com/Papers/Foresight97/Foresight97.htm.

2803. T.A. Jung, R.R. Schlitter, J.K. Gimzewski, H. Tang, C. Joachim, "Controlled Room-Temperature Positioning of Individual Molecules: Molecular Flexure and Motion," Science 271(12 January 1996):181-184.

2804. Olivier Mongin, Albert Gossauer, "Tripodaphyrins, a New Class of Porphyrine Derivatives Designed for Nanofabrication," Tetrahedron Lett. 37(1996):3825-3828.

2805. B.C. Stipe, M.A. Rezaei, W. Ho, "Inducing and Viewing the Rotational Motion of a Single Molecule," Science 279(20 March 1998):1907-1909.

2806. T.R. Ramachandran, C. Baur, A. Bugacov, A. Madhukar, B.E. Koel, A. Requicha, C. Gazen, "Direct and controlled manipulation of nanometer-sized particles using the non-contact atomic force microscope," Nanotechnology 9(September 1998):237-245. See also: C. Baur, A. Bugacov, B.E. Koel, A. Madhukar, N. Montoya, T.R. Ramachandran, A.A.G. Requicha, R. Resch, P. Will, "Nanoparticle manipulation by mechanical pushing, underlying phenomena and real-time monitoring," Nanotechnology 9(December 1998):360-364.

2807. R. Resch, C. Baur, A. Bugacov, B.E. Koel, A. Madhukar, A. Requicha, P. Will, "Building and manipulating 3-D and linked 2-D structures of nanoparticles using scanning force microscopy," 9 March 1998, Laboratory for Molecular Robotics website at: http://alicudi.usc.edu:80/~lmr.

2808. MinFeng Yu, Mark J. Dyer, George D. Skidmore, Henry W. Rohrs, Xue Kun Lu, Kevin D. Ausman, James Von Ehr, Rodney S. Ruoff, "3 Dimensional Manipulation of Carbon Nanotubes under a Scanning Electron Microscope," paper presented at the Sixth Foresight Nanotechnology Conference, November 1998; see also: Robert F. Service, "AFMs Wield Parts for Nanoconstruction," Science 282(27 November 1998):1620-1621; and http://www.foresight.org/Conferences/MNT6/Papers/Yu/index.html.

2809. J.M. Neumeister, W.A. Ducker, "Lateral, normal, and longitudinal spring constants of atomic force microscopy cantilevers," Rev. Sci. Instrum. 65(1994):2527-2531.

2810. Hiroshi Morishita, Yotaro Hatamura, "Development of Ultra Micro Manipulator System Under Stereo SEM Observation," Proc. 1993 IEEE/RSJ Intl. Conf. on Intelligent Robots and Systems, 26-30 July 1993, Yokohama, Japan, Volume 3, pp. 1717-1721.

2811. Robert E. Tuzun, Karl Sohlberg, Donald W. Noid, Bobby G. Sumpter, "Docking envelopes for the assembly of molecular bearings," Nanotechnology 9(March 1998):37-48.

2812. M.S. Dresselhaus, D. Dresselhaus, K. Sugihara, I.L. Spain, H.A. Goldberg, Graphite Fibers and Filaments, Springer-Verlag, New York, Vol. 5, Springer Series in Materials Science, 1988.

2813. T. Itoh, T. Suga, "Development of a force sensor for atomic force microscopy using piezoelectric thin films," Nanotechnology 4(1993):218-224. See also: T. Itoh, T. Suga, "Scanning force microscope using a piezoelectric microcantilever," J. Vac. Sci. Technol. B 12(1994):1581-1585; T. Itoh, T. Ohashi, T. Suga, "Scanning force microscope using piezoelectric excitation and detection," IEICE Trans. Electron. E78-C(1995):146-151.

2814. M. Tortonese, H. Yamada, R.C. Barrett, C.F. Quate, "Atomic force microscopy using a piezoresistive cantilever," Digest of Technical Papers, Sixth Intl. Conf. Solid-State Sensors and Actuators, Transducers '91, San Francisco, CA, 24-28 June 1991, pp. 448-451. See also: M. Tortonese, R.C. Barrett, C.F. Quate, "Atomic resolution with an atomic force microscope using piezoresistive detection," Appl. Phys. Lett. 62(22 February 1993):834-836.

2815. N. Blanc, J. Brugger, N.F. de Rooji, U. Durig, "Scanning force microscopy in the dynamic mode using microfabricated capacitive sensors," paper presented at the 8th Intl. Conf. Scanning Tunneling Microscopy/Spectroscopy and Related Techniques, STM '95, Snowmass Village, CO, 23-28 July 1995. See also: J. Brugger, R.A. Buser, N.F. de Rooij, "Micromachined atomic force microprobe with integrated capacitive readout," J. Micromech. Microeng. 2(1992):218-220.

2816. Fumiya Watanabe, Makoto Arita, H. Murayama, Teruaki Motooka, Ken Okano, Takatoshi Yamada, "Diamond Tip Arrays for Parallel Processing of Microelectromechanical Systems," Japan J. Appl. Phys. 37(1998):L562-L564.

2817. Toshihiro Itoh, Takahiro Ohashi, Tadatomo Suga, "Piezoelectric Cantilever Array for Multiprobe Scanning Force Microscopy," MEMS-9, 1996, pp. 451-455.

2818. S.C. Minne, Ph. Flueckiger, H.T. Soh, C.F. Quate, "Atomic force microscope lithography using amorphous silicon as a resist and advances in parallel operation," J. Vac. Sci. Technol. B 13(May/June 1995):1380-1385.

2819. S.C. Minne, S.R. Manalis, C.F. Quate, "Parallel atomic force microscopy using cantilevers with integrated piezoresistive sensors and integrated piezoelectric actuators," Appl. Phys. Lett. 67(1995):3918-3920.

2820. S.R. Manalis, S.C. Minne, C.F. Quate, "Atomic force microscopy for high speed imaging using cantilevers with an integrated actuator and sensor," Appl. Phys. Lett. 68(1996):871-873.

2821. S.R. Manalis, S.C. Minne, A. Atalar, C.F. Quate, "Interdigital cantilevers for atomic force microscopy," Appl. Phys. Lett. 69(1996):3944-3946.

2822. K. Wilder, H.T. Soh, S.C. Minne, S.R. Manalis, C.F. Quate, "Cantilever arrays for lithography," Naval Research Reviews 49(1997):35-48.
2823. C.F. Quate, "Scanning probes as a lithography tool for nanostructures," Surface Science 386(1997):259-264.
2824. S.C. Minne, S.R. Manalis, A. Atalar, C.F. Quate, "Independent parallel lithography using the atomic force microscope," J. Vac. Sci. Technol. B 14(1997):2456-2461.
2825. S.C. Minne, G. Yaralioglu, S.R. Manalis, J.D. Adams, J. Zesch, A. Atalar, C.F. Quate, "Automated parallel high speed atomic force microscopy," Appl. Phys. Lett. 72(1998):2340-2342.
2826. Kathryn Wilder, Calvin F. Quate, Bhanwar Singh, David F. Kyser, "Electron beam and scanning probe lithography: A comparison," J. Vac. Sci. Technol. B 16(November/December 1998):3864-3873.
2827. K. Wilder, D. Adderton, R. Bernstein, V. Elings, C.F. Quate, "Noncontact nanolithography using the atomic force microscope," Appl. Phys. Lett. 73(1998):2527-2529.
2829. S.C. Minne, J.D. Adams, G. Yaralioglu, S.R. Manalis, A. Atalar, C.F. Quate, "Centimeter scale atomic force microscope imaging and lithography," Appl. Phys. Lett. 73(1998):1742-1744.
2830. J. Jason Yao, Susanne C. Arney, Noel C. MacDonald, "Fabrication of High Frequency Two-Dimensional Nanoactuators for Scanned Probe Devices," J. Microelectromech. Syst. 1(March 1992):14-22.
2831. Z. Lisa Zhang, Noel C. MacDonald, "A RIE process for submicron, silicon electromechanical structures," J. Micromech. Microeng. 2(March 1992):31-38.
2832. Z. Lisa Zhang, N.C. MacDonald, "Integrated Silicon Process for Micro-Dynamic Vacuum Field Emission Cathodes," J. Vac. Sci. Technol. B 11(November/December 1993):2538-2543.
2833. S. Arney, N.C. MacDonald, "Formation of Submicron Silicon on Insulator Structures by Lateral Oxidation of Substrate-Silicon Islands," J. Vac. Sci. Technol. B 6(January/February 1988):341-345.
2834. J.P. Spallas, N.C. MacDonald, "Self-aligned Silicon Field Emission Cathode Arrays formed by selective, lateral thermal oxidation of silicon," J. Vac. Sci. Technol. B 11(March/April 1993):437-440.
2835. Scott A. Miller, Kimberly L. Turner, Noel C. MacDonald, "Microelectromechanical scanning probe instruments for array architectures," Rev. Sci. Instrum. 68(November 1997):4155-4162. See also: http://www.news.cornell.edu/releases/March98/nanoprobe.bs.html.
2836. Robert F. Service, "Scanning scopes go parallel," Science 274(1 November 1996):723.
2837. Alfons van Blaaderen, Rene Ruel, Pierre Wiltzius, "Template-directed colloidal crystallization," Nature 385(23 January 1997):321-324.
2838. J.J. McClelland, R.E. Scholten, E.C. Palm, R.J. Celotta, "Laser-Focused Atomic Deposition," Science 262(5 November 1993):877-879.
2839. M.-O.Mewes, M.R. Andrews, D.M. Kurn, D.S. Durfee, C.G. Townsend, W. Ketterle, "Output Coupler for Bose-Einstein Condensed Atoms," Phys. Rev. Lett. 78(27 January 1997):582-585.
2840. M.R. Andrews, C.G. Townsend, H.-J. Miesner, D.S. Durfee, D.M. Kurn, W. Ketterle, "Observation of Interference Between Two Bose Condensates," Science 275(31 January 1997):637-641.
2841. K.S. Johnson, J.H. Thywissen, N.H. Dekker, K.K. Berggren, A.P. Chu, R. Younkin, M. Prentiss, "Localization of Metastable Atom Beams with Optical Standing Waves: Nanolithography at the Heisenberg Limit," Science 280(5 June 1998):1583-1586.
2842. Michael D. Ward, "Design of Self-Assembling Molecular Systems: Electrostatic Structural Enforcement in Low-Dimensional Molecular Solids," in B.C. Crandall, James Lewis, eds., Nanotechnology: Research and Perspectives, MIT Press, Cambridge MA, 1992, pp. 67-101.
2843. A.F. Wells, Three-Dimensional Nets and Polyhedra, John Wiley and Sons, New York, 1977.
2844. W.A. Goddard III, "Computational Chemistry and Nanotechnology," presentation at the Fourth Foresight Conference on Molecular Nanotechnology, November 1995.
2845. T. Cagin, A. Jaramillo-Botero, G. Gao, W.A. Goddard III, "Molecular mechanics and molecular dynamics analysis of Drexler-Merkle gears and neon pump," Nanotechnology 9(September 1998):143-152. See at: http://www.wag.caltech.edu/foresight/foresight_1.html.
2846. B.F. Hoskins, R. Robson, "Design and Construction of a New Class of Scaffolding-like Materials Comprising Infinite Polymeric Frameworks of 3D-Linked Molecular Rods. A Reappraisal of the $Zn(CN)_2$ and $Cd(CN)_2$ Structures and the Synthesis and Structure of the Diamond-Related Frameworks $[N(CH_3)_4][Cu[I]Zn[II](CN)_4]$andCu[I][4,4',4'',4'''-tetracyanotetraphenylmethane $]BF_4{}^{*}xC_6H_5NO_2$," J. Am. Chem. Soc. 112(1990):1546-1554.
2847. K.E. Drexler, "Directions in Nanotechnology," presentation at the Fourth Foresight Conference on Molecular Nanotechnology, November 1995.
2848. C. Park, J.L Campbell, W.A. Goddard III, "Protein Stitchery: Design of a Protein for Selective Binding to a Specific DNA Sequence," Proc. Natl. Acad. Sci. USA 89(1 October 1992):9094-9096.
2849. Boris I. Yakobson, "Dynamics of Buckyshuttle as a 1-bit memory device," poster presentation at the Fifth Foresight Conference on Molecular Nanotechnology, November 1997; see at: http://www.foresight.org/Conferences/MNT05/Abstracts/Yak2abst.html.
2850. Markus Krummenacker, "Steps Towards Molecular Manufacturing," Chem. Design Autom. News 9(January 1994):1, 29-39; see also: http://www.ai.sri.com/~kr/nano/cda-news/cda-news.html.
2851. Bernd Mayer, "Specifications and Design of a Self-Assembled Biodevice," poster presentation at the Fifth Foresight Conference on Molecular Nanotechnology, November 1997; see at: http://www.foresight.org/Conferences/MNT05/Abstracts/Mayeabst.html.
2852. Tahir Cagin, Jianwei Che, Michael N. Gardos, Amir Fijany, William A. Goddard III, "Simulation and Experiments on Friction and Wear of Diamond: A Material for MEMS and NEMS Applications," paper presented at the Sixth Foresight Conference on Molecular Nanotechnology, November 1998. See at: http://www.wag.caltech.edu/foresight/papers/Cagin/Caginpap.html. See also: "Diamond and Polycrystalline Diamond for MEMS Applications: Simulations and Experiments," in Arthur H. Heuer, S. Joshua Jacobs, eds., Materials Science of Microelectromechanical Systems (MEMS) Devices, 1999.
2853. William A. Goddard III, Tahir Cagin, Stephen P. Walch, "Atomistic Design and Simulations of Nanoscale Machines and Assembly," 1996; see at: http://www.wag.caltech.edu/gallery/nano_comp.html.
2854. A. Fijany, T. Cagin, A. Jaramillo-Botero, W.A. Goddard III, "Novel Algorithms for Massively Parallel, Long-Term Simulation of Molecular Dynamics Systems," Advances in Engineering Software 29(1998):441-450; "A Fast Algorithm for Massively Parallel, Long Term Simulations of Complex Molecular Dynamics Simulations," in E.H. D'Hollander, G.R. Joubert, F.J. Peters, U. Trottenberg, eds., Parallel Computing: Fundamentals, Applications and New Directions, 1998, pp. 505-515.
2855. C.-H. Kiang, W.A. Goddard III, R. Beyers, D.S. Bethune, "Structural Modification of Single-Layer Carbon Nanotubes with an Electron Beam," J. Phys. Chem. 100(1996):3749-3752.
2856. W. Utsumi, T. Yagi, "Light-Transparent Phase Formed by Room-Temperature Compression of Graphite," Science 252(1991):1542-1544.
2857. C.-H. Kiang, W.A. Goddard III, R. Beyers, J.R. Salem, D.S. Bethune, "Catalytic Synthesis of Single-Layer Carbon Nanotubes with a Wide Range of Diameters," J. Phys. Chem. 98(1994):6612-6618.
2858. K. Eric Drexler, Ralph C. Merkle, "Simple Pump Selective for Neon," http://www.imm.org/Parts/Parts1.html. See also at: http://science.nas.nasa.gov/Groups/Nanotechnology/gallery/pump/pumpWhite.jpg.
2859. K. Eric Drexler, Ralph C. Merkle, "A Fine-Motion Controller for Molecular Assembly," http://www.imm.org/Parts/Parts2.html. See also at: http://science.nas.nasa.gov/Groups/Nanotechnology/archive/Drexler/fineMotionController/whiteBackground.jpg.
2860. Foresight Institute, "Feynman Grand Prize," http://www.foresight.org/GrandPrize.0.html.
2861. Geoff Leach, "Advances in molecular CAD," Nanotechnology 7(September 1996):197-203. See also: Geoff I. Leach, Ralph C. Merkle, "Crystal Clear: A Molecular CAD Tool," Nanotechnology 5(1994):168-171; and see at: http://www.cs.rmit.edu.au/~gl/research/nano/crystal.html.
2862. Yaron Rosenfeld Hacohen, Enrique Grunbaum, Reshef Tenne, Jeremy Sloan, John L. Hutchison, "Cage structures and nanotubes of $NiCl_2$," Nature 395(24 September 1998):336-337.
2863. Chemical Abstracts Service (CAS) Registry; see at: http://www.cas.org/cgi-bin/regreport.pl.
2864. Herb Bowie, Why Die?: A Beginner's Guide to Living Forever, Power Surge Publications, 1998.
2865. Iwao Fujimasa, Micromachines: A New Era in Mechanical Engineering, Oxford Science Publications, 1997.
2866. P.A. Serena, N. Garcia, Nanowires, NATO ASI Series, Vol. 340, Kluwer Academic Publishers:Dordrecht, The Netherlands, 1997.
2867. David A. Meyer, "Quantum Strategies," Phys. Rev. Lett. 82(1999):1052-1055.
2868. Ralph C. Merkle, "Design considerations for an assembler," Nanotechnology 7(September 1996):210-215. See at: http://nano.xerox.com/nanotech/nano4/merklePaper.html.
2869. Ralph C. Merkle, "Convergent assembly," Nanotechnology 8(1997):18-22.
2870. J. Storrs Hall, "Architectural Considerations for Self-Replicating Manufacturing Systems," paper presented at the Sixth Foresight Conference on Molecular Nanotechnology, November 1998; see also: http://www.foresight.org/Conferences/MNT6/Papers/Hall/index.html.
2870. J. Storrs Hall, "Architectural Considerations for Self-Replicating Manufacturing Systems," paper presented at the Sixth Foresight Conference on Molecular Nanotechnology, November 1998; see also: http://www.foresight.org/Conferences/MNT6/Papers/Hall/index.html.
2871. Moshe Sipper, "Fifty Years of Research on Self-Replication: An Overview," Artificial Life 4(Summer 1998):237-257, in "Special Issue on Self-Replication." See also: Moshe Sipper, "The Artificial Self-Replication Page," http://lslwww.epfl.ch/~moshes/selfrep/.
2872. Ralph C. Merkle, "Self-replicating systems and low cost manufacturing," in M.E. Welland, J.K. Gimzewski, eds., The Ultimate Limits of Fabrication and Measurement, Kluwer, Dordrecht, 1994, pp. 25-32. See at: http://nano.xerox.com/nanotech/selfRepNATO.html.
2873. Ralph C. Merkle, "Self replication and nanotechnology," see at: http://nano.xerox.com/nanotech/selfRep.html.

2874. Ralph C. Merkle, "Some Links to the (Robert Morris, Jr.) Internet Worm Incident of 1988," see at: http://nano.xerox.com/nanotech/worm.html.

2875. Myles Axton, "Regulation of a Runaway Replicator," at: http://www.outbreak.org/cgi-unreg/dynaserve.exe/Ebola/ebola-replication.html.

2876. National Center for Genome Resources, "*Mycoplasma capricolum*," 13 October 1998, see at: http://www.ncgr.org/microbe/mcapricolum.html.

2877. Stanley B. Prusiner, "The Prion Diseases," Scientific American 272(January 1995):48-57.

2878. Ramanujan S. Hegde et al., "A Transmembrane Form of the Prion Protein in Neurodegenerative Disease," Science 279(6 February 1998):827-834.

2879. L.S. Penrose, R. Penrose, "A Self-Reproducing Analogue," Nature 179(8 June 1957):1183.

2880. L.S. Penrose, "Mechanics of Self-Reproduction," Ann. Human Genetics 23(1958):59-72.

2881. L.S. Penrose, "Self-Reproducing Machines," Scientific American 200(June 1959):105-114.

2882. Homer Jacobson, "On Models of Reproduction," Amer. Sci. 46(1958):255-284.

2883. Harold J. Morowitz, "A Model of Reproduction," Amer. Sci. 47(1959):261-263.

2884. J.B.S. Haldane, "The origin of life," New Biol. 16(1954):12.

2885. Jason D. Lohn, Gary L. Haith, Silvano P. Colombano, "Two Electromechanical Models of Self-Assembly," presentation at the Sixth Foresight Conference on Molecular Nanotechnology, November 1998; see also: http://www.foresight.org/Conferences/MNT6/Abstracts/Lohn/index.html.

2886. Jason D. Lohn, "Self-Replicating Systems," see at: http://ic.arc.nasa.gov/ic/people/jlohn/srs.html.

2887. "Custom DNA Synthesis" and "Custom Oligonucleotide Order Form," Ransom Hill Bioscience, Inc. (P.O. Box 219, Ramona CA 92065), 4 October 1995; see also: http://www.ransomhill.com/custom.html.

2888. See: Alpha DNA, "Custom DNA Synthesis," (http://www.alphadna.com/catalog.html); Bioline, "Custom Oligonucleotides," (http://www.bioline.com/oligo.htm); Keystone Laboratories, Inc., "Custom Oligo Synthesis," (http://www.keydna.com/product_frame.htm); Midland (http://www.mcrc.com/products-dna.html); Oligos-U-Like (http://www.path.cam.ac.uk/oligo/custom.html); Pacific Oligos, "Custom Oligonucleotide Prices," (http://www.oligo.com.au/prices.html).

2889. Edward A. Rietman, Enabling Technologies for Molecular Nanosystems, AIP Series, Springer-Verlag, New York, 1999.

2890. George O. Gey, Ward D. Coffman, Mary T. Kubicek, "Tissue Culture Studies of the Proliferative Capacity of Cervical Carcinoma and Normal Epithelium," Cancer Res. 12(1952):264-265.

2891. American Type Culture Collection, "ATCC Serum-Free Cell Lines: HeLa/SF [serum free derivative of HeLa (ATCC CCL-2)]," 14 May 1998; see at: http://www.atcc.org/hilights/serum-free.html.

2892. X. Bu, P. Feng, G.D. Stucky, "Large-cage zeolite structures with multidimensional 12-ring channels," Science 278(19 December 1997):2080-2085.

2893. Peidong Yang, Tao Deng, Dongyuan Zhao, Pingyun Feng, David Pine, Bradley F. Chmelka, George M. Whitesides, Galen D. Stucky, "Hierarchically Ordered Oxides," Science 282(18 December 1998):2244-2246.

2894. W.M. Lomer, "A Dislocation Reaction in the Face-Centered Cubic Lattice," Phil. Mag. 42(November 1951):1327-1331. See also: A.S. Nakekdar, J. Narayan, "Atomic Structure of Dislocations in Silicon, Germanium, and Diamond," Phil. Mag. A 61(1990):873-891.

2895. Gary Stix, "Waiting for Breakthroughs," Scientific American 274(April 1996):94-99.

2896. Jacqueline Krim, "Friction at the Atomic Scale," Scientific American 275(October 1996):74-80.

2897. Robert Crawford, "Japan Starts a Big Push Toward the Small Scale," Science 254(29 November 1991):1304-1305.

2898. T.E. Schaffer, J.P. Cleveland, F. Ohnesorge, D.A. Walters, P.K. Hansma, "Studies of vibrating atomic force microscope cantilevers in liquid," J. Appl. Phys. 80(1996):3622-3627.

2899. J.A. Darsey, B.K. Rao, B.G. Sumpter, D.W. Noid, "Molecular Dynamics and Ab Initio SCF-MO Modeling of Nanogenerator and Nanologic Circuit Molecules," paper presented at the Fifth Foresight Conference on Molecular Nanotechnology, November 1997; see abstract at: http://www.foresight.org/Conferences/MNT05/Abstracts/Darsabst.html. See also: Polymer Preprints 39(January 1998):363-364.

2900. R.R. Reeber, "Lattice dynamical prediction of the elastic constants of diamond," Mat. Res. Soc. Symp. Proc. 453(1997):239-243.

2901. S.B. Sinnott, R.J. Colton, C.T. White, O. Shenderova, D.W. Brenner, J.A. Harrison, "Atomistic Simulations of the Nanometer-Scale Indentation of Amorphous Carbon Thin Films," J. Vac. Sci. Technol. A 15(May/June 1997):936-940. See also: Judith A. Harrison, Donald W. Brenner, "Simulated Tribochemistry: An Atomic-Scale View of the Wear of Diamond," J. Am. Chem. Soc. 116(1995):10399-10402; J.A. Harrison, C.T. White, R.J. Colton, D.W. Brenner, "Investigation of the atomic-scale friction and energy dissipation in diamond using molecular dynamics," Thin Solid Films 260(15 May 1995):205-211; and J.A. Harrison, C.T. White, R.J. Colton, D.W. Brenner, "Effect of Atomic-Scale Surface Roughness on Friction: A Molecular Dynamics Study of Diamond Surfaces," Wear 168(1993):127 et seq.

2902. E.M. Sevick, D.R.M. Williams, "Polymer Brushes as Pressure-Sensitive Automated Microvalves," Macromolecules 27(1994):5285-5290. See also: S. Adiga, D.W. Brenner, "Atomistic Simulation of Shear-Induced Polymer Brush Swelling," at: http://www.mse.ncsu.edu/CompMatSci/index.html.

2903. D.H. Robertson, D.W. Brenner, C.T. White, "Temperature Dependent Fusion of Colliding C_{60} Clusters from Molecular Dynamics Simulations," J. Phys. Chem. 99(1995):15721-15724.

2904. S.B. Sinnott, C.T. White, D.W. Brenner, "Properties of Novel Fullerene Tubule Structures: A Computational Study," Mat. Res. Symp. Proc. 359(1995):241-246.

2905. S.B. Sinnott, O.A. Shenderova, C.T. White, D.W. Brenner, "Mechanical Properties of Nanotubule Fibers and Composites Determined from Theoretical Calculations and Simulations," Carbon 36(1997):1-9.

2906. B.I. Dunlap, D.W. Brenner, G.W. Schriver, "Symmetric Isomers of $C_{60}H_{36}$," J. Phys. Chem. 98(17 February 1994):1756-1757.

2907. Michael Page, Donald W. Brenner, "Hydrogen Abstraction from a Diamond Surface: Ab Initio Quantum Chemical Study using Constrained Isobutane as a Model," J. Am. Chem. Soc. 113(1991):3270-3274.

2908. J.D. Schall, O.A. Shenderova, D.W. Brenner, M.R. Falvo, R. Superfine, R.M. Taylor, "Prediction of Band Gap and Relative Conductivity of Carbon Nanotubules as Function of Strain," paper presented at the Fifth Foresight Conference on Molecular Nanotechnology, November 1997; see at: http://www4.ncsu.edu/~jdschall/Papers/bending2.html. See also: J.D. Schall, O.A. Shenderova, D.W. Brenner, "Novel Nanoscale Straingauge Design using Carbon Nanotubes," 20 May 1998; see at: http://www4.ncsu.edu/~jdschall/Papers/nanostraingauge.htm.

2909. D.W. Brenner, J.D. Schall, J.P. Mewkill, O.A. Shenderova, S.B. Sinnott, "Virtual Design and Analysis of Nanometer-Scale Sensor and Device Components," J. Brit. Interplanet. Soc. 51(1998):137-144. Presentation at the Fifth Foresight Conference on Molecular Nanotechnology, November 1997; see abstract at: http://www.foresight.org/Conferences/MNT05/Abstracts/Brenabst.html.

2910. C. Kiskoti, J. Yarger, A. Zettl, "C_{36}, a new carbon solid," Nature 393(25 June 1998):771-774.

2911. R. Glas, M. Bogyo, J.S. McMaster, M. Gaczynska, H.L. Ploegh, "A proteolytic system that compensates for loss of proteasome function," Nature 392(9 April 1998):618-622.

2912. Q. Liu, S.S. Gross, "Binding sites of nitric oxide synthases," Methods Enzymol. 268(1996):311-324.

2913. L. Jia, C. Bonaventura, J. Bonaventura, J.S. Stamler, "S-nitrosohaemoglobin: A dynamic activity of blood involved in vascular control," Nature 380(21 March 1996):221-226.

2914. Fernando I. Rodriguez, Jeffrey J. Esch, Anne E. Hall, Brad M. Binder, G. Eric Schaller, Anthony B. Bleecker, "A Copper Cofactor for the Ethylene Receptor ETR1 from Arabidopsis," Science 283(12 February 1999):996-998.

2915. Elke Geier, Gunter Pfeifer, Matthias Wilm, Marian Lucchiari-Hartz, Wolfgang Baumeister, Klaus Eichmann, Gabriele Niedermann, "A Giant Protease with Potential to Substitute for Some Functions of the Proteasome," Science 283(12 February 1999):978-981.

2916. K. Tanaka, T. Tamura, T. Yoshimura, A. Ichihara, "Proteasomes: Protein and gene structures," New Biologist 4(March 1992):173-187.

2917. M. Rechsteiner, L. Hoffman, W. Dubiel, "The multicatalytic and 26 S proteases," J. Biol. Chem. 268(25 March 1993):6065-6068.

2918. C. Nathan, "Nitric oxide as a secretory product of mammalian cells," FASEB J. 6(September 1992):3051-3064.

2919. S. Moncada, A. Higgs, "The L-arginine-nitric oxide pathway," New Eng. J. Med. 329(30 December 1993):2002-2012.

2920. G.C. Brown, C.E. Cooper, "Nanomolar concentrations of nitric oxide reversibly inhibit synaptosomal respiration by competing with oxygen at cytochrome oxidase," FEBS Lett. 356(19 December 1994):295-298.

2921. Stephen S.-Y. Chui, Samuel M.-F. Lo, Jonathan P.H. Charmant, A. Guy Orpen, Ian D. Williams, "A Chemically Functionalizable Nanoporous Material $[Cu_3(TMA)_2(H_2O)_3]_n$," Science 283(19 February 1999):1148-1150.

2922. Vinzenz M. Unger, Nalin M. Kumar, Norton B. Gilula, Mark Yeager, "Three-Dimensional Structure of a Recombinant Gap Junction Membrane Channel," Science 283(19 February 1999):1176-1180.

2924. Shigeru Ikeda et al., "Mechano-catalytic overall water splitting," Chem. Commun. (21 October 1998):2185-2186.

2925. C.V. Saba, P.A. Barton, M.G. Boshier, I.G. Hughes, P. Rosenbusch, B.E. Sauer, E.A. Hinds, "Reconstruction of a Cold Atom Cloud by Magnetic Focusing," Phys. Rev. Lett 82(18 January 1999):468-471. See also: Andrew Watson, "Videotape Brings Atoms To a Focus," Science 283(29 January 1999):626-627.

2926. A.N. Cleland, M.L. Roukes, "A Nanometer-Scale Mechanical Electrometer," Nature 392(12 March 1998):160-162; "Fabrication of high frequency nanometer scale mechanical resonators from bulk Si crystals," App. Phys. Lett. 69(28 October 1996):2653-2655. See also: http://www.cmp.caltech.edu/~roukes/nanomechanics.html.

2927. A.N. Cleland, M.L. Roukes, "External control of dissipation in a nanometer-scale radio frequency mechanical resonator," Sensors and Actuators A 72(16 February 1999):256-261.

2928. M.L. Roukes, "Yoctocalorimetry: phonon counting in nanostructures," Physica B 263-264(March 1999):1-15.

2929. B.J. Suh, P.C. Hammel, Z. Zhang, M.M. Midzor, M.L. Roukes, J.R. Childress, "Ferromagnetic Resonance Imagine of Co Films using Magnetic Resonance Force Microscopy," J. Vac. Sci. Technol. B. 16(July/August 1998):2275-2279.
2930. W.E. Paul, R.A. Seder, "Lymphocyte responses and cytokines," Cell 76(28 January 1994):241-251.
2931. M.L. Dustin et al., "A novel adaptor protein orchestrates receptor patterning and cytoskeletal polarity in T-cell contacts," Cell 94(4 September 1998):667-677.
2932. M. Beier, F. Reck, T. Wagner, R. Krishnamurthy, A. Eschenmoser, "Chemical Etiology of Nucleic Acid Structure: Comparing Pentapyranosyl-(2'-4') Oligonucleotides with RNA," Science 283(29 January 1999):699-703.
2933. Terry M. Tritt, "Holey and Unholey Semiconductors," Science 283(5 February 1999):804-805.
2934. Th. Zemb, M. Dubois, B. Deme, Th. Gulik-Krzywicki, "Self-Assembly of Flat Nanodiscs in Salt-Free Catanionic Surfactant Solutions," Science 283(5 February 1999):816-819.
2935. E. Ravussin, S. Lillioja, T.E. Anderson, L. Christin, C. Bogardus,"Determinants of 24-hour energy expenditure in man. Methods and results using a respiratory chamber," J. Clin. Invest. 78(December 1986):1568-1578.
2936. F. Zurlo, R.T. Ferraro, A.M. Fontvielle, R. Rising, C. Bogardus, E. Ravussin, "Spontaneous physical activity and obesity: Cross-sectional and longitudinal studies in Pima Indians," Am. J. Physiol. 263(August 1992):E296-E300.
2937. James A. Levine, Norman L. Eberhardt, Michael D. Jensen, "Role of Nonexercise Activity Thermogenesis in Resistance to Fat Gain in Humans," Science 283(8 January 1999):212-214.
2938. Corinna Wu, "A Nonconformist Compound," Science News 155(20 February 1999):120-121.
2939. N. Seppa, "Prospects Dim for Live AIDS Vaccine," Science News 155(13 February 1999):100.
2940. M.P. Krafft, J.G. Riess, "Highly fluorinated amphiphiles and colloidal systems, and their applications in the biomedical field: A contribution," Biochimie 80(May/June 1998):489-514.
2941. F. Frezard, C. Santaella, P. Vierling, J.G. Riess, "Permeability and stability in buffer and in human serum of fluorinated phospholipid-based liposomes," Biochim. Biophys. Acta 1192(1 June 1994):61-70.
2942. C. Guedj, B. Pucci, L. Zarif, C. Coulomb, J.G. Riess, A.A. Pavia, "Vesicles and other supramolecular systems from biocompatible synthetic glycolipids with hydrocarbon and/or fluorocarbon chains," Chem. Phys. Lipids 72(8 August 1994):153-173.
2943. F. Guillod, J. Greiner, J.G. Riess, "Vesicles made of glycophospholipids with homogeneous (two fluorocarbon or two hydrocarbon) or heterogeneous (one fluorocarbon and one hydrocarbon) hydrophobic double chains," Biochim. Biophys. Acta 1282(25 July 1996):283-292.
2944. L. Clary, V. Ravily, C. Santaella, P. Vierling, "Transmembrane pH-driven Na^+ permeability of fluorinated phospholipid-based membranes," J. Controlled Release 51(12 February 1998):259-267.
2945. Healthway Online, "Propane/Poison," see at: http://www.healthanswers.com/database/ami/converted/002836.html.
2946. Flogas Ireland Ltd., "Flogas LPG/Propane/Butane Safety Data Sheet," see at: http://www.flogas.ie/flopds.html.
2947. Active Propane Co. Inc., "Material Safety Data Sheet," 1 December 1998, see at: http://www.lpg.com/safety/msds.html.
2948. "DuPont Suva(R) refrigerants: SUVA HP81 (R402B)," revised 25 October 1996, MSDS Number 6000FR, DuPont Corporate MSDS Number DU005603; see at: http://www.dupont.com/suva/na/usa/sa/techinfo/msds/6000frsuvahp81.html.
2949. B.A. Cornell, G.C. Fletcher, J. Middlehurst, F. Separovic, "The lower limit to the size of small sonicated phospholipid vesicles," Biochim. Biophys. Acta 690(25 August 1982):15-19.
2950. Stephen L. Gillett, "Near-term nanotechnology: The molecular fabrication of nanostructured materials," Nanotechnology 7(September 1996):168-176.
2951. Young-Kyun Kwon, David Tomanek, Sumio Ijima, "Bucky Shuttle Memory Device: Synthetic Approach and Molecular Dynamics Simulations," Phys. Rev. Lett. 82(15 February 1999):1470-1473.
2952. P.S. Virk, E.W. Merrill, H.S. Mickley, K.A. Smith, E.L. Mollo-Christensen, "The Toms Phenomenon: Turbulent Pipe Flow of Dilute Polymer Solutions," J. Fluid Mech. 30-32(1967):305-328.
2953. R. Sureshkumar, Robert A. Handler, Antony N. Beris, "Direct numerical simulation of the turbulent channel flow of a polymer solution," Physics of Fluids 9(1997):743-755. See also: Michael Schneider, "Stretchy Molecules in Low-Drag Solutions," at: http://access.ncsa.uiuc.edu/CoverStories/StretchyMolecules/gasol_1.html.
2954. Kevin D. Ausman, Henry W. Rohrs, MinFeng Yu, Rodney S. Ruoff, "Nanostressing and Mechanochemistry," paper presented at the Sixth Foresight Nanotechnology Conference, November 1998; see at: http://www.foresight.org/Conferences/MNT6/Papers/Ausman/index.html.
2955. Al Globus, John Lawton, Todd Wipke, "Automatic molecular design using evolutionary techniques," paper presented at the Sixth Foresight Nanotechnology Conference, November 1998; see at: http://www.foresight.org/Conferences/MNT6/Papers/Globus/index.html.
2956. Tad Hogg, "Robust Self-Assembly Using Highly Designable Structures," paper presented at the Sixth Foresight Nanotechnology Conference, November 1998; see at: http://www.foresight.org/Conferences/MNT6/Papers/Hogg/index.html.
2957. D. Pierson, C. Richardson, B.I. Yakobson, "Symmetry-dependent strength of carbon nanotubes," presentation at the Sixth Foresight Nanotechnology Conference, November 1998; see at: http://www.foresight.org/Conferences/MNT6/Abstracts/Pierson/index.html.
2958. Carol Pickering, "Silicon Man Lives: Just Ask Peter Cochrane," Forbes ASAP (22 February 1999)82.
2959. Peter Cochrane, Tips for Time Travelers, McGraw-Hill, New York, 1998. See also: http://btlabs1.labs.bt.com/people/cochrap/index.htm.
2960. C.A. Angell, H. Kanno, "Density Maxima in High-Pressure Supercooled Water and Liquid Silicon Dioxide," Science 193(17 September 1976):1121-1122.
2961. A. Bejan, P.A. Tyvand, "The Pressure Melting of Ice Under a Body With Flat Base," Trans. ASME J. Heat Transfer 114(May 1992):529-531; P.A. Tyvand, A. Bejan, "The Pressure Melting of Ice Due to an Embedded Cylinder," Trans. ASME J. Heat Transfer 114(May 1992):532-535.
2962. P.W. Bridgman, "The Pressure-Volume-Temperature Relations of the Liquid, and the Phase Diagram of Heavy Water," J. Chem. Phys. 3(October 1935):597-605. See also: P.W. Bridgman, Collected Experimental Papers, Harvard University Press, Cambridge MA, 1964.
2963. Felix Franks, ed., Water: A Comprehensive Treatise, Volume 7, Water and Aqueous Solutions at Subzero Temperatures, Plenum Press, New York, 1982.
2964. G.P. Johari, Andreas Hallbrucker, Erwin Mayer, "Isotope and impurity effects on the glass transition and crystallization of pressure-amorphized hexagonal and cubic ice," J. Chem. Phys. 95(1 November 1991):6849-6855.
2965. H. Kanno, R.J. Speedy, C.A. Angell, "Supercooling of Water to -92°C Under Pressure," Science 189(12 September 1975):880-881.
2966. John S. Tse, "Mechanical instability in Ice Ih: A mechanism for pressure-induced amorphization," J. Chem. Phys. 96(1 April 1992):5482-5487.
2967. C. Cavazzoni, G.L. Chiarotti, S. Scandolo, E. Tosatti, M. Bernasconi, M. Parrinello, "Superionic and Metallic States of Water and Ammonia at Giant Planet Conditions," Science 283(1 January 1999):44-46.
2968. Philip Ball, The Self-Made Tapestry: Pattern Formation in Nature, UOP, 1999.
2969. M. Saura, C. Zaragoza, A. McMillan, R.A. Quick, C. Hohenadl, J.M. Lowenstein, Charles J. Lowenstein, "An antiviral mechanism of nitric oxide: Inhibition of a viral protease," Immunity 10(January 1999):21-28.
2970. Kurt Bachmaier, Nikolaus Neu, Luis M. de la Maza, Sukumar Pal, Andrew Hessel, Josef M. Penninger, "Chlamydia Infections and Heart Disease Linked Through Antigenic Mimicry," Science 283(26 February 1999):1335-1339.
2971. Brian J. Balin, Alan P. Hudson, et al., "Identification and localization of *Chlamydia pneumoniae* in the Alzheimer's brain," Med. Microbiol. Immunol. 187(June 1998):23-42.
2972. John Desmond Bernal, The World, the Flesh, and the Devil: An Enquiry into the Future of the Three Enemies of the Rational Soul, reprint of the 1929 essay, Indiana University Press, Bloomington, 1969. See also at: http://www.hia.com/pcr/bernal.html.
2973. Ben Bova, Immortality: How Science Is Extending Your Life Span—and Changing the World, Avon Books, New York, 1998.
2974. J.D. Watson, F.H.C. Crick, "Molecular structure of nucleic acids," Nature 171(1953):737-738.
2975. James D. Watson, The Double Helix, Atheneum Publishers, New York, 1968.
2976. D. Rudman et al., "Effects of human growth hormone in men over 60 years old," New. Engl. J. Med. 323(1990):1-6.
2977. Ronald Klatz, Frances A. Kovarik, eds., Advances in Anti-Aging Medicine, Volume I, Mary Ann Liebert Press, 1996.
2978. Ronald Klatz, Robert Goldman, Bob Goldman, Don R. Bensen, Stopping the Clock, Keats Publ, 1996.
2979. Ronald Klatz, Carol Kahn, Grow Young with HGH, HarperCollins, New York, 1997.
2980. Bob Goldman, Ronald Klatz, Lisa Berger, Robert Goldman, Brain Fitness, Doubleday, New York, 1998.
2981. "American Academy of Anti-Aging Medicine," see at: http://www.worldhealth.net/a4m/overview.html.
2982. Marvin Minsky, The Society of Mind, Simon and Schuster, New York, 1985.
2983. Julian Jaynes, The Origin of Consciousness in the Breakdown of the Bicameral Mind, Houghton Mifflin, Boston, 1976.
2984. Sigmund Freud, A General Introduction to Psychoanalysis, Buni and Liveright, New York, 1920. See also: The Complete Psychological Works of Sigmund Freud, translated by James Strachey in collaboration with Anna Freud, Hogarth, London, 1961.
2985. Carl G. Jung, Analytical Psychology, Moffat & Yard, New York, 1916. See also: Psychological Types, Harcourt, Brace & World, New York, 1933.
2986. Otto Rank, The Trauma of Birth, Robert Brunner Publ., New York, 1952.
2987. G.W. Allport, H.S. Odbert, "Trait-names: A psycho-lexical study," Psychological Monographs 47(1936):1-171.
2988. Paul M. Churchland, Matter and Consciousness, revised edition, MIT Press, Cambridge MA, 1988. See also: A Neurocomputational Perspective, MIT Press, Cambridge MA, 1989; The Engine of Reason, the Seat of the Soul, MIT Press, Cambridge MA, 1995.

2989. Patricia S. Churchland, Neurophilosophy: Toward a Unified Science of the Mind-Brain, MIT Press, Cambridge MA, 1986.
2990. Gerald M. Edelman, Bright Air, Brilliant Fire: On the Matter of Mind, BasicBooks, New York, 1992.
2991. Alexander Sasha Chislenko, "Intelligent Information Filters and Enhanced Reality," Extropy #16, Qtr I, 1996, pp. 13-17, 26. See also: http://www.lucifer.com/~sasha/EnhancedReality.html.
2992. Max More, "Technological Self-Transformation," Extropy #10, Winter/Spring 1993, pp. 15-24.
2993. Max More, "Beyond the Machine: Technology and Posthuman Freedom," Proc. Ars Electronica 1997, Ars Electronica Center, Springer, Wien, New York, 1997.
2994. Bradley Rhodes, Seum-Lim Gan, "Collab97 Project Proposal: The Direction Bump," see at: http://rhodes.www.media.mit.edu/people/rhodes/collab97.proposal.html.
2995. Association for Unmanned Vehicle Systems International, "Aerial Robotics Competition," see at: http://avdil.gtri.gatech.edu/AUVS/IARCLaunchPoint.html.
2996. David Brin, The Transparent Society, Addison-Wesley, Reading MA, 1998.
2997. Allergy Internet Resources, "Food Allergies," see at: http://www.immune.com/allergy/allabc.html.
2998. The Genome Database, "Genetic Disorders by Chromosome," last updated 21 February 1999; see at: http://gdbwww.gdb.org/gdbreports/GeneticDiseases.html.
2999. Beverly Merz, "Blazing A Genetic Trail: Reading the Human Blueprint," A Report from the Howard Hughes Medical Institute, July 1998; see at: http://www.hhmi.org/GeneticTrail/reading/read.htm.
3000. Hans P. Moravec, Robot: Mere Machine to Transcendent Mind, Oxford University Press, Cambridge, 1998.
3001. Jon A. Wolff, ed., Gene Therapeutics: Methods and Applications of Direct Gene Transfer, Springer-Verlag, New York, 1994.
3002. J.B. Griffiths, Raymond E. Spier, eds., Animal Cell Biotechnology, Volume 6, Academic Press, New York, 1994.
3003. Michael G. Kaplitt, Arthur D. Loewy, eds., Viral Vectors: Gene Therapy and Neuroscience Applications, Academic Press, New York, 1995.
3004. Jeff Lyon, Peter Gorner, Altered Fates: Gene Therapy and the Retooling of Human Life, W.W. Norton and Company, 1995.
3005. John E. Smith, Biotechnology, Cambridge University Press, New York, 1996.
3006. George Morstyn, William Sheridan, eds., Cell Therapy: Stem Cell Transplantation, Gene Therapy, and Cellular Immunotherapy, Cambridge University Press, New York, 1996.
3007. P.R. Lowenstein, L.W. Enquist, eds., Gene Transfer in Neuroscience: Towards Gene Therapy of Neurological Disorders, John Wiley and Sons, New York, 1996.
3008. H. Wekerle, H. Graf, J.D. Turner, eds., Cellular Therapy, Springer-Verlag, New York, 1997.
3009. Wayne A. Marasco, ed., Intrabodies: Basic Research and Clinical Gene Therapy Applications, Springer-Verlag, New York, 1998.
3010. Peter J. Quesenberry, Gary S. Stein, Bernard Forget, eds., Stem Cell Biology and Gene Therapy, Wiley-Liss, New York, 1998.
3011. Edmund C. Lattime, Stanton L. Gerson, eds., Gene Therapy of Cancer: Translational Approaches from Preclinical Studies to Clinical Implementation, Academic Press, New York, 1998.
3012. K.D. Cummings, R.C. Frye, E.A. Rietman, "Using a neural network to proximity correct patterns written with a Cambridge electron beam microfabricator 10.5 lithography system," Appl. Phys. Lett. 57(1 October 1990):1431-1433.
3013. "Electroactive Polymer Actuators (Artificial Muscles)," NDEAA Group Website at NASA/JPL, see at: http://eis.jpl.nasa.gov/ndeaa/nasa-nde/lommas/aa-hp.htm.
3014. Glen A. Evans, "The 'Jurassic Park' Paradigm for the Construction of Synthetic Organisms," talk given at the Genome Sequencing and Analysis Conference IX, Hilton Head, South Carolina, 16 September 1997.
3015. Robert J. Bradbury, "Paths to Immortality," talk given at EXTRO3, The Future of the Body and Brain / Future Infrastructure, Third Conference of the Extropy Institute, 9-10 August 1997, San Jose, CA. See also: http://www.extropy.com/ex3/extro3.htm.
3016. Per Bro, "Chemical Reaction Automata: Precursors of Synthetic Organisms," talk delivered to the American Chemical Society, Central New Mexico Section, 25 April 1997; see announcement at: http://www.nm.org/~acs/archive/news0497.html.
3017. Charles Ostman, Nanobiology—Where Nanotechnology and Biology Come Together," see at: http://www.biota.org/ostman/nchip.htm.
3018. Fred Rieke, David Warland, Rob de Ruyter van Steveninck, William Bialek, Spikes: Exploring the Neural Code, MIT Press, Cambridge MA, 1996.
3019. Michael A. Arbib, ed., The Handbook of Brain Theory and Neural Networks, MIT Press, Cambridge MA, 1998.
3020. James M. Bower, David Beeman, The Book of GENESIS: Exploring Realistic Neural Models with the GEneral NEural SImulation System, Springer-Verlag, New York, 1998.
3021. Christof Koch, Idan Segev, Methods in Neuronal Modeling: From Ions to Networks, MIT Press, Cambridge MA, 1998.
3022. Christof Koch, Biophysics of Computation: Information Processing in Single Neurons, Oxford University Press, 1998.
3023. Philippe Poncharal, Z.L. Wang, Daniel Ugarte, Walt A. de Heer, "Electrostatic Deflections and Electromechanical Resonances of Carbon Nanotubes," Science 283(5 March 1999):1513-1516. See also: http://www.gtri.gatech.edu/res-news/BALANCE.html.
3024. A.M Cassell, W.A. Scrivens, J.M. Tour, "Assembly of DNA/Fullerene Hybrid Materials," Angew. Chem. Int. Ed. Engl. 37(1998):1528-1531.
3025. Keith F. Lynch, "Brain Backup Proposal," see at: http://www.clark.net/pub/kfl/les/cryonet/3326.html.
3026. S. Mark Halpin et al., Voltage and Lamp Flicker Issues, "Part Five: Case Studies Using the IEC Flickermeter," see at: http://www.powerclinic.com/flicker5.htm. See also: "Electricity Supply Voltage Requirements and Problems" at: http://genesisauto.com.au/voltage.htm; and Combustion in Energy and Transformation Industries, Figure 5, "Load variation and arrangement of power plants according to the voltage regulation characteristic," at: http://www.eea.eu.int/aegb/cap01/b111_123.htm.
3027. NIST Time and Frequency Division, "NIST Time and Frequency FAQ," see at: http://www.bldrdoc.gov/timefreq/faq/faq.htm; see also "NIST Network Time Service," at: http://www.bldrdoc.gov/timefreq/service/nts.htm.
3028. Fouad G. Major, The Quantum Beat: The Physical Principles of Atomic Clocks, Springer-Verlag, 1998.
3029. Jo Ellen Barnett, Time's Pendulum: The Quest to Capture Time — From Sundials to Atomic Clocks, Plenum Press, 1998.
3030. Yojiro Kawamura, Morley Kare, eds., Umami: A Basic Taste: Physiology, Biochemistry, Nutrition, Food Science, Food Science and Technology Series, Volume 20, Marcel Dekker, New York, 1987.
3031. Shizuko Yamaguchi, "Basic properties of umami and effects on humans," Physiol. and Behav. 49(1991):833-841.
3032. S. Fuke, Y. Ueda, "Interactions between umami and other flavor characteristics," Trends in Food Sci. Technol. 7(1996):407-411.
3033. Chaudhari et al., "The taste of monosodium glutamate: membrane receptors in taste buds," J. Neurosci. 16(1996):3817-3826.
3034. K. Kurihara, M. Kashiwayanagi, "Introductory remarks on umami taste," Ann. N.Y. Acad. Sci. 855(30 November 1998):393-397.
3035. International Food Information Council Foundation, "Glutamate and Monosodium Glutamate: Examining the Myths," August 1997, see at: http://ificinfo.health.org/review/ir-msg.htm. See also: "Everything You Need To Know About Glutamate And Monosodium Glutamate," January 1997, see at: http://ificinfo.health.org/brochure/msg.htm.
3036. S.A. Kiselev, S.R. Bickham, A.J. Sievers, "Properties of Intrinsic Localized Modes in One-Dimensional Lattices," Comments Cond. Mat. Phys. 17(1995):135-173.
3037. Carleen Hawn, "Counting Sheep," Forbes 163(8 February 1999):102.
3038. John M. Pawelek, K. Brooks Low, David Bermudes, "Tumor-targeted *Salmonella* as a Novel Anticancer Vector," Cancer Research 57(15 October 1997):4537-4544. See also: Alexandra Alger, "Fighting Disease With Disease," Forbes 162(16 November 1998):240; and: Vion Parmaceuticals, "Tumor Amplified Protein Expression Therapy," see at: http://www.vionpharm.com/TAPET_splash.html.
3039. B. Cornell, V. Braach-Maksvytis, L. King, P. Osman, B. Raguse, L. Wieczorek, R. Pace, "A biosensor that uses ion-channel switches," Nature 387(5 June 1997):580-583; see also "Tethered Lipid Bilayer Membranes: Formation and Ionic Reservoir Characterization," Langmuir 14(14 January 1998):648-659.
3040. Australian Membrane and Biotechnology Research Institute (AMBRI), "The ICS Biosensor," see at: http://www.ambri.com.au/institute/technology/ics/index.html.
3041. Cheng-Hsien Liu, "Micromachined Tunneling Accelerometer," Stanford Micro Structures and Sensors Lab, September 1998; see at: http://www.standford.edu/~chliu/MTA.html.
3042. Peter Gumbsch, Huajian Gao, "Dislocations Faster than the Speed of Sound," Science 283(12 February 1999):965-968.
3043. A.R. Williams, "Effects of Ultrasound on Blood and the Circulation," in Wesley L. Nyborg, Marvin C. Ziskin, eds., Biological Effects of Ultrasound, Churchill Livingstone, New York, 1985, pp. 49-65.
3044. F.S. Foster, H. Obara, T. Bloomfield, L.K. Ryan, G.R. Lockwood, "Ultrasound Backscatter from Blood in the 30 to 70 MHz Frequency Range," 1994 IEEE Ultrasonics Symposium, pp. 1599-1602.
3045. Barbara L. Golden, Anne R. Gooding, Elaine R. Podell, Thomas R. Cech, "A Preorganized Active Site in the Crystal Structure of *Tetrahymena* Ribozyme," Science 282(9 October 1998):259-264.
3046. Qinyu Wang, S.R. Challa, D.S. Sholl, J.K. Johnson, "Quantum sieving in carbon nanotubes and zeolites," Phys. Rev. Lett. 82(1 February 1999):956-959.
3047. Larry D. Partain, ed., Solar Cells and Their Applications, John Wiley and Sons, New York, 1995.
3048. Life Plus, Product Information Sheet No. 8058, "L-Salivarius Plus Other Beneficial Microflora," see at: http://www.galicia.simplenet.com/salivarex.com.
3049. Alka-Line Products, "Alkadophilus: The Non-Refrigerated Acidophilus," see at: http://www.homeopathiccenter.com/acido.htm.
3050. "Microbial Life in the Digestive Tract," in Laura Austgen, R.A. Bowen, Pathophysiology of the Digestive System, hypertextbook at: http://arbl.cvmbs.colostate.edu/hbooks/pathphys/digestion/basics/gi_bugs.html.
3051. L. Chong, B. van Steensel, D. Broccoli, H. Erdjument-Bromage, J. Hanish, P. Tempst, T. de Lange, "A Human Telomeric Protein," Science 270(8 December 1995):1663-1667.

3052. D. Broccoli, A. Smogorzewska, L. Chong, T. de Lange, "Human telomeres contain two distinct Myb-related proteins, TRF1 and TRF2," Nature Genet. 17(October 1997):231-235.

3053. Susan Smith, Izabela Giriat, Anja Schmitt, Titia de Lange, "Tankyrase, a Poly(ADP-Ribose) Polymerase at Human Telomeres," Science 282(20 November 1998):1484-1487.

3054. A.A. Avilion, L.A. Harrington, C.W. Greider, "*Tetrahymena* telomerase RNA levels increase during macronuclear development," Dev. Genet. 13(1992):80-86.

3055. Joachim Lingner, Timothy R. Hughes, Andrej Shevchenko, Matthias Mann, Victoria Lundblad, Thomas R. Cech, "Reverse Transcriptase Motifs in the Catalytic Subunit of Telomerase," Science 276(25 April 1997):561-567.

3056. J. Travis, "Tick, tock, enzyme rewinds cellular clock," Science News 153(17 January 1998):37.

3057. J.W. Shay, S. Bacchetti, "A survey of telomerase activity in human cancer," Eur. J. Cancer 33(April 1997):787-791. See also: S. Bacchetti, C.M. Counter, Int. J. Oncol. 7(1995):423-432.

3058. Nam W. Kim, Mieczyslaw A. Piatyszek, et al., "Specific Association of Human Telomerase Activity with Immortal Cells and Cancer," Science 266(23 December 1994):2011-2015. See also: Lisa Seachrist, "Telomeres Draw a Crowd at Toronto Cancer Meeting," Science 268(7 April 1995):29-30.

3059. A. Bodnar, N.W. Kim, R.B. Effros, C.-P. Chiu, "Mechanism of telomerase induction during T cell activation," Exp. Cell Res. 228(10 October 1996):58-64.

3060. C.-P. Chiu, W. Dragowska, N.W. Kim, H. Vaziri, J. Yui, T.E. Thomas, C.B. Harley, P.M. Lansdorp, "Differential expression of telomerase activity in hematopoietic progenitors from adult human bone marrow," Stem Cells 14(March 1996):239-248.

3061. W.E. Wright, M.A. Piatyszek, W.E. Rainey, W. Byrd, J.W. Shay, "Telomerase activity in human germline and embryonic tissues and cells," Dev. Genet. 18(1996):173-179.

3062. M. Engelhardt, R. Kumar, J. Albanell, R. Pettengell, W. Han, M.A. Moore, "Telomerase regulation, cell cycle, and telomere stability in primitive hematopoietic cells," Blood 90(1 July 1997):182-193.

3063. D. Broccoli, J.W. Young, T. de Lange, "Telomerase activity in normal and malignant hematopoietic cells," Proc. Natl. Acad. Sci. USA 92(26 September 1995):9082-9086.

3064. C.M. Counter, J. Gupta, C.B. Harley, B. Leber, S. Bacchetti, "Telomerase activity in normal leukocytes and in hematologic malignancies," Blood 85(1 May 1995):2315-2320.

3065. H. Tahara, T. Nakanishi, M. Kitamoto, R. Nakashio, J.W. Shay, E. Tahara, G. Kajiyama, T. Ide, "Telomerase activity in human liver tissues: comparison between chronic liver disease and hepatocellular carcinomas," Cancer Res. 55(1 July 1995):2734-2736.

3066. Andrea G. Bodnar, Michel Ouellette, et al., "Extension of Life-Span by Introduction of Telomerase into Normal Human Cells," Science 279(16 January 1998):349-352.

3067. D.S. Chance, M.K. McIntosh, "Hypolipidemic agents alter hepatic mitochondrial respiration in vivo," Comp. Biochem. Physiol. C. Pharmacol. Toxicol. Endocrinol. 111(June 1995):317-323.

3068. D.P. Jones, "Intracellular diffusion gradients of O_2 and ATP," Am. J. Physiol. 250(May 1986):C663-C675.

3069. P. van der Valk, J.J. Gille, A.B. Oostra, E.W. Roubos, T. Sminia, H. Joenje, "Characterization of an oxygen-tolerant cell line derived from Chinese hamster ovary. Antioxygenic enzyme levels and ultrastructural morphometry of peroxisomes and mitochondria," Cell Tissue Res. 239(1985):61-68.

3070. L.A. del Rio, L.M. Sandalio, J.M. Palma, "A new cellular function for peroxisomes related to oxygen free radicals?" Experientia 46(15 October 1990):989-992.

3071. K. Kremser, W. Kovacs, H. Stangl, "Peroxisomal diseases — oxygen and free radicals," Wien Klin Wochenschr. 107(1995):690-693. In German.

3072. I. Singh, "Mammalian peroxisomes: Metabolism of oxygen and reactive oxygen species," Ann. N.Y. Acad. Sci. 804(27 December 1996):612-627.

3073. A.M. Kogelnik, M.T. Lott, M.D. Brown, S.B. Navathe, D.C. Wallace, "MITOMAP: An update of the human mitochondrial genome database," Nucleic Acid Res. 25(January 1997). See also: http://www.gen.emory.edu/mitomap.html.

3074. P.R. Kennedy, R.A. Bakay, "Restoration of neural output from a paralyzed patient by a direct brain connection," Neuroreport 9(1 June 1998):1707-1711.

3075. J.W. Gofman, Radiation and Human Health, Pantheon, New York, 1983.

3076. V. Beir, Health Effects of Exposure to Low Levels of Ionizing Radiation, National Research Council, National Academy Press, Washington, 1990.

3077. J.K. Shultis, R.E. Faw, Radiation Shielding, Prentice Hall, Upper Saddle River, New Jersey, 1996.

3078. E.L. Alpen, Radiation Biophysics, Second Edition, Academic Press, San Diego, 1998.

3079. T. Moriizumi, "Biosensor, Electronics, and Biorobot," Tanpakushitsu Kakusan Koso 43(July 1998):1303-1309. In Japanese.

3080. R.D. Beer, H.J. Chiel, R.D. Quinn, R.E. Ritzmann, "Biorobotic approaches to the study of motor systems," Curr. Opin. Neurobiol. 8(December 1998):777-782.

3081. University of Washington Biorobotics Laboratory, see at: http://rcs.ee.washington.edu/BRL/index.html; Harvard BioRobotics Laboratory, see at: http://hrl.harvard.edu/hrsl/; Miura-Shimoyama Laboratory for Autonomous Biorobotics, see at: http://www.leopard.t.u-tokyo.ac.jp/researchProjects/AB.html.

3082. H. Bielefeldt-Ohmann, "Analysis of antibody-independent binding of Dengue viruses and Dengue virus envelope protein to human myelomonocytic cells and B lymphocytes," Virus Res. 57(September 1998):63-79.

3083. Alexander Ferworn, Deborah A. Stacey, "Inchworm Mobility — Stable, Reliable and Inexpensive," see at: http://hebb.cis.voguelph.ca/~alex/research/inchworm.html. See also: Burleigh Instruments Inc., "Inchworm Motors," at: http://www.burleigh.com/_vti_bin/shtml.exe/IWmotors.htm/map.

3084. Lal Tummala, Dean Aslam, Sridhar Mahadevan, Ranjan Mukherji, John Weng, Ning Xi, "Reconfigurable Adaptable Micro-Robots," see at: http://www.egr.msu.edu/microrobot/fr-main.htm.

3085. Karen Thomas, "Coiled again: Slinky still takes the stairs after turning 50," 4 December 1995, see at: http://detnews.com/menu/stories/27228.htm. See also: "Slinky Operating Instructions," at http://www.cit.nepean.uws.edu.au/~rocky/fun/slinky.html; and "The Creation of the Slinky," at: http://www.yippeee.com/what/slinky.html.

3086. K. Ikeuchi, K. Yoshinaka, S. Hashimoto, N. Tomita, "Locomotion of Medical Micro Robot with Spiral Ribs Using Mucus," 7th Intl. Symp. on Micro Machine and Human Science (MHS'96), 2-4 October 1996.

3087. Richard Nakka, personal communication, 26 March 1999. See also: "Experimental Rocketry Web Site," 27 February 1999, at: http://members.aol.com/~ricnakk/dex.html; and "glucose burning test report" at: http://members.aol.com/ricbnakk/soft/dexrpt.zip.

3088. Sidney B. Lang, "Pyroelectric Effect in Bone and Tendon," Nature 212(12 November 1966):704-705. See also: "Thermal expansion coefficients and the primary and secondary pyroelectric coefficients of animal bone," Nature 224(22 November 1969):798-799.

3089. Robert O. Becker, Andrew A. Marino, Electromagnetism and Life, State University of New York Press, Albany, 1982. See at: http://www.ortho.lsumc.edu/Faculty/Marino/EL/ELTOC.html.

3090. Eiichi Fukuda, Iwao Yasuda, "On the Piezoelectric Effect of Bone," J. Phys. Soc. Japan 12(1957):1158-1162.

3091. C. Andrew L. Bassett, Robert O. Becker, "Generation of Electric Potentials by Bone in Response to Mechanical Stress," Science 137(1962):1063-1064.

3092. Morris H. Shamos, Leroy S. Lavine, Michael I. Shamos, "Piezoelectric Effect in Bone," Nature 197(5 January 1963):81.

3093. J.H. McElhaney, "The charge distribution on the human femur due to load," J. Bone Joint Surg. 49(December 1967):1561-1571.

3094. J.C. Anderson, C. Eriksson, "Piezoelectric properties of dry and wet bone," Nature 227(1 August 1970):491-492.

3095. A.A. Marino, R.O. Becker, S.C. Soderholm, "Origin of the piezoelectric effect in bone," Calcif. Tissue Res. 8(1971):177-180.

3096. Philippa J.R. Uwins, Richard I. Webb, Anthony P. Taylor, "Novel nano-organisms from Australian sandstones," American Mineralogist 83(November/December 1998):1541-1550. See also: http://www.uq.edu.au/nanoworld/uwins.html; and "Nanobiology" at http://naturalscience.com/ns/links/nanobiol.html.

3097. "Global Temperature Trends: 1998 Global Surface Temperature Smashes Record," see at: http://www.giss.nasa.gov/research/observe/surftemp/. See also: "Rise in Temperature Suggests a Connection," at: http://www.csmonitor.com/durable/1997/12/03/feat/temperature.html.

3098. Arthur D. Moore, Electrostatics: Exploring, Controlling and Using Static Electricity, Including the Dirod Manual, 2nd Edition, Laplacian Press, CA, 1997. See also the "Electrostatic Applications Website," at: http://www.garlic.com/electro/index.html.

3099. G. Sessler, R. Gerhard-Multhaupt, eds., Electrets, 3rd Edition, Volumes I and II, Laplacian Press, CA, 1999.

3100. Howard A. Wilcox, Hothouse Earth, Praeger Publishers, New York, 1975.

3101. S.A. Kaplan, ed., Extraterrestrial Civilizations: Problems of Interstellar Communication, Nauka Press, Moscow, 1969; translated from the Russian by IPST Jerusalem, 1971 (IPST Cat. No. 5780); NASA Technical Translations F-631.

3102. H. Royer, Arch. Physiol. Normale Pathol. 7(1895):12.

3103. C. Balny, R. Hayashi, S. Shimada, P. Masson, High Pressure and Biotechnology, Volume 224, Colloques INSERM/John Library Eurotext Ltd., France, 1992.

3104. R. Hayashi, High Pressure Bioscience and Food Science, San-Ei Publishing Co., Japan, 1993. In Japanese.

3105. B.H. Hite, West Virginia Univ. Agric. Expt. Station Bull. 58(1899):15.

3106. R. Hayashi et al., "High Pressure Food Processing," see at: http://cc.usu.edu/~josephi/highpres/highpres.html.

3107. M. Gross, R. Jaenicke, "Proteins under pressure. The influence of high hydrostatic pressure on structure, function and assembly of proteins and protein complexes," Eur. J. Biochem. 221(1994):617-630.

3108. V. Hill, D.A. Ledward, J.M. Ames, "Influence of high hydrostatic pressure and pH on the rate of Maillard browning in a glucose-lysine system," J. Agric. Food Chem. 44(1996):594-598. See also: "The Maillard Reaction," at: http://www.fst.reading.ac.uk/people/aamesjm/maillard.htm.

3109. Alan Bruzel, "Chemistry — Maillard Reaction," 28 December 1998, at: http://chemistry.miningco.com/library/weekly/aa122898.htm; and Dairy Management Inc., "Lactose: Browning," 1998, at: http://www.doitwithdairy.com/ingredients/lactose/lacfunbro.htm;

3110. "Nonenzymatic Browning," see at: http://courses.che.umn.edu/97fscn8311-1f/nonenzymatic_browning.htm.

3111. Charlie Scandrett, "Maillard Reactions 101: Theory," 4 April 1997, see at: http://brewery.org/brewery/library/Maillard_CS0497.html.

3112. J. Zhou, "Inactivation, recovery, nucleic acid leakage and cell disruption of *Escherichia coli* by high hydrostatic pressure," M.S. Thesis, Washington State University, 95 pages; reported at: http://impact.wsu.edu/proj_25.htm.

3113. E. Kowalski, H. Ludwig, B. Tauscher, "Behavior of organic compounds in food under high pressure: Lipid peroxidation," in R. Hayashi, C. Balny, eds., High Pressure Bioscience and Biotechnology, Progress in Biotechnology, Volume 13, 1996, pp. 473-478.

3114. Allied Healthcare Products, Inc., "Oxygen Equipment Safety Information," see at: http://www.life-assist.com/recallinfo.html.

3115. Air Liquide, "Specific Safety Precautions: Vessel with Liquid Oxygen," 1997, see at: http://www.medtek.lu.se/Svensk/Utbildning/oxygenterapi/eng/specsec.htm.

3116. Canadian Center for Occupational Health and Safety, "Prevention and Control of Hazards: How Do I Work Safely With Cryogenic Liquids?" 27 November 1997, see at: http://www.ccohs.ca/oshanswers/prevention/cryogens.html.

3117. "NASA Glenn Safety Manual, Chapter 5 — Oxygen Propellant," July 1997, see at: http://www-osma.lerc.nasa.gov/lsm/lsm5.htm.

3118. "UMIST Safety Manual, Part 2, Cryogenics," see at: http://www.trades.umist.ac.uk/safety/safman2a_10.htm.

3119. George Goble, "Cooking HKN Hamburgers and Lighting the Grill," see at: http://ghg.ecn.purdue.edu/.

3120. Brian Carusella, "The Sugar Cube Page: The Burning Sugar Cube Trick," see at: http://freeweb.pdq.net/headstrong/sugar.htm. See also: "Ash Catalyzes the Combustion of Sugar," at: http://chemlearn.chem.indiana.edu/demos/AshCata.htm.

3121. Niels Birbaumer et al., "A spelling device for the paralysed," Nature 298(25 March 1999):297-298.

3122. Roger A. Laine, "A calculation of all possible oligosaccharide isomers, both branched and linear yields 1.05 x 10^{12} structures for a reducing hexasaccharide: The isomer barrier to development of single-method saccharide sequencing or synthesis systems," Glycobiology 4(1994):1-9. See also: "The Information Storing Potential of the Sugar Code," at: http://chrs1.chem.lsu.edu/~wwwbc/laine/biologic.html.

3123. Walter M. Elsasser, "Earth," Encyclopedia Britannica 7(1963):845-852.

3124. L.B. Lockhart, Jr., ed., The NRL Program on Electroactive Polymers, First Annual Report, GPO, Washington, D.C., 1979; R.B. Fox, The NRL Program on Electroactive Polymers, Second Annual Report, GPO, Washington, D.C., 1980.

3125. F. Gutmann, L.E. Lyons, Organic Semiconductors, John Wiley and Sons, New York, 1967; see also F. Gutmann, H. Keyzer, L.E. Lyons, R.B. Somoano, Organic Semiconductors, Krieger Publ. Co., Malbar, FL, 1983.

3126. J.E. Katon, ed., Organic Semiconducting Polymers, Marcel Dekker, New York, 1968.

3127. Ya. M. Pushkin, T.P. Vishnyakova, A.F. Lunin, S.A. Nizova, Organic Polymeric Semiconductors, John Wiley and Sons, New York, 1968.

3128. J. Simon, J.-J. Andre, Molecular Semiconductors, Photoelectrical Properties and Solar Cells, Springer-Verlag, New York, 1985.

3129. E.A. Rietman, "Electrical Properties of α-Cyclodextrine Metal Iodide Inclusion Compounds," Mat. Res. Bull. 25(1990):649-655.

3130. Michael Lesk, "How Much Information Is There In the World?" at: http://www.lesk.com/mlesk/ksg97.ksg.html.

3131. Lernout and Hauspie, "Connecting People and Machines through Speech and Language," at: http://www.lhsl.com/.

3132. Dragon Systems, Inc., "The Natural Speech Company," at: http://www.dragonsys.com/.

3133. James Brent Wood, personal communication, 1998. See also: "The Cephalopod Page," 1995-1999, at: http://is.dal.ca/~ceph/TCP/index.html.

3134. Trygg Engen, The Perception of Odors, Academic Press, New York, 1982.

3135. Piet A. Vroon, Paul Vincent, Anton Van Amerongen, Smell: The Secret Seducer, Farrar Straus & Giroux, New York, 1997.

3136. Biological Asymmetry and Handedness, Ciba Foundation Symposia Series No. 162, John Wiley and Sons, New York, 1991.

3137. Stanley Coren, G.E. Stelmach, P.A. Vroon, Left-Handedness: Behavioral Implications and Anomalies, North-Holland, 1990.

3138. The *C. elegans* Sequencing Consortium, "Genome Sequence of the Nematode *C. elegans*: A Platform for Investigating Biology," Science 282(11 December 1998):2012-2018.

3139. Stephen A. Chervitz et al., "Comparison of the Complete Protein Sets of Worm and Yeast: Orthology and Divergence," Science 282(11 December 1998):2022-2028.

3140. Malcolm G. Parker, ed., Nuclear Hormone Receptors: Molecular Mechanisms, Cellular Functions, Clinical Abnormalities, Academic Press, San Diego, 1991.

3142. Julian M. Sturtevant, "The Enthalpy of Hydrolysis of Acetylcholine," J. Biol. Chem. 247(10 February 1972):968-969.

3143. Jack R. Cooper, Robert H. Roth, Floyd E. Bloom, The Biochemical Basis of Neuropharmacology, Oxford University Press, Cambridge, 1996.

3144. D. Welch et al., "High reliability, high power, single mode laser diodes," Electronics Lett. 26(1990):1481-1482.

3145. D. Botez et al., "66% CW wallplug efficiency from Al-free 0.98 micron-emitting diode lasers," Electronics Lett. 32(10 October 1996):2012-2013.

3146. D.G. Hardie, Biochemical Messengers: Hormones, Neurotransmitters and Growth Factors, Chapman and Hall, 1991.

3147. N. Shiina, Y. Gotoh, E. Nishida, "A novel homo-oligomeric protein responsible for an MPF-dependent microtubule-severing activity," EMBO J. 11(December 1992):4723-4731.

3148. F.J. McNally, R.D. Vale, "Identification of katanin, an ATPase that severs and disassembles stable microtubules," Cell 75(5 November 1993):419-429.

3149. J.J. Thwaites, N.H. Mendelson, "Mechanical properties of peptidoglycan as determined from bacterial thread," Int. J. Biol. Macromol. 11(August 1989):201-206.

3150. W.J. Becktel, W.A. Baase, "A lysoplate assay for *Escherichia coli* cell wall-active enzymes," Anal. Biochem. 150(1 November 1985):258-263.

3151. J.J. Thwaites, U.C. Surana, A.M. Jones, "Mechanical properties of *Bacillus subtilis* cell walls: Effects of ions and lysozyme," J. Bacteriol. 173(January 1991):204-210.

3152. S. Makino, N. Ito, T. Inoue, S. Miyata, R. Moriyama, "A spore-lytic enzyme released from *Bacillus cereus* spores during germination," Microbiology 140(June 1994):1403-1410.

3153. T.F. Deuel, R.M. Senior, J.S. Huang, et al., "Chemotaxis of monocytes and neutrophils to platelet-derived growth factor," J. Clin. Invest. 69(1982):1046-1049.

3154. M.E.A. Churchill, T.D. Tullius, N.R. Kallenbach, N.C. Seeman, "A Holliday Recombination Intermediate is Twofold Symmetric," Proc. Natl. Acad. Sci. USA 85(1988):4653-4656. See also: M. Susman, B. Engels, "Strand Exchange and Translation of Holliday Junction," 27 July 1997, see at: http://www.wisc.edu/genetics/Holliday/holliday3D.html.

3155. Dana H. Ballard, Christopher M. Brown, Computer Vision, Prentice-Hall, Englewood Cliffs, NJ, 1982. See also: Guy Robinson, "12.4.1 Oct-Trees," 1 March 1995, at: http://www.netlib.org/utk/lsi/pcwLSI/text/node279.html.

3156. TopoMetrix Home Page at: http://www.topometrix.com; merged with Park Scientific to form ThermoMicroscopes, at: http://www.thermomicro.com.

3157. R.J. Tillyard, The Biology of Dragonflies, Oxford University Press, Cambridge, 1917.

3158. Brian Hocking, "The intrinsic range and speed of flight of insects," Trans. Roy. Entomol. Soc. London 104(1953):225-345.

3159. J.F. Butler, 1994; cited as personal communication in J.H. Byrd, "University of Florida Book of Insect Records, Chapter 1: Fastest Flyer," 31 May 1994, at: http://gnv.ifas.ufl.edu/~tjw/chap01.htm.

3160. R.C. Wilkerson, J.F. Butler, "The Immelmann Turn, a pursuit maneuver used by hovering male *Hybomitra hinei wrighti*," Ann. Entomol. Soc. Am. 77(1984):293-295.

3161. R.K. Josephson, R.C. Halverson, "High frequency muscles used in sound production by a katydid: Organization of the motor system," Biol. Bull. 141(1971):411-433.

3162. D. Young, R.K. Josephson, "Mechanisms of sound-production and muscle contraction kinetics in cicadas," J. Comp. Physiol. 152(1983):183-195.

3163. W. Linss, C. Pilgrim, H. Feuerstein, "How thick is the glycocalyx of human erythrocytes?" Acta Histochem. 91(1991):101-104. In German.

3164. K.A. Haldenby, D.C. Chappell, C.P. Winlove, K.H. Parker, J.A. Firth, "Focal and regional variations in the composition of the glycocalyx of large vessel endothelium," J. Vasc. Res. 31(January-February 1994):2-9.

3165. M. Ogata, K. Araki, T. Ogata, "An electron microscopic study of *Helicobacter pylori* in the surface mucous gel layer," Histol. Histopathol. 13(April 1998):347-358.

3166. T.M. Chen, M.J. Dulfano, "Mucus viscoelasticity and mucociliary transport rate," J. Lab. Clin. Med. 91(March 1978):423-431.

3167. C.S. Kim, M.A. Greene, S. Sankaran, M.A. Sackner, "Mucus transport in the airways by two-phase gas-liquid flow mechanism: continuous flow model," J. Appl. Physiol. 60(March 1986):908-917. See also: C.S. Kim, C.R. Rodriguez, M.A. Eldridge, M.A. Sackner, "Criteria for mucus transport in the airways by two-phase gas-liquid flow mechanism," J. Appl. Physiol. 60(March 1986):901-907.

3168. M.A. Sleigh, J.R. Blake, N. Liron, "The propulsion of mucus by cilia," Am. Rev. Respir. Dis. 137(March 1988):726-741.

3169. M. King, M. Agarwal, J.B. Shukla, "A planar model for mucociliary transport: effect of mucus viscoelasticity," Biorheology 30(January-February 1993):49-61.

3170. A. Silberberg, "On mucociliary transport," Biorheology 27(1990):295-307.

3171. E.A. Evans, "Structure and deformation properties of red blood cells: Concepts and quantitative methods," Methods Enzymol. 173(1989):3-35.

3172. R. Waugh, E.A. Evans, "Thermoelasticity of red blood cell membrane," Biophys. J. 26(April 1979):115-131.

3173. E.W. Hagley, L. Deng, M. Kozuma, J. Wen, K. Helmerson, S.L. Rolston, W.D. Phillips, "A Well-Collimated Quasi-Continuous Atom Laser," Science 283(12 March 1999):1706-1709. See also: David Voss, "Atom Lasers Get More Laserlike," Science 283(12 March 1999):1611-1613.

3174. "Nobel Chemist on Nanotechnology," Foresight Update #20, 1 February 1995, p. 1.

3175. Phil Scott, "A Bug's Lift," Scientific American 280 (April 1999):51, 54.

3176. B. Jack Copeland, Diane Proudfoot, "Alan Turing's Forgotten Ideas in Computer Science," Scientific American 280(April 1999):98-103.

3177. Lan Bo Chen, "Mitochondrial Membrane Potential in Living Cells," Annu. Rev. Cell Biol. 4(1988):155-181.
3178. J. Bereiter-Hahn, "Behavior of Mitochondria in the Living Cell," Int. Rev. Cytol. 122(1990):1-63.
3179. Michael P. Yaffe, "The Machinery of Mitochondrial Inheritance and Behavior," Science 283(5 March 1999):1493-1497.
3180. J. Bereiter-Hahn, M. Voth, "Dynamics of Mitochondria in Living Cells: Shape Changes, Dislocations, Fusion, and Fission of Mitochondria," Microsc. Res. Techniq. 27(15 February 1994):198-219.
3181. V. Iota, C.S. Yoo, H. Cynn, "Quartzlike Carbon Dioxide: An Optically Nonlinear Extended Solid at High Pressures and Temperatures," Science 283(5 March 1999):1510-1513.
3182. Johannes Denschlag, Donatella Cassettari, Jorg Schmiedmayer, "Guiding Neutral Atoms with a Wire," Phys. Rev. Lett. 82(8 March 1999):2014-2017. See also: Alexander Hellemans, "Attractive Wire Guides Atoms Out of Trap," Science 283(12 March 1999):1614.
3183. J.J. Paggel, T. Miller, T.-C. Chiang, "Quantum-Well States as Fabry-Perot Modes in a Thin-Film Electron Interferometer," Science 283(12 March 1999):1709-1711.
3184. Adam F. Carpenter, Apostolos P. Georgopoulos, Giuseppe Pellizzer, "Motor Cortical Encoding of Serial Order in a Context-Recall Task," Science 283(12 March 1999):1752-1757.
3185. Jocelyn Kaiser, "Windup Computers?" Science 283(19 March 1999):1811.
3186. Elizabeth Pennisi, "Academic Sequencers Challenge Celera in a Sprint to the Finish," Science 283(19 March 1999):1822-1823.
3187. James C. Mullikin, Amanda A. McMurray, "Sequencing the Genome, Fast," Science 283(19 March 1999):1867-1868; errata, Science 284(11 June 99):1776.
3188. Hany Aziz, Zoran D. Popovic, Nan-Xing Hu, Ah-Mee Hor, Gu Xu, "Degradation Mechanism of Small Molecule-Based Organic Light-Emitting Devices," Science 283(19 March 1999):1900-1902.
3189. M. Switkes, C.M. Marcus, K. Campman, A.C. Gossard, "An Adiabatic Quantum Electron Pump," Science 283(19 March 1999):1905-1908.
3190. T. Ogawa, K. Tomita, T. Ueda, K. Watanabe, T. Uozumi, H. Masaki, "A Cytotoxic Ribonuclease Targeting Specific Transfer RNA Anticodons," Science 283(26 March 1999):2097-2100.
3191. Daoguo Zhou, Mark S. Mooseker, Jorge E. Galan, "Role of the *S. typhimurium* Actin-Binding Protein SipA in Bacterial Internalization," Science 283(26 March 1999):2092-2095.
3192. "Images From the History of Medicine," at: http://wwwihm.nlm.nih.gov.
3193. Michel Grandbois, Martin Beyer, Matthias Rief, Hauke Clausen-Schaumann, Hermann E. Gaub, "How Strong Is a Covalent Bond?" Science 283(12 March 1999):1727-1730.
3194. Robert F. Service, "Watching DNA at Work," Science 283(12 March 1999):1668-1669.
3195. W.E. Moerner, Michel Orrit, "Illuminating Single Molecules in Condensed Matter," Science 283(12 March 1999):1670-1676.
3196. Shimon Weiss, "Fluorescence Spectroscopy of Single Biomolecules," Science 283(12 March 1999):1676-1683.
3197. E. Schrodinger, "Are There Quantum Jumps? Part II," British J. Philos. of Science 3(1952-1953):233-242.
3198. R. Yasuda, Hiroyuki Noji, Kazuhiko Kinosita Jr., Masasuke Yoshida, "F_1-ATPase Is a Highly Efficient Molecular Motor that Rotates with Discrete 120° Steps," Cell 93(26 June 1998):1117-1124.
3199. Dennis Normile, "Building Working Cells in Silico," Science 284(2 April 1999):80-81.
3200. James K. Gimzewski, Christian Joachim, "Nanoscale Science of Single Molecules Using Local Probes," Science 283(12 March 1999):1683-1688.
3201. Karel Svoboda, Christoph F. Schmidt, Bruce J. Schnapp, Steven M. Block, "Direct observation of kinesin stepping by optical trapping interferometry," Nature 365(21 October 1993):721-727.
3202. H. Kojima, E. Muto, H. Higuchi, T. Yanagida, "Mechanics of single kinesin molecules measured by optical trapping nanometry," Biophys. J. 73(October 1997):2012-2022.
3203. Wei Hua, Edgar C. Young, Margaret L. Fleming, Jeff Gelles, "Coupling of kinesin steps to ATP hydrolysis," Nature 388(24 July 1997):390-393.
3204. Mark J. Schnitzer, Steven M. Block, "Kinesin hydrolyses one ATP per 8-nm step," Nature 388(24 July 1997):386-390.
3205. Immanuel Bloch, Theodor W. Haensch, Tilman Esslinger, "Continuous atom laser beam," Phys. Rev. Lett. (12 April 1999):In press.
3206. Richard Martel, Herbert R. Shea, Phaedon Avouris, "Rings of single-walled nanotubes," Nature 398(25 March 1999):299.
3207. Bettina Malnic, Junzo Hirono, Takaaki Sato, Linda B. Buck, "Combinatorial Receptor Codes for Odors," Cell 96(5 March 1999):713-723. See also: John Travis, "Making Sense of Scents," Science News 155(10 April 1999):236-238.
3208. K. Eric Drexler, "Molecular Nanomachines: Physical Principles and Implementation Strategies," Annu. Rev. Biophys. Biomol. Struct. 23(1994):377-405.
3209. J.F.V. Vincent, Structural Biomaterials, John Wiley and Sons, New York, 1982.
3210. F. Oosawa, S. Asakura, Thermodynamics of the Polymerization of Protein, Academic Press, London, 1975.
3211. F.M. Richards, "Areas, volumes, packing, and protein structure," Annu. Rev. Biophys. Bioeng. 6(1977):151-176.
3212. Farida Darkrim, Dominique Levesque, "Monte Carlo simulations of hydrogen adsorption in single-walled carbon nanotubes," J. Chem. Phys. 109(1998):4980-4984.
3213. Ifadat Ali Khan, K.G. Ayappa, "Density distributions of diatoms in carbon nanotubes: A grand canonical Monte Carlo study," J. Chem. Phys. 109(1998):4576-.
3214. Qinyu Wang, J. Karl Jonhson, "Molecular simulation of hydrogen adsorption in single-walled carbon nanotubes and idealized carbon slit pores," J. Chem. Phys. 110(1999):577-586.
3215. Qinyu Wang, J. Karl Jonhson, "Computer Simulations of Hydrogen Adsorption on Graphite Nanofibers," J. Phys. Chem. B 103(1999):277-281.
3216. P. Douglas Tougaw, Craig S. Lent, "Logical devices implemented using quantum cellular automata," J. Appl. Phys. 75(1 February 1994):1818-1825.
3217. Islamshah Amlani, Alexei O. Orlov, Geza Toth, Gary H. Bernstein, Craig S. Lent, Gregory L. Snider, "Digital Logic Gate Using Quantum-Dot Cellular Automata," Science 284(9 April 1999):289-291.
3218. N.S. Isaacs, M. Coulson, "The effect of pressure on processes modelling the Maillard reaction," in R. Hayashi, C. Balny, eds., High Pressure Bioscience and Biotechnology, Progress in Biotechnology, Volume 13, 1996, pp. 479-484.
3219. M.R. Falvo et al., "Manipulation of individual viruses: friction and mechanical properties," Biophysical J. 72(March 1997):1396-1403.
3220. Lucy Cusack, S. Nagaraja Rao, Donald Fitzmaurice, "Heterosupramolecular Chemistry," in M. Moskovits, V. Shalaev, eds., Nanostructural Materials: Clusters, Composites, and Thin Films, ACS Symposium Series 679, American Chemical Society, Washington DC, 1997, pp. 17-28.
3221. Sridhar Komarneni, John C. Parker, Heinrich J. Wollenberger, eds., Nanophase and Nanocomposite Materials II, Symposium Proceedings, Volume 457, Materials Research Society, Pittsburgh PA, 1997.
3222. Avery N. Goldstein, ed., Handbook of Nanophase Materials, Marcel Dekker, NY, 1997.
3223. Henry Harris, The Birth of the Cell, Yale University Press, 1999.
3224. Rajesh S. Gokhale, Stuart Y. Tsuji, David E. Cane, Chaitan Khosla, "Dissecting and Exploiting Intermodular Communication in Polyketide Synthases," Science 284(16 April 1999):482-485.
3225. H.N. Schulz, T. Brinkhoff, T.G. Ferdelman, M. Hernandez Marine, A. Teske, B.B. Jorgensen, "Dense Populations of a Giant Sulfur Bacterium in Namibian Shelf Sediments," Science 284(16 April 1999):493-495.
3226. Phillip Belgrader, William Benett, Dean Hadley, James Richards, Paul Stratton, Raymond Mariella Jr., Fred Milanovich, "PCR Detection of Bacteria in Seven Minutes," Science 284(16April 1999):449-450.
3227. Min Ge et al., "Vancomycin Derivatives That Inhibit Peptidoglycan Biosynthesis Without Binding D-Ala-D-Ala," Science 284(16 April 1999):507-511.
3228. Galina S. Kachalova, Alexander N. Popov, Hans D. Bartunik, "A Steric Mechanism for Inhibition of CO Binding to Heme Proteins," Science 284(16 April 1999):473-476.
3229. Max N. Yoder, "Diamond: What, When, and Where," in A.J. Purdes et al., Proc. Second Intl. Symp. on Diamond Materials, Proceedings Volume 91-8, The Electrochemical Society, Pennington NJ, 1991, pp. 513 et seq.
3230. B.T. Kelly, Physics of Graphite, Applied Science Publishers, 1981.
3231. S.M. Sze, Physics of Semiconductor Devices, Second Edition, John Wiley and Sons, New York, 1981.
3232. E. Richard Cohen, Barry N. Taylor, "The Fundamental Physical Constants," Physics Today 48(August 1995):BG9.
3233. The extermination speed (against in vivo pathogens) using medical nanorobots is described in Chapter 19 and depends upon many factors. Deployment of nanorobots from in vivo storage allows in sanguo migration to within a few cell widths of almost any infected site within at most one blood circulation time (<60 sec); alternatively, direct transdermal insertion by medical personnel allows on site deployment near well-localized infections in 5-10 sec (e.g. duration of a small injection). Recognition of a pathogenic cell type may occur in ~2 millisec (Section 8.5.2.2); a nanorobot concentration of 10^{-3} micron^{-3} at the infected site allows positive identification of all microbes located inside the 1000 micron^3 patrol volume of each nanorobot within ~90 sec (Section 8.4.4). Once recognized, mechanical killing and disposal of a virus particle requires ~0.1 sec of processing time (Section 10.4.2.4.2); mechanical killing and disposal of a bacterial pathogen requires ~50 sec (Section 10.4.2.5.3). Typical extermination time for well-localized infections thus ranges from 100-200 sec. Chapter 19 further explores eradication statistics as a function of pathogen population and distribution, especially for less localized infections; cell and chromosome repair or replacement following infiltration by exogenous viral genetic material is described in Chapters 20 and 21.
3234. For example, see "Section 5. Safety and Biocompatibility" at: http://www.foresight.org/Nanomedicine/Respirocytes.html.
3235. L. Lehr, M.T. Zanni, C. Frischkorn, R. Weinkauf, D.M. Neumark, "Electron Solvation in Finite Systems: Femtosecond Dynamics of Iodide-$(Water)_n$ Anion Clusters," Science 284(23 April 1999):635-638.
3236. Evelyn Strauss, "A Symphony of Bacterial Voices," Science 284(21 May 1999):1302-1304.
3237. David A. Relman, "The Search for Unrecognized Pathogens," Science 284(21 May 1999):1308-1310.

3238. Ray H. Baughman et al., "Carbon Nanotube Actuators," Science 284(21 May 1999):1340-1344.
3239. Meher Antia, "Imaging Living Cells The Friendly Way," Science 284(28 May 1999):1445.
3240. A. Yu. Kasumov et al., "Supercurrents Through Single-Walled Carbon Nanotubes," Science 284(28 May 1999):1508-1511.
3241. Forrest Bishop, "Description of the Cell Rover," see at: http://www.iase.cc/html/cellrover.html.
3242. Geoffrey B. West, James H. Brown, Brian J. Enquist, "The Fourth Dimension of Life: Fractal Geometry and Allometric Scaling of Organisms," Science 284(4 June 1999):1677-1679.
3243. Gang He, Martin H. Muser, Mark O. Robbins, "Adsorbed Layers and the Origin of Static Friction," Science 284(4 June 1999):1650-1652.
3244. Konrad Spindler, The Man in the Ice: The Preserved Body of a Neolithic Man Reveals the Secrets of the Stone Age, Harmony Books, 1994. See also: John Noble Wilford, "Peek Into the Iceman's Prehistoric Medicine Kit," at: http://home.earthlink.net/~marksiporen/reference/NCR-iceman.html.
3245. William L. Ditto, "Computing with Leeches," see at: http://www.physics.gatech.edu/chaos/leeches/. See also: "Biological computer born," at http://news.bbc.co.uk/hi/english/sci/tech/newsid_358000/358822.stm.
3246. Henry Bortman, "Whirlybugs," New Scientist 162(5 June 1999); see also: http://www.newscientist.com/ns/19990605/whirlybugs.html.
3247. Ehud Shapiro, "A Mechanical Turing Machine: Blueprint for a Biological Computer," paper presented at the 5th Intl. Meeting on DNA Based Computers, MIT, 14-15 June 1999; see at http://www.wisdom.weizmann.ac.il/~udi/DNA5/turing5.html.
3248. Tom Knight, "Microbial Engineering Home Page," see at: http://www.ai.mit.edu/people/tk/ce/microbial-engineering.html.
3249. A. Krammer, H. Lu, B. Isralewitz, K. Schulten, V. Vogel, "Forced unfolding of the fibronectin type III module reveals a tensile molecular recognition switch," Proc. Natl. Acad. Sci. USA 96(16 February 1999):1351-1356.
3250. Fedor N. Dzegilenko, Deepak Srivastava, Subhash Saini, "Simulations of carbon nanotube tip assisted mechano-chemical reactions on a diamond surface," Nanotechnology 9(December 1998):325-330.
3251. Cees J.M. van Rijn, Gert J. Veldhuis, Stein Kuiper, "Nanosieves with microsystem technology for microfiltration applications," Nanotechnology 9(December 1998):343-345.
3252. Joseph Alper, "Lobbing Nanobombs at Pathogens," Science 284(11 June 1999):1754-1755.
3253. Roger M. Knutson, Furtive Fauna: A Field Guide to the Creatures Who Live on You, Ten Speed Press, Berkeley, CA, 1996.
3254. Roger M. Knutson, Fearsome Fauna: A Field Guide to the Creatures Who Live in You, W.H. Freeman and Company, New York, 1999.
3255. O. Painter, R.K. Lee, A. Scherer, A. Yariv, J.D. O'Brien, P.D. Dapkus, I. Kim, "Two-Dimensional Photonic Band-Gap Defect Mode Laser," Science 284(11 June 1999):1819-1821.
3256. Timothy Stowe, Thomas Kenny, Daniel Rugar, David Botkin, Koichi Wago, Kevin Yashimura, "Force Detection with Atto-Newton Precision," reported at the American Physical Society March Meeting, 17-21 March 1997, Kansas City, MO. See Physics News Report at: http://www.aip.org/enews/physnews/1997/physnews.313.htm and press release at: http://www.eurekalert.org/E-lert/current/public_releases/deposit/atto-newton.html.
3257. "Web Elements," at: http://www.shef.ac.uk/chemistry/web-elements/fr-define/isotope-nucl-mag-moment.html.
3258. "Japanese Introduce Ant-Size Robot," Associated Press report, 21 June 1999; see at: http://www.salonmagazine.com/tech/log/1999/06/21/robot/index.html.
3259. R.G. Mayer, Embalming: History, Theory, and Practice, Appleton and Lange, Norwalk CT, 1990.
3260. L. Lopez, W.G. Sannita, "Glucose availability and the electrophysiology of the human visual system," Clin. Neurosci. 4(1997):336-340.
3261. Michael Gross, Travels to the Nanoworld: Miniature Machinery in Nature and Technology, Plenum Press, New York, 1999.
3262. Gregory Timp, ed., Nanotechnology, Springer-Verlag, New York, 1999. See also: Arthur ten Wolde, ed., Nanotechnology: Towards a Molecular Construction Kit, Netherlands Study Centre for Technology Trends (STT), New World Ventures, 1998; executive summary at: http://www.stt.nl/textE/sv60.htm.
3263. John Travis, "One small bacterial genome, to go," Science News 155(12 June 1999):377.
3264. A. John Appleby, "The Electrochemical Engine for Vehicles," Scientific American 281(July 1999):74-79.
3265. Stephen C. Woods, Randy J. Seeley, Daniel Porte Jr., Michael W. Schwartz, "Signals That Regulate Food Intake and Energy Homeostasis," Science 280(29 May 1998):1378-1383.
3266. David Tomanek, Peter Kral, Phys. Rev. Lett. (1999):In press. Reported in: Michael Brooks, "Drawing A Fine Line," New Scientist 162(26 June 1999); see also: http://www.newscientist.com/ns/19990626/newsstory2.html.
3267. S. Backhaus, G.W. Swift, "A thermoacoustic Stirling heat engine," Nature 399(27 May 1999):335-338.
3268. Michael H. Dickenson, Fritz-Olaf Lehmann, Sanjay P. Sane, "Wing Rotation and the Aerodynamic Basis of Insect Flight," Science 284(18 June 1999):1954-1960.
3269. Erich Sackmann et al., Phys. Rev. Lett. (21 June 1999):In press. Reported in: Phil Ball, "Swimming lessons for micro-bubbles," Nature 399(24 June 1999); see at: http://helix.nature.com/nsu/990624/990624-10.html.
3270. Jerry Emanuelson, The Life Extension Manual, Colorado Futurescience, Inc., 1991-1997; see at: http://www.futurescience.com/cfsc/leintro.html.
3271. "Biomaterials Properties Table Listing: Yield Strength," April 1996, see at: http://www.lib.umich.edu/libhome/Dentistry.lib/Dental_tables/Yieldstr.html.
3272. James G. Hamilton, "Needle Phobia: A Neglected Diagnosis," J. Family Practice 41(August 1995):169-175. See also "Needle Phobia Page" at: http://www.futurescience.com/cfsc.needles.html.
3273. V.P. Stupnitskii, G.M. Zarakovskii, "Phenomenology of behavior and unusual mental states of operators during forced wakefulness," Kosm. Biol. Aviakosm. Med. 25(May-June 1991):7-11. In Russian.
3274. Andre Thiaville, Jacques Miltat, "Small Is Beautiful," Science 284(18 June 1999):1939-1940.
3275. Julia Uppenbrink, "Completing the Cycle," Science 284(18 June 1999):1942.
3276. P.M. Platzman, M.I. Dykman, "Quantum Computing with Electrons Floating on Liquid Helium," Science 284(18 June 1999):1967-1969.
3277. Vlado Valkovic, "Is Aluminum An Essential Element for Life?" Origins of Life 10(September 1980):301-305.
3278. R.G. Pina, C. Cervantes, "Microbial interactions with aluminum," Biometals 9(July 1996):311-316.
3279. K. Zaman, A. Zaman, J. Batcabe, "Hematological effects of aluminum on living organisms," Comp. Biochem. Physiol. C 106(October 1993):285-293.
3280. G.F. van Landeghem, M.E. de Broe, P.C. D'Haese, "Al and Si: Their Speciation, Distribution, and Toxicity," Clin. Biochem. 31(July 1998):385-397.
3281. W.J. Lukiw, H.J. LeBlanc, L.A. Carver, D.R. McLachlan, N.G. Bazan, "Run-on gene transcription in human neocortical nuclei. Inhibition by nanomolar aluminum and implications for neurodegenerative disease," J. Mol. Neurosci. 11(August 1998):67-78.
3282. V.D. Appanna, R. Hamel, "Aluminum detoxication mechanism in *Pseudomas fluorescens* is dependent on iron," FEMS Microbiol. Lett. 143(1 October 1996):223-228.
3283. J. Jo, Y.S. Jang, K.Y. Kim, M.H. Kim, I.J. Kim, W.I. Chung, "Isolation of ALU1-P gene encoding a protein with aluminum tolerance activity from *Arthrobacter viscosus*," Biochem. Biophys. Res. Commun. 239(29 October 1997):835-839.
3284. M.L. McDermott, H.F. Edelhauser, H.M. Hack, R.H. Langston, "Ophthalmic irrigants: A current review and update," Ophthalmic Surg. 19(October 1988):724-733.
3285. Makoto Fujita, Norifumi Fujita, Katsuyuki Ogura, Kentaro Yamaguchi, "Spontaneous assembly of ten components into two interlocked, identical coordination cages," Nature 400(1 July 1999).
3286. J.G. Humble, W.H.W. Jayne, R.J.V. Pulvertaft, "Biological Interaction Between Lymphocytes and Other Cells", Brit. J. Haemat. 2(1956):283-294.
3287. Harry L. Ioachim, "Emperipolesis of Lymphoid Cells in Mixed Cultures", Lab. Investig. 14(October 1965):1784-1794.
3288. F.M. Reid, G.P. Sandilands, K.G. Gray, J.R. Anderson, "Lymphocyte emperipolesis revisited. II. Further characterization of the lymphocyte subpopulation involved," Immunology 36(February 1979):367-372.
3289. J. Thiele, R. Krech, H. Choritz, A. Georgii, "Emperipolesis — a peculiar feature of megakaryocytes as evaluated in chronic myeloproliferative diseases by morphometry and ultrastructure," Virchows Arch. B. Cell Pathol. Incl. Mol. Pathol. 46(1984):253-263.
3290. L. Chyczewski, W. Debek, J. Dzieciol, J.K. Kirejczyk, J. Niklinski, S. Sulkowski, "Influence of brain hypoxia on megakaryocytic emperipolesis in rats," Folia Histochem. Cytobiol. 32(1994):187-190.
3291. M. Tanaka, Y. Aze, T. Fujita, "Adhesion molecule LFA-1/ICAM-1 influences on LPS-induced megakaryocytic emperipolesis in the rat bone marrow," Vet. Pathol. 34(September1997):463-466.
3292. K. Samii, E. Pasteur, "Images in hematology: Emperipolesis," Am. J. Hematol. 59(September 1998):64.
3293. V. Deshpande, K. Verma, "Fine needle aspiration (FNA) cytology of Rasai-Dorfman disease," Cytopathology 9(October 1998):329-335.
3294. "Study Looks to Nuclear Energy as Micro-Scale Fuel," University of Wisconsin, Madison, Press Release, 29 June 1999; see at: http://www.news.wisc.edu/thisweek/Research/Engr/Y99/micro_nuclear.html.
3295. D.A. Muller, T. Sorsch, S. Moccio, F.H. Baumann, K. Evans-Lutterodt, G. Timp, "The electronic structure at the atomic scale of ultrathin gate oxides," Nature 399(24 June 1999):758-761. See also: Max Shultz, "The end of the road for silicon?" Nature 399(24 June 1999):729-730.
3296. V. Argiro, M.B. Bunge, M.I. Johnson, "A quantitative study of growth cone filopodial extension," J. Neurosci. Res. 13(1985):149-162.
3297. Martin L. Sternberg, Mary E. Switzer, American Sign Language Dictionary: Unabridged Edition, Harper Reference, New York, 1998.
3298. J.A. Gerlt, F.H. Westheimer, J.M. Sturtevant, "The enthalpies of hydrolysis of acyclic, monocyclic, and glycoside cyclic phosphate diesters," J. Biol. Chem. 250(10 July 1975):5059-5067.

3299. A.U. Yap, G. Ong, "An introduction to dental electronic anesthesia," Quintessence Int. 27(May 1996):325-331.
3300. D.J. Estafan, "Invasive and noninvasive dental analgesia techniques," Gen. Dent. 46(November-December 1998):600-603.
3301. Peter Kind, "Personnel Status Monitor (PSM) System," at: http://www.sainc.com/arpa/abmet/sarcos.htm. See also: Richard Satava, "Combat Casualty Care," at: http://www.darpa.mil/arpatech-96/transcripts/satava.html.
3302. "What is UTC?" 14 August 1998, see at: http://wwwghcc.msfc.nasa.gov/utc.html. See also: "Systems of Time," at: http://tycho.usno.navy.mil/systime.html, and "NIST Time and Frequency Services" at http://physics.nist.gov/GenInt/Time/boulder.html.
3303. M.C. Mazzoni, T.C. Skalak, G.W. Schmid-Schonbein, "Structure of lymphatic valves in the spinotrapezius muscle of the rat," Blood Vessels 24(1987):304-312.
3304. J.F. Stoltz, S. Gaillard, G. Thibault, J.C. Puchelle, R. Herbeuval, "Study of the rheological properties of human lymph," Biorheology 13(February 1976):83-84. In French.
3305. G. Miserocchi, "Physiology and pathophysiology of pleural fluid turnover," Eur. Respir. J. 10(January 1997):219-225.
3306. A. Milosevic, L.J. Dawson, "Salivary factors in vomiting bulimics with and without pathological tooth wear," Caries Res. 30(1996):361-366.
3307. C. Reppas, J.H. Meyer, P.J. Sirois, J.B. Dressman, "Effect of hydroxypropylmethylcellulose on gastrointestinal transit and luminal viscosity in dogs," Gastroenterology 100(May 1991):1217-1223.
3308. J.G. Ruseler-van Embden, L.M. Van Lieshout, D.J. Binnema, M.P. Hazenberg, "Isolation and characterization of the viscous, high-molecular-mass microbial carbohydrate fraction from faeces of healthy subjects and patients with Crohn's disease and the consequences for a therapeutic approach," Clin. Sci. (Colch) 95(October 1998):425-433.
3309. H.J. Ehrlein, J. Prove, "Effect of viscosity of test meals on gastric emptying in dogs," Q. J. Exp. Physiol. 67(July 1982):419-425.
3310. R.O. Dantas, W.J. Dodds, "Influence of the viscosity of the swallowed food bolus on the motility of the pharynx," Arq. Gastroenterol. 27(October-December 1990):164-168. In Portuguese.
3311. F.M. Larsen, M.N. Wilson, P.J. Moughan, "Dietary fiber viscosity and amino acid digestibility, proteolytic digestive enzyme activity and digestive organ weights in growing rats," J. Nutr. 124(June 1994):833-841.
3312. S. Hamlet, J. Choi, M. Zormeier, F. Shamsa, R. Stachler, J. Muz, L. Jones, "Normal adult swallowing of liquid and viscous material: scintigraphic data on bolus transit and oropharyngeal residues," Dysphagia 11(Winter 1996):41-47.
3313. C.H. Smith, J.A. Logemann, W.R. Burghardt, T.D. Carrell, S.G. Zecker, "Oral sensory discrimination of fluid viscosity," Dysphagia 12(Spring 1997):68-73.
3314. M.C. Lin, T.C. Tsai, Y.S. Yang, "Measurement of viscosity of human semen with a rotational viscometer," J. Formos. Med. Assoc. 91(April 1992):419-423.
3315. K. Okazaki, Y. Yamamoto, K. Ito, "Endoscopic measurement of papillary sphincter zone and pancreatic main ductal pressure in patients with chronic pancreatitis," Gastroenterology 91(August 1986):409-418.
3316. G.I. Leitch, S.A. Harris-Hooker, I.A. Udezulu, "Movement of *Entamoeba histolytica* trophozoites in rat cecum and colon intact mucus blankets and harvested mucus gels," Am. J. Trop. Med. Hyg. 39(September 1988):282-287.
3317. R.D. Pullan, "Colonic mucus, smoking and ulcerative colitis," Ann. R. Coll. Surg. Engl. 78(March 1996):85-91.
3318. E. Aizenman, H. Engelberg-Kulka, G. Glaser, "An *Escherichia coli* chromosomal `addiction module' regulated by guanosine 3',5'-bispyrophosphate: a model for programmed bacterial cell death," Proc. Natl. Acad. Sci. (USA) 93(11 June 1996):6059-6063.
3319. R.E. Bishop, B.K. Leskiw, R.S. Hodges, C.M. Kay, J.H. Weiner, "The entericidin locus of *Escherichia coli* and its implications for programmed bacterial cell death," J. Mol. Biol. 280(24 July 1998):583-596.
3320. H. Engelberg-Kulka, M. Reches, S. Narasimhan, R. Schoulaker-Schwarz, Y. Klemes, E. Aizenman, G. Glaser, "RexB of bacteriophage lambda is an anti-cell death gene," Proc. Natl. Acad. Sci. (USA) 95(22 December 1998):15481-15486.
3321. L. Snyder, "Phage-exclusion enzymes: a bonanza of biochemical and cell biology reagents?" Mol. Microbiol. 15(February 1995):415-420.
3322. T. Georgiou, Y.N. Yu, S. Ekunwe, M.J. Buttner, A. Zuurmond, B. Kraal, C. Kleanthous, L. Snyder, "Specific peptide-activated proteolytic cleavage of *Escherichia coli* elongation factor Tu," Proc. Natl. Acad. Sci. (USA) 95(17 March 1998):2891-2895. See also: Andy Coghlan, "Suicide squad," New Scientist 163(10 July 1999).
3323. Ian Anderson, "Radio transmitters keep tabs on players," New Scientist 162(5 June 1999).
3324. Robert Uhlig, "Meet Mr. Cyborg: half-husband, half-machine," 27 August 1998, at: http://www.telegraph.co.uk:80/; see also: "Technology gets under the skin," 25 August 1998 at: http://news.bbc.co.uk/hi/english/sci/tech/newsid_158000/158007.stm.
3325. I.G. Bloomfield, I.H. Johnston, L.E. Bilston, "Effects of proteins, blood cells and glucose on the viscosity of cerebrospinal fluid," Pediatr. Neurosurg. 28(May 1998):246-251.
3326. M. Blank, O. Denisova, G. Cornelissen, F. Halberg, "Enhanced circasemiseptan (about 3.5-day) variation in the heart rate of cancer patients?" Anticancer Res. 19(January-February 1999):853-855.
3327. P.J. Brown, R.A. Dove, C.S. Tuffnell, R.P. Ford, "Oscillations of body temperature at night," Arch. Dis. Child 67(October 1992):1255-1258.
3328. M. Miura, J. Okada, "Non-thermal vasodilation by radio frequency burst-type electromagnetic field radiation in the frog," J. Physiol. (London) 435(April 1991):257-273.
3329. A. Weydahl, F. Halberg, "Daily spot-checking versus chronobiologic monitoring of human differential surface (rib versus breast) temperature," Prog. Clin. Biol. Res. 227A(1987):483-491.
3330. R.J. Seymour, W.E. Lacefield, "Wheelchair cushion effect on pressure and skin temperature," Arch. Phys. Med. Rehabil. 66(February 1985):103-108.
3331. G.D. Callin, "A shower spray facility for accurate control and rapid changes of skin temperature," J. Appl. Physiol. 40(April 1976):641-643.
3332. S.J. Park, H. Tokura, "Effects of different types of clothing on circadian rhythms of core temperature and urinary catecholamines," Japan J. Physiol. 48(April 1998):149-156; "Effects of two types of clothing on the day-night variation of core temperature and salivary immunoglobilin A," Chronobiol. Int. 14(November 1997):607-617.
3333. R.R. Freedman, D. Norton, S. Woodward, G. Cornelissen, "Core body temperature and circadian rhythm of hot flashes in menopausal women," J. Clin. Endocrinol. Metab. 80(August 1995):2354-2358.
3334. J.W. Doust, "Periodic homeostatic fluctuations of skin temperature in the sleeping and waking state," Neuropsychobiology 5(1979):340-347.
3335. F.S. Mohler, J.E. Heath, "Oscillating heat flow from rabbit's pinna," Am. J. Physiol. 255(September 1988):R464-R469.
3336. J. Poschl, T. Weiss, C. Diehm, O. Linderkamp, "Periodic variations in skin perfusion in full-term and preterm neonates using laser Doppler technique," Acta Paediatr. Scand. 80(November 1991):999-1007.
3337. K. Krauchi, A. Wirz-Justice, "Circadian rhythm of heat production, heart rate, and skin and core temperature under unmasking conditions in men," Am. J. Physiol. 267(September 1994):R819-R829.
3338. G. Yosipovitch, G.L. Xiong, E. Haus, L. Sackett-Lundeen, I. Ashkenazi, H.I. Maibach, "Time-dependent variations of the skin barrier function in humans: transepidermal water loss, stratum corneum hydration, skin surface pH, and skin temperature," J. Invest. Dermatol. 110(January 1998):20-23.
3339. L.G. Durand, P. Pibarot, "Digital signal processing of the phonocardiogram: review of the most recent advancements," Crit. Rev. Biomed. Eng. 23(1995):163-219.
3340. F. Debiais, L.G. Durand, P. Pibarot, R. Guardo, Z. Guo, "Time-frequency analysis of heart murmurs," Med. Biol. Eng. Comput. 35(September 1997):474-479, 480-485.
3341. S.H. Kim, H.J. Lee, J.M. Huh, B.C. Chang, "Spectral analysis of heart valve sound for detection of prosthetic heart valve disease," Yonsei Med. J. 39(August 1998):302-308.
3342. M. Cozic, L.G. Durand, R. Guardo, "Development of a cardiac acoustic mapping system," Med. Biol. Eng. Comput. 36(July 1998):431-437.
3343. W.H. Fishman, "Clinical and biological significance of an isozyme tumor marker —PLAP," Clin. Biochem. 20(December 1987):387-392.
3344. D.W. Mercer, "Serum isoenzymes in cancer diagnosis and management," Immunol. Ser. 53(1990):613-629.
3345. E.J. Nouwen, M.E. De Broe, "Human intestinal versus tissue-nonspecific alkaline phosphatase as complementary urinary markers for the proximal tubule," Kidney Int. Suppl. 47(November 1994):S43-S51.
3346. K. Sudo, "Progress in biotechnology and its clinical application to isozyme diagnosis," Nippon Rinsho 53(May 1995):1119-1123. In Japanese.
3347. E.G. Krause, G. Rabitzsch, F. Noll, J. Mair, B. Puschendorf, "Glycogen phosphorylase isoenzyme BB in diagnosis of myocardial ischaemic injury and infarction," Mol. Cell Biochem. 160-1(July-August 1996):289-295.
3348. D.H. Smith, J.W. Bailey, "Human African trypanosomiasis in south-eastern Uganda: clinical diversity and isoenzyme profiles," Ann. Trop. Med. Parasitol. 91(October 1997):851-856.
3349. F. Levato, R. Martinello, C. Campobasso, S. Porto, "LDH and LDH isoenzymes in ovarian dysgerminoma," Eur. J. Gynaecol. Oncol. 16(1995):212-215.
3350. H.J. Huijgen, G.T. Sanders, R.W. Koster, J. Vreeken, P.M. Bossuyt, "The clinical value of lactate dehydrogenase in serum: a quantitative review," Eur. J. Clin. Chem. Clin. Biochem. 35(August 1997):569-579.
3351. A.M. Rajnicek, "Bacterial galvanotropism: mechanisms and applications," Sci. Prog. 77(1993-94):139-151.
3352. W. Takken, "Synthesis and future challenges: The response of mosquitos to host odours," Ciba Found. Symp. 200(1996):302-312, 312-320(discussion).
3353. N. Calander, K.A. Karlsson, P.G. Nyholm, I. Pascher, "On the dissection of binding epitopes on carbohydrate receptors for microbes using molecular modelling," Biochemie 70(November 1988):1673-1682.
3354. P.V. Balaji, P.K. Qasba, V.S. Rao, "Molecular dynamics simulations of asialoglycoprotein receptor ligands," Biochemistry 32(30 November 1993):12599-12611; "Molecular dynamics simulations of high-mannose oligosaccharides," Glycobiology 4(August 1994):497-515; "Molecular dynamics simulations of hybrid and complex type oligosaccharides," Int. J. Biol. Macromol. 18(February 1996):101-114.
3355. T. Peters, B.M. Pinto, "Structure and dynamics of oligosaccharides: NMR and modeling studies," Curr. Opin. Struct. Biol. 6(October 1996):710-720.
3356. J. Beuth, H.L. Ko, G. Uhlenbruck, G. Pulverer, "Lectin-mediated bacterial adhesion to human tissue," Eur. J. Clin. Microbiol. 6(October 1987):591-593.

3357. L.G. Baum, J.C. Paulson, "Sialyloligosaccharides of the respiratory epithelium in the selection of human influenza virus receptor specificity," Acta Histochem. Suppl. 40(1990):35-38.
3358. I.J. Rosenstein, C.T. Yuen, M.S. Stoll, T. Feizi, "Differences in the binding specificities of *Pseudomonas aeruginosa* M35 and *Escherichia coli* C600 for lipid-linked oligosaccharides with lactose-related core regions," Infect. Immun. 60(December 1992):5078-5084.
3359. Itzhak Ofek, Ronald J. Doyle, Bacterial Adhesion to Cells and Tissues, Chapman and Hall, New York, 1993.
3360. L. Hansson et al., "Carbohydrate specificity of the *Escherichia coli* P-pilus papG protein is mediated by its N-terminal part," Biochim. Biophys. Acta 1244(9 June 1995):377-383.
3361. N. Sharon, H. Lis, "Lectins — proteins with a sweet tooth: functions in cell recognition," Essays Biochem. 30(1995):59-75.
3362. Ronald J. Doyle, Itzhak Ofek, eds., Adhesion of Microbial Pathogens, Methods in Enzymology, Vol. 253, Academic Press, New York, 1995.
3363. B. Poolman et al., "Cation and sugar selectivity determinants in a novel family of transport proteins," Mol. Microbiol. 19(March 1996):911-922.
3364. W.I. Weis, K. Drickamer, "Structural basis of lectin-carbohydrate recognition," Annu. Rev. Biochem. 65(1996):441-473.
3365. M. Mouricout, "Interactions between the enteric pathogen and the host. An assortment of bacterial lectins and a set of glycoconjugate receptors," Adv. Exp. Med. Biol. 412(1997):109-123.
3366. Hans-Joachim Gabius, Sigrun Gabius, eds., Glycosciences: Status and Perspectives, Chapman and Hall, New York, 1997.
3367. K.J. Yarema, C.R. Bertozzi, "Chemical approaches to glycobiology and emerging carbohydrate-based therapeutic agents," Curr. Opin. Chem. Biol. 2(February 1998):49-61.
3368. M. Jacques, S.E. Paradis, "Adhesin-receptor interactions in *Pasteurellaceae*," FEMS Microbiol. Rev. 22(April 1998):45-59.
3369. K.A. Karlsson, "Meaning and therapeutic potential of microbial recognition of host glycoconjugates," Mol. Microbiol. 29(July 1998):1-11; "Microbial recognition of target-cell glycoconjugates," Curr. Opin. Struct. Biol. 5(October 1995):622-635.
3370. C.A. Lingwood, "Oligosaccharide receptors for bacteria: A view to a kill," Curr. Opin. Chem. Biol. 2(December 1998):695-700.
3371. E. Arnold, M.G. Rossmann, "Analysis of the structure of a common cold virus, human rhinovirus 14, refined at a resolution of 3.0 A," J. Mol. Biol. 211(20 February 1990):763-801.
3372. L. Haarr, S. Skulstad, "The herpes simplex virus type 1 particle: Structure and molecular functions," APMIS 102(May 1994):321-346.
3373. A.C. Steven, B.L. Trus, F.P. Booy, N. Cheng, A. Zlotnick, J.R. Caston, J.F. Conway, "The making and breaking of symmetry in virus capsid assembly: glimpses of capsid biology from cryoelectron microscopy," FASEB J. 11(August 1997):733-742.
3374. Allan Granoff, Robert G. Webster, eds., Encyclopedia of Virology, Second Edition, Academic Press, New York, 1999.
3375. "Family: Animal virus proteins, mammalian viruses, protein domains," http://strucbio.biologie.uni-konstanz.de/scop-1.37/data/scop.1.002.008.001.004.html.
3376. W. Silva, H. Maldonado, G. Chompre, N. Mayol, "Caveolae: a new subcellular transport organelle," Bol. Asoc. Med. P. R. 90(January-March 1998):30-33.
3377. A. Schlegel et al., "Crowded little caves: structure and function of caveolae," Cell Signal 10(July 1998):457-463.
3378. T. Fujimoto, H. Hagiwara, T. Aoki, H. Kogo, R. Nomura, "Caveolae: From a Morphological Point of View," J. Electron. Microsc. (Tokyo) 47(1998):451-460.
3379. D. Sviridov, "Intracellular cholesterol trafficking," Histol. Histopathol. 14(January 1999):305-319.
3380. P.M. Harrison, P. Arosio, "The ferritins: Molecular properties, iron storage function and cellular regulation," Biochim. Biophys. Acta 1275(31 July 1996):161-203.
3381. L.B. Kong, A.C. Siva, L.H. Rome, P.L. Stewart, "Structure of the vault, a ubiquitous cellular component," Structure 7(April 1999):371-379.
3382. D.C. Chugani, L.H. Rome, N.L. Kedersha, "Evidence that vault ribonucleoprotein particles localize to the nuclear pore complex," J. Cell Sci. 106(September 1993):23-29.
3383. L.M. Grimm, B.A. Osborne, "Apoptosis and the proteasome," Results Probl. Cell Differ. 23(1999):209-228.
3384. Immo E. Scheffler, Mitochondria, John Wiley and Sons, New York, 1999.
3385. D.B. Callerio, P. Revelant, L. Di Filippo, "Cristae of a triangular aspect in the mitochondria of the corneal cells," Boll. Ist. Sieroter Milan 54(1975):492-499. In Italian.
3386. B. Fernandez, I. Suarez, C. Gianonatti, "Fine structure of astrocytic mitochondria in the hypothalamus of the hamster," J. Anat. 137(October 1983):483-488.
3387. P.J. Lea, R.J. Temkin, K.B. Freeman, G.A. Mitchell, B.H. Robinson, "Variations in mitochondrial ultrastructure and dynamics observed by high resolution scanning electron microscopy (HRSEM)," Microsc. Res. Tech. 27(1 March 1994):269-277.
3388. F.P. Prince, "Mitochondrial cristae diversity in human Leydig cells: A revised look at cristae morphology in these steroid-producing cells," Anat. Rec. 254(1 April 1999):534-541.
3389. F.A. Steinbock, G. Wiche, "Plectin: A Cytolinker by Design," Biol. Chem. 380(February 1999):151-158. See also: G. Wiche, "Role of plectin in cytoskeleton organization and dynamics," J. Cell. Sci. 111(September 1998):2477-2486.
3390. C. Ruhrberg, F.M. Watt, "The plakin family: versatile organizers of cytoskeletal architecture," Curr. Opin. Genet. Dev. 7(June 1997):392-397.
3391. J.A. Guttman, D.J. Mulholland, A.W. Vogl, "Plectin is concentrated at intercellular junctions and at the nuclear surface in morphologically differentiated rat Sertoli cells," Anat. Rec. 254(March 1999):418-428.
3392. K. Andra, B. Nikolic, M. Stocher, D. Dreckhahn, G. Wiche, "Not just scaffolding: plectin regulates actin dynamics in cultured cells," Genes Dev. 12(1 November 1998):3442-3451.
3393. B.J. Foets, J.J. van den Oord, V.J. Desmet, L. Missotten, "Cytoskeletal filament typing of human corneal endothelial cells," Cornea 9(October 1990):312-317.
3394. I. Bruderman, R. Cohen, O. Leitner, R. Ronah, A. Guber, B. Griffel, B. Geiger, "Immunocytochemical characterization of lung tumors in fine-needle aspiration," Cancer 66(15 October 1990):1817-1827.
3395. B. Czernobilsky, "Intermediate filaments in ovarian tumors," Int. J. Gynecol. Pathol. 12(April 1993):166-169.
3396. W. Gotz, M. Kasper, G. Fischer, R. Herken, "Intermediate filament typing of the human embryonic and fetal notochord," Cell Tissue Res. 280(May 1995):455-462.
3397. J. Southgate, P. Harnden, L.K. Trejdosiewicz, "Cytokeratin expression patterns in normal and malignant urothelium: a review of the biological and diagnostic implications," Histol. Histopathol. 14(April 1999):657-664.
3398. K.L. Vikstrom, S.H. Seiler, R.L. Sohn, M. Strauss, A. Weiss, R.E. Welikson, L.A. Leinwand, "The vertebrate myosin heavy chain: Genetics and assembly properties," Cell Struct. Funct. 22(February 1997):123-129.
3399. M.H. Stromer, "The cytoskeleton in skeletal, cardiac and smooth muscle cells," Histol. Histopathol. 13(January 1998):283-291.
3400. B.M. Millman, "The filament lattice of striated muscle," Physiol. Rev. 78(April 1998):359-391.
3401. S.R. Todd, J.A. Kitching, "Cultivation of *Acanthamoeba castellanii*, Neff Strain, at high hydrostatic pressures," J. Protozool. 22(February 1975):105-106.
3402. N.S. Wang, "Anatomy and physiology of the pleural space," Clin. Chest Med. 6(March 1985):3-16.
3403. N. Pante, U. Aebi, "Molecular dissection of the nuclear pore complex," Crit. Rev. Biochem. Mol. Biol. 31(April 1996):153-199.
3404. L.F. Pemberton, G. Blobel, J.S. Rosenblum, "Transport routes through the nuclear pore complex," Curr. Opin. Cell Biol. 10(June 1998):392-399.
3405. D. Stoffler, B. Fahrenkrog, U. Aebi, "The nuclear pore complex: From molecular architecture to functional dynamics," Curr. Opin. Cell Biol. 11(June 1999):391-401.
3406. H. Ris, "High-resolution field-emission scanning electron microscopy of nuclear pore complex," Scanning 19(August 1997):368-375.
3407. S.A. Rutherford, M.W. Goldberg, T.D. Allen, "Three-dimensional visualization of the route of protein import: the role of nuclear pore complex substructures," Exp. Cell Res. 10(April 1997):146-160.
3408. N. Pante, U. Aebi, "Sequential binding of import ligands to distinct nucleopore regions during their nuclear import," Science 273(20 September 1996):1729-1732.
3409. V.C. Cordes, H.R. Rackwitz, S. Reidenbach, "Mediators of nuclear protein import target karyophilic proteins to pore complexes of cytoplasmic annulate lamellae," Exp. Cell Res. 237(15 December 1997):419-433.
3410. C. Cremer et al., "Nuclear architecture and the induction of chromosomal aberrations," Mutat. Res. 366(November 1996):97-116.
3411. P.C. Park, U. De Boni, "A specific conformation of the territory of chromosome 17 locates ERBB-2 sequences to a DNase-hypersensitive domain at the nuclear periphery," Chromosoma 107(May 1998):87-95.
3412. L.G. Koss, "Characteristics of chromosomes in polarized normal human bronchial cells provide a blueprint for nuclear organization," Cytogenet. Cell Genet. 82(1998):230-237.
3413. D. Zink, H. Bornfleth, A. Visser, C. Cremer, T. Cremer, "Organization of early and late replicating DNA in human chromosome territories," Exp. Cell Res. 247(25 February 1999):176-188.
3414. A.E. Visser, R. Eils, A. Jauch, G. Little, P.J. Bakker, T. Cremer, J.A. Aten, "Spatial distributions of early and late replicating chromatin in interphase chromosome territories," Exp. Cell Res. 243(15 September 1998):398-407
3415. D. Zink, T. Cremer, R. Saffrich, R. Fischer, M.F. Trendelenburg, W. Ansorge, E.H. Stelzer, "Structure and dynamics of human interphase chromosome territories in vivo," Hum. Genet. 102(February 1998):241-251.
3416. L. Solovjeva et al., "Conformation of replicated segments of chromosome fibres in human S-phase nucleus," Chromosome Res. 6(December 1998):595-602.
3417. C. Munkel et al., "Compartmentalization of interphase chromosomes observed in simulation and experiment," J. Mol. Biol. 285(22 January 1999):1053-1065.
3418. P. Loidl, A. Eberharter, "Nuclear matrix and the cell cycle," Int. Rev. Cytol. 162B(1995):377-403.
3419. M.A. Mancini, D. He, I.I. Ouspenski, B.R. Brinkley, "Dynamic continuity of nuclear and mitotic matrix proteins in the cell cycle," J. Cell Biochem. 62(August 1996):158-164.
3420. J.R. Davie, "Nuclear matrix, dynamic histone acetylation and transcriptionally active chromatin," Mol. Biol. Rep. 24(August 1997):197-207.

3421. J.P. Bidwell, M. Alvarez, H. Feister, J. Onyia, J. Hock, "Nuclear matrix proteins and osteoblast gene expression," J. Bone Miner. Res. 13(February 1998):155-167.
3422. J.H. Hughes, M.B. Cohen, "Nuclear matrix proteins and their potential applications to diagnostic pathology," Am. J. Clin. Pathol. 111(February 1999):267-274.
3423. S.K. Keesee, J.V. Briggman, G. Thill, Y.J. Wu, "Utilization of nuclear matrix proteins for cancer diagnosis," Crit. Rev. Eukaryot. Gene Expr. 6(1996):189-214.
3424. P.T. Moen Jr., K.P. Smith, J.B. Lawrence, "Compartmentalization of specific pre-mRNA metabolism: an emerging view," Human Mol. Genet. 4(1995):1779-1789.
3425. R.C. Gibbs, "Fundamentals of dermatoglyphics," Arch. Dermatol. 96(Dece,ber 1967):721-725.
3426. H. Shiono, "Dermatoglyphics in medicine," Am. J. Forensic Med. Pathol. 7(June 1986):120-126.
3427. B.A. Schaumann, J.M. Opitz, "Clinical aspects of dermatoglyphics," Birth Defects Orig. Artic. Ser. 27(1991):193-228.
3428. Chris C. Plato, Ralph M. Garruto, Blanka A. Schaumann, Dermatoglyphics: Science in Transition, John Wiley and Sons, New York, 1991.
3429. T. Togawa, "Non-contact skin emissivity: Measurement from reflectance using step change in ambient radiation temperature," Clin. Phys. Physiol. Meas. 10(February 1989):39-48.
3430. A. Boylan, C.J. Martin, G.G. Gardner, "Infrared emissivity of burn wounds," Clin. Phys. Physiol. Meas. 13(May 1992):125-127.
3431. Newport Electonics, "Table of Total Emissivity: Non-Metals," 26 January 1999, see at: http://www.newport2.com/Databook/table2.htm.
3432. "PharmaSeq, Inc.," see at: http://www.PharmaSeq.com/. See also: Vicki Glaser, "Trends in Pharmacogenomics," Gen. Eng. News 19(15 June 1999):17, 34.
3433. P. Duchamp-Viret, M.A. Chaput, A. Duchamp, "Odor Response Properties of Rat Olfactory Receptor Neurons," Science 284(25 June 1999):2171-2174.
3434. Charles A. Czeisler et al., "Stability, Precision, and Near-24-Hour Period of the Human Circadian Pacemaker," Science 284(25 June 1999):2177-2181.
3435. Eduardo Perozo, D. Marien Cortes, Luis G. Cuello, "Structural Rearrangements Underlying K^+-Channel Activation Gating," Science 285(2 July 1999):73-78.
3436. Benoit Roux, Roderick MacKinnon, "The Cavity and Pore Helices in the KcsA K^+ Channel: Electrostatic Stabilization of Monovalent Cations," Science 285(2 July 1999):100-102.
3437. Bojan Zagrovic, Richard Aldrich, "For the Latest Information, Tune to Channel KcsA," Science 285(2 July 1999):59-61.
3438. Dieter Britz, Chemistry Department, Aarhus University, "Britz's Cold Nuclear Fusion Bibliography," see at: http://kemi.aau.dk/~db/fusion/.
3439. A. Rambourg, Y. Clermont, "Three-dimensional electron microscopy: structure of the Golgi apparatus," Eur. J. Cell Biol. 51(April 1990):189-200.
3440. M.S. Ladinsky, D.N. Mastronarde, J.R. McIntosh, K.E. Howell, L.A. Staehelin, "Golgi structure in three dimensions: functional insights from the normal rat kidney cell," J. Cell Biol. 144(22 March 1999):1135-1149.
3441. R.D. Klausner, J.G. Donaldson, J. Lippincott-Schwartz, "Brefeldin A: insights into the control of membrane traffic and organelle structure," J. Cell Biol. 116(March 1992):1071-1080. See also: J.G. Donaldson, D. Finazzi, R.D. Klausner, "Brefeldin A inhibits Golgi membrane-catalysed exchange of guanine nucleotide onto ARF protein," Nature 360(26 November 1992):350-352.
3442. J.B. Helms, J.E. Rothman, "Inhibition by brefeldin A of a Golgi membrane enzyme that catalyses exchange of guanine nucleotide bound to ARF," Nature 360(26 November 1992):352-354.
3443. B.S. Glick, T. Elston, G. Oster, "A cisternal maturation mechanism can explain the asymmetry of the Golgi stack," FEBS Lett. 414(8 September 1997):177-181.
3444. A.A. Mironov, A. Luini, R. Buccione, "Constitutive transport between the trans-Golgi network and the plasma membrane according to the maturation model: A hypothesis," FEBS Lett. 440(27 November 1998):99-102. See also: A. Mironov Jr., A. Luini, A. Mironov, "A synthetic model of intra-Golgi traffic," FASEB J. 12(February 1998):249-252.
3445. Bernard B. Allan, William E. Balch, "Protein Sorting by Directed Maturation of Golgi Compartments," Science 285(2 July 1999):63-66.
3446. Steven L. Garrett, "Thermoacoustic Refrigerators and Engines," see at: http://www.arl.psu.edu/techareas/acsrefrige/acsrefrige.html.
3447. J. Scheuer, M. Orenstein, "Optical Vortices Crystals: Spontaneous Generation in Nonlinear Semiconductor Microcavities," Science 285(9 July 1999):230-233.
3448. M. Marsh, A. Helenius, "Adsorptive endocytosis of Semliki Forest virus," J. Mol. Biol. 142(25 September 1980):439-454.
3449. I. Gaidarov, F. Santini, R. Warren, J.H. Keen, Nature Cell Biol. 1(1999):1 et seq.
3450. C.J. Smith, N. Grigorieff, B.M. Pearse, "Clathrin coats at 21 A resolution: a cellular assembly designed to recycle multiple membrane receptors," EMBO J. 17(1 September 1998):4943-4953.
3451. A. Musacchio, C.J. Smith, A.M. Roseman, S.C. Harrison, T. Kirchhausen, B.M. Pearse, "Functional organization of clathrin in coats: combining electron cryomicroscopy and X-ray crystallography," Mol. Cell 3(June 1999):761-770.
3452. M. Marsh, H.T. McMahon, "The Structural Era of Endocytosis," Science 285(9 July 1999):215-220.
3453. Arash Grakoui, Shannon K. Bromley, Cenk Sumen, Mark M. Davis, Andrey S. Shaw, Paul M. Allen, Michael L. Dustin, "The Immunological Synapse: A Molecular Machine Controlling T Cell Activation," Science 285(9 July 1999):221-227.
3454. Bernard Malissen, "Dancing the Immunological Two-Step," Science 285(9 July 1999):207-208.
3455. S. Valitutti, S. Muller, M. Cella, E. Padovan, A. Lanzavecchia, "Serial triggering of many T-cell receptors by a few peptide-MHC complexes," Nature 375(11 May 1995):148-151.
3456. C.V. Harding, E.R. Unanue, "Quantitation of antigen-presenting cell MHC class II/peptide complexes necessary for T-cell stimulation," Nature 346(9 August 1990):574-576.
3457. J.O. Schmidt, S. Yamane, M. Matsuura, C.K. Starr, "Hornet venoms: Lethalities and lethal capacities," Toxicon 24(1986):950-954.
3458. A.N. Santana et al., "Partial sequence and toxic effects of granulitoxin, a neurotoxic peptide from the sea anemone *Bundosoma granulifera*," Braz. J. Med. Biol. Res. 31(October 1998):1335-1338.
3459. A.E. Eno, R.S. Konya, J.O. Ibu, "Biological properties of a venom extract from the sea anemone, *Bunodosoma cavernata*," Toxicon 36(December 1998):2013-2020.
3460. H. Rochat et al., "Maurotoxin, a four disulfide bridges scorpion toxin acting on K^+ channels," Toxicon 36(November 1998):1609-1611.
3461. D.M. Gill, "Bacterial toxins: A table of lethal amounts," Microbiol. Rev. 46(March 1982):86-94.
3462. L.C. Sellin, "The action of botulinum toxin at the neuromuscular junction," Med. Biol. 59(February 1981):11-20.
3463. O. Fodstad, S. Olsnes, A. Pihl, "Toxicity, distribution and elimination of the cancerostatic lectins abrin and ricin after parenteral injection into mice," Br. J. Cancer 34(October 1976):418-425.
3464. V.J. Christiansen, C.H. Hsu, K.J. Dormer, C.P. Robinson, "The cardiovascular effects of ricin in rabbits," Pharmacol. Toxicol. 74(March 1994):148-152.
3465. T. Fu, C. Burbage, E.P. Tagge, T. Brothers, M.C. Willingham, A.E. Frankel, "Ricin toxin contains three lectin sites which contribute to its in vivo toxicity," Int. J. Immunopharmacol. 18(December 1996):685-692.
3466. A.A. Lugnier, E.E. Creppy, G. Dirheimer, "Ricin, the toxic protein of the castor-oil plant (*Ricinis communis L*). Structure and properties," Pathol. Biol. (Paris) 28(February 1980):127-139.
3469. Johnson Matthey Company, "Sapphire Properties: Sapphire Technical Data," 3 December 1997, see at: http://www.jmcrystar.com/sapphire.htm.
3470. W.A. Hagins, P.D. Ross, R.L. Tate, S. Yoshikami, "Transduction heats in retinal rods: tests of the role of cGMP by pyroelectric calorimetry," Proc. Natl. Acad. Sci. USA 86(February 1989):1224-1228.
3471. E.A. Liberman, "Analog-Digital Molecular Cell Computer," Biosystems 11(August 1979):111-124.
3472. C.J. Tourenne, "A model of the electric field of the brain at EEG and microwave frequencies," J. Theoret. Biol. 116(October 1985):495-507.
3473. K.R. Foster, E.D. Finch, "Microwave Hearing: Evidence for Thermoacoustic Auditory Stimulation by Pulsed Microwaves," Science 185(19 July 1974):256-258.
3474. J.C. Lin, "Microwave-induced hearing: some preliminary theoretical observations," J. Microwave Power 11(September 1976):295-298; "Microwave auditory effect — a comparison of some possible transduction mechanisms," J. Microwave Power 11(March 1976):77-81.
3475. W.T. Joines, "Reception of microwaves by the brain," Med. Res. Eng. 12(1976):8-12.
3476. J.C. Lin, R.J. Meltzer, F.K. Redding, "Microwave-evoked brainstem potentials in cats," J. Microwave Power 14(September 1979):291-296.
3477. A.H. Frey, E. Coren, "Holographic Assessment of a Hypothesized Microwave Hearing Mechanism," Science 206(12 October 1979):232-234. See also: C.K. Chou, A.W. Guy, K.R. Foster, R. Galambos, D.R. Justesen, "Holographic Assessment of Microwave Hearing," Science 209(5 September 1980):1143-1145.
3478. J.A. D'Andrea, "Microwave radiation absorption: behavioral effects," Health Phys. 61(July 1991):29-40.
3479. R.L. Seaman, R.M. Lebovitz, "Auditory unit responses to single-pulse and twin-pulse microwave stimuli," Hear. Res. 26(1987):105-116.
3480. R.L. Seaman, R.M. Lebovitz, "Thresholds of cat cochlear nucleus neurons to microwave pulses," Bioelectromagnetics 10(1989):147-160.
3481. L. Puranen, K. Jokela, "Radiation hazard assessment of pulsed microwave radars," J. Microwave Power Electromagn. Energy 31(1996):165-177.
3482. I. Tasaki, K. Kusano, P.M. Byrne, "Rapid mechanical and thermal changes in the garfish olfactory nerve associated with a propagated impulse," Biophys. J. 55(June 1989):1033-1040.
3483. J.V. Howarth, R.D. Keynes, J.M. Ritchie, A. von Muralt, "The heat production associated with the passage of a single impulse in pike olfactory nerve fibres," J. Physiol. (London) 249(July 1975):349-368.
3484. J.V. Howarth, J.M. Ritchie, "The recovery heat production in non-myelinated garfish olfactory nerve fibres," J. Physiol. (London) 292(July 1979):167-175.
3485. J.V. Howarth, J.M. Ritchie, D. Stagg, "The initial heat production in garfish olfactory nerve fibers," Proc. R. Soc. Lond. B. Biol. Sci. 205(31 August 1979):347-367.
3486. Peter Coy, "A steam engine smaller than an ant's whisker," Business Week (18 October 1993):67.

3487. Corbett Merrill, "Will Nanotechnology, the Manufacturing of Objects Atom by Atom, be a Feasible Medical Breakthrough?" 12 June 1995; see at: http://www.cslab.vt.edu/~comerril/Strand.htm.

3488. Steven C. Vetter, "Oak Ridge National Laboratory's Dr. Noid Describes Simulation Software to Minnesota Study Group," Foresight Update No. 23, 30 November 1995, p.9.

3489. B.E. Nordenstrom, "Impact of biologically closed electric circuits (BCEC) on structure and function," Integr. Physiol. Behav. Sci. 27(October-December 1992):285-303; "The paradigm of biologically closed electric circuits (BCEC) and the formation of an International Association (IABC) for BCEC," Eur. J. Surg. Suppl. 574(1994):7-23.

3490. B.E. Nordenstrom, A.C. Kinn, J. Elbarouni, "Electric modification of kidney function. The excretion of radiographic contrast media and adriamycin," Invest. Radiol. 26(February 1991):157-161.

3491. B.E. Nordenstrom, "Electrical pulses appear in the inferior vena cava and abdominal aorta at contraction of leg muscles," Physiol. Chem. Phys. Med. NMR 24(1992):147-152; B.E. Nordenstrom, H. Larsson, M. Lindqvist, "Potential differences in the inferior vena cava and between cava and extravascular electrode at leg contraction in man," Physiol. Chem. Phys. Med. NMR 24(1992):153-158.

3492. V. Parsonnet, L. Gilbert, I.R. Zucker, R. Werres, T. Atherly, M. Manhardt, J. Cort, "A decade of nuclear pacing," Pacing Clin. Electrophysiol. 7(January 1984):90-95.

3493. M.R. Shorten, "The energetics of running and running shoes," J. Biomech. 26(Suppl. 1, 1993):41-51.

3494. A. Forner, A.C. Garcia, E. Alcantara, J. Ramiro, J.V. Hoyos, P. Vera, "Properties of shoe insert materials related to shock wave transmission during gait," Foot Ankle Int. 16(December 1995):778-786.

3495. T. Fahraeus, L.O. Almquist, "Cellular telephones may interfere with cardiac stimulators. Yuppie telephones and alarms are hazardous for patients with pacemakers," Lakartidningen 92(25 October 1995):4009-4010. In Swedish.

3496. K.A. Ellenbogen, M.A. Wood, "Cellular phones and pacemakers: urgent call or wrong number?" J. Am. Coll. Cardiol. 27(May 1996):1478-1479.

3497. W. Irnich, "Mobile telephones and pacemakers," Pacing Clin. Electrophysiol. 19(October 1996):1407-409.

3498. M. Roelke, A.D. Bernstein, "Cardiac pacemakers and cellular telephones," N. Engl. J. Med. 336(22 May 1997):1518-1519. See also: B.D. Zuckerman, M.J. Shein, J.T. Danzi, "Cardiac pacemakers and cellular phones," N. Engl. J. Med. 337(2 October 1997):1006-1008.

3499. Urless Norton Lanham, "Why Do Insects Have Six Legs?" Science 113(8 June 1951):663.

3500. Keir Pearson, "The Control of Walking," Scientific American 235(December 1976):72-86.

3501. F.V. Paladino, J.R. King, "Energetic cost of terrestrial locomotion: biped and quadruped runners compared," Rev. Can. Biol. 38(December 1979):321-323.

3502. E. Foth, U. Bassler, "Leg movements of stick insects walking with five legs on a treadwheel and with one leg on a motor-driven belt," Biol. Cybern 51(1985):313-318, 319-324.

3503. M.H. Raibert, "Trotting, pacing and bounding by a quadruped robot," J. Biomech. 23(Suppl. 1, 1990):79-98.

3504. R.J. Full, M.S. Tu, "Mechanics of six-legged runners," J. Exp. Biol. 148(January 1990):129-146; "Mechanics of a rapid running insect: two-, four- and six-legged locomotion," J. Exp. Biol. 156(March 1991):215-231.

3505. C.D. Zhang, S.M. Song, "A study of the stability of generalized wave gaits," Math. Biosci. 115(May 1993):1-32.

3506. P. Nanua, K.J. Waldron, "Energy comparison between trot, bound, and gallop using a simple model," J. Biomech. Eng. 117(November 1995):466-473.

3507. R. Kram, B. Wong, R.J. Full, "Three-dimensional kinematics and limb kinetic energy of running cockroaches," J. Exp. Biol. 200(July 1997):1919-1929.

3508. W.H. Ko, B.P. Bergmann, R. Plonsey, "Data acquisition system for body surface potential mapping," J. Bioeng. 2(April 1978):33-46.

3509. A.U. Igamberdiev, "Foundations of metabolic organization: coherence as a basis of computational properties in metabolic networks," Biosystems 50(April 1999):1-16.

3510. W.H. Ko, S.P. Liang, C.D. Fung, "Design of radio-frequency powered coils for implant instruments," Med. Biol. Eng. Comput. 15(November 1977):634-640.

3511. Erich Hausmann, Edgar P. Slack, Physics, U.S. Naval Academy Edition, D. van Nostrand Company, New York, 1944.

3512. G. Fontenier, M. Mourot, "Coating evolution with an implantable biological battery," Biomed. Eng. 11(August 1976):273-277.

3513. C.L. Strohl Jr., R.D. Scott, W.J. Frezel, S.K. Wolfson Jr., "Studies of bioelectric power sources for cardiac pacemakers," Trans. Am. Soc. Artif. Intern. Organs 12(1966):318-328.

3514. J.A. Armour, O.Z. Roy, W.B. Firor, R.W. Wehnert, D.C. MacGregor, K. Sindhavananda, W.G. Bigelow, "A batteryless biological cardiovascular pacemaker," Surg. Forum 17(1966):164-165.

3515. C.C. Enger, F.A. Simeone, "Biologically energized cardiac pacemaker: in vivo experience with dogs," Nature 218(13 April 1968):180-181.

3516. G. Benkert, W. Fabian, "Can an electric pacemaker be powered by the body's own energy? A medico-technical speculation," Fortschr. Med. 99(27 August 1981):1211-1213.

3517. W. Greatbatch, "Implantable Power-Sources: A Review," J. Med. Eng. Technol. 8(March-April 1984):56-63.

3518. T.B. Fryer, "Power sources for implanted telemetry systems," Biotelemetry 1(1974):31-40.

3519. M.A. Acker, R.L. Hammond, J.D. Mannion, S. Salmons, L.W. Stephenson, "Skeletal Muscle as the Potential Power Source for a Cardiovascular Pump: Assessment In Vivo," Science 236(17 April 1987):324-327.

3520. C. Li, J. Odim, A. Zibaitis, C. Desrosiers, R.C. Chiu, "Pulmonary artery counterpulsation with a skeletal muscle power source," ASAIO Trans. 36(July-September 1990):M382-M386.

3521. T. Doi, T. Mitsui, S. Matsushita, T. Tsutsui, M. Hori, "Efficacy of a biomechanical counterpulsation device powered by skeletal muscle for right heart assist," ASAIO Trans. 36(July-September 1990):M389-M392.

3522. M.E. Talaat, J.H. Kraft, R.A. Cowley, A.H. Khazei, "Biological Electrical Power Extraction from Blood to Power Cardiac Pacemakers," IEEE Trans. Biomed. Eng. 14(October 1967):263-265. See also: J.J. Konikoff, "Comments on `Biological Electric Power Extraction from Blood to Power Cardiac Pacemakers'," IEEE Trans. Biomed. Eng. 15(July 1968):232.

3523. J.F. Antaki, G.E. Bertocci, E.C. Green, A. Nadeem, T. Rintoul, R.L. Kormos, B.P. Griffith, "A gait-powered autologous battery charging system for artificial organs," ASAIO J. 41(July-September 1995):M588-M595.

3524. Robert Goff, "Aurora Borealis in a Rock," Forbes 163(5 April 1999):158-159.

3525. M.M. van Greevenbroek, T.W. de Bruin, "Chylomicron synthesis by intestinal cells in vitro and in vivo," Atherosclerosis 141(December 1998):S9-S16; see related papers, pp. S25-S107.

3526. H.T. Tien, Z. Salamon, A. Ottova, "Lipid bilayer-based sensors and biomolecular electronics," Crit. Rev. Biomed. Eng. 18(1991):323-340.

3527. E. Weidlich, G. Richter, F.V. Sturm, J.R. Rao, "Animal experiments with biogalvanic and biofuel cells," Biomater. Med. Devices Artif. Organs 4(1976):277-06.

3528. V.P. Satinsky, J. Cassel, A. Salkind, "Cardiac pacemakers powered by biogalvanic cells," Surg. Forum 22(1971):156-158.

3529. J.K. Cywinski, A.W. Hahn, M.F. Nichols, J.R. Easley, "Performance of implanted biogalvanic pacemakers," Pacing Clin. Electrophysiol. 1(January 1978):117-125.

3530. M.M. Misro, H. Kaur, S. Mahajan, S.K. Guha, "An intravasal non-occlusive contraceptive device in rats," J. Reprod. Fertil. 65(May 1982):9-13.

3531. H. Vais, I. Ardelean, D.G. Margineanu, "Biolelectrical conversion in sensors with living cells," Physiologie 26(October-December 1989):349-353.

3532. X. Hu, A. Damjanovic, T. Ritz, K. Schulten, "Architecture and mechanism of the light-harvesting apparatus of purple bacteria," Proc. Natl. Acad. Sci. USA 95(1998):5935-5941. See also: "Reviews on light-harvesting complex II of purple bacteria," 1 April 1999, at: http://metallo.scripps.edu/PROMISE/LH2PB_REV.html.

3533. Mark Caldwell, "The Amazing All-Natural Light Machine," Discover (December 1995); see also: http://www.discover.com/archive/index.html.

3534. R.D. Hoffman, S.E. Woosley, "Stellar Nucleosynthesis Data. Table 5B. Reactions Included Below 12C," Tables of Reaction Rates for Nucleosynthesis Charged Particle, Weak, and Neutrino Interactions, Version 92.1, 1992, see at: http://ie.lbl.gov/astro/hw92_1.html.

3535. L.R. Gavrilov, Tsirulnikov, I.A. Davies, "Application of focused ultrasound for the stimulation of neural structures," Ultrasound Med. Biol. 22(1996):179-192.

3536. K. Holmberg, U. Landstrom, B. Nordstrom, "Annoyance and discomfort during exposure to high-frequency noise from an ultrasonic washer," Percept. Mot. Skills 81(December 1995):819-827.

3537. A. Wright, I. Davies, J.G. Riddell, "Intra-articular ultrasonic stimulation and intracutaneous electrical stimulation: evoked potential and visual analogue scale data," Pain 52(February 1993):149-155.

3538. A.R. Williams, J. McHale, M. Bowditch, D.L. Miller, B. Reed, "Effects of MHz ultrasound on electrical pain threshold perception in humans," Ultrasound Med. Biol. 13(May 1987):249-258.

3539. T.G. van Leeuwen, C. Borst, "Fundamental laser-tissue interactions," Semin. Interv. Cardiol. 1(June 1996):121-128; see related papers, pp. 129-171.

3540. E.E. Manche, J.D. Carr, W.W. Haw, P.S. Hersh, "Excimer laser refractive surgery," West. J. Med. 169(July 1998):30-38.

3541. C.P. Collier, E.W. Wong, M. Belohradsky, F.M. Raymo, J.F. Stoddart, P.J. Kuekes, R.S. Williams, J.R. Heath, "Electronically Configurable Molecular-Based Logic Gates," Science 285(16 July 1999):391-394, 313-314 (discussion).

3542. Daniel Coore, Radhika Nagpal, "Implementing Reaction Diffusion on an Amorphous Computer," 1998 MIT Student Workshop on High Performance Computing in Science and Engineering, MIT/LCS/TR-737; see at: http://www-swiss.ai.mit.edu/~switz/amorphous/papers/Coore_Nagpal.ps.gz, and see abstract at: http://www-swiss.ai.mit.edu/~switz/amorphous/paperlisting.html.

3543. Ron Weiss, George Homsy, Radhika Nagpal, "Programming Biological Cells," paper presented at the 8th International Conference on Architectural Support for Programming Languages and Operating Systems (ASPLOS '98), Wild and Crazy Ideas Session, San Jose, CA, 1998; see at: http://www-swiss.ai.mit.edu/~rweiss/bio-programming/asplos98-talk.ps, and see abstract at: http://www-swiss.ai.mit.edu/~switz/amorphous/paperlisting.html.

3544. Ron Weiss, George Homsy, Thomas F. Knight, "Toward in vivo Digital Circuits," paper presented at Dimacs Workshop on Evolution as Computation, Princeton, NJ, January 1999; see at: http://www-swiss.ai.mit.edu/~rweiss/bio-programming/dimacs99-evocomp.ps (postscript version) or http://www-swiss.ai.mit.edu/~rweiss/bio-programming/dimacs99-evocomp-talk (html version), and see abstract at: http://www-swiss.ai.mit.edu/~switz/amorphous/paperlisting.html.
3545. P. Tandon, S.L. Diamond, "Hydrodynamic effects and receptor interactions of platelets and their aggregates in linear shear flow," Biophys. J. 73(November 1997):2819-2835.
3546. R.H. Yoon, B.S. Aksoy, "Hydrophobic Forces in Thin Water Films Stabilized by Dodecylammonium Chloride," J. Colloid. Interface Sci. 211(1 March 1999):1-10.
3547. A. Pierres, H. Feracci, V. Delmas, A.M. Benoliel, J.P. Thiery, P. Bongrand, "Experimental study of the interaction range and association rate of surface-attached cadherin 11," Proc. Natl. Acad. Sci. USA 95(4 August 1998):9256-9261.
3548. J.Z. Xia, T. Aerts, K. Donceel, J. Clauwaert, "Light scattering by bovine alpha-crystallin proteins in solution: hydrodynamic structure and interparticle interaction," Biophys. J. 66(March 1994):861-872.
3549. M. Tomoeda, M. Inuzuka, T. Date, "Bacterial sex pili," Prog. Biophys. Mol. Biol. 30(1975):23-56.
3550. R.D. Allen, R.W. Wolf, "Membrane recycling at the cytoproct of *Tetrahymena*," J. Cell Sci. 35(February 1979):217-227.
3551. K. Ogawa, "Four ATP-binding sites in the midregion of the β heavy chain of dynein," Nature 352(15 August 1991):643-645.
3552. C.J. Brokaw, "Mechanical components of motor enzyme function," Biophys. J. 73(August 1997):938-951.
3553. C. Shingyoji, H. Higuchi, M. Yoshimura, E. Katayama, T. Yanagida, "Dynein arms are oscillating force generators," Nature 393(18 June 1998):711-714.
3554. I. Minoura, T. Yagi, R. Kamiya, "Direct measurement of inter-doublet elasticity in flagellar axonemes," Cell Struct. Funct. 24(February 1999):27-33.
3555. M.J. Sanderson, M.A. Sleigh, "Ciliary activity of cultured rabbit tracheal epithelium: beat pattern and metachrony," J. Cell Sci. 47(February 1981):331-347.
3556. K.J. Ingels, F. Meeuwsen, H.L. van Strien, K. Graamans, E.H. Huizing, "Ciliary beat frequency and the nasal cycle," Eur. Arch. Otorhinolaryngol. 248(1990):123-126.
3557. K.J. Ingels, H.L. van Strien, K. Graamans, G.F. Smoorenburg, E.H. Huizing, "A study of the photoelectrical signal from human nasal cilia under several conditions," Acta Otolaryngol. (Stockholm) 112(September 1992):831-838.
3558. S. Gueron, K. Levit-Gurevich, "Computation of the internal forces in cilia: application to ciliary motion, the effects of viscosity, and cilia interactions," Biophys. J. 74(April 1998):1658-1676.
3559. K.M. Paknikar, "Bacterial catalytic processes for transformation of metals," Hindustan Antibiot. Bull. 35(February-May 1993):183-189.
3560. D.P. Kelly, J.K. Shergill, W.P. Lu, A.P. Wood, "Oxidative metabolism of inorganic sulfur compounds by bacteria," Antonie Van Leeuwenhoek 71(February 1997):95-107.
3561. B.E. Jones, W.D. Grant, A.W. Duckworth, G.G. Owenson, "Microbial diversity of soda lakes," Extremophiles 2(August 1998):191-200.
3562. J.L. van de Vossenberg, A.J. Driessen, W.N. Konings, "The essence of being extremophilic: the role of the unique archaeal membrane lipids," Extremophiles 2(August 1998):163-170.
3563. A. Matin, "pH homeostasis in acidophiles," Novartis Found. Symp. 221(1999):152-163, 163-166 (discussion).
3564. T. Wilson, J.W. Hastings, "Bioluminescence," Annu. Rev. Cell Dev. Biol. 14(1998):197-230.
3565. N. Duran, M.C. Marcucci, M.P. De Mello, A. Faljoni-Alario, "Enzymatically generated electronically excited molecules induce transformation of 4-thiouridine to uridine," Biochem. Biophys. Res. Commun. 117(28 December 1983):923-929.
3566. R.C. Allen, "Role of oxygen in phagocyte microbial action," Environ. Health Perspect. 102(Suppl. 10, December 1994):201-208.
3567. Y.F. Li, P.F. Heelis, A. Sancar, "Active site of DNA photolyase: tryptophan-306 is the intrinsic hydrogen atom donor essential for flavin radical photoreduction and DNA repair in vitro," Biochemistry 30(25 June 1991):6322-6329.
3568. S.T. Kim, P.F. Heelis, T. Okamura, Y. Hirata, N. Mataga, A. Sancar, "Determination of rates and yields of interchromophore (folate-flavin) energy transfer and intermolecular (flavin-DNA) electron transfer in *Escherichia coli* photolyase by time-resolved fluorescence and absorption spectroscopy," Biochemistry 30(26 November 1991):11262-11270.
3569. R.C. Venema, D.H. Hug, "Activation of urocanase from *Pseudomonas putida* by electronically excited triplet species," J. Biol. Chem. 260(5 October 1985):12190-12193.
3570. G.L. Indig, G. Cilento, "Peroxidase-promoted aerobic oxidation of 2-nitropropane: mechanism of excited state formation," Biochim. Biophys. Acta 923(19 March 1987):347-354.
3571. E. Cadenas, "Lipid peroxidation during the oxidation of haemoproteins by hydroperoxides. Relation to electronically excited state formation," J. Biolumin. Chemilumin. 4(July 1989):208-218.
3572. G. Cilento, A.L. Nascimento, "Generation of electronically excited triplet species at the cellular level: a potential source of genotoxicity," Toxicol. Lett. 67(April 1993):17-28.
3573. P.F. Heelis, A. Sancar, T. Okamura, "Excited quartet states in DNA photolyase," J. Photochem. Photobiol. B 16(December 1992):387-390.
3574. A.L. Nascimento, J.A. Escobar, G. Cilento, "The peroxidative metabolism of tenoxicam produces excited species," Photochem. Photobiol. 57(February 1993):362-366.
3575. Z. Karni, W.Z. Polishuk, A. Adoni, Y. Diamant, "Newtonian viscosity of the human cervical mucus during the menstrual cycle," Int. J. Fertil. 16(1971):185-188.
3576. D.P. Wolf, L. Blasco, M.A. Khan, M. Litt, "Human cervical mucus. II. Changes in viscoelasticity during the ovulatory menstrual cycle," Fertil. Steril. 28(January 1977):47-52.
3577. Y. Lotan, Y.Z. Diamant, "The value of simple tests in the detection of human ovulation," Int. J. Gynaecol. Obstet. 16(1978-79):309-313.
3578. H. Winet, S.R. Keller, "Spirillum swimming: theory and observations of propulsion by the flagellar bundle," J. Exp. Biol. 65(December 1976):577-602.
3579. R. Skalak, M. Sugihara-Seki, "Transient relative motion of two cells in a channel flow," Biorheology 25(1988):181-189.
3580. S.F. Goldstein, N.W. Charon, "Motility of the spirochete *Leptospira*," Cell Motil. Cytoskeleton 9(1988):101-110.
3581. D.B. Dusenbery, "Minimum size limit for useful locomotion by free-swimming microbes," Proc. Natl. Acad. Sci. USA 94(30 September 1997):10949-10954.
3582. D.B. Dusenbery, "Fitness landscapes for effects of shape on chemotaxis and other behaviors of bacteria," J. Bacteriol. 180(November 1998):5978-5983.
3583. M.D. Levin, C.J. Morton-Firth, W.N. Abouhamad, R.B. Bourret, D. Bray, "Origins of individual swimming behavior in bacteria," Biophys. J. 74(January 1998):175-181.
3584. M. Ramia, D.L. Tullock, N. Phan-Thien, "The role of hydrodynamic interaction in the locomotion of microorganisms," Biophys. J. 65(August 1993):755-778.
3585. K.C. Chen, R.M. Ford, P.T. Cummings, "Mathematical models for motile bacterial transport in cylindrical tubes," J. Theoret. Biol. 195(21 December 1998):481-504.
3586. M.V. Wright, M. Frantz, J.L. Van Houten, "Lithium fluxes in *Paramecium* and their relationship to chemoresponse," Biochim. Biophys. Acta 1107(30 June 1992):223-230.
3587. B. Foliguet, E. Puchelle, "Apical structure of human respiratory cilia," Bull. Eur. Physiopathol. Respir. 22(January-February 1986):43-47.
3588. G.J. Sibert, C.A. Speer, "Fine structure of nuclear division and microgametogony of *Eimeria nieschulzi Dieben*, 1924," Z. Parasitenkd. 66(1981):179-189.
3589. J. Bailey, D. Gingell, "Contacts of chick fibroblasts on glass: results and limitations of quantitative interferometry," J. Cell Sci. 90(June 1988):215-224.
3590. A.M. Romanenko, "Ultrastructural diagnostic markers of the urinary bladder precancer," Bull. Assoc. Anat. (Nancy) 73(March 1989):31-35.
3591. G.B. Schneider, S.M. Pockwinse, S. Billings-Gagliardi, "Binding of concanavalin-A to critical-point-dried and freeze-dried human lymphocytes," Am. J. Anat. 156(September 1979):121-129.
3592. G.A. Langer, "The structure and function of the myocardial cell surface," Am. J. Physiol. 235(November 1978):H461-H468.
3593. R.H. Adamson, G. Clough, "Plasma proteins modify the endothelial cell glycocalyx of frog mesenteric microvessels," J. Physiol. London 445(January 1992):473-486.
3594. D.E. Sims, M.M. Horne, "Non-aqueous fixative preserves macromolecules on the endothelial cell surface: an in situ study," Eur. J. Morphol. 32(March 1994):59-64, 31(December 1993):251-255.
3595. P.A. Santi, C.B. Anderson, "A newly identified surface coat on cochlear hair cells," Hear. Res. 27(1987):47-65.
3596. J. Nanduri, J.E. Dennis, T.L. Rosenberry, A.A. Mahmoud, A.M. Tartakoff, "Glycocalyx of bodies versus tails of *Schistosoma mansoni* cercariae. Lectin-binding, size, charge, and electron microscopic characterization," J. Biol. Chem 266(15 January 1991):1341-1347. See also: C.P. Chiang, J.P. Caulfield, "*Schistosoma mansoni*: ultrastructural demonstration of a miracidial glycocalyx that cross-reacts with antibodies raised against the cercarial glycocalyx," Exp. Parasitol. 67(October 1988):63-72; J.C. Samuelson, J.P. Caulfield, "The cercarial glycocalyx of *Schistosoma mansoni*," J. Cell Biol. 100(May 1985):1423-1434.
3597. G.K. Yates, D.L. Kirk, "Cochlear electrically evoked emissions modulated by mechanical transduction channels," J. Neurosci. 18(15 March 1998):1996-2003.
3598. Y.N. Shvarev, B. Canlon, "Receptor potential characteristics during direct stereocilia stimulation of isolated outer hair cells from the guinea-pig," Acta Physiol. Scand. 162(February 1998):155-164.
3599. R.S. Carvalho, J.E. Scott, D.M. Suga, E.H. Yen, "Stimulation of signal transduction pathways in osteoblasts by mechanical strain potentiated by parathyroid hormone," J. Bone Miner. Res. 9(July 1994):999-1011.
3600. D.M. Salter, J.E. Robb, M.O. Wright, "Electrophysiological responses of human bone cells to mechanical stimulation: evidence for specific integrin function in mechanotransduction," J. Bone Miner. Res. 12(July 1997):1133-1141.
3601. C.D. Toma, S. Ashkar, M.L. Gray, J.L. Schaffer, L.C. Gerstenfeld, "Signal transduction of mechanical stimuli is dependent on microfilament integrity: identification of osteopontin as a mechanically induced gene in osteoblasts," J. Bone Miner. Res. 12(October 1997):1626-1636.
3602. M. Wright, P. Jobanputra, C. Bavington, D.M. Salter, G. Nuki, "Effects of intermittent pressure-induced strain on the electrophysiology of cultured human chondrocytes: evidence for the presence of stretch-activated membrane ion channels," Clin. Sci. (Colch.) 90(January 1990):61-71.

3603. K. Kada, K. Yasui, K. Naruse, K. Kamiya, I. Kodama, J. Toyama, "Orientation change of cardiocytes induced by cyclic stretch stimulation: time dependency and involvement of protein kinases," J. Mol. Cell. Cardiol. 31(January 1999):247-259.

3604. C.R. Jacobs, C.E. Yellowley, B.R. Davis, Z. Zhou, J.M. Cimbala, H.J. Donahue, "Differential effect of steady versus oscillating flow on bone cells," J. Biomech. 31(November 1998):969-976.

3605. J.H. Yang, W.H. Briggs, P. Libby, R.T. Lee, "Small mechanical strains selectively suppress matrix metalloproteinase-1 expression by human vascular smooth muscle cells," J. Biol. Chem. 273(13 March 1998):6550-6555.

3606. M. Sokabe et al., "Mechanotransduction and intracellular signaling mechanisms of stretch-induced remodeling in endothelial cells," Heart Vessels 12(Suppl. 1997):191-193.

3607. C.T. Brighton et al., "The biochemical pathway mediating the proliferative response of bone cells to a mechanical stimulus," J. Bone Joint Surg. Am. 78(September 1996):1337-1347.

3608. H. Wang, W. Ip, R. Boissy, E.S. Grood, "Cell orientation response to cyclically deformed substrates: experimental validation of a cell model," J. Biomech. 28(December 1995):1543-1552.

3609. O.R. Rosales, B.E. Sumpio, "Changes in cyclic strain increase inositol triphosphate and diacylglycerol in endothelial cells," Am. J. Physiol. 262(April 1992):C956-C962.

3610. J. Klein-Nulend, E.H. Burger, C.M. Semeins, L.G. Raisz, C.C. Pilbeam, "Pulsating fluid flow stimulates prostaglandin release and inducible prostaglandin G/H synthase mRNA expression in primary mouse bone cells," J. Bone Miner. Res. 12(January 1997):45-51.

3611. O. Thoumine, A. Ott, "Time scale dependent viscoelastic and contractile regimes in fibroblasts probed by microplate manipulation," J. Cell Sci. 110(September 1997):2109-2116.

3612. M. Takeuchi, H. Miyamoto, Y. Sako, H. Komizu, A. Kusumi, "Structure of the erythrocyte membrane skeleton as observed by atomic force microscopy," Biophys. J. 74(May 1998):2171-2183.

3613. P.Y. Jay, C. Pasternak, E.L. Elson, "Studies of mechanical aspects of amoeboid locomotion," Blood Cells 19(1993):375-386, 386-388 (discussion). See also: D. Bray, J.G. White, "Cortical Flow in Animal Cells," Science 239(19 February 1988):883-888.

3614. J.C. Brown, R. Timpl, "The collagen superfamily," Int. Arch. Allergy Immunol. 107(August 1995):484-490.

3615. W.D. Donachie, S. Addinall, K. Begg, "Cell shape and chromosome partition in prokaryotes or, why *E. coli* is rod-shaped and haploid," Bioessays 17(June 1995):569-576.

3616. F. Mayer, "Principles of functional and structural organization in the bacterial cell: 'Compartments' and their enzymes," FEMA Microbiol. Rev. 10(April 1993):327-345.

3617. W.D. Donachie, "The cell cycle of *Escherichia coli*," Annu. Rev. Microbiol. 47(1993):199-230.

3618. W. Firshein, P. Kim, "Plasmid replication and partition in *Escherichia coli*: Is the cell membrane the key?" Mol. Microbiol. 23(January 1997):1-10.

3619. J.P. Bouche, S. Pichoff, "On the birth and fate of bacterial division sites," Mol. Microbiol. 29(July 1998):19-26.

3620. G.B. Calleja, B.Y. Yoo, B.F. Johnson, "Fusion and erosion of cell walls during conjugation in the fusion yeast (*Schizosaccharomyces pombe*)," J. Cell Sci. 25(June 1977):139-155.

3621. W.P. Hoekstra, A.M. Havekes, "On the role of the recipient cell during conjugation in *Escherichia coli*," Antonie Van Leeuwenhoek 45(1979):13-18.

3622. A. Kitamura, T. Sugai, Y. Kitamura, "Homotypic pair formation during conjugation in *Tetrahymena thermophila*," J. Cell Sci. 82(June 1986):223-234.

3623. F. Cross, L.H. Hartwell, C. Jackson, J.B. Konopka, "Conjugation in *Saccharomyces cerevisiae*," Annu. Rev. Cell Biol. 4(1988):429-457.

3624. A. Tozeren, "Cell-cell, cell-substrate adhesion: theoretical and experimental considerations," J. Biomech. Eng. 112(August 1990):311-318.

3625. E. Lanka, B.M. Wilkins, "DNA processing reactions in bacterial conjugation," Annu. Rev. Biochem. 64(1995):141-169.

3626. W.A. Klimke, L.S. Frost, "Genetic analysis of the role of the transfer gene, traN, or the F and R100-1 plasmids in mating pair stabilization during conjugation," J. Bacteriol. 180(August 1998):4036-4043.

3627. K. Hiwatashi, "Conjugation in protozoa," Tanpakushitsu Kakusan Koso 43(March 1998):337-345.

3628. G.M. Dunny, B.A. Leonard, P.J. Hedberg, "Pheromone-inducible conjugation in *Enterococcus faecalis*: interbacterial and host-parasite chemical communication," J. Bacteriol. 177(February 1995):871-876.

3629. H.W. Kuhlmann, C. Brunen-Nieweler, K. Heckmann, "Pheromones of the ciliate *Euplotes octocarinatus* not only induce conjugation but also function as chemoattractants," J. Exp. Zool. 277(1 January 1997):38-48.

3630. K.G. Anthony, C. Sherburne, R. Sherburne, L.S. Frost, "The role of the pilus in recipient cell recognition during bacterial conjugation mediated by F-like plasmids," Mol. Microbiol. 13(September 1994):939-953.

3631. E. Plumper, M. Freiburg, K. Heckmann, "Conjugation in the ciliate *Euplotes octocarinatus*: Comparison of ciliary and cell body-associated glycoconjugates of non-mating-competent, mating-competent, and conjugating cells," Exp. Cell Res. 217(April 1995):490-496.

3632. P.M. Silverman, "Towards a structural biology of bacterial conjugation," Mol. Microbiol. 23(February 1997):423-429.

3633. H.J. Apell, "Electrogenic properties of the Na,K pump," J. Membr. Biol. 110(September 1989):103-114.

3634. R.W. Van Dyke, "Acid transport by intracellular vesicles," J. Intern. Med. Suppl. 732(1990):41-46.

3635. H. Wieczorek, "The insect V-ATPase, a plasma membrane proton pump energizing secondary active transport: molecular analysis of electrogenic potassium transport in the tobacco hornworm midgut," J. Exp. Biol. 172(November 1992):335-343.

3636. G.A. Gerencser, K.R. Purushotham, H.B. Meng, "An electrogenic chloride pump in a zoological membrane," J. Exp. Zool. 275(1 July 1996):256-261. See also: G.A. Gerencser, "The chloride pump: a Cl(-)-translocating P-type ATPase," Crit. Rev. Biochem. Mol. Biol. 31(1996):303-337.

3637. W.F. Boron, P. Fong, M.A. Hediger, E.L. Boulpaep, M.F. Romero, "The electrogenic Na/HCO3 cotransporter," Wien. Klin. Wochenschr. 109(27 June 1997):445-456. See also: V.F. Boron, M.A. Hediger, E.L. Boulpaep, M.F. Romero, "The renal electrogenic Na^+:HCO^-_3 cotransporter," J. Exp. Biol. 200(January 1997):263-268.

3638. P. Dimroth, "Bacterial energy transductions coupled to sodium ions," Res. Microbiol. 141(March-April 1990):332-336.

3639. A.A. Eddy, P. Hopkins, R. Shaw, "Proton and charge circulation through substrate symports in *Saccharomyces cerevisiae*: non-classical behaviour of the cytosine symport," Symp. Soc. Exp. Biol. 48(1994):123-139.

3640. A.J. Miller, S.J. Smith, F.L. Theodoulou, "The heterologous expression of H(+)-coupled transporters in *Xenopus* oocytes," Symp. Soc. Exp. Biol. 48(1994):167-177.

3641. T.J. Jacob, M.M. Civan, "Role of ion channels in aqueous humor formation," Am. J. Physiol. 271(September 1996):C703-C720.

3642. W.D. Stein, "Energetics and the design principles of the Na/K-ATPase," J. Theor. Biol. 147(21 November 1990):145-159.

3643. F.G. Martin, W.R. Harvey, "Ionic circuit analysis of K^+/H^+ antiport and amino acid/K^+ symport energized by a proton-motive force in *Manduca sexta* larval midgut vesicles," J. Exp. Biol. 196(November 1994):77-92.

3644. R.L. Jungas, M.L. Halperin, J.T. Brosnan, "Quantiative analysis of amino acid oxidation and related gluconeogenesis in humans," Physiol. Rev. 72(April 1992):419-448.

3645. P.C. Maloney, "The molecular and cell biology of anion transport by bacteria," Bioessays 14(November 1992):757-762.

3646. T. Clausen, "Potassium and sodium transport and pH regulation," Can. J. Physiol. Pharmacol. 70(1992):S219-S222.

3647. A. Lepier, M. Azuma, W.R. Harvey, H. Wieczorek, "K^+/H^+ antiport in the tobacco hornworm midgut: the K(+)-transporting component of the K^+ pump," J. Exp. Biol. 196(November 1994):361-373.

3648. P.C. Maloney, R.T. Yan, K. Abe, "Bacterial anion exchange: reductionist and integrative approaches to membrane biology," J. Exp. Biol. 196(November 1994):471-482.

3649. D.K. Kakuda, C.L. MacLeod, "Na(+)-independent transport (uniport) of amino acids and glucose in mammalian cells," J. Exp. Biol. 196(November 1994):93-108.

3650. G.I. Bell et al., "Molecular biology of mammalian glucose transporters," Diabetes Care 13(March 1990):198-208; see related papers, pp. 6-11, 209-243.

3651. S.A. Baldwin, "Molecular mechanisms of sugar transport across mammalian and microbial cell membranes," Biotechnol. Appl. Biochem. 12(October 1990):512-516.

3652. M.J. Lentze, "Molecular and cellular aspects of hydrolysis and absorption," Am. J. Clin. Nutr. 61(April 1995):946S-951S.

3653. K. Takata, "Glucose transporters in the transepithelial transport of glucose," J. Electron. Microsc. Tokyo 45(August 1996):275-284.

3654. B.B. Kahn, "Glucose Transport: Pivotal Step in Insulin Action," Diabetes 45(November 1996):1644-1654.

3655. M.J. Tanner, "The major integral proteins of the human red cell," Baillieres Clin. Haematol. 6(June 1993):333-356.

3656. D.M. Malchoff, V.G. Parker, R.G. Langdon, "Reconstitution of the glucose transport activity of rat adipocytes," Biochim. Biophys. Acta 817(25 July 1985):271-281.

3657. K.M. Dus, C. Grose, "Multiple regulatory effects of varicella-zoster virus (VZV) gL on trafficking patterns and fusogenic properties of VZV gH," J. Virol. 70(December 1996):8961-8971.

3658. R.J. Hessler, R.A. Blackwood, T.G. Brock, J.W. Francis, D.M. Harsh, J.E. Smolen, "Identification of glyceraldehyde-3-phosphate dehydrogenase as a Ca^{2+}-dependent fusogen in human neutrophil cytosol," J. Leukoc. Biol. 63(March 1998):331-336.

3659. T. Shangguan, C.C. Pak, S. Ali, A.S. Janoff, P. Meers, "Cation-dependent fusogenicity of an N-acyl phosphatidylethanolamine," Biochim. Biophys. Acta 1368(19 January 1998):171-183.

3660. R.A. Blackwood, A.T. Transue, D.M. Harsh, R.C. Brower, S.J. Zacharek, J.E. Smolen, R.J. Hessler, "PLA2 promotes fusion between PMN-specific granules and complex liposomes," J. Leukoc. Biol. 59(May 1996):663-670.

3661. B. Dale, M. Iaccarino, A. Fortunato, G. Gragnaniello, K. Kyozuka, E. Tosti, "A morphological and functional study of fusibility in round-headed spermatozoa in the human," Fertil. Steril. 61(February 1994):336-340.

3662. Z.W. Yu, P.J. Quinn, "The modulation of membrane structure and stability by dimethyl sulphoxide," Mol. Membr. Biol. 15(April-June 1998):59-68; and "Dimethyl sulphoxide: A review of its applications in cell biology," Biosci. Rep. 14(December 1994):259-281.

3663. A.L. Kindzelskii, H.R. Petty, "Early membrane rupture events during neutrophil-mediated antibody-dependent tumor cell cytolysis," J. Immunol. 162(15 March 1999):3188-3192.

3664. X.Y. Xie, J.N. Barrett, "Membrane resealing in cultured rat septal neurons after neurite transection: evidence for enhancement by Ca(2+)-triggered protease activity and cytoskeletal disassembly," J. Neurosci. 11(October 1991):3257-3267.

3665. P.L. McNeil, S. Ito, "Gastrointestinal cell plasma membrane wounding and resealing in vivo," Gastroenterology 96(May 1989):1238-1248.

3666. G.Q. Bi, J.M. Alderton, R.A. Steinhardt, "Calcium-regulated exocytosis is required for cell membrane resealing," J. Cell Biol. 131(December 1995):1747-1758. See also: G.Q. Bi, R.L. Morris, G. Liao, J.M. Alderton, J.M. Scholey, R.A. Steinhardt, "Kinesin- and myosin-driven steps of vesicle recruitment for Ca^{2+}-regulated exocytosis," J. Cell Biol. 138(8September 1997):999-1008.

3667. M. Terasaki, K. Miyake, P.L. McNeil, "Large plasma membrane disruptions are rapidly resealed by Ca^{2+}-dependent vesicle-vesicle fusion events," J. Cell Biol. 139(6 October 1997):63-74.

3668. T. Togo, J.M. Alderton, G.Q. Bi, R.A. Steinhardt, "The mechanism of facilitated cell membrane resealing," J. Cell Sci. 112(March 1999):719-731.

3669. P.A. Raj, M. Johnsson, M.J. Levine, G.H. Nancollas, "Salivary statherin. Dependence on sequence, charge, hydrogen bonding potency, and helical conformation for adsorption to hydroxyapatite and inhibition of mineralization," J. Biol. Chem. 267(25 March 1992):5968-5976.

3670. B.L. Slomiany, V.L. Murty, J. Piotrowski, A. Slomiany, "Salivary mucins in oral mucosal defense," Gen. Pharmacol. 27(July 1996):761-771.

3671. C. Hagberg, "Electromyography and bite force studies of muscular function and dysfunction in masticatory muscles," Swed. Dent. J. Suppl. 37(1986):1-64. See also: C. Hagberg, G. Agerberg, M. Hagberg, "Regression analysis of electromyographic activity of masticatory muscles versus bite force," Scand. J. Dent. Res. 93(October 1985):396-402.

3672. M. Bakke, L. Michler, K. Han, E. Moller, "Clinical significance of isometric bite force versus electrical activity in temporal and masseter muscles," Scand. J. Dent. Res. 97(December 1989):539-551.

3673. E. Hellsing, C. Hagberg, "Changes in maximum bite force related to extension of the head," Eur. J. Orthod. 12(May 1990):148-153.

3674. Helim Aranda-Espinoza, Yi Chen, Nily Dan, T.C. Lubensky, Philip Nelson, Laurence Ramos, D.A. Weitz, "Electrostatic Repulsion of Positively Charged Vesicles and Negatively Charged Objects," Science 285(16 July 1999):394-397.

3675. J.D. Veldhuis, "The hypothalamic pulse generator: the reproductive core," Clin. Obstet. Gynecol. 33(September 1990):538-550.

3676. W. Wuttke, H. Jarry, C. Feleder, J. Moguilevsky, S. Leonhardt, J.Y. Seong, K. Kim, "The neurochemistry of the GnRH pulse generator," Acta Neurobiol. Exp. (Warsz) 56(1996):707-713.

3677. R.I. Weiner, "Cellular basis of the GnRH pulse generator," Nippon Sanka Fujinka Gakkai Zasshi 48(August 1996):573-577.

3678. M. Nishihara, Y. Takeuchi, T. Tanaka, Y. Mori, "Electrophysiological correlates of pulsatile and surge gonadotrophin secretion," Rev. Reprod. 4(May 1999):110-116.

3679. C. Bolger, S. Bojanic, N.F. Sheahan, D. Coakley, J.F. Malone, "Dominant frequency content of ocular microtremor from normal subjects," Vision Res. 39(June 1999):1911-1915; "Ocular microtremor in oculomotor palsy," J. Neuroophthalmol. 19(March 1999):42-45.

3680. B. Wilhelm, H. Wilhelm, P. Streicher, H. Ludtke, M. Adler, "Pupillography as an objective attention test," Wien Med. Wochenschr. 146(1996):387-389. In German.

3681. L.S. Gray, B. Winn, B. Gilmartin, "Accommodative microfluctuations and pupil diameter," Vision Res. 33(October 1993):2083-2090.

3682. K. Niwa, T. Tokoro, "Influence of spatial distribution with blur on fluctuations in accommodation," Optom. Vis. Sci. 75(March 1998):227-232.

3683. K. Toshida, F. Okuyama, T. Tokoro, "Influences of the accommodative stimulus and aging on the accommodative microfluctuations," Optom. Vis. Sci. 75(March 1998):221-226.

3684. K. Ukai, K. Tsuchiya, S. Ishikawa, "Induced pupillary hippus following near vision: increased occurrence in visual display unit workers," Ergonomics 40(November 1997):1201-1211.

3685. R.E. Yoss, N.J. Moyer, R.W. Hollenhorst, "Hippus and other spontaneous rhythmic pupillary waves," Am. J. Ophthalmol. 70(December 1970):935-941.

3686. W.H. Meck, "Neuropharmacology of timing and time perception," Brain Res. Cogn. Brain Res. 3(June 1996):227-242; errata, 6(January 1998):233.

3687. S.C. Hinton, W.H. Meck, "The internal clocks of circadian and interval timing," Endeavor 21(1997):82-87.

3688. B.C. Rakitin, J. Gibbon, T.B. Penney, C. Malapani, S.C. Hinton, W.H. Meck, "Scalar expectancy theory and peak-interval timing in humans," J. Exp. Psychol. Anim. Behav. Process 24(January 1998):15-33.

3689. J.R. Wild, S.J. Loughrey-Chen, T.S. Corder, "In the presence of CTP, UTP becomes an allosteric inhibitor of aspartate transcarbamoylase," Proc. Natl. Acad. Sci. USA 86(January 1989):46-50.

3690. F. Van Vliet et al., "Heterotropic interactions in aspartate transcarbamoylase: turning allosteric ATP activation into inhibition as a consequence of a single tyrosine to phenylalanine mutation," Proc. Natl. Acad. Sci. USA 88(15 October 1991):9180-9183.

3691. P. England, G. Herve, "Synergistic inhibition of *Escherichia coli* aspartate transcarbamylase by CTP and UTP: binding studies using continuous-flow dialysis," Biochemistry 31(13 October 1992):9725-9732.

3692. T.T. Lee, R.L. Momparier, "Inhibition of uridine-cytidine kinase by 5-azacytidine 5'-triphosphate," Med. Pediatr. Oncol. 2(1976):265-270.

3693. N.M. Samuels, B.W. Gibson, S.M. Miller, "Investigation of the kinetic mechanism of cytidine 5'-monophosphate N-acetylneuraminic acid synthetase from *Haemophilus ducreyi* with new insights on rate-limiting steps from product inhibition analysis," Biochemistry 38(11 May 1999):6195-6203.

3694. E. Perel, K.H. Stolee, L. Kharlip, M.E. Blackstein, D.W. Killinger, "The intracellular control of aromatase activity by 5 alpha-reduced androgens in human breast carcinoma cells in culture," J. Clin. Endocrinol. Metab. 58(March 1984):467-472.

3695. T.H. Xia, R.S. Jiao, "Studies of glutamine synthetase from *Streptomyces hygroscopicus* var. jinggangensis," Sci. Sin. B 29(April 1986):379-388.

3696. C.A. Woolfolk, E.R. Stadtman, "Regulation of glutamine synthetase. 3. Cumulative feedback inhibition of glutamine synthetase from *Escherichia coli*," Arch. Biochem. Biophys. 118(20 March 1967):736-755.

3697. C. Biswas, H. Paulus, "Multivalent feedback inhibition of aspartokinase in *Bacillus polymyxa*. IV. Arrangement and function of the subunits," J. Biol. Chem. 248(25 April 1973):2894-2900.

3698. V.Y. Hook, E.F. LaGamma, "Product inhibition of carboxypeptidase H," J. Biol. Chem. 262(15 September 1987):12583-12588.

3699. C.L. Boyajian, D.M. Cooper, "Potent and cooperative feedback inhibition of adenylate cyclase activity by calcium in pituitary-derived GH3 cells," Cell Calcium 11(April 1990):299-307.

3700. S. Zhang, G. Pohnert, P. Kongsaeree, D.B. Wilson, J. Clardy, B. Ganem, "Chorismate mutase-prephenate dehydratase from *Escherichia coli*. Study of catalytic and regulatory domains using genetically engineered proteins," J. Biol. Chem. 273(13 March 1998):6248-6253.

3701. Warren D. Smith, "DNA computers in vivo and vitro," DIMACS Series in Discrete Mathematics and Theoretical Computer Science, American Mathematical Library, Vol. 27, 1996, pp. 121-185. See abstract at: html://www.neci.nj.nec.com/homepages/wds/dnaarticle.abstract; full paper and missing figures are available at: html://www.neci.nj.nec.com/homepages/wds/journalpubs.html.

3702. Maurice Chittenden, David Lloyd, "007 Implant to Protect Kidnap Victims," The Sunday Times (London), 12 October 1998; see at: http://www.freerepublic.com/forum/a36226f323946.htm.

3703. P. Rusmee, "Pressure Vessel," 29 December 1998, see at: http://www.mech.utah.edu/~rusmeeha/labNotes/pressure.html.

3704. G.D. Shockman, L. Daneo-Moore, R. Kariyama, O. Massidda, "Bacterial walls, peptidoglycan hydrolases, autolysins, and autolysis," Microb. Drug Resist. 2(Spring 1996):95-98.

3705. R.B. Jensen, K. Gerdes, "Programmed cell death in bacteria: proteic plasmid stabilization systems," Mol. Microbiol. 17(July 1995):205-210.

3706. T. Franch, K. Gerdes, "Programmed cell death in bacteria: translational repression by mRNA end-pairing," Mol. Microbiol. 21(September 1996):1049-1060.

3707. A. Hochman, "Programmed cell death in prokaryotes," Crit. Rev. Microbiol. 23(1997):207-214.

3708. S. Asoh, K. Nishimaki, R. Nanbu-Wakao, S. Ohta, "A trace amount of the human pro-apoptotic factor Bax induces bacterial death accompanied by damage of DNA," J. Biol. Chem. 273(1 May 1998):11384-11391.

3709. S.I. Ahmad, S.H. Kirk, A. Eisenstark, "Thymine metabolism and thymineless death in prokaryotes and eukaryotes," Annu. Rev. Microbiol. 52(1998):591-625.

3710. R. Kolter, D.A. Siegele, A. Tormo, "The stationary phase of the bacterial life cycle," Annu. Rev. Microbiol. 47(1993):855-874.

3711. F. Rallu, A. Gruss, E. Maguin, "*Lactococcus lactis* and stress," Antonie Van Leeuwenhoek 70(October 1996):243-251.

3712. M.P. Spector, "The starvation-stress response (SSR) of *Salmonella*," Adv. Microb. Physiol. 40(1998):233-279.

3713. N.J. Talley, "Irritable bowel syndrome: disease definition and symptom description," Eur. J. Surg. Suppl. 583(1998):24-28.

3714. S.M. Browning, "Constipation, diarrhea, and irritable bowel syndrome," Prim. Care 26(March 1999):113-139.

3715. S.M. Collins, G. Barbara, B. Vallance, "Stress, inflammation and the irritable bowel syndrome," Can. J. Gastroenterol. 13(March 1999):47A-49A.

3716. C. Scarpignato, I. Pelosini, "Management of irritable bowel syndrome: novel approaches to the pharmacology of gut motility," Can. J. Gastroenterol. 13(March 1999):50A-65A.

3717. A.J. Barsky, J.F. Borus, "Functional somatic syndromes," Ann. Intern. Med. 130(1 June 1999):910-921.

3718. E. Stubblefield, M. Pershouse, "Direct formation of microcells from mitotic cells for use in chromosome transfer," Somat. Cell Mol. Genet. 18(November 1992):485-491.

3719. J. Fulka Jr., R.M. Moor, "Noninvasive chemical enucleation of mouse oocytes," Mol. Reprod. Dev. 34(April 1993):427-430.

3720. L. Karnikova, M. Horska, M. Tomanek, J. Kanka, F. Urban, R. Moor, J. Fulka Jr., "Chemically enucleated mouse oocytes: ultrastructure and kinetics of histone H1 kinase activity," Reprod. Nutr. Dev. 38(November-December 1998):643-651.
3721. Y. Mori, H. Akedo, T. Matsuhisa, Y. Tanigaki, M. Okada, "Extrusion of nuclei of murine suspension culture cells with microtubule poisons," Exp. Cell Res. 153(August 1984):574-580.
3722. S.P. Xue, S.F. Zhang, Q. Du, H. Sun, J. Xin, S.Q. Liu, J. Ma, "The role of cytoskeletal elements in the two-phase denucleation process of mammalian erythroblasts in vitro observed by laser confocal scanning microscope," Cell Mol. Biol. 43(September 1997):851-860.
3723. D.G. Newell, U. Jayaswal, J. Smith, S. Roath, "Unusual lymphocyte morphology in a case of chronic lymphatic leukaemia: apparent nuclear extrusion," Acta Haematol. 59(1978):25-30.
3724. R.W. Jack, J.R. Tagg, B. Ray, "Bacteriocins of Gram-positive bacteria," Microbiol. Rev. 59(June 1995):171-200.
3725. F.J. van der Wal, J. Luirink, B. Oudega, "Bacteriocin release proteins: mode of action, structure, and biotechnological application," FEMS Microbiol. Rev. 17(December 1995):381-399.
3726. T. Baba, O. Schneewind, "Instruments of microbial warfare: bacteriocin synthesis, toxicity and immunity," Trends Microbiol. 6(February 1998):66-71.
3727. Nikhil Hutheesing, "Worker bees," Forbes 164(26 July 1999):248.
3728. Richard Brodie, Virus of the Mind, Integral Press, Seattle WA, 1996. See also: Richard Dawkins, The Selfish Gene, Oxford University Press, NY, 1976. Chapter 11 "Memes".

INDEX

A

B

C

D

E

F

G

H

I

J

K

L

M

N

Q

R

S

T

U

V

W

X

Y

Z

Printed and bound by CPI Group (UK) Ltd, Croydon, CR0 4YY
23/10/2024
01777685-0018